Discovery after Discovery, We Are Making Contraceptive Choices Simpler

At Wyeth, a consistent history of discoveries has made our ongoing contribution to hormonal contraception innovative and productive.

We are proud to once again be taking part in the World Congress of Gynecology and Obstetrics — an eminent forum for the exchange of the most recent and exciting advances in obstetrics and gynecology. As participants, we would like to extend a warm welcome to you on the occasion of the 11th annual meeting of this distinguished assembly…and invite you to share in some of the discoveries that have made Wyeth a world leader in female health.

Wyeth International Limited

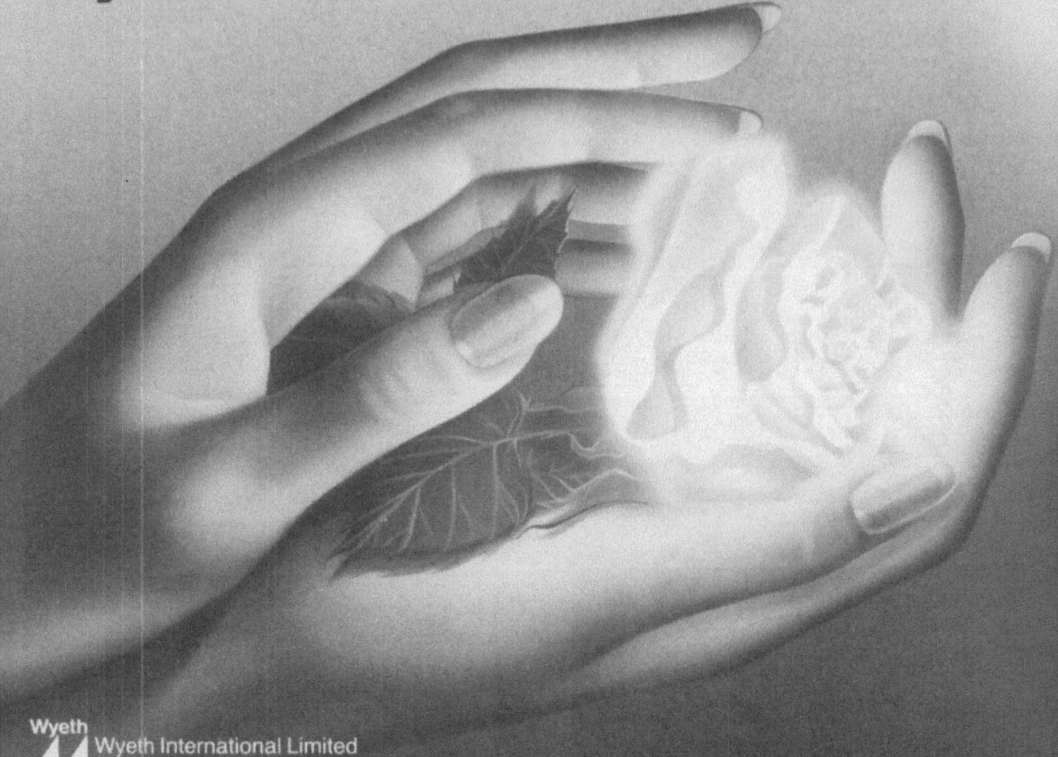

Archives of Gynecology
Organ of the Deutsche Gesellschaft für Gynäkologie und Geburtshilfe

Since 1921 (Vol. 117) "Archiv für Gynäkologie" has been the organ of the Deutsche Gesellschaft für Gynäkologie und Geburtshilfe. Founded in 1870. Edited by K. Credé, A. Gusserow, E. Bumm, A. Döderlein, R. Meyer, C. Kaufmann, G. A. Wagner, and others. Vols. 1–114 (1920) published by August Hirschwald, Berlin; Vols. 115–175 by Springer, Berlin; as of Vol. 176 (1948) by J. F. Bergmann, Munich. Published under the English title "Archives of Gynecology" as of Vol. 226 (1978).

Manuscripts and inquiries may be addressed to:

Prof. Dr. H. A. Hirsch
Universitäts-Frauenklinik
Schleichstrasse 4
D-7400 Tübingen, FRG

Dr. F. E. Loeffler, F.R.C.S., F.R.C.O.G.
St. Mary's Hospital
Praed Street
London W2, England

Prof. Dr. H. Ludwig
Universitäts-Frauenklinik
Schanzenstrasse 46
CH-4031 Basel
Switzerland

Prof. Dr. K.-H. Wulf
Universitäts-Frauenklinik
Josef-Schneider-Strasse 4
D-8700 Würzburg, FRG

Other Regulations

Authors publishing in this journal can, under certain conditions, benefit from library and photocopy fees collected by VG WORT. Authors of German nationality and those resident in the Federal Republic of Germany or Berlin (West), as well as citizens of Austria, Switzerland and member countries of the European Community may apply to Verwertungsgesellschaft WORT, Abteilung Wissenschaft, Goethestraße 49, D-8000 München 2, for detailed information.

Subscription Information

Volume 237–238 (4 issues each) will appear in 1985.

North America. Annual subscription rate: Approx. US $ 201.00 (single issue price: approx. US $ 30.00) including carriage charges. Subscriptions are entered with prepayment only. Orders should be addressed to:

Springer-Verlag New York Inc.
Service Center Secaucus
44 Hartz Way
Secaucus, NJ 07094, USA
Tel. (201) 348-4033, Telex 0023-125994

All Other Countries. Annual subscription rate: DM 532.00 plus carriage charges. Volume price: DM 266.00, single issue price:

DM 79.80, plus carriage charges. Airmail delivery on request only. Carriage charges for SAL (Surface Airmail Lifted) to Japan, India, Australia and New Zealand are available on request. Orders can either be placed with your bookdealer or sent directly to

Springer-Verlag, Heidelberger Platz 3, D-1000 Berlin 33, Tel. (0) 30/8207-1, Telex 1-83319

Changes of Address. Allow six weeks for all changes to become effective. All Communications should include both old and new addresses (with Postal Codes) and should be accompanied by a mailing label from a recent issue.

Back Volumes. Prices are available on request.

Microform. Microform editions are available from:
University Microfilm International
300 N. Zeeb Road
Ann Arbor, MI 48106, USA

Production and responsibility for advertisements, only for Supplement, to Vol. 237, Abstracts

Günther Sachs, Karin Berkholz
Congress Project Management GmbH
Letzter Hasenpfad 61
D-6000 Frankfurt 70
Federal Republic of Germany

Printers

Satz: Daten- und Lichtsatz-Service, Würzburg
Druck und Einband:
Graphischer Betrieb,
Konrad Triltsch, Würzburg

ISBN 978-3-662-38962-1
ISBN 978-3-662-39916-3 (eBook)
DOI 10.1007/978-3-662-39916-3

01.13.01

Current concepts in the etiology and treatment of dysmenorrhea: Dawood, M Y. Dept. Obstet. and Gyn., Univ. of Illinois, Chicago, IL, USA

Dysmenorrhea is either primary (when there is no visible pathology) or secondary (when a visible pathology is present and responsible). Primary dysmenorrhea occurs with ovulatory cycles. Prevailing data indicate that in primary dysmenorrhea there is abnormal and increased uterine activity during the menstrual phase of the cycle, often of prostaglandins (PG). Preliminary evidence implicates changes in menstrual fluid prostanoids and possibly increased release of circulating vasopressin in primary dysmenorrhea but sequential measurements are needed. In secondary dysmenorrhea due to intrauterine device (IUD) use, the pain is due to increased endometrial PG levels secondary to the inflammatory response induced by the IUD: The role of PG in dysmenorrhea associated with endometriosis is unestablished. The treatment of choice for primary dysmenorrhea is an effective nonsteroidal anti-inflammatory drug (NSAID) which inhibits cyclo-oxygenase and therefore PG biosynthesis. Likewise, the secondary dysmenhorrhea due to the IUD is relieved with NSAID but other causes of secondary dysmenorrhea are best corrected by treating the underlying pathology. Primary dysmenorrhea can also be relieved with oral contraceptive (OC) but this should be prescribed only to patients who want the OC as a contraceptive. Both NSAID and OC will suppress the menstrual fluid PG; the former inhibits cyclo-oxygenase while the latter suppresses endometrial growth and development and thereby reduces the PG levels.

01.13.02

The clinical pharmacology of piroxicam: Guttadauria, M. Pfizer International, NY, USA

Piroxicam is the first of the oxicam class of nonsteroidal anti-inflammatory drugs. It is a potent inhibitor of prostaglandin biosythesis via inhibition of cyclo-oxygenase. It is rapidly asorbed in humans with significant blood levels within 1 or 2 hours and a serum half-life of about 50 hours allowing once daily dosing. After chronic dosing with 20 mg, daily steady state plasma levels are usually achieved within 1 to 2 weeks. When given at a dose of 40 mg daily for 2 days followed by 20 mg daily, steady state plasma levels are similar to those achieved with the 20 mg daily dose. However, 75% of steady state is attained immediately after the second 40 mg dose, a level achieved only after 8 days with the daily 20 mg dose. These observations provide the rationale for the use of the 2 day 40 mg loading dose in acute conditions. A single 40 mg dose of piroxicam has been demonstrated to rapidly reduce uterine contractility in dysmenorrheic women. Piroxicam (Feldene) has been available for the last 5 years for the treatment of a wide range of acute musculoskeletal and chronic rheumatic conditions around the world. Extensive clinical trials in these acute and chronic conditions demonstrate that Feldene is as affective as aspirin 3.5–5 gms daily and indomethacin 75–150 mg daily but better tolerated and that it is as effective and as well tolerated as diclofenac 75–150 mg daily and naproxen 500–1000 mg daily.

01.13.03

A comparative crossover study of piroxicam versus mefenamic acid and diclofenac in France: Serfaty, D. Hosp. Saint-Louis, Paris

Ninety-one patients with primary dysmenorrhea participated in this randomized comparative study. The comparative agents were piroxicam versus either mefenamic acid or diclofenac. Patients were treated during four menstrual cycles: the first two cycles they received either piroxicam or one of the two agents against which it was being compared; the treatments were reversed during the third and fourth cycles. The efficacy assessment was statistically in favour of piroxicam over both of the comparative drugs. The toleration of all three drugs was good. The study made it obvious that piroxicam, an antiprostaglandin NSAID (non-steroidal anti-inflammatory drug), is active in countering uterine contractility and consequently is efficacious in the treatment of primary dysmenorrhea.

01.13.04

Worldwide studies comparing piroxicam and naproxen: Plantema, F. St. Liduina Stichting, The Netherlands

Results of double blind crossover studies performed in several countries around the world comparing the efficacy and toleration of piroxicam and naproxen in the treatment of primary dysmenorrhea will be presented. In one such study conducted in Sweden, 83 patients were treated for one menstrual cycle with each drug for up to 5 days. Piroxicam was given in a dose of 40 mg once daily for the first 2 days followed by 20 mg once daily. Naproxen sodium 500 mg was given twice daily for the entire treatment period. With both agents treatment commenced at the onset of menstrual pain. There were no statistically significant differences between the drugs for any of the efficacy parameters which included daily assessment of menstrual pain intensity, effect of medication on pain, need for rescue analgesics and ability to perform usual work. However, piroxicam was judged by patients to be overall the more effective drug in reducing the symptoms of dysmenorrhea ($p < 0.01$). Patient preference was in favour of piroxicam. Both drugs were well tolerated with no patient reporting serious side-effects or needing to discontinue medication due to side-effects.

01.14.01

Maternal intake of highly refined carbohydrates and fetal growth: Yla-Outinen, A, Tuimala, R, Visala, T. Inst. Clin. Sci., Univ. of Tampere, Finland

In order to study the association between fetal growth and maternal intake of different foodstuffs during pregnancy, 739 non-diabetic parturients who had given birth to a singelton baby filled up a questionnaire concerning their dietary habits during pregnancy. Mothers were divided into three groups according to the birth weight of the infant: small-for-gestational age (SGA), average-for-gestational age (AGA) and large-for-gestational age (LGA) groups. Differences in the consumption of various foodstuffs between these groups were further analysed by using multiple discriminant analysis. The mean number of warm meals or sandwiches, or the frequency of most foodstuffs consumed during pregnancy seemed not to differ between these three groups. However, the summarized variable of foodstuffs containing highly refined carbohydrates (cookies, candies, free sugar etc.) presented weak but significant ($p < 0.05$) discriminative power between these three groups with higher frequency of use in AGA and LGA groups. Our results thus suggest an association between frequent use of highly refined carbohydrates and enhanced fetal growth.

01.14.02

Zinc and copper concentration in Egyptian women during normal and complicated pregnancy and its impact on the newly born: Kandil, O, Fahmy, A, El-sheikha, Z, Fahim, M, Zaki, K. Dept. Obstet. and Gyn., Fac. Med., Al-Azhar Univ., Cairo, Egypt

Serum zinc and copper were determined in 208 subjects including normal pregnancy, pre-eclampsia, diabetic patients, and spontaneous first and second trimesters abortion, using the atomic absorption. A control group of healthy non-pregnant premenstrual women was included for comparison. A gradual significant decline of zinc in contrast to a significant rise in serum copper in all pregnant patients was found. In spontaneous abortion serum zinc and copper levels were significantly lower when compared to normal pregnancy. Parity significantly decreased serum zinc. Premature rupture of membranes caused a significant decrease in maternal and neonatal zinc and maternal copper. Pre-term neonates had significantly lower serum zinc accompanied by a significant decrease in birth weight.

01.14.03

Antepartum death of one twin: Lumme, R, Saarikoski, S. Dept. Clin. Sci., Univ., Tampere and Dept. Obstet. and Gyn., Univ., Kuopio, Finland

Twenty-two cases with antepartum death of one twin were identified in 909 twin pregnancies treated in Tampere Central Hospital during the years 1964–1980. Antenatal diagnosis was made in 16 cases. In six delivery was immediate because of spontaneous labor. In three labors was likewise spontaneous but after a time interval of one to 16 weeks between the diagnosis and delivery. In five labors was induced after confirmation of the diagnosis. In two amniocentesis was performed. When pulmonary maturity was confirmed delivery was carried out. The mode of delivery was Cesarean section in six mothers. The placenta was monochorionic in 11 pregnancies and five stillborn fetuses had a velamentous insertion of the umbilical cord. Five stillborn fetuses were delivered as a fetus papyraceus, 11 had severe and six no maceration. One monochorionic co-twin of a fetus papyraceus had multiple structural defects, otherwise the neonatal morbidity was not increased if the low gestational age averaging 34 weeks is taken in account. One co-twin was lost because of immaturity. These results suggest that antepartum death of one twin is not an indication for labor induction unless antenatal surveillance of the living co-twin is suggestive of fetal compromise.

01.14.04

The problem with magnesium therapy during pregnancy: Mund-Hoym, S, Schlebusch, H.* Univ.-Frauenklin., Köln, Univ.-Frauenklin., Bonn*

In a longitudinal study 220 measurements by atomic absorptions of plasma magnesium levels were made in healthy, pregnant women. The results were as follows:

	x	s
< 8.–14. gestational weeks:	0.81	± 0.05 mmol/l
15.–18. gestational weeks:	0.78	± 0.05 mmol/l
19.–23. gestational weeks:	0.78	± 0.06 mmol/l
24.–27. gestational weeks:	0.79	± 0.06 mmol/l
28.–31. gestational weeks:	0.78	± 0.06 mmol/l
32.–35. gestational weeks:	0.77	± 0.06 mmol/l
36.–41. gestational weeks:	0.77	± 0.06 mmol/l

These results indicate a significant lowering of plasma magnesium levels around the 15th week of pregnancy after which a stabilisation is achieved. A broader range of magnesium variability is seen in the erythrocyte intracellular magnesium measurements. In contrast, lower plasma levels were found in 145 samples of women with pathologic pregnancy (diabetics and gestosis). The magnesium levels of diabetics were not related to their serum glucose. These findings call into question which is the clinically relevant compartment for magnesium measurement as well as the wisdom of widespread magnesium substitution as is currently practiced in the Federal Republic of Germany.

01.14.05

Influence of the combination therapy β_2-stimulation + β_1-blockade on water and electrolyte balance during tocolysis: Grospietsch, G, Engelmann, A, Kuhn, W. Dept. Obstet. and Gyn., Univ., Göttingen

The development of pulmonary edema during betamimetic tocolysis has a multifactorial origin. The principal mechanism is water retention during medication. The combination of Fenoterol (F) and Metoprolol (M) has been found to be useful during tocolysis because of its cardioprotective effects. This study was undertaken to clarify the effects on kidney function of this combination. – Methods: Two groups of patients were studied during 24 hr intravenous tocolysis and bed-rest. The F-group (n = 10) received Fenoterol only and the F/M-group (n = 15) received the combination of Fenoterol with Metoprolol. Hgb, Hct, Na, K, creatinine, osmolality, renin and aldosterone were determined in blood. Urinary output, Na, K, creatinine and osmolality were also determined. – Results: In the F-group the well-known changes were observed: decrease in urinary output, decline in Hgb, Hct, aldosterone and creatinine clearance as well as an increase in renin. In contrast the M/F-group showed no change in the urinary output, Hgb, Hct, creatinine clearance or renin. – Discussion: These results demonstrate that the reduction in kidney function and influence on the water and electrolyte balance during betamimetic tocolytic therapy is for the most part caused by a residual β_1-activity.

01.14.06

Cervical collagen concentration; A predictor of labor delivery time: Ulmsten, U, Ekman, G, Uldbjerg, U. Dept. Obstet. and Gyn., Malmö, Sweden and Pharmacol, Århus, Denmark

Spontaneous cervical ripening at term is accompanied by biochemical changes in the cervical connective tissue (1). The aim of the present study was to establish a possible relation between cervical collagen content and cervical dilatation during labor and to find out if locally applied PGE_2 induces a collagen break-down in patients with unripe cervices similar to that seen in spontaneous ripening. – Material and methods: Collagen and collagenase were quantitated (1) in cervical biopsies from three groups of patients: Group A, 10 term pregnant women with favorable cervices and spontaneous labor; Group B, 12 term pregnant women with unripe cervices given 0.5 mg PGE_2 in gel intracervically for cervical ripening and labor induction; Group C, 5 term pregnant women with unripe cervices and spontaneous labor. – Results: Women in Group C had longer cervical dilatation times (18 hours) compared to women in Group A (6.7 hours) and in Group B (5.0 hours) (p < 0.001). In line with that the cervical collagen concentration was higher in Group C, 8.58 μg/mg wet weight compared to 6.7 μg/mg in Group A and 5.47 μg/mg in Group B (p < 0.001). The collagenolytic activity was also significantly higher in PGE_2-treated patients of Group B (530 U/100 mg) compared to women in Group A (380 U/100 mg) (p < 0.05). – Conclusion: This study provides clear evidence of a closed correlation between the biochemical composition of the cervix and the clinical course of delivery. Local application of PGE_2 seems to mimic spontaneous cervical ripening in both clinical and biochemical terms.

(1) *Uldbjerg, N.* Am. J. Obstet. Gyn. **147**, 662 (1983)

01.14.07

A new modality for treatment of threatened abortion (Solcoseryl) "A preliminary report": Khairy, M, Kandil, O, Abdel Razik, M, El Gazzar, A. Benha Fac. Med., Cairo, Egypt

Fifty cases of first trimester threatened abortion manifested by vaginal bleeding with or without low backache and/or lower abdominal colics had been included in this study. These were randomly divided into two groups after delicate clinical evaluation of the cervix and ultrasonic confirmation of viable gestation. The Solcoseryl group included 25 cases and were treated with 10 mls. of Solcoseryl in 500 mls. of 25% glucose i. v. slowly daily with bed rest. The control group included 25 cases and were advised to get bed-rest and only given 500 ccs. of 25% glucose i. v. slowly daily. The pregnancy continuation rate for the Solcoseryl group was 80% in comparison to 52% in the control group which was statistically significant (p < 0.05). Among the continued pregnancies, there was no increased risk of congenital anomalies nor intra-uterine growth retardation in either group. Unlike the control group, there were no pre-term deliveries reported in the Solcoseryl group. As a continuation for our successful trials in treatment of IUGR with Solcoseryl, also possible promising results are developing in threatened abortion treatment.

01.14.08

Extraperitoneal Cesarean section – a mode of coexistence with transperitoneal approach: Zaczek, T, Skręt, A, Piela, A. Dept. Obstet. and Gyn., District Hosp., Rzeszów, Poland

Extraperitoneal Cesarean section (ESC) has been previously presented as alternative to transperitoneal Cesarean section (TSC). In this report we purposely relinquished stereotype comparison of ESC and TSC to present our own system of Cesarean section procedure with "built in" extraperitoneal technic. In this system, based on pre-operative and intraoperative selection of patients to ESC, during a 4-year period a total of 1640 Cesarean sections (1162 primary and 478 secondary) were performed. Pre-operative selection disqualified 538 (32.8%) patients due to: 1. indications for immediate delivery (56), 2. need of abdominal cavity inspection/operation (61), 3. poorly developed low uterine segment (96), 4. unavailability of personel trained in extraperitoneal technic. In this group of patients "elective TSC" was performed. Remaining 1102 (67.2%) patients were qualified to trial of ESC, thus 933 ESC were managed without opening of peritoneal cavity while 66 operations resulted in little peritoneal entry (fenestration). In 103 cases extraperitoneal

3

technic was abandoned because of failure of access to Bogros space or unintentional wide peritoneal entry, which resulted in "enforced TSC". The presented mode of coexistence of ESC and TSC, similar to well-known system of vaginal/abdominal approach in hysterectomy may enable understanding of ESC as adjunct procedure to TSC and facilitate wider clinical proliferation of this much discussed procedure.

01.14.09
Effects of labor on serum glycoprotein; Comparison with those of gynecological operation: Hashimoto, S, Harada, T, Terada, S, Akasofu, K, Nishida, E. Dept. Obstet. and Gyn., Kanazawa Univ., Kanazawa, Japan
In order to investigate the effects of labor on serum glycoprotein fractions, the concentrations of 40 serum protein components were measured during the period of late gestation, labor and puerperium. Sera were sampled in series from the period of late gestation to the 30th post partum day. The concentrations of serum glycoproteins slightly changed during labor. And after delivery several glycoprotein fractions increased remarkably, and some of the other protein fractions decreased. The serum protein fractions which increased after delivery included α_1-acid glycoprotein, haptoglobin, α_1-antichymotrypsin, C-reactive protein, and 9.5S-α_1-glycoprotein. Conversely serum concentrations of α_2-AP-glycoprotein and α_2-HS-glycoprotein decreased after delivery. In addition, serum protein fractions, α_1-antitrypsin, ceruloplasmin, immunoglobulin M, did not show any significant change during early puerperium. The effects on serum glycoproteins of labor were compared with those of gynecological operation. The changing patterns of 20 glycoprotein components after delivery were very similar to those of gynecological operation. These changing patterns were classified into three groups, increased, decreased and unchanged patterns. The effects on glycoproteins of labor were also compared with those of estrogen administration.

01.14.10
Semi-quantitative evaluation of the intrapartum variable deceleration of FHR pattern and its association with umbilical cord blood gas analysis: Nishida, T, Chen, S, Koike, S, Mori, H, Kigawa, T. Dept. Obstet. and Gyn., Oita Med. Coll., Oita, Japan
Variable deceleration of FHR pattern was semi-quantitatively evaluated to establish the diagnostic value of variable deceleration for fetal distress. FHR charts of 55 normal deliveries by direct monitoring were analysed and SDA (Sum of Dip Area) was calculated using following equation: $SDA = \Sigma$ duration of dip (sec.) $\times$ depth of dip (bpm.) and correlation between SDA and umbilical cord blood gas analysis was obtained. Significant correlation was observed between SDA of the last one hour of delivery and cord blood gas data. PHua: $r = -0.524$ ($p < 0.005$), PO_2ua: $r = -0.332$ ($p < 0.05$); BEua: $r = -0.461$ ($p < 0.005$), PHuv: $r = -0.336$ ($p < 0.02$); PO_2uv: $r = -0.468$ ($p < 0.005$), BEuv: $r = -0.47$ ($p < 0.005$). In 14 cases which showed prolonged variable deceleration (PVD), significant correlation was observed between SDA of PVD and PH of umbilical venous blood (UV): PHuv $= 7.425 - 0.000774$ SDA ($r = -0.756$, $p < 0.005$), whereas in 17 cases with severe variable deceleration (SVD) no significant correlation was seen between the SDA of SVD and the PH of UV. These results suggest that SDA value is helpful for evaluation of variable deceleration during labor.

01.14.11
Studies on prostanoids in streptozotocin-induced diabetic pregnancy in the rat: Katou, K, Matsumoto, T, Sugiyama, Y. Dept. Obstet. and Gyn., Mie Univ., School Med., Mie, Japan
It has been reported that prostacyclin (PGI_2), in contract to thromboxane A_2 (TxA_2), play an important part in the maintenance of the blood flow. In this study we measured 6-keto-$PGF_{1\alpha}$ and TxB_2, metabolites of these prostanoids, in tissues of the pregnant rats with diabetes mellitus induced by streptozotocin to elucidate the relationship between fetal growth and prostanoids. Maternal aorta, placenta, fetal lung and liver in the STZ treated pregnant rats were collected on days 20 of pregnancy. PGI_2 activity was evaluated as inhibition of collagen-induced platelet aggregation according to the bioassay proposed by *Okuma*. The concentration of 6-keto-$PGF_{1\alpha}$ and TxB_2 in tissues were measured by RIA after extraction and silicic acid chromatographic procedures according to the modified Jaffe's method. PGI_2 formation from the aorta in the STZ treated pregnant group was 0.44 ± 0.15 nmol/mg wet tissue/h which tended to be lower than in the normal pregnant group. The prostanoid levels in the placenta were; 6-keto-$PGF_{1\alpha}$, 205.9 ± 38.9 pg/mg protein; and TxB_2, 105.3 ± 24.0 pg/mg protein in the STZ treated pregnant group. These were significantly lower than those of the normal pregnant group. These results suggest that fetoplacental blood flow may be disturbed when a diabetic mother is not favorably controlled, and this may eventually lead to a delay in fetal growth.

01.14.12
Luteolytic effects of the uterus in the pregnant rat: Nanjo, K, Kato, H, Numa, F, Wataki, K, Torigoe, T. Dept. Obstet. and Gyn., Yamaguchi Univ., School Med., Kogushi, Ube, Japan
It has been reported that the pituitary or the uterus exerts the luteolytic effect in pregnant rats (Endocrinology 111, 2020, 1982; 112, 1678, 1983). The present study was designed to show when and how the uterus could influence the luteal function. S-D pregnant rats were laparotomized on day 7 of pregnancy, and the number of conceptuses was adjusted to one by aspirating all but one conceptus (Asp-group). The rats were divided into five subgroups and the non-gravid part of the uterus, except that contained a single conceptus,

4

was removed on day 7, 8, 9, 10, or 12 of pregnancy (Hyst-group). Serum progesterone levels were significantly increased after day 15 in the D7-Hyst- and D8-Hyst groups as much well as those normally observed in the intact pregnant rats with full conceptuses, whereas there were no such rises in serum progesterone levels in rats whose uterus was removed after day 9. Interestingly, hypophysectomy in the Asp-group on day 12 of pregnancy induced significant increases in serum progesterone levels after day 15 of pregnancy. Daily treatment with estradiol plus placental luteotrophins (in a form of day-12 pregnant rat serum) between day 12–17 of pregnancy did not show any differences in the changes of serum progesterone levels between the Asp-group and the D7-Hyst group, which indicated that there would not be any essential differences in the nature of the CL between these two groups. It was concluded that the presence of the uterus between day 7–9 of pregnancy induced the luteolysis after day 12, probably mediated through the pituitary.

01.14.13

Immunohistochemical study of fetal and maternal endocrine pancreas in streptozotocin-induced diabetic rats: Tanaka, Y, Toyoda, N, Murata, K, Yamamoto, T, Sugiyama, Y. Dept. Obstet. and Gyn., Mie Univ., School Med., Mie, Japan

It has been suggested that functional changes of maternal endocrine pancreas could play important roles in the fetal growth as well as her own metabolism during pregnancy. In order to clarify the structural changes of endocrine pancreas induced by pregnant status complicated diabetes mellitus, we investigated the distribution of A, B and D cells in the islets of Langerhans in normal and streptozotocin (STZ)-induced diabetic pregnant rats. STZ-induced diabetic female Sprague-Dawley (SD) rats were mated with normal male SD rats. After decapitation on day 20 of pregnancy, maternal and fetal pancreas were obtained and fixed immediately in Bouin's solution and embedded in paraffin for light microscopic examination. Sternberger's PAP method was employed for the detection of A, B and D cells in the islets. Both in normal and diabetic states, islets of Langerhans increased in size and number of its component cells during pregnancy, although B cell numbers were remarkably reduced by STZ administration in nonpregnant state. A and D cell numbers were greater in the diabetic rats than in the normal rats both in pregnant and nonpregnant states. However, they had no remarkable changes during pregnancy. Fetal B cell numbers were somewhat greater in normal rats than in diabetic rats. Fetal D cell numbers were slightly greater in diabetic rats than in normal rats. Fetal A cell numbers had no significant difference between the two groups. These findings suggest that not only normal but also diabetic islets of Langerhans can adapt themselves to metabolic changes induced by pregnancy.

01.14.14

Leukotriene D_4 found in experimental amniotic fluid embolism: Azegami, M, Mori, N. Dept. Obstet. and Gyn., Miyazaki Med. Coll., Miyazaki, Japan

The mechanism of amniotic fluid embolism (AFE) is still unknown. *Steiner* and *Lushbaugh* have emphasized the importance of anaphylactoid reaction. In anaphylactic shock, slow reacting substance (SRS) was found and thought to be an important mediator. Recently, SRS has been identified as a member of newly discovered group of substances, leukotrienes (LTs), and has been shown to consist of LTC_4, LTD_4 and LTE_4. The purpose of this study is to examine an occurrence of LTs in the lungs of experimental AFE models as possible inducers of the symptoms in AFE. The adjusted human amniotic fluid was injected into marginal ear vein of rabbits (amniotic fluid group). Control group was injected with saline. Extract from lungs of the amniotic fluid group showed biological activities like LTs on guinea pig ileums with the concentration of $42 \pm 8.5\,\text{ng/g}$ ($n=10$) of LTD_4, and the contraction was reversed with FPL55712, selective LTs inhibitor, at low concentration of $10^{-6}\,\text{M}$. Reversed phase high performance liquid chromatography of samples from the amniotic fluid group indicated the presence of a peak cochromatographing with synthetic LTD_4 ($n=10$). However, the control group showed neither biological activities nor peaks of LTs. The results suggested the possibility that LTs contribute to the clinical and pathophysiological features of AFE.

01.14.15

Study on experimental intracranial hemorrhage and cerebral blood vessel structure in rat newborns: Kawai, N, Yamaguchi, S, Nishijima, S, Koshino, T, Murooka, H. Dept. Obstet. and Gyn., First Hosp. of Nippon Med. School, Japan

Purpose: Intracranial hemorrhage in neonates is considered to be mainly due to the immaturity in fetuses with fetal hypoxia. Therefore, we tried to study the cause of this disease from the aspect of its cerebral blood vessel structure and to make use of the results in clinical practice. – Method: The rat newborns were divided into following four groups. Group 1: rat newborns 22 days of gestation (term rat newborns); Group 2: rat newborns 22 days of gestation with IUGR; Group 3: premature rat newborns 19 days of gestation; Group 4: premature rat newborns 17 days of gestation. Indian ink or latex was injected into the jugular vein or umbilical vein of rat newborns in each group, and then each group was divided into nonhypoxia group and hypoxia group. And, the occurrence of intracranial hemorrhage and the cerebral blood vessel structure were observed on each sample of rat newborns with binocular magnifier. – Results: (1) ICH was not observed in rat newborns 22 days of gestation, rat newborns 22 days of gestation with IUGR or rat newborns 19 days of gestation. (2) In rat newborns 17 days of gestation, ICH was frequently observed in the hypoxia group. At this stage, the undevelopment of the circle of Willis was observed in the cerebral blood vessel structure. As a result, it was suggested that ICH is associated with the immaturity of cerebral blood vessels. It is, therefore, considered to be most important for the prevention of neonatal intracranial hemorrhage that the pregnancy should be maintained until full term of gestation.

01.14.16
A study of the mechanism regulating the onset of labor: the interaction of rat amniotic membrane and fetal lung in the synthesis of prostaglandin E$_2$: Furuya, K, Yoshida, T, Fukui, Y. Nihon Univ. School Med. **Tokuyama, T.** Tokuyama Clin. **Fujimoto, J.** Fujimoto Clin., Tokyo, Japan
Prostaglandin E$_2$ (PGE$_2$) is found in high concentration in the amniotic fluid in late pregnancy and thought to have various biological activities. However, the site of synthesis and the regulatory mechanism of PGE$_2$ in the amniotic fluid are not yet fully understood. Therefore, we attempted to elucidate the fetal membrane activities in synthesizing PGE$_2$ under the influence of other fetal organs, such as, lung, liver and kidney. The fetal membranes, fetal lung, liver and kidney were obtained from Wistar strain rats. The fetal membranes were cultured in 5% CO$_2$ in air for 24 hours followed by an additional 24 hours of incubation with fetal organs. The supernatant was evaluated by RIA to determine the PGE$_2$ synthesis. The cultures of the fetal membranes for 24 hours showed a decrease of PGE$_2$. However, addition of the other fetal tissues to the culture followed by a further 24 hours of culture showed an increase of PGE$_2$. It is concluded that fetal tissues are making a contribution to the PGE$_2$ synthesis by fetal membranes.

01.14.17
Effects of pregnancy and hormone treatments on the pressor response to angiotensin II in the conscious rat: Nakamura, T, Matsui, K, Ito, M, Yoshimura, T, Maeyama, M. Dept. Obstet. and Gyn., Kumamoto Univ. Med. School, Kumamoto, Japan
The increased refractoriness to the pressor effects of angiotensin II (A-II) that accompanies normal human pregnancy is lost rapidly following delivery. This finding prompts us to speculate that hormones of placental origin which are rapidly cleared from plasma immediately postpartum may be responsible for the normal pregnancy-associated refractoriness to the pressor effects of A-II. Based on this observation, a comparison was made between the pressor responses to A-II in conscious rats during different stages of the pregnancy, the castrated rats following estrogen and progesterone treatment and the rats after human chorionic gonadotropin (hCG) treatment. The rats were placed in the restricted cage and blood pressure was measured with the polygraph by cannulation of the femoral artery. Pregnancy was found to diminish the pressor response to A-II as well as human. Progesterone treatment also diminished the pressor response to A-II as compared to the castrated (control) rats. However, no evidence for an effect of estrogen on the pressor response to A-II was found. Furthermore, hCG induced the elevation of endogenous progesterone level which was followed by the remarkable decrease of the pressor response to A-II. From these observations, we suggest that the refractoriness to the pressor effect of infused A-II which characterizes normal pregnancy may be mediated, at least in part, by the action of progesterone.

01.14.18
Plasma immunoreactive β-endorphin in early puerperium and during breast-feeding: Tulenheimo, A, Laatikainen, T. Dept. I Obstet. and Gyn., Helsinki Univ. Centr. Hosp., Helsinki, Finland
Changes in the plasma concentration of immunoreactive β-endorphin + β-lipotropin (β-ELI) were studied in early puerperium and during breast-feeding. In five women in whom spontaneous labor had begun at 38 to 40 weeks of gestation, the mean level of β-ELI decreased from 282 pg/ml at the time of delivery to 72 pg/ml at 10 min, 51 pg/ml at 30 min, and 19 pg/ml at 60 min after the delivery of the newborn. The mean level of β-ELI was still higher during the first 6 days of puerperium (23.4 ± 3.8 pg/ml) than was found in nonpregnant healthy women (12.4 ± 0.8 pg/ml, p < 0.01) suggesting that endorphin secretion from the maternal hypophysis remains increased in the early puerperium. The effect of suckling stimulus on plasma concentration of β-ELI was studied in five additional women for three to six days after delivery when breast-feeding had already been established. The mean concentration of β-ELI, 33.4 pg/ml, at the beginning of breast-feeding, did not differ statistically significantly from those during or after the breast-feeding being 31.4, 32.2, 26.8, and 30.3 pg/ml 10, 30, 60, and 120 min respectively, after the start of breast-feeding. Thus we were not able to demonstrate any effect of the suckling stimulus on the maternal endorphin secretion. The rapid withdrawal of endorphins from the maternal circulation after delivery might, however, predispose the development of various psychic symptoms common in the early puerperium.

01.14.19
Gastrointestinal regulatory peptides in human lactation: Haukland, H H (1), Holst, N (1), Jenssen, T G (2), Burhol, P G (2), Jorde, R (2), Maltau, J M (1), Haug, E (3). (1) Dept. Obstet. and Gyn. and (2) Dept. Intern. Med. Labor. Gastroent., Inst. Clin. Med., Univ., Tromsø, Norway; (3) Hormone Labor., Aker Hosp., Oslo, Norway
The circulating levels of prolactin (PRL), vasoactive intestinal polypeptide (VIP), somatostatin (SRIH), cholecystokinin (CCK), pancreatic polypeptide (PP), insulin, motilin and blood-glucose were measured in nine nursing women 27 to 40 days after delivery, to establish the possible role of some gastrointestinal regulatory peptides in human lactation. During the last 20 minutes of lactation a significant (p < 0.05)

increase in serum PRL was observed concomittantly with a significant decrease in plasma SRIH levels ($p < 0.05$ at 20 min and $p < 0.01$ at 30 min). There was a highly significant inverse correlation between the mean plasma concentrations of PRL and SRIH during the first 30 minutes of lactation ($r = -0.996$, $p < 0.001$). This suggests a physiological role for SRIH in the hormonal control of PRL secretion in human lactation. PP increased significantly ($p < 0.01$) during nursing, possibly due to cephalic-vagal mechanisms. There were no significant changes in the other gastrointestinal regulatory peptides studied.

01.14.20

Evaluation of serum β-hCG and sonograms in ectopic pregnancy in comparison with abnormal intrauterine pregnancy: Söderqvist, G, Lundström, V, Marsk, L. Dept. Obstet. and Gyn., Karolinska Hosp., Stockholm, Sweden

Two hundred and two early abnormal pregnancies were evaluated with clinical data and β-hCG in serum as well as ultrasound examination. Final diagnosis of ectopic pregnancy was obtained in 54 cases, continuing intrauterine pregnancy in 26 cases and spontaneous abortion in 82 cases. No definite diagnosis of complete spontaneous abortion or early tubal pregnancy could be made in the remaining 40 cases, in which the diagnosis of a pregnancy was based on a β-hCG assay in serum. Rapid clinical improvement concomitant with a falling β-hCG to low levels did not indicate laparoscopy or dilatation and evacuation. The majority of cases with ectopic pregnancy had β-hCG levels below 6000 IU/l and ultrasound was then of uncertain value. The appearance of an adnexal mass on ultrasound strengthened the suspicion of ectopic pregnancy in nine cases. Rapidly increasing β-hCG in serum with the existence of an intrauterine sac above the β-hCG level 6000 IU/l verified an ongoing intrauterine pregnancy. However, the major diagnostical problems are between missed abortion and ectopic pregnancy where rapidly falling β-hCG in serum more likely indicates a complete spontaneous abortion. The appearance of an intrauterine sac in cases with β-hCG in the range below 6000 IU/l indicated missed abortion in eight cases while no ectopic pregnancy presented this sign.

01.14.21

Microchemical measurement of phosphates in amniotic fluid (AF): Relationship to antibacterial activity: Tomblin, J, Larsen, B, Charles, D. Dept. Obstet. and Gyn., Marshall Univ. School Med., Huntington, USA

In vitro addition of phosphate to term AF of healthy women diminishes the activity of an antibacterial factor responsible for suppressing the growth of E. coli, providing presumptive evidence of the presence of phosphate-sensitive antibacterial factor. Investigation of the role of endogenous phosphates in regulating such activity would be facilitated by a simple and reliable procedure requiring minimal sample. Therefore, adaptation of the malachite green complexometric assay (Clin. Chem. Acta. **14**, 361, 1966) for determination of inorganic and organic phosphate in AF was undertaken, and phosphate in these samples correlated with bacterial growth inhibiting activity. Growth inhibition was determined by viable plate counts of E. coli ATCC 33908 in AF. 10^4 washed bacteria were placed in 1 ml of AF and incubated at $36°C$ for 24 hours. Phosphate was determined by absorbance at 600 nm after combining the sample with malachite green-ammonium molybdate color reagent. Lipid phosphates were extracted with organic solvents. Trichloroacetic acid was used to precipitate protein and nucleic acid phosphates. Wet ashing liberated organically bound phosphate from the samples. The malachite green method was found to be as accurate as, and more sensitive than the Fiske-Subbarow method. We analyzed 23 AF samples for phosphates and antibacterial activity. Free phosphate was the most abundant form of phosphate in AF, but its concentration only weakly correlated with bacterial growth. It is concluded that phosphate is only indirectly related to growth inhibition and that additional factors may be involved in the antibacterial effect.

01.14.22

Mother-to-infant transmission of Chlamydia trachomatis in perinatal period: Yasuda, J, Yamamoto, T, Kanao, M, Okada, H. Dept. Obstet. and Gyn., Kyoto Prefect. Univ. Med., Kyoto, Japan

Chlamydia trachomatis is recognized as one of the common etiologic agents of STD. Its true incidence is difficult to quantify, since chlamydial infections are not formally reported. The infections may progress to more severe diseases such as endometritis, salpingitis and PID, and it may be transmitted to newborn infants, resulting in neonatal conjunctivitis and respiratory infections. The transmission rate of chlamydia from infected mother to infants has not been precisely studied, but is assumed to be approximately 50%. This paper aimed to study the incidence of chlamydial infection in Japanese women and transmission from mother to newborn infants. The infection of chlamydia was diagnosed through the demonstration of chlamydial inclusions within McCoy cells stained by Giemsa, and immunofluorescent antibody technic. Clinical specimens were obtained from the cervix, conjunctiva and pharyngeal swabs. The incidence of infection of pregnant women (36–40 WG) before delivery was 4.9% (8/161), whereas 32.4% in STD clinic. Three infants delivered from the infected women (8) were diagnosed to have chlamydial infection in the conjunctiva. The transmission rate from infected mother to newborn infant at delivery was 37.5%. Perinatal care of infected women is significantly important.

01.14.23

Antibiotic chemoprophylaxis in Cesarean section (c.s.); Our experience with 570 cases: Sprefico, P, Scian, A, Scalambrino, S, Regallo, M, Bonazzi, C. Dept. Obstet. and Gyn., S. Gerardo Hosp., Monza, Italy
This study is a retrospective analysis of the efficacy of different schedules of antibiotic prophylaxis of infections after c.s. From October 81 to November 84 570 women underwent c.s.; according to four subsequent schedules of antibiotic prophylaxis they received: 1) from October 81 to April 83 Cephalexin 2 g i. v. at the end of operation, or nothing (237), 2) from May 83 to December 83 Cephalexin 2 g i. v. at the end of operation, 5 hours and 12 hours later (all pts at risk for infection, 48) or nothing (pts without risk, 94), 3) from January 84 to May 84 Ceftezole 2 g i. v. at the end of operation, 5 hours and 12 hours later (patients at risk, 37) or nothing (pts without risk, 53), 4) from June 84 to November 84 and further on, Ceftezole 2 g i. v. 30 min before operation, 5 hours and 12 hours later (all patients, 101). A prophylactic failure was defined by the occurrence of hyperpyrexia ($>38°$ C for two days at least, the operative day excepted) or by clinical evidence of infection. Whenever available, samples from the site of infection were collected for a complete microbiological evaluation. We had prophylactic failures: 1) 15/75 (20%) vs 29/162 (17.9%), 2) 8.3% vs 28.7%, 3) 18.9% vs 32% between prophylaxis and control groups; 4) 9.9%. Ceftezole administered perioperatively showed itself useful in preventing infections.

01.14.24

Search for possible routes of vertical and horizontal transmission of adult T-cell leukemia virus: Nakano, S, Ando, Y, Ichijo, M, Moriyama, S I, Saito, K. Dept. Obstet. and Gyn., Nara Med. Univ., Nara, Japan
ATL in Japan is remarkably clustered in humans in ATLV-endemic areas, such as the Kyushu and Okinawa areas, and this limited distribution and other epidemiological analysis have strongly suggested the possibility of familial spreading of ATLV. We are interested in whether ATLV can be transmitted from mother to child via the placenta and/or breast milk and also from husband to wife via semen. We collected serum samples from healthy pregnant women in the Ginowan and Urasoe districts, Okinawa prefecture, during 1983 and 1984. The sera were tested for anti-ATLA (ATLV-specific antigens). The antibodies were found in sera of 90 (6.4%) of 1405 healthy pregnant women. Next, we examined possible placental transmission of ATLV to neonates from anti-ATLA positive mothers. We collected samples of the mothers' blood and cord blood of neonates immediately after birth. A monoclonal antibody GIN-14 to ATLV p19 and p28 was used for detection of ATLA. We examined 35 pairs (neonate and mother) for the appearance of ATLA in the cultured cells. ATLA was definitely demonstrated in the cells from 29 mothers. However, no ATLA-positive cells were detected among the cells from any of the neonates tested. We have similarly examined the mononuclear cells of breast milk from anti-ATLA antibody positive pregnant women. We found all specimens from 12 individuals tested to be ATLA-positive. We observed the expression of ATLA from the semen of one of the three ATLA-positive males.

01.14.25

The role of prostaglandins in relation to the initiation of labor: Makimura, N, Kato, K, Nagata, I, Seki, K, Furuya, K. Dept. Obstet. and Gyn., Nat. Defense Med. Coll., Japan
The purpose of this study is to elucidate the role of prostaglandins (PGs) in relation to the mechanism of labor onset. Placenta which showed the highest PGs content before and after labor onset among the tissues of pregnant rabbit was used to observe the PGs production and the influence of sex steroids on it. – Materials: Rabbit placenta in late pregnancy and human placenta at the time of Cesarean section was used for this study. – Methods: The effect of arachidonate on PGs production in human placenta at different stages of labor were observed by superfusion and incubation techniques. PGs were acidified and extracted with ethylacetate, and PGs concentration was measured by RIA. – Results: Placental PGE increased toward the term of pregnancy and showed the highest value at the time of onset of labor. It decreased thereafter. $PGF_{2\alpha}$ showed high value after the onset of labor. The highest PGs production was observed in the placenta before the onset of labor as compared with the other stages of labor. PGs production decreased in the placenta before labor onset by the additon of progesterone. – Conclusion: PGs has an important role on the mechanism of parturition. PGE production increased in the placenta when progesterone decreased. It is supposed that PGE acts as a trigger for the onset of labor, on the other hand, $PGF_{2\alpha}$ assists the uterine contraction.

01.14.26

The effect of intracervical PGE_2-gel on plasma levels of 13,14-dihydro-15-keto-PGE_2 (PGEM) in women at term: Noah, M L, Kimball, F A, Ruppel, P L, de la Fuente, P*, Decoster, J M. The Upjohn Company, Kalamazoo, MI, USA; *Residence Sanitaria, 1° de Octubre-Maternidad, Madrid, Spain
Patients undergoing preinduction cervical softening were randomized to receive no treatment (controls) or 0.5 mg PGE_2-triacetin gel. Plasma samples containing PGEM collected 4 hrs post-treatment and converted to the stable bicyclo degradation product (bicyclo-PGEM) were assayed by RIA (*Bothwell* et al. J. Pharmacol. Ther. **220**, 229, 1982). Positive clinical effect (responders) during 12 hrs after treatment (Bishop score increase ≥ 3 in labor or delivered) was assessed. All evaluations were blind. In nonresponders (n = 35), the means of the bicyclo-PGEM variables (mean, maximum, area under the curve) were all about 18% higher in gel-treated patients (n = 6) than controls (n. s.). In responders (n = 38), the variables were all about

80% higher in gel-treated women (n = 32) than controls (p < .01). In controls (n = 35), the responders (n = 6) had 50% higher levels than nonresponders (n. s.). In the gel-treated women (n = 38), responders (n = 32) had about 140% higher levels than nonresponders (p < .01). The results suggest that both exogenous and endogenous bicyclo-PGEM were measured. Differences in pairwise comparisons suggest that there may be substantially less exogenous bicyclo-PGEM in the gel nonresponders than in gel responders or substantially more endogenous bicyclo-PGEM in gel responders than in control-responders.

01.14.27

Myometrial activity after local application of PGE_2-gel for cervical ripening and term labor induction: *Ekman, G, **Uldbjerg, N, *Ulmsten, U. *Dept. Obstet. and Gyn., Malmö Univ. Hosp., Malmö, Sweden and **Dept. Pharmacol., Univ., Århus, Denmark
Local application of prostaglandin E_2 (PGE_2) in gel has been found effective for cervical ripening and labor induction. Since myometrial hyperstimulation has been reported it is essential to evaluate the risk of inducing unwanted uterine activity and how to avoid it. – Material: Twelve nulliparous term pregnant women with unripe cervices participated in the study. In four women 0.5 mg PGE_2 in 2 ml gel was applied strictly within the cervical canal. In another four the PGE_2-gel was allowed to escape into the extra-amniotic space. In the remaining four women 4 mg PGE_2 was applied vaginally. Thirty minutes before the gel application external cardiotocography was started. For proper recording of the myometrial activity a microtip transducer was at the same time introduced into the extra-amniotic space via the cervical canal. The pressure signals obtained were amplified and registered on a pen recorder. The recordings lasted for at least 4 hours. – Results: Strict intracervical application of PGE_2-gel induced minimal or sporadic myometrial activity whereas regular uterine contractions were recorded within five minutes of extra-amniotic application. After intravaginal application regular contractions were recorded within 30 minutes. – Conclusion: With strict intracervical application of a low dose (0.5 mg) PGE_2 in gel the risks for myometrial hyperstimulation seem to be minimized or avoided. Extra-amniotic or vaginal application of PGE_2-gel seems on the other hand to induce a prompt activation of the myometrium.

01.14.28

Induction of labor with prostaglandin-E_2: Ponnath, H, Weitzel, H. Hosp. Gyn. and Obstet., FU, Berlin
The medically indicated termination of pregnancy in cases of underdeveloped vaginal findings is a problem which has not as yet been conclusively solved. Oxytocin which is used as standard medication, only produces satisfactory results if the myometrium is adequately sensitive, which normally requires favorable vaginal findings. In the meantime, our clinic has established a series of indications for which prostaglandine-E_2 (PGE_2) is given the preference over oxytocin. We use PGE_2 to induce labor in pregnant women with unfavorable cervix or gestoses as well as in so-called oxytocin failures. We give PGE_2 intravenously, since the dosage can be adapted precisely to the need despite possible systemic side-effects. We start with a dose of $0.25 \mu g/min.$ which, depending on its effect, is increased up to a maximal dose of $2.5 \mu g/min.$ This method has so far been successfully used in over 150 pregnant women. In most cases, it was possible to achieve a spontaneous or operative-vaginal delivery. In 21% of the cases, pregnancy had to be terminated by Cesarean section; but only in one fourth caused by imminent asphyxia. Assessment of the partograms show that the effect of PG takes a typical course. After a long period in which the only detectable alteration is a softening of the cervix, there is a rapid opening of the cervical os. If necessary, the PG-induced contractions can be counteracted by fenoterol. The APGAR values and the pH-level of the umbilical artery indicated no negative influence on the newborns. It must, however, be emphasized that the relationship of PG to oxytocin should be regarded as supplementary rather than competitive.

01.14.29

The influence of maternal position on duration of labor: Ahmed L T, Bouchetara, K. Algeria
This study from January 1983 to September 1983 measured the time in active labor of 80 patients who met ten criteria and were divided randomly into two groups of 40. Group A subjects were placed in the usual supine position and group B subjects were allowed to be in a sitting position. The mean time in the active phase of labor for group B, 3.21 hr., was not significantly less than group A, 3.29 hr.; but the patients' comfort was higher in the B group throughout labor.

01.14.30

β-endorphin in maternal and umbilical cord plasma at elective Cesarean section and after spontaneous labor: Räisänen, I, Laatikainen, T. Dept. I Obstet. and Gyn., Helsinki Univ. Centr. Hosp., Helsinki, Finland
Concentration of β-endorphin (β-E) in relation to the mode of delivery and of anesthesia was studied in maternal and cord plasma in 30 healthy women at term pregnancy using a specific assay (*Laatikainen* et al. Clin. Chem. **31**, 134, 1985). The mean maternal β-E level at elective Cesarean section under epidural anesthesia rose from 9.8 ± 2.7 (S. E.) pmol/l before induction to 15.5 ± 3.7 pmol/l at the time of delivery (p < 0.02). Under general anesthesia the mean β-E level rose more, from 14.6 ± 7.2 to 34.4 ± 7.8 pmol/l reaching the mean β-E value of the second stage of normal labor, 39.4 ± 7.0 pmol/l. In the cord plasma, the mean β-E level did not differ in relation to the mode of anesthesia. The mean β-E value in cord arterial

9

and venous plasma was significantly higher after spontaneous labor (40.9 $\pm$ 11 and 40.1 $\pm$ 9.2 pmol/l, respectively) than at elective Cesarean section under epidural (14.3 $\pm$ 1.9 and 12.4 $\pm$ 3.6 pmol/l, respectively) or general anesthesia (11.9 $\pm$ 2.2 and 13.4 $\pm$ 2.2 pmol/l, respectively). Thus Cesarean section under general anesthesia proved to be more stressful to the mother than that under epidural anesthesia if β-E release is used as a measure of stress. The mode of anesthesia did not seem to influence of the plasma β-E level in the newborn infant. Normal delivery by vaginal route increased the release of β-E both to the maternal and to the fetoplacental circulation.

01.14.31

Changes in serum 5α dihydroprogesterone (5αDHP) prior to normal parturition: Löfgren, M, Bäckström, T, Joelsson, I. Dept. Obstet. and Gyn. and Physiol., Univ., Umeå, Sweden

It has been shown that (5αDHP) in serum closely follows the concentration of progesterone during human pregnancy with a ratio of 1 : 4 (1). Metabolism of progesterone to 5αDHP has been verified in placental tissue (2). Little is known, however, about 5αDHP production around parturition. In the present study eight women with uncomplicated pregnancy were followed with blood sampling twice weekly from 36 weeks of gestation to parturition. Progesterone and 5αDHP were analysed utilizing earlier described RIA methods (3). Non parametric statistics were used. 5αDHP decreased significantly during the last week of pregnancy. The mean 5αDHP serum concentration decreased from 133 $\pm$ 36 nmol/l at one week prior to parturition to 101 $\pm$ 19 nmol/l at the day of parturition (p < 0.01). The ratio progesterone/5αDHP increased with high statistical significance (p < 0.005) during the two last weeks of pregnancy. No significant change occurred in serum progesterone during the observation time. These results suggest a change in progesterone metabolism and 5αDHP production preceding the onset of spontaneous labor.

(1). *Millewitch, Gomez-Sanchez, Madden* and *McDonald.* Gyn. Invest. **6**, 291 (1975).
(2). *Millewitch, Grant, Schwartz, Shen* and *McDonald.* Am. J. Obstet. Gyn. **133**, 611 (1979).
(3). *Bäckström, Andersson, Baird, Selstam.* Acta endocr. (Kbh.), Suppl. **756**, 257 (1983).

01.14.32

Studies of coagulable-fibrinolytic and kallikrein-kinin systems in the utero-placental circulation and amniotic fluid: Mutoh, S, Teh, A, Shimoji, Y, Nishi, N, Saitoh, M. Dept. Obstet. and Gyn., Tokyo Med. and Dent. Univ., School Med., Tokyo, Japan

In 40 cases of full term pregnancy Cesarean section performed before and during onset of labor, the amniotic fluid and blood samples from the uterine artery, uterine vein and the peripheral vein were collected and the changes of FPA, FPB$_\beta$15-42, HMW-kg, LMW-kg, glandular kallikrein and kinin were studied. The levels of FPA in UA increased significantly during onset of labor as compared to the increase in UV and PV and although the UA level of FPB$_\beta$15-42 also showed the same pattern of increase during labor but the increase was not so sharp. Levels of HMW- and LMW-kg gradually decreased during onset of labor but no significant differences among UA, UV and PV were found. Level of kinin in UA increased significantly during labor but remained unchanged in UV. In the amniotic fluid, the levels of FPA, FPB$_\beta$15-42, and HMW-kg increased gradually while that of kinin increased significantly and decreases of glandular kallikrein and LMW-kg were seen during labor. These findings suggested that with the increased consumption of HMW- and LMW-kg and kinin during labor, the uteroplacental circulation exhibited a state of hypercoagulability secondary to hyperfibrinolytic activity resulting in the increase in vascular permeability to the amniotic fluid and increased production of kinin.

01.14.33

Outcome after myomectomy during pregnancy: Kiyota, Y, Ichimaru, S, Chiga, M, Motomatsu, S, Doi, Y. Kumamoto Red Cross Hosp., Kyushu, Japan

Recently the tendency of growth of uterine myomata in early reproductive life is slightly increasing. For the past nine years in our clinic, 15 cases of myomectomy during pregnancy were carried out because of seriously complicated subserous and intramural myomata producing symptomatic signs such as uterine irritability and contractility which thought to interrupt pregnancy. These patients were recommended therapeutic abortion or hysterectomy by other surgeons. They were all primigravidas except one and desired to continue pregnancy. In this series myomectomy was performed after 12 weeks of pregnancy. Blood loss during myomectomy was well controlled. No abortion was noticed after the operation. Fourteen (93.3%) out of 15 cases gave birth to mature term babies vaginally. Blood loss at delivery was within normal limits. One case had Cesarean section due to fetal distress after PROM. In nine of our cases, subsequent pregnancies were also followed up to term. All of them delivered normal mature term babies vaginally without any evidence of recurrence of myomata. In one case, the third pregnancy was followed to term. She had a normal mature baby vaginally. Finally 15 cases of myomectomy during pregnancy delivered a total of 24 normal mature babies (96%) vaginally.

01.14.34

Work during pregnancy and birth weight: Langhoff-Roos, J, Jansson, S, Gebre-Medhin, M, Lindmark, G. Uppsala Univ., Dept. Obstet. and Gyn. and Dept. Pediat., Akad. Sjukh., Uppsala, Sweden

Strenous working conditions during pregnancy have been shown to be associated with adverse outcomes of pregnancy, including reduced birth weight. The situation in Sweden is unique with respect to both a very high proportion of mothers working professionally and generous possibilities for paid absence from work during pregnancy. This means that especially those women who have physically hard jobs, can leave early. 500 consecutive term pregnancies were studied with a questionnaire. 400 of these had professional work outside their home. 77 continued working up to term, but the rest were absent from work at a mean two weeks in first trimester and 2.5 and 6 weeks in second and third trimester respectively. The number of weeks at work had no association with birth weight, but there was a mean difference of 150 g between infants whose mothers had been working full time and half time. The results show that the majority of pregnant women need extra rest in the last period of pregnancy, and that the social security system can compensate to a great extent for differences in working conditions.

01.14.35

Prognosis of low birth weight infants: Hiratsuka, K, Koresawa, M. Perinat. Ctr., Saiseikai Shimonoseki Gen. Hosp., Shimonoseki, Japan

The present paper shows the outcome in 80 infants with birth body weight of 500–1500 g. The survival rate of these 80 cases was 85%. The survival rate was particularly greater in a group of infants with birth weight of more than 700 g (92.3%, 60/65 cases) than those of 700 g or smaller (53.3%, 8/15 cases). A group of infants born at the 25th week of gestation or later also showed a significantly greater survival rate (91.3%, 63/69 cases) than those born before the 24th week (45.5%, 5/11 cases). In 41 cases who were followed for at least one year after birth, one case had cerebral palsy, two had major handicaps (e. g., deafness and/or blindness), and two had minor neurological handicaps. The main factors which caused the neonatal death or complications in these high risk group of infants were severe respiratory distress syndrome and intracranial hemorrhage. The possible role of Cesarean section in achieving the improvement of survival rate is also discussed.

01.14.36

Elderly smokers are at higher risk than younger smokers for developing fetal growth disturbances: Cnattingius, S, Axelsson, O, Eklund, G, Lindmark, G. Dept. Obstet. and Gyn., Uppsala Univ., Uppsala, Sweden

A prospective clinical study from an unselected area-based population was performed in order to study the influence of different factors on birth weight for gestational age (standardized birth weight), with special respect to risk factors for intrauterine growth retardation. Smoking was the most important risk factor: Sixteen per cent of the mothers smoked at least ten cigarettes per day and the influence of smoking on standardized birth weight was highly significant. Although maternal age in itself had no effect on standardized birth weight, among smokers, the reduction in standardized birth weight was hardly significant among younger mothers but very marked among mothers above the age of thirty. Long-term smoking has previously been reported to increase the risk of severe placental complications. This study emphasizes that elderly smokers also must be considered to be at a higher risk than younger smokers for developing fetal growth disturbances.

01.14.37

Intensive plasma exchange in severe rhesus isoimmunized pregnant woman: effect of antibody eliminated autologous plasma: Ukita, M, Takakura, K, Emi, N, Yagiri, Y*, Ueda, Y*, Ueda, M*, Yamada, N*, Ikeda, Y*. Dept. Obstet. and Gyn., Blood Serv. Ctr.*, Kurashiki Centr. Hosp., Kurashiki, Japan

Intensive plasma exchange (PE), using autologous plasma which absorbed anti-D antibody with D positive red cells, was given to a severe Rh immunized woman. In her 3rd and 4th pregnancy, PE started at 29 and 16 weeks gestation and she received 7 and 34 times of PE, respectively. Antibody titers (AHG-T) altered from 1 : 512 to 1 : 4096. Fetal conditions were estimated by amnion fluid examinations, USG, and non stressed FHR-monitoring. The 3rd infant weighed 2150 gr (33 weeks) with cord Hb 11.2 gr/dl, while the 4th 1280 gr (28 weeks) with 6.7 gr/dl. Both required exchange transfusions and did well. The procedure for selective antibody absorption is as follows: maternal plasma separated by IBM 2997 was incubated with D positive washed packed red cells at 37°C for 5 minutes. Mix ratio of plasma and packed red cells was settled to 3 : 1. Incubated mixture was separated by Haemonetics Model 30, and collected plasma was frozen at −65° C immediately and was used as the replacement fluid for next PE. Residual red cell counts in the processed plasma were 2.6 to 4.2 per mm^3, and this seemed to be negligible as the cause of reimmunization. We think that PE using processed autologous plasma is the most physiological, and is preventive against hepatitis, and economical.

01.14.38

State of acidity as an indicator of quality care in obstetrics: Regalia, A, Molina, P, Del Bo, R, Bottino, S. Dept. Obstet. and Gyn., S. Gerardo Hosp., Monza, Italy

Increasingly, excellence in obstetric care is not just measured by perinatal mortality, but also by the ratio of the infants born with acidosis. From September 1983 to February 1985 we performed routine determination of the state of acidity in the newborns of high risk labors (meconium stained liquor, pathological CTG, operative deliveries either V. E. either C. S. for fetal distress). We analyzed in 577 samples the relation between Apgar scores and the acid-base status of the babies at birth and the different predictivity of these two indices on the subsequent need of neonatal intensive care. The results will be discussed.

01.14.39

Diagnosis of prenatal deformity: Kupka, K, Wagner, K H, Simoens, W. Frauenklin., Städt. Klin., Kassel
In many cases the obstetrician is also the first physician who is confronted with congenital deformities and has to deal with them. We have had a critical look at the congenital anomalies, within the total of births which took place between 1980 and 1984 (6899 births/70 malformations). The high incidence of intestinal malformations (38) is striking. Next in order of frequency (28) are the malformations of the head and the rump ("Pole deformities") and the deformities of the extremities. In the course of our prenatal investigations we found one microcephalus and one huge lymphangiectatic hygroma (the so-called "Nackenblasen-fetus"). There was also a coarctation of the aorta, as well as hypoplasia and retarded maturation of the ovaries. This clinical picture represents a fetal Turner's syndrome. Because of its rarity, there is little in the literature about the prenatal diagnosis of cases of this sort.

01.14.40

Prenatal diagnosis of fetal ascites: Diagnostic and therapeutic problems: Hüneke, B, Carstensen, M H, Kitschke, H-J. Univ.-Frauenklin., Hamburg-Eppendorf
Ultrasound has become an invaluable help in the assessment of fetal abnormalities such as fetal ascites. With decreasing frequency of rh-isoimmunization the nonimmune hydrops fetalis (NIHF) has become the more important form of hydrops. From 1981 to 1984 30 cases of hydrops fetalis were seen in our department: 16 were caused by hemolytic diseases and treated with prenatal transfusion. 14 cases of NIHF were diagnosed primarily using ultrasound (4 before, 10 after 24 weeks gestation). In addition blood typing, antibody screening, serology, fetal echocardiography, clinical examination and amniocentesis were performed. The following conditions were associated with NIHF: chromosomal anomalies (2), hypophospha-tasia (1), multiple congenital anomalies (3), hypoproteinemia (2). Two of the NIHF patients without congenital or chromosomal anomalies were delivered healthy without therapy after spontaneous disappearance of the ascites. One fetus died after delivery by Cesarean section at the 33rd week of gestation in spite of prenatal therapy with digitalis. Pregnancies with multiple anomalies or chromosomal anomalies were terminated. – Conclusion: Even with extensive prenatal diagnostic measures and therapy, the prognosis of NIHF is worse than that of immunological cases.

01.14.41

Osaka birth defects monitoring program, initial report: Suehara, N, Kurachi, K, Takemura, T, Teramura, S, Fukui, M, Ogita, S. Dept. Obstet. and Gyn., Osaka Univ. Med. School, Osaka Med. Ctr. Maternal and Child Hlth., Osaka Med. Ass., Osaka Soc. Obstet. and Gyn., Osaka Municip. Maternity and Infant Ctr., Osaka, Japan
The Osaka Birth Defects Monitoring Program was started in December 1981, as a population-based monitoring system, in Osaka Prefecture. The 22 maker malformations and other major malformations were monitored for all live-births and still-births (over 24th gestational week and/or over 500 grams) within seven days after birth. In the first 34 months, 169,046 records were collected from 305 obstetric hospitals and clinics. Those records were corresponding to about 60% of the annual births in Osaka Prefecture. Among the 169,046 births, the incidence of still-birth was 0.67% and the average of all maternal age was 28.03 years. The incidence of low birth weight (less than 2500 grams) was 5.40% and premature births, 4.45%. The overall incidence of total malformations in all births was 1.06% and that in still-births was 15.7% and maternal diabetus mellitus, 4.61%. The incidence of anencephalus (per 10,000 births) was 7.7, hydrocephalus, 3.5, cleft lip (with or without cleft palate), 13.8, cleft palate, 5.5, spina bifida, 3.4, omopha-locele, 2.8, atresia ani, 3.8, hypospadias (among male), 4.0 and Down's syndrome, 6.2 The monthly transitions were monitored for each maker malformations. The incidence of anencephalus and cleft lip had a higher point than 90% line of the Poisson distributions in the early period of this program. Most cases of anencephalus and about one half of the cases of encephalocele were diagnosed prenatally.

01.14.42

Obstetric problems in the prophylaxis of the respiratory distress syndrome: Hadjiev, A, Mirkov, K. Inst. Obstet. and Gyn., Med. Acad., Sofia, Bulgaria
On the basis of 1983 tests of amniotic fluid obtained from 101 patients, a model of normal values of the L/S ratio during pregnancy has been built up beginning from the 29th, up to the 42nd week of gestation. The model includes the limit of $\pm$ 2 SD. Several groups of pregnant women with complicated pregnancies have been investigated and the trends in the maturation of the fetal lung maturity have been followed up. For stimulation of the fetal lung maturity we used Celestone (betamethasone). There is a statistically significant increase in the L/S ratio in comparison with the values before administration of the drug. The observation in cases with spontaneous rupture of membranes showed that there is a statistically significant increase in the L/S ratio in the period after the amniotic fluid escapes. The immature fetuses (29 to 33 w. g.) are more sensitive to the stimulating effect of the rupture of the membranes. The main increase of the L/S ratio occurs about the third day after the rupture of membranes. The factor "rupture of amniotic membranes" requires certain "latent period" after which the corresponding system of the fetus begins to synthesize surfactants.

01.14.43

Chemotherapy of squamous carcinoma of the cervix: Lahousen, M, Pickel, H. Geburtshilfl.-Gyn. Univ.-Klin., Graz, Austria

Thirty-nine patients with advanced and/or recurrent squamous cell carcinoma of the cervix were treated with a combination of mitomycin, vincristin, bleomycin and cis-platinum recommended by *Alberts* et al. (Cancer Clin. Trials **4**, 313, 1981). Six patients (15.4%) showed a complete response lasting between three and 33 months. Twelve patients (30.7%) had a partial response to the chemotherapy lasting between two and 11 months. The response rate for patients with radiation ($n = 22$) before chemotherapy was lower 45.5%) than for patients ($n = 17$) without prior radiation (59%). Even the mean survival times were significantly lower for patients with a history of radiation (six months) versus patients with no prior radiation (12 months). This chemotherapy regimen was well tolerated. It is concluded that this four drug chemotherapy has some effect in advanced and recurrent squamous cell carcinoma of the cervic uteri.

01.28.01

Follicular fluid-regulators of estrogen secretion: Daume, E, Sturm, G, Chari, S. Women's Hosp., Dept. Gyn. Endocr., Univ., Marburg

Previous studies have shown that ovarian function is controlled not only by steroids but also by ovarian non-steroidal regulators (*Daume* et al. In: Inadequate Luteal Phase. Ed: *H. D. Taubert* and *H. Kuhl,* MTP press LTD, 7, 1984). Human ovarian follicular fluid (hFF) was subjected successively to gel permeation, ion-exchange and dye-affinity chromatographies. The protein(s) that bound to the dye (Orange A) possessed the ability to inhibit dose-dependently the amounts of estrogen secreted by porcine granulosa cells *in vitro,* during 3 hr incubation at 37° C. *In vivo* it inhibited hMG-induced E_2 secretion in immature female rats. This substance also exhibited inhibin-activity (inhibition of FSH secretion) when tested *in vivo,* in castrated female rats, and *in vitro,* by cultured rat pituitaries. The proteins that did not bind to Orange A dose-dependently stimulated the release of E_2 by porcine granulosa cells *in vitro.* No demonstrable inhibin-activity was found in this unbound-fraction. Human serum proteins purified in a similar manner had no effect in the biological test systems indicating the specificity of the biological activities of the hFF-proteins. The data suggest that the FF-inhibitors/stimulators may play an important role in the local regulation of estrogen biosynthesis.

01.28.02

Purification of porcine follicular fluid inhibin: Fukuda, M, Miyamoto, K, Nomura, M, Hasegawa, Y, Igarashi, M, Kangawa, K*, Matsuo, H*. Dept. Obstet. and Gyn., Gunma Univ., School Med., Maebashi, Gunma, Japan; *Dept. Biochem., Miyazaki Med. Coll., Miyazaki, Japan

The most pressing need in inhibin research is to isolate and characterize this molecule. We have tried to isolate ovarian inhibin from porcine follicular fluid (pFF) and purified it to an apparent homogeneity. Biological activities of inhibin preparations were estimated from suppressions of spontaneous FSH release from cultured rat anterior pituitary cells. Thirteen liters of pFF were collected from 20,000 ovaries and used as a starting material. Concentrations causing half maximal inhibition (ED_{50}) were used to assess potency of the various fractions. An ED_{50} value of the starting material was 6 $\mu g/ml$ medium. Purification was performed by successive chromatographies using Matrex gel Red A, Phenyl Sepharose, Sephacryl S-200, DEAE-Sepharese CL-6B and reverse-phase HPLC. Results of the purification starting from 1L of pFF were listed below.

	protein (mg)	ED_{50} (ng/ml)	specific activity	yield %
pFF	67700	6000	1	100
Phenyl Seph.	3060	440	13.5	64
DEAE-Seph.	3.8	6.25	960	5.4
RP-HPLC	0.5	1.2	5000	3.7

The final preparation after RP-HPLC showed a single band on a SDS-polyacrylamide gel electrophoresis under a non-reduced condition, and the bioactivity was associated with the protein band. This preparation did not contain steroid hormones, i. e. estradiol, progesterone, or testosterone, and suppressed FSH but not LH or PRL in our bioassay system.

01.28.03

Lipids and apolipoproteins in human follicular fluid: Enk, L, Crona, N, Hillensjö, T. Dept. Obstet. and Gyn., Sahlgrenska Hosp., Göteborg, Sweden

Lipoproteins (LP) play an important role in the production of steroids in the adrenals, placenta and corpus luteum (CL) in the human. LP are internalised into the steroid-producing cells by receptor-mediated mechanisms, and cholesterol (CH) is utilised as substrate. In these organs synthesis of CH is quantitatively insignificant. In previous studies LDL (low density LP) has been shown to stimulate progesterone production in isolated CL and in luteinised granulosa cells *in vitro,* while HDL (high density LP) was reported to inhibit luteinisation and progesterone synthesis. A study on non-preovulatory follicles has indicated that the levels of LDL and VLDL in follicular fluid (FFl) are low. We obtained FFl by ultrasound guided puncture shortly prior to ovulation in 17 women participating in the *in vitro* fertilisation program. Follicular maturation had been induced by clomiphene, followed by hMG and hCG injections according to the routine procedure of our clinic. Serum from the patients was obtained simultaneously and the levels of CH, triglycerides (TG) and phospholipids (PL), apolipoprotein A1 (apo-A1) and -B (apo-B) assayed in serum and in the FFl. The level of apo-A1 in the FFl was 56% of that of serum, while apo-B was virtually absent. Apo-A1 is the major protein constituent of HDL and not present in other LP, while apo-B is present in VLDL and LDL but not in HDL. The levels of CH, TG and PL in the FFl were approximately half of the levels in HDL in normal serum, and correlated very well with apo-A1 in FFl. These data therefore indicate that HDL is present in these preovulatory follicles while LDL and VLDL are not. Thus it appears that the "blood-follicle barrier" exists also in the late preovulatory follicle.

01.28.04
Granulosa-cell growth factor in oocyte and its transport systems: Takaoka, H, Satoh, H, Makinoda, S, Moriya, S, Ichinoe, K. Dept. Obstet. and Gyn., Hokkaido Univ. School Med., Sapporo, Japan
The possible existence of granulosa-cell growth factor (GGF) in the oocyte has been investigated using the labelling index (LI) with ^{3}H-thymidine and the mitotic index (MI) of granulosa cells (G-cells) in mice. The following results were obtained: (1) In preantral follicles the LI increased with the development of the oocyte until its diameter reached the maximum (approximately 90 μm). In preantral follicles with the oocyte diameter below 69 μm, the LI was low (9.5 $\pm$ 1.7%) and the follicular diameter was small. As the oocyte developed, the LI increased and reached the maximum value (20.3 $\pm$ 3.8%) when the follicular diameter was approximately 200 μm. Then it decreased a little but maintained a high value. The antrum formation was seen when the follicular diameter was about 300 μm showing no change in LI. (2) In preantral follicles with the oocyte diameter over 80 μm the G-cell near the oocyte had a much higher LI than the distant one. After the antrum formation, the LI and MI of cumulus layers adjacent to the oocyte were three times as great as those of the mural layers. (3) Among the mural cell layers in the antral follicle the layer adjacent to the antrum showed remarkably high LI in comparison with the distant layers. These results suggest that GGF, which seems to play a role in the formation of cumulus, is secreted with the development of the oocyte and is transported through the follicular fluid in addition to through the G-cell gap-junction.

01.28.05
Steroidogenesis by theca and granulosa cells in combined monolayer culture from preovulatory human ovarian follicles: Tamaoka, Y, Katayama, E, Nakamura, Y, Sawada, T, Higuchi, Y. Dept. Obstet. and Gyn., School Med., Keio Univ., Tokyo, Japan
Cellular interaction on steroidogenesis by two cell types of ovary has been suggested by previous studies. To verify this, we studied steroidogenesis of theca and granulosa cells, separated or combined, using two cell combined monolayer culture method. Granulosa and theca cells were harvested from preovulatory follicles of women with normal menstrual cycles. RIA measurements of steroidogenesis revealed as follows: 1) Estradiol (E_2) production of granulosa cells after 24 hr culture was significantly higher than theca cells, but rapidly declined after 48 hr. 2) Theca cells are major site of androstenedione (Δ_4) biosynthesis during early culture period. 3) E_2 production of combined culture after 24 hr and 48 hr was significantly higher than the sum of E_2 production of each separated culture. 4) Δ_4 production of combined culture after 24 hr was significantly lower than the sum of Δ_4 production of each separated culture. 5) E_2 production of combined culture revealed higher values than Δ_4 – added granulosa cell culture after 24 hr. These data suggest that cellular interaction between two cell on E_2 biosynthesis exists not only as aromatase substrate (Δ_4), supply from theca to granulosa cells but also as some intercellular stimulating factor.

01.28.06
Enzyme-histochemical studies on localization of 17β-estradiol in follicular oocytes and granulosa cells: Satoh, H, Makinoda, S, Takaoka, H, Moriya, S, Ichinoe, K. Dept. Obstet. and Gyn., Hokkaido Univ. School Med., Sapporo, Japan
Previous studies showed the possible existence of granulosa cell growth factor and luteinizing inhibitory factor in the oocyte. In this study, localization of 17β-estradiol, which is speculated to be one of the granulosa cell growth factors, was investigated using the labelled antigen method in rat ovaries. Ovaries were fixed with 8% paraformaldehyde or 10% formalin, embedded in polyethyleneglycol and thinly sliced. Preparations were incubated in rabbit-anti 17β-estradiol-6-BSA, and then treated with peroxidase-labelled goat anti-rabbit IgG, and stained with diamine benzidine (DAB). Stain intensity was estimated by microscope photometer. The following results were obtained: (1) A significant quantity of 17β-estradiol was detected in follicular oocytes and corpus luteum but was minimal in granulosa cells. (2) Oocytes of preantral and small antral follicles, in which granulosa cells actively proliferate, revealed a strong intensity of 92.3%. (3) On the other hand oocytes in primordial follicles showed weak intensity. (4) In large antral follicles, the strong intensity rate of the oocytes reduced to 41.7%. On the basis of the results of this study, we suggest that 17β-estradiol is present in rat follicular oocytes and that it plays an important role in follicular development.

14

01.32.01

Comparison of the zona-free hamster egg sperm penetration test and human *in vitro* fertilization: Awaji, H, Inoue, M, Kobayashi, Y, Honda, I, Fujii, A. Dept. Obstet. and Gyn., School Med., Tokai Univ., Isehara, Japan

We have developed a sensitive zona-free hamster egg sperm penetration test (ZSPT) by the use of Ca ionophore A23187, which is useful for the assessment of fertility potential of men with abnormal semen. In the present study, we compared the penetration rate in the ZSPT with the *in vitro* fertilization (IVF) of human eggs, to further assess the accuracy of this bioassay. ZSPTs were performed on sperm from 46 husbands prior to IVF of human eggs. Thirty-two men with normal ZSPT ($\geq 70\%$) showed high penetration rates (group mean $95.7 \pm 1.6\%$), and fertilized most of their wives' eggs in 58 inseminations, resulting in an overall fertilization rate of 88.6% (101/114 eggs). Of seven men with subnormal ZSPT (30–70%), three failed to fertilize human eggs, but 21 (80%) out of 26 eggs used were fertilized in this group. Seven men with abnormal ZSPT ($< 30\%$) whose mean penetration rate was 5.3 ± 4.3, ranging from 0% to 28.1%, showed a very poor fertilization performance, and only 1 (3.4%) of 29 eggs were fertilized in 12 inseminations. These results indicate that the ZSPT using Ca ionophore A23187 correlates highly with the fertilization of human egg *in vitro*.

01.32.02

Comparative study of hamster-test and human *in vitro* fertilization: Kubo, H, Abe, Y, Rin, K, Katayama, S. 1st Dept. Obstet. and Gyn., Toho Univ. School Med., Tokyo, Japan

It is important to evaluate the fertilizing capacity of gametes *in vitro* for the analysis of sterility. The present study was designed to evaluate the reliability of hamster-test (HT) comparing with the results of human *in vitro* fertilization (IVF). Both human eggs and semen were collected from sterile couples. Hamster oocytes were obtained by the induction of superovulation (PMS + HCG). Recovered human eggs were precultured 5–72 hrs before insemination. Semens were centrifuged twice (395 g, 5 min), sperm pellet was overlaid with Ham F10 + 10% inactivated human serum, then incubated for 30 min in an atmosphere of 5% CO_2, 5% O_2, 90% N_2 at 37°C. Insemination was performed with the final concentration of $0.5–1 \times 10^5$ sperms. In male sterility, although results of HT showed only $35.4 \pm 27.8\%$ of hamster ova penetration rate, 53.3% (8/15) of human eggs were fertilized in IVF. In idiopathic sterility, although HT showed $88.2 \pm 10.7\%$ of ova penetration, only 41.6% (5/12) of human eggs were fertilized. In the other female sterility, HT showed $83.5 \pm 24.5\%$ of penetration rate, and IVF showed 79.2% (19/24) of eggs were fertilized. In conclusions, HT is reliable in some of male factor sterility, but in idiopathic female sterility, no correlation is obvious between penetration rates of HT and the results of human IVF.

01.32.03

Results of zona-free hamster egg sperm penetration tests from 1082 infertile couples: Kobayashi, Y, Inoue, M, Honda, I, Uchimura, M, Fujii, A. Dept. Obstet. and Gyn., School Med., Tokai Univ., Isehara, Japan

We have established a sensitive zona-free hamster egg sperm penetration test (ZSPT) by the use of Ca ionophore A23187, and reported that this bioassay is useful for evaluating sperm fertilizing ability, particularly in patients with abnormal semen parameters, based on 817 ZSPTs from 549 infertile couples (Acta. obstet. gyn. jap. **36**, 2466, 1984). We extended these studies and analysed the ZSPTs performed to date, in order to determine if it is possible to evaluate quantitatively, male fertility potential, using this bioassay. From February 1980 through January 1985, 1167 ZSPTs were performed on 1082 infertile couples. Liquefied semen was processed in a standard two-step wash sequence, using BWW medium. After 1 hour pre-incubation, sperm suspensions (1 ml) were treated with 10 μm A23187 for 60 min. at 37°C. They were washed again, and then used for insemination. About 30 zona-free hamster eggs were scored per sample. In this communication, the results are presented in detail, and a relationship between the penetration rate and subsequent fertility is discussed.

01.32.04

The enhancement of sperm quality and the penetration rates in the hamster oocyte system by various pharmacological substances and the effects of IVF: Argiriou, C, Langenbucher, H, Riedel, H-H, Mettler, L. Dept. Obstet. and Gyn., Univ., Kiel

The zona pellucida hamster oocyte penetration test established in 1976 by *Yanagimachi* can not replace andrological examination of ejaculates. It must be taken into consideration that there is no sufficient correlation between the system of zona-free hamster oocytes and *in vitro* fertilization in the human system as already published by *Hall* in 1981. In the course of the *in vitro* fertilization program at our Department we saw some correlation between the results of the hamster oocyte penetration test and the andrological diagnosis. We also investigated the increase in quality (morphology, mortility) of infertile men's sperm by addition of L-ascorbic-acid, kallikrein and caffeine. Further we evaluated the influence of these substances on the penetration capability of spermatozoa in the zona-free hamster cell system. These data serve to improve the *in vitro* fertilization rate of men coming for further treatment after one unsuccessful trial of *in vitro* fertilization.

15

01.32.05

Effects of addition of serum albumin on penetration of human spermatozoa into zona-free hamster eggs:
Kyono, K, Tsuiki, A, Furuhashi, N, Suzuki, M. Dept. Obstet. and Gyn., Tohoku Univ., School Med., Sendai, Japan

Since *Yanagimachi* et al. (1976) suggested that human spermatozoa were capable of penetrating zona-free hamster eggs, this *in vitro* assay has been used to analyse the fertilizing ability of human spermatozoa. Serum albumin is an important constituent of the medium used for the assay. However, a great variation in the rate of sperm penetration was observed in the use of different albumin preparations at different concentrations. Therefore we examined the effects of three different kinds of albumin preparations on the rate of human sperm penetration into zona-free hamster eggs. The percentages of eggs being penetrated by spermatozoa from three fertile donors A, B, and C were assessed. When Fraction V, Globulin Free and Fatty acid Free albumin preparations were tested at a concentration of 3.5% (W/V) by the assay using sperm from donor A, penetration rates were 13.3%, 97.4%, and 8.7% respectively. Dilution of the albumin concentration to 0.3% considerably changed the penetration rates to 64.4%, 78.8%, and 12.1% in that order. In cases B and C, penetration rates showed the same tendency as in case A. It is concluded that use of the same preparation of good quality is mandatory for human sperm penetration tests using zona-free hamster eggs to evaluate the results with reproducibility and accuracy.

01.41.01

The effect of ritodrine infusion on prostacyclin, thromboxane and norepinephrine in mother and infant in
Cesarean section: Ekblad, U, Erkkola, R, Uotila, P, Scheinin, M. Dept. Obstet. and Gyn., Physiol. and Pharmacol., Univ., Turku, Finland

Ritodrine is widely used for inhibition of uterine contractions. However, its metabolic effects on the mother and infant are still insufficiently understood. In this study we measured the concentrations of prostacyclin (PGI_2), thromboxane (Thx), and norepinephrine (NE) in eight mothers, when ritodrine infusion was started before Cesarean section at term and finished when the umbilical cord was closed. Sampling was performed at the beginning of infusion and at the closure of the umbilical cord and the samples from the newborn were taken simultaneously with the last maternal samples. Eight mothers receiving infusion of physiological saline served as controls. Due to ritodrine infusion, the level of Thx decreased significantly in the mother while the PGI_2 level remained unchanged. NE level in the mother was also significantly increased. No differences were observed in the levels of prostanoids in cord plasma when the ritodrine treated group was compared to the control group. NE levels in newborns after ritodrine treatment were significantly increased.

01.41.02

The influence of beta-2-mimetic drugs on the blood flow velocity in the fetal descending aorta: Vetter, K, Baer,
S, Fallenstein, F, Huch, R, Huch, A. Dept. Obstet. and Gyn., Univ., Zurich, Switzerland

The accidental observation of an increased mean blood flow in the fetal descending aorta as a consequence of an increased mean blood flow velocity under tocolytic therapy with beta-2-mimetic drugs led to the hypothesis of a systematic effect of these drugs on the fetus. Eight pregnant women between 31 and 37 weeks of pregnancy were studied before and during or after tocolytic therapy respectively. Blood flow measurements were carried out by means of a Kranzbuehler 8130/8105 ultrasound duplex combination with a 3 MHz realtime scanner and a 2 MHz pulsed doppler. The Doppler signals were analysed in opposite directions simultaneously with a two-channel spectrum analyser. All fetuses had an elevated mean blood flow velocity under fenoterol given either orally or intravenously. The median was 40 cm/sec compared to 32.5 cm/sec before or after therapy. These results show that beta-2-mimetic drugs given to pregnant women to stop premature labor do have a distinct effect on the fetal circulation with the well-known rise in basal fetal heart rate and a significant elevation of the mean blood flow velocity.

01.41.03

Fetal cardiac responsiveness to clenbuterol and fenoterol: Resch, B A, Papp, J G. Dept. Obstet. and Pharmacol., Univ. Med. School, Szeged, Hungary

Intrinsic responsiveness to clenbuterol and fenoterol, two beta-adrenergic agonists with predominant action on $beta_2$-adrenoceptors and used in obstetric practice for their tocolytic activity, was studied in human isolated fetal hearts obtained at legal terminations of pregnancy, utilizing a complex method as described earlier (*Resch, B A, Papp, J G.* Am. J. Obstet. Gyn. **146**, 231, 1983). Both clenbuterol and fenoterol exerted an age- and concentration-dependent increase in sino-atrial rate and ventricular contractility in hearts from the first and second trimester of gestation. The attainable maximum chronotropic and inotropic response to clenbuterol was, however, significantly smaller than that to fenoterol. At high concentrations ($> 10^{-6}$ mol/l) the cardio-stimulant actions of clenbuterol, but not those of fenoterol, were considerably diminished. Cardiac dysrhythmias were not observed in the presence of clenbuterol, whereas in six out of 24 hearts arrhythmia was induced by fenoterol. The results seem to indicate that on the basis of intrinsic responsiveness less adverse cardio-stimulant effects might be expected in the human fetus following maternal exposure to clenbuterol than observed after administration of fenoterol.

01.41.04

Neonatal hypoglycemia after tocolytic therapy (ritodrine-chloride): Dordević, M, Stanulović, M, Nikoloć, L, Aleksić, S. Dept. Obstet. and Gyn., Novi Sad, Yugoslavia

Tocolytic drugs (ritodrine-chloride) cause myometrial relaxation and are clinically useful in the inhibition of premature labor. In addition to the effects on smooth muscle relaxation, the beta-sympathomimetic agents have significant metabolic effects on both the mother and the fetus. The effect of oral beta-sympathomimetic tocolytic therapy (ritodrine-chloride) on neonatal serum glucose concentrations in the first several hours after delivery was examined in 60 newborns, and was sustained over at least a 30-minute period in 25 newborns. The group with sustained hypoglycemia had a higher cord serum insulin concentrations, a lower serum glucose ratio and a more rapid initial rate of serum glucose decrease than those newborns with normal glycemia or transient hypoglycemia. Sustained hypoglycemia was observed in 25 out of 30 newborns delivered within two days of the termination of tocolytic therapy but it was not present in 30 newborns delivered five or more days after the end of the tocolytic therapy.

01.41.05

Treatment of polyhydramnios with indomethacin: Cabrol, D, Soubrane, O, Uzan, M, Poli, G, Sureau, C. Clin. Univ. Baudelocque, Paris, France

The poor results of the usual management of polyhydramnios (P. H.) led us to the therapeutic use of prostaglandin synthetase inhibitors in order to decrease the amniotic fluid volume and prevent premature labor in such cases. From January 1983 to February 1984 we used indomethacin for seven patients with P. H. (four diabetes and three without known maternal or fetal disease) after having obtained an informed consent. Indication for indomethacin treatment was specific: a definite P. H., both ultrasonographically and clinically and associated complications after elemination of fetal anomalies incompatible with extrauterine existence (ultrasonography, karyotyping) and this could be the main difficulty. Indomethacin was given in tablets and/or suppositories at a dose 3 mg per kg per day. Treatment began at 30.1 ± 3.7 weeks and ended at 35.1 ± 0.5 weeks. Care was taken to postpone delivery for at least one week after the end of treatment. Results were based on: daily clinical data (decrease of maternal symptoms and uterine contractions, measure of fundal height and umbilical circumference) and weekly ultrasonography in order to approximate amniotic fluid volume, measure fetal growth, hourly urine output and fetal renal volume. If under treatment an oligohydramnios or an interruption of fetal urinary flow was observed, indomethacin treatment was decreased or discontinued. We observed a definite effect on amniotic fluid volume in each of our treated cases: Clinically, fundal height and umbilical circumference decreased confirmed by ultrasonographic data, with normal fetal growth. Gestational age at delivery was 38.6 ± 1.7 weeks. There were no premature delivery and all the infants were found to be normal based on physical examination and laboratory data during the neonatal period and at six months after delivery. Although we were able to decrease amniotic fluid volume and avoid premature delivery, our cohort is too small to draw definite conclusions. Indomethacin seems to be effective and convenient in the treatment of P. H. and the risk benefit ratio may justify clinical use in specific circumstances.

01.42.01

Improved intrauterine contraception with copper IUDs: Kurz, K H. Int. Res. Inst. Reproduct., Düsseldorf

The uncontrolled increase in human population is the main problem of mankind. Intrauterine devices are the most popular form of contraception world-wide. About 100 million women, including those of the Peoples Republic of China are using this method. Improved technology, such as the more exact measurement of length and width of the individual uterine cavity and the use of medicated, not too rigid and not too flexible IUDs in various sizes, has reduced the occurrence of unwanted side effects, such as pain, bleeding, expulsion and infection, without decrease of effectiveness. The film shows current techniques in intrauterine contraception and associated problems, caused mainly by dimensional incompatibility between the IUD and the individual uterine cavity. New techniques are demonstrated, such as the measurement of the uterine cavity with the Cavimeter, the use of adapted IUDs or those of different standard sizes, the pain-free insertion of an IUD with paracervical block, the prevention of "initial" or "late" infection by the use of Betadine solution prior to insertion and the intracervical shortening of the control-threads. Check-ups of the positions of IUDs using ultrasound and the simple extraction of an IUD without visible threads are demonstrated. There is no need to accept the whole new technology demonstrated by this film. Parts of it may be used to improve IUD programs.

01.42.02

Microsurgery in the tubal infertility. What is to be done: Tran, D K. Hosp. Annexe République, Univ., Nice, France

In this film, all the personal techniques of microsurgical tubal reconstruction are described. These techniques were used in 400 operations between 1978 and 1983. After sterilization, when the discrepancy in the caliber of the segments to be anastomosed is great, we section the smaller segment into two valves which increase the surface of anastomosis. Microsurgery restores the mobility and the morphology of the Fallopian tubes. We describe our techniques of salpingolysis, tubuloplasty and a personal technique: the isthmo-ostial reimplantation.

02.02.01

Tumors of the ovary. A ten-year review: Volakis, M, Mantzavinos, T, Botsis, D, Zourlas, P A. 2nd Dept. Obstet. and Gyn., Athens Univ., Areteion Hosp., Athens, Greece

Two hundred and seven cases with ovarian tumors were analysed retrospectively in the second Department of Obstetrics and Gynecology of the University of Athens in a 10-year period from 1975 to 1984. One hundred and forty-two were benign and sixty-five malignant tumors. Benign tumors showed mainly pelvic pain in 67% and malignant in 37% plus ascites in 30%. The age of the patients of the first group was between 20–40 in 70%, and in the second group in 60% between 40–60. The PAP-smear in the second group was class I or II in 30% of the patients and class III in 57%. 12% of the patients showed class IV. Surgery was used in all the patients with benign tumors and in 38% of them total abdominal hysterectomy was performed. In patients with malignant tumors laparotomy was done in 70% and in 50% total abdominal hysterectomy was advised. Co-treatment was applied in 50% of the patients and chemotherapy in 27% of the patients. The staging of the disease was: Stage I: 2 cases, stage II: 31 cases, stage III: 24 cases and stage IV: 8 cases. The pathology report of the benign tumors was: endometrial cysts 43, dermoid cysts 29, serous cystadenoma 31, and simple serous cysts 20. The pathology of the malignant tumors was reported: mucinous cystadeno-Ca 30, serous cystadeno-Ca 26, and other types 9. The follow-up of the patients with malignant tumors showed five years survival rate 60% for stage I, 15% for stage II, 5% for stage III, and none for stage IV.

02.02.02

A 15 years review of the ovarian cancer: Mantzavinos, T, Botsis, D, Volakis, M, Zourlas, P A. 2nd Dept. Obstet. and Gyn., Athens Univ., Areteion Hosp., Athens, Greece

Ninety-three patients with cancer of the ovaries were studied retrospectively for a period of fifteen years from 1970 to 1984. All the patients were managed in the Second Department of Obstetrics and Gynecology of the University of Athens. The symptoms of the patients were: pelvic pain in 38%, ascites in 30%, metrorrhagia in 22% and weight loss in 11%. Fifty-five per cent of the patients were between 40 to 60 years old and 63% were menopause. The PAP-smear in 40% was class I or II, in 47% was class III, and in 13% was class IV–V. The stage of the disease was: 2 patients stage I, stage II 33, stage III 38 and 20 stage IV. No patients had stage 0. The treatment which was applied: Laparotomy in 60 patients from which 48 had total abdominal hysterectomy, forty-six patients had Co-treatment and 23 patients chemotherapy. The pathology report was: mucinous cystadeno-Ca in 35% of the cases, serous cystadeno-Ca in 33%, solid tumors in 16% and 15% other types of malignant tumors. The follow-up of the patients showed. A five-year survival rate in 60% for stage I, 15% for stage II, 5% for stage III, and none for stage IV.

02.02.03

Epidemiological study of ovarian cancer in Israel – survey of 17 years: Anteby, S O, Mor Yosef, S, Schenker J G. Dept. Obstet. and Gyn., Hadassah Univ. Hosp., Jerusalem, Israel

A total of 2658 cases of ovarian cancer in Israel during 17-year period is screened. The incidence was found to be between 17 to 19/100,000 women over age 15. Seventy-five per cent were between the ages of 45 and 74. The majority of patients were diagnosed in stage III and stage IV. Five years survival rate was improved from 15% during the period of 1960–1965 to 31% in 1972–1976. The continent of birth was found to be a major factor in the incidence of the disease. Women of European/American origin had three times higher incidence than women of Asian/African background. In the adolescent (under the age of 20) the incidence between the various ethnic groups did not differ. The difference in histological type and stage of malignancy between adult and young will be presented. Moreover, prognostic factors in different types of tumors will be discussed.

02.02.04

Malignant ovarian tumors in adolescence: Bastos, A C, Souen, J S, Salvatore, C A, Bagnoli, V R. Gyn. Clin. Med. School, Univ., São Paulo, Brazil

Twelve of 45 ovarian tumors diagnosed in adolescent girls were malignant (26.6%). The histologic diagnosis of such tumors were as follows: Germ cell tumors–Malignant teratoma five, Dysgerminoma two, Endodermal sinus tumor one, Mixed form (Malignant teratoma + Endodermal sinus tumor) one. Sex-cord stromal tumors – androblastoma two. Epithelial tumors – mucinous cystadenocarcinomal. The most frequent malignant ovarian tumors at adolescence are the germ cell tumors and among them the malignant teratoma. The malignant teratoma and the Endodermal sinus tumor are both highly malignant. Radical surgery has not avoided poor results. Non-radical surgery is possible in stage Ia of malignant ovarian tumors in teenagers.

02.02.05

Ovarian carcinoma in the reproductive years (age 18–40): Tserkezoglou, A, Fotiou, S, Fertakis, E, Aravantinos, D. 1st Dept. Obstet. and Gyn., Univ., Athens, Greece

During a 5-year period (April 1978 to April 1983), 190 patients were treated for primary ovarian carcinoma, at the University Maternity Hospital "Alexandra" in Athens. Of these cases, 22 patients (11.6%) were between 18–40 years of age and were studied as a group while 168 were older patients. Certain features favoring a better prognosis were noticed in the younger group. Stage I disease was quite common (59%)

and 60% of the epithelial tumors (86.4%) were well differentiated. In two cases, conservative surgical management was chosen, after careful evaluation. Menstrual disorders (36%) and more frequent routine examinations led the patients to the doctor and contributed to early detection of the disease. In two of the cases diagnosis was made during pregnancy and in a third, the disease was accidentaly found during Cesarean section performed for obstetrical reasons. The survival in this group of patients was better than that reported for all ages. These observations suggest that a conservative surgical approach can be considered for these patients, in stage Iai, grade I disease.

02.02.06

Ovarian tumors in postmenopausal women: A clinicopathological study of 205 cases: Sarin, A R, Singla, P, Gupta, S. Govt. Med. Coll. and Hosp., Patiala, India
We did a comparative study of 205 cases of ovarian tumors in 2645 postmenopausal women seen in our Gynecology Division over eight years (Feb. 77–Dec. 84) as such a large study in this age group has not been reported earlier from India. Clinical studies and histopathology of ovarian tumors and endometrium were done in all cases. Ovarian tumors were found in 7.7% cases. The clinical features were abdominal mass (58.8%), postmenopausal bleeding (41.2%), abdominal pain (1.9%), etc. Benign tumors (65.8%) were more common than malignant (34.2%), and were mostly cystic (77.7%). Malignant tumors were mostly solid (80%), bilateral in 18.5%, and commoner (7.8%) in women with postmenopausal bleeding than in non-bleeding cases (2.2%). In benign tumors endometrium was commonly atrophic (50.4%) while it was mostly (51.1%) hyperplastic in malignant ones. The subtypes of benign and malignant tumors were similar to earlier reports. Contrary to the usual belief, we find that in postmenopausal women benign tumors were more common. The similarity in total incidence and subtypes of ovarian tumors in this series with reports from other countries indicates that racial, socio-economic and geographical factors are not operative as opposed to cervical and endometrial carcinoma.

02.02.07

Echography in the early diagnosis of cancer of the ovary, preliminary results: Pinotti, J A, Marussi, E F, Zeferino, L C, Franzin, C M. Dept. Obstet. and Gyn., State Univ., Campinas, Brazil
Diagnostic procedures for early detection of ovarian tumors, are not yet effective enough. This fact explains the current situation of poor prognosis. The echography appears in this area like an alternative method. The results of 30,749 echographies and pelvic examinations in the same 14,525 women are presented. 553 small (larger than 3 cm) ovarian tumors were diagnosed through echography, 73% of which were not detected through pelvic examination. In 97 patients who underwent operation, the echographic diagnosis was confirmed. Three out of the six cases that presented ovarian cancer were detected only through echography. The results show that a good echographic examination can be better than a pelvic one in some circumstances. Echography can complement pelvic examination in the diagnosis of small ovarian tumors, increasing the possibility of early detection of ovarian cancer.

02.02.08

Computed tomography prior to surgery for ovarian carcinoma: Simon, A, *Fields, S, Schenker, J G, Anteby, S O. Dept. Obstet. and Gyn. and *Dept. Radiol., Hadassah Univ. Hosp., Jerusalem, Israel
The value of investigation of patients with ovarian carcinoma by pre-operative computed tomography scan was evaluated in all the patients operated on in the last two years. Twenty-two patients were included in this study and evaluated. In 11 patients the scan was performed prior to the primary operation and in the other 11 patients before a second look following chemotherapy. CT scan was found to be highly sensitive in detecting ascites, pelvic wall extension and spread or involvement of the uterus. Peritoneal and omental spread was detected in only half of the patients before primary surgery. Prior to second look operation CT scan was effective in excluding liver metastasis, ascites, para-aortic lymph node enlargement, pelvic wall extension and pelvic residual tumor. Generally, CT scan failed to detect peritoneal and omental spread. It is an important tool for pre-operative evaluation of the extension of the disease and planning of surgery, but still, the final staging requires explorative laparotomy.

02.02.09

Primary carcinoma of the fallopian tube: Mogensen, H, Pfeiffer, P, Honoré, E, Amtrup, F. Denmark
From 1978–1983 60 cases of primary carcinoma of the fallopian tube (PTC) were diagnosed in Denmark (Danish Cancer Register). The average observation time of these patients is 42 months. At the time of the operation, 24 of the patients were registered as stage I (tumor strictly limited to the tube). Of these patients 14 are either dead, or alive with metastases. Ten patients in stage I were given primary postoperative radiotherapy (PPR) without improvement of survival. Thirty-six patients were in stage II–IV. Although all of them received PPR, 27 had died within 42 months. Tumor extension through the serosa of the tube, at the time of operation, seems to be the most important prognostic factor. No connection between prognosis, tumor histology, age and parity was seen. The literature is dominated by case reports and a few surveys covering decades, using none or different stages. Comparisons of treatment and prognosis is therefore difficult. PPR has been recommended for 50 years, but you find no evidence that PPR improves survival. At the time of diagnosis PTC is often metastasized. The frequency and pathways of spread are partly unknown. During the last 5–10 years effect of chemotherapy is described and evaluated by second-look

operation. As treatment we propose a standardized tumor including lymphadenectomy eventually, followed by chemotherapy. In this way there may be a hope of improving the survival rate and of increasing the knowledge of the spread of this tumor.

02.02.10

In vivo effect of oil in promotion of tumorigenesis of ovarian carcinoma: Rotmensch, J, Holt, J, Herbst, A. Div. Gyn. Oncol., Dept. Obstet. and Gyn., Univ., Chicago, IL, USA

Evidence from epidemiologic studies have implicated dietary fats and oils as a factor in the promotion of ovarian carcinoma. A variety of mechanisms, direct and indirect, have been proposed. The purpose of this study is to investigate the direct effect of oil on tumorigenesis in ovarian carcinoma using the nude mouse model, OVCAR III. The study was designed to investigate this hypothesis in the nude mouse model. Twenty-four 28-to-32-day old castrated male nu/nu mice were injected intraperitoneally with 4.69×10^7 cells of human ovarian adenocarcinoma (OVCAR III). Twelve mice (Group A) were injected using normal saline as a vehicle and twelve mice (Group B) were injected using sesame oil. All mice died with ascites producing tumor within 60 days in both groups. The median survival in Group A was 42 days (range 35–55 days); the median survival in Group B was 29 days (range 20–35 days) (p < .05). The monoclonal antibody CA 125, a biological marker for epithelial ovarian carcinoma, was measured serially until the death of the animals. The median CA 125 production in Group A was 23,000 U/ml (range 3,900–52,000 U/ml) and 138,000 U/ml (range 3,900–152,000 U/ml) in Group B. The data indicates that sesame oil potentiated the growth of OVCAR III cell in nude mice. This study suggested that oils may have a promoting effect on tumorigenesis of ovarian carcinoma.

02.02.11

Ferritinemia in ovarian cancer and its clinical significance: Yuan, C C, Ng, H T, Yeh, S H. Dept. Obstet. and Gyn., Vet. Gen. Hosp., Taiwan

Ferritin was found elevated in the serum and tissue of ovarian cancer (*Borisenko, S. A.* Vop. Onkol. **29**, 45, 1983). Serum ferritin was studied by using the liver-ferritin radioimmunoassay, and divided into three groups: (1) 51 ovarian cancers, (2) 110 healthy controls, (3) 51 benign gynecologic tumors. The titer of the first group (436.7 + 619.8 ng/ml, range: 19.9 to 2896 ng/ml) was significantly higher than others, with a stage-dependent characteristic. This study demonstrated that 12 of 17 patients with ferritin greater than 300 ng/ml had liver metastases, while the false negative rate was 20% (3/15). Whereas, for the 42 patients with epithelial cancers, the false positive and false negative rate for liver metastases were 21.4% and 15.4% respectively. Prospectively in the study of several patients, serum ferritin greater than 300 was found and correlated well with the findings of CAT scan and sonography of liver, might proved to be with better sensitivity. It did differentiate a subdiaphragmatic mass from true liver metastases in a young patient with germ cell tumor of ovary. Our conclusion is that ferritin might be a good marker for detecting liver metastases and should be measured regularly in all ovarian cancers.

02.02.12

Serum copper levels in ovarian carcinoma: Margalioth, E J, Udassin, R, Maor, J, Schenker, J G. Dept. Obstet. and Gyn., Hadassah Univ. Hosp., Jerusalem, Israel

Serum copper levels (SCL) were determined prior to any diagnostic procedure or treatment in forty women admitted for the investigation of a pelvic mass. Twenty-two were found to have ovarian carcinoma, four had pelvic metastases of breast or colon carcinomas and fourteen had benign ovarian disease. The mean copper level of the patients with ovarian carcinoma was 195 µg/dl. Of the 22 patients only one had SCL of less than 150 µg/dl. The patients with pelvic metastases of colon or breast carcinomas had a mean SCL of 198 µg/dl, while the patients with the benign lesions had a mean of 130 µg/dl which was significantly lower than the patients with ovarian malignancy. An SCL of 150 µg/dl clearly separated patients with a pelvic mass on the basis of ovarian carcinoma and those with benign lesions. It is suggested that SCL be included as a member of the screening panel of biological tumor markers in general and in ovarian carcinoma in particular.

02.02.13

The histologic types of primary ovarian cancer in Iran: Izadian, N, Behjatnia, Y, Aflatoony, M, Shirin-Sokhan, M. Dept. Obstet. and Gyn., Mirzakuchak-Khan Hosp., Teheran, Iran

Previous studies have been shown that malignant neoplasms produced by human and animal carcinogens are frequently limited to a single organ with a specific histologic type. Histologic patterns may be important in the evaluation of possible causal relationship (*H. Rothschild.* Cancer **49**, 1874, 1982). Prenatal exposure to synthetic estrogens has been linked to clear cell carcinoma of the vagina and cervix in patients 7 to 29 years of age (*A. Herbst.* New Engl. J. Med., **284**, 878, 1971). Our present study examines the age relation of the individual of histologic types with the hope of making a introductory etiologic separation of types. The major histologic types of primary ovarian cancer was examined. All types of ovarian cancer tumors except endometroid and clear cell tumors increased in frequency until fifth of life, after which the frequency decreased. The frequency of epithelial cancer tumors was much more higher than nonepithelial tumors. The peak frequency for epithelial cell tumors was in fifth decades, while the peak frequency for nonepithelial was among young women.

02.02.14

Comparison and correlation of lactic dehydrogenase levels in serum and ovarian tissue – malignant and benign: Awais, G M, Shamberger, R J. Cleveland Clin. Found., Cleveland, OH, USA

The purpose of this study is to explore further the significance of serum lactic dehydrogenase in the diagnosis of carcinoma of the ovary. I have reported that serum lactic dehydrogenase is elevated in the presence of carcinoma of the ovary. Particularly in ovarian dysgerminoma, lactic dehydrogenase was highly elevated and dropped sharply to normal levels after treatment. (*Awais, G. M.*, Carcinoma of the ovary and serum lactic dehydrogenase levels. Surgery **146**, 893–895, 1978. Dysgerminoma and serum lactic dehydrogenase levels. *Awais, G. M.* Obstet. Gyn. **61**, 99–101, 1983.) In the present study, levels of lactic dehydrogenase in serum and ovarian tissue were determined and compared. Results indicate that in the presence of ovarian carcinoma, the levels of lactic dehydrogenase are elevated, both in the serum and in ovarian tissue. Results also show that in metastatic carcinoma in which the ovary is secondarily involved and the primary is elsewhere, lactic dehydrogenase is not elevated. The conclusion is that lactic dehydrogenase levels are important in the diagnosis of primary carcinoma of the ovary.

02.03.01

Means and measures of German technical cooperation in family planning: The MCH and FP project Munshiganj, Bangladesh: Boss, R M, Merk, G, Korte, R. Dtsch. Ges. Techn. Zusammenarbeit GTZ, Eschborn

Rapid population growth is one of the main constraints hampering the development of Third World countries. It is simultaneously the major challenge for Technical Cooperation projects concerned with Family Planning. In german technical cooperation we adopt an approach which integrates Family Planning into overall developmental efforts and especially into Primary Health Care System. Since 1979 GTZ has been carrying out the Integrated MCH-FP Project Dacca Munshiganj in Bangladesh in cooperation with the Ministry of Health and Population Control. Its main target is to implement the National Population Programme of Bangladesh in a district near Dacca to serve as a model for other areas, by using the existing infrastructure of the National Health Organisation. Financial inputs and commodity aid are kept as low as possible to avoid the creation of another structure parallel to the existing one which would stop working after conclusion of the foreign contribution. By increasing the administrative and management capacity of the health administration, the project tries to enhance the efficiency of the FP Programme. The project was able to identify constraints and bottlenecks and to give valuable recommendations to overcome them. Two main areas of activity should be mentioned – Service delivery, which covers the unmet demand for FP-measures, – Community oriented activities, which create demand for FP. The effects of the project activities were a significant increase of the Contraceptive Prevalence Rate in the intervention areas.

02.03.02

Factors related to unplanned pregnancies: Farnot, U. Fac. Med. Sci., Havana, Cuba

We defined "unplanned pregnancy" as one occurring in mothers who although unwilling or being afraid to become pregnant, do not use some form of contraception. A study about the factors related to unplanned pregnancies was carried out over a period of six months in ten maternity hospitals, where questionnaires were filled in by 13,173 mothers with single births some hours after delivery, recording demographic biological and social data, the characteristics of their pregnancy, labor and the circumstances under which the present pregnancy occurred in relation to contraceptive use. The possible answers were: 1) contraception used when pregnancy occurred (failure of contraceptive); 2) contraception stopped in order to become pregnant; 3) contraception stopped for other reasons; 4) no contraception used in order to become pregnant; 5) no contraception used, but pregnancy feared or unwanted. 13,038 mothers responded to the questionnaire: 4345 had used contraceptives, 7485 had never used them because they wanted children, 1208 had never used them although they did not want children. This last group was considered as one of "Unplanned Pregnancies". A statistical analysis was made of the common factors present in these mothers, utilizing the chi-square test. Unplanned pregnancies were significantly higher in: 1) mothers 17 years or less; 2) mothers 35 years or more; 3) mothers who had previously had at least two children and specially in mothers who had four or more children; 4) mothers with low to median educational levels; 5) unmarried mothers (widows, divorcees, etc.) specially single ones. Others factors such as low income per capital, bad living conditions or overcrowded homes were significantly associated with the lack of family planning.

02.03.03

Physician attitudes and practices regarding family planning in Nigeria: Otolorin, E O. Univ. Coll. Hosp., Ibadan, Nigeria; **Covington, D L.** Family Hlth. Int., North Carolina, USA

Contraceptive use is low in Nigeria. With no organized Family Planning program, physicians are major providers of services. Consequently, their attitudes and practices have a major impact on family planning use. In October–December 1984, a sample of 750 physicians was interviewed. While they expressed favorable attitudes, only half of those in marital union used contraceptives themselves, and of these about one-third used rhythm or withdrawal. Most of the respondents recommended contraceptives (85%), but only half provided them. OB/GYNs and general practitioners (GPs) were most likely to provide (84%) and other physicians least likely (28%). The main methods provided were orals, IUDs and tubal ligations. Although illegal, 41% of OB/GYNs and 36% of GPs said they performed abortions. Barrier methods were the only methods which physicians approved for distribution by non-physicians. Over 50% disapproved of non-physicians distributing IUDs, 68% orals, 76% injectables and 96% disapproved of non-physicians performing vasectomies or tubal ligations.

02.03.04
Implementation in a developed country: Andolšek, L. Obstet. Gyn. Dept., Univ. of Ljubljana, Yugoslavia

Yugoslavia is multinational community with many regional, ethnic and cultural diversities in its population of 22 424 711 inhabitants (1981 census), living on area of 255 804 square kilometres. Different historical development in individual regions as well as the influence of different civilizations and culture on Yugoslav nations and nationalities have created considerable regional differences in terms of local socioeconomic development and demographic trends. In Yugoslavia the family planning movement developed from the early movement for abortion liberalization. Although contraception was introduced in the entire country as a part of public health on the primary health care level as early as the second half of the 1950s, it won different affirmation in various regions. The awareness gradually spread that family planning implied much more than just giving advice on contraception or performing an abortion. Family planning began to be seen as a part of an interrelated social system. The concept of family planning as a human right is developing also alongside. Long lasting endeavours were given an official recognition by the Resolution on Family Planning adopted in 1969 and in the 1974 Yugoslav Constitution. This defines free decision-making on childbirth (which includes also the right of abortion) as a human right. The implementation of this right is within the competence of republics and provinces, the educational system and the social welfare system. Despite impressive achievements in family planning in some regions the medical termination of pregnancy is still one of the most used method of fertility regulation.

02.03.05
Some specific gynecological complaints of women working in different branches of industry: Lambreva, T. 1st Workers Hosp., Sofia, Bulgaria

The results of ten years observations are given. Working women have happened to complain of frequent pains in the genital sphere, accompannied by local and general vegetative disorders. The complaints were mostly due to phlogistic, static or neoplastic alterations in genitals, the pelvic muscular floor and injuries of the locomotor system. The lowest per cent of complaints was found in women without morphological and functional alterations. In terms of contemporary neuro-vegetology this complex morbidity should be regarded as a diencephalic syndrome. On the other hand the complaints are mostly characteristic for women working under higher occupational strain, with a longer length of service and many deliveries, whereas women engaged with administrative work have seldom raised similar complaints. That complex malady should be considered as a result of higher occupational strain. A number of prophylactic medicinal and social recommendations appear expedient.

02.03.06
Long-acting intrauterine contraceptive devices: El Mahgoub, S. Fac. Med., Ain Shams Univ., Cairo, Egypt

Two main types of long-acting contraceptive device were tried in more than 1700 subjects for three years. 1. The levonorgestrel intrauterine and intracervical T, Nova-T, and Mini-T devices, releasing 10 or 20 mcg/day. These devices are expected to have an effective life time over seven years. 2. The copper-T 380 Ag (TCU 380 Ag) devices which are expected to have an active life span of more than ten years. Both devices proved to be highly effective with pregnancy rates of only 0.3 per 100 per year. The levonorgestrel devices were associated with marked reduction in the menstrual blood and the number of days of bleeding. The Mini-T intracervical device can be used in subjects with septate or bicornuate uterus. These devices produce their effect through local action on the endometrium and cervical mucus. The effects of these devices on the blood pressure, plasma lipids, serum immunoglobulins phospholipids and liver function tests were studied. After three years no changes suggestive of malignancy were encountered. These two devices are highly recommended to be used in fertility control.

02.03.07
Preliminary report of a new IUD with tubal occlusion properties: Cimber, H S, Dreher, E. Dept. Obstet. and Gyn., Univ., Bern, Switzerland

Over a period of up to 2 years 75 cases have been evaluated since 1982. The new IUD is tolerated by nulli- and multiparas as are the previously known types. There are not enough data yet to reach a satisfactory statistical evaluation with regard to the Pearl index. Four hundred further cases will be clinically tested in the near future. The main advantages over the known IUDs are: 1) occlusion of the tubes thus eliminating the possibilities of ectopic pregnancy, one of the most serious complication of the known IUDs. 2) The soft, round, 4.5 mm plastic occlusion bodies at the end of the T-bar are less traumatic to the uterine lining than the relatively sharp ends of the known ones. Occasionally IUDs have been known to cause infertility secondary to infection which is possibly due to partial or total perforation. 3) In utero the occlusion bodies can be easily visualized by ultrasound, an additional safety factor beside the distance of the IUD from the fundus (< 2 cm). Ultrasound localisation of the IUD became the method of choice. It could be proven by comparison with previous used methods like hysterogram (40), Douglas puncture for sperm presence (10), and tubal insufflation (22) that tubal occlusion occurs if the new IUD has a correct uterine position. So far two pregnancies occurred shortly after removal of the IUD approximately one and one and a half years. There were no unwanted pregnancies. The uterine introduction of the IUD can be easily achieved with a new dilating laminaria called Lamicel.

02.03.08

The intrauterine corrosion process of copper and copper-silver wires: Koch, U J, Stichel, W*, Stange, J*. *Bundesanstalt für Materialprüfung (BAM), Berlin (West)

The intrauterine corrosion process, which is combined with the desired copper release into the uterine secretions, is dependent on the copper mass and surface, the quantity and quality of the secretory activity of the endometrium and the intensity of the endometrial bleeding. The copper corrosion was investigated by metallographic cross-section-measurements, mass-loss-estimations and scanning electron microscopy using the IUDs ML Cu 250 (standard), ML Cu 250 Ag (Internload) and Nova-T (Ag). Up to eight years of IUDs usage examinations of the corrosion process were performed. In order to characterize the corrosion process, a correlation between the length of usage and the loss of copper mass was attempted by using a regression analysis. Due to the asymmetrical corrosion process of the copper wire of the ML Cu 250, the wire retains its stability for more than five years of usage; the corrosion process is extremely reduced near the vertical stem of this IUD. The process of corrosion is time-dependent in a linear function. Therefore, the life span of IUDs with thicker wires is longer than with thinner wires. The "copper reservoir" of the ML Cu 250 is sufficient for long-term usage; normally more than 50% of the copper is uncorroded after a period of five years; corrosive fragmentation is extremely rare and without clinical relevance. The corrosion layer of the copper wires with the silver core is identical with that of the pure copper wires in the first years of usage. But an increased copper corrosion takes place during exposure of the silver core in long-term usage due to the development of an electrical charge.

02.03.09

A further communication of a New Zealand study of fertility after the use of an intrauterine device: Wilson, J. St Helens Hosp., Auckland, New Zealand

This is a further report of a prospective all New Zealand study of patients having an intrauterine device (IUD) removed to conceive, commenced March 24, 1982. Since November 1982, all patients who have had an IUD out for any complication have been entered into a prospective trial. After one year, whether they have tried to conceive was determined. The cut off date was November 7, 1983 with continuing observation until analysis by modified life-table on November 7, 1984, so that a true one year rate of conception could be determined. 95% confidence limits were calculated for net event rates.

Patients	At 1 year:		At 2 years:	
	Total	conceived%	Total	conceived%
All	768	87.0 ± 0.9	618	92.7 ± 0.6
Nulliparous	219	82.2 ± 2.1	203	89.3 ± 1.4
Parous	476	89.0 ± 0.9	415	94.5 ± 0.5

The difference between the nulliparous and parous conception rates at 1 and 2 years was significant $p < 0.0001$.

At two years fertility outcome

Patients	Ectopic	Miscarriage	Term Birth	Premature	Still Pregnant
All	0.5 ± 0.5	12.2 ± 2.6	82.2 ± 3.5	1.1 ± 0.9	4.0 ± 1.5

At one year, in the complicated fertility study 94 (75.1%) had conceived out of a total of 125 patients. The use of an IUD does not appear to affect fertility adversely.

02.03.10

Intracervical, contraceptive device: Katz, Z, Lancet, M, Hiber, S. Dept. Obstet. and Gyn., Kaplan Hosp., Rehovot, Israel (Affil. to the Hadassah-Hebrew Univ. School Med.)

Contraceptive methods in use today, whether hormonal, spermicidal, barrier or intrauterine, may cause local or systemic side-effects or complications, and most are not fully effective. Their use may depend on the age, state of health and habits of the couple, and due consideration must be given to any pathology of the genital organs or systemic diseases of the woman. Most of these problems can be circumvented by the use of an intracervical contraceptive device, which can be used when such problems arise. The authors present a preliminary report on a reversible contraceptive method using a small device which is easily inserted into the cervical canal by an introducer, and contains a one-way valve. The valve prevents the penetration of spermatozoa into the canal, but allows free flow of menstrual blood or uterine debris. The device is left *in situ,* and can be removed by the physician upon the patient's request. It is now being used by twelve married women who had at least two normal deliveries in the past, the last one not less than three years before the insertion. The age range is 34 to 41 (mean: 38 years), and the device has been in place for between 12 and 17 cycles, for a total of 156 women-months. Pap smears before and one year after the introduction of the valve were normal. No pregnancies have occurred. This is a novel approach to contraception and looks very promising. Large-scale studies are necessary to prove its efficacy and the lack of complications due to its use.

02.03.11
Experience of contraception, reasons for abortion and need for follow-up among women applying for legal abortion in Sweden: Claesson, U, Kvint, S, Svanberg, B. Dept. Gyn. and Obstet., Centr. Hosp., Skövde, Sweden
Approximately 25% of the pregnancies in Sweden are, on demand by the women, interrupted by legal abortion. Among those young women who have had one abortion performed, 40% will have a second abortion within five years. 202 women applying for abortion were interviewed and offered a follow-up three months later. Teenagers and women over 39 years of age, represented in this material 14% each. One third were nulliparous. The most frequent motives were: family planning 39%, age 38%, work or education 22% and relation problems 20%. One out of four hesitated in their decision. 79% of the women had earlier experiences of contraceptive pills and/or IUD but had ceased because of side-effects. At the present conception 45% used no contraception, 36% used barrier methods, 9% chemical methods or interrupted intercourse, 7% pills and 3% IUD. At the time of abortion 46% of the women planned to use pills, 35% IUD and 11% wanted sterilization. At the follow-up three months later nearly half needed further contraceptive advice. The continuation rates for the pill and IUD were only 80%. Minor psychological problems were experienced by 39%. In women who were ambivalent in their decision to have abortion performed 57% had psychological problems. – Conclusion: Women applying for abortion have great and bad experiences of different contraceptive methods. Follow-up after abortion is of value in improving the contraceptive advice and in handling the psychological problems in connection with the abortion.

02.03.12
The value of volumetric changes in cervico-vaginal fluid to detect the fertile phase of the menstrual cycle: Flynn, A M Docker, M, McCarthy, A M, Royston, J P. Dept. Obstet. and Gyn., Birmingham Matern. Hosp., UK
A precise knowledge about the fertile phase of the cycle by simple techniques suitable for home use would enable couples using natural methods of family planning (NFP) to reduce the days of abstinence required to avoid a pregnancy; it would also benefit subfertile couples to optimize their chances of achieving a pregnancy by indicating the highly fertile days in the cycle. Recent studies have shown that volumetric changes in cervico-vaginal fluid (CVF) which can be measured by women using a self-applicable vaginal aspirator showed a good correlation with serum E_2, LH and progesterone (*Usala* et al. Fertil. and Steril. **39**, 304–305, 1983). We studied 20 women, using the sympto-thermic method of NFP, who measured and recorded their CVF volumes daily over 60 cycles. They also recorded the usual clinical indicators (BBT, mucus, cervix, mittelschmerz) on the same graph. Six of these women over 18 cycles had daily ultrasonic examination of the ovaries and follicular tracking from day 6 of the cycle until ultrasonic evidence of ovulation occurred. In addition, these women also used, at home, the ovustick urine LH kit to detect the LH surge indicating high fertility. The data obtained were analysed and appropriate algorithms used to determine the reliability of the CVF to detect the onset of the potential pre-ovulatory fertile phase and the day of maximal fertility relative to the ultrasonic urinary and sympto-thermal indicators of fertility. The results and their implication for fertility will be presented and discussed.

02.03.13
Factors affecting choice of traditional birth attendant (daya): Galal, S. Commun. Med. Dept., Fac., Med., El-Azhar Univ., Cairo, Egypt
Traditional medicine and modern medicine are two systems providing primary health care in Egypt. At least 50% of deliveries are carried out through traditional birth attendants (dayas), despite the availability and accessibility of health centers all over the country (*Galal*, 1982). In urban areas patients have the option between seven formal health care delivery systems, but they still decide to choose dayas particularly for delivery. Intensive interviews were carried through with 14 dayas in poor socio-economic areas in Cairo to gather information about age, socio-economic conditions, services and fees provided, professional activities, their opinion about their work and qualitites necessary for it. Participant observation during three deliveries was possible. One hundred and three mothers of childbearing age (15–45 years) with children till five years in private mostaw-safat and other organizations hospitals were interviewed by questionnaire about their socio-economic conditions, former deliveries, reasons for dayas choice and for choice of other formal services, their seeking help behaviour etc.

02.04.01
A new approach to tubal sterilization (when, where and how?): Van Steeter, D P. St. Mark's Hosp., Univ. of Utah, Salt Lake City, UT, USA
This communication recommends a new approach to the method of pelviscopic tubal sterilization. The world literature and statistics are summarized including the author's 1400 procedures. Particular attention is paid to the method and site of occlusion which relates to the success rate and to subsequent ectopic pregnancies. All electrical and mechanical methods for tubal sterilization are discussed with slides and

ultimate results. The only known failure in the author's series was a rare (previously unpublished) tubal-peritoneal-tubal fistula (1) which resulted in an intrauterine pregnancy (X-rays and slides). Endosalpingo-blastosis (2) is discussed as a cause for fistulas and ectopic pregnancies. Based on the information presented a recommendation is made for a single thorough bipolar coagulation on the middle one-third of the tube. (1) *Van Steeter, D P:* Tubal peritoneal fistula – an unusual sterilization failure, Am. Ass. Gyn. Laparosco-pists, Presentation Hong Kong, Aug. 1984. (2) *McCaulsand, A M:* Endosalpingoblastosis following lapar-oscopic tubal coagulation as an etiologic factor of ectopic pregnancy. Am. J. Obstet. Gyn. **143**, 12, 1982.

02.04.02
Objective evaluation of menstrual blood loss (MBL) after four methods of tubal sterilization: El Sahwi, S, El Einein, M A, Gaweesh, S, Toppozada, M, Anwar, M, Kamel, M. Alexandria, Egypt
One hundred females requesting tubal ligation were randomly divided into four groups (25 subjects each). Group I: had laparoscopic Falope ring application, Group II: had laparoscopic tubal fulguration (biopo-lar), Group III: had laparoscopic Hulka clip application, Group IV: had Pomeroy tubal ligation through minilaparotomy. All subjects fulfilled the criteria of being at least six months post-partum, or post abortive, with regular menstruation, moderate monthly bleeding, not using hormonal contraception for at least six months and with no gross pelvic pathology. The MBL was objectively measured by the alkaline hematin method with rapid mechanical extraction of the sanitary pads using the stomacher lab-blender 3500 to ensure rapid extraction of the alkaline hematin. The MBL in each subject was estimated one cycle prior to the operation (control) and repeated at 3, 6 and 12 months after sterilization. The females subjective assessment of MBL during each visit was also recorded. The results indicated that the MBL at 3, 6 and 12 months post-ligation did not change significantly compared to the pre-ligation MBL in the four groups. Though the mean post-sterilization increase in MBL was highest after electrocoagulation, lowest after Pomeroy ligation and Falope ring and lowest after clip application the differences among the four groups were not statistically significant. The patient's subjective evaluation of her menstrual blood loss did not correlate with the actual volumes of blood as measured objectively by the alkaline hematin method.

02.04.03
A prospective comparison of three methods for female sterilization: Ladehoff, P, Hansen M K, Larsen, S, Sørensen, T. Dept. Gyn. and Obstet., Odense Univ. Hosp., Denmark
Previous studies have demonstrated that female sterilization may cause menstrual disturbances, abdominal pain and climacteric symptoms. Therefore, we have compared three procedures for sterilization: Cornual resection (CR) via laparotomy, laparoscopic Hulka-Clips (HC) and laparoscopic Falope-Ring (FR). All women referred for sterilization were selected randomly for laparoscopic or laparotomy sterilization, which was carried out as a cornual resection of the uterus. The laparoscopic group was randomized in a FC-group and a HC-group. The patients were interviewed prior to and twelve months after the operation. – Results: Within and between the three groups of patients no significant difference was demonstrated in the heaviness and length of bleedings, and length of cycles before and twelve months after operation. In the CR-group (n = 157) none, in the HC-group (n = 99) four, and in the FR-group (n = 101) one woman became pregnant. No significant difference in the frequency of lower abdominal pain, dyspareunia, nervousness, depression, palpitation, hot flushes and sweats at nights was found between the groups. But female sterilization as a whole was found to decrease the number of patients with dispareunia (p < 0.001) and nervousness (p < 0.005), and increased the number of women with a "high" libido (p < 0.0005). In the CR-group five · women, in the HC-group none, and in the FR-group two women regretted the sterilization. In conclusion, CR was the most effective method for female sterilization, but the admission time was about twice as long as for the laparoscopic groups. The pregnancy rate in the HC-group (4%) is unacceptable.

02.04.04
Ectopic pregnancy subsequent to female sterilization: Park, C M, Bai, B C, Kwak, H M, Whang, Y W. Korean Association for Voluntary Sterilization, Seoul
This study was undertaken for the clinico-statistical analysis of 822 women with ectopic pregnancies after tubal sterilization, who had been treated by 303 hospitals under the support of the Korean government during the last three years. The following features were the result of the study: 1) The median age of these 822 patients was 32.3 years. The average gravidity and number of living children were 4.1 and 2.7 respectively. 2) 25.2% of the total patients presented themselves within one year of their operation and 50.6% presented after two years of their operation, with the mean interval being 2 years 5 months. 3) 88.9% of the total patients were correctly diagnosed pre-operatively, while 9.1% were diagnosed after explolapar-otomy. Culdocentesis was performed in 80.7% of the total paients. 4) The most frequent implantation site of ectopic pregnancy was the Fallopian tube (90.0%) and 69.9% were located in the distal and fimbrial segment. 5) In the types of sterilization preceding ectopic pregnancy, the greatest number, 88.8%, under-went laparoscopy coagulation method, 9.4% laparoscopy banding method, 1.4% mini-lap, and 0.4% post-partum tubal ligation. 6) The surgeons reported the cause of ectopic pregnancy as 44.2% fistula formation, 22.9% tubal recanalization, 21.3% inadequate occlusion, and 11.9% unknown. 7) 38.2% of the patients underwent sterilization associated with pregnancy termination at the same time and the majority of them presented within two years of their operation, with the mean interval being 1 year 7 months.

02.04.05

Sterilization failure after laparoscopic endothermic coagulation: Pellicer, A, Martinez, L, Aviñó, J, Millet, A, Perez, M, Tortajada, M, Boni, F. Dept. Obstet. and Gyn., Hosp. Clin., Valencia, Spain

During the period January, 83 to May, 84, 282 women were sterilized in our clinic by laparoscopy. In 164 cases (58%) the endothermic technique was used; in 94 (33.3%) bipolar electrocoagulation; in 17 (6%) monopolar electrocoagulation and 5 (1.77%) by Yoon rings. Between three and six months after laparoscopy, a HSG was performed in 200 patients as control. After at least ten months of follow-up, ten pregnancies occurred, nine with the endothermic technique and one with monopolar cautery; the general pregnancy rate is 3.5% and 5.5% of all endothermic coagulations became pregnant. No pregnancy occurred with the bipolar technique. Five HSG were performed in the group of pregnancies and all tubes were occluded. From the other 272 cases, four HSG showed total patency of fistulae (three monopolar and one Yoon ring).

02.04.06

The post-sterilization syndrome in 567 patients: Desrosiers, J. Univ. Montréal, Canada

In 1982, at the San Francisco FIGO meeting, we presented a partial report on a prospective study made on more than 550 patients who underwent sterilization between 1978 and 1981 included: we could then demonstrate that 60 patients or 11% presented a pathology ranging from a small fibroid, PID, or ovarian tumors to endometritis etc. We then proposed to make a follow-up of these 60 patients to see their medical fate a few years after. The whole study was in relation to assess the so called "Post-Sterilization Syndrome" so we could prove that the sterilization per se does not create a new pathology as certain could think of. We compared the group of pathologic patients to the remaining group of patients we could trace back as of today to find out that no additional pathology developed in the remaining group in direct relation to their sterilization, while the fate of those who had fibroids or PID developed their disease so they had to suffer more procedures but still in a small percentage of the cases.

02.04.07

Our experience with the Falope ring banding under local anesthesia for female sterilisation in Bihar (India): Saha, T C. Patliputra Med. Coll., Dhanbad, Bihar, India

The complications inherent with the cautery laparoscopic sterilisation procedure is well known. With a view to avoiding thermal injuries, non-electrical methods were developed such as Falope ring & Hulka clips. Falope ring is by far the most commonly used procedure. The introduction of this technic has made tremendous impact on the sterilisation programme in India. Between March '82 to February '85 more than three hundred thousand female sterilisation by this method have been performed in the state of Bihar in north east India. This includes the author's own series of eleven thousand cases. All these operations were done in camps organised at Primary health centres (PHC), sub-divisional, district and medical college hospitals. The percentage achievement of sterilisation target went very high in the first year (84.24%) after the introduction of this technic. This figure on comparison with the achievements of the past few years points to the patient acceptance of this new method which inflicts minimum invalidity on the part of the acceptors. Various aspects of the procedure have been discussed in detail in the text. The purpose of this communication is to ventilate the impact of multifocal approach in curbing the population growth effectively.

02.04.08

Postpartum tubal ligation by nurse-midwives in Thailand: A long-term follow-up: Dusitsin, N, Tasanapradit, P, Onthuam, Y, Satayapan, S. Inst. Hlth. Res., Chulalongkorn Univ. and Ministry of Publ. Hlth., Bangkok, Thailand

Between 1979–1980, thirty-three operating-room nurses, recruited from various parts of Thailand, were trained in a standardized 3-month course to perform postpartum tubal ligation. By the end of September 1984, twenty-eight of these nurses had provided postpartum tubal sterilization services for a 2–6 year period under medical supervision to a total of 46,534 women. Twenty of these nurses operated regularly and covered 52% of all cases done in their hospitals. The major operative complications reported in the first year of their practice out of a total number of 7067 operations included injury to the bladder two, injury to the small bowel one, tear of the mesosalpinx three and postoperative internal hemorrhage one. All these incidents were promptly recognized by the nurses and were properly managed by the supervising physicians. No serious complications were encountered in subsequent years of the nurses' practice. The study of the attitudes of the chiefs of departments of obstetrics and gynecology and the head-nurses of the operating-rooms under whom the trained nurses worked, was very favorable regarding the trained nurses' roles and performance.

02.04.09

Hydrogelic tubal occlusion with the P-block – an alternative to abdominal sterilization: Brundin, J. Dept. Obstet. and Gyn., Karolinska Inst., Danderyd Hosp., Danderyd, Sweden

The hysteroscopical technique of hydrogelic blocking of the human oviduct under local anesthesia will be presented. Long-term animal (rabbit) experiments have shown no significant, inadvertent side-effects with hematology, blood chemistry, organ weights, macro- and micropathological studies. Microscopical studies of human oviducts after three years of blocking with P-blocks have shown an similar lack of inadvertent reaction (*Brundin & Sandstedt,* Acta path. microbiol. scand., Sect. A, in press 1985). The improvement of the hysteroscopical insertion technique into the intramural part of the human oviduct is described in detail together with the evolution of the shape of the hydrogelic tubal blocking device – the P-block. The present data declare a high rate of successful insertions and retentions when a comparatively stiff polyvinyl chloride catheter, containing only 12% of softener was used. The hysteroscopical, transcervical, intramural occlusion of the human oviduct with a hydrogelic occlusion device – the P-block has developed into an alternative to abdominal sterilization in women.

02.04.10

An evaluation of the FEMCEPT/MCA system for out-patient female sterilization: Richart, R M, Neuwirth, R S., New York, USA

We have previously described a system through which it is possible on an out-patient basis to inject methylcyanoacrylate (MCA) through a delivery system known as the FEMCEPT device. This system has been tested in over 1500 women to date and has produced a bilateral closure rate as determined by hysterosalpingography of 70% on a single application and 90% on two-application. The success in closure is related to uterine size and uterine position, but it appears to be relatively skill independent as most investigators obtain similar results. A new instrument to test tubal patency, the FEMTEST device, has also been devised to be used in conjunction with the FEMCEPT/MCA system. The FEMTEST device utilizes a balloon-containing cannula to block the uterine outflow of a premeasured quantity of carbon dioxide gas which is instilled in the uterine cavity under constant conditions. Patency and non-patency are indicated by a sliding pointer built into the handle. It is believed that a combination of the FEMCEPT/MCA system and the FEMTEST system will enable the practitioner to sterilize women on an out-patient basis with relative ease, safety, and cost-effectiveness.

02.04.11

Nonsurgical female sterilization by quinacrine hydrochloride pellets – a four year follow-up: Bhatt, R V, Waszak, C S. BM Amin Hosp., Baroda, India

Surgical female sterilization is an effective method. Many women are afraid of operation and would prefer an alternative. There may be difficulty in providing surgical expertize. Eighty-four women were admitted to a study in Baroda, India, designed to evaluate the efficacy of three transcervical insertions of quinacrine hydrochloride pellets one month apart to produce occlusion of the oviduct. Four year follow-up has been completed for all of the women. Three women became pregnant during the time between the first and the third administrations were complete. Of the 81 women remaining in the study after administrations were complete, three became pregnant during the four year follow-up period, resulting in a cumulative life table pregnancy rate of 3.7 at 48 months. The results of this study indicate that intrauterine insertion of quinacrine pellets can be a safe, effective, nonsurgical sterilization procedure.

02.06.01

Cervical uterus cancer as a public health problem – study and evaluation: Aguirre Lewis, A. Guayaquil, Ecuador

Gynecology mission to prevent oncology problems, social level, sanitary in women. Objective: positive examination of every woman and emphasize in dangerous ages – complete control ages 30 and 60 years obligatory. Known methods and amply and follow-up according to the case. To protect the women with public health laws including in sanitary code. Oncology and gynecology chaper like in other diseases such as tuberculosis with abreughraphy system at least screening with Papanicolaou colposcopy and periodical endometrical biopsy. To maintain the concept when a woman died from cancer cervix some body is blameful. What we advise is a global systematic examination unscreening to every women without and with pathology since the former programs are restricted and oriented when there is a genital pathology or clinical history and despite the programs of detaining the cervical uterus cancer still in Ecuador and in Latin America when women come to gynecology and oncology center Hospital with an advanced pathology of a bad prognosis and lethal at a short-term notwithstanding the methods of surgery advanced and sophisticated treatment. Our statist since 25 years from my post degree in Oncology Practice in Madrid Botella LL and Berlin Prof. Herbert Lax. The cervical cancer is the most frequent in the death of women in Ecuador 15 years ago 4000 women died from cancer in the year in a country of 8,000,000 inhabitants. With obligatory test, with control of the Governments of each Country provide priority for control and treatment at a level of public health until, determine programs, factors, genesis, heredity factor with influence in the development. That we on the basis of incentive FIGO-FLASOg UICC. To try and find out the priority at a level of Public Health in Ecuador in Latin America is pathology occupy the second place as cause of the death.

02.06.02

Epidemiological evaluation of early cervical cancer detection in Slovenia up to 1980: Pompe Kirn, V, Vrščaj Uršič, M, Kovačič, J, Primic Žakelj, M. Inst. Oncol. and Gyn. Dept., Univ. Clin. Ctr., Ljubljana, Yugoslavia

Cervical cancer screening is performed in whole Slovenia in connection with normal clinical practice since

1960. Only in three selected gynecological centers smears were taken before. The evaluation is based on the data of the Cancer Registry of Slovenia. The incidence of invasive cervical cancer (CC) has been decreasing since 1962 with an average annual percentage change of 3%, in 1980 it was 18.5/100,000. The incidence of *in situ* CC is increasing; in 1980 it was 25/100,000, but only among younger women up to the age of 40, and is much better in three-commune aggregates around the three selected gynecological centers. All 307 cases of stage I invasive CC diagnosed in the period 1975–1980, treated at the Gynecological department of the University Clinical Center (UCC), at the Institute of Oncology Ljubljana, and in the General Hospital Maribor were classified according to FIGO classification into Ia and Ib stages. In comparison with all stages, the cases from the three selected commune aggregates had a greater percentage of Ia stage. The Ia stage was agglomerated more in the age 20–39 and there was no peak of the Ib stage evident in the age 40–49. The agglomeration of the Ia stage was even more evident after exclusion of the Maribor region, where also a greater ratio of Ib stage in the age 20–39 was observed. The question to be solved is whether the greater ratio of Ib stage in young women in Maribor is due to a greater number of rapidly growing tumors or a less efficient early detection.

02.06.03
Cervical carcinoma below age 35 – a clinicopathological study: Chen, H F, Hu, W M. Dept. Obstet. and Gyn., Chang Gung Memo. Hosp., Taipei, Taiwan
From 1979 to 1983, 52 cases of Cx Ca below age 35 were collected. Epidemiology including education, age of sexual exposure and marriage, frequency and hygiene of sexual life were studied. When compared with control group, early sexual exposure, low educational class and multigravida seem to be risk factors. Pathology was reviewed also, cell type, grading, L-N metastasis rate and early recurrent rate were analysed. Poor differentiation is the major grading of young age group, L-N metastasis and early recurrence rate (< 18 months) are higher in young age group.

02.06.04
The significance of serial neopterin determinations for monitoring patients with cervical cancer during follow-up: Hetzel, H, Richler, A, Reibnegger, G, Wachter, H. Dept. Obstet. and Gyn., Univ., Innsbruck, Austria
The value of the pretherapeutic neopterin levels in patients with genital cancer was demonstrated by Bichler (see abstract 7696/11490). The purpose of this paper is to show the significance of serial neopterin determinations during the follow-up in patients with cervical cancer. The relative risks of a patient for the critical event relapse, metastasis and death according to different neopterin levels during follow-up as well have been assessed by the means of the "proportional hazards" model with time-dependent variables (Cox DR). We found the first significant neopterin elevation in patients with cervical cancer 150 days before death from cancer, 60 days before the clinico-radiological diagnosis of metastasis, 30 days before the clinico-radiological diagnosis of tumor recurrence. Based on our data, we can conclude that a neopterin elevation during the follow-up is an early indicator for a tumor recurrence or metastasis in patients with cervical cancer. Our results confirm us that the neopterin determination during the follow-up is a very useful indicator for monitoring patients with cervical cancer.

02.06.05
The serum lactic dehydrogenase levels in patients with cervical carcinoma: Friedman, M, Peretz, B A, Paldi, E. Dept. Obstet. and Gyn. "B", Rambam Med. Ctr., Technion, Fac. Med., Haifa, Israel
Cancer cells have increased glycolysis, leading to an increased synthesis of lactate. Lactic dehydrogenase is a glycolytic enzyme with an increased activity in malignant tissue. Lactic dehydrogenase (LDH) activity in serum was studied serially in 110 patients suffering from carcinoma of the uterine cervix, 28 patients with cervical carcinoma *in situ* (CIS) and 25 healthy women (control group). In the first group of patients the levels of LDH were measured before, during and after irradiation therapy, and every six months during the follow-up period. The overall incidence of elevated LDH levels was 76.8%, while only 10.7% and 4% in the CIS and control group respectively. There was a positive correlation between the incidence of raised LDH and the clinical stage of disease. No correlation between enzyme activity and the histological grade of tumor was found. The elevated LDH levels dropped during the course of the therapy in the majority of cases. An additional group of patients who presented with widespread recurrence was evaluated. In 87.5% of them the LDH levels were abnormal. A retrospective analysis of serum LDH activity in this group showed that in more than half of these patients the pretreatment levels of this enzyme were higher than normal. This study indicates that serial LDH measurements in serum of patients with cervical carcinoma may be of value in the management of this disease.

02.06.06
Usefulness of serial CEA determinations in follow-up during radiotherapy for squamous cell carcinoma of the cervix: Matsuzawa, M, Hasumi, K, Takahashi, M, Shiromizu, K, Ishihara, M. Dept. Gyn., Saitama Ca Ctr., Japan
Fifty-seven patients with squamous cell carcinoma of the cervix undergoing radiation therapy were followed by serial plasma CEA measurements. CEA levels were determined weekly by the radio-immunoassay (Sandwich method), plasma CEA value of 2.5 ng/ml was taken as the upper limit of normal. Thirty-nine

patients with negative CEA values on diagnosis had unchanged CEA levels during irradiation. In 12 out of 18 patients with positive CEA values on diagnosis, irradiation to the pelvis resulted in a reduction in circulating CEA levels and subsequently their CEA values reverted to the normal within four weeks of irradiation. Four patients out of these 12 developed a recurrence within two years of therapy. Elevated CEA titers in the remaining six patients decreased partially or at all in spite of a complete regression of pelvic tumors. In these patients, distant metastasis or liver cirrhosis were found a short time after radiotherapy.

02.06.07

In vivo and in vitro induction of TA-4 in a uterine cervical epidermoid cancer cell line (SKG-IIIa): Nozawa, S, Kojima, M, Tsai, D Z, Sakayori, M, Kurihara, S. Dept. Obstet. and Gyn., School Med., Keio Univ., Tokyo, Japan

In order to investigate whether a tumor maker can be induced by an antitumor agent, experiments *in vitro* and *in vivo* were carried out. Newly established uterine cervical epidermoid cancer cell line (SKG-IIIa), was used, which was proved to produce TA-4 (a tumor antigen of squamous cell carcinoma purified by Dr. *Kato*). *In vitro* experiment, when the cells become nearly confluent, peplomycin (10 μg/ml) was added to the culture medium and TA-4 content in the medium and cultured cells were measured by RIA. Immunocytochemical TA-4 staining of cultured cells was also performed by PAP method. *In vivo* experiment, peplomycin was administrated to SKG-IIIa transplanted nude rats by osmotic infusion pump, and serum TA-4 level was measured. *In vitro* study, total TA-4 content and the proportion of TA-4 positive cells increased $2 \sim 3$ times after five days peplomycin treatment compared to the control. *In vivo* study, transient elevations of serum TA-4 level during peplomycin administration were observed in several rats. From these data, it was suggested that peplomycin stimulated TA-4 production or release *in vivo* and *in vitro*.

02.06.08

Cytoplasmic and nuclear steroid receptors in squamous cancer of the cervix: Soutter, W P, Ginsberg, R, Corbett, P J, Sharp, F. Dept. Gyn., Univ. Sheffield, UK

All the component tissues of the human cervix clearly respond to estrogens. In particular, the growth of cervical squamous epithelium is stimulated by estrogen and contains estrogen and progesterone receptors (*B. M. Sanborne* et al., J. Steroid Biochem. **9**, 951, 1978). The presence of these receptors in both the cytoplasm and the nucleus of breast cancers indicates an improved prognosis and the likelihood of response to endocrine treatment whether given for recurrent disease (*R. E. Leake* et al., Brit. J. Cancer **43**, 59, 1981) or as an adjuvant to surgery (*B. Fisher* et al., New Engl. J. Med. **305**, 1, 1981). If steroid receptors are present in cervical cancers they might indicate a hitherto little explored role for ovarian hormones in the biology and management of the second most common cancer in women worldwide (*D. M. Parkin* et al., Bull. WHO **62**, 162, 1984). There is wide uncertainty as to the proportion of squamous cervical cancers containing steroid receptors (*W. P. Soutter* et al., Cancer of the Uterine Cervix, eds *McBrien & Slater*, 295, 1984). This study confirms that more than 40% of these tumors contain both cytoplasmic and nuclear receptors. Furthermore, these data suggest that when the receptor mechanism becomes abnormal in the tumor, it does so in the underlying stroma also. This suggests a role for the stroma in the development of cervical cancers.

02.06.09

Role of X-ray CT in estimating prognosis of cervical cancer: Yamada, E, Kojima, Y, Yamauchi, I, Takahashi, K, Suzuki, M. Dept. Obstet. and Gyn., Kyorin Univ. School Med., Tokyo, Japan

The authors have studied endometrial cancers with the intention of classifying CT findings and evaluating the effect of radiotherapy on cancers. The present paper reports studies on the relationship of CT findings prior to treatment of the cervical cancer to the prognosis. The CT equipment used was EMI-5005 or CT/T, and the CT findings were evaluated according to the classification reported previously. Fifty-six patients who had been followed for at least three years were evaluated. The CT findings have been proved to have a significant relationship to prognosis as a result of study on findings such as enlargement of cervices, high density of parametria and images of lymphadenopathy larger than 2 cm. This established relationship will assure the CT examination of possibility of its application to clinical staging of cervical cancer, and play an important part in determination of the methods of treatment.

02.06.10

The value of computed tomography (CT) in cervical carcinoma: Botsis, D, Gregoriou, O, Tsarouchis, C, Zourlas, P A. 2nd Dept. Obstet. and Gyn., Athens Univ., Areteion Hosp., Athens, Greece

The purpose of our study was to determine the value of computed tomography (CT) in relation to the local spread of cervical carcinoma and possible invasion of the pelvis and the retroperitoneal space. Fifty-two patients treated for cervical carcinoma during the period 1980–1984 were included. Histologic diagnosis of the disease was done by punch cervical biopsy and diagnostic curettage. The investigation of all patients included intravenous pyelography, opaque enema, bone and liver scanning and computed tomography. Our results demonstrate a correlation between CT data and anatomopathologic evidence in 85%. Computed tomography must be considered as a dependable method for staging cervical carcinoma.

02.06.11

A study of ovarian function after surgical transposition of the ovaries and pelvic irradiation in patients with uterine cervical cancer: Mok, J-E. Kyung Hee Univ. Hosp., Seoul, Korea

It has been accepted as inevitable that pre-menopausal women receiving therapeutic doses of pelvic irradiation will invariably become sterile and amenorrheic if the ovaries are not protected in some way. It was the aim of this study to investigate whether ovaries transpositioned away from the irradiated field would continue to function normally. The ovaries were transpositioned to the parietal peritoneum overlying the kidney on 21 cervical cancers under age of 40, in 89 radical hysterectomies. The effect of ovarian transposition on gonadal function was investigated in seven women. After pelvic irradiation, the ovarian function of the study group had confirmed by radioimmunoassay as estradiol above 30 pgm/ml, LH under 15.4 mIU/ml and FSH below 8.0 mIU/ml. The control group consisted of five patients without ovarian transposition but pelvic irradiation. There were higher LH and FSH (67.2–87 mIU/ml, 87.1–109 mIU/ml) but lower estradiol (under 30 pgm/ml). Symptoms related to failed or decreased ovarian function were higher. Thus, transposition of the ovary preceding radiotherapy is an effective means of preserving ovarian secretion in young women in whom malignancies of the pelvic region demand irradiation.

02.06.12

Uterine cancer. Vagina border of section: importance of its study in the operative specimen: López de la Osa Gonzalez, E, Recio Sanchez, S, López de la Osa Garcés, L, López García, N. Instituto Nacional de Oncología, Madrid, Spain

We describe the extraordinary importance of the histopathologic study of the border of the vagina's free section, in the operative specimen resulting from the surgical treatment of uterine cancer, cervical carcinoma as well as endometrial carcinoma. We also indicate the number of tumor cells found in the section border mentioned, the complementary treatment and the existing analogy with the discovery of a tumor nidus in the vaginal part extirpated during the second surgical exploration.

02.06.13

Colposcopy on adenocarcinoma of the uterine cervix: Hasegawa, T, Akiba, R, Kiguchi, K, Tsutsui, F, Kurihara, S. Dept. Obstet. and Gyn., School Med., Keio Univ., Tokyo, Japan

To clarify colposcopic features of cervical adenocarcinoma colposcopic findings were studied on 38 consecutive cases. The following seven groups were observed; group 1, findings of atypical transformation zone only, two cases; group 2, large abnormal vessels in transformation like findings, five cases; group 3, pleomorphic abnormal vessels in yellowish background with abundant mucus, two cases; group 4, findings of atypical vessels, four cases; group 5, polyp or papilloma-like findings, two cases; group 6, frank invasion with irregular surface, pleomorphic vascular pattern, partly necrotic membrane and partly mucus secretion, 15 cases and group 7, unsatisfactory colposcopic findings, eight cases. As for relation between colposcopic group and histology group 2 revealed three of four mucus secretion type. Well differentiated type (18 cases) distributed widely and 13 out of 14 moderately differentiated type corresponded to group 6 and 7. Group 3 and 6 revealed one poorly differentiated and one clear cell type respectively. In conclusion colposcopic features of cervical adenocarcinoma are pleomorphic abnormal vessels and mucus secretion in yellowish background representing group 2 to 5. Mucus secretion type revealed typical findings.

02.06.14

Rectosonography of local recurrences of gynecologic tumors: Its use in diagnosis and treatment: Wischnik, A*, Hoetzinger, H**. * Dept. Gyn., Rot-Kreuz-KH, München. **Dept. Rad., Staedt. KH, Passau

Rectosonography is a new diagnostic procedure which allows the visualization of the internal female genitalia, especially of lesions near the transducer. The method seems to be of great value for detection of postoperative local recurrences of gynecologic tumors (carcinomas of the cervix, the corpus uteri and the ovaries). Thirty patients with local postoperative recurrences were scanned, the results were verified cytologically and by the clinical course. The tumor masses appeared in 100% as areas of low echogenicity. The extension could be correctly defined in correlation to CT in all cases. The therapy of local recurrences presents great problems because in most cases neither a new operation is possible, nor is percutaneous radiotherapy effective. Rectosonography, however, allows the use of local brachytherapy with ultrasound guided installation of afterloading needles. Up till now 13 cases have been treated. The procedure is presented.

02.07.01

The staging process and therapeutic choices in breast cancer: Teixeira, L C, Alvarenga, M, Zeferino, L C, Pinotti, J A. Dept. Obstet. and Gyn., State Univ., Campinas, Brazil

The staging of breast cancer is related to the choice of the primary and adjuvant therapeutic approach and to the prognosis. 330 pts with Stages I to IIIa were reviewed. 70 were submitted to a quadrantectomy (QUA), 60 to Radical Mastectomy (RM) with an Immediate Reconstruction (IR) and the other 200 to MRM. A modified mastectomy is achieved if the tumor is smaller than 5 cm and if the intrasurgical frozen section examination of the axilla is negative. Tumors larger than 5 cm had 50% (5/10) of muscle involvement and 15% (15/33) of local recurrence. This rate was 1.9% (1/52) if a Halsted operation was performed. There were 11 cases (18.3%) of re-utilization of the nipple-areola complex (NAC) in IR. When the presurgical examination of the NAC was normal there were 10% of invasive carcinoma, with 47% of involvement if the tumor's diameter was more than 51 mm and 51% if it had more than six positive nodes in the axilla. 18% of invasive carcinomas in the NAC were found when there was vascular invasion of the dermis. One pt (1.4%) was submitted to a QUA and four pts (6.6%) treated by RMIM had dermal lymphatic carcinomatosis. There was 62.9% (112/178) of accuracy in the clinical evaluation of the axilla. We observed a change in staging in 27 pts (8.19%) with 74.0% and 92.5% of accuracy if the clinical staging was I or IIIa, respectively. It is recommended to return to the traditional presurgical biopsy and to achieve the intrasurgical staging whenever necessary.

02.07.02

Operable breast cancer: The experience at the Universitäts-Frauenklinik Heidelberg: Kubli, F, Kaufmann, M, Schmid, H, v. Fournier, D, Müller, A. Univ. Hosp., Dept. Obstet. and Gyn., Heidelberg
The present study is a retrospective analysis of 1609 patients (pts) with operable breast cancer out of 2004 cases treated at the Univ.-Frauenklinik Heidelberg from 1971 to the end of 1983. Purpose of this review is to describe therapy strategy during this 13-year period and to analyse the prognosis of these patients. The study population includes 1417 pts treated with a modified radical mastectomy and 192 pts with conservative breast surgery. Histologically examined radical axillary lymphonodectomy resulted in 965 node negative and 644 node positive cases. Clinical data include age, menopausal status, tumor size, number of involved lymph nodes, and steroid hormone receptor status. Therapeutic outcome is analysed for disease free and overall survival. Surgical procedures became more aggressive during this analysed time period – especially for axillary clearance (level I, II, III). On the other side surgical treatment was minimalized in T1 and clinically node negative pts. The use of postoperative radiotherapy decreased and changed to a systematic use of adjuvant chemo- and/or endocrine therapy. The variety of primary surgical and postoperative treatment is therefore analysed for different time periods. Effects of better histologically proven diagnosis and risk adapted therapy including adjuvant cytotoxic and/or endocrine treatment are discussed as well as treatment failures.

02.07.03

Multiple primary malignant neoplasms in breast cancer patients in Israel: Schenker, J G, Levinsky, R, Ohel, G. Dept. Obstet. and Gyn., Hadassah Univ. Hosp., Jerusalem, Israel
Multiple primary malignant neoplasms seem to be increasing in frequency. As breast carcinoma is the most prevalent malignancy in Israeli women, we chose to study multiple primary malignancies in this population. During the 18-year period of study 12,302 cases of breast carcinoma were diagnosed, and, of these, 984 patients (8%) had multiple primary malignant tumors. Forty-seven of these patients developed two multiple primary cancers. A significantly higher than expected incidence of second primary cancers occurred at the following five sites: the opposite breast, salivary glands, uterine body, ovary, and thyroid. Cancers of stomach and gall bladder were fewer than expected. Treatment of the breast cancer by irradiation was associated with an increased risk of subsequent cancers of lung and hematopoietic system. The prognosis was mainly influenced by the site and malignancy of the second primary cancer. The incidence of multiple primary malignancies justifies a high level of alertness to this possibility in the follow-up of breast cancer patients.

02.07.04

Radical mastectomy with immediate reconstruction of the breast: Keppke, E M, Teixeira, L C, Pinotti, J A. Dept. Obstet. and Gyn., State Univ., Campinas, Brazil
Breast Reconstruction (BR) is usually performed some years after the primary operation. To evaluate the role of BR in the disease-free interval and survival, we treated 60 pts with tumors $T_{1a-2a,1b-1a}$ by Radical Mastectomy and Immediate Reconstruction with rectus abdominis muscle. Pts were submitted to a modified mastectomy, if the intrasurgical frozen section examination of the axillary nodes was negative. The plastic surgeon's team works concomitantly, preparing the dissection of abdominal flap. Pts with positive lymph nodes were treated with postsurgical radiotherapy. The adjuvant treatment was chemotherapy (CMF) and antiestrogen (tamoxifen). The nipple-areola complex (NAC) was re-used in 11 pts (18.3%). 28 immediate complications (46.6%) were observed: 15% of seroma, 10% of partial necrosis of NAC and 10% of surgical scar infections. There were 16 late complications (26.6%): fat necrosis (15%) and abdominal herniation (11.6%), with mean time for complications of 7.6 and 6.9 months respectively. There was one (1.6%) local recurrence and three (5%) distant metastases. The psychological aspects of these pts tested before and after operation show the superiority of the emotional recuperation of the pts that had BR.

02.07.05

The lower transverse rectus abdominis musculocutaneous (TRAM) flap, an alternative for breast reconstruction: Brunnert, K, Schermann, J. Frauenklin., Klinikum Karlsruhe
The lower TRAM flap is performed in a two stage operation. First, the transfer of the flap from the abdominal to the chest wall via a tunnel. Second, scar revision and reconstruction of the nipple-areola approx. three months later. Ten pts underwent 12 breast reconstructions, 8 pts with unilateral breast reconstruction, one pt with single stage bilateral breast reconstruction and one pt with single stage unilateral breast reconstruction and contralateral subcutaneous mastectomy, using the dissected half of the

lower TRAM flap, instead of an alloplastic implant. Average pt age was 42 years (28 to 49 years). Medium follow-up is 9.5 months. All pts had undergone mastectomy for breast cancer, two pts had undergone radical mastectomy, eight pts modified radical mastectomy. Two pts suffered from skin damage, due to previous radiation. All breast reconstructions were performed without using an alloplastic implant. No major vascular problems were observed, except one case in which, due to insufficient vascularity of the flap, another technique for reconstruction was used. In four pts the flap showed minor tip loss which healed satisfactorily by secondary intention. No weakening of the abdominal wall was observed. With careful patient selection, the lower TRAM flap is an excellent alternative for breast reconstruction.

02.07.06

Stage III breast cancer treatment: Souza, J B, Souza, A Z, Hegg, R, Fonseca, A M, Salvatores, C A. Gyn. Clin., São Paulo Univ. Med. School, Brazil

Between 1979–83, 55 patients with stage III (TNM-UICC) breast cancer were treated at São Paulo University Medical School. Twenty-two (40%) pre-menopausal women underwent a bilateral ovariectomy before starting this schedule. According to modality of stage III breast cancer, two different trials were undertaken in these patients. Thirty-three (60%) underwent radiotherapy as basic procedure before chemo-therapy plus total mastectomy. Twenty-five (75.8%) of these patients were alive and free of disease after 48.9 months. The remaining twenty-two (40%) were submitted to preliminary chemotherapy during 4 months before total mastectomy plus radiotherapy. Thirteen (59.1%) were alive and free of disease after the same period of follow-up. The average number of chemotherapy series was 21 for both schedules. Radiotherapy dosage varied between 4000 to 5000 rads. Based upon these data the authors propose radiotherapy and or chemotherapy as the main therapeutic procedures, according to the modality of stage III. Surgical treatment (total mastectomy) should be considered of secondary importance, unless as a hygienic procedure.

02.07.07

Simultaneous adjuvant chemotherapy (CT) and irradiation (I) (combined modality) in "high risk" breast cancer (HR-BR): Suchy, B R, Mayr, A C, Koch, K. Oncol. and Radiother. Dept., Rudolf-Virchow-Hosp., Berlin

Simultaneous adjuvant CT and I requires good cooperation between medical oncologist and therapeutic radiologist. We treated 27 "high risk" women with combined modalities (08/82–12/84). Indications: $pT_{2b/3/4}$ (n=17) pT multilocular a/o unknown nodal status (n=7); pT_2 medial quadrant histologically positive nodes (N+) and family history of BC (n=3); inflammatory BC (n=5); tumor enucleation with N+ (n=5). CT: six monthly courses of VCMFP. I: high energy electrons to chest wall and axillary nodes 40 Gy + supraclavicular 30 Gy/fractionation weekly 4 Gy (d 60–150). – Results: 30 pts received more than 85% of calculated dosage. In one pt platelets fell to a nadir of 5/nl after the third course but eventually had 88% of dosage. One pt got 88% of the proposed dosage, but skipped irradiation after 22 Gy for personal reasons. Seven pts received less than 85% of calculated amount because of prolonged leucopenia. Nonmyelotoxic side-effects: all pts had marked reversible alopecia. One pt lost 5 kg of weight, 32 pts gained weight between 0.6 kg and 14 kg. There was no death or severe complication during therapy. In pts with BC this adjuvant combined modality was well tolerated and feasible.

Combination schedule of chemotherapy and irradiation

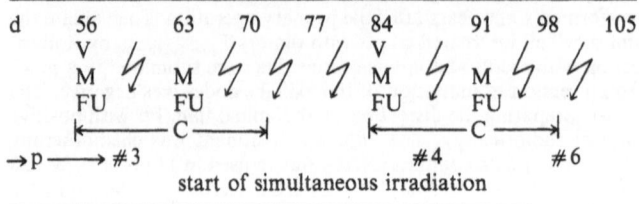

start of simultaneous irradiation

02.07.08

Pregnancy after breast carcinoma: Centonze, M, Centonze, A. Div. Gin. Obstet., Osp. S. Martino. Genova, Italy

In Jan. 1976 a solid alveolar duct carcinoma of the breast (T2a N0) was discovered in a 35-year-old patient (G.M. No. 4519/76), who came for consultation on a problem of sterility. Radical mastectomy (Halsted) was performed in our department. Two months after the operation the woman became pregnant and we allowed the pregnancy to run its course. The woman wanted this too, but some endocrinologists and oncologists we talked with did not agree. In the aftermath the patient developed uterine fibromyomas and another baby was delivered in 1978 by Cesarean section with total hysterectomy and bilateral oophorec-tomy. So far mother and children are fine. The follow-up continues. Although the epidemiologists have demonstrated that obstetrical factors are strictly bound to risk carcinoma of the breast, endometrium and ovary, we agree with the majority of the authors who think that fertility must be preserved in young patients treated for cancer and that termination of the pregnancy must be considered in cases of breast carcinoma with metastases in the lymph-nodes or when an embryotoxic therapy must be administred. It is not often that we have to deal with a pregnancy after surgical treatment for cancer of the breast. This case in living memory shows that sometimes we can judge our behaviour only after many years, and then we know if a decision we were required to take promptly was right or not.

02.08.01

Functional development of regulatory mechanisms in human fetal heart rate, using a factor analysis: Koyanagi, T, Nakahara, H, Nakano, H. Dept. Gyn. and Obstet., Fac. Med., Kyushu Univ., Fukuoka, Japan
To elucidate the functional development of the mechanisms which regulate fetal heart rate (FHR), we devised a mathematical model involving factor analysis and a computer system. The study was made on various sets of the instantaneous FHR values (bpm) in sequence for three continuous hours, obtained from fetuses at around 20 to 42 weeks of gestation. Factor analysis was employed on the matrix with absolute FHR values (bpm) ranging from 116 to 175 bpm and the corresponding beat-to-beat differences between ± 15 bpm, respectively in columns and rows. It was evident that there were at least three different and independent components of FHR regulation which may drive an individual FHR pattern. The first component acts as an accelerator, the second as decelerator and the third as "fluctuation" varying symmetrically around zero within ± 3 bpm of the beat-to-beat differences. The former two became clear by 30 week's gestation, while the latter was seen throughout pregnancy, suggesting the function of bias for maintaining so-called baseline heart rate. In conclusion, a human fetus endeavors to obtain the mechanisms of heart rate regulation by 30 week's gestation and starts to function at that period. The fact that results merely obtained by the mathematical model are well comparable with those by physiological experimental models indicates that the mathematical analysis may propose the stepping stone for the study of human fetus as one of the available methodologies.

02.08.02

Ante-partum fetal heart rate recording – rapid digital distance telemetry: Dawson, A J, Gough, N A J, Tompkins, T. Dept. Obstet., Univ. of Wales Coll. Med., Cardiff, UK
An analogue real time system for telephonic ante-partum fetal heart rate monitoring from patient's homes was reported in 1983 (*Dalton, K J*, Brit. med. J. **286**, 1545, 1983). This was followed by a digital system (*Gough, N A J*, Fetal and Neonatal Physiological Measurements, 1984, Butterworths, in press); recordings could be made at the patient's convenience and the digital values representing fetal heart beat-to-beat intervals later rapidly transmitted to the hospital for processing and immediate expert reporting. However, there was no reliable method of checking the quality of the heart signal during the recording session. There was a test for the corruption of data by noise on the telephone line, but the resulting gaps could not be accurately quantified. Our new system, MicroTel, developed in this centre, uses a compact and portable dedicated microprocessor unit in the patient's home communicating with the central computer in the hospital after the recording has been made. It now provides data reduction while recording is in progress, and automatically protected data transmission to the central computer over a period of about 20 seconds for a full half hour recording. The system is likely to be of value for long-term intensive domiciliary surveillance of high-risk pregnancies.

02.08.03

A computerized system for fetal home telemetry: Dalton, K J, Currie, J, Manning, K, Dripps, J. Dept. Obstet., Univ., Cambridge; Signal Processing Group, Dept. Electrical Engineering, Univ., Edinburgh, UK
We have developed a computerised system whereby the fetal heart rate is recorded telemetrically from patients' homes, transmitted over conventional public telephone lines, and displayed in real time in hospital. We transmitted over 100 telemetric recordings from home by February 1985. Patients use a Sonicaid D206 fetal monitor at home, and they simply telephone its audible output signal directly into the Rosie Maternity Hospital in Cambridge. There it is digitally processed using a Motorola 68,000 microprocessor in association with a Hewlett Packard computer. All our patients have been able to transmit a 30 minute recording to hospital without direct home supervision. A broad beam ultrasonic transducer is easier to use than a narrow one, and it gives half the signal loss. Such losses need be little more than 10%, and we are trying to improve this further. We have made a detailed study of the home circumstances during recording sessions, and thereby we have been able to optimise the recording situation. All patients claim to have found the whole experience most enjoyable and emotionally satisfying. Our method permits safe antenatal monitoring of the fetal heart, whilst avoiding the expense and social trauma of hospital admission. We minimise operating costs by using only one digital processing unit centrally, and by loaning patients monitors which are robust and relatively cheap (about 400 US$). We can also change software centrally whenever required. These economic advantages should be attractive in the U.S. where local telephone calls are often free, and in developing countries where maintenance of electronic equipment may be expensive.

33

02.08.04

Fully portable perinatal database system using handheld microcomputer with itemized keyboard: Yanagita, Y. Tokyo Maternity Clin., Tokyo, Japan

As the Japanese obstetricians/midwives are not well acquainted with typewriter-type keyboard, they meet with considerable difficulties in inputting the data. Also in obstetrics, a patient moves from private room to labor room then to delivery room when labor progresses, so that the portable computer with itemized keyboard has a very good place in use at the delivery floor in Japan. The architecture of this database system consists of HC-40 (CPU), PF-10 (floppy disk drive), and P-80K (printer). They are all battery operated and are portable. On admission of the patient to the delivery floor, all physical findings are recorded. Thereafter procedures and treatment as well as physical findings are recorded with their times by a single touch on an itemized keyboard. 120 data of 10 patients are recorded on 38 KB RAM files in CPU. As the CPU is made of CMOS, it can hold the data when the switch is cut-off. As there are 64 itemized keys, one can assign one time on one key. The data on RAM files can be transmitted to 3.5 inches microdisk, which is later brought back to CPU for statistical analysis. A microfloppy disk can accommodate data from 120 patients. 95% of nurses have learned how to use this computer in only 15 minutes, and the total expense for this system is less than 1200 US$. – Conclusion: This small portable perinatal data anywhere, can be used by anybody after 15 minutes of practice and it can record and store the data big enough to cover that of small community hospital.

02.08.05

On the equality of several variability indices: Kubo, T, Inaba, J, Shigemitsu, S, Koresawa, M, Shibata, J, Iwasaki, H. Inst. Clin. Med., Univ. of Tsukuba, Ibaraki, Japan

Many variability indices, which have been proposed to represent quantitatively both short-term variability ($=$STV) and long term variability ($=$LTV), were analysed mathematically and the following static property was obtained. All of the approximate expectations for indices developed by TARLO, KERO, DALTON, HEILBRON and CABAL assumed the same formula $\kappa\sqrt{1-\varrho\sigma}$ (κ: constant, ϱ: correlation coefficient between the beat-to-beat interval T_i and the adjacent interval T_{i+1}, σ: standard deviation of T_i), and were identical except for the constants. Those values for de Haan's and Yeh's indices were $\kappa\sqrt{1-\varrho\sigma}/T_0$ (T_0: mean of T_i), while those for Modanlou's, Wade's, and Organ's indices were $\kappa\sqrt{1-\varrho\sigma}/T_0^2$ respectively. Hence, all of these indices represented the same quantity in essence when the mean beat-to-beat interval was constant. The expected value for de Haan's and Heilbron's LTV indices was approximately $\kappa\sqrt{1+\varrho\sigma}$ (κ: constant), while those for Yeh's, Organ's, and Cabal's ITV indices were essentially the standard deviation ($=\sigma$) of T_i. From these results, it can be concluded that measuring STV and LTV according to those formulae means evaluating ϱ and σ at the same time. Hence there may be little significance in measuring them individually if ϱ changes little. That is, it may suffice merely to measure the standard deviation ($=\sigma$) of T_i as a quantity of variability.

02.08.06

Data processing system in obstetric practise: Nakahara, H, Koyanagi, T, Nakano, H. Dept. Gyn. and Obstet., Fac. Med., Kyushu Univ., Fukuoka, Japan

Medical data obtained during pregnancy include various forms of information; symptoms, physical and laboratory data. These data are accumulated on each patients' visit. It is necessary to devise a method for processing large amounts of data. Since the conventional medical charts do not serve prompt retrieval, for the purpose, we devised a data processing system using a Local area network (LAN). With this system of LAN, terminal microcomputers in different areas of the same department, outpatient department, nurse center, delivery room and neonatal room, are connected to the central control unit. The data which are input by the medical staffs at any terminal are immediately stored in the data base of the central control unit, and all staff members have free access to the data base at any terminal. We also attempted to make a connection between one terminal of the LAN and the Computer center of Kyushu University through a definite communication channel, because a mass storage system is needed for permanent storage of the data. Furthermore, this LAN is capable of operating at the national level. This LAN we designed is a very compact system, because it is based on the microcomputer system, and it needs no special training in use. This system is most useful not only for assessment of medical care, but also for medical training.

02.08.07

The quantitative relationship between the spectral analysis of CTG and other various indices for LTV: Hara, K, Jimbo, T, *Grothe, W, *Rüttgers, H, *Kubli, F. Kagawa Med. School, Japan; *Univ. Heidelberg

Concerning the amplitude of STV and LTV, we reported that there is a close relationship among indices of various methods and have the same mean for clinical use. As for the frequency of LTV, relationship among these remained unclear. The spectral analysis (SPA) is known as a good method for the analysis of irregular signals. In this study, the frequency of LTV was quantitatively compared using the SPA method. – Methods: A mini-computer HP1000 and hard disc of 20 Mbite were used. The FECG signals from HP8040A was digitalized (4/sec) and divided into small particles of 48 sec which were calculated according to each formula of LTV and SPA. As for the amplitude, peak to peak method, SD of FHR and another three features were compared to that of SPA: As we reported, the correlation coefficients for the amplitude were sufficiently high (0.735–0.877). As for the frequency, peak to peak method, 0 cross of 24 and 48 sec of floating mean and 48 sec of fixed mean methods were compared to that of SPA. The correlations coefficients among these were extremely low (0.196–0.672). These phenomena depend on the different characteristics of the measurements. The high frequency components ar emphasized by peak to peak method, conversely low frequency components are emphasized by the 0 cross method. SPA is the best method for the frequency of LTV.

02.08.08

PERGYN: Perinatal gynecological information system. Part I: Haller, U, Frielingsdorf, B, Nievergelt, E, Ehrsam, A, Litschgi, M. Dept. Obstet. and Gyn., Kantonsspit., St. Gallen, Switzerland

PERGYN is a scientific research project of a purely medical nature. Its goal is to procure and evaluate the entire body of obstetrical and gynecological data in all its complexity. This system, for which the ground-work has been laid during the past four years by the cooperation of medical doctors and informatic scientists was developed on the base of a medical data model, course tree concept, transaction program for the acquisition, mutation and output of medical data. The system will permit the evaluation of all the collected medical data and their coherencies, e. g.: trend-recognition in diagnosis and therapy, procurement of a statistical basis for answer in current perinatal and gynecological questions, complications and side-effects of therapies and surgical proceedings, setting up of cost profile analysis and risk benefit analysis etc. The dialog processing is self-explanatory, so that only a short training period, without further subpro-grams of the data system including the statistical evaluation are presented: Input processes in gynecological surgery, intraoperative complications, obstetrical and gynecological diagnosis input processes.

02.08.09

PERGYN: Perinatal gynecological information system. Part II (engineering): Frielingsdorf, B, Haller, U, Nievergelt, E, Ehrsam, A, Litschgi, M. Dept. Obstet. and Gyn., Kantonsspit., St. Gallen, Switzerland

The informatical basis of the information system PERGYN is a data model. The most important entity-types are "patient", "treatment", "medical term", "admitting agent", "relator", "cause" and "course". Data models and programs (algorithms) together created PERGYN databank. Entity-types are here filed for (disk-)stored data. In file "medical term" are stored over 7000 terms from SNOMED (College of American Pathologists: Systematized Nomenclature of Medicin, SNOMED; Chicago 1976). The terms were selected for PERGYN's special purposes from the SNOMED-categories: "procedure", "diseases", "etiology", "morphology", "function" and self-created term-groups: "findings", "ICD-diagnoses" and "medicament". The medical data input to an in-patient starts with those standardized SNOMED-terms. Certain terms are therefore connected with a predefined process, called "course-tree". A course-tree is a recursively data structure, materialized as fixed-length data-records in file "course"; it contains for men-machinery-interactions a chained sequence with medical questions and if possible, proper proposals for reply. A question-complex can be multiphase. Those objects are a product of knowledge engineering. Course-tree's nodes determine what is to happen in a single dialog phase. Hence software is data structure orientated and works like a determinated finitely recognizing automatic machine. New on that computer-dialog-technic are full semantical dialog-phases, in error cases stepwise invertible. That kind of dialog processing allows occasional users and informatical novices computer-handling in their own special subject.

02.09.01

The trophoblast and monoclonal antibodies: Barbati, A, Cosmi, E V. Inst. Gyn. and Obstet., Univ., Perugia, Italy

Previous studies have shown that certain human tumor tissues and cell lines express antigens otherwise found only in placental trophoblast and absent from other normal non-malignant tissues and cells (*Faulk* et al., Proc. Nat. Acad. Sci. **75**, 1947, 1978; *Loke* et al., Int. J. Cancer, **25**, 459, 1980). Such membrane antigens may represent the product of de-repression or enhancement of fetal genetic loci normally quiescent in adult tissues; they could play a role in the mechanism of evasion of both tumor cells and the feto-placental unit from rejection by their respective immunologically-competent hosts (*Johnson* et al., Am. J. Repr. Immun. **1**, 83, 1981). These "oncotrophoblast" membrane antigens were originally identified by using polyclonal xenogenic antisera raised against isolated human placental syncytiotrophoblast microvil-lous plasma membrane (StMPM) preparations. In the last years, in order to investigate oncotrophoblast membrane antigenic specificities in detail, we have used mouse monoclonal antibodies (McAb) produced following initial immunisation of mouse Balb/c with isolated human placental StMPM preparation. The aim of this study was to monitor possible changes in the expression of membrane antigens of trophoblastic cells from early to term pregnancy and to detect immunological differences in spontaneous abortions responsible for impaired maternal-fetal relationship. Of 19 positive clones, we have studied the characteris-tics of three McAb: H315, H316, H317. H315 and H317 reacted with trophoblast antigenic determinants. These McAb may be useful to monitor some human tumors.

02.09.02

Trophoblastic disease. Treatment, results in 200 cases: Akrivos, T, Keramopoulos, A, Giorgiotis, D, Leonar-dos, V, Aravantinos, D. 1st Dept. Obstet. and Gyn., Univ. of Athens, Maternity Hosp. of Alexandra, Athens, Greece

Since in 1979, 200 cases of Trophoblastic Disease (T. D.) were examined and followed at the Trophoblastic

Disease Center (T.D.C.) of Alexandra maternity hospital. The incidence rate was 1/200 pregnancies. In 56 cases (28%) chemotherapy was given while in the remaining 144 cases (72%) spontaneous remission was observed in 4–12 weeks. The criteria for chemotherapy in these 56 cases were, (1) Metastatic T. D. (8 cases), (2) High risk group (β-HCG > 100,000 IU/l after the primary evacuation of the uterus, delayed diagnosis and T. D. after full term pregnancy) (16 cases), (3) Marked cellular atypia and hyperplasia or choriocarcinoma (14 cases) and (4) Persistants of high titers of β-HCG or plateau or increase during the follow-up period (18 cases). Monotherapy (methotrexate) was used in 46 cases while triple drug therapy (methotrexate, actinomycin-D, cyclophosphamide) was given in eight cases and two cases received multiple drug treatment (C.H.A.M.O.M.A.). Fifty-one of 56 cases received 100% of the doses. In five cases slight modifications of treatment was needed. The β-HCG titers reached the normal level in 55 out of 56 cases in 3–11 weeks after the beginning of the treatment. One woman died from liver rupture. Thirteen of the above 56 cases had normal pregnancies and deliveries and two had normal pregnancy but spontaneous abortion. It is believed that these good results have been reached by the intensive follow-up and the immediate administration of the proper treatment.

02.09.03

The incidence of trophoblastic disease in south-eastern part of Turkey: Erman, O, Turfanda, A, Bengisu, E, Uyar, H, Akkaya, A. Dept. Obstet. and Gyn., Dicle Univ., Diyarbakir, Turkey

Among 20,701 pregnant patients from south-eastern part of Turkey, 200 (0.97%) were found to have hydatiform mole, and 12 (0.06%) choriocarcinoma; thus hydatiform mole was encountered once in every 100, and choriocarcinoma once in every 1725 deliveries. Trophoblastic diseases have been found to occur more frequently in the younger age groups especially between ages 20 and 30, with 40%. The occurrence rate of trophoblastic disease were higher in multiparous women (86.5%) than in primiparous women (13.5%). In 41.66% of cases choriocarcinoma was found to follow hydatiform mole, in 33.3% normal pregnancy, in 16.66% abortions and in 8.33% ectopic pregnancy. Environmental, cultural, socio-economic and genetic factors and poor nutrition were held responsible for the high incidence of trophoblastic disease in this part of Turkey; since most of the patients were from the poor urban areas, where early marriage is more common, no birth control is used, and the socio-economic and the cultural level of the people is very low.

02.09.04

Trophoblastic disease in Spain. Analysis of the national incidence: Herruzo, A[1], Miranda, J A[1], Gonzalez, F[2], Hernandez, F[1], Rodriguez-Escudero, F[3], Lopez, N[4]. 1: Hosp. Maternal de la S. S. Granada; 2: Hosp. Clin., Granada; 3: C. S. "Enrique Sotomayor", Bilbao; 4: Inst. Nac. Oncol., Madrid, Spain

The analysis is introduced about the national incidence of Trophoblastic Disease (T.D.), made by the Oncology Section of the Spain Gynecology Association, founded in the retrospective collection of 55 hospitals in all the country during the period of years 1962–1984. 1663 cases was collected in 1,110,493 referencied deliveries which gave a frequency of one case of E.T., for every 958 deliveries with a range between 1/530 and 1/1250 depending of the different regions. In the analysis we can see that the frequency of T.D. is high in women of more than 40 years, but this not occurred among teenagers. The 2.5% of the patients had suffered a T.D. before. Almost all the cases happened after a uterine gestation, and its diagnosis was made between 8 and 20 weeks, but only in the 41% of the cases was produced before the expulsion, with a tendency to increase in the last years (53%), by the echography development. The 86% of the cases finished by curettage (nearly all of the cases by "D" and "C"). The 6.6% of the cases there was a stormy course. The most of the cases were treated by monochemotherapy (methotrexate). The rate of mortality in the cases of persistent E.T. or of stormy course, was of 5% in direct relation–with the more advanced ages and stages.

02.09.05

Gestational trophoblastic tumors – a ten-year experience: Pagadalla, R, Mhaskar, A, Chakravarthy, B, Asha, O. JIPMER, Pondicherry, India

In the past three decades, trophoblastic tumors have attracted world-wide attention for various reasons. Geographical distribution of these tumors showed that they are common in Asia. The higher incidence in these areas may be due to poor socio-economic conditions and malnutrition. We present experience from Department of Obstetrics and Gynecology, Jawaharlal Institute of Postgraduate Medical Education & Research from 1972 to 1981. The incidence of mole was found to be 1 in 143 deliveries and that of choriocarcinoma was 1 in 513. Early diagnosis, proper management and close follow-up are the sheet anchors in the successful treatment of trophoblastic tumors. The overall remission rate for gestational trophoblastic tumors (GTT) has touched 92% (*Goldstein*, 1972, *Lurain* et al., 1982). The high curability rate depends on the sensitivity of GTT to chemotherapeutic agents, availability of laboratory techniques and aggressive use of chemotherapeutic agents. However, the aggressive use of chemotherapeutic agents may prove fatal in patients who are already malnourished like ours. Therefore new effective regimens that are less toxic but curative should be evolved. We present our experiences.

02.09.06

The natural history of gestational trophoblastic neoplasia in Riyadh, Saudi Arabia: Chattopadhyay, S K, Sengupta, B S, Muharram, H H, Burhan, Y E. Fac. Med., King Saud Univ. and Maternity and Children Hosp., Riyadh, Saudi Arabia

Retrospective analysis of 302 cases of gestational trophoblastic neoplasia treated at Maternity and Children Hospital, Riyadh, during the period 1978 through 1983, shows an incidence of 1 in 427 deliveries for hydatidiform mole and 1 in 5725 deliveries for choriocarcinoma. This relative higher incidence in spite of country's economic affluence is difficult to explain merely on the basis of early marriage and childbirth. Approximately 75% of patients were 30 years and 70% were less than para 5. Consanguinity was present in only 50% of benign tumors while 80% of choriocarcinoma patients were consanguineous. Blood group 0 was noted in 60% of benign lesions and 55% of choriocarcinoma. Irregular vaginal bleeding (85%) was the predominant symptom following 9–20 weeks amenorrhea. Uterine size was larger than suggested date in 61% cases and 16% cases it was smaller than dates. Ultrasound scanning was diagnostic in 94% cases and gave false positive results in 5% cases. Suction evacuation followed 5–7 days later by a second curettage was the standard treatment. All patients with choriocarcinoma were treated with methotrexate of 6–8 courses. Hysterectomy was performed in only four patients with benign GTN and in two with choriocarcinoma although 30% of patients were grand multiparae. Only 62% of patients could be followed for up to eight weeks and 32% up to one year. Prophylactic chemotherapy was given in 36 patients and perhaps indicated in all patients to overcome poor follow-up, yet we cannot consider this to be ideal. Our social situation demands a continuum of reproductive functions as it is considered a hallmark of femininity. Careful follow-up which involve enforced contraception and frequent check-ups are unwelcome interruptions. Ideally, what we need is a tumor marker of precise prognostic value in order to minimise long years of suspense and longer months of nonproductive reproductive function.

02.09.07

A highly sensitive colorimetric enzyme immunoassay for hCG using specific antibodies against the CTP of the β-hCG: Sato, Y, Hirohashi, T, Sudo, Y, Takeuchi, S. Dept. Obstet. and Gyn., Niigata Univ., Japan

A highly sensitive enzyme immunoassay (EIA) for hCG was newly developed. The Fab' fragment of rabbit anti-whole hCG antibody was conjugated with horse radish peroxidase (HRP) using the hydroxysuccinimide ester of N-(4-carboxycyclohexylmethyl) maleimide. Polystyrene balls were coated with the hCG specific antibody, directed against the C-terminal portion of β-hCG, which was purified from anti-β-hCG bovine thyroglobulin sera by sequential affinity chromatography. This EIA was found to detect as little as 0.2 mIU/ml of hCG without the interference by human LH coexisting at a concentration of 200 mIU/ml. The levels by the assay was closely correlated with those of RIA assay for β-hCG (r = 0.92, y = 1.27χ + 1.8). The assay has been used in management of hydatidiform mole, invasive mole, choriocarcinoma and other gynecological malignancies, indicating its usefulness in follow-up practice because of increase in sensitivity roughly ten times as great as β-hCG RIA system.

02.09.08

The determination of the recognition site of an antiserum detecting desialylation on O-glycosidic carbohydrates of hCG and its clinical applications: Takeuchi, Y, Matsuura, S, Nishimura, R, Mochizuki, M. Univ. Kobe, Japan

Human chorionic gonadotropin (hCG) is a specific tumor marker for trophoblastic disease. It contains 4 asparagine-linked and 4 serine-linked carbohydrate units. Recently, variations in the carbohydrate moieties of hCG in choriocarcinoma have been suggested. So, we attempted to assess the possibility of establishing a radioimmunoassay system which can detect malignant transformational change in serine-O-glycosidically linked carbohydrate units of hCG. An antiserum generated against the enzymatically cleaved, desialylated hCG β COOH-terminal peptide by toepad immunization method was existensively characterized. This antiserum reacts with asialo-hCG better than with native hCG. It does not bind with synthetic COOH-terminal peptides nor monosaccharides such as N-acetyl-D-galactosamine and D-galactose. Beta subunit gains its binding capability to the antiserum only upon desialylation, while native α and β subunits do not react. The antiserum has high specificity toward asialo-hCG in which particular O-glycosidic carbohydrate units are desialylated. With a radioimmunoassay system using this, 29 patients with various trophoblastic diseases were analysed. Asialo-hCG immunoactivity was insignificant in all patients with hydatidiform mole, invasive hydatidiform mole and persisted trophoblastic disease. However, asialo-hCG was found in two out of six cases of choriocarcinoma. The existence of asialo-hCG may be related to the advancement of disease. Therefore, the immunological detection of malignant transformational changes induced in carbohydrate moieties of hCG would be valuable for the early diagnosis and management of choriocarcinoma.

02.09.09

Determinent-differences in hydatidiform mole and choriocarcinoma: Sathiavathy, N. S.A.T. Hosp., Med. Coll., Trivandrum, Kerala, India

In recent years, study of trophoblastic tumors has attained special interest due to better diagnostic and treatment facilities. It was observed as early as 1951, by *Acosta-Sisin* et al. that the geographic and racial differences are the two important determinents responsible for the variation in the incidence of trophoblastic tumors. Along with these, the socio-demographic characteristics viz. age, parity, religion etc. and ABO blood group were looked into, in the present study for hydatidiform and choriocarcinoma separately, in order to find out the determinent differences in either group. A total of 115 cases of trophoblastic diseases were registered during the calendar years 1983 and 1984 in the S.A.T. Hospital, Medical College, Trivandrum, of which 103 were hydatidiform mole and 12 choriocarcinoma. Thus the incidence was found to be 1 : 206 in hydatidiform mole and 1 : 1771 in choriocarcinoma. A significant increase in the incidence of choriocarcinoma was noticed in the age group 35–49 years and in parity 4 and above. But no such remarkable difference was observed in the case of vesicular moles. The religious status of patients was also found to be very much associated with the higher incidence of choriocarcinoma and the difference was statistically significant (p < .01). As regards, the ABO blood group of patients, the present study showed a higher incidence in B group patients contrary to some other previous studies. Thus the risk of development of choriocarcinoma was found to be very high among Christians in Kerala, compared to other religions and the age and parity established a positive correlation. However, all these determinents showed no significant association as far as the vesicular mole cases were concerned.

02.10.01
Some epidemiologic factors of the mosaic cervical image on colposcopy: de la Fuente, F, Jurado, M, González Falcó, J, Madamba, A M, Oriol, A. Dept. Gyn. Univ. Clin. of Navarre, Pamplona, Spain
We compared the age, menarche, menopause, menstrual formula and cycle duration characteristics of women with mosaic cervical pattern with another group without mosaic. For this, we reviewed 10,051 clinical histories of women with routine colposcopic and cervical cytology exams, natives of Navarre, one of the areas with the lowest incidence of cancer of the uterine cervix in the world. There were 195 cases with mosaic (1.94%), a frequency similar to those areas with a greater incidence of squamous carcinoma of the cervix. Patients with mosaic pattern had an earlier menarche (12.84 ± 1.3) than the control group (13.4 ± 1.5) (p < 0.01), and a later menopause (51.2 ± 3.3), control (47.4 ± 5.8) (N.S.), the duration of the menstruation was 4.3 ± 1.27 days, control 4.1 ± 1.25 (p < 0.05). There were no significant differences in cycle lengths between both population groups. Patients with mosaic were significantly younger (mean age 30.9 ± 8.1) than the control groups (mean age 38.9 ± 12.5), (p < 0.0001) being most frequent in the 25–30 years age group (4.2%). After 40 years of age, the frequency of the mosaic patterns falls to a minimum (0.65%), however, it is important to take note that just before this decrease, in the 35–40 years age group, the mosaic pattern is associated with its maximum frequency (57%). These data speak in favor of a hormonal predisposing factor in the genesis of mosaic. Its gradual decrease in frequency after 30 years of age suggests that there may be two types of populations with mosaic, one which is cured spontaneously while the other progresses to dysplasia.

02.10.02
The importance of the epidemiologic factors – in the management of the pré-invasive carcinoma of the cervix: Salvatore, C A. Gyn. Clin., Univ. of São Paulo Med. School, São Paulo, Brazil
The management of the pre-invasive carcinoma of the uterine cervix cannot be the same for patients of the high risk group and low risk group.The follow-up of 328 cases of carcinoma *in situ* of the cervix and the high incidence (8 to 10%) of new carcinoma *in situ* in the patients of the high risk group, after two to five years of cervical amputation and total hysterectomy shows that in this group of patients, the conservative treatment should be possible only in well selected cases.

02.10.03
An initial report of a prospective study of 130 teenage girls with abnormal first cervical smears with regard to the long-term development of intra-epithelial neoplasia: Usherwood, M, Wolfendale, M, Symonds, M. Stoke Mandeville Hosp., Aylesbury, Bucks., UK
Out of 3500 teenage girls having first time cervical smears, we have found 130 with abnormal cytology. These girls have the characteristics of being heavier smokers, starting intercourse earlier and having more sexual partners than those with normal smears. They underwent colposcopy and viral investigation for wart virus (HPV), herpes virus and cytomegalovirus (CMV). They were randomly allocated to two groups; one was biopsied and treated with cryotherapy or laser vaporisation, and the other was followed up only cytologically. Colposcopy showed that there were 78% with the appearance of HPV infection. Herpes studies showed a 97% incidence of antibodies to herpes simplex virus. Of those biopsied one had invasive adenocarcinoma and 50% had CIN abnormalities with koilocytosis. Early results of follow-up question the need, however, for laser treatment of these teenage girls.

02.10.04
Cervical intra-epithelial neoplasia: The impact of long-term oral contraceptive use and smoking habits. Hellberg, D, Valentin, J, Nilsson, S. Dept. Obstet. and Gyn., Falun Hosp., Uppsala Univ. and Nat. Inst. Radiat. Protection, Uppsala, Sweden
Long-term use of oral contraceptives and smoking have both been associated with an increased frequency of cervical intra-epithelial neoplasia (CIN). It has been questioned if these effects are confounding with other risk factors for CIN. This case-control study includes 420 pregnant women, 140 with CIN, and two matched controls for each case. A questionnaire, which included 17 potential risk factors for CIN was

answered by 95% of all women. 155 women, who had recently used oral contraceptives (OC), answered also another questionnaire with details about their OC use. The initial statistical analyses with crude significance tests and analysis of variance revealed that only age at first intercourse, number of sexual partners and smoking were significantly associated with CIN. OC use in general tended to occur more frequently with CIN, but not significantly. Frequency of CIN increased by duration of OC use, and was significant with more than 60 months of OC use. Log-linear analyses, which included sexual factors, smoking and long-term OC use, only left number of sexual partners and smoking as significant and independent risk factors of CIN. The association between CIN and long-term OC use diminished when simultaneous adjustment was made for number of sexual partners and smoking, and vanished when use of barrier methods also was statistically controlled for. Sexual behavior and smoking in this study appear to be the only true risk factor of CIN, and the association between long-term OC use and CIN seems to be coincidental.

02.10.05
Cervical intra-epithelial neoplasia found by colposcopy in patients with negative cervical cytology and inflammatory changes: Kirkman R J E, Peel, J, Sharp, F. Centr. Hlth Clin., Sheffield, UK

Patients with cervical smears which show persistent "inflammatory" changes present a management problem in population screening. There are too many to refer to specialist colposcopy sessions, and repeated smear tests distress the patient and do not advance the diagnosis. Use of a colposcope with polaroid camera allows the work of a relatively inexperienced doctor in an outlying community clinic to be checked and supervised by a hospital-based specialist. Findings including Colpophotographs will be presented from a session screening patients with "negative" cytology but some abnormality not serious enough to have been referred to hospital. So far over 100 patients have been seen. In 66 the Index smear was "inflammatory" and of these 6 had CIN – 2 grade 1, 3 grade 2, 1 grade 3. In 23 out of the first 100 patients colposcopy confirmed no pre-malignancy and the patient was returned to routine (3 or 5 yearly) frequency of screening. The session is cost effective as a further screening procedure when the smear test is unhelpful, permitting a relatively inexperienced doctor to identify and refer to the Specialist those who require treatment, and cut down the unnecessary repeat smear tests on those confirmed to have no pre-malignant changes. The pick-up rate of CIN was high in a group who would not otherwise have had further investigation.

02.10.06
New colposcopic grading system in the diagnosis of early cervical neoplasia: Ahn, W S, Namkoong, S E, Lee, H Y, Kim, S J. Dept. Obstet. and Gyn., Cath. Med. Coll., Seoul, Korea

A colposcopic grading system for evaluation of severity of the transformation zone in the diagnosis of early cervical neoplasia was presented by several authors and reported good correlation between the histology of the directed biopsies and usual colposcopic grading, grade I, II and III. But it is difficult to obtain more detailed interpretation of grade I lesion between inflammation and dysplasia. This study was focused on the differentiation of chronic inflammatory disorders and dysplastic lesions of the cervix by using our new grading system, grade 0, I, II and III. Colposcopic grading was made according to vascular pattern, intercapillary distance, surface pattern and color tone opacity, clarity of demarcation (Grade 0; Benign squamous metaplasia, Grade I; Mild dysplasia, Grad II; Moderate dysplasia, Grade III; Severe dysplasia or more severe lesion). Total number of analysed biopsies performed at Precancerous Lesion Detection Clinic of Kangnam St. Mary's Hospital was 1517 cases, consisting of 944 cases of benign (62.1%), 347 cases of dysplastic lesion (22.8%) and 226 cases of more severe lesion (14.9%). The diagnostic accuracy of colposcopically directed biopsy, the final diagnosis did not differ by more than one grade from that of the directed biopsy diagnosis, was 97% in patients with benign lesion, 87.5% in mild dysplasia, 82.2% in moderate dysplasia and 90.1% in severe and more than severe dysplasia.

02.10.07
Colposcopy in the prospective follow-up of cervical human papilloma virus (HPV) lesions: Väyrynen, M, Syrjänen, K, Saarikoski, S, Castrén, O, Mäntyjärvi, R. Kuopio Univ. Centr. Hosp., Kuopio, Finland

As a part of the long-term prospective follow-up study conducted for women with cervical HPV (human papilloma virus) infections (either with or without CIN) to assess their natural history, the colposcopic data on 292 consecutive patients with the mean follow-up of 16 months are reported. The results are based on 786 colposcopies performed at 6-month intervals. Colposcopic findings are categorized into one of the following patterns: normal, warty, punctation, mosaicism, leukoplakia and combination. Colposcopic patterns bore an excellent correlation with the natural history of the HPV lesions, in that colposcopy was normal in 75% of the regressor (RE) lesions, in 38% of the persistors (PE), and in only 16% of the progressors (PR). The percentage of RE increased in parallel with the frequency of normal pattern. Leukoplakia and combination were the two most frequent (55.7%) patterns in PR lesions, as compared with only 16.4% in RE and in 33.2% of the PE. The same was true with the 15 lesions which progressed into (CIS), and were treated by cone. In the PR lesions, an abnormal colposcopic pattern was disclosed in 65% to 100%, as compared with 14% to 35% only in the RE group. In conclusion, the present study provides evidence that colposcopy is an applicable and accurate diagnostic method in assessing the cervical HPV lesions. Colposcopy also seems to have prognostic value in the follow-up of HPV lesions, in that a normal colposcopic pattern is frequently associated with regression and leukoplakia and combination are encountered more frequently than others in HPV lesions with CIN, shown to be more prone to progress.

02.10.08
Microcolpohysteroscopy and cone biopsy of the cervix in the management of cervical intra-epithelial neoplasia: Nava, G, Jordan, J A, Chan, K K, Wade-Evans, T. Birmingham & Midland Hosp. Women, Birmingham, UK
Cone biopsy of the cervix is widely used to treat cervical intra-epithelial neoplasia. Cone biopsy has complications. There is evidence that these are related directly to the length of the cone. If a method can be found whereby the position of the squamocolumnar junction (SCJ) in the endocervical canal can be assessed then the length of the cone biopsy can be tailored accordingly. Unnecessarily long cone biopsies could therefore be avoided and the complication rate reduced. Microcolpohysteroscopy (MCH) may allow one to assess location of the SCJ. This assertion was tested in the following study. 47 consecutive patients presenting with abnormal cervical cytology in whom the SCJ was not visible on colposcopic examination had MCH performed before cone biopsy of the cervix. The distance from the SCJ to the endocervix was successfully measured in 42 of these patients. The same measurements were made blindly on the histological specimen. Measurements at MCH correlate significantly with those on histology (Pearson product moment co-efficient 0.68, 0.75, $p < 0.001$). There were no complications attributable to MCH. It was concluded that (1) the method was simple to use; (2) it could accurately estimate the position of the SCJ; (3) it had no complications; (4) it could be used to tailor the length of the cone biopsy so a minimal amount of endocervical tissue would be removed; (5) the results of this study confirm the similar findings reported by *Soutter* et al. (*Soutter, W P, Fenton, D W, Gudgeon, P, Sharp, F.*, Brit. J. Obstet. Gyn. **91**, 712–715, 1984) in 13 patients.

02.10.09
Dynamics of epithelial atypicality with "FIAE" finding on cervix uteri: Kišmanov, M, Boškovski, R. Clin. Gyn. and Obstet. Med. Fac., Univ., Skopje, Yugoslavia
The dynamics of the epithelial atypicality with "FIAE" finding depends on the degree of the epithelial atypicality. Analysis is carried out on the material of colposcopy for the period of 1961 to 1979 on registered 2714 cases with "FIAE" on cervix uteri. Stagnation as a biological feature of basic hyperplasia is stated in 50% cases with this morphological change, dysplasia epithelialis gradus levioris stagnated in 50.44% cases, dysplasia epithelialis gradus gravis stagnated in 38.57% cases. The progression noticeably depended more on the degree of epithelial atypicality, in this way the basic hyperplasia progressed to dysplasia epithelialis gradus levioris and mediocris in 11.53% cases. The progression of dysplasia epithelialis gradus levioris in dysplasia epithelialis gradus mediocris and gravis is stated in 7.07% cases. In the same way the regression depended on the degree of epithelial atypicality. The cases of "FIAE" with basic hyperplasio in 38.46% regressed, dysplasia epithelialis gradus levioris in 42.47% cases, dysplasia epithelialis gradus mediocris spontaneously regressed in a lower degree of epithelial atypicality or disappeared in 15.5% cases, dysplasia epithelialis gradus gravis regressed in 11.42% cases. It can be concluded that the progression of morphological material of "FIAE" regions, noticeably depended on the degree of epithelial atypicality, while the regression was in inverse proportion to the degree of epithelial atypicality.

02.11.01
Update on hormonal effects: Goldzieher, J W. Baylor Coll. Med., Dept. Obstet. and Gyn., Houston, USA; **Hammerstein, J.** Abt. F. Gyn. Endokr., Sterilität & Familienplanung, Frauenklin. Klinikum Steglitz, FU, Berlin
There has been a reevaluation of the cardiovascular hazards attributed to all contraceptive uses. Careful reanalysis of the epidemiologic methods employed suggests major biases for confounded results. When reanalyzed, cardiovascular hazards seemed to be limited exclusively to smokers over 35. The whole question of thromboembolic disease must be reexamined because the error in clinical diagnosis vitiates all results obtained to date. Changes in plasma lipoproteins may be statistically significant but rarely exceed the normal range and the clinical significance is questionable. For any contraceptive method, risks and benefits must be evaluated with respect to age, reproductive status, diseases and psychological conditions as well as ethnic, geographic and political variables. Selected methods of contraception, including oral contraceptives, must be put into perspective within this framework, taking into consideration any beneficial extra-contraceptive effects. In selecting oral contraceptives, low-dose formulations should usually be given preference. In the authors' opinion, the pill is currently under-rated rather than over-rated in the majority of countries.

02.12.01
Epidemiology of hypertension in pregnancy: The effect of maternal age, marital status and gravidity: Newcombe, R G, Dalton, K J, Coles, E C. Dept. Obstet., Univ., Cambridge; Dept. Med. Statist. & Computing, Univ. of Wales Coll. Med., Cardiff, UK
Because some of the better-known epidemiological studies of hypertension in pregnancy are now relatively dated, we decided to take a fresh look at how its incidence relates to maternal age, to marital status and to gravidity. We have used the 55,142 pregnancies recorded by the Cardiff Birth Survey in 1970–79, and

such a large number of pregnancies has permitted effective separation from each other of these three inter-related factors. The CBS database is truly population-based, and it has few missing data (only 1.9%). We found that the incidence of hypertension in pregnancy increases with advancing maternal age, but decreases with advancing parity or gravidity. Irrespective of age, older women are at more risk of hypertension in pregnancy than are younger women, and teenagers have the lowest incidence of all. Irrespective of age, the incidence of hypertension is lowest in those previously delivered, and indeed the younger the woman the more does a previous delivery protect against hypertension. Previous abortions generally confer some protection against hypertension, though not as much as previous deliveries. It is interesting that in teenagers a previous abortion has virtually no protective effect against hypertension, whereas in the forties a previous abortion is as protective as is previous delivery itself. The incidence of hypertension is higher in the ever-weds than in the never-weds, and it also changes if a patient conceiving pre-nuptially is led to marry in haste.

02.12.02

The role of prostaglandine in the pathogenesis of EPH-gestotis: Katsoulov, A, Melamed, V, Milanov, S, Milkov, V, Kourtev, I. Inst. Obstet. and Gyn., Med. Acad., Sofia, Bulgaria
One of the latest aspects in the pathogenesis of EPH-gestosis, studied recently, is the role of prostaglandins (Pg): PgE_2 and PgF_2, and the compounds related to them – prostacyclin and thromboxine. The first studies showed that PgE_2 showed a decreased concentration, while PgF_2 showed an increased concentration in various substrates taken from pregnant women with EPH-gestosis (placenta, amniotic fluid, amniotic membranes, the umbilical cord, blood serum, urine). Later studies (*K. Hiller, M. Smith*) showed, however, that the placenta synthesized equal quantities of PgE_2 in normal pregnancies as well as in pregnancies with EPH-gestosis. These contradictory data gave grounds for the authors to study the PgE_2 concentration in different substrates (placenta, amniotic fluid, amniotic membranes) of pregnant women with and without EPH-gestosis. On the basis of the results obtained, the authors discuss the role of PgE_2 in the pathogenesis of EPH-gestosis.

02.12.03

6-keto prostaglandin F1a, thromboxane B2 and lipid peroxide levels in EPH-gestosis: A correlation with disease activity. Tsukatani, E, Haga, K, Itoh, K, Suzuki, H, Kunimoto, K, Nishiya, I. Dept. Obstet. and Gyn., Iwate Med. Univ., Morioka, Iwate, Japan
We studied the pathology of EPH-gestosis from the aspect of the relationship between prostaglandin (PG), prostanoid and lipid peroxide (MDA). Simultaneously, with the determination of 6-keto-PGF1a and thromboxane B2 (TxB2) in each stage of gestation and EPH-gestosis. Blood MDA was determined as index for abnormality in the metabolism of lipid which include abnormal PG metabolism, and the relationship between them was studied. The levels of 6-keto PGF1a, TxB2 was determined by RIA and identified by Gas-Mass. MDA was measured with Yagi's method. TxB2 and MDA showed a considerable increase. In contrast levels of 6-keto PGF1a are increased. The presently observed correlation between plasma MDA, TxB2 level and activity of EPH-gestosis is involved in these regulators of vascular tissues. In case EPH-gestosis, it shows significant increase with 6.63 ng/ml compared with mean levels at the tenth month of gestation. The difference being statistically significant at 5% level. Generally, TxB2 level tend to increase simultaneously with the onset of EPH-gestosis and decrease with time thereafter to became stabilized. However, in serious cases, 6-keto PGF1a was low compared with the mean value.

02.12.04

Plasma prostaglandin concentration and urinary immunoreactive prostaglandin levels of normal and pre-eclampsia: Yamaguchi, M, Mori, N. Dept. Obstet. and Gyn., Miyazaki Med. Coll., Miyazaki, Japan
Our previous studies (*Yamaguchi, M, Mori, N.*, Am. J. Obstet. Gyn., in press) have shown suppressed 6-keto $PGF_{1\alpha}$ levels in pre-eclamptic patients. However, urinary level of prostaglandins (PGs) is not definite in pregnant women. The purpose of this study is to investigate plasma and urinary levels of PGs. The blood samples were collected from 23 normotensive women and 15 pre-eclamptic patients. Urinary samples were collected from 23 normotensive women and 9 pre-eclamptic patients. Plasma PGs were extracted with etyhl acetate, purified by thin layer chromatography (TLC) and measured by specific radioimmunoassay (RIA). Urinary PGs were absorbed with Bondelut C18 column, eluted with 60% methyl alcohol, purified by TLC and measured by RIA. Urinary creatinine (cre) was also measured. Plasma 6-keto $PGF_{1\alpha}$ levels were 318.6 ± 58.0 pg/ml of normotensive pregnant women and 118.8 ± 16.4 pg/ml of pre-eclamptic patients. Plasma 6-keto $PGF_{1\alpha}$ level was significantly lower in pre-eclamptic patients than normotensive women. Urinary immunoreactive 6-keto $PGF_{1\alpha}$ level of pre-eclamptic patients was 105.3 ± 28.2 pg/cre, which was significantly lower than normotensive women (211.2 ± 33.8 pg/cre). Plasma and urinary thromboxane B_2 level showed no significant difference between normal and pre-eclamptic women. Although origin of urinary PGs is still controversial, our results may indicate an involvement of PGs in the pathophysiology of pre-eclampsia.

02.12.05

Is decidua affected in toxemia? Iino, K, Sjöberg, J*, Seppälä, M*. Dept. Obstet. and Gyn., Keio Univ., Tokyo, Japan; *Dept. I Obstet. and Gyn., Univ. Centr. Hosp., Helsinki, Finland
It is well-known that the placenta can be affected in toxemia. Little attention has been paid to decidual

disorders. Placental protein 12 (PP12) was recently shown to be synthesized by the decidua, but not by the placenta (*Rutanen* et al. Endocrinology, in press). We report here that the circulating levels of PP12 are elevated in toxemia. PP12 was measured by radioimmunoassay in the serum of 73 Finnish and 35 Japanese apparently healthy pregnant women between 32 and 40 weeks, and the results were compared with those of 33 patients with toxemia at similar weeks. There was no significant difference in the serum PP12 concentrations between Finnish and Japanese pregnant women. In toxemia, the serum PP12 values were significantly elevated in both the Finnish and the Japanese groups. Our results point to a decidual disorder in toxemia.

02.12.06
Immunologic studies in pregnant women with EPH-gestosis: Kozhuharova, M, Bogdanov, N, Mantov, S, Liniova, V A, Mirkov, K. Med. Acad., Ctr. Cardiovasc. Dis., 3rd City Hosp., Sofia, Bulgaria
Thirty-six women with normal pregnancy and 25 women with EPH-gestosis were studied for circulating antitissue antibodies, immunoglobulins and complement, using the antiglobulin-consumption test by *Steffen* and immunodiffusion by *Mancini*. The mean age of the patients was 23.7 ± 3.8 and 24.5 ± 4.7. The mean arterial pressure was $15.99/10.43$ kPa and $22.42 \pm 1.22/14 \pm 1.61$ kPa. The lowering of the values of IgG and the increasing of the values of IgD was significant in the group of pregnant women with EPH-gestosis and elevated level of $CH_{50} - 102.5$ HE/ml of complement factor C_3. The same patients were with higher of circulating immune complex and high per cent of circulating tissue antibodies (93.62%). The established immunological changes of pregnant women with EPH-gestosis are giving grounds for discussion of maternal-fetal immunological conflict.

02.12.07
A study on prolactin in toxemia of pregnancy: Lee, T Y, Huang, S C, Yang, Y S, Yang, K H. Dept. Obstet. and Gyn., Coll. Med., Nat. Taiwan Univ., Taipei, Taiwan
The present study investigates the relationship between prolactin levels and toxemia of pregnancy, and evaluates the usefulness of prolactin measurement in early pregnancy as a predictor of future development of toxemia of pregnancy. The clinical materials include 229 normal singleton pregnancies between the 6th and 40th weeks of gestation and 35 patients with toxemia of pregnancy. This included simultaneous assays of prolactin in maternal blood, cord blood and amniotic fluids in 19 patients with toxemia of pregnancy. Multiple pregnancy is frequently associated with manifestations of toxemia of pregnancy, therefore, six patients with twin pregnancy were also studied for comparison. The prolactin level was measured by radioimmunoassay. The prolactin levels in normal pregnancies were used to calculate the 10th, median and 90th centile of the normal range. The prolactin level increased with the progress of gestation, and reached a plateau after 31st week (ca. 120 ng/ml, median). The prolactin levels in toxemia of pregnancy seemed higher than those in normal pregnancy of corresponding gestation weeks, but the prolactin levels in twin pregnancy seemed to be similar to those of normal pregnancy. In summary, the prolactin seemed to be associated with the occurrence of toxemia of pregnancy, and higher prolactin levels were noted in toxemia of pregnancy.

02.12.08
The spectrum of renal lesions in pregnancies complicated by toxemia: Deniz, Y, Turfanda, T, Turfanda, A, Koçak, N, Babuna, C. Dept. Obstet. and Gyn., Istanbul Med. Fac., Istanbul, Turkey
The renal biopsies from 30 toxemic patients who presented with proteinuria, high blood pressure and edema during their repeated pregnancies have been reviewed. Biopsies were carried out to determine the nature of the underlying renal disease or to assess the severity of lesions and the chances of successful pregnancy in the future. Among these patients a biopsy diagnosis of underlying glomerulonephritis had been made in 16, chronic pyelonephritis in six, and pure pre-eclamptic toxemia in eight. All 22 patients with underlying chronic glomerulonephritis and pyelonephritis were found to have persisting clinical findings, urine abnormalities, and deteriorated renal functions after pregnancy which confirmed the diagnosis; whereas, patients with pure toxemia showed the return of normal renal functions and disappearance of urine abnormalities and clinical findings. Histological analysis of patients with glomerulonephritis revealed nine mesangioproliferative and membranoproliferative and three simple proliferative glomerulonephritis. Whereas in patients with pure pre-eclampsia seven showed mesangioproliferative and only one membranoproliferative changes. In six patients toxemia was found to be superimposed on a biopsy proven chronic pyelonephritis. In conclusion it can be said that the mesangioproliferative nephropathia is the most common histological lesion seen in both pure toxemia and in toxemias superimposed on an underlying renal disease.

02.12.09
Maternal serum levels of SP_1 in pregnant women with EPH-gestosis; Maticki, M. Dept. Obstet. and Gyn., Novi Sad, Yugoslavia
Maternal serum levels of a pregnancy specific beta-1 glycoprotein (SP_1) were measured by radial-immunodiffusion in 105 normal pregnancies in the period over 28 weeks of gestation. The control group was made of 142 pregnant women with EPH-gestosis distributed into weak, moderate and serious forms of the disease by Goeck's index. The results obtained indicate significant difference between the mean value

of maternal serum levels of SP_1 of the control group and each form of EPH-gestosis. Significantly decreased maternal serum levels of SP_1 were registered in all the forms of EPH-gestosis in pregnant women whose newborn infants demonstrated the signs of the retarded intrauterine growth while compared with the control group. Maternal serum SP_1 assay as an indicator of the retarded intrauterine growth in pregnant women with EPH-gestosis, suggests the limit value of the serum SP_1 of 140 mg/l SP_1. By estimation of the statistical data of the test efficiency, we found that sensitivity was 72.97%, prognostic value 62.69% while the relative risk was 6.30.

02.12.10
Urinary N-acetyl B-D glucosaminidase (NAG) levels in normal and hypertensive pregnancies: Beydoun, S N, Penso, C, Steele, B W, Abuhamed, A, Paz, J. Univ. of Miami, FL, USA
NAG is a lysosomal hydrolase that is elevated in urines with renal tubular damage. Urinary NAG levels in pregnancy have not been reported. The purpose of this study is to determine its levels in pregnancy, and to see if it can predict the development of pre-eclampsia. Urinary NAG levels were obtained in 12 non-pregnant, 55 presumed normal pregnant patients in the 2nd and 3rd trimesters, and in nine patients with clinical diagnosis of pre-eclampsia on $MgSO_4$ in labor. The levels obtained (in nmole hr^1creatinine^{-1}) were (non-pregnant 59.08 ± 28.4, 2nd trimester 122.2 ± 40.0, 3rd trimester 217.5 ± 100.2, and pre-eclamptic 498.25 ± 498.1). NAG levels were significantly lower in non-pregnant than in pregnant, and in 2nd trimester than in 3rd ($p < .01$). No significant difference was present between 3rd trimester and pre-eclamptics. The results obtained suggest: (1) Urinary NAG levels progressively increase in normal pregnancy suggesting that the physiologic hydronephrosis may be associated with transient renal tubular damage. (2) Are elevated above normal pregnancy values in those that develop pre-eclampsia as early as the 2nd trimester suggesting that renal tubular damage precedes hypertension and proteinuria (3) can, if obtained then, predict pre-eclampsia with a sensitivity of 100%, specificity of 94% and a predictive value of 75%.

02.12.11
Serum cortisol levels in hypertensive pregnancy patients: Tanaka, M, Furuhashi, N, Suzuki, M, Kyono, K, Kohno, H. Dept. Obstet. and Gyn., Tohoku Univ. School Med., Sendai, Japan
There has been no systematic study of hypertensive pregnancy in relation to the levels and physical state of serum cortisol, although serum cortisol levels in pregnancy have been studied. In this study, we measured the serum cortisol levels in 15 normal and eight hypertensive pregnancy primigravidas. The cortisol level of normal primigravida ($n = 15$, 47.1 ± 14.7 μg/dl, mean $\pm$ S.D.) was significantly ($p < 0.04$) higher than that of hypertensive pregnancy patients ($n = 8$, 33.8 ± 9.4 μg/dl). Especially, four severe hypertensive pregnancy patients had a significant ($p < 0.03$) lower cortisol level ($n = 4$, 32.5 ± 10.5 μg/dl) than that of normal. The lower maternal cortisol level of hypertensive pregnancy patients became more significant with the severity of clinical symptoms of hypertensive pregnancy. After the onset of labor, the cortisol levels of hypertensive pregnancy patients did not rise compared with normal pregnancy. These data suggests that in the hypertensive pregnancy patient the responsibility of the adrenal cortex to adrenocorticotropic hormone (ACTH) may be weak or the cortisol production in the adrenal cortex may decrease because of the insufficient tissue circulation due to hypertensive pregnancy.

02.12.12
Weight gain during pregnancy and perinatal mortality: Barreto, M G, Sabatino, H, Herrman, V, Pinotti, J A. Dept. Obstet. and Gyn., State Univ., Campinas, Brazil
The pregnant women were distributed into three groups according to weight gain during pregnancy. Group 1: 413 deliveries with a perinatal mortality rate of 9.7%. Female patients included: from 14 kg lost up to a weight gain of 5 kg. Group 2: 779 deliveries with a prenatal mortality of 6%. Gain with between 6 to 10 kg. Group 3: 742 deliveries with a perinatal mortality of 1.6%. Gain weight of 11 kg or more. The difference between these groups were highly significant ($p < 0.001$). When a correlation between these three groups and the 21 selected intermediary variables is made, we observed a statistically significant relationship between weight gain and: maternal height, prenatal care, twin births, method of delivery; clinical gestational age; newborn weight, newborn height, and weight of the placenta. Not considered significant was the relationship of the variables indicated below: weight gain versus age of mother, marital status, schooling of the mother, intergestational period, amniotic fluid, Apgar score at 1, 5 to 10 minutes; neonatal morbidity, fetal heart rate, the umbilical cord around the neck of the newborn. We concluded that there is an important relationship between weight gain and perinatal mortality in female patients belonging to the lower social classes but some intermediary variables could have influenced these results.

02.12.13
The correlation of renal functions to serum protein compositions and proteinuria in hypertensive disorders of pregnancy: Turfanda, A, Turfanda, T, Babuna, C, Karahan, U, Sivas, A. Dept. Obstet. and Gyn., Istanbul Med. Fac., Istanbul, Turkey
The correlation of renal functions to proteinuria and plasma protein composition have been studied by electrophoresis in 14 cases of toxemia and six cases of pregnancy complicated by chronic renal disease. No significant correlation had been found between the renal functions and the degree of proteinuria and plasma protein composition. But a positive correlation was found between the degrees of proteinuria and

the plasma protein composition; as the proteinuria gets more severe, the changes in plasma protein composition become more prominent. Total plasma protein concentration had been found to decline from 6.75 g/100 ml in normal pregnancy to 6.12 g/100 ml in mild and to 5.50 g/100 ml in severe pre-eclampsia. Albumin concentration also decreased from 3.10 g/100 ml to 2.55 g/100 ml in mild, and to 1.80 g/100 ml in severe pre-eclampsia. Whereas alpha 1 globulin concentration was about 0.46 g/100 ml both in normal and mild pre-eclampsia and increase to 0.60 g/100 ml in severe pre-eclampsia. Alpha 2 globulin also showed a sharp increase from 0.78 to 1.07 g/100 ml in mild and 1.28 g/100 ml in severe pre-eclampsia. Beta globulins decreased from 1.22 g/100 ml to 0.95 g/100 ml in mild and to 0.69 g/100 ml in severe cases. Gamma globulins have been found to decline to lower levels than those detected in normal pregnancies i.e. from 0.60 to 0.40 g/100 ml. Alpha 2 globulins have been found to be excreted in large amounts in the urines of all the patients with pre-eclampsia. No differences in the plasma protein composition were observed from those of normal pregnancy, in the patients with chronic renal disease of non-nephrotic type.

02.12.14
Serum lipids and lipoproteins in women with emesis gravidarum as compared to non-affected pregnant subjects and non-pregnant controls: Samsioe, G, Eriksson, B, Järnfelt-Samsioe, A, Mattson, L-Å. Dept. Obstet. and Gyn., Sahlgren's Hosp., East Hosp. and Nordic School Publ. Hlth., Göteborg Univ., Sweden
In the first trimester of pregnancy, nausea and vomiting or emesis gravidarum is so frequent that the condition is accepted as a symptom of pregnancy. The specific cause of this disorder is still unknown, but endocrine factors have been considered. A significant proportion of women who use oral contraceptives develop nausea. In this study we examined serum lipid and lipoprotein concentrations in 102 healthy pregnant women in early and late pregnancy. 62 subjects complained of emesis gravidarum. As pregnancy advanced serum cholesterol, triglycerides and phospholipids were elevated in all subjects due to an increase in all lipoprotein classes. Low-density lipoproteins (LDL) and high-density lipoproteins (HDL) were relatively enriched in triglycerides. In early pregnancy the lipid content of HDL was significantly lower in women with emesis gravidarum. In contrast, during the last trimester the total lipid content in all fractions was higher in women who had suffered from nausea and vomiting in early pregnancy. Thus, a metabolic difference between the nauseated, emetic women and non-affected subjects persisted throughout pregnancy. It is suggested that emesis gravidarum is related to a "functional stress" on the liver induced by hormones.

02.13.01
The pathogenic mechanisms of gonococcal salpingitis: Woods, M L, McGee, Z A. Univ. of Utah, Salt Lake City, UT, USA
Despite available effective antimicrobials and public health programs, gonococcal infections including salpingitis remain a major world-wide problem resulting in significant rates of infertility. Using an experimental model of infected human Fallopian tubes in organ culture examined by light, scanning an transmission electron microscopy, basic pathogenic interactions between the Fallopian tube and the gonococcus have been elucidated. These include attachment, damage, and invasion. Attachment appears to result from interaction of gonococcal pili and the tips of microvilli of nonciliated cells. After gonococcal attachment occurs, Fallopian tube damage is evident with loss of ciliary activity and sloughing of ciliated cells. The mediators of this damage appear to be gonococcal lipopolysaccharide which is released from the surface of the organism in outer membrane blebs and monomeric units of peptidoglycan which are elaborated by the organism. Gonococcal attachment appears to initiate phagocytosis by nociliated epithelial cells. Gonococci are transported to the base of the cell and are released into the subepithelial space. This may lead to local disease (salpingitis) or disseminated disease (dermatitis-arthritis). Understanding the molecular mechanisms by which gonococci attach to, damage or invade the Fallopian tube mucosa may identify ways of preventing gonococcal infections and their sequealae.

02.13.03
Sulbactam-ampicillin versus metronidazole-gentamicin in the treatment of obstetric and gynecologic infections: Crombleholme, W*, Landers, D, Ohm-Smith, M, Robbie, M O, Hadley, W K, DeKay, V, Dahrouge, D, Sweet, R L. Univ. of California, San Francisco, CA, USA
The clinical efficacy and safety of Sulbactam/Ampicillin (SA) versus Metronidazole/Gentamicin (MG) were evaluated in a comparative, randomized, prospective study. Thirty-nine patients were treated: SA in 20 and MG in 19. There were 30 cases of severe acute PID with peritonitis, 3 tubo-ovarian abscesses (TOAs), 4 endomyometritis, and 2 post hysterectomy pelvic cellulitis. Aerobic and anaerobic cultures from the sites of infection yielded 259 microorganisms from 38 patients; an average of 6.8 bacteria per infection (3.9 anaerobes and 2.9 aerobes). The most frequent isolates were Bacteroides sp. 21, B. bivius 13, B. disiens 8, Fusobacterium sp. 9, Peptostreptococcus anaerobius 15, P. asaccharolyticus 8, anaerobic gram pos. cocci 17, G. vaginalis 24, N. gonorrhoeae 14, alpha-hemolytic streptococci 6, and E. coli 3. Clinical cure was noted in 19/20 SA treated and 16/19 MG treated patients. The sulbactam-ampicillin failure was a PID patient with a positive C. trachomatis culture who required anti-chlamydial therapy. The metronidazole-gentamicin failures include a tubo-ovarian abscess requiring surgical drainage and 2 chlamydia positive PID patients requiring anti-chlamydia treatment. No adverse hematologic, renal, or hepatic effects were noted with either regimen.

02.13.04

A single blind comparative study of parenteral sublactam/ampicillin versus clindamycin/gentamicin in female patients with serious pelvic infection: Gunning, J E. Harbour/UCLA Med. Ctr., Torrance, CA, USA

The purpose of this study is to determine the efficacy and safety of sublactam and ampicillin coadministered *i. v.* in treatment of polymicrobial infection and to compare it to a standard therapeutic regimen of clindamycin and gentamicin. The diagnosis of salpingitis with or without pelvic abscess was established by clinical symptoms and signs, culdecentesis revealing purulent meterial, and ultrasound. Peritoneal fluid was cultured for aerobes and anaerobes. The cervix was cultured for GC and chlamydia. All isobates were tested for sensitivity to the study drugs. Sixty patients were randomized into the two treatment regimens. In the sublactam/ampicillin group, 19 of 20 (95%) evaluable patients had bacteriological cure and 27 of 30 (90%) had clinical cure. In the clindamycin/gentamicin group, 19 of 19 (100%) evaluable patients had bacteriological cure and 28 of 30 (93%) had clinical cure. No serious adverse side-effects were noted in either group. Sublactam/ampicillin is equally as effective as clindamycin/gentamicin as a treatment regimen for patients with serious pelvic infection.

02.13.05

Sulbactam/Ampicillin vs. cefoxitin in gynecological infections: Senft, H-H[1], Stiglmayer, R, Eibach, H W, Körner, J. [1]Malteserkrankenhaus, Bonn

Sulbactam (S) is a betalactamase inhibitor which expands the spectrum of Ampicillin (A) to most betalactamase producing strains. A randomized clinical trial comparing Sulbactam/Ampicillin (S/A) with Cefoxitin (CXT) was performed. This report deals with the preliminary results of 49 female patients suffering from gynecological infections including pelveoperitonitis, endometritis, salpingitis, tuboovarialabscess. The dosage of S/A was 1 g S and 2 g A t.i.d. and that of CXT 2 g t.i.d. Clinical cure was achieved in 22/25 (88%) patients with S/A and 18/24 (75%) with CXT. Improvement in 3/25 (12%) with S/A and 2/24 (8,3%) with CXT. There was no clinical failure with S/A and 4/24 (16%) with CXT. Most frequent organisms were S. faecalis, E. coli and Staphylococci. In microbiological testing there were found 2 Staphylococci, 2 E. coli, 1 Enterobacter, 1 Klebsiella resistant to A but susceptible to S/A. 7 strains were susceptible to CXT but resistant to A. However, 18 S. faecalis, 4 E. coli and 2 Streptococci were resistant to CXT but susceptible to A. Side-effects were observed: diarrhoea (3 CXT), transient eosinophilia (2 S/A, 1 CXT), transient elevation of transaminases (1 S/A, 2 CXT), candida colpitis (3 S/A, 3 CXT), pruritus (1 S/A) and transient exanthema in 4 patients treated with S/A. Other laboratory tests remained normal including serum creatinine and Quick's value. The results confirmed that S/A is an effective and well tolerated treatment of gynecological infections and may also be used in infections caused by bacteria that are resistant to A alone.

02.13.06

Sulbactam-ampicillin in the treatment of obstetric and gynecologic infections: Hemsell, D L. Univ. of Texas Hlth. Sci. Ctr., Parkland Memo. Hosp., Dallas, TX, USA

Although effective as a therapeutic regimen for women with milder forms of obstetric and gynecologic pelvic infections, ampicillin alone is not effective in the treatment of more serious or complicated pelvic infections. A major reason for this is that many of the pathogens of these polymicrobial infections have as a major mechanism of resistance the production of β-lactamase enzymes. Addition of a β-lactamase inhibitor to an inexpensive but susceptible β-lactam antibiotic such as ampicillin should significantly increase efficacy. Sulbactam, a penicillanic acid sulphone derivative, has no antibacterial activity by itself, with the notable exception of Neisseria genorrhoeae, and has been shown to be an irreversible inhibitor of several important β-lactamases. (*Retsema, J A* et al., Antimicrob. Agents Chemother. **17**, 615, 1980; *Greenwood, D* and *Eley, A,* J. Antimicrob. Agents Chemother. **10**, 117, 1982). Enhancement of the *in vitro* activity of ampicillin against 272 anaerobic strains, including 70 Bacteroides fragilis, by the addition of sulbactam was reported by *Wexler* et al. (Antimicrob. Agents Chemother. **27**, 876, 1985). Susceptibility increased from 76.2% to 99.6% at 16 μg/ml. The combination of sulbactam and ampicillin has been given to women with pelvic infections in several different medical centers. Comparative control regimens evaluated have included metronidazole and gentamicin, clindamycin and gentamicin, and cefoxitin. Data from these prospective, randomized, comparative clinical trials will be summarized.

02.14.01

Prenatal ultrasonic diagnosis of umbilical cord pathology and fetal sex: Pelosi, M A. Univ. of Med. and Dent., New Jersey Med. School, NJ, USA

This scientific exhibit illustrates and demonstrates that pathologic condition of the umbilical cord (cord prolapse, true knots, nuchal cord, cord hematoma, cysts of the cord, and single umbilical artery) can be easily detected in the prenatal period by ultrasound as an office procedure and that the physiopathologic effects can be confirmed by the nonstress test. The exhibit emphasizes the foreknowledge value in the clinical management and was based upon 3000 patients from the author's private practice. In addition, the second section of the exhibit illustrates ultrasonographic techniques used in the determination of fetal sex in each trimester of pregnancy.

02.14.02

Application of reflectance spectrophotometry to the monitoring of fetal oxygenation during labor: Shimizu, K, Sato, N, Kawano, S, Tanizawa, O. Perinat. Ctr. & 1st Dept. Med., Osaka Univ., Osaka, Japan
The reflectance spectrophotometer which is equipped with a bifurcated optical fiber and a linear array photodiode allows one to analyse coloration of the living tissues non-invasively. Using this device, we have already succeeded in estimating oxygen saturation of the fetal presenting part from the absorption spectrum of hemoglobin in the tissue capillaries. (*Shimizu, K* et al. In: Transcutaneous Blood Gas Monitoring. ed. by *Huch & Huch, Dekker,* 1983). An application of this device for fetal monitoring was tested by comparing the values measured photo-optically from the fetal tissues and those measured in the blood collected from the umbilical vessels. For the reflectance spectrophotometry, TS-200 Tissue Spectrum Analyser, Sumitomo Elect. Co., Osaka and MCPD-200 Multichannel Spectroanalyser, Union Giken Co., Osaka, for the blood gas analysis, Combi Analysator MT-A100 Eschweiler, Kiel and OSM2 Hemoximeter, Radiometer Copenhagen were used. As the levels of fetal tissue oxygenation were observed to fluctuate widely in relation to the uterine contractions, the highest value observed 30 minutes before delivery was chosen as the representative for the levels of fetal oxygenation (F). The value F was found to have a good correlation both to oxygen saturation ($r = 0.67$, $n = 44$, $p < 0.01$) and to pH ($r = 0.61$, $n = 44$, $p < 0.01$) of the umbilical artery. These results suggest that the device could be used for the screening of fetal hypoxia during labor.

02.14.03

Pan-endomicroscopy for diagnosis in gynecology: Ohkawa, K, Ohkawa, R. Kanagawa, Japan
Atempts have been made with a special Pan-endomicroscope using high magnification to study cells *in vivo* without biopsy. – Material and methods: Pan-endomicroscopes permit forward and lateral observation and are 8 mm diameter and 360 mm long, made by Machida Co. For supervital staining of nuclei the cresyl violet acetate and thionin were used. – Results: In pan-endomicroscopic findings of vulva, vaginal wall, and portio vaginalis, 22,520 cases were tested. In these cases 22,140 cases of ectopy, inflammation and transformation were found. In 580 cases of pan-endomicropy of cervix canal 44 cases of dysplasia and 22 cases of cancer were found. In the 259 cases of pan-endomicroscopy of endometrium, 52 cases of cancer, and 207 of hyperplasia and bleeding were found. In 260 cases of pregnancy the pan-endomicroscopic findings of abortion, atrophy, chorioadenoma and choriocarcinoma were found. – Conclusion: With miniature pan-endomicroscope which can be inserted into various sites within the body, it is practicable to make microscopic observation of the surface of tissue. The cresyl violet acetate is remarkably useful for the purpose of diagnosis.

02.14.04

Advances in research, training, application and control of methods for fertility regulation. Support for reproductive health care projects: Kurz, K H. IRIR, Int. Res. Inst. Reprod., Düsseldorf
The organization in 1981 founded has the following innovations: Foldable gyne-chair of 8 kg weight, Cavimeter to measure length and widths of the individual uterine cavity prior to insertion of more fitting IUDs, IUD-Remover, endometrial biopsy clamp, battery lit Miniscope to detect intracervically divided IUD threads or the intrauterine presence of an IUD, improved specula and tenaculum for easy application of paracervical block and IUD insertion, jet-injector for low-risk-application of paracervical block, IPPIF-System, Immediately Post-Partum IUD Fixing System, female pelvic phantom with uterine models of several sizes and flexions for training of personnel for inserting IUDs, film and videofilm on improved intrautrine contraception, cell-count chamber for counting cells e. g. leucocytes in secretion, to detect infection of the female upper genital tract. IRIR periodically conducts education and training courses on all methods of fertility regulation including diagnosis, treatment and prevention of infertility. IRIR supports family planning projects in developing countries e. g. by delivering know-how, training facilities and means for contraception on the base of social marketing. IRIR is a registered non-profit-making organization.

02.14.05

Extradural analgesia in patients showing high obstetric risk (bupivacaine, 0.75%): Ulloa-Muñoz, O. Santiago Chile
Introduction: This work, which intends only to have an illustrative nature, concerns the measures we adopt in order to prevent multiple changes that often occur in the "high obstetric risk" group, which might produce problems during anesthesia, both to the mother and to the newborn baby. The study will serve as the basis for an evaluation survey on "high risk in obstetrics" in patients, confined after the earthquake which took place on March 3, 1985 in Chile. – Summary: Epidural analgesia is a very valuable technique used in Cesarean sections. Results therefrom could be improved as arterial hypotension affecting the mother is avoided and local anesthetic agents with higher analgesic action are used, which present the least possible severe fetal repercussion. We now present the results of epidural analgesia in a sample of 800 patients showing high obstetric risk, scheduled for elective Cesarean section during the years 1983 and 1984 (i. e., prior to the earthquake of March 3, 1985 in Chile). This programme involved in-patients of similar clinical characteristics who belong to a definite social stratum and had been covered by a maternity preventive programme. The anesthetic agent used bupivacaine, 0.75% ("Bupivan", Abbott), a monodrug

with no adrenaline content. Special attention was given to prophylaxis, detection and prompt treatment of maternal hypotension. "Syntocinon" (a synthetic oxytocin) was used. The analgesia had excellent results in all patients. Surgical conditions were satisfactory in the opinion of the surgeons involved. Both vital condition and tolerance level in respect of maternal stress upon the newborn children were rated as "high" according to the APGAR score. – Comments (Referred to the patient's socio-economic context): It is very hard to disregard the socio-economic and emotional conditions affecting patients after an earthquake of the magnitude and intensity of the one which recently affected Chile (March 1985), with a view to consider pregnancy and anesthesia as isolated events which offer no explanation. A great number of mothers who live in conditions of extreme poverty count with very few possibilities to come out of it without any help, since they can hardly cover their daily minimum needs (housing, health, nutrition, etc.). Solutions become every day more unattainable; they finally learn to live in this deficient condition and this learning process is transmitted from one generation to the next. The poverty cycle is thus originated, which is increasingly more difficult to break. A mother who is poor will always have poor children; these poor children need from the very moment they are conceived, adequate feeding if it is intended that they start their life in similar conditions to the children of mothers belonging to the medium or high segments of population. If this is not the case, they may start their lives affected by brain handicaps which will rarely allow them later on to integrate themselves to human society in a normal way. Adolescent mothers who belong to the same minimum acceptable living conditions to those of the groups of women who have a lower quality level of life are affected by a more severe situation due to the social abandonment. Thus the habit is acquired towards a form of life full of permanent difficulties which definitely hinder their basic needs. The positive results of eradicating the high risk are not achieved through merely understanding the problem or through emphasizing the importance of a maternal prevention programme. It is imperative to apply a different strategy which comes closer to each individual patient. With a view to uprooting the high risks at their descendance level, it is necessary to give the same opportunities to all pregnant women, in order that their children are born in good condition, as happens with other women who belong to better economic strata. Family integration is the best means we envisage so that mothers who are in an irregular affective situation (adolescents, couples who live together but are not married or others who are affected by extreme poverty) may satisfactorily face their pregnancy and their children may enjoy a normal development, instead of allocating costly budgets to social prevention plans.

02.28.01

Correlation between the ultrasound and hormonal findings in induced ovulations: Bogdanov, S, Empy, Palčevski, G, Sahpazov, M. Obstet. and Gyn. Clin., Univ., Skopje, Yugoslavia

The growth of the human ovarian follicle has been observed by 58 patients, who were treated for sterility. In the earlier cycle it has been proved that there was no growth of the follicle. The stimulation has been executed by Clomiphen, Pergonal and HCG. The longest and the shortest diameter from the internal side of the follicle were measured and their number as well, starting on the eight day of the cycle. At the same time the E_2 was observed everyday. Comparing the ultrasound findings and the E_2 observations we came to the conclusion that they are in linear correlations and two days after their maximum (21 – 23 mm follicle and 450 ± 20 nmol/l) the ovulation appeared. The BT has been measured in all patients and it was biphasic. Working in this way we could control the growth of the follicle, the hypo/hyperstimulation and determine precisely the fertility day.

02.28.02

Ultrasonic and hormonal evaluation of dysfunctional ovarian cyst as a cause of infertility in regularly cycling women: Eissa, M K, Hudson, K, Sawers, R S, Newton, J R. Dept. Obstet. and Gyn., Birmingham Maternity Hosp., Birmingham, UK

Serial ultrasound monitoring of ovarian follicular growth in a group of regularly cycling but infertile women detected abnormal patterns of follicular growth. Scanning and venepuncture for hormone estimation were performed daily from menstrual day 7 until the mid-luteal phase. In 15 cycles in 11 patients, the leading follicle failed to rupture at mid-cycle and continued to grow, forming a cyst in the luteal phase. The hormone profiles of follicle stimulating hormone (FSH) luteinizing hormone (LH) estradiol (E_2) and progesterone (P), when compared with those of 17 conception cycles showed a marked reduction in the E_2 and P surges. The studies so far show that ultrasound can easily detect this abnormality and it can be differentiated from other dysfunctions as luteinized unruptured follicles. Also it seems that this abnormality is not entirely persistent.

02.28.03

Importance of simultaneous serum estradiol measurement and sonography to recognize multiple follicular maturation in ovulation induction by HMG and clomiphen: Steffen, R, Birkhäuser, M H, Wiget, D, Huber, P R, Eppenberger, U. Dept. Obstet. and Gyn., Univ. of Basle, Kantonsspit., Basle, Switzerland

One hundred and ten human menopausal gonadotropin (HMG) and 70 clomiphen citrate induced cycles have been regularly controlled by sonography and by serum estradiol determination. The day before ovulation, real time ultrasound measurement revealed in the gonadotropin group one dominant follicle (DF) in 54%, 2 DF in 29% and 3 DF in 17%; the respective data for the clomiphen citrate group were 61%, 30% and 9%. In both groups serum estradiol levels showed significant differences in the extent of the preovulatory increase according to the maturation of 1, 2 or 3 dominant follicles. In the gonadotropin group, mean serum estradiol values were 2.3 nmol/l in the patient group showing 1 DF, 4.8 nmol/l in the group showing 2 DF respectively 6.0 nmol/l in the group showing 3 DF ($p < 0.01$), showing a parallelism of serum estradiol and ultrasound examination in patients with high risk of potential multiple pregnancy. Thus the rise of serum estradiol allowed the differentiation between mature follicles and functionless cystic formations. From these data it can be concluded that combined monitoring by ultrasound and serum estradiol measurements may be essential to reduce the multiple pregnancy rate consecutive on stimulation of follicular maturation.

02.28.04

Prospective diagnosis of the ovulation by ultrasound: Mendes Pereira, D H, Souza, A Z, Salvatore, C A. Gyn. Clin., Univ. of São Paulo Med. School, São Paulo, Brazil

The author has investigated fifteen eumenorrheic infertile patients and the proposition of this research was: (1) The accuracy of the pelvic echography in the diagnosis of ovulation. (2) The medium follicular diameter on the day preceding ovulation. (3) The relation between the medium follicular diameter and the E-3 plasma concentrations. (4) The analysis of the basal body temperature chart in relation to the follicular eclosion. The method devised for this study was: serial pelvic echography in the follicular, peri-ovulatory and luteal phases; plasmatic FSH, and E-2 determinations in the peri-ovulatory period and progesterone dosage in the luteal phase; cervical mucus and basal body temperature chart evaluation. The analysis of the results led to the following conclusions: (1) The serial pelvic echography was the best method for detecting ovulation when compared to the hormonal determinations, the basal body temperature chart and the cervical score. The total collapse of the follicle was observed in 76.5% of the cycles and the partial collapse in 23.5% of them. (2) The medium follicular diameter on the day preceding ovulation was $22.6\% \pm 1.7$ mm, ranging from 18.6 mm to 26.0 mm.

02.28.05

Monitoring of ovulation induction by measurement of vaginal fluid volume: Broer, K H, Scholze, R, Schumacher G F B. Dept. Obstet. and Gyn., Cologne-Porz

Earlier investigations using the method of cervico-vaginal fluid aspiration have shown a good correlation between the hormonal levels of estradiol, LH, progesteron during the pre- and post-ovulatory period and the volume charges of cervico-vaginal secretion. Using the especially designed fluid aspirator, which is self-administered by the woman, we studied the volume profile during ovulation induction therapy including treatment of HMG/HCG, clomiphen, bromocriptine. In combination with ultrasound-folliculometry, E_2, LH and progesteron the cervico-vaginal fluid aspiration served as a method to monitor the effect of treatment. There was a statistically good correlation between these parameters in 60 observed cycles. Especially the increase of E_2 during the pre-ovulatory phase of HMG/HCG induction correlated well with the increasing volume of the cervico-vaginal fluid. It was possible to predict the occurrence of ovulation in untreated and the treated cycles as well. These results of our investigation based on the data of 60 cycles indicate, that the method of cervico-vaginal fluid self-measurement will be a useful approach to the monitoring of the hormonal events and will therefore be a time- and cost-saving procedure since it allows a reduction in the number of serum hormone determinations.

02.28.06

Endocrine and echographic patterns in pulsatile Gn-Rh induced ovulatory cycles: Mancuso, S, Caruso, A, Lanzone, A, Fulghesu, A M, Pilloni, D, Massidda, M, Depau, L. Dept. Obstet. and Gyn., Univ., Cagliari, Italy

Ovulation induction in five patients with primary hypogonadotropic amenorrhea (PHA) was carried out by i. v. pulsatile Gn-Rh (15 cycles of treatment) with doses ranging from 2.5 to 12.5 µg every 90 min. Follicular development was monitored by daily ultrasound scanning and plasma E_2 assay. Ovulation occurred during Gn-Rh treatment in eight cycles (A) or after i. m. HCG administration (5,000–10,000 IU) (B; n = 7). HCG was also given after ovulation with the purpose of maintaining the function of corpus luteum. For pregnancies (A = 2; B = 2) were obtained. Our data show: (1) Ovulatory follicular diameter was 19.7 ± 63 mm; no difference between conceptive (C) and non-conceptive (NC) (17.6 ± 49 vs 19.0 ± 60 mm) or A and B cycles (17.5 ± 74 vs 21.8 ± 47 mm) was observed; (2) E_2 preovulatory levels were similar in A and B, although a greater variability in B was seen (311 ± 86 vs 442 ± 274 pg/ml); (3) Ovulation occurred in 16.8 ± 6.3 days (d) and, in relation to Gn-Rh doses, the time employed was: $2.5 \mu g$–12.3 ± 2.5 d; $5 \mu g$–15.7 ± 6.6 d (NC = 19.2 ± 4.9; C = 13.3 ± 0.5): 10–$12.5 \mu g$: 21 ± 10.8 d ($p < 0.5$ NS); (4) No complication or ovarian hyperstimulation was observed. Our data indicated that pulsatile Gn-Rh is a "physiological" way of inducing ovulation in PHA patients. Furthermore no significant difference between C and NC or A and B cycles was noted.

02.28.07

Possible relationship between the pre-ovulatory follicle size and the abortion rate in HMG/HCG induced pregnancies: Ben-Nun, I, Gruber, A, Abramowicz, J, Fejgin, M, Altaras, M, Ben-Aderet, N. Dept. Obstet. and Gyn. "A", Sapir Med. Ctr., Kfar Saba, Israel

The outcome of HMG/HCG induced pregnancies using a newer treatment protocol is reviewed. The gonadotropin treatment was monitored by estrogen measurements and ovarian sonography, but the estimation of follicular maturation and the timing of ovulation induction based exclusively on ultrasonic follicular measurements (dominant follicle ≥ 19 mm). In general there was a poor correlation between the dominant follicle size and estrogen secretion. HMG dosage was individually adjusted in an effort to balance estrogen rise with pace of follicular development. Estrogen levels at the time of ovulation induction ranged between 348 and 3000 pg/ml E_2. So far in a series of 23 pregnancies 15 were delivered (one set of quadruplets, 6 sets of twins and 8 singletons). Eight women are still pregnant in various gestational ages. These preliminary results are in contrast with the high abortion rate (25%–30%) following gonadotropin therapy in which cervical score and/or estrogens are used for estimation of follicular maturity. It appears that the use of follicular measurement as an index of maturity may improve the rate of success of gonadotropin therapy.

02.28.08

The significance of the different parameters for detection of ovulation: Rabinowitz, R, Malaach, D, Yarkoni, S, Schenker, J G. Dept. Obstet. and Gyn., Hadassah Univ. Hosp., Jerusalem, Israel

In search for the best method for detection of the estimated day of ovulation, 47 spontaneously ovulating women were studied. Serum E_2, LH and progesterone levels were measured every one to two days together with basal body temperature, cervical mucus arborization and follicular measurement by ultrasonography. Ovulation was found to occur 33 hrs ± 3.8 SEM after the peak of estradiol (E_2), 25.9 hrs ± 1.64 SEM after LH surge and 33.2 hrs ± 4.4 SEM after BBT rise. Peak serum E_2 was 278.1 pg/ml ± 17.4 SEM, mid-luteal progesterone was 6.4 ng/ml ± 0.6 SEM. Maximal cervical mucus arborization was observed on the estimated day of ovulation in 64.5% of the women. Peak follicular diameter, as observed on ultrasound, was 21.5 cm ± 0.7 SEM. The good correlation between follicular diameter and serum E_2 renders this combination a most reliable method for detection of ovulation in spontaneously ovulating women.

02.28.09

Assessment of follicular maturation by plasma estradiol levels and ultrasound in the normal and clomiphene stimulated menstrual cycles: Chang, Y S, Lee, J Y, Moon, S Y, Lim, Y T. Dept. Obstet. and Gyn., Seoul Nat. Univ., Seoul, Korea

Follicle monitoring in the normal and clomiphene cycles was analysed in the Seoul IVF Program. Ovarian follicular diameter was measured by real-time sector scanner and plasma estradiol levels were assayed radioimmunologically. There was a good statistical correlation between the mean follicular diameters and the plasma estradiol levels in normal and clomiphene cycles. The mean diameters of leading follicles in clomiphene and normal cycle were 21.3 ± 3.4 mm and 19.2 ± 0.8 mm, respectively. The peak levels of plasma estradiol in clomiphene and normal cycle were 1053.8 ± 553.6 pg/ml and 298.3 ± 39.6 pg/ml, respectively. Daily growth rates of follicular diameter in clomiphene and normal cycle were 2.1 mm and 1.9 mm, respectively. Mean follicle numbers of clomiphene and normal cycle were 2.3 ± 1.1 and 1.1 ± 0.2, respectively. Plasma estradiol level per follicle was 461.8 ± 24.1 pg/ml in the clomiphene cycle. Our data revealed that mean follicular diameter and estradiol level prior to hCG administration in IVF & ET should reach 17.8 ± 3.0 mm and 949.4 ± 487.1 pg/ml in the clomiphene cycle. Ultrasound was shown to be complementary to plasma estriol levels in the assessment of follicular maturation because the number and diameter of ovarian follicles could be measured by daily ultrasound monitoring.

02.28.10

Prediction of conception in induced cycles by periovulatory serum 17β estradiol pattern: Brzezinski, A, Navot, D, Laufer, N, Margalioth, E, Birkenfeld, A, Schenker, J G. Hadassah Univ. Hosp., Dept. Obstet. and Gyn., Jerusalem, Israel

Recently it has been demonstrated that a high degree of correlation exists between the periovulatory pattern of serum 17β estradiol (E_2) secretion and the conception rate in patients undergoing in vitro fertilization. The present study was undertaken in order to assess prospectively the association between the periovulatory serum E_2 pattern and conception in hMG-hCG induced cycles of anovulatory infertile women. Thirty women treated with hMG were daily monitored for serum E_2 levels starting three days before the day of hCG administration (day 0) and up to three days later. Fifty cycles of treatment were studied. The patients were divided, according to their response to hMG-hCG into two groups of E_2 patterns: group A – an increase of E_2 levels on the day following hCG administration (day +1); group B – a decrease of E_2 levels on day +1. Sixteen pregnancies were achieved from the 50 cycles of treatment (32%), of which 14 (88%) occurred in women responding in an A pattern. High response pattern (A_1) occurred in 11 (69%) of the pregnancies. Of the 34 infertile cycles 20 (59%) demonstrated pattern B. In summary, unlike the events occurring in the spontaneous ovarian cycle, in which E_2 declines after the LH surge, we demonstrated that in induced cycles women responding in an A pattern, i.e. an increase in E_2 after hCG administration, have the highest rate when compared to group B pattern.

02.28.11

Changes in the breast telethermography during the cycle as a predictor of ovulation: Aviño, J, Pellicer, A, Bonilla-Musoles, F, Martinez, P. Med. School, Valencia, Spain

Shah et al. demonstrated an increase of the temperature of a selective point in the breast related to an increase in the E_2 production during the cycle. Our purpose was to evaluate this finding as a monitoring test to predict ovulation in programs of induced pregnancies (AID & IVF). Twenty-five women from our IVF program and 15 from AID, were subjected daily to breast temperature measurements at four different points until they have ovulated and one to two times during the luteal phase. These results were compared with the other monitoring methods (BT, E_2, ultrasound). We noted an increase in breast temperature near ovulation (E_2 peak) but no values were found to predict ovulation like E_2-peak or LH-Sir.

02.28.12

Ultrasonography in 1019 women with menstrual problems: Zaidi, S. Ultrasound Clin., Nazimabad, Karachi, Pakistan

Ultrasonography was performed on 1019 women referred because of various menstrual problems. These included: 35 girls (3.43%) with primary amenorrhoea, 94 women (9.22%) with secondary amenorrhoea, 435 (42.88%) with menorrhagia, 51 (5%) with polymenorrhagia, 154 (15.11%) with hypo- and oligomenorrhoea, 25 (2.45%) with postmenopausal bleeding, and the rest with other menstrual disturbances. Of girls with primary amenorrhoea, 9 (25.71%) had no uterus, 15 (42.86%) had small uteri, and 1 (2.86%) had haematocolpos. Of women with menorrhagia, 175 (40%), and of those with polymenorrhagia 17 (33.33%), had uterine fibroids; of those with post-menopausal bleeding, 3 (12%) had ovarian tumors, and another 3 (12%) had cystic ovaries. A detail of the ultrasound findings of these patients, and their follow-up is presented. Ultrasound was found valuable in primary and secondary amenorrhoeas, where the presence and size of the uterus and ovaries could be determined, often rendering unnecessary an invasive procedure such as laparoscopy. In menorrhagia and polymenorrhagia, fibroids could be confirmed or excluded, though small ones, especially on the posterior wall were at times missed.

02.32.01

Toxic effect on spermatozoa of peritoneal fluid from infertile patients: Dorez, F, Wahl, P, Bajolle, F, Quereux, C. Dept. Obstet. and Gyn., C.H.U., Reims, France

This study is based on a group of 28 infertile patients and nine fertile patients. The peritoneal fluid is collected during laparoscopy, which is carried out between the 12th and 22nd day of the menstrual cycle. Male gametes are rapidly immobilized upon contact with peritoneal fluid from infertile patients. Nine of the eleven peritoneal samples taken from infertile patients with endometriosis showed this toxic effect, all samples from patients with inflamed of infected pelvis and the two cases of infertile patients having normal pelves. Samples from fertile patients retained spermatozoa mobility. The participation of antibodies, complement is eliminated. The mechanism of unexplained infertility especially when accompanied by endometriosis, infection or normal pelvis seems elucidated.

02.32.02

Clinical significance of sperm recovery from peritoneal fluid at diagnostic laparoscopy: Murakami, M, Inoue, M, Kobayashi, Y, Honda, I, Fujii, A. Dept. Obstet. and Gyn., School Med., Tokai Univ., Kanagawa, Japan

Sperm recovery from peritoneal fluid is an unequivocal evidence of successful sperm transport to the site of fertilization. In the present study, we attempted peritoneal sperm recovery from 109 infertile patients at diagnostic laparoscopy, to see whether this kind of sperm migration test does have a diagnostic validity in infertility workup. Laparoscopy was scheduled for the estimated day of ovulation, based on the previous menstrual history. The patients were instructed to have coitus on the morning of admission. The peritoneal fluid was aspirated 26–30 h after coitus. Alliquot of each aspirate was treated with 0.01% saponin solution to lyse contaminating red blood cells and centrifuged. The pellet was resuspended in 10% KOH and centrifuged again. A small amount of distilled water was added to the sediment and the suspension was examined for the presence of spermatozoa. Sperm recovery was recorded in 21 patients (19%). Of 87 patients who were followed up at least one year, 37 (43%) achieved pregnancy. The pregnancy rate of sperm positive group (63%) was significantly higher than that of sperm negative one (38%). These results indicate that peritoneal sperm recovery is useful for predicting subsequent fertility in selected patients.

02.32.03

The variability of sperm penetration in cervical mucus from normal women between different days and cycles in relation to mucin content and serum hormonal levels: Jonsson, B, Landgren, B-M, Eneroth, P, Fleetwood, L, Nordström, L*, Svanborg, K. Dept. Obstet. and Gyn. and *Clin. Chem., Karolinska Hosp. Stockholm, Sweden

Although the *in vitro* sperm penetration test by *Kremer* has been widely used, no studies have been performed on the variability of test results on different pre-ovulatory days and different cycles in normal women. In this study, we have collected cervical mucus from 15 normally menstruating women without fertility problems. Sample collecting started on the 8th cycle day and continued until ovulation had occurred. This was repeated during three different menstrual cycles. Sperm penetration tests were performed (Kremer tests) using two different fresh ejaculates. The cervical mucus was also used for measurement of trace elements, prostaglandins F and E, mucin and albumin. The results of the Kremer tests were evaluated using a scoring system: excellent performance 7–9, acceptable 4–6 and bad 0–3. Results: The results of the Kremer tests were found to vary considerably between cycle days and showed no clear-cut correlation with serum hormone levels. Maximal sperm penetration was usually seen once around mid-cycle but with a few women the test gave the highest score on a couple of days. For each woman the outcome of the test was similar during the three cycles investigated. The relative content of magnesium in cervical secretions was high. Of the two prostaglandins, those belonging to the F series predominated. Certain correlations between analysates and Kremer test results were found.

02.32.04
Laser-Doppler spectroscopy – a new device for assessment of sperm motility: Uses and clinical results in an *in vitro* fertilization-program: Pusch, H H. Univ. Hosp. Gyn. and Obstet., Graz, Austria
Sperm motility is considered as an important factor for the penetration of oocytes *in vivo* and *in vitro*. As long as conventional microscopic assessment of motility had to be used, no reliable and reproduceable results could be gained. Objective measurement of sperm-motility is possible now by means of Laser-Doppler Spectroscopy. This new and accurate technic has been used for motility determinations in our *in vitro* fertilization program. The device determines sperm density, total sperm motility and mean sperm velocity. Results of motility determinations are related to different spermiogram diagnoses and results of *in vitro* fertilization. Mean spermatozoal velocity is a new and important factor for the evaluation of fertilizing capacity in human ejaculate. Normospermic men had a mean velocity of 56 μm/sec. In cases of asthenozoospermia, 32 μm/sec could be measured. In teratozoospermia 24 μm/sec have been reached, the mean velocity of oligospermic men was 15 μm/sec. Special attention is laid on the group of oligospermic men, working out additional prognostic criteria for this problem group in IVF by exact motility determinations.

02.32.05
Acrosome reaction after medical stimulation *in vitro*: Mizutani, T, Kihira, M, Matsuzawa, K, Suzuki, M, Tomoda, Y. Dept. Obstet. and Gyn., Nagoya Univ., School Med., Nagoya, Japan
Many physiological and pharmacological substances have stimulating effects on human sperm motility *in vitro* (*W.-B. Schill*, Andrologia **11**, 77, 1979; *T. Mizutani* et al., Andrologia, in press), but little is known about the influence on the acrosome reaction (AR) following medical stimulation. The purpose of our pilot study was to get the information, first, how the motility and velocity of washed human sperm will be improved by different compounds and second, what percentage of acrosome reacted sperm increase within 24 hours. Multiple exposure photography (*A. Makler*, Fertil. and Steril. **30**, 192, 1978) with bradykinin, kallikrein, angiotensin I, II, acetylcarnitine, prolactin, LH, FSH, caffeine and arginine after 30-minute incubation period at 22°C, 33°C and 37°C and a triple-stain method (*Talbot* et al., J. exp. Zool. **215**, 201, 1981) and an electron microscope were used. Since each sample showed its own stable reaction pattern, i.e. achieving time to maximum and a rate of AR with and without substances, three different types of donors were examined intensively. Mainly four compounds make an increase of AR rate of +7 to +18% (p < 0.05) but one donor's showed no improvement. Our *in vitro* studies indicate that distinct compounds directly stimulate sperm motility and the mode of their effects was rather time, temperature and donor dependent. This preliminary work shows that more detailed studies of the mechanism of medical stimulation are necessary and much attention to the individual difference in sperm reaction should be given, before its possible clinical applications e.g. optimal preincubation time determination of artificial insemination and IVF program.

02.32.06
Acrosome reaction and movement characteristics of human spermatozoa after incubation *in vitro*: Sato, H, Töpfer-Petersen, E, Schill, W-B, Kobayashi, T, Iizuka, R. Dept. Obstet. and Gyn., Ise Keio Univ. Hosp., Mie-Pref. Japan and Univ., Munich
Acrosome and acrosome reaction of human spermatozoa were assessed using a triple stain method (*P. Talbot, R. S. Chacon*, J. exp. Zool. **215**, 201, 1981) and an immunofluorescent method. Movement characteristics of spermatozoa during incubation were examined using a multiple exposure photography method (*A. Makler*, Fertil. and Steril. **30**, 192, 1978). Percentage of acrosome reaction increased after one hour incubation from 30.8% to 43.5%, being stable at time level six hours. Progressive spermatozoa that show greater than 10 μm lateral head displacement increased significantly after one and three hours incubation. Furthermore, different stages of acrosome reaction were observed by indirect immunofluorescence. These results show that vigorous swimming behavior of spermatozoa seem to occur coincidently with the acrosome reaction.

02.32.07
Sperm velocity and percentage of motility in the presence of a varicocele: Papaloucas, A, Vlassis, G, Marga-ritis, B, Makedos, G, Moysatat, J, Panidis, D. 2nd Dept. Obstet. and Gyn., Aristotelian Univ., Thessa-loniki, Greece
Semen specimens from 100 men with varicocele, aged 32.1 ± 5.2 years, were analysed by the multiple exposure photography method. The purpose of this study was: a) the assessment of the parameters of the spermiogram (including objective evaluation of motility) in men with varicocele, and b) the correlation between the more significant parameters of semen, namely motility, morphology and sperm density. The results (mean ± SD) were as follows: motile spermatozoa, 30.9% ± 20.3; spermatozoal velocity,

30.5 μm/sec $\pm$ 5.6; motility index, 10.5 μm/sec $\pm$ 7.1; normal forms, 29.0% $\pm$ 16.9; sperm concentration, 35.0 $\times$ 10^6/ml $\pm$ 41.4. Moderate significant correlations were found between number of spermatozoa/ml, normal forms, percentage of motility, and spermatozoal velocity the first hour after ejaculation. Furthermore, highly significant correlations were found between percentage of motility, spermatozoal velocity and normal forms. Finally, moderate significant correlation was found between normal forms and spermatozoal velocity.

02.32.08

Hormonal profile in oligospermic patients: Koudounarakis, J, Sarris, S, Comninos, A. "Marika Eliadi" Maternity Hosp., Athens, Greece

This work was done in oligospermic patients with no clinical symptoms – thyroid pathology, hypogonadism, hyperprolactinemia or chromosomal abnormalities. The level of FSH (follicle stimulating hormone), LH (luteinizing hormone), T (testosterone), PRL (prolactin), E_2 (estradiol), and SHBG (sex hormone binding globulin) and their variations were studied in oligospermic patients. Investigation showed that (1) There is an inverse relationship of FSH with number of spermatozoa and the degree of activity of the spermatic epithelium. (2) LH shows also the same inverse relationship but the numerical values obtained are within normal limits. (3) There is a decrease of testosterone values only in cases of severe damage of the spermatic epithelium. (4) Prolactin shows a decrease in oligospermic patients but not statistically significant. (5) Estradiol shows a small increase but also not statistical significant. (6) SHBG demonstrates a minor but non-significant rise in all cases of oligospermia. From the above it can be concluded that the FSH levels are a good index for assessing the activity of the spermatic epithelium.

02.32.09

The effects of traditional herbal medicine, Shakuyaku-Kanzo-To (S-K-T), for lowering serum testosterone (T) levels on female rats: Takeuchi, T, Nishii, O, Takahashi, M, Okamura, T, Yaginuma, T, Kobayashi, T. Dept. Obstet. and Gyn., Fac. Med., Univ. of Tokyo at Mejirodai, Tokyo, Japan

S-K-T contains equivalently Shakuyaku, extract of Paeoniae Radix, and Kanzo, extract of Glycyrrhizae Radix. In the previous studies we reported that S-K-T lowered high serum T levels in oligomenorrheic women. In the present study, adult androgen-sterilized rats showing anovulatory persistent estrus were given orally 11.25, 22.5, 45, 90, 180 mg/kg of S-K-T in water daily for two weeks, and the controls only water. The dose of 22.5 mg/kg was the same as the women was given ordinarily. The weight of pituitary, adrenal and uterus was not affected by S-K-T. The ovarian weight and serum T levels were significantly dose-dependently (p < 0.001 at both) decreased. Serum FSH and LH levels did not significantly decreased. There was a significant positive correlation between the serum T levels and the weight of ovary or the serum LH levels (r = 0.88 or r = 0.81, respectively, p < 0.01 at both). These results suggested that S-K-T could lower serum T levels by direct effects at least on ovaries.

02.32.10

Ligation of the vas deferens: Histologic consequences on the rat testis: Sengos, C, Leonardos, V, Nicolaou, P, Mesogitis, S, Tserkezoglou, A, Aravantinos, D. 1st Dept. Obstet. and Gyn., Univ. of Athens, "Alexandra" Hosp., Athens, Greece

A hundred and eighty-eight male Wistar rats were divided into three main groups according to their age, 3, 6 and 12 months old, and underwent laparotomy and bilateral ligation of the vas deferens. The animals were further divided in four subgroups (a, b, c, d) in regard to the duration of ligation, 3, 6, 12, and 18 months respectively. At the end of the period appropriate for each subgroup, the testes were removed and histologically examined. Johnsen's method was used for the evaluation of the criteria which were: a) spermatogenesis, b) diameter of the seminal tubes, c) hyalinoid differentiation of the vas deferens wall, d) number and size of Leydig cells. Statistical analysis of the results lead to the following conclusions: a) No statistically significant difference (S.S.D.) in the microscopic image of the test is in the three main age groups (p > 0.1). b) No S.S.D., but nevertheless measurable difference in the increase of the diameter of the seminal tubes between subgroups c, d and subgroups a, b (p < 0.1). c) S.S.D. regarding all other criteria between subgroups c, d and subgroups a, b (p < 0.05). d) S.S.D. regarding spermatogenesis between subgroup c and d. In conclusion, rat fertility rate diminishes in accordance with the duration of ligaton of the vas deferens.

02.32.11

Peritoneal sperm migration (PSM) test: Influence of timing: Hammerstein, J, Stäbler, G. Abt. Gyn., Klinikum Steglitz, FU, Berlin

Sperm migration up to the abdominal cavity after homologous intracervical insemination has been routinely checked at laparoscopy in 1153 sterile couples since the introduction of the PSM test in 1972 by *Koch* et al. (Arch. Gyn. **219**, 610, 1976). The present study was conducted to determine the influence of varying time intervals between insemination and fluid collection from the pouch of Douglas. 521 consecutive PSM tests in women with patent tubes were evaluated. The tests were grouped according to the time intervals as follows: Group A 60–119 min (n = 79); Group B 120–179 min (n = 115); Group C 180–240 min (n = 120); Group D 241–450 min (n = 207). The over-all results do not indicate any differences in sperm migration depending on the time interval:

Sperm migration up to:	Group A	B	C	D	Interpretation
Pouch of Douglas	29.1	27.0	28.3	33.8%	test positive
Uterine cavity	32.9	37.4	32.5	34.8%	migration reduced
None	38.0	35.6	39.2	31.4%	test negative

When only cases with normal sperm quality are considered (n = 280), again no differences were found between groups A and D (42.5% vs. 46.6% positive tests): Cases with poor sperm quality (n = 51), i. e. density below 10 mill/ml, less than 30% motility and/or less than 30% normal-shaped sperm, gave positive tests in 12.5% (group A) and 12.6% (group D) only. Unlike the cases with normal sperm, half of the peritoneal sperm in group D were immotile. Intermediate results were seen in the remaining 190 cases with mild subfertility, but without an increase in immotile peritoneal sperm with time. Conclusion: No bias is introduced into the test by neglecting the time interval between insemination and fluid collection within the limits of 1 to 7½ h. Survival of peritoneal spermatozoa appears to be distinctly longer than 7½ h unless sperm quality is poor.

02.41.01

Computerized quality control in an obstetrical department: Backe, B. Norweg. Inst. Hosp. Res., Trondheim, Norway

A concept for quality control in obstetrics was introduced in 1980 by *Bergsjø, Bakketeig* and *Buhaug* (Gynecology and Obstetrics, International Congress Series No. 512, Excerpta Medica, 1980, 867–870). From May 1984 a modified version has been implemented in the Regional Hospital of Trondheim, Norway. This concept is based upon the assumption that each unit has its own level of quality, and that this can be measured and monitored over time by the relative incidence of selected process and outcome variables. Control charts are used for monthly feedback to the clinicians. Control limits are set corresponding to 10% and 90% levels using the cumulative binomial level of probability. Based upon clinical considerations, the patients are grouped into five groups by parity, onset of labor, planned mode of delivery and presentation. The variables selected for processing were tested by discriminant analysis, which confirmed the relevance of the grouping. The control charts processed so far have shown, among others, significant variations in the rates of instrumental deliveries and inductions. After one year's experience with the present registration, some fields for improvement of clinical practice have been clearly indicated. Continuous recording and analysis of clinical activities are valuable for clinicians in facilitating a critical approach to their routines.

02.41.02

Risk factor scoring as an index of maternal and child health care: Shah, N A. King Edward Med. Coll., Lahore, Pakistan

Perinatal mortality has always been an important measure of obstetric efficiency. Perinatal death rates are at excessive levels in Punjab villages of Pakistan, 80 per 1000 deliveries. Neonatal death rates are more than four times those of economically favored countries. Deaths in later months of infancy are still more excessive, 78 per 1000 live births in the post neonatal period compared with a usual 5 per 1000 in advanced countries. These observations led to the present study which has the purpose of identifying high risk obstetric patients. Recently I began to apply the Nesbitt-Aubry maternal and Child Care Index to every registrant in the General Obstetric Clinic. An index was made out at the patient's first registration and was based entirely on the patient's history, physical and initial laboratory findings. The index was then filed away until 500 cases had been accumulated. The patient's care was given in the usual fashion and was not dictated specifically by the results of the index. The outcome of each pregnancy was then analysed in detail and the index score sheets were collated with corresponding clinical records and the investigation of all possible association was made between the score and the obstetrical results. The results of this study are discussed in detail. The perinatal concept of risk factor scoring approach should and can be utilized.

02.41.03

Perinatal aspects of adolescent women in Cartagena, Colombia: Barrios-Amaya, J, Ramos-Olier, A, Soto-Yances, A. Dept. Obstet. and Gyn., School Med., Univ. Cartagena, Colombia

We reviewed 18,559 patients accepted for the first time at the Maternity Clinic "Rafael Calvo C" of the University of Cartagena, during a period of three years. Of these cases, 2070 (11.2% of the total) were of women under 18 years of age. Of these adolescent women, 73.6% came from the urban area and 22.4% came from the rural area. The mean age for the menarche was 12.4 years, and 90% menstruated for the first time between 11 and 15 years, with limit ages of 7 and 17 years. 70% were unmarried, 23% were married, and we have no information about the remaining 7%. They started marital life at a mean age of 14 years, with a limit age of 11 years. Their obstetrical life started at a mean age of 16 years, with a limit age of 11 years. 90.5% were primigravidae. 27.2% of the cases had complications during pregnancy, being the most frequent: Hypertensive disease of pregnancy; Premature rupture of membranes; Hypodynamia; Premature delivery; Cephalopelvic disproportion. Of the cases 89.4% had normal vaginal delivery, and

53

6.2% had Cesarean section. The remaining cases had complicated deliveries. The weight of the newborns was between 2500 and 3500 gm in 69% of the cases, and 10.3% weighed less than 2500 gm.

02.41.04
Grandmultipartiy; An obstetric enigma: Malhotra, P, Malhotra, R M, Malhotra, N, Malhotra, J. Nursing Maternity Home, Agra, India

A review of 5000 confinements in Malhotra Nursing and Maternity Home, Agra, India was carried out with special reference to grandmultipartiy. Its incidence in our series was 7.8%. The mean age of patient was between 30–38 years. Four of our patients were 14th paras Muslims formed 19.38%, Hindus 5.5%. Education plays an important part. The high rate of multipartiy in an educated patient was for want of a male child. The delivery pattern in our series of 390 grandmultis was spontaneous delivery 50%, ventouse delivery 30%, Cesarean section 11%, assisted breech delivery 6%, forceps delivery 3%. Complications met with were obstetrical, surgical and medical. The main obstetric complication was antepartum hemorrhage 14.79%. The second main complication met with was malpresentations 10.56%. – Conclusion: In todays modern era the picture of a harassed women who stands badly, walks badly, eats indifferently and does not get enough sleep, should be wiped out completely by effective family planning measures and removal of adverse social stigmas. I come from the city of Taj. The monument of love. Built on death of Mumtaj Mahal who died bearing her 14th child.

02.41.05
Performance of gravid mothers with previous reproductive wastage: Balasubramaniam, N, Ravikumar, H, Jadhav, M. Christian Med. Coll. and Hosp., Vellore, India

Five hundred consecutive gravid patients with previous Bad Obstetric History, who attended the antenatal, labor and neonatal services from the Department of Obstetrics/Gynecology and Child Health, Christian Medical College and Hospital, Vellore during a period of three years (4800 deliveries per year) were studied as regards their reproductive performance in subsequent pregnancy and labor. The results were analysed with an emphasis on, (1) the chance of recurrence of the same condition, (2) fetal wastage – in early and late gestation, (3) type of labor, (4) complications like prematurity/placental insufficiency, (5) early neonatal outcome, (6) place of timely termination – induction/Cesarean section, monitoring the biophysical and biochemical factors. In this study, "Bad Obstetric History" (BOH) is taken as those cases when the previous fetal wastage either due to maternal and fetal causes has made an alteration in the management of pregnancy and labor in question. The results show that recurrence rate of the same condition was not so high as expected and that the overall fetal salvage rate was quite satisfactory. The paper rightfully stresses the crucial role played by the Neonatal Team of Physicians, in achieving this outcome.

02.41.06
Outcome of pregnancy following previous abortion and premature labor: Gun, K M. Dept. Obstet. and Gyn., Med. Coll., Calcutta, India

The author and his colleagues in Medical College, Calcutta, and N.R.S. Medical College, Calcutta, treated 840 cases with a history of two or more previous abortions. In addition 72 cases with a history of two or more preterm deliveries were also treated during a period of 11 years between January 1973 and December 1983. These 912 cases had 2227 past pregnancies with only 189 surviving babies (8.4%). About twothirds of cases (608) belonged to lower socio-economic class. Ninety-two cases (10.08%) were doing some jobs which involved commuting from home to place of work. Four hundred and twenty-eight cases (50.09%) had first trimester abortions and the remaining 412 cases a combination of first and second trimester abortions. Two hundred and twelve cases (23.2%) had a history of one or more induced abortions followed by preterm labor or spontaneous abortion. Surgical treatment prior to fresh pregnancy undertaken in 23 cases included trachelorrhaphy, myomectomy and utriculoplasty. Of the etiological factors, no cause was found in 632 cases (69.3%); cervical incompetence in 237, diabetes in 19, hypertension 12, cardiac disease nine, and syphilis three cases. Prolonged antenatal admission in hospital was necessary in 662 cases. Pregnancy was monitored mainly by clinical parameters. Synthetic progestogens and isoxsuprine were used in selected cases. Encirclage was performed for incompetence. Outcome of pregnancy was successful in 862 cases (94.5%). Cesarean section rate was 60.5%.

02.41.07
Prolonged pregnancy: Das, B, Batabyal, S K, Naskar, S C. Calcutta

Naegeles rule remains the standard procedure in calculating the expected date of confinement. Its value is that it is quite inexpensive. The main drawback has been found that most of the patients (55.69%) of Chittaranjan Seva Sadan, Calcutta, did not know their last menstrual date. Health education from marriage life in this regard might improve accuracy and could prevent many associated complications of pregnancy. Multigravidas have been found less keen to have their pregnancies prolonged (*Browne*, 1963). Fetal distress and meconium in the liquor amnii have been found increasingly as pregnancy became more and more prolonged and the incidence was more in primigravidas and in induced group. Vaginal delivery (33.33%) in the induced group has been found much less than in the non-induced group (84.81%). The instrumental delivery and Cesarean section have been found approximately five times more frequently in the induced group than in the non-induced group. Maternal serum alpha fetoprotein (AFP) steadily decreases up to the expected date of delivery from its peak value at 36 weeks of gestation. After the expected

54

date of delivery the value has been found still lower and continued to fall significantly as the postdate progressed. Again much higher values of AFP was observed in fetal distress and the highest concentration was recorded into uterine fetal death (*Ruoslahti* and *Seppala*, 1971).

02.41.08

Management of prolonged pregnancy: Samayoa, E O, Fortín, B, Romero, A, Gonzáles, O. Hosp. Centr. Inst. Hondureño de Segur. Soc., Tegucigalpa, D.C. Honduras, C.A.

Prolonged pregnancy (PP) is a serious problem in the prenatal clinic. Several procedures have been used to afford a fetal well being. Because of financial shortages we selected a very practical procedure: the daily maternal autocontrol of fetal movements and the weekly NST and/or OCT. PP was considered when the amenorrhea was more than 42 weeks. In the period from July 1, 1981 to June 30, 1982, 370 prolonged pregnancies were seen among a total of 4773 deliveries in that period of time. One hundred cases were blindly selected for presentation, 58% had more than 42.5 weeks, 42% had more than 43 weeks, up to 49 weeks. There were six cases with hypoactive fetal movements detected by the mother. 14% NST were non-reactive, 5% OCT were positive, 15% of the newborns were meconium stained, but no Clifford II or III were found. Only five had Apgar 1–5 at one minute with a good recovery at five minutes. There was 21% of Cesarean sections. There were no perinatal deaths in the 379 PP. A control group of 22 affected newborns with Clifford syndrome in the same period of time were reviewed; none of the mothers were seen by us, 15 mothers had no prenatal clinic control. There were three perinatal deaths, eight babies had Clifford II, eleven had Clifford I and two had Clifford III, one had congenital heart defect. There were no perinatal deaths among the PP controlled by MF and NST/OCT.

02.41.09

Outcome of post-term pregnancy: Manimekalai, P, Nafeesa Beebi, A, Sujatha, K. Inst. Obstet. and Gyn., Madras, South India

This is a retrospective analysis of 550 cases of post-term labor during January 1983 to December 1984 at Government Women and Children Hospital, Egmore, Madras. Incidence, relation to parity, mode of delivery, perinatal mortality and morbidity of post-term labor (42–44 weeks) were compared to those of 315 women carrying 41 weeks as control. Incidence of post-term labor is 1.6%. Out of 550 cases, 70.5% delivered at 42 weeks, 25.3% at 43 weeks, and 4.2% at 44 weeks. 45.8% were primi, 24.7% second gravida, 19.3% third gravida. At 41 weeks 48.6% were primi, 28.2% second gravida, 14.2% third gravida. Primigravida tended more to be post dated and post-term. 82.5% of post-term gravidae had normal onset of labor and 13% had induction. There was not much difference in the mode of delivery of post-term labor in the "normal onset group" and "induced group". Thus routine induction is not very beneficial. At 41 weeks the Cesarean section rate was 64% i. e. double that of post-term 32%, which is due to increase of repeat Cesarean sections at 41 weeks. The incidence of Cesarean section rate done for fetal distress increased according to weeks. Perinatal mortality reached 21.7% at 44 weeks. Thus, close observation and selective intervention is sufficient to assure optimal perinatal outcome in post-term labor.

02.41.10

No perinatal mortality in post date pregnancy, achieved by active management: Wiknjosastro, G, Sianturi, M H R, Zega, Y. Perinat. Subdiv., Dept. Obstet. and Gyn., Fac. Med., Univ. of Indonesia, Jakarta

Fetal distress and meconium aspiration syndrome might increase the perinatal mortality in post date pregnancy. Changing of management showed a significant decrease of mortality in 162 cases. Active management of post date pregnancy (> 42 weeks) consisted of: a) stress test, b) amnioscopy, c) induction of labor. A negative stress test showed 97.4% of specificity for a negative fetoplacental dysfunction. If pelvic score 4 or less, we inserted Foley catheters (no 24) to ripen the cervix and oxytocin infusions were given in case the women were not in labor. Cesarean sections (15.4%) were done for fetal distress and failed progress of labor. There was a no perinatal mortality (corrected for two cases with lethal congenital malformation).

02.41.11

Pregnancy out-come after the "Body-Mind-Breath exercise work-out" during the third trimester of pregnancy: Bansal, R. Bansal's Mangalde Nursing Home, Agra, **Sarkar, B.** Sarkar Nursing Home, Agra, India

Pregnancy is a period of stress and strain but yet a woman can derive full benefits from the harmonious relationship between herself and the fetus, affect an easy delivery and a speedy recovery thereafter, if she indulges in the "Body-Mind-Breath exercise work-out" during the antenatal period. This requires the participation of the body in the form of a very good therapeutic program during the antenatal period, of the mind in the way of increased body awareness and that of the breath in better oxygenation and relaxation of the body. The following study was carried out on 400 women attending antenatal clinics. Out of these 200 cases were kept as control and 200 were subjected to an hour of exercises, breathing and relaxation technics every day during the third trimester of pregnancy. It was found that the patients in the study group were in peak physical condition during the antenatal period, had relatively easy delivery and readily "bounced back" to their normal figure and life routine. Thus we can conclude that through the body-mind-breath system of participation during the antenatal period the expectant mothers can limber and liven up their entire body to become better aligned, in balance, more lithe and flexible to nourish the fetus, and enjoy good health before, during and after delivery.

02.41.12

Benign intracranial hypertension and subarachnoid block for Cesarean section: Ali, V, Abouleish, E. Obstet. and Gyn. and Anesth., Univ. of Texas Med. School, Houston, TX, USA

BIH is defined as a syndrome of elevated intracranial pressure without clinical and laboratory or radiologic evidence of a focal lesion such as hydrocephalus. In 50% of cases the conditions can get worse during pregnancy with invariable resolution after abortion or delivery. Permanent damage to vision is the main threat which occurs in 5–10% of cases. In literature the anesthetic management of obstetric patients with BIH is rare. Spinal anesthetic in a BIH pregnant patient can be advantageous. It is both therapeutic, by way of relieving tension, and diagnostic too. This case report is about a 31-year-old, black female, G2, P1, who was diagnosed as having BIH prior to her first pregnancy in 1981. She had an intrauterine death at term needing a Cesarean section under general anesthesia for a big baby. Her BIH reverted to normal after the pregnancy. Her second pregnancy was complicated by class "A" diabetes which was managed by diet alone. Her BIH recurred. She had an elective Cesarean section at term under spinal anesthesia. Opening pressure was 250 mm H_2O. The dose of analgesic drug was comparable to a patient with normal CSF pressure. Baby's Apgar score was 8/9. Use of spinal anesthesia can be informative of the intracranial pressure, is therapeutic and also be used for the purpose of obstetric anesthesia.

02.41.13

Management of abnormal cervical cytology in pregnancy by conization and pregnancy outcome: Eleftheriadis, P, Weitzel, H. Dept. Obstet. and Gyn., Hosp. Oststadt and Henriettenstiftung, Univ. School Med., Hannover

Prenatal cervical cytologyc screening and conization have been recommended since 1960 (Obstet. Gyn. **16**, 521, 1960). The available literature data from the last 25 years, regarding epidemiology of pre- and invasive cervical neoplasia (CN) among 259,970 pregnancies and pregnancy outcome after conization of 986 cases, were studied comparatively with control groups of obstetric population 1970–1981. The study showed: a) no different incidence of CN 2.72‰. (1.07–8.75‰.) among pregnant women and a relatively young average age 29.71 (20–41) years; b) increased (p<0.001) maternal obstetric complications after conization (55.57%), which are associated with higher (p<0.001) rates of early (15.21%) and late (5.05%) spontaneous abortions, prematurity (18.06%) and perinatal mortality (5.60%); and c) a limited diagnostic effectivity of conization in a high percentage 44.55% (19–68%) by residual tumor. It is concluded that: a) prenatal cervical cytologic screening should be wide recommended, b) pregnant women subjected to conization during pregnancy belong to high risk group and require intensive prenatal care, and c) conizations performed in pregnancy should be reduced by providing of other alternative less tissue destructive diagnostic methods, e. g. multiple biopsies under colposcopy.

02.42.01

Advantages of the use of the partographic chart: Panella, M, Gulisano, A S, Fichera, M, Pep, F, Tarascio, A, Torrisi, G. Gyn. and Obstet. Dept., Univ., Catania, Italy

The speaker illustrates the enclosed model of the partographic chart in use since 1970 in the Obstetrics and Gynecology Department of the University of Catania. After the adoption of the partographic chart, the perinatal mortality rate per 25,025 births was reduced from 30‰ to 15‰. In the years 1982 and 1983 we have adopted the systematic use of the norms listed in the partographic chart in 5,082 births. Perinatal mortality rates have decreased from 15‰ to 11.21‰. The percentage of Cesarean sections has not increased (15.82%). A significant difference has been noted, in particular, between perinatal mortality rate in physiological labor (7.28‰) and perinatal mortality in conducted labor (3.93‰), which follow the criteria illustrated in our chart: elective and active treatment of labor. – Supported by Grants CNR (Italy).

02.42.02

Fetal behaviour during active labor: Zimmer, E Z, Divon, M Y, Vadas, A, Peretz, B A, Paldi, E. Dept. Obstet. and Gyn., Rambam Med. Ctr., Haifa, Israel

The relationship between fetal activity and heart rate patterns is of great value in the antenatal period. The aim of our study was to evaluate the correlation between heart rate, short-term beat to beat variability and fetal trunk movements in labor. Seventeen healthy parturients with normal fetuses were scanned and monitored using a computerized system which was developed in our department. Our conclusions were: (1) 88% of fetuses performed body movements in labor. (2) The probability of occurrence of fetal movements is greater during contractions than between contractions. (3) 30% of contractions were accompanied by fetal movements. (4) Fetal heart rate beat to beat variability is increased during contractions. (5) Fetal heart rate accelerations are frequently accompanied by fetal movements. (6) Accelerations during contractions are usually caused by fetal movements. (7) There is a time-lag between the beginning of acceleration and start of fetal movements.

02.42.03

Fetal heart rate patterns and vibro-acoustic stimulation in labor: Ohel, G, Simon, A, Evron, S, Granat, M, Beyth, Y, Sadovsky, E. Dept. Obstet. and Gyn., Hadassah Univ. Hosp., Jerusalem, Israel

Sound evoked FHR accelerations have been shown to correlate with good fetal outcome. In the present study we have assessed the FHR response to vibro-acoustic stimulation of 300 fetuses. Three types of FHR responses were characterized: type I, acceleration; type II, tachycardia of duration longer than two minutes; type III, combined acceleration-deceleration response. All fetuses demonstrating any of these three types of responses including cases with abnormal FHR tracings, had good outcome at birth. In some exceptional cases, the abnormal FHR patterns suggestive of a "stressed fetus" have changed abruptly to normal following the stimulation and good outcome has followed. This may be explained by the vigorous fetal movement induced by the stimulation and possibly release of cord compression. In four cases with low Apgars and acidotic state, in which vibro-acoustic stimulation was applied before delivery, the characteristic FHR response did not occur. The potential use of vibro-acoustic stimulation in the assessment of fetal condition in labor awaits further clinical confirmation.

02.42.04

Consideration technic about the lactate dosage and mother-fetus changes in normal labor: Navarrete, L, Clavero, P, Gilabert, T, Bueno, M, González Gómez, F. Univ. Granada, Spain
When blood lactate modifications are very rapid it is difficult to get true outcome with classic enzymatic methods. The use of new method enzymo-amperometer allows to analyse immediately. When, on the other hand we use one sample of 100 microliter it is possible to utilize blood samples of fetus scalp. The tune a technique has allowed that we can calculate normal range in maternal and fetus blood during the labor. After numerous studies we conclude that the best method is from hemolysed and deproteinized total blood, because: (1) The result did not change with the time. (2) It permits us to measure the intra- and extracellular lactate. Once standardized the best method we have analysed the result got in 71 cases with normal pregnancy, – labor and newborn. We made 21 scalp, a 71 umbilical cord (vein and artery) and 92 mother analyses.

The results are:

| | Cervix dilatation | | | Umbilical | After labor: |
	3–5 cm	6–8 cm	9–10 cm	artery	1.5 hour
Fetus	1.9 ± 0.5	2.1 ± 0.6	2.3 ± 0.6	2.7 ± 0.8	1.8 ± 0.3
Mother	1.7 ± 0.8	2.3 ± 0.5	2.8 ± 0.7	3.3 ± 1.1	——

With this result we can conclude that lactate critical level is 3.9 mmol/litre for 95% confidence.

02.42.05

Endorphinergic pain modulation during pregnancy and delivery: Rust, M, Keller, M, Egbert, R, Graeff, H. Depts. Anesthesiol. and Obstet. and Gyn., TU, Munich
It has been suggested that endorphins exert an antinociceptive action during pregnancy. *Gintzler* (Science 1980) demonstrated a naloxone-reversible increase of pain threshold (PTH) in pregnant rats. A similar rise of PTH in human pregnancy was found by *Rust* et al. (Arch. Gyn. 1983). Our aim was to assess endorphinergic pain modulation related to parturition. PTH (°C) was tested by radiant heat stimulation in dermatomes C_1 or S_1. The effect of pethidine (50 mg i. m.) placebo (0.9% NaCl i. m.) and naloxone (1.2 mg i. v.) on PTH was examined in three non-pregnant control groups. Eleven women with and without pethidine (50 mg i. m.) were tested during labor. Placebo vs. naloxone (1.2 mg i. v.) was evaluated in seven women shortly after delivery. Placebo for postoperative analgesia did not alter mean PTH in non-pregnant controls. Pethidine for premedication produced a rise of PTH for 3–4 hours showing significant elevations after 60 minutes and 130 minutes and an intermediate decrease after 105 minutes. Naloxone did not alter normal PTH. In unsupplemented women there was no further rise of elevated PTH during labor, whereas pain intensity increased with cervical dilatation. Pethidine for labor pain had only minimal effect on PTH and pain intensity. Post-partum placebo had no effect, but naloxone induced a rapid, highly significant fall of PTH in the same women. We conclude that there is an endorphin-mediated diminution of pain sensitivity in women during pregnancy and delivery.

02.42.06

Cord compression: Malpartida, E. Perinat. Res. Unit, Mease Hosp, Dunedin, FL, USA
Every labor is associated with some degree of cord compression, but in the majority of cases, this has no clinical significance. Some cases of cord compression cause changes in the fetal monitor, but few produce fetal distress. From a group of 200 patients in labor, 46 cases (23%), showed signs of cord compression on the fetal monitor, and from this group only 6 (3%) developed fetal distress. The cases with clinical significance are usually associated with fetal respiratory acidosis and when this occurs, the alteration in blood gases depend upon the intensity and duration of this condition. (1) Mild cord compression: usually does not produce significant alterations. (2) Moderate cord compression: produces mild hypoxia, mild hypercapnia, and mild changes in hydrogen ion concentration (H^+). Usually there is no alteration on buffer base (BB), this is respiratory acidosis. (3) Severe cord compression: produces frank changes in blood gases: deep hypoxia, high hypercapnia and acidosis. If the compression is intense, prolonged and present during each uterine contraction for a long time base deficit (BD) becomes evident. This is a metabolic acidosis.

02.42.07

The significance of the prolonged early deceleration: Stewart, K S, Khan, M. Roy. Infirm., Stirling, Scotland

In the second stage of labor because of increased head compression and increased placental compression the fetal heart rate (FHR) pattern can become very erratic and cause considerable concern. It is necessary, therefore, to establish the normal second stage FHR pattern and so reduce alarm and avoid unnecessary intervention. Fifty cardiotographic traces were examined. Each second stage was normal with no cord complications. The duration of pushing contractions was less than 45 mins (mean 30 mins) and the Apgar scores were > 9. Mean fetal scalp pH at beginning of second stage was 7.30 and umbilical artery pH 7.24. In all cases the base line was normal; in 85% variability was normal and in 15% there was flattening. The FHR patterns were grouped together. Accelerations occurred with 6% of the total number of contractions. Decelerations were observed with 73% of contractions of which 52% were prolonged early. The other 16% were early and 5% late. Repeated early and prolonged early decelerations, therefore, are normal to the correctly timed second stage. The prolonged early deceleration is a combination of the early head compression deceleration and the late placental insufficiency deceleration. It is the same as the prolonged early deceleration associated with the head compression and marked moulding found in the first stage of labor in the presence of cephalopelvic disproportion, described by *Stewart* and *Philpott* (Brit. J. Obstet. Gyn. **87**, 641–651, 1980). The prolonged early deceleration starts early, there is no time-lag and it ends late in relation to the contraction.

02.42.08

Doppler ultrasound in human fetal circulation dynamics: Kurz, C S[1], Klosa, W[2], Graf, H P[3]. [1]Dept. Obstet. and Gyn., Univ., Essen and [2]Freiburg, [3]Dept. Radiol., Univ., Freiburg

Introduction: Recordings of fetal blood flow (FBF) using real-time-scan and pulsed Doppler provides problems due to inaccuracies caused by technical and physiological factors (*Hasaart* et al., 1984; *Kurz* et al., 1985). Contrary to clinical data there is little in the literature about reproducibility and technical influence upon the estimated datas. – Material and methods: The aim of this study was to simulate FBF volume under varying experimental conditions by using an *in vitro* model and by thus examining and comparing different pulsed Doppler equipments. – Results: There existed a correlation between defined and estimated volume flow rates. However, particularly low flow rates resulted in relatively too high blood flow volumes when using high pass "thump" filtering to avoid Doppler signals from the vessel wall. These deviations are explained by the different instrument technics and fetal movements, as well as changes in fetal thoracic and abdominal pressure. Using high pass filters the measuring failure amounts to 50–170 ml/min. – Conclusions: These, to our knowledge, first systematic estimations showed that quantitative FBF has to be interpreted with great care according to the documented results. The effect of high pass filtering and fetal activity states have to be taken into account.

02.42.09

Evaluation of a PGE$_2$ analogue for pre-operative cervical dilatation: Eder, S, Chatterjee, M, Salvio, C. Dept. Obstet. and Gyn., UMDNJ-New Jersey Med. School, Newark, NJ, USA

PGE$_2$ has been shown to be effective in dilating the gravid uterine cervix. To our knowledge no studies have done to show the effects of prostaglandin (PG) on the non-pregnant cervix. The efficacy and complication rate of meteneprost potassium (9-deoxo-16,16, dimethyl-9-methylene PGE$_2$) was studied using a randomized double blind placebo controlled protocol. Three hours prior to a dilatation and curettage procedure a suppository, containing either 10 mg of experimental drug or a placebo, was placed in the posterior fornix of the vagina. Assessment of cervical dilation was done by determining resistance to graduated Hegar dilators at the time of suppository insertion and again after general anesthesia was induced. The mean age in the study (n = 14) and control (n = 15) population were 31.5 ± 2.1 and 34.6 ± 2.6 years respectively (p = 0.37). Both groups showed a mean cervical dilation of 3.6 mm. A significant percentage (8/14) of the study group (57%) reported nausea, vomiting, abdominal cramping, or diarrhea as compared to the placebo group (2/15; 13.3%) (p < 0.013). A correlation was observed between obesity and side-effects. Study patients with a body mass index (WT/HT2) > 25 had a significantly higher incidence (p = 0.021) than the non-obese. Meteneprost potassium does not appear to be effective in dilating the nonpregnant uterine cervix. Side-effects of this PG appear to be related to weight. Adipose tissue might retard elimination of the PG through binding. On the other hand PG might activate as yet unidentified enzymatic systems in lipocytes producing gastrointestinal side-effects. – Study supported by Upjohn, Kalamazoo, MI.

02.42.10

Fetuses of smoking mothers have higher heart rate variability during labor than controls: Rosti, J, Kariniemi, V. Dept. Obstet. and Gyn., Salo District Hosp., Salo, Finland

Previous studies of our group have demonstrated that maternal smoking and chewing nicotine-containing gum have an acute, decreasing effect on fetal heart rate variability (FHRV). The present study was undertaken to measure the possible chronic effect of smoking on intrapartum FHRV. All mothers admitted to Salo District Hospital for labor were asked whether they had smoked during pregnancy and how much. The differential indices (DI) measuring the short-term, and the interval indices (II), measuring the long-term component of FHRV were computed in ten minute epochs of abdominal or direct fetal electrocardio-gram by special-purpose computers throughout labor. The mothers who admitted any alcohol consumption during pregnancy were excluded (13%). The study group consisted of 41 smokers and 281 were controls. The differences of means were compared by Student's t-test in cases of equal variances and by Welch's t-test in cases of unequal variances. The DIs were normally distributed. DIs of the study group tended to be higher than controls throughout labor, but they were significantly higher only during the last hour of the first stage ($p < 0.001$). The IIs of smokers also tended to be higher among smokers than among controls, but the differences did not reach significance. The study and control groups did not differ in terms of gestational weeks at birth (40.0 vs 40.5), duration of labor (8.5 vs 8.3 h), birthweight (3628 vs 3738 g), head circumference (34.8 vs 35.2 cm) and placental weight (574 vs 565 g). The observed differences of the beat-to-beat variation of FHR among smokers and nonsmokers presumably represent a chronic excitatory effect of nicotine on the fetal autonomous nervous system.

02.42.11
Thermal aspect of pelvic soft tissues and their effect on fetal heat flux: Rudelstorfer, R, *Simbruner, G, Bernaschek, G, Janisch, H. II. Univ.-Frauenklin. and *Kinderklin., Vienna, Austria
Heat flux (HFX) from the fetus is a biological variable which can be easily measured during active labor until delivery. It mainly relates to the placental capability of eliminating heat which is generated by the fetal metabolism. First studies have shown that low HFX values were correlated with low umbilical artery pH and low Apgar scores (Arch. Gyn. **233**, 85, 1983). We continued our search for factors which influence fetal HFX. The purpose of this study was to measure the temperatures of the pelvic soft tissues during the gradual descent of the fetal head and their effect on HFX. In 20 vertex deliveries we measured the HFX from the fetal head and the temperatures of the surrounding pelvic tissues by means of a thermistor mounted on the HFX-transducer. – Results: Pelvic soft tissues temperatures at levels of the inlet, midpelvis and outlet were not significantly different (Mean $T = 37.6 \pm 0.2$, 37.7 ± 0.4, 37.7 ± 0.2 degree C). During uterine contractions soft tissue temperatures fell and resulted in an increased HFX from the fetal head. The changes were significant ($r = 0.5964$ $p < .01$, Analysis of variance). Axillary temperature was found to be only a rough approximation to pelvic soft tissues temperatures ($p < .05$). We speculate that these temperature changes could be brought about by a local reduction in blood perfusion. We conclude that they have to be taken into account when HFX is used for fetal monitoring.

02.42.12
Dynamic evaluation of CTG patterns from newborns with severe or prolonged acidosis: Stummvoll, W, Wiebogen, L, Prestel, A, Nagl, F. Dept. Obstet., Krankenh. d. Barmh. Schwestern, Ried i. I., Austria
In 1975–1984, despite an invasive monitoring rate of 80% and the use of additional diagnostic methods like fetal scalp sampling and maternal acid balance, 145 acidoses below pH art. 7.10 occurred among 9087 newborns on our ward, i. e. 1.6%. The highest rate was 4.6% in 1976, the lowest 0.9% in 1984. In 100 cases CTG tracings of more than 90 min before delivery were available. For every 30 min evaluation was done using the score described by *Hammacher*. 0–30 min before delivery (b. d.) it showed a pathologic (55%) or prepathologic (38%) score in 90% of all cases, while 7% were classified as suspicious and none as normal. 30–60 min b. d. the figures were 21%, 35%, 33%, 11%, 60–90 min b. d. 6%, 27%, 44%, 23%. The average score in the last half hour b. d. was 8.1 points, 30–60 min b. d. 5.4 points and 60–90 min b. d. 4.1 points. Most pathologic signs were seen evaluating the floating line, followed by pathology of oscillation and much less in the base line. CTG deterioration in cases with pathological increased uterine contractility was shown to occur faster than in cases with umbilical cord problems or chronic placental insufficiency. This may be a vote for doing internal pressure measurement, as well as frequent scoring of suspicious patterns, as well as prepathologic ones.

02.42.13
Transcutaneous carbon dioxide tension (tcP_{CO_2}) of fetus and mother during delivery: Kurz, C S. Dept. Obstet. and Gyn., Univ., Essen
Introduction: Measurement of tcP_{CO_2} with heated Severinghouse type electrodes have shown fair correlations to arterial values although a lot of problems affecting the electrode function are not yet understood (*Hansen* et al., 1979; *Herrell* et al., 1980). – Material and methods: Continuous tcP_{CO_2} monitoring was carried out in 15 deliveries according to *Kurz*, 1983, 1984 with tcP_{CO_2} electrodes (Dräger). – Results: The mean fetal tcP_{CO_2} in between labor and fetal heart rate (FHR) alterations was 52 mm Hg. Registration time varied between 30 min and 9 h. The range of maternal tcP_{CO_2} varied between 24 and 37 mm Hg. During labor maternal hyperventilation led to a significant maternal tcP_{CO_2} decrease of about 3 mm Hg. During labor fetal tcP_{CO_2} increased significantly for about 6 mm Hg and decreased in the pause in between labor. A fetal tcP_{CO_2} increase could be recognized in FHR decelerations as well as accelerations. During maternal supine position fetal tcP_{CO_2} increased analogous to the known tcP_{CO_2} decrease. Correlating the fetal tcP_{CO_2} measurements with micro blood analysis (MBA) from the fetal scalp tcP_{CO_2} values at 44° C were higher than those estimated by MBA. Between maternal and fetal tcP_{CO_2} existed a significant relationship ($p < 0.001$). During delivery acute fetal complications were always clearly indicated by a tcP_{CO_2} increase. – Conclusions: Continuous blood gas monitoring is of great scientific value and is able to reduce unnecessary operative intervention for terminating labor on account of to fetal indications.

02.79.01

Termination of early pregnancy by the antiprogestin RU 486: Swahn, M L, Bygdeman, M. Dept. Obstet. and Gyn., Karolinska Hosp., Stockholm, Sweden

RU 486 is a synthetic steroid which acts as an antiprogestin at the receptor level. Recently we have shown that oral administration of RU 486 effectively terminates early pregnancy but that the frequency of complete abortion was unsatisfactory (61%). The outcome of the therapy was not dose-related, at least not within the dose range of 50 to 200 mg daily for four days. The aims of the present study were to evaluate the pharmacokinetics of the compound, the effect of the drug on spontaneous uterine contractility and sensitivity to prostaglandin (PG) and if a sequential therapy of RU 486 and PG could increase the frequency of complete abortion. Following oral administration of RU 486 the peak plasma level was reached within 1 to 2 hours and the half-life time was approximately 24 hours. The resulting plasma levels were approximately dose-related. The blockage of the progesterone receptor resulted in an increased coordinated uterine activity and a pronounced increased sensitivity to PG. Treatment with RU 486, 50 mg daily for four days, supplemented with a low dose of a PGE analogue on the last day was found to be highly effective in terminating early pregnancy (appr. 95% complete abortion) and associated with few side-effects. The results indicate that the lack of dose effect (complete abortion) is not due to a poor bioavaliability, that the withdrawal of the intrinsic uterine suppressor progesterone will result in increased uterine activity and sensivity to PG and that a sequential therapy with RU 486 and PG gives a better prospect as a nonsurgical method of terminating early pregnancy than if either compond is used alone.

02.79.02

Clinical effects of RU 486, 50 mg × 2, for seven days in early pregnancy: Birgerson, L, Odlind, V, Johansson, E D B. Dept. Obstet. and Gyn., Univ., Uppsala, Sweden

RU 486 is a steroid with progesterone and glucocorticoid receptor antagonistic properties. In the present study RU 486, 50 mg × 2, was given for seven days to 30 healthy women, applying for legal abortion before the end of the seventh week of pregnancy. Out of the 30 patients treated, all responded with some bleeding. In five patients, however, the bleeding was very scanty and the patients were considered as non-responders and had a surgical termination. In the remaining 25 patients 22 were considered to have had a complete abortion as judged by a history of heavy bleeding, passage of products of conception, followed by the finding of a normal sized uterus and disappearance of hCG/s. Three patients had an incomplete abortion and had a curettage performed. In these patients the involution of the uterus was inadequate and the hCG/s remained elevated. The mean duration of bleeding in the women with complete abortion was 10.9 days (range 7 to 18 days). A slight decrease in hemoglobin was found at the first follow-up visit on treatment day seven. No woman, however, required blood transfusion or admission to hospital. A significant increase within the normal range of serum levels of cortisol was found on treatment day seven. One week after termination of treatment serum cortisol was back to pretreatment levels. The only side-effects reported were slight nausea and fatigue. It is concluded that RU 486 is a potent abortifacient in very early pregnancy, with a rate of complete abortions close to 80%, and is very well tolerated by the women.

02.79.03

Interruption of early pregnancy by an anti-progestational agent – RU 486: Haspels, A A, Vervest, H A M. State Univ., Utrecht, The Netherlands

RU 38-486 (17β-hydroxy-11β-(4-dimethylaminophenyl)-17α-(1-propynyl) estra-4,9-dien-3-one), an anti-progestational compound which acts by a competitive binding at the site of the progesterone and cortisol receptor. The antiprogesterone was given to 44 women, seeking termination of pregnancy. The patients were divided into two groups, 35 patients in group I with an amenorrhea up to 7 6/7 weeks = 55 days and 9 patients in group II 8–10 weeks amenorrhea. The patients received 200 mg RU 486 daily for four days. The start, duration and amount of bleeding were determined for 14 days. β-HCG, plasma progesterone, estradiol and cortisol were determined at day 0 and day 7. All patients started to bleed during treatment. Frequency of complete abortion was 83% (29 out of 35 patients) in group I. In nulliparous women a complete expulsion occurred in 17 out of 19 women (89%). In group II 33% (3 out of 9 patients). Most of the patients experienced only minor side-effects in terms of mild uterine pain and bleeding as in a spontaneous abortion. However, two patients suffered from heavy bleeding, requiring blood transfusion and curettage. Both in group II 8 resp. 9 2/7 weeks amenorrhea. In the patients with complete abortion, β-HCG, estradiol and progesterone decrease significantly within one week. Cortisol concentrations remained within the normal range at day 0 and day 7. Treatment with TU 486 provide and acceptable method of early abortion, especially in women who refuse operative treatment and prefer a "spontaneous abortion".

02.79.04

Post-coital interception by an anti-progestational compound RU 486: van Santen, M R, Haspels, A A. State Univ., Utrecht, The Netherlands

Post-coital interception started in the early sixties with the administration of large doses of estrogens: 50 mg di-ethyl stilbestrol for 5 days by *Morris* and *Van Wagenen* in the U.S. or 5 mg ethinyl-estradiol (E. E.) for five days by *Haspels* in Europe. Recently a double blind study compared the original hormonal therapy of 5 mg E. E. for 5 days with a combination with 1 mg DL-Norgestrel of which 2 doses are given, the second

12 hours after the first. This method was equally effective in preventing pregnancy. Moreover it resulted in less nausea and vomiting. These methods can be used up to 72 hours post-coitum. Post-coital use of intra-uterine devices can be used as an alternative up to six days post-coitum. Later during the cycle up till recently no method of interception was available and the women had an anxious wait for her next period. RU-486 (17β-hydroxy-11β-(4-dimethylaminophenyl)-17α-(1-propynyl) estra-4,9-dien-3-one) is an antiprogestational compound which acts by a competitive binding at the site of the progesterone and cortisol receptor. This antiprogesterone was administered to 22 patients from day 25 to 28 of the cycle as a late "morning-after pill" in a dosage of 100 mg daily. All women except one started to bleed before day 28 and observed a normal menstrual period. One woman stayed amenorrhoeic for two months, she was not pregnant but had an anovulatory cycle with a low progesterone level. β-HCG and progesterone levels will be presented. With th use of RU 486 side-effects were observed.

02.79.05

Effects of RU 486 on endometrial morphology: Uem, J F H M van, Chillik, C F, Hsiu, J G, Acosta, A A, Hodgen, G D. Dept. Obstet. and Gyn. and Dept. Path. Eastern Virginia Med. School, Norfolk, VA, USA

RU 486 antagonizes P_4 activity at the endometrial receptor level. To investigate the morphologic consequences of this action, the endometrium of 12 normal cycling rhesus monkeys was studied. In six monkeys, receiving 10 mg/kg/day RU 486 IM from cycle D3 (n = 3) or D7 (n = 3) until D24, ovulation was induced with hMG/hCG to avoid any central inhibitory action of RU 486 on gonadotropin secretion during the follicular phase. In the remaining monkeys, 5 mg RU 486/kg/day (n = 3) or placebo (n = 3) was administered from D21 until D24. In all monkeys an endometrial biopsy or hysterectomy was performed on D25. Femoral blood for RIA of LH, LH, E_2 and P_4 was obtained daily. Ovulation was confirmed based on stigma formation, presence of corpus luteum and elevated serum P_4 levels. When RU 486 was administrated starting in the follicular phase, only anovulatory proliferative endometrium without bleeding was found (average thickness 0.6 mm) despite dynamic E_2 and P_4 elevations. RU 486 induced menses in 84 h in all monkeys receiving the drug in luteal phase only. Histologic evaluation showed severe and homogeneous shedding of the secretory endometrium to the basalis (average thickness 1.34 mm). The controls did not bleed and the average thickness of the secretory endometrium was 3.38 mm. We conclude that the administration of RU 486 in the follicular phase inhibits endometrial proliferation as well as its transformation into the secretory stage. Further, when administered in the midluteal phase RU 486 induces a severe and uniformly sloughing of the endometrium. These data indicate a potential application of RU 486 for control of estrogen-induced endometrial mitogenesis and as a contraceptive agent.

03.13.01

Fungicidal action of various antifungals in relation to times of exposure: Rumler, W, Heins, S. Childrens Univ. Hosp., Martin-Luther-Univ., Halle-Wittenberg

The conventional methods for testing the susceptibility of microorganisms to inhibition by antibiotics or antimycotics allow the estimation of concentration-effect relations. In clinical microbiology the mostly used parameter is the minimum inhibitory concentration (MIC) of a given drug-organism combination. But, how much time of contact between an antifungal and, for example, Candida cells is necessary to reach the maximum of these concentration-depended inhibitory effects? It has been shown by us, that these optimal times of exposure are only short, from some minutes (clotrimazole and other azole-derivatives) up to 1 hour (5-fluorocytosine and others). Using a two-step cultivation method (1st step: incubation of the microorganisms for various times with various drug concentrations; 2nd step: measurement of cell multiplication after growth in antimycotic free broth) we found, that a prolongation of exposure does not lead to an increased effect, both in respect of cell multiplication (Mykosen **26**, 216 and 293, 1983) and of germ tube formation (Mykosen 1985 in press). So, short time peak levels should be more efficacious than long lasting median drug levels.

03.13.02

Candida albicans attachment and growth in monolayer cultures of epithelial cells from the human cervix uteri; Effects of azole antifungal agents: Hawkins, D F, Farrell, S M. Inst. Obstet. and Gyn., Hammersmith Hosp., Univ., London, England

Primary cultures of epithelial explants taken from the cervix yield monolayers of epithelial cells which can be grown for up to 9 days, Candida albicans spores added to the cultures on the 7th day appear to attach to the epithelial cells, and produce hyphae within 2 h. The hyphae then penetrate the cells, weaving in and out of the cytoplasm. Within 24 h the monolayer has been completely disrupted. The cultures can be repeatedly washed with phosphate-buffered saline and then the number of Candida spores which have attached per unit area of monolayer assessed. Alternatively, cultures can be fixed at various times after inoculation and examined by scanning electron microscopy. These methods are being employed to assess the effect of clotrimazole, bifonazole and ketoconazole on the attachment, production of hyphae and penetration of cells by Candida.

03.13.03

Clotrimazole plasma levels in pregnant and non-pregnant patients with candida vaginitis after a single dose of 500 mg: Ritter, W. Bayer AG, Inst. Clin. Pharmacol., Wuppertal

Previous studies in healthy volunteers have shown that the concentrations of clotrimazole in blood plasma after a single vaginal treatment with 500 mg were lower than 10 ng per ml (*W. Ritter* et al., Chemotherapy **29** Suppl. 1, 37, 1982). Recently, investigations on the clotrimazole plasma levels were initiated in pregnants and in patients with vaginal candidiasis. The results so far obtained demonstrate that the clotrimazole plasma levels in pregnants and in patients after treatment with a single vaginal dose of 500 mg are not different from those in healthy volunteers.

03.13.04

Overview of single-dose administration of clotrimazole in the treatment of Candida vaginitis: Fleury, F, Hughes, D, Floyd, R, Guess, E, Hester, L, Hodgson, C. Springfield, IL; Philadelphia, PA; Stanford, CA; Los Angeles, CA; Charleston, SC; West Haven, CT, USA

A series of double-blind studies involving 200 patients with clinically and mycologically documented vulvovaginal candidiasis compared single-dose treatment with a 500 mg clotrimazole vaginal tablet to either 3-day treatment with two 100 mg clotrimazole vaginal tablets administered daily or to treatment with a placebo vehicle. Patients were reassessed 5 to 10 days (visit 2) and at least 27 days (visit 3) post-treatment. Treatment with one 500 mg clotrimazole tablet was successful in 75% of patients and in no patients receiving placebo. Three of the 203 patients included in the drug safety evaluation reported treatment-related emergent signs and symptoms during the study period. These clinical trials indicate that the 500 mg clotrimazole vaginal tablet offers safe, effective, and convenient treatment of vulvovaginal candidiasis.

03.13.05

Topical and oral treatment of vaginal mycoses: Cohen, L. Cardiff Roy. Infirm., Cardiff, UK

Based on the results obtained during the course of six separate trials into the effectiveness of different topical antifungal preparations in different dosage regimes, a comparison has been made between local and oral antifungal therapy in the management of acute vulvovaginal fungal infection. Several reliable clinical trials carried out into the effect of oral ketoconazole have been drawn upon to make this comparison. The parameters used to compare the two routes of treatment were: Effectiveness, acceptability, compliance, cost, side and toxic effects. Statistically, a five day course of ketoconazole, 200 mgs b. d. was found to be as effective as a single 500 mg tablet of intravaginal clotrimazole. There was no difference in patients' acceptability, but compliance was greater in the single dose topical preparation. The cost of the single dose intravaginal treatment was almost half that of the comparable oral regime. No difference was found in the local side-effects produced by either regime, but the potential irreversible hepatotoxicity that might be caused by the ketoconazole, in the authors' view, totally precludes the use of this oral treatment for which a safe alternative exists.

03.13.06

Double-blind comparison of the efficacy and safety of single dose intravaginal treatment with clotrimazole and five days oral treatment with ketoconazole in vulvovaginal candidiasis: Loendersloot, E W*, Goormans, E**, Van Kempen, P J H*, Branolte, J H***. Pieter Pauw Ziekenhuis, Wageningen*, Ziekenhuis Leyenburg, The Hague**, Bayer Nederland B. V., Mijdrecht***, The Netherlands

Candida albicans, is the most common cause of vulvovaginal infections. The efficacy of single dose treatment with one vaginal tablet containing 500 mg clotrimazole proved to be very high in a number of trials: 89% respectively 82% of the patients had negative mycological cultures 1 and 4 weeks after treatment. In a bicentric trial 120 non-pregnant patients with vulvo-vaginal candidiasis (approximately ⅔ with primary and ⅓ with recurrent infections) will be randomly assigned to one of the following treatment schedules: one vaginal tablet of 500 mg clotrimazole and five days treatment with oral placebo twice daily; one vaginal placebo tablet and five days treatment with oral ketoconazole twice daily 200 mg. At the time of compilation of this abstract more than half of the envisaged number of patients has been included in the trial. At this moment it can be remarked that the mycological cure rate is satisfactory and that only few side effects are reported. Comparative results can only be calculated when the trial has been concluded and the code can be broken. An inquiry among the patients treated so far showed no preference for either the five days oral treatment or the single dose topical treatment.

03.41.01

Radical pelvic surgery: Reconstruction of the pelvic floor with myocutaneous gluteus-maximus flaps: Knapstein, P G, Bickmann, H J, Guth, U, Idel, P, Wiegand, U. Städt. Frauenklin., Krefeld

In a 62-year-old patient recurrence of vulva carcinoma occurred nine years after radical vulvectomy and postoperative irradiation. Treatment of the recurrent tumor, invading the rectum, consisted in resection of the total pelvic floor including parts of the urethra and vagina and the entire rectum. Primary covering of the large tissue defect is achieved by bilateral myocutaneous flaps with the gluteus maximus muscles. The technique is demonstrated in a 12-minute film (16 mm). The results of six cases are excellent even in far advanced tumors in older patients. The method can also be used in total exenteration for cancer of the vagina or cervix.

03.41.02

Dr. Nadakarni's sleeve excision and the anastomosis of the cervix in prolapse with supravaginal elongation of the cervix: Nadkarni, R M. V. S. Hosp. & K. M. School Post Grad. Med. & Res., Ahmedabad, India

Indisputable is the importance of the portio vaginalis of the cervix in the sex life and in the process of fertilization. The management of a prolapse with supravaginal elongation of the cervix in the child-bearing period poses a big problem. The procedure of amputation of portio cervix in the management of prolapse as suggested by *Sturmdorf* (1916) is helplessly used everywhere in spite of a consciousness of its disadvantages and esthetically giving a hideous appearance. The present film shows the procedure independently adopted and successfully carried out to solve the problem of supravaginal elongation of the cervix in cases of prolapse during the child-bearing age. The procedure mainly cosists of stepts of sleeve excision of the elongated supravaginal part of the cervix and end-to-end anastomosis of the two segments. It has resulted in an incrased rate of pregnancy and normal deliveries.

03.41.03

"Mitra Operation" for cancer of the cervix: Extraperitoneal pelvic lymphadenectomy et radical vaginal hysterectomy: Chowdhury, N N R. Med. Coll., Calcutta, India

Description of Film: Exact length: 900 ft., width: 16 mm (colour), projection time: 30 minutes, language of film: English, number of reels for film: two. The film demonstrates systematic bilateral removal of pelvic nodes extraperitoneally together with ligature of ovarian and uterine vessels and blunt dissection of parametria. The vaginal part demonstrates the steps of radical vaginal hysterectomy with massive removal of parametria.

03.41.04

Vaginal hysteretomy with and without prolapse: Joel-Cohen, S J. Beilinson Med. Ctr., Tel-Aviv Univ., Israel

The film demonstrates two complete operations, one with prolapse and one without prolapse. There is an insert demonstrating an easy method of removing ovaries vaginally; also shown are two extra inserts demonstrating the method of operating in the absence of prolapse. The method of urethral and anal dilatation demonstrated in the film, greatly reduce the need for post-operative catheterisation and reduce post-operative pain.

03.42.01

Gynecologic endoscopy–hysteroscopy. Part I: Technique: Vancaillie, T, Schmidt, E H. Frauenklin., Diakonissenanstalt, Bremen

This film is divided into two parts. The first half deals with the apparatus as e. g. the distention media used and their instillation rate. The handling of the hysteroscope itself is explained in detail. The second part of the film shows some examples, which firstly illustrate the diagnostic aims of the method and secondly put emphasis on systematic progress and on the mine of information got if one looks at every detail. The purpose is primarily to instruct those not familiar with and perhaps therefore sceptical towards this medical examination.

03.42.02

Needlescopic sterilization: McKenzie, E N. Darlington Memo. Hosp., Darlington, UK

This video film emphasises the use of miniaturised laparoscopy combined with miniaturised instrumentation. The objective is to help the patient in a painless and atraumatic fashion to achieve a pleasing cosmetic result. In addition discharge from hospital is possible on a day case basis. The method works well and has been performed on over 600 cases. In this series no case needed re-admission for internal bleeding or infection. The claim to safety is emphasised because there was no damage from burning to adjacent organs. This technique is simple and quick but should only be performed by experienced laparoscopists. This work has stimulated the development of a series of miniaturised gynecological telescopes. The important feature of these optical instruments is their excellent optical performance.

03.42.03

New approach to semen analysis: Makler, A, Neil, J, MacLusky, P, DeCherney, A, Heaseltine, F. Infertility Inst., Rambam Med. Ctr, Haifa, Israel, Yale Univ., USA

This video describes a new $10\,\mu m$ counting chamber which can be used for semen analysis as a rapid office procedure instead of the multiple steps and time-consuming technique where hemocytometer, ordinary slide and dry stained smears are used. In addition the chamber can be used for the more elaborated multiple exposure-photography (MEP) technique for objective semen motility determination in clinical and research studies. Samples placed in this chamber are photographed while being illuminated by stroboscopically 6-light pulses. Images of photographed sperm are projected on a magnetic tablet and information is fed with the aid of a digitizer into an ordinary home computer. In this way sperm concentration, percentage of motility, average velocity, frequency distribution of sperm velocities as well as percentage of abnormal forms are immediately shown upon the screen or provided as hard copy. One of the main advantages of this technique is that information can be stored in the film and re-evaluated when required.

03.42.04

Microsurgery of the cornual portion of the tube: Pellicer, A, Bonilla-Musoles, F. Med. School, Valencia, Spain

We present some different operations under microscope at the intramural portion of the tube. Our technique of cornual anastomosis is described.

03.42.05

Vacuum laparoscopy: Hengstberger, M. Frühdiagnosezentrum, Privatklin., Vienna, Austria

The vacuum laparoscopy permits a fast and safe diagnosis on outpatients, performed in laparoscopy centers or in specialist's practices which are especially equipped for this purpose. It also allows a risk-free trocar puncture during surgical laparoscopies. A vacuum bell was developed which permits aspiration and safe lifting of the abdominal walls prior to the trocar puncture. The puncture is performed with an acoustic safety trocar which has a diameter of only 3 mm for diagnostic purposes. Postoperative wound dressing is thus not required and there is practically no scar. The telescope for the quick laparoscopic diagnosis is inserted through the trocar sleeve. Only a minimal CO_2-insufflation is required. In diagnostic laparoscopy it only serves to compensate for the vacuum produced by lifting the abdominal walls. The acoustic safety trocar which I newly designed has an installed automatic Veres system for three trocar sizes (3 mm, 5 mm and 10 mm diameter) and indicates the correct position of the trocar tip in the intraperitoneal region by means of an acoustic signal. An intervention according to this method takes only two to three minutes, therefore a short anesthesia is sufficient and the patient can leave the hospital after one or two hours. I see excellent chances for the future of early diagnosis of ovarian cancer thanks to a reduced risk and simplification of the laparoscopy. The film shows a quick diagnostic laparoscopy and a sterilisation desired by the patient and carried out according to this method.

03.42.06

Systematic surgical procedure for external endometriosis with extensive adhesion: Nagata, I, Furuya, K, Kato, K. Dept. Obstet. and Gyn., Nat. Defense Med. Coll., Saitama, Japan

Radical operations for advanced endometriosis including chocolate cyst and frozen pelvis is occasionally very difficult especially for beginners because of the extensive adhesion. We devised a systematic surgical procedure always applicable to these cases. This video shows the procedure. The essential points of the procedure are as follows: 1. The abdominal wall is incised transversely or longitudinally and the peritoneal cavity is entered. 2. Peritoneal fluid is taken for cytology. 3. The endometrical cyst is aspirated. 4. The peritoneum is incised bilaterally between the round and infundibulopelvic ligaments. 5. The ureters are visualized or mobilized. 6. The infundibulopelvic ligaments are dissected. 7. Adhesions between the posterior wall of the cyst and pelvic peritoneum are separated with gentle digital or sharp dissection. 8. Bilateral pararectal spaces are dissected medially to the ureters. 9. The uterine arteries and upper parts of the lateral cervical ligaments are cut and ligated. 10. The anterior vagina is opened and the vaginal vault is amputated. 11. The residual cervical ligaments are clamped and ligated bilaterally from the already opened vaginal fornix upward. 12. The remaining adhesion between the cervix and rectum is sharply cut from below upward under direct vision and the uterus is removed. 13. The vaginal stump is closed with absorbable suture material. 14. The posterior peritoneum is not necessarily reattached. 15. Peritoneal cavity is irrigated with 2000 ml of warm saline. 16. The abdomen is then closed in two or three layers.

04.02.01

Evaluation of interferon alpha$_2$ in the treatment of condyloma acuminatum: Hatch, K D, Bart, B, Hansen, R, Reichman, R. Univ. of Alabama, Birmingham, AL, Hennepin County Med. Ctr, Minneapolis, MN, Univ. of Arizona, Tucson, AZ, Rochester NY

A multi-center, double-blind, placebo controlled, parallel-group study of the efficacy and safety of interferon alpha$_2$ in the treatment of condyloma acuminatum was conducted enrolling 114 patients. A single wart on each patient was injected with .01 ml 10^6 units interferon, 10^5 units interferon, or a placebo, three times weekly for three weeks and then followed for an additional nine weeks. Efficacy was evaluated by measuring change in size and overall change in disease status of the test wart relative to initial condition. In the high dose treatment group the mean percentage improvement in lesion size was 70.9% at 12 weeks versus 22.5% and 16.7% for low dose interferon and placebo respectively ($p < .05$). Complete clearing of the treated wart occurred in 53% of the high dose interferon group versus 10% and 14% of the low dose interferon and placebo groups respectively ($p < .01$). Adverse reactions were mild and limited in duration. Flu-like symptoms were present in 57% of high dose, 29% of low dose and 23% of placebo patients. Alpha$_2$ interferon at a dose of 10^6 units injected intralesionally three times a week for three weeks was highly efficacious in the treatment of condylomata acuminata with excellent safety.

04.02.02

Genital herpes in different groups of female populations: Briones, H, Suarez, M, Dubinovsky, S, Bernal, J, Maggi, L. Obstet. and Gyn. Dept., Microbiol. and Parasit. Dept., Fac. Med., Student Hlth Serv., Univ. of Chile, Santiago

We have studied different groups (g) of female populations comparing clinical symptoms with two laboratory tests: 1. Viral isolation, practiced in samples of the patient's lesion, or vaginal pouch or uterine cervix using Vero cell line. 2. Serologic investigation to determine the type, titers and evolution of the anti-herpes simplex virus antibodies, utilizing indirect hemagglutination and index value II/I was done on serum samples from acute and convalescent period (*Suarez, M*. et al. Rev. Med. Chile **111**, 771, 1983). In the first g. with clinical evidences of genital herpes, we found 55% of positive viral isolation (28/51). Serological analysis was negative in six cases, titers between 1/32–1/64 in 28 patients (55%) and titers ≧ 1/128 in 4 cases. Seroconversion was observed in three occasions. In the second g., 378 asymptomatic university students, 20–29 years old, three positive viral isolations (0.79%) were found. In the third g. with 500 asymptomatic multiparas of a Family Planning Clinic, we found 1% of viral isolation. In the fourth g. we testet 200 patients under Prenatal Care and we detect 2% of herpes infection. In the fifth g. we selected 400 prostitutes and we found a prevalence of 4.5% positive viral isolation. These results show a good correlation between clinical and laboratory diagnosis. The different groups have the prevalence that we could expect as compared with international values for similar groups of age and sexual habits.

04.02.03

Herpes simplex virus: Treatment with cimetidine (Tagamet): Peretz, B A, Friedman, M, Paldi, E. Dept. Obstet. and Gyn. "B", Rambam Med. Ctr, Haifa, Israel

Thymus-dependent T lymphocytes have H_2-receptors. Theoretically it is therefore possible for H_2-receptor antagonists, such as cimetidine, to modify cell-mediated immune responses. The importance of immune mechanisms in preventing herpes virus infections is well known. Tagamet was used in treating patients with Herpes Simplex infection. Six patients had herpes labialis (HL) infection, and 23 genital herpes (HG). In the latter group 17 women presented with recurrent disease and five with primary infection. Prior to treatment the relapse frequency varied from 3–4 weeks to 2–3 months. Herpes Simplex virus was isolated from each patient. The dosage schedule of the drug was derived empirically from the standard regimen recommended for the treatment of peptic ulcers. Duration of treatement was consistent for all patients. The efficacy of the treatment resulted in improving the clinical status in four aspects: 1. improvement of symptoms, 2. reduction of disease duration, 3. reduction of disease intensity with each subsequent reactivation (in respect to dimension and number of lesions), 4. decrease in the recurrence rate. Best results were achieved in the HL group, all but one patient noted marked improvement. 76.4% of the HG group benefited by the treatment. In the primary GH infection group the following improvements were noted: a) Tagamet had an analgesic effect on all five patients. b) Three patients showed an accelerated healing rate. The mean duration of the disease dropped to five days from the expected 14–17 days. Further studies on the efficacy of cimetidine against herpes virus need to be performed.

04.02.04

Cervical intra-epithelial neoplasm in specific AMCR vaginosis: Plantema, F H F., Voojis, P G. Dept. Gyn., St. Liduina Hosp., Boxtel; Vooijs, PG, Inst. Path. Anat., Univ., Nijmegen, The Netherlands

Anaerobic motile curved rods (AMCR) play an important role in female discharge. Patients with an AMCR vaginosis have few complaints. Phase-contrast bacterioscopic screening of the vaginal flora in a direct wet preparation of a flagellotrophic solution enables one to specify the vaginal discharge in patients with a so-called nonspecific vaginitis (NSV). AMCR adhere to epithelial cells by a glycocalyx resulting in a "Comma-cell". In a group of 990 women who visited in a trimester a general gynecological practice for diverse reasons, the vaginal flora was screened by phase-contrast microscopy and a flagellotrophic solution. Forty-four women were positive for AMCR. In 384 of the 990 women routine cervix-cytologic examination was carried out. The results of the cytologic study are discussed in comparison with bacteriological features of the AMCR positive group. The positive group shows 2.5 × more atypical vaginal epithelial cells and 2.5 × more atypical metaplastic squamoid cells. Light and moderate dysplasia were found respectively two and seven times more frequently. Atypical columnar epithelial cells were also found six times more frequently, than in the AMCR negative group.

04.02.05

Vaginal trichomoniasis treatment by immunization with lactobacillus acidophilus vaccine: Azevedo, E M M, Fonseca, A M, Souza, A Z, Bagnoli, V R, Salvatore, C A. Gyn. Clin., São Paulo Univ. Med. School, São Paulo, Brazil

Clinical efficacy and tolerance of Solcotrichovac vaccine (inactivated lactobacilli) were evaluated in patients with symptomatic vaginal trichomoniasis. The average age of the patients was 38, from 19 to 58 years old. The main symptoms were vaginal discharge (100.0%), vaginal pruritus (78.3%), pelvic pain (41.6%) and dyspareunia (53.3%). Gynecologic examination showed: edema (18.3%), erythema (38.3%) and cervicitis (18.3%). Trichomonas vaginalis was identified through direct microscopic examination in wet smears in all patients. Thirty patients were vaccinated with Solcotrichovac in four intramuscular injections, the first one given at diagnosis and the rest at 2 and 4 weeks, and 12 months later. Meanwhile, thirty patients taking placebo in the same schedule, formed the control group. The main results obtained after 15 months were: 1) The patients treated with Solcotrichovac showed marked relief of symptoms and improvement of clinical findings compared with placebo group. 2) Trichomonas vaginalis was identified in 1 (3.3%) patients treated with Solcotrichovac and 6 (20.0%) of the placebo group. 3) In the vaccinated group, antibodies titers distribution was different from placebo group. This result could be an explanation for the clinical influence on vaginal trichomoniasis.

04.02.06

Management of trichomonas vaginalis resistant to 5-nitroimidazoles: Forssman, L, Milsom I, Forsgren, A. Dept. Obstet. and Gyn., Univ. of Göteborg, East Hosp., Göteborg and Dept. Clin. Bacteriol., Univ. of Lund, Malmö Gen. Hosp., Malmö, Sweden

The efficacy of Trichomonas vaginalis treatment improved significantly with the advent of the 5-nitroimidazoles. The existence of Trichomonas vaginalis strains resistant to 5-nitroimidazoles is at present an uncommon problem. Since 1978 we have been able to identfy three unrelated cases of Trichomonas vaginalis resistant to 5-nitroimidazoles. Minimal trichomonicidal concentrations were between 40 and 160 μg/ml as opposed to normal values of $< 10 \mu$g/ml. Reinfection, deficient drug absorption and local drug inactivation could be excluded as a cause of persistent infection. The vaginal microflora was dominated by anaerobes and Group B β-hemolytic streptococci. One of the patients had only mild symptoms and was left untreated. Five years later the infection had healed spontaneously. The other two patients had troublesome symptoms which were reduced by local 5-nitroimidazole treatment. However, the trichomonads were not eliminated. Continuous treatment with 5-nitroimidazoles for a period of years is not be recommended. Local application of albothyl (Nelex®, Byk Gulden) was effective as symptomatic treatment. During this treatment anaerobes and Group B streptococci disappeared and lactobacilli became dominant. Regular intermittent treatment with albothyl appears to offer means of symptomatic relief in resistant cases.

04.02.07

Colposcopic study of 50 cases of systemic schistosomiasis: Aguiar, L M, Souza, A Z, Fonseca, A M, Hegg, R. Gyn. Clin., Univ. of São Paulo Med. School, São Paulo, Brazil

Cervical infestation by Schistosoma mansoni was detected four times among 95,128 patients screened by colposcopy in the prevention service of the clinic in the period from 1952–1980. The colposcopic appearances were characterized by polypoid spiry red tumoration, bleeding easily on the surface. In order to get a more detailed knowledge about this matter, 50 women registered in the Dept. of Infectious and Tropical Diseases of the Medical School, University of São Paulo, all of them suffering from systemic schistosomiasis, were subjected to colposcopic investigation; in three of these patients schistosomiasis granulomata of the uterine cervix could be diagnosed. In two of them there was a large typical dotting with a more generalized red zone. The third patient presented a thickened epithelium, associated with other changes which could be interpreted as a intra-epithelial carcinoma. Although this screening study was performed only in 50 patients with systemic schistosomiasis one 'may conclude that the uterine cervix only achieves any clinical importance in about 6.0% of the women suffering from this infestation.

04.02.08

Actinomyces israelii in the female genital tract – microbiological and immunological studies: Persson, E, Holmberg, K. Karolinska Inst., Danderyd Hosp. and Nat. Bacteriol. Labor., Stockholm, Sweden

The occurrence of Actinomyces israelii in the genital tract of women was studied by culture and by direct microscopy, including immunofluorescence techniques. Examination of samples from the endocervix, IUDs and uterine secretions of asymptomatic women revealed the bacterium in approximately 5% of the material. The same results were obtained in a longitudinal study when cervical samples were analyzed. Vaginal colonization was then found to occur in 13% an perineal colonization in 24% of the sampling occasions. No co-variation was found in the occurrence of A.israelii and different parameters studied, such as phase of menstrual cycle. A. israelii was defined as a part of the indigenous genital flora. IUD use per se was not found to increase the prevalence of A. israelii and duration of such IUD use was also found insignificant for colonization. A serological test system comprising two techniques for electroimmunoprecipitation in gel was used for detecting antibodies against A. israelii. No serological immune response was detected to A. israelii colonization in the lower genital tract. The serological test system was proven to be a valuable tool for detecting cases of genital actinomycosis. Precipitation reactions were also found when analyzing uterine secretions from IUD users. A hypothesis of a local immune response was suggested.

04.02.09

Recurrent periclitoral abscess: A case report and review of literature: Inoue, H, Fukushima, Y. Chigasaki Tokushukai Med. Ctr, Japan

A large abscess with disabling symptoms, adjacent to the clitoris is called a periclitoral abscess. Only six instances of recurrent periclitoral abscess habe been recorded in the literature between 1975 and 1984. The review of the cases, as well as features of the patient therein reported, will serve as the basis for presenting a clinical profile of this disease and for appropriate management. One case of recurrent periclitoral abscess treated by marsupialization is presented here. In the course of our five years' obstetric and gynecological practice, only one case of recurrent periclitoral abscess has been encountered. – Case history: A 49-year-old female, gravida-1, para-1, was seen at our clinic on January 5, 1982, complaining of throbbing pain and swelling in the genital region of five days' duration. The abscess was incised and drained. Two months later, swelling and intolerable pain recurred. Consequently, she had repeated episodes of the abscess in the same area on six occasions from January 1982 to December 1984. This patient was admitted to our hospital on December 1, 1984, and on the same day marsupialization of the periclitoral abscess was performed. Since then the patient has had no recurrence of the episode.

04.03.01

Plasma concentrations of gestoden and endogenous sexual hormones in a 21-day treatment cycle with the new oral contraceptive and in two further treatment cycles with defined 2-day breaks in treatment in 6 young women: Düsterberg, B, Hassan, S H, Matthes, H. Schering AG, Berlin

Design of study: After a treatment-free preliminary cycle, six young women received a daily oral dose of 75 μg gestoden (G) and 30 μg ethinylestradiol for 21 days in the first treatment cycle. In the following second treatment cycle the doses in the 6th and 7th day and in the third treatment cycle the doses on the 11th and 12th day were not taken. Plasma concentrations of G, progesterone, 17β-estradiol, FSH and LH were estimated by RIA. In addition, the plasma concentrations of SHBG were determined in the preliminary cycle and treatment cycle I. – Results: 0.8 ± 0.3 h after the first oral dose the plasma level of G reached a max. of 3.8 ± 2.8 ng/ml. The drug level fell with half-lives of 1.6 ± 1.4 and 10.6 ± 6.0 h. The area under the drug concentration curve was 24 ± 20 ng/ml × h. During daily oral admin. the plasma concentration of G (24 h after each admin.) rose, reaching peak values of 8.06 ± 5.6 ng/ml between the 14th and 19th day. No further increase in G level was observed during the last days of the treatment cycle. 1.3 ± 1 h after the 21st dose a mean peak plasma concentration of 9.72 ± 3.4 ng/ml was measured. The G level fell with half-lives of 1.5 ± 1 and 18.2 ± 4.2 h. The area under the drug concentration curve from 0 to 24 h after the 21st admin. was 136 ± 58 ng/ml × h. A marked elevation of SHBG concentration in the first treatment cycle was found in comparison to the preliminary cycle. The interruptions of treatment led to a clear reduction in drug levels. The course of the progesterone and 17β-estradiol levels showed that ovulation had no taken place in any of the treatment cycles. FSH an LH levels showed considerable fluctuations during the treatment cycles; in some cases the peak concentration attained values found in the preovulatory phase in the preliminary cycles. In four of the subjects temporary increases in gonadotrophin levels were observed which could be attributed to the dosage interruptions in treatment. In the other two women LH and FSH peaks were only seen during the normal treatment-free period. With two exceptions, the two-day dosage interruptions always resulted in intermenstrual bleeding.

04.03.02

Metabolic effects and blood coagulation under oral contraception with a gestoden-containing low dose combined pill and a levonorgestrel-containing combined pill: Rabe, T, Waibel S, Kiesel, L, Runnebaum, B, Kohlmeier, M*, Harenberg, J*, Weicker, H**. Dept. Obstet. and Gyn., *Dept. Int. Med., **Dept. Int. Med., Pathophys. and Sports Med., Univ., Heidelberg

Sixty healthy female volunteers (18 to 35 years of age), without oral contraception for at least six months participated in a within patient trial and were randomly divided into two groups (n = 30). Metabolic effects of a gestoden containing combined pill (ethinylestradiol 30 μg/gestoden 75 μg) and of a levonorgestrel-containing combined pill (30 μg ethynylestradiol/150 μg levonorgestrel) (Microgynon® = German brand name) is investigated during a 24 month administration period and compared with basal values before OC administration. At the beginning of the study glucose tolerance test was performed in each patient between day 18–22 of two consecutive menstrual cycles without OC treatment. Carbohydrate metabolism was evaluated by measuring serum glucose, insulin and HbA_{1c} before, one and two hours after oral glucose loading (oligosaccharides corresponding to 100 g) (Boehringer, Mannheim). In addition blood samples were taken for lipid and blood coagulation analysis and fibrinolysis. Furthermore testosterone, free testosterone, SHBG, thyroid and adrenal cortex hormones were determined. After the two pre-treatment cycles, OCs were given and tests were performed after 3, 6, 12, 18 and 24 months of OC use. An interim analysis will be performed after 3 and 6 months of OC treatment and data will be analysed as regards metabolic data on other contraceptive steroids published in the literature.

04.03.03

Endocrine-pharmacological profile of gestoden: Elger, W, Steinbeck, H, Schillinger, E, Losert, W, Beier, S. Berlin (West)

17α-Ethynyl-13-ethyl-17β-hydroxy-4,15-gonadien-3-on (gestoden, GES) is a new gestagen for use in OCs. In rats and rabbits GES exhibited about 3–10 times more gestagenic effect than levonorgestrel (LN) which is structurally related. The same applies to its anti-estrogenic and anti-ovulatory activity. GES has 59% binding affinity to the androgen receptor in the rat prostate (^{3}H-5α-DHT = 100%). GES displayed some androgenic activity in the accessory sex glands of castrated male rats. However, when the more potent gestagenic action of GES, as compared to LN and other 19-nonsteroids, is taken into account. the androgenic and gestagenic potencies of GES can be seen to be dissociated by a factor of approx. 3 to 5. GES showed no estrogenic or anti-androgenic activity. Receptor studies demonstrated the affinity of GES for the mineralocorticoid receptor, thus causing slight anti-mineralocorticoid action in rats. In conclusion, GES is a potent gestagen which offers a greater dissociation of androgenic and gestagenic efficacy. Further investigations are necessary to elucidate the biological significance of the anti-mineralocorticoid activity.

04.03.04

Estrogen antagonizing effect of gestoden at the pituitary level: Baumgarten, S, Römmler, A, Hammerstein, J. Abt. Gyn. Endocr., UFK Steglitz, Berlin

It is well established that ethynylestradiol (EE) raises the pituitary responsiveness to GnRH. In contrast, synthetic progestins may counteract this effect depending on their structure and dosage (*Römmler* et al.

Contraception **25**, 1982). To define the pharmacological potency of progestins at the hypophyseal level the GnRH-double-stimulation test serves as a useful and sensitive model. The present investigation compares the potency of L-norgestrel (50-75-125 µg/day – tristep) with that of a new progestin gestoden (50-70-100 µg/day) in antagonizing the EE-induced (30-40-30 µg/day) rise of pituitary responsiveness to GnRH. In six women taking L-norgestrel + EE (Triquilar®) and gestoden + EE a GnRH-double-stimulation test was performed on the last day of each treatment cycle. The max. net increase of LH and FSH after the first (Δ_1) and 2nd (Δ_2) GnRH-stimulation served as indicator for hypophyseal function. – Under medication with gestoden + EE Δ_1 and Δ_2 of both gonadotrophins (LH: Δ_1 20.4 ± 18.5; Δ_2 25.2 ± 18.6; FSH: Δ_1 2.8 ± 2.7 Δ_2 4.8 ± 4.9 mean-SD, mIU/ml) remained below the values obtained under Norgestrel + EE (LH: Δ_1 27.1 ± 20.6; Δ_2 49.1 ± 16.2; FSH: Δ_1 2.9 ± 1.9; Δ_2 6.4 ± 4.7) (p < 0.05). – Conclusion: The new progestin gestoden reveals a stronger antagonistic influence on the EE-induced rise in pituitary responsiveness to GnRH than L-norgestrel. This indicates the higher anti-estrogenic potency of gestoden at the hypophyseal level.

04.03.05

Comparison of the effects of levonorgestrel and gestoden on pituitary function, follicular development and cervical mucus: Eyong, E, Elstein, M. Dept. Obstet. and Gyn., Univ. of South Manchester, Manchester, UK
Levonorgestrel was compared with a new progestogen, gestoden (Δ^{15} levonorgestrel). Three groups of five women of reproductive age were studied, prior to hysterectomy for benign disease. In the first menstrual cycle the serum levels of FSH and LH were measured on alternate days and follicular growth monitored by ultrasound pelvic scanning. The cervical score (*Insler, V* et al., Int. J. Gyn. Obstet. **10**, 223–228, 1972) and the sperm penetration of mucus (*Kremer, J*, Int. J. Fertil. **10**, 205–215, 1965) were quantified at mid-cycle. During days 8–18 of th next cycle, one group received 75 µg levonorgestrel daily, one received 75 µg gestoden and the trial group acted as a control. Similar measurements were made to those performed in the first cycle and preliminary data indicate a greater suppressive action by gestoden compared to levonorgestrel. After this course of treatment, hysterectomy was performed and the biochemical effect of these progestins on the endometrium investigated (see *Chantler* et al., this meeting).

04.03.06

Inhibition of ovulation with Δ^{15}-levonorgestrel (gestoden): Spona, J. 1st Dept. Obstet. and Gyn., Univ., Vienna, Austria
The aim of the present investigation was to study gestoden (Δ^{15}-levonorgestrel) action in females with normal cycles. Furthermore, modulation by gestoden of LH-RH stimulated gonadotropin release was studied in a rat model system and in cell culture. In addition, gestoden receptor interaction was investigated. Gestoden affected both basal as well as LH-RH stimulated LH and FSH serum levels in the ovariectomized rat. Data indicate a 3-times greater potency than levonorgestrel. Additionally, 3×10^{-8} M gestoden suppressed LH and FSH release at ED_{50} of LH-RH to 50 and 70%, resp., in a pituitary cell culture system. Results of these experiments suggest greater biological potency of gestoden than levonorgestrel. Borderline dose of gestoden for inhibition of ovulation was studied in 16 females. Daily treatment with 10 and 20 µg of gestoden resulted in luteal insufficiency, whereas 30 µg caused inhibition of ovulation in three and follicular maturation without ovulation in eight out of 12 subjects. These results were derived from estimations of hormone serum levels, cervical score data and karyopyknotic index. These results were corroborated by studies on inhibition of ovulation in 20 females who were given 75 µg gestoden plus 30 µg ethynylestradiol (EE$_2$) and 75 µg levonorgestrel plus 30 µg EE$_2$, resp., through 21 days. Additional studies on receptor interactions indicate that gestoden is not different from other progestagens in current use in its androgen residual potency. No interaction with the estrogen receptor was observed. Present data combine to suggest that gestoden is a new generation progestogen with enhanced biological activity. Ratio between progestogen and androgen activity is better than that of progestagens in current use.

04.03.07

Endometrial receptor response to two progestogens, levonorgestrel and gestoden: Chantler, E, Sharma, R, Eyong, E, Elstein, M. Dept. Obstet. and Gyn., Univ. Hosp. of South Manchester, Manchester, UK
Fifteen women of reproductive age undergoing hysterectomy for menorrhagia were tested for the progestational effect of a new contraceptive steroid, gestoden, which is considered to be more potent than levonorgestrel. Two groups of five patients received orally either 75 µg gestoden daily for 10 days, starting on days 8–10 of the menstrual cycle, when estradiol levels were near their maximum. A third group of five patients received no exogenous steroids. Following hysterectomy on day 20, the endometrium was removed, snap-frozen in liquid nitrogen and then stored at −70°C. To compare the uterine response to the two synthetic gestogens, the nuclear estradiol receptor and cytosolic 17β-hydroxysteroid dehydrogenase were measured. The cytosol of the homogenized endometrium was incubated with H-estradiol and nicotinamide adenine dinucleotide (NAD), and the resultant ^{3}H-estrone estimated. The nuclear receptor concentration was measured by Scatchard analysis of the levels of bound estradiol, in the presence of diethylstilbestrol. Both of these systems are known to be influenced by gestogens, when the endometrium has previously been

exposed to estrogens, causing a decrease in the concentration of nuclear estrogen receptor levels and inducing production of 17β-hydroxysteroid dehydrogenase (which converts estradiol to estrone). By measuring these variables both in the normal woman and those using either of the two gestogens, the uterine response to the gestogens may be quantified.

04.03.08

Phase II + III clinical trials with a combined pill containing gestoden and ethinylestradiol: Unger, R. Schering AG, Berlin

The aim of the trial was to demonstrate the contraceptive reliability of the preparation, the acceptable cycle control and the good tolerance in a large patient population. 707 women were recruited under strict observation of the contraindications. The treatment period covered 24 cycles and no pregnancies were recorded in the course of 9947 cycles monitored. Cycle length, duration and intensity of the withdrawal bleedings were within normal range. When the "intermenstrual" bleeding rates in individual cycles are compared it becomes apparent that the rate decreases with the passage of time. For example, spotting was reported in the control cycle by 6.2% of the women. Without taking errors in tablet-taking into account the spotting rate in the first treatment cycle was 10.9% but had sunk to 6.9% by the sixth cycle. Sharp increases in the spotting rate in response to forgotten tablets are obvious. Break-through bleeding maintained relatively low rates throughout all the treatment cycles. The figure for amenorrhea was 0.6%. Diastolic blood pressure values in normotensive women remained practically uninfluenced throughout the entire period of the trial. The body weight was uninfluenced even after 24 cycles in 80.5% of the trial population. The subjective side-effects reported under therapy were comparable to those known from other OC preparations also. Available results clearly show that this extremely low-dosed trial preparation fulfills all the criteria listed above.

04.03.09

Comparative studies of low-dose estrogen oral contraceptives combined with levonorgestrel, gestoden and desogestrel in monophasic and triphasic formulations: Bonnar, J, Daly, L, Carroll, M E. Trinity Coll. Dept. Obstet. and Gyn., St. James' Hosp. and Rotunda Hosp., Dublin, Ireland

Women taking combined estrogen-progestogen oral contraceptives (OC) have an increased risk of venous and arterial thrombo-embolic disease. This excess risk has been shown to relate to the dosage of estrogen and progestogen, smoking, advanced age and prolonged usage. Consistent findings in women taking the combined OC are a raised level of fibrinogen and factor VII activity, changes in factors II, VIII, IX and X, antithrombin III and platelet function have also been shown. Fibrinolytic activity is usually increased with the OC and this should counteract the increased activity of the coagulation factors and the greater propensity of fibrin formation. Serial studies of blood coagulation factors, fibrinolysis and platelets are in progress in 120 women taking Logynon®, Marvelon®, Trinordiol® and SHD 415G (gestoden) The effect of the estrogen is modified by the progestogen used in combination as shown by the changes in levels of factor X, antifactor Xa, plasminogen, fibrinolytic activity and platelet aggregation. The aim should be to develop formulations which induce the least hemostatic changes. This may reduce or eliminate the increased risk of thrombo-vascular complications in women taking oral contraceptives.

04.03.10

Clinical and cytoendometrial aspects in women treated with triphasic OC (SHD 415 G) with gestoden: Palumbo, G, Russo, I, Cianci, A, Asero, S, Riillo, S. 2nd Dept. Obstet. and Gyn., Univ., Catania, Italy

The study has been performed on 26 women aged between 21 and 35 years, treated with a new estroprogestinic association in a triphasic formulation for contraceptive purpose. This estroprogestinic association contains a new gestagenic compund such as gestoden (Δ^{15}-L-norgestrel) given orally in the following doses: 5 tablets containing 0.030 mg of ethynylestradiol +0.050 mg of gestoden; 6 tablets containing 0.030 ethynylestradiol +0.070 mg of gestoden; 10 tablets containing 0.030 mg of ethynylestradiol +0.100 mg of gestoden. The protocol consisted of six months of treatment with the following clinical examinations at cycles 0, 3, 6. These examinations consisted of clinical evaluation of the features of the menstrual cycles, hormonal and metabolic measurements and evaluation of microhysteroscopical, histological and cytological aspects. During the treatment the authors did not see any remarkable variation in the metabolic and hormonal features. For what concerns histological and cytological aspects, they seem to be well correlated to each other. Nevertheless these aspects do not seem absolutely constant. In fact the degree of glandular hypoplasia and stromal hyperplasia is quite variable. The authors think that the variability of these aspects could be due to the influence of residual ovarian activity on the endometrial histomorphology.

04.03.11

Clinical experience with a new triphasic oral contraceptive containing gestoden: Gammi, L, Flamigni, C. Serv. Fisiopat. Riprod., Catt. Endocr. Gin., Univ. Bologna, Italy

Oral contraception with triphasic preparations is increasingly more appreciated as the latest outcome of pharmacological research on estro-progestogen contraceptives. A double-blind study on 30 patients was carried out administering two triphasic preparations the first containing levonorgestrel and the second the new progestagen gestoden (Δ^{15} levonorgestrel). 720 cycles of administration were observed and monitored according to the usual clinical and hematochemical protocols. This confirmed, as already in previous studies, the 100% contraceptive efficacy as well as the excellent acceptability of both preparations, as well as the important advantage of "normalising" the menstrual cycle particularly in terms of timing and duration. Spotting and/or BTB were found to be negligible and with levels lower then those reported for low dosed monophasic preparations. Side-effects were rare and of very minor importance. For these reasons, in spite of their recent development, triphasic oral contraceptives have reached the ranking of drugs of choice in female hormonal contraception.

04.04.01

In vitro chemosensitivity testing of gynecologic tumors with two different cell viability tests and ³H-thymidine incorporation: Jakkula, H, Kivinen, S, Stenbäck, F, Silvennoinen-Kassinen, S, Tiilikainen, A. Dept. Med. Microbiol., Gyn and Path., Univ., Oulu, Finland

The aim was to develop a reliable in vitro method for tumor cell chemosensitivity. The tumor specimen was divided into three parts: One for pathologist, one for mouse subrenal capsule assay and one for in vitro assays. In vitro assay: Dissociated cancer cells were exposed to antineoplastic drugs, except control cells, for 18 h, washed and cultured 10^5 cells per culture well. Three assays were employed. Drug effect was measured by comparison to untreated control cells. 1) The cell proliferation was followed with 72 h ^{3}H-thymidine incorporation. 2) Cell viability was determined with trypan blue exclusion after 24 and 72 h and also the total cell number was counted. 3) In the method of *Weisenthal* et al. (1983) the cells were cultured three days after drug exposure and stained with Fast green (FG), sedimented onto cytocentrifuge slides and counterstained with hematoxylin-eosin. FG stained dead cells were calculated as a percentage of control based on the relative numbers of living tumor cells, living non-tumor cells and dead cells. ^{3}H-thymidine incorporation reveals proliferation capacity and cytostatic effect of drugs. Trypan blue exclusion measures cytotoxic effects revealing numbers of dead cells; only the follow-up of total cell numbers reveals the amount of completely destroyed cells. The Weisenthal method provides a distinction between tumor and non-tumor cells and the relative numbers of dead cells. Thus, only one method gave no full information about drug effect on our 18 samples tested so far.

04.04.02

Chemotherapeutic studies on rat ovarian cancer (the 2nd report): Sugiyama, T, Nishida, T, Oda T, Yakushiji, M, Kato, T. Dept. Obstet. and Gyn., Kurume Univ., Japan

Following direct application of 7,12-dimethylbenz(a)anthracene (DMBA) to the ovary of Wistar rats, the incidence of tumorigenesis was 48% and the tumorigenic lesions were concomitant adenocarcinomas showing both glandular and solid elements. The DMBA-induced cancers were transplantable, caused ascites, and were similar morphologically and biologically to human counterpart. Chemotherapy-induced changes of tumor tissue have been observed and reported in the primary autochthonous ovarian cancers in our series. In this presentation we evaluated morphological comparison of anticancer effects between the original autochthonous tumor and its transplanted counterpart. Anticancer agents used were cis-DDP and iphosphamide. Histologic and microangiographic investigation were performed. Transplanted tumor appeared much more homogenous solid pattern with obvious vascular development than was seen in the original tumor, and the effect of the chemotherapy was more evident. All of the transplanted tumors decreased in size and 20 out of 100 tumors were completely eradicated. Histologic effects were also remarkable with the reduction of the intratumoral neovascularizations. The combination procedure of these in vivo models appeared to be available for assay of anticancer agents and effects.

04.04.03

Morphological evaluation of synergistic efficacy in combination of a bacterial pyrogen and cytotoxic agent on a transplantable ovarian cancer: Oda, T, Sugiyama, T, Yakushiji, M, Kato, T. Dept. Obstet. and Gyn., Kurume Univ., Japan

Bacterial pyrogen as a biological response modifier (BRM) has still not obtained a certain place in the practical cancer therapy. To evolve the therapeutic significance of bacterial BRM, the synergistic effect of a streptococcal pyrogen in combination with cis-diamminedichloroplatinum (DDP) was evaluated on a transplantable cancer in rat. The tumor line was obtained from a rat ovarian adenocarcinoma induced by local application of 7,12-dimethylbenz(a)anthracene. After serial transplantations throughout 15 generations, the tumor tissue has a definite growth rate and is able to kill the host within five weeks from the inoculation. The pyrogen used was OK432, which is regarded as a non-specific immunostimulant in Japan. Twenty rats with the tumor received 10 mg/kg of DDP as an intravenous administration three weeks after the transplantation. A half of them also received 0.3 KE (Klinische Einheit) of OK432 intravenously. None of the rats in DDP alone group could survive up to fifth week from the treatment. Although the size of the tumors in this group on the increase, however, the cytotoxic effect of DDP was histologically evident, showing a large central necrosis in the tumor. All of the pyrogen-treated rats did not die within nine weeks from the combination therapy. The tumor sizes decreased gradually and, of interest, one of the tumors was completely eradicated. Histologically, remarkable histiocytic infiltrations were noted in the damaged tumor tissue. From these, the enhanced efficacy of DDP in OK432 combined therapy was suggested and recommendations were made for clinical trials for DDP plus OK432 treatment.

04.04.04

Evaluation of the effect of ten standard anticancer agents on human ovarian tumors by use of the Human Tumor Colony Forming Assay (HTCFA): Schieder, K, Bieglmayer, C, Csaicsich, P, Kölbl, H, Breitenecker, G, Szepesi, T, Nowotny, C, Janisch, H. 2nd Dept. Gyn. and Obstet., Univ., Vienna, Austria

Fifty-three tumor specimens from 36 patients suffering from malignant ovarian tumors of different clinical stages were tested for their sensitivity to ten standard anticancer agents by the HTCFA. Number and size of the grown colonies were evaluated by an optical image analyser (Omnicon 3000). In 79% of the assays there was a growth of colonies greater than 60 μm in diameter, whereas a sufficient number of colonies for a statistically significant evaluation (more than 30 colonies per control group) was only found in 49%. Plating efficiency ranged from 0.011–0.35%. The coefficient of variation for control growth was with the exception of four cases less than 30%. Eleven tumor specimens from nine patients (2 patients had a previous treatment with anticancer drugs, one a previous irradiation therapy) proved to be resistant against all tested drugs. In 15 specimens of 13 patients (one had a previous cytostatic therapy) a sensitivity of the Tumor Colony Forming Units (TCFUs) against one or several anticancer substances was found. In three cases we could compare chemosensitivity of two different specimens (peritoneal washing-primary tumor, ascites-metastasis of the omentum, pleural effusion-ascites). We found discordant dry effects of the TCFUs, a possible expression of the tumor heterogeneity. Mitomycin (7/26), endoxan (6/22), methotrexate (6/26) and tamoxifen (6/26) were identified as the most effective drugs.

04.04.05

Chemosensitivity testing using subrenal capsule assay for ovarian cancer: Mashiba, H, Matsunaga, K, Jimi, S, Watanabe, Y, Kurano, A. Nat. Kyushu Ca Ctr., Fukuoka, Japan

Selection of antitumor drugs is very important to obtain excellent results in chemotherapy of cancer. In this study, subrenal capsule assay in mice was used to evaluate chemotherapeutic agents. A 1-mm cube fragment of tumor tissue was implanted into the subrenal capsule of normal immunocompetent ddY mice. Treatment was started the day after implantation and continued on every day for five days. When spontaneous mammary tumors of C3H mouse were implanted into male mice, growth of the tumor was inhibited compared with that in female mice. Six patients with ovarian cancer were examined. The maximally tolerated dose of antitumor drugs was employed as reported. Degree of responsiveness was various in an individual case. Cyclophosphamide and etoposide were effective in all cases, and tumor size was decreased compared with that before treatment. Rate of cases in which cis-DDP or adriamycin was effective was 66.7% and 83.3%, respectively. Oral administration of tegafur (1.25 mg/day) was also effective. Relation of chemosensitivity to clinical response was examined. Drugs effective in this assay were used for treatment of ovarian cancer of a recurrent case and partial response was observed. This assay seems to be beneficial to predict clinical response and to decide on ranking of antitumor drugs in clinical use.

04.04.06

Antitumor effect of "Two Route Chemotherapy" (TRC) on experimental peritoneal dissemination: Kamura, T, Matsuyama, T, Tsukamoto, N, Nakano, H. Dept. Gyn. & Obstet., Fac. Med., Kyushu Univ., Fukuoka, Japan

Recently, sodium thiosulfate (STS) has been reported to be an antagonist of cisplatinum (CDDP). As a treatment of peritoneal dissemination of ovarian cancer, antitumor effect and toxicity of TRC, which consists of intraperitoneal (ip) CDDP and intravenous (iv) STS were evaluated using an animal model. Highly inbred DDD mice and Ehrlich ascites tumor (EAT) were used. LD50 value of ipCDDP was 20 mg/kg, while ivSTS showed no toxicity up to a dose of 2000 mg/kg. 1500 mg/kg of ivSTS completely rescued from toxic death mice simultaneously given 20 mg/kg of ipCDDP. Histologically, kidneys of the mice given 20 mg/kg of ipCDDP showed serious changes; dilatation of tubules and flattened tubular epithelium, whereas TRC gave no changes. In terms of weight loss, toxicity of 10 mg/kg of ipCDDP was mild and equal to that of simultaneously use of 20 mg/kg of ipCDDP and 1500 mg/kg of ivSTS (simultaneous TRC). As for an antitumor effect on ip EAT in mice, 8 of 10 mice were cured with the simultaneous TRC, while 5 of 10 with ipCDDP alone. Plasma concentration of platinum following ipCDDP reached maximum at an interval of 10 min. Sequential administration of ipCDDP and ivSTS at an interval of 10 min. showed a serious toxicity, whereas at an interval of 5 min. the antitumor effect was higher than the simultaneous TRC and the toxicity was mild. In conclusion, first, TRC showed higher antitumor effect on experimental peritoneal dissemination than ipCDDP alone, without any increase of acute toxicity. Secondly, sequential administration increased an efficacy of TRC. Clinical evaluation of TRC and search for other combinations are now going on.

04.04.07

Immunohistochemical demonstration of HNK-1-defined antigen in gynecologic tumors with argyrophilia: Ueda, G, Abe, Y, Tanizawa, O. Dept. Obstet. and Gyn., Osaka Univ. Med. School, Osaka, Japan

Gynecologic tumors with argyrophilia were tested immunohistochemically for reactivity with HNK-1 antibody which had been shown to detect normal and neoplastic cells derived from the neuroectodermal and the APUD system. They included six small cell carcinomas and four adenocarcinomas of the cervix, 23 adenocarcinomas of the endometrium (13 with type I and 10 with type II argyrophil cells), 11 mucinous tumors (three benign, three borderline and five malignant), eight endometrioid carcinomas (four with type I and four with type II argyrophil cells), and two carcinoid tumors (one insular and one strumal type) of the ovary. HNK-1 reactive cells were found in four small cell carcinomas and two adenocarcinomas of the cervix, 11 adenocarcinomas of the endometrium, and four mucinous, two endometrioid and two carcinoid tumors of the ovary. Some of the type I or similar argyrophil cells were corresponding to HNK-1 reactive cells, but others were not. Also, non-argyrophilic tumor cells were partly HNK-1 positive. Although argyrophilia is not necessarily almighty to detect APUD nature, the significance of such discrepant reactivities with HNK-1 antibody requires to be further investgated.

04.04.08

Localization of monoclonal antibody (791T/36) in gynecological tumors: Powell, M C, Perkins, A, Pimm, M, Symonds, E M, Baldwin, R W. Univ. Hosp., Nottingham, England

The use of radiolabelled anti-tumor antibodies for the detection of malignancies has been increasing over the past few years. The antibody 791T/36 originally prepared against osteogenic sarcoma tumor cells has been shown to localize successfully in primary osteogenic sarcoma, primary and secondary breast and colonic carcinoma, and more recently, ovarian tumors. Studies in this latter group have now been extended and consist of 18 patients with ovarian carcinoma, 13 with cervical carcinoma and 11 with carcinoma of the body of the uterus. Both ^{111}In and ^{131}I have been used as antibody radio labels and their efficiency compared. External imaging studies showed a true positive rate of 94% and a true negative rate of 78% with ovarian tumors. True positive rates of 50% and 73% were found in the cervical and corpus tumors respectively. Tumor to non-tumor count rates were calculated per gram of tissue and autoradiographical and immunoperoxidase techniques applied to determine the site of localization at a cellular level. The monoclonal antibody 791T/36 offers potential for determining sites of recurrent disease and imaging studies support the use of cytotoxic drug conjugates particularly in the treatment of ovarian carcinoma.

04.04.09

Visualisation of ovarian cancer tissue by external scintigraphy using radiolabelled monoclonal antibodies: Pateisky, N, Skodler, W, Philipp, K, Hamilton, G, Burchell, J. 1st Dept. Obstet. and Gyn., Univ., Vienna, Austria

The production of specific monoclonal antibodies by the Hybrid-Technique provides the basis for a non-invasive visualisation of primary and metastatic tumor sites by Radioimmunoscintigraphy (RIS). 400 μg of the antibody HMFG-2 (raised against a tumor-associated antigen) were labelled by 2 mCi radioactive J-123 and subsequently injected intravenously into the patient. Static scintigrams up to 24 hours were then carried out to search after malignant tissue in the abdominal cavity. 35 patients with the suspicion of having either primary (n = 14) or metastatic ovarian cancer (n = 21) were investigated by RIS. 27 out of the 35 patients underwent primary or second look operation a few days after carrying out RIS, so that the scan findings could be compared in these 27 cases with the histological diagnosis. The scan results of the remaining eight patients were compared by other diagnostic procedures. In 31 of the 35 patients (88.5%), the scan findings turned out to be correct. In six out of the 21 patients with a known history of ovarian carcinoma tumor sites could be detected, that could not be found or classified concerning their nature by any pre-operative performed investigation method, including computed tomography. Regarding our results, RIS appears to offer a new clinical tool for precise tumor location in the human body, even when tumor identification by other clinical methods has failed.

04.04.10

Studies of ovarian cancer patients – using the monoclonal antibody Ca 12-5: Kitschke, H J, Stegner, H E, Schippling, K. Dept. Obstet. & Gyn., Univ., Hamburg

The murine monoclonal antibody CA 12-5 reacts with most epithelial ovarian carcinomas. By the radio-immunoassay 78% of 42 patients with ovarian carcinomas had serum Ca 12-5 levels above 65 U/ml. In contrast, 8% of breast cancer patients and 16% of patients with benign ovarian tumors had elevated levels of antigens. 91% of all patients with non-mucinous cystadenocarcinomas had antigen levels above 65 U/ml. Determination of Ca 12-5 levels may aid in monitoring response to treatment in patients with epithelial ovarian carcinomas.

04.06.01

Mass screening of the uterine cancer with the automated cell image analyzer: Kuwabara, S, Sugiura, K, Takabayashi, H, Ishima, T, Mukawa, A. Dept. Obstet. and Gyn., Kanazawa Med. Univ., Ishikawa, Japan

The automated cell image analyser was evaluated for mass screening on the uterine cervical cancer. The system equipped with a two stage flying spot scanner slide changer, an X-Y stage, diagnostic classifier, 1/0 devices and controller. The diagnostic logic uses four parameters; nuclear/cytoplasmic (N/C) ratio, nuclear size, nuclear optical density and nuclear shape. Selected features from about 300 cells of each slide are analyzed statistically and both atypical and distribution patterns are compared to that of normal and malignant cases. The results are printed out as normal, suspicious and reject. The fixed smears were stained by the standard method of Papanicolaou and double checked by three pathologists. In present paper, both results on 10,549 cases from 1977 to 1981 and that of 9010 cases from 1981 to 1984 after improvement of the system were compared. According to the reformed apparatus assessment, the false positive rate was reduced from 41.8% to 28.2% while the reject increased slightly from 4.3% to 7.0%. True positive rate of assessment for 28 cases and 7 cases of abnormal-suspicious in two groups were 100%. Present study disclosed that our automated analyser is useful for mass screening of uterine cancer and able to eliminate at least 70% of the work of cytoscreener with a reasonable accuracy.

04.06.02
Results of ten years of cytological screening for cervical carcinoma and its precursors: Soost, H-J, Ruffing, B. Inst. Clin. Cytol., TU, Munich

Within the German national screening program for women 742 445 cytological examinations of 277 118 women have been carried out at the Cytological Institute of the Bavarian Cancer Society in Munich. The participation was highest among women between 30 and 54 years. About one half of the patients had at least one repeat smear. The frequency of positive findings was 4.8‰ at the first examination and dropped to 1.4‰ at the second, 0.9‰ at the third and 0.4‰ at the fourth examination. In cases of repeated examination the frequency of positive findings rises again when the interval gets longer. The number of invasive carcimonas detected cytologically and confirmed histologically totalled 335 cases, that of carcinoma *in situ* and severe dysplasia 1235 cases. In relation to the number of patients examined in each age group the age distribution for carcinoma *in situ* showed a maximum between the 30th and the 34th year of age. For invasive carcinomas the curve rose up to the highest age groups. From 1971 to 1980 the rate of histologically confirmed invasive cervical carcinomas dropped from 0.9‰ to 0.2‰, the rate of carcinoma *in situ* and severe dysplasia dropped from 3.5‰ to 1.4‰.

04.06.03
Evaluation of the effect of Papanicolaou screening in Sweden. Record linkage between a central screening register and the National Cancer Register: Pettersson, F, Näslund, I, Malker, B. Dept. Gyn. Oncol, Radiumhemmet, Karolinska Sjukh., and the Swedish Ca Registry, Nat. Board Hlth and Welfare, Stockholm, Sweden

The outcome with regard to development of *in situ* or invasive carcinoma of the uterine cervix was studied among 930 127 women reported to a Swedish central screening register through a record linkage between that register and the National Cancer Register. The relative protection against cervical cancer after one negative smear calculated on incidence level prior to screening amounts to 14.5 times the first year and drops to 3.4 the fifth year after the screening occasion. The relative protection after two or more negative smears is considerably higher the first three years, but then drops to the same level as after one negative smear.

04.06.04
Evaluation of screening for cervical cancer in Sweden. Trends in incidence and mortality 1958–1980: Björkholm, E, Pettersson, F, Näslund, I. Dept. Gyn. Oncol., Radiumhemmet, Karolinska Sjukh., and Swedish Ca Registry, Nat. Board Hlth and Welfare, Stockholm, Sweden

Papanicolaou-smear screening for cancer of the uterine cervix was introduced in Sweden in the late 1950s. Screening programmes covering the age groups 30–49 years were organized in various counties between 1965 and 1973. The approximate number of smears rose from 100 000 in 1960 to one million in 1970, in a female population of four millions. Almost 60 000 cases of *in situ* carcinoma and 17 100 invasive carcinomas of the uterine cervix were registered in Sweden between 1958 and 1980. The age-standardized incidence of invasive carcinoma fell in this period by about 40%. Within the screened cohorts and age groups, the incidence was reduced by two-thirds and there was a parallel fall in mortality from the disease. At least part of these reductions seemed to be explained by the intensity of screening.

04.06.05
Mass screening for cervical cancer in Iceland: Sigursson, K, Geirsson, Tulinius, H. The Icelandic Cancer Society, Reykjavik, **Day, N**, IARC, Lyon, France

Mass screening for cervical cancer started in June 1964. The aim was to lower the incidence and mortality rate by screening all women in the age group 25–69 at two to three years intervals. The total attendance rate since 1964 has been 89% but the 3 year attendance rate has been 68%. During the time period 1964–79 there was an initial increase in both rates. The five year survival rate more than doubled at the same time as there was an increase in stage IA and IB tumors and decrease in all more advanced tumors. Further the mortality among the unscreened population was more than tenfold higher than among the screened population. During the five-year period 1980–84 there has been a new increase in the incidence rate and the mortality has stopped falling. 77 new cases were diagnosed during this time period. 30% of these (23 women) had more advanced disease than stage I and of these 80% had not attended the screening the last three years before diagnosis. An analysis of the screening history of the cases diagnosed since 1980 revealed that 68% had never attended (32 women) or not attended the last three years before diagnosis (20 women). Of the 25 women screened during the last three years before diagnosis 13 women had earlier some abnormalities in the smear that had not been followed up according to the working rules. Of the 12 women followed according to the working rules five patients had adeno- or adenosquamous cancer and five patients had stage IA with 1 to 2 mm invasion. In the light of the experience gained it is concluded that mass screening is a powerful tool to lower both the incidence and the mortality rate. With effective central steering, well functioning data handling system, well defined working rules and reliable diagnostic methods it should be possible in a well defined population to limit the cervix cancer to cases of stage IA and cases of adeno- and adenosquamous cancer.

04.06.06
The importance of vaginal cytology in the diagnosis of invasive cancer of the cervix uteri. Tronstad, S-E, Berge, T. Dept. Gyn. & Path., Centr. Hosp., Skövde, Sweden
Signs, symptoms and methods of diagnosis of invasive cancer of the cervix uteri in one decade (A, 1959–1968) without and one decade (B, 1969–1978) with organized cytological screening in Skaraborg Couty were studied. Vaginal cytology for routine diagnosis was introduced in the late sixties, and screening was offered to all women aged 30–50 from 1969. 346 cases of invasive cancer were diagnosed during the whole period. We found stage I cancer in 37%, stage II in 39%, stage III in 17.5% and stage IV in 6.5%, of which 88% were squamous epithelial and 12% adenocarcinomas. – Results: There was no difference in incidence, stage or differentiation of cancer or age of patients between the periods. Adenocarcinoma increased significantly (p < 0.05) from 7.2% in period A to 15.7% in period B. There was a significant difference (p < 0.00001) in the number of asymptomatic patients: 4 (2.5%) in period A compared to 38 (23%) in period B. The rest of the women had one or more symptoms: vaginal bleeding (80%), vaginal discharge (36%), pain (6.5%), poor general condition (12%) and symptoms from the urinary tract (7.5%), without difference between the periods. Presenting symptom and the duration of symptoms were similar in both periods. Marked differences in diagnostic methods were found: atypical smears caused diagnostic biopsy in 21 patients (8%) in period A, compared to 65 patients (32%) in period B. All asymptomatic patients' smears indicated cancer. – Conclusion: One out of four patients found to have invasive cancer of the cervix uteri in the last decade (1969–78) was asymptomatic. A vaginal smear is therefore a most important tool for diagnosis of invasive cancer of the cervix.

04.06.07
Colposcopic yielding in patients with macroscopic cervical pathology: Mor-Yosef, S, Anteby, S O, Bercovici, B, Schenker, J G. Dept., Hadassah Univ. Hosp., Jerusalem, Israel
Colposcopic evaluation of 775 women with macroscopical cervical lesion was performed in the years 1980–1984. The indications for referral by out-patients' physicians were: A. 561 patients with an erosion-like lesion, in this group of patients only 72 had previous or documented cytological cervical C.I.N. B. 74 patients with tumor appearance lesions. The majority were papillary growth. C. 72 patients with unhealed cervical infections at the squamo-columnar junction. D. 68 patients had abnormal vaginal bleeding with suspicion of cervical origin. Every patient had a complete physical examination, cervical pap smear and colposcopy. Cervical biopsy was performed according to abnormal colposcopy findings. The prevalence of abnormal cytology in this low risk population will be presented. The effect of age, gravity, parity, methods of birth control on colposcopic appearance of the cervical pathology will be reported. The above with correlation to cytological and histological findings emphasize the value of colposcopy as a primary screening procedure.

04.06.08
The value of screening colposcopy in detection of cervical cancer in a low risk population: Markov, S, Goldberger, S B, Fejgin, M, Cohen-Alloro, J, Ben-Nun, I, Ben-Aderet, N. Dept. Obstet. and Gyn. "A", Meir Gen. Hosp., Sapir Med. Ctr., Kfar-Sava, Israel
The Jewish population is proven to be at low risk for cervical cancer. Six-hundred and seventy patients were colposcopically examined at the screening colposcopy unit at Meir hospital from June 1983 through January 1985. All the patients had a cervical Papanicolaou smear taken in addition to a careful colposcopy examination. This retrospective study was designed to evaluate the benefits of routine first visit colposcopy in a population which does not enjoy the privileges of outpatient cervical smear screening system. The examination revealed 15 patients who suffered from moderate dysplasis and only two patients in whom severe dysplasia/CIS was diagnosed. We therefor conclude that screening colposcopy is not cost-effective in a low risk population, and a routine outpatient cervical Papanicolaou smear is safely sufficient for early detection of cervical pathology.

04.06.09
A system of uterine cervix-cancer prevention (UCCP) in Czechoslovakia: Kanka, J, Svoboda, B, Beková, A, Havránková. Dept. Obstet. and Gyn., Charles Univ., Prague, Czechoslovakia
A new two-step system in UCCP has been proposed and tested during the past eight years and is now being introduced in the whole country. The basis of this system is the center of cervical cancer prevention which consists of a colposcopic and a cytologic unit and is directed by a highly qualified gynecologist specially trained in colposcopy and preventive oncology. The center is responsible for a district of about 200 000 inhabitants and covers the second step of prevention. The first step is represented by all gynecologists working in this district. Every woman visiting her district gynecologist for the first time is examined colposcopically and cytologically. Women with a negative cervical finding are followed up and treated (if necessary) as out-patients in his office. All women with significant findings are recommended to the centre

where adequate therapy of the given cervical lesion is decided upon (cone-biopsy, cryosurgery, electrodia-thermy, coagulation etc.). Patients with bioptically verified CIN are followed-up in the center for the period required. This system corresponds to the present situation when not all gynecologists are sufficiently trained in colposcopy as well as in preventive gynecological oncology. The suggested procedure makes it possible to prevent cervical cancer in a large population of women, on a high professional level, to introduce new methods in therapy and to abandon outmoded treatment, i.e. to avoid overtreatment.

04.06.10

Diagnostic certainty in out-patient cervical curettage using conventional and vabra curettage of the cervix: Hald, F, Kristoffersen, S E, Hariri, J, Hansen, M K. Inst. Obstet. and Gyn. and Inst. Path., Univ., Odense, Denmark

The purpose of the investigation was to examine the diagnostic certainty using conventional cervix curett-age and vabra cervix curettage in the diagnosis of cervical intraepithelial neoplasia (CIN). Among 316 consecutive out-patients referred for CIN, 298 patients entered the investigation and were randomly allocated to one of two groups. The first group underwent vabra curettage and immediately after conven-tional cervix curettage. The second group had the same two procedures in the reverse order. Among the 298 patients 114 patients were found to have CIN in the cervix mucosa. In the first group of 55 patients who first underwent vabra curettage ten patients had normal histology at the first procedure and CIN at the second. Diagnostic certainty with vabra: 80%. In the second group of 59 patients who had conventional curettage first, 30 patients had normal histology at the first procedure and CIN found secondly with vabra. Diagnostic certainty with conventional cervix curettage: 49%. There were no per- or post-operative complications. Pain and discomfort were recorded. The vabra procedure seems to cause less pain than conventional cervix curettage. – Conclusions: the diagnostic certainty using vabra curettage is significantly better than conventional cervical curettage in the diagnostic procedure of CIN of the cervix (p < 0.00004), and causes less discomfort.

04.06.11

Adenocarcinoma of the uterine cervix: Nasu, I*, Higashiiwai, H*, Yonemoto, Y*, Sato, A**, Kaneta, N**. *Tohoku Teishin Hosp., **Miyagi Cancer Society, Sendai, Japan

During the five-year period from 1979 to 1983, 639 993 screenings were performed in Miyagi Prefecture, Japan, and a total of 624 cases of cervical neoplasia including carcinoma *in situ* were detected. Thirty-three were classified as adenocarcinoma of the cervix, and consisted of five cases of adenocarcinoma *in situ*, one case of microinvasive adenocarcinoma and twenty-seven cases of invasive adenocarcinoma. Invasive adenocarcinoma constituted 8.8% of all cases of invasive cervical carcinoma. Only 15.2% of the cases of adenocarcinoma were detected in stage 0, while 41.8% of the cases of squamous carcinoma were detected in this stage. There were three cases of advanced adenocarcinoma overlooked by previous screening because the tumor cells were well-differentiated and difficult to distinguish. Repeat biopsies including cone biopsies were often necessary for correct diagnoses of early stage adenocarcinoma. Most of the adenocar-cinomas *in situ* (four out of five cases) were associated with co-existing squamous neoplasia and screened because of atypical squamous cells in the initial cytological specimens. When atypical squamous cells exist in cytological specimens, careful examinations of gland cells are required for the detection of early cervical adenocarcinoma.

04.06.12

Carcinoma of the uterus: S. B. Radosavljević. Gyn. Obstet. Clin., Niš, Yugoslavia

Results of early discovery of carcinoma of the uterus in operated patients and patients treated with X-ray are analysed. In the period of seven years, between 1978 and 1984, there were surgeries in 4643 cases and there were examined by method of Papanicolaou 5989 cases, of which Pa III was found in 324 cases (0.05%) and Pa IV and V in 121 cases (0.02%). Cervical carcinoma was discovered by histopathological examina-tion. Histopathological examination of materials by punch biopsy and conisation found dysplasia of mild degree in 6 cases, of medium degree in 18 cases (0.002%) and of severe degree in 17 cases (0.002%). Cervical carcinoma was discovered in a total of 136 cases, as follows: carcinoma *in situ* in 25 cases (0.18%) which were surgically treated – cervical carcinoma of I degree in 32 cases (0.23%) and IIa degree in 21 cases (0.15%) that were surgically treated and cervical carcinoma of II-a and II-b degree in 15 cases (0.11%) treated by X-ray. We found 202 cases of endometrial carcinoma. Of these 139 cases (0.68%) were surgically treated and the remaining 63 cases (0.31%) by X-ray, because of different contra-indications for surgery, such as heart failure, diabetes mellitus, kidney disease, arterial hypertension, etc. Besides above cases, there were 6 cases (0.02%) of endometrial sarcoma and 3 cases (0.01%) of adenoacanthoma.

04.07.01

Immunological states and their changes during the course of disease in breast cancer (BC), stages I and II (preliminary communication): Contreras Ortiz, O, Stoliar, A, Tapia, J C. Gyn. Dept. Segba, Buenos Aires, Argentina

The specific-cellular αhumoral- and nonspecific-phagocytosis-immunity was investigated in 14 BC patients, same social level, 50–70 years old, stages I (2)αII (12) (international classification), belonging to multipara-metrical longitudinal investigation protocol. The samples were made before operation (S1), free of treatment, 3α6 months postoperation (S2αS3) of modified radical surgery and TCT and/or PQT, correlating S1 with 20 normal controls (N) of the same level and age, and S2αS3 with their respective S1. In peripheral blood we determined: T lymphocytes (TL) through total E (E) and active E (aE) rosettes; killer cells, antibody dependent cytotoxicity through EA rosettes (EA); blastic transformation with phytohemagglutinin (IT); serum immunoglobulins (Ig) G, A, M; phagocytosis (P) and intracellular killing (K); leucocyte migration inhibition (LMI) with autologous tumor extract and homologous controls. Student's t test was used for statistical analysis. The absolute mean/mm$^3 \pm$ DS statistically relevant found in each sample were: S1-I: E increased (i), 1955 ± 12 (N: 1398 ± 346 $p < .02$;-II: EA i, 493 ± 409 (N: 202 ± 51) $p < .05$; IT decreased (d), 16 ± 11 (N: 27 ± 6), $p < .02$; IgG i, 2128 ± 276 (N: 1200 ± 120), $p < .001$, A i, 276 ± 69 (N: 210 ± 55), $p < .01$; K d, 59 ± 23 (N: 74 ± 7), $p < .05$. S2-I: E d, 493 ± 93 $p < .05$;-II: aE d, 326 ± 95, $p < .001$; EA d, 169 ± 44, $p < .001$; IT d, 6 ± 3, $p < .001$. S3-II: aE d, 502 ± 228, $p < .05$. The LMI made in immediately postoperative, S2αS3 showed sensitiveness to tumor antigen $p < .001$ in I: 16, 15, 23% and II: 37, 39, 45%. We conclude: 1) these patients show quantitiative and functional alterations of immune system referring to normal population and type of stadium and are related to the disease development; 2) i EA, d function TL, B lymphocytes and phagocytosis alteration, may constitute a prognostic, independently of pre-operative clinical classification, confirmed or not in the postoperative; 3) in IαII, sensitivity and recognition to tumoral antigen during checking time was found.

04.07.02

Cellular immunological status in patients with operable breast cancer – prognostic value of different subclasses and the influence of adjuvant chemo- and/or hormonotherapy: Schmid, H, Kaufmann, M, Heinrich, D, Kubli, F. Dept. Obstet. and Gyn., Univ. Hosp., Heidelberg
In 64 patients with primary breast cancer (T1-3, nodal neg. and pos.) and no evidence of distant metastases the cellular immunological status was determined with commercially available monoclonal antibodies (MAB). Leucocytes were determined with an Anti-Leucocyte-MAB, T-helper-lymphocytes with the Anti-Leu 3, T-suppressor-lymphocytes with the Anti-Leu 2, natural-killer-cells with two different MAB (Anti-Leu 7+11), B-lymphocytes with the Anti-Leu 12 and macrophages/monocytes with the Anti-Leu M3. Median follow-up time of all 64 patients has been 11 months. The immunological status was determined before and after operation, during and after adjuvant chemo- and/or hormonotherapy (CMF/AC and/or tamoxifen). Within the short period of follow-up it can be demonstrated for some cases with early recurrence that changes of the rations of T-helper-/T-suppressor-cells and macrophages/B-cells have prognostic value. The influence of different anticancer drugs on the cellular immune system will be discussed with regard to th possible immunological prognostic factors.

04.07.03

Validity of adjuvant chemo- and hormone therapy for breast cancer: A randomized controlled clinical trial: Salzer, H, Kubista, E, Smekal-Stempel, G, Langer, M, Sevelda, P. 1st Dept. Obstet. and Gyn., Univ., Vienna, Austria
The validity of an adjuvant chemo- or hormone-therapy of breast cancer was assessed in a prospective randomized controlled trial. 218 patients, 71 of them premenopausal, 147 postmenopausal, were controlled in the trial since 1979 after they had undergone modified radical mastectomy. Patients were stratified according to menopausal status, estrogen receptor (ER) status and the presence of axillary lymph node (LN) involvement. Patients either received six cycles of chemotherapy (CMF-scheme, cyclophosphamide-methotrexate, 5-FU, standard dosage) and/or tamoxifene (20 mg per day). In premenopausal patients tamoxifene was administered only if ER was positive, postmenopausal patients received tamoxifene regardless of receptor status. We evaluated the probability of achieving a 3-year relapse-free interval for the respective subgroups: premenopausal vs. postmenopausal: 70 vs 72%, ER pos. vs. ER neg.: 77 vs 66% $p < 0.05$, LN neg vs. LN pos.: 83 vs 63%, $p < 0.02$. Premenopausal patients with positive LN and negative ER (therapy: 6 cycles CMF) had a significantly lower percentage of 3 year relapse free interval than all other branches of the study ($p < 0.05$). Tamoxifene proved to benefit postmenopausal patients, as both if given in addition to chemotherapy (65 vs 80%, $p < 0.03$) or as single agent (no therapy vs. Tam 78 vs 90%). This finding was more pronounced in the ER pos group than in the ER neg group. Observation time being too short to draw final conclusions, we may yet state already that adjuvant tamoxifene may result in a significant improvement of 3 year relapse-free interval.

04.07.04

Morphological features of breast carcinomas related to tamoxifen treatment results: Schnürch, H-G, Bender, H G, Lehmann, R, Matthiessen, H v. Dept. Obst. and Gyn., Univ., Düsseldorf
Receptor status is an accepted criterion with prognostic value for the response to hormonal treatment. Hormone receptor contents of breast carcinomas on the other hand show more or less clear correlation to morphological features of the primary tumor. We tried to find out a direct correlation between histological and cytological criteria of tumor tissue and response to tamoxifen in case of relapse in 81 patients with breast cancer. We looked for the subcriteria of the WHO-grading and of the nuclear grading according to BLACK: tubule formation, anisonucleosis, hyperchromastism and mitoses, size of nuclei and nucleoli, chromatin crumping. Although we found some well known relationships between tumor differentiation and other prognostic factors such as duration of disease-free interval and site of metastases there was no

statistically significant correlation found between morphology and response to tamoxifen treatment. Our data lead to the conclusion that the morphological analysis of the primary tumor cannot give conclusive hints for the prediction of response rate to hormonal therapy with tamoxifen in case of relapse.

04.07.05
Determination of tamoxifen, 4-hydroxy-tamoxifen and N-desmethyl-tamoxifen serum levels in 50 postmenopausal mammary tumor patients: Grill, H J, Kreienberg, R, Westermann, R, Pollow, K. Dept. Exp. Endocr., Dept. Obstet. and Gyn., Johannes Gutenberg-Univ., Mainz

Tamoxifen (TAM) is currently the compound of choice for hormonal treatment of metastasic human breast cancer. In a collective of 50 postmenopausal patients suffering from metastasizing breast cancer and treated with 20 mg Tamoxifen per day were the serum levels of TAM and the two metabolites 4-hydroxy-tamoxifen (OHT) and N-desmethyl-tamoxifen (NDT) quantified. The serum samples were extracted using Sep-Pak C_{18} cartridges and the extracts chromatographed on a CN reversed phase column ($5\,\mu$) using HPLC. To the end of the chromatographic column was connected a PTFE capillary tube wound in 10 cm distance around a high pressure mercury lamp (150 W) for photocyclisation of TAM and its metabolites to the corresponding phenanthrene derivatives. Those were ultimately detected in a fluorescence monitor ($_{\cdot\cdot EX}=236$ nm, $_{\cdot\cdot EM}=375$ nm). The mobile phase consisted of acetonitrile – 0.3 mol/l H_3PO_4 – 10 mmol/l KH_2PO_4 (380:50:280) at a flow rate of 2 ml/min. From most of the patients the estrogen and progesterone receptor content of the primary tumor were known. It is the aim of this investigation to evaluate the serum level profiles of TAM and its two well characterized metabolites of 50 advanced breast cancer patients during daily dose TAM treatment by mouth, with respect to the clinical response.

04.07.06
High dose medroxyprogesterone acetate therapy in mammary carcinoma patients: Clinical and biochemical results: Pollow, K, Kreienberg, R, Grill, H J. Dept. Exp. Endocr., Dept. Obstet. and Gyn., Johannes Gutenberg-Univ., Mainz

Medroxyprogesterone acetate (MPA), a potent synthetic progestagen, has been widely used in the hormonal treatment of advanced breast cancer, but with varying dose schedules at present. The availability of a sensitive RIA-method for determination of serum MPA has stimulated the reearch on MPA serum levels in patients after repeated MPA administration. The aim of this study was to assay blood level profiles of MPA as well as of cortisol, ACTH, DHEA-sulphate, androstendione and prolactin during repeated high dose orally administered MPA. 85 patients with metastatic breast cancer were enrolled in this study. The dosage regimen was based on the daily oral administration of 1,000 mg MPA. During MPA treatment a decrease of cortisol, DHEA-sulfate and androstendione serum levels was observed in nearly all patients. Within the observation time of 10 months 18% responded to the therapy (complete and partial response). No change was observed in 36% and progression in 46% of the patients. Within the remission group (CR and PR), a good correlation between persisting serum levels above 150 ng/ml and remission was observed. But in the no change and in the progression group no such correlation could be observed. There seem to be several modes of high dose MPA treatment: 1) progestin effects via progesterone receptor, 2) glucocorticoid effects of MPA itself, 3) antiestrogen effects by reducing adrenal androgen synthesis (precursors of estrogens), 4) direct cytotoxic effects as measured in cell cultures.

04.07.07
Analysis of individual medroxyprogesterone, cortisol- and tumor marker plasma levels under high dose MPA-therapy in advanced breast cancer: Kreienberg, R, Grill, H-J, Melchert, F, Pollow, K. Dept. Obstet. and Gyn., Univ.-Hosp., Mainz

For several years medroxyprogesterone (MPA) has been used in the therapy of metastatic breast cancer. The MPA-therapy has mainly been administered intramuscularly. In this study we are reporting on our experience with a high-dose i. m. and peroral MPA-therapy. 76 patients with metastatic breast cancer were treated with MPA (i. m. 1000 mg/die for 2 weeks, then 1000 mg/week or per os 1000 mg/die continuously). In 37% of patients under i. m. MPA-therapy (n = 30) we observed a distinct clinical response (CR, PR, no change). 63% of patients showed progressive tumor growth. Regarding the MPA- and cortisol-plasmalevels of this group of patients it becomes evident that those cases with remissions show significantly higher MPA-serum-level (> 100 ng/ml) than patients in the "no change" or "progression" group (< 100 ng/ml). With rising MPA-plasma-levels cortisol is increasingly suppressed. However, the individual variations of the cortisol-plasma-levels are rather great. On the other hand 65% of patients under peroral MPA-therapy (n = 46) demonstrated a clinical response (CR.PR.NC). This clinical success was combined with an early rise of the MPA-plasma-levels over 100 ng/ml. Patients with tumor progression showed distinctly lower MPA-plasma-concentrations (< 50 ng/ml). Our data demonstrate: 1) only MPA-plasma-levels of > 100 ng/ml show a therapeutic effect; 2) peroral MPA-therapy leads to distinctly higher MPA-plasmalevels within a shorter time; 3) plasma cortisol is increasingly suppressed with rising MPA-plasmacencentrations. On account of the observed individual variations the cortisol-plasma-level, however, seems to be unsuitable for monitoring the efficacy of the MPA-therapy.

04.07.08

Clinical and endocrinological aspects of pharmacokinetics and pharmacodynamics of high-dose MPA therapy in metastatic breast cancer: Schmidt-Rhode, P, Schulz, K-D, Sturm, G. Dept. Obstet. and Gyn., Univ., Marburg

Many clinical trials have clearly pointed out the effectiveness of high-dose medroxyprogesterone acetate (MPA) therapy in advanced breast cancer. Just a small number of studies is reported on the pharmacokinetics and pharmacodynamics of this drug. Furthermore there exists a considerable vagueness with regard to the method of MPA-plasma determination. For this reason we performed measurements of plasma MPA levels by GC-MF controlled Radioimmunoassay. RIA-determinations were made without (dir. RIA) and after petroleum ether extraction (extr. RIA) and correlated to endocrinological parameters (ACTH, cortisol, FSH, LH, prolactin, estrogens and androgens) and the clinical progress of the disease. MPA-plasma levels after oral administration of 1000 mg MPA/d slowly increased within 2 to 4 weeks to a median concentration of 130 ng/ml measured by RIA after petroleum ether extraction. Determination by direct RIA showed fairly big amounts of MPA to a concentration of 800 to 1000 ng/ml which may be caused by cross reacting of MPA metabolites. There was no great difference between the GC-MF and the extracted RIA measurements. Parallel to increase of MPA concentrations the gonadotropin, estrogen and androgen plasma levels declined to nearly 20% of their pre-therapeutic levels. As a sign of adrenal suppression cortisol plasma values decreased to approximate 10% of the pre-therapeutic level. Patients with advanced breast cancer, who responded well to MPA treatment generally demonstrated high MPA-plasma levels with a marked decline of cortisol level. In patients with primary or secondary progression lower plasma MPA levels and less suppressed cortisol values were observed.

04.07.09

Megestrol acetate in stage IV-breast cancer: Hegg, R, Souza, A Z, Souza, J B, Tomioka, E, Salvatore, C A. Gyn. Clin., São Paulo Univ. Med. School, São Paulo, Brazil

During 1983–84, 30 post-menopausal patients with progressive advanced (stage IV) breast cancer were treated with megestrol acetate orally as palliative therapy. A careful study of the disease including chest x-ray, bone scan, liver scan, liver ultrasound, hepatic enzyme profile were performed before the hormonal therapy. Lesions previously irradiated, cytotoxic chemotherapy and hormonal therapy in the last sixty days, CNS involvement, bone marrow and pulmonary lymphangitis were criteria of exclusion. 40 mg of megestrol acetate was given four times a day, total dose 160 mg p. o., at least for sixteen weeks. The main results were: 1) none had complete objective response; 2) two (6.6%) showed partial objective response; 3) twenty-three (76.8%) showed no progression of disease; 4) five (16.6%) had progression of disease; 5) Twenty-five (83.3%) showed subjective response; 6) only major side-effect observed was genital bleeding; 7) minor side-effects, such as weight gain, nausea, and vomiting, anorexia, occurred with no discontinuation of the treatment.

04.08.01

Cardiac disease in pregnancy: Jairaj, P, Tony, E L. CMC Hosp., Vellore, India

Review of 203 pregnancies with cardiac disease, admitted to Christian Medical College Hospital during 1972 July to 1983 June is presented. Of these 164 had Rheumatic Valvular disease (VD), 36 had congenital lesions and 43 had correcitve cardiac surgery. The mitral valve was involved in all but six (VD) of rheumatic origin and stenosis was the predominant lesion. The common congenital lesions were septal defects and tetralogy of Fallot. Incidence of cardiac Grade III and IV (New York Heart Association) was seen to increase with age reaching 90–100% at and above 35 years. Increasing parity worsened functional capacity. With multivalvular involvement and multiple lesions cardiac function deteriorated. Effective antenatal care and surgical correction prior to pregnancy improved functional capacity. Complications during pregnancy included pregnancy induced hypertension, anemia and recurrent respiratory infection. The incidence of preterm labor and small-for-dates babies, perinatal mortality and morbidity was increased. Cardiac complications included atrial fibrillation, thromboembolic phenomena, congestive cardiac failure (CCF) and acute pulmonary edema. There were two maternal deaths in patients with rheumatic multi-valvular lesions with CCF who had no antenatal care and died undelivered. In this review of 203 pregnancies with cardiac disease prognostic factors and obstetric performance are discussed.

04.08.02

An analysis of a clinical group of mothers with heart disease: Poňuch, A, Blaškovà, O, Sorelová, D, Pohlová, G, Sasko, A, Šutta, I, Petrenko, M, Redecha, M. Dept. Gyn. and Obstet., Med. Fac., Comenius Univ., Bratislava, Czechoslovakia

During a five-year period 140 women with a heart disease gave birth to their children in our department. Within the group 43 women had congenital defects, 41 women had acquired valvular defects, 20 women have had heart operations and 36 women had other heart diseases. Pregnant women were regularly checked with prenatal care. They were admitted to hospital in every case of impairment of internal or obstetric status and at the latest in the last month of pregnancy. The pregnancies terminated in 62.9% spontaneously, in 20% by vacuum extractor, in 0.7% by low forceps and on 16.4% Cesarean section was performed. In the type of delivery, cardiologic and obstetric status were decisive. By the intensive prenatal and perinatal care (cardiologist, obstetrician, anesthesiologist and pediatrician) we got 1.1% mortality and 2.2% perinatal morbidity. No mother died. Every patient with heart disease should plan conception after consulting her health condition with the cardiologist and obstetrician.

04.08.03

Maternal and neonatal outcome of pregnancy in 110 patients with organic heart disease: Katz, M, Luria, S. Div. Obstet. and Gyn., Soroka Med. Ctr, Fac. Hlth Sci., Ben-Gurion Univ. of the Negev, Beer-Sheba, Israel

The decrease of maternal mortality from obstetric causes during the past quarter of this century may account for the fact that heart disease is today one of the leading causes of maternal death. The outcome of pregnancy for mother and newborn is related to the functional capacity of the cardiovascular system, and the more symptomatic is the patient, the poorer the prognosis. Even in mild cases of heart disease – babies of cardiacs are found to be growth retarded and premature more often than those of healthy mothers. The present study, 110 cardiac disease parturients of which 100 were of class I and II, and 10 class III and IV of New York Heart Association Functional Classification are evaluated. The variables analysed included type of heart disease, past and present obstetric history, hematocrit levels, duration of hospital stay, maternal and neonatal outcome. The average birth weight of babies in class I and II patients was 3340 ± 853.5 grams, in class III and IV 2945 ± 171.9 grams. The average birth weight in 110 control babies matched for ethnic origin, gestational age and sex, was 3427 ± 148.7 grams – and was not statistically different from the study population. There was no maternal mortality and perinatal mortality was 4.2%. The present study suggests that the perinatal outcome in patients with organic heart disease is similar to that of control group. This is most probably due to the strict protocol of management which included liberal hospitalization as well as avoiding anemia or infection in those patients.

04.08.04

Pregnancy following renal transplantation in Saudi Arabia: Sabagh, T O, Al Khader, A, Abomelha, M, Jawdat, M. Armed Forces Hosp., Riyadh, Saudi Arabia

This paper describes nine pregnancies in seven patients. Five of the patients have had transplantation in the Armed Forces Hospital, Riyadh and two of the patients have had transplantation in the United States of America. All pregnancies have been carried out successfully. The renal function during pregnancy and the details of the babies born are described. There are eight Tables which contain the renal function for pregnancy, during pregnancy and after pregnancy, the maternal course of pregnancy and the time of transplantation and pregnancy and the creatinine clearance during pregnancy. The Table(s) also describe the mode of delivery and the complications which occur during pregnancy and after pregnancy, the management of the patients during pregnancy; the mean gestational age at which all babies were delivered; the weight of the babies; Apgar score and the sex of the babies. It makes comparison also to other applications about renal transplantation and pregnancy.

04.08.05

A study on serological markers of hepatitis B virus in sera of parturients and in cord blood: Kim, H, Je, G H. Inje Med. Coll., Paik Hosp., Pusan, Korea

The authors investigated the serological markers of hepatitis B virus in 1813 cases of parturients and 1605 cord blood samples by means of R-PHA and PHA methods for HBsAg and anti-HBs: RIA or EIA for HBeAg, anti-HBe and anti-HBc, respectively. The results obtained were summarized as follows: 1. Positive rates of serum HBsAg and anti-HBs were 6.4% and 21.2% in pregnant women, and 2.2% and 17.0% in cord blood, respectively. 2. Positive rates of serum HBsAg was 21.6% in cord blood of neonates born to asymptomatic HBsAg positive pregnant women, and that of serum anti-HBs was 58.2% in cord blood of those born to anti-HBs positive pregnant women. 3. Positive rates of serum HBeAg and anti-HBe were 38.7% and 37.8% in asymptomatic HBsAg positive pregnant women, and 75.0% and 12.5% in HBsAg positive cord bloods. 4. HBsAg positive rate was 34.2% in cord sera of the neonates born to HBeAg positive pregnant women and 15.0% in cord sera of those born to anti-HBe positive ones. 5. HBeAg positive rates of cord sera were significantly higher in the neonates born to HBsAg positive pregnant women, as compared to those in the neonates born to anti-HBs and HBeAg positive ones. Anti-HBe positive rates of cord sera showed no significant difference between neonates born to anti-HBs positive pregnant women with positive anti-HBe and those born to anti-HBs positive pregnant women with negative anti-HBe. On the basis of the results obtained, it can be concluded that all serological markers of hepatitis B virus pass through the placenta with or without decrease in their titers.

04.08.06

Immunological responses to total dose iron infusion: Stabile, I, Nysenbaum, A M, Gutteridge, C, Duley, L, Price, K, Newland, A, Grudzinskas, J G, Teisner, B. Dept. Obstet. and Gyn. and Haemat., London Hosp. Med. Coll., London, UK; Inst. Med. Microbiol., Univ., Odense, Denmark

Clinical, humoral and cellular immunological events were observed before, during and after an intravenous infusion of iron-dextran in pregnant and non-pregnant individuals with anemia due to iron deficiency. Evidence of profound activation of the complement system was observed in all patients who had an intrainfusion adverse reaction. Analyses of C3, C4 and C3 and C4 split product levels implied that the activation was not mediated via the classical pathway. Patients undergoing a delayed reaction were generally observed to have an elevation of C3, C4 levels or other acute phase proteins. Hematological and other cellular phenomena wre unrelated to the events observed in patients with acute or delayed reactions. The significance of these data will be discussed in the context of usage of total iron infusions during pregnancy.

04.08.07

Value of serum ferritin in the diagnosis of anemia in pregnant women: Ulmer, H U, Goepel, E, Neth, R D. Gyn. Dept./Dept. Clin. Chem., Univ. Hosp., Hamburg

In West Germany, anemia in the final stage of pregnancy occurs in about 20–50% of cases, depending on the diagnostic criteria applied; 90% of these are hypoferric anemias. 150 women were examined for hemoglobin, MCH value and serum ferritin predominantly at the end pregnancy. The concentration of serum ferritin is proportional to the ferritin concentration on the whole and can therefore be taken as proportional to the iron reserves in the body. 58% of the pregnant women investigated had hemoglobin values of below 12 g/dl; the MCH-values as a sign of disturbed hemoglobin synthesis were below 28 pg in 47%, and the serum ferritin values were shown to be under the minimum of 20 g/l in 70% of cases. The object of the investigation was to find possible correlations between anemic parameters such as Hb, MCH and ferritin and the clinical criteria such as weight of the newborn child, Apgar score and pregnancy complications like gestosis and infections and the occurrence of premature labor. Premature labor was found to be closely correlated with low ferritin values; other correlations were not found.

04.08.08

Desferrioxamine in pregnancy: Christiaens, G C M L[1], Rijksen, G[1], Marx, J[1], Pott Hofstede, D[2], Staal, G E J[1]. [1]Univ. Hosp., Utrecht; [2]Diakonessen Hosp., Hilversum

Desferrioxamine (R° Desferal) is an iron chelating agent used to prevent and treat chronic or acute iron overload in primary hemochromatosis, in several disorders with secondary hemochromatosis and in acute iron poisoning. Its teratogenicity in laboratory animals and its chelating capacity for other elements such as zinc have been reason to suggest induced abortion in case of pregnancy during drug exposure. We report a case with successful pregnancy outcome where desferrioxamine was administred intramuscularly in a dosage of 1000 mg once in 2 days during the first 10 5/7 weeks of gestation in a patient with hexokinase deficiency. We describe the management of the underlying disease after discontinuation of the drug. The outcomes of other cases of desferrioxamine use during pregnancy reported to the manufacturer are reviewed and recommendations for future management are made for the most frequent diseases where desferrioxamine treatment may be necessary, such as transfusion dependent thalassemia and hemolytic anemias.

04.08.09

Plasma ferritin status in anemic Indian pregnant women: Raman, L, Subbalaxmi, P V, Narasinga Rao, B S. Nat. Inst. Nutr., Hyderabad, India

Anemia in pregnancy due to iron deficiency is widely prevalent in the Indian population. It is known that plasma ferritin decreases significantly in iron deficiency anemia and is thus a reflection of iron stores. To study the iron stores, plasma ferritin was measured by radioimmunoassay in Indian pregnant women in different trimesters of pregnancy. Also the effect of iron supplementation (oral and parenteral) was studied on plasma ferritin levels at term and six months after delivery. It was observed that 60–70% of pregnant women had plasma ferritin < 10 ng/ml at the onset of pregnancy. Parenteral iron raised the ferritin from a level of 9.4 ng/ml at 20 weeks to 57.3 ng/ml at term (p < 0.001), which was maintained at high level (40 ng/ml) even six months after delivery. With oral iron (60 mg elemental during the last 100–120 days of pregnancy) there was only a marginal incrase in serum ferritin (13.5 ng/ml to 30.6 ng/ml at term) which returned to basal level six months after delivery. Thus it would appear that in the existing wide prevalence of iron deficiency in pregnancy, oral prophylactic iron supplements alone may not be adequate to build up the iron stores in pregnant Indian women. It may be necessary to provide depot iron (as parenteral iron 500 mg) to all the pregnant women followed by oral iron if one wishes to maintain the iron stores in the Indian population.

04.08.10

Medical complications of pregnancy – case report: Pregnancy and functional paraganglioma: Verstraeten, P R, Boer, R de. Groot Ziekengasthuis, 's Hertogenbosch, The Netherlands

A 23-year-old primigravida was first seen at 14 weeks gestation because of a heart murmur. She was admitted at 21 weeks with a severe hypertension. Urinary VMA values were elevated and the presence of a catecholamine-producing tumor was cofirmed by elevated plasma catecholamines. Norepinephrine/ epinephrine ratio suggested an extra-adrenal localisation. Hypertension was controlled by metroprolol and later by phentolamine. At 31 weeks gestation amniocentesis showed sufficient fetal lung maturity and a 1040 g female infant was delivered by Cesarean section under general anesthesia. Subsequent abdominal exploration revealed a 112 g para-aortic paraganglioma, which was successfully removed. Postoperative course was uneventful, with normal urinary and plasma catecholamines. Malignancy of paragangliomas and pheochromocytomas cannot be excluded on histological basis, therefore a scintigraphic investigation will take place using ^{131}I meta-iodobenzylguanidine. The case report is well documented and offers an opportunity to present the most recent methods for diagnosis, localisation and management of these tumors during and after pregnancy.

04.09.01
Warning – could be a mole! Valle, G A, Mendoza, I, Montaño, A. Dept. Obstet. and Gyn., Gen. Hosp., Mexico, D. F.

We studied 9519 patients that entered the hospital during one year, of which 2924 were spontaneous abortion of the first trimester and 96 (3.17%) molar pregnancy, a total of 3020 (31.72%). Of the 2924 patients, 66 (2.25%) were reported as microscopic moles, that were not diagnosed clinically or surgically. Of the group of molar abortion and the group of microscopic moles nine (0.29%) developed into choriocarcinoma. Among the patients with molar abortion, 20 were selected at random, 16 (80%) had arterial hypertension 160/100 or 190/100; simlar data as the severe eclampsia patients, a fact that demanded the performance of renal biopsy. The biopsy of these patients was compared with the biopsy in eclampsia patients (both groups of biopsies were studied by regular microscopy, immunofluorescence and electron microscopy), the results were very similar. These findings made us study systematically every patient with abortion during the first trimester, either by measuring fraction B of HCG, as well as using the anticarboxybeta HCG system, suggested by other authors. 1) Every patient with spontaneous abortion, the study of fraction B of HCG should be made. 2) In those patients with negative results of the fraction HCG, the study of the system anti-carboxy-beta-HCG, should be performed. 3) Renal changes in the mole patients were similar to the ones obtained in eclampsia patients.

04.09.02
Prognostic scoring system in prophylactic chemotherapy for molar pregnancy: Lahiri, B C. Med. Coll., Calcutta, India

From 1976 to 1983, 238 cases of GTN were treated of which 205 were of benign mole, 10 invasive mole and 23 choriocarcinoma out of 100,336 obstetric admissions giving an incidence of 1 in 489 for benign mole and 1 in 4362 for choriocarcinoma. 21 patients with a benign mole developed malignancy within 1–5 years during follow-up (10.3%). 35 cases of benign mole received prophylactic treatment, 21 hysterectomy, eight by chemotherapy and six by hysterectomy with chemotherapy. The rate of malignancy was lower in the group with prophylactic treatment – 8.5% compared to 10.5% in a control group. The risk was found to be increased with age, parity, uterine size, gross ovarian enlargement, higher hCG values, size of villi, trophoblastic proliferation and patients with blood group A. As a guide to selective prophylactic chemotherapy, a scoring system based upon above data before evaluation was worked out and scores allocated to each of these prognostic factors. The total score of each patient is determined by adding the actual values to each prognostic factor. All patients with malignant sequelae had score value of 7 or more and no malignancy occurred in patients with scores less than 7. If a score value of 7 is taken as the selective point and those with scores of 7 or above are treated with prophylactic chemotherapy, all 18 with malignant sequelae would have been treated prophylactically. This selection of high risk patients by the above scoring system and treating them with prophylactic chemotherapy appears to be a good screening procedure for selective prophylaxis.

04.09.03
Cytogenetic, morphological and clinical studies on partial hydatidiform moles: Ueda, K, Okamoto, E, Nomura, K, Ohama, K, Fujiwara, A. Dept. Obstet. and Gyn., Hiroshima Univ. School Med., Hiroshima, Japan

In order to establish the clinical management of partial moles, cytogenetic, morphological and clinical studies of 57 partial moles including three twin cases were performed. 1) The karyotypes of the 54 singletons were 46 triploid and 8 diploid. By examination of genetic markers, two of the diploid moles were proved to be derived from normally fertilized conceptuses. 2) In two of the twin cases, the molar tissue and a normal placenta with a fetus were delivered separately. Both of these cases proved to be binovular twins in which the molar tissues (46,XX) were androgenetic in origin while the other parts were derived from normally fertilized conceptuses. 3) An embryo (or a fetus) (26.9%) or just an umbilical cord (9.6%) was found in some triploid and diploid moles. Vessels with erythroblasts were also recognized in most cases. Additionally, there was positive correlation between cyst formaton and gestational length in triploid conceptuses. These findings suggest that triploid partial moles are an altered form of missed abortion. 4) Forty-eight patients were followed up for at least one year. The mole became invasive in one twin case with an androgenetic mole, but the remaining cases had uneventful courses. These results indicate that partial moles can be divided into three groups: 1. triploid, 2. diploid derived from normally fertilized conceptus, 3. binovular twin with androgenetic mole, and that, except for those in group 3, partial moles have no malignant potential and require no intensive follow-up.

04.09.04
Significance of negative α-fetoprotein in the interstitial area of mole tissues: Yoshimatsu, N, Munakata, S, Sugawara, N, Fukushima, T. Dept. Obstet. and Gyn., Fukushima Med. Coll., Fukushima, Japan

The presence of a fetal component is an important factor in explaining the mechanism of occurrence of total moles and partial moles. On the other hand, α-fetoprotein (AFP) has been considered to be produced by the fetal component alone. Fetuses at the early period of pregnancy, the umbilicus, normal villi, villi after abortion, partial moles and total moles were investigated from the viewpoint of this concept. Paraffin sections of the villi, liver and umbilicus, which were obtained by artificial termination of pregnancy between 5 and 10 weeks, and the villi after natural abortion, partial moles and total moles were examined for the presence of AFP by the peroxidase-anti-peroxidase method. – Results: (1) In normal pregnancy, the fetal liver, the gelatinous area of the umbilicus and the interstitial area of the villi were AFP positive, and the epithelial area of the villi was negative. (2) The interstitial areas of the villi after abortion, from which it is difficult to identify a fetus, were positive. (3) The interstitial areas of both normal and abnormal villi of partial moles, from which it is difficult to identify a fetus, were positive. (4) The interstitial areas of the total moles were negative. These results suggested that the villous interstitial area derived from the mesoblast was AFP positive if the fetus survived for a given period. From the observation that only the interstitial area of total moles was negative, it was considered that genesis of the embryo component of a total mole could not have taken place or was discontinued at an early period.

04.09.05
Molar pregnancy evacuation by interavenous infusion of sulprostone and its follow-up: Pastorfide, G B, Granados, S, Engo, M, Zapatos, C. Cardinal Santos Memo. Hosp., Metro Manila, Philippines
Sulprostone, a prostaglanding E_2 derivative, was used to terminate 14 molar pregnancies of 8–32 weeks gestation. No absolute failures occurred and no severe systemic complications were observed. The mean infusion time was 11.7 hours. Follow-up of these patients consisted of periodic hCG determinations. The use of intravenous infusion of sulprostone was not associated with any proliferative trophoblastic sequelae, either noninvasive, locally invasive or metastatic.

04.09.06
Sex chromatin in hydatidiform moles and abortions: Moegni, E M, Chan, M S N, Barnas, B, Samil, R S. Dept. Obstet. and Gyn., Med. Fac. of Indonesia/Dr. Cipto Mangunkusumo Hosp., Jakarta, Indonesia
Based on recent studies it can be concluded that hydatidiform moles cytogenetically are of three types. Incomplete or partial moles are triploid and unlikely subsequently to develop malignant trophoblastic neoplasm. Complete moles are diploid and the majority are homozygous, karyotype XX. Some of complete moles are heterozygous, karyotype XX or XY, with more risk for the subsequent development of malignant trophoblastic neoplasm than homozygous complete moles. An examination of sex chromatin was already conducted in 83 histopathological slides of hydatidiform moles patients, in the Department of Obstetrics and Gynecology – Dr. Cipto Mangunkusumo Hospital, during the period of January, 1, 1981 until December 31, 1981. Data of patients age, parity, education, subsequent development of malignancy and follow-up during two years, were also collected. As control group was examined the histopathological slides of 83 patients with abortion during the same period. It became evident that sex chromatin in hydatidiform moles was dominant that in abortions (p < 0.05). There seems to be a tendency that the higher the amount of cytotrophoblast cells which contain sex chromatin, the more possibility that it will develop into malignant trophoblastic neoplasm. Based on this studies, it is suggested to do a closer observation on patients with hydatidiform moles whose cytotrophoblast cells contain 15% or more sex chormatin.

04.09.07
High risk of choriocarcinoma following hydatidiform mole in older patients: Soma, H, Takayama, M, Matayoshi, K. Dept. Obstet. and Gyn., Tokyo Med. Coll., Shinjuku, Tokyo, Japan
The increased risk of hydatidiform mole in older women has been emphasized. In the older patients with hydatidiform mole, the risk of choriocarcinoma or invasive mole after removal of the mole is significantly higher than that of malignant progression following hydatidiform mole for 38 women in the 40 to 54-year age is discussed. Results: 1) The age distribution of 38 patients consists of 11 cases over 50 years of age, 16 in the 45–49 years of age and 11 from 40 to 44 years old. 2) In 23 of the older patients, a diagnosis was made by evacuation of the mole and 14 cases were misdiagnosed as uterine myoma. Although hysterectomy was performed in nine cases, in three of them invasive moles were found in the uterus. 3) Of those patients, 16 cases developed into eight choriocarcinomas and eight invasive moles, and eight had pulmonary metastases, thereafter two cases died of extensive metastases. 4) HCG levels in older patients on admission to hospital ranged widely from 491,000 iu/l to 2400 iu/l, and it took about two to six months until the hCG titer fell to LH level following chemotherapy. 5) Since hCG titer hardly fell to LH level, even after chemotherapy was given for 2 to 10 courses after removal of the mole, four patients had undergone hysterectomy, at which small tumor foci remained in the myometrium. A 49-year-old patient had choriocarcinoma in the uterus removed only 17 days after evacuation of the mole. In conclusion, it should be stressed that in patients over 40 years of age with a hydatidiform mole there is a greater risk of choriocarcinoma.

04.09.08
Hydatidiform mole: Dizygotic twin gestations by diploid androgenesis and normal fertilization: Vejerslev, L O. Dept. Med. Genet., J. F. Kennedy Inst., Glostrup/Copenhagen; **Dueholm, M.** Dept. Gyn. and Obstet., Randers County Hosp.; **Hassing Nielsen, F.** Dept. Gyn. and Obstet., Horsens Hosp., Denmark
About 1 : 160 deliveries in Denmark include dizygotic twins. In 1984 52 hydatidiform moles (HM) were

observed (1 : 961 deliveries). Thus, the probability of HM in a dizygotic twin pregnancy would be about 1 : 75,400 deliveries, i. e. one case about every $1^1/_2$ years. During the first year of the current Danish study on HM (initiated January 1984) two twin gestations with HM were observed. In case 1 evacuation in the 22nd week of gestation revealed a homogeneous placental mass with macroscopically visible cystic swelling of the villi and wihtout fetal parts. Karyotyping and genetic marker analyses of cultured cells revealed two cell lines: 46,XX consistent with diploid androgenesis and 46,XY, an apparently normal conception. In case 2 spontaneous abortion occurred in the 22nd week of gestation, as repeated ultrasound scans showed both a cystic placental mass of increasing size, and a live fetus. Cultured cells from cystic villi had the karyotype 46,XX, markers being consistent with diploid androgenesis. Cultured fetal fibroblasts showed the same karyotype 46,XX originating from a chromosomally normal conception. In both cases contamination by maternal fibroblasts could be excluded. Dizygotic twin gestation with HM and a normal conceptus might be a distinct entity in which the risk of malignant sequelae could be elevated in spite of the observation of fetal parts. Maybe the basic mechanism involved in production of HM increases the probability of a concomitant second conception.

04.09.09
The prevention of trophoblastic disease by early detection of blighted ovum: Džikov, Z, Kalamaras, E, Jovkovski, V, Dimitrova, M. Univ. Clin. Obstet. and Gyn., Skopje, Yugoslavia
Sonographic findings of a blighted ovum, confirmed twice in two weeks period required admission of the patient, instrumental evacuation of the uterus and follow-up of HCG level afterwards. For a period of almost three years 20 cases of hydatidiform moles in different stages of development have been diagnosed and histologically confirmed. What is the total number of patients with blighted ovum is not known, since all patients with such a sonographic finding have not undergone the clinical observation. Pathohistologic finding was usually partial molar transformation or hydropic degeneration of villi stroma with deficit or less of blood vessels and proliferation of trophoblastic epithelium. In combination with this morphologic finding in the villi, deposits of fibrin in intervillous spaces and calcification were found. Early diagnosis of hydatidiform mole in some patients with blighted ovum has a great significance in their further diagnostic and therapeutic management. For the mentioned period of time there was a brisk reduction of trophoblastic disease in the clinical material.

04.10.01
Cervical dysplasia in female partners to men with genital warts: Rådberg, T, Jonassen, F, Löwhagen, G B. Dept. Gyn. and Dermatovener., Sahlgren's Hosp., Univ., Göteborg, Sweden
Human papilloma virus (HPV), causing genital warts, are much discussed as a possible cause of cervical dysplasia (CIN) and cancer of the cervix. Therefore, the female partners to men with genital warts attending a venereal disease clinic were examined by vaginal cytology and colposcopy. All women with pathological findings underwent biopsies for histopathological diagnosis. The women, who were screened by vaginal cytology at a family planning clinic when consulting for contraceptive aid served as controls. Among the 51 partners 18 (35%) had visible external condylomata and 17 (33%) had pathological cytology compared to 28 out of 639 controls. The prevalence of moderate and severe CIN was 14 out of 51 (27%) in partners but only 12 out of 639 (2%) in controls. When all degrees of CIN were considered, CIN was almost as frequent in partners without visible condylomata as in women with genital warts (36% and 39%, respectively). Furthermore, CIN seems to be at least ten times as frequent in partners to men with genital warts as in the normal, sexually-active female population of comparable ages (p < 0.0001). Thus, women exposed to HPV, as e. g. by having a regular partner treated for genital warts, need a close attention to the risk of developing cervical dysplasia.

04.10.02
The cervical tumor associated antigen (AG-4/ICP-10) is encoded by the tumorigenic region of HSV-2 DNA: Iwasaka, T, Smith, C C, Aurelian, L, Sugimori, H. Div. Biophys., Johns Hopkins Med. Inst., Baltimore, MD, USA and Dept. Obstet. and Gyn., Saga Med. School, Saga, Japan
Bgl II fragment C mapping between 0.416 and 0.580 map units (m.u.) on the herpes simplex virus type 2 (HSV-2) genome causes neoplastic transformation of normal diploid mammalian cells. Sequences mapping between 0.419–0.525 m. u. cause cellular immortalization. However, sequences within 0.525–0.580 m. u. are required for the acquisition of tumorigenic potential (*Jariwalla* et al., Proc. nat. Acad. Sci. **80,** 5902–5906, 1983). Here we show that RNA homologous to the Bgl II C fragment directs the synthesis of three proteins with approximate molecular weights of 144,000, 52,000 and 27,000. The 27,000 dalton protein is encoded by sequences within the Hind III/EcoRI AE fragment (0.419–0.525 m. u.) that overlap the immortalizing sequences within Bgl II C. The 144,000 (144K) and 52,000 dalton proteins are encoded by sequences within the BamHI "e" fragment of HSV-2 DNA (0.535–0.585 m. u.). The 144K protein is the only species translated *in vitro* from mRNA hybrid-selected from cells arrested in the "early" (β) phase of viral protein synthesis. Immunoprecipitation by anti-ICP-10 serum and monoclonal antibody 48S and tryptic peptide analysis revealed that this translated 144K protein is antigenically and structurally similar to ICP-10 that was antigenically identified in Bgl II C transformed cells and was shown to be immunologically identical to the cervical tumor associated antigen AG-4.

04.10.03

Human papilloma virus infection and cervical neoplasia: A colposcopical approach: Barrasso, R*, Coupez, F**, Ionesco***, de Brux, J***. *Dept. Obstet. and Gyn. II, Univ., Bologna, Italy. ** Ctr Hosp. Intercommun., Créteil, France. ***IPECA, Paris, France

A study was undertaken to evaluate the accuracy of some colposcopical criteria to differentiate cervical atypias with and without papilloma virus (PV)-related features. One hundred and twelve patients with atypical cytology underwent colposcopy and colposcopically directed biopsies. Colposcopically, irregular surface contour of the atypical transformation zone, asperities and irregular response to the Schiller Test, as previously described (*Coupez, F.*, Gynécologie **24**, 177, 1983) were tentatively considered PV-related features. Of 82 cases with two or three PV-related features on colposcopy, 72 (87.8%) were diagnosed as CIN, with features of condyloma; ten (12.2%) simply as CIN. Of 30 cases with one or no PV-related features on colposcopy, only four (13.3%) were diagnosed as CIN with features of condyloma; 26 (86.7%) simply as CIN. Moreover, in 23 cases we observed a peripheral pattern with PV-related features both on colposcopy and histology, which merged into a high grade lesion (CIN III) showing only lesser degrees of koilocytotic atypia in histology, without any identifiable PV marker on colposcopy. Some colposcopic changes seem to be related to the papilloma virus infection, but no clear demarcation line exists between cervical atypias, papilloma virus-related and not. Moreover, our observations suggest that at least some PV-induced lesions may progress to high grade CIN. Nevertheless, the possibility that these high grade lesions could be biologically different from true CIN, or that PV infection and CIN simply co-exist, could not be excluded.

04.10.04

Detection of HSV-1 and HSV-2 by monoclonal antibodies in cervical cancer patients: Nicolaou, C, Fotiou, S, Nocolaou, P, Pavlatou, M, Patramani, I, Aravantinos, D. 1st Dept. Obstet. and Gyn., "Alexandra" Hosp., Univ., Athens, Greece

The possible association of cervical cancer with type HSV-2 infection has been widely investigated. Numerous seroepidemiological studies in many countries, have shown an increased prevalence of HSV-2 antibodies in patients with carcinoma of the cervix than in matched controls. Such differences have not been observed in all geographic areas nor socioeconomic classes. However, the results reported in many of these studies give a crude measure of past infection by HSV-2 since the serological assays used detected antibodies to both type-common and type-specific antigens. The production of monoclonal antibodies presented the laboratory with a sensitive, rapid and reliable method for the measurement of type specific antibodies and the typing of the virus. Eighty-four women with cervical cancer were tested by immunofluorescence with monoclonal antibodies. We used: 1) Anti-herpes simplex virus I (non-cross reactive with HSV2, CMV, or EBV) for the detection of HBV-1 specific proteins (antibody class IgG1K). 2) Anti-herpes simplex virus 2 for the detection of HSV-2 specific proteins (antibody class IgG1K). The results showed a positive relation between HSV and cervical cancer. Women with an herpetic infection of the genital tract should be considered as a group of high risk and be followed frequently.

04.10.05

Levels of anti-HSV-VCA circulating antibodies in women with papova virus genital infection: *Guglielmino, S, **Corbino, N, **Nuciforo, G, **Petrina, M, *Tempera, G, *Garozzo, A, *Castro, A, **Cianci, S. *Inst. Microbiol., **Inst. Clin. Obstet. and Gyn. IIa, Univ., Catania, Italy

Serum levels of anti-HSV-VCA Ig were measured in 148 women with evidence of dyskeratosis on PAP-test. 112 healthy subjects from medical staff and nurses served as controls. Levels of IgM plus IgG detected by complement deviation assay in patients were below 1/64 in 12.8% and over in 87.2% while in controls the corresponding figures were 81.2% and 18.8%. Levels of IgA detected by immunofluorescent assay in patients were below 1/64 in 54% and over in 46% while in controls the corresponding figures were 97.2% and 2.8%. Values are statistically significant. Immunofluorescent assay of HSV- and HPV-VCA on cervicovaginal exfoliated cells showed that in patient group 8.1% were HSV$^+$HPV$^-$, 39,1% were HSV$^-$HPV$^+$, 41.8% were HSV$^+$HPV$^+$ and 11% were HSV$^-$HPV$^-$. Levels of IgA in HSV$^+$HPV$^+$ were over 1/64 in 100%. Infecting HSV was isolated from 8% of patients. Strains typing revealed HSV1 in 37% and HSV2 in 63%. Cytological examinations showed that koilocytosis was associated in 16%, dysplasia was detected in 7% and metaplasia in 20%. Colposcopy revealed mosaic in 30%, white epithelium in 12%, atypical regenerating areas in 9%, condyloma in 9%. 40% of patients had a negative colposcopy. High levels of IgA anti-HSV-VCA are detectable only in patients with double infection of genital tract by herpes and papova virus.

04.10.06

HPV-standardization and DNA-cytophotometry in dysplasia of the cervix uteri: Göppinger, A, Birmelin, G, Ikenberg, H, Hillemanns, H G, Hilgarth, M. Univ. Women's Hosp., Freiburg/Br.

Recent studies on dysplasia of the cervix uteri indicate that human papilloma virus (HPV) infections might play a causal role in the pathogenesis of a cervical intra-epithelial neoplasia or an invasive carcinoma. Viruses of the HPV group 16/18 were found among malignant changes on the cervix uteri, whereas viruses of the HPV group 11 could only be singled out in cases of slightly dysplastic changes. The results from 300 patients were studied by comparing the isolated virus types with the degree of severity of the histological and cytological changes. Cytophotometric DNA measurements were additonally made in 30 cases of slight to moderate dysplasia, as earlier studies have confirmed the prognostic value of the DNA distribution pattern in the evaluation of the nature of cervical dysplasia.

04.10.07

Papilloma virus (HPV) infections of the lower genital tract detected by DNA *in situ* hybridization: Schneider, A[1], Schumann, R A[1], Gissmann, L[2]. 1 Dept. Gyn. and Obstet., Univ. Ulm; 2 German Ca Res. Inst., Heidelberg
Analysis of the prevalence and follow-up data of HPV-infections in cytological positive and negative gynecological smears, correlation of the HPV-types (6)11 and 16/18 to benign, premalignant or malignant changes of the uterine cervix and detection of penile lesions in partners of HPV – positive women were the prupose of this study. HPV-DNA was identified in gynecological smears using the method of molecular *in situ* hybridization. In more than two-thirds of women with positive cervical smears HPV-DNA could be detected, showing a decrease of HPV (6)11 and an increase of HPV 16/18 prevalence through the stages of precancer towards cancer. Histological examination confirmed this distribution. Follow-up examination of cytological and HPV-positive women over a period up to nine months showed regression in all HPV (6)11 cases unless an infection with HPV 16/18 was acquired additionally. 50% of all HPV 16/18-associated lesions reverted to negative, 50% persisted. 1169 cytological negative women showed HPV-DNA in 6.5% and HPV 16/18 was recognized twice as frequently in pregnant women compared to non-pregnant. Reexamination of cytological negative, HPV-positive women showed HPV-associated changes in a high percentage using colposcopy and cytology. Male partners of cytological and HPV-positive women were scrutinized and in 25% HPV-positive lesions were identified – including cases of bowenoid papulosis. The distribution of different HPV-types and their correlation to cytology during follow-up corresponded with the biological potential of cervical lesions. HPV-positive lesions in asymptomatic male partners emphasized the need for their detection and proper treatment in respect to their infecting and preneoplastic potential.

04.10.08

Identification of the human papilloma virus (HPV) as an etiologic factor in cervical intra-epithelial neoplasia (CIN): Meandzija, M, Locher, G W, Beretta, K R. Dept. Obstet. and Gyn., Univ., Bern, Switzerland
Infection of the lower genital tract with HPV is closely linked to premalignant and malignant disease in that area, particularly the cervix. To evaluate this hypothesis, we screened 588 patients (pts) with suspect PAP smears over 36 months using a specially designed questionnaire. Part 1 consisted of epidemiological and socio-economic questions, and Part 2 of questions related to colposcopic, light microscopic (cytologic and histologic), and specific virus identification techniques. There was no statistically significant correlation between colposcopic and light microscopic features for viral involvement of metaplastic and squamous epithelium. There was, however, a strong correlation between colposcopic criteria for viral involvement and its detection in the tissue using immunocytochemic and/or hybridization techniques. We also observed the persistence of the virus in the epithelium of the genital tract in 22% of pts who underwent local tissue destruction or superficial abrasion of these lesions. Early identification of the virus, using one standardized epidemiological and clinical protocol worldwide, is now imperative in order better to screen out those individuals in the population at large who are at risk of developing invasive cervical and other genital cancers.

04.10.09

Sister chromatid exchanges in lymphocytes of patients with cervical intra-epithelial neoplasia: Moon, H, Kim, K T, Kim, D S, Paik, Y K*. Dept. Obstet and Gyn. and Dept. Genet.*, School Med., Hanyang Univ., Seoul, Korea
The frequency of sister chromatid exchanges (SCE) was investigated in cultured lymphocytes from 20 women with cervical intra-epithelial neoplasia (CIN) together from ten control women. For scoring CSE, 40 second-and/or third cycle metaphases were analyzed from each subject. The mean frequencies of SCE per metaphase were 6.29 ± 0.23 and 5.16 ± 0.16 in CIN cases and controls, respectively. The average increase of SCE was about 22% in CIN cases, and the difference was significant ($p < 0.01$). The individual frequency of SCE (based on the number of SCEs in 40 metaphases) of control subjects was relatively constant compared with that of CIN, and the variance of SCE frequency in controls was significantly smaller than that of CIN cases ($p < 0.025$). The frequency of SCE in seven cases of CIN I and II were found to be similar to that of controls, but in 13 cases of CIN III (severe dysplasia and carcinoma *in situ*) the frequency was significantly higher than that of controls ($p < 0.001$). The lymphocytes responding to phytohemagglutinin (PHA-M) in cultures from CIN cases showed no sign of delay in cell cycle in comparison to those of controls. The possibility of using SCE as a preclinical marker for early detection of cervical cancer is suggested.

04.10.10

Study of onco-fetal antigens (CEA & AFP) in cervical intra-epithelial neoplasia: Saraiya, U B, Joshi, S. Cama & Albless Hosp. and Breach Candy Hosp., Bombay, India
Onco-fetal antigens were studied in tissue and serum in 120 cases of CIN. Serum CEA levels were studied by RIA Kits using a one step sandwich method in 70 cases. Forty-three showed negative levels wheras 14

were borderline and 13 were positive. Only five cases were positive for AFP. CEA in tissue was studied by the indirect triple bridge immunoperoxidase method in formalin fixed paraffin embedded tissue in 50 cases. The presence of CEA could be reliably assessed by brown staining in atypical epithelial cells. CEA positivity increased from 50% in dysplasia to 63.6% in carcinoma *in situ* and to 84.2% in invasive cancer. From our experience it is tempting to speculate that CEA positivity in dysplasia reflects a malignant potential. In patients with treated carcinoma of the cervix continued normal levels of serum CEA affirms the absence of the disease whereas development of an elevated level is highly suspicious of recurrence. Tumor markers and hormone receptors have widened the horizons of clinical oncology. Since carcinoma of the cervix has an easily detectable precancerous phase it is a good model for studying the role of tumor markers. This field will continue to grow in the near future and has possibilities of being used in routine clinical practice.

04.11.01
Choice of the type of hysterectomy in urgent gynecological-obstetric intervention: Vuković, D, Colaković, B. Obstet. & Gyn. Dept., Clin. Hosp., Titograd, Yugoslavia
Urgent hysterectomies are often performed in an easier manner for the patient and the surgeon, without regard whether this easier kind of operation is also in reality an adequate surgical intervention. The subtotal hysterectomy is more simple than the total one, but leaving the cervix behind is already long ago not acknowledged as a method for a definite healing. In urgent cases supravaginal amputation has to be used, but the remaining cervix must also additionally be removed. A modern solution of this problem approves only an extirpation of the uterus "in toto" as an adequate gynecological intervention and final healing. During the period of 15 years (1970–1984) we carried out 989 abd. hysterectomies, of which 22 were supravaginal (2.23%). Urgent hysterectomies were 37 (3.74%). Urgent total hysterectomies were executed 24 (64.87%), and subtotal 13 (35.13%). During the first five years seven urgent subtotal hysterectomies were performed; in the next five years five, and during the last period of five years only one. On four patients we executed afterwards an extirpation of the cervix. From the data we review it can be concluded that also in cases of urgent hysterectomies we attempt by all means to avoid a supravaginal amputation of the uterus. Although we for programmed hysterectomies most often use intrafascial hysterectomy by *Aldridge* on account of the benignancy of the disease, we consider that for all urgent cases the classic uterus extirpation is the right method of choice.

04.11.02
Gynecological operation on women 80 years of age or over: Jaluvka, V, Post, K-G, Weitzel, H. Dept. Obstet. and Gyn., Klinikum Steglitz, FU, Berlin
Between the years 1970 and 1984 in 18 gynecological departments of West Berlin 2806 operations were performed on women 80 years of age or over. Out of 1460 "major" operations 285 were done on genital displacement, 743 on malignant tumors, 401 on benign tumors, 17 on other gynecological and 14 on other surgical diseases. Out of 1346 "minor" interventions 23 were performed on genital displacement (removal of pessary), 131 on malignant tumors, 35 on benign tumors, 1140 on other gynecological diseases an 17 on other surgical diseases. During the same 15-year period 110 women (3.8%) 90 years of age or over were operated for the following reasons: 14 genital displacements, 40 malignant tumors, 21 benign tumors, 32 other gynecological diseases and 3 other surgical diseases. No correlation was found between the extent of the intervention and the postoperative mortality, which, on the other hand, seems to correlate positively with higher stages of malignant tumors. In conclusion, the analysis of the postoperative mortality in women 80 or more years old shows, that 1) cancer prevention examinations on elderly women have to be intensified, 2) there should be a broader indication in some selected cases for abdominal hysterectomy with bilateral salpingo-oophorectomy despite the somewhat higher postoperative mortality, and that 3) in cases of genital displacement colpohysterectomy seems to have become the method of choice.

04.11.03
Computer-based quality assessment in operative gynecology: Braeutigam, H H, Hegerfeld, R. Dept. Obstet. and Gyn., Marienkrankenhaus, Hamburg
For ethical and economical reasons hospital based medicine should be obliged to exert an effective quality assessment program. This program must be proved in daily routine hospital surgery. We established a quality assessment study using on-line structure with the aid of a video display terminal which for practical use is located in the operation room area. The hospital administration supplies all relevant personal patient data. The doctor who is the user of the terminal is responsible for the input of all surgical data such as pre-operative risks, kind of operation, indications and diagnosis. To evaluate patients outcome all neces-sary data such as postoperative complications and patient's and treatment related data are given into the terminal. Nine different statistical programs were computerized and reliable data on postoperative outcome were produced. Combined with morbidity statistics which are printed every four weeks efficiency statistics are available to demonstrate the work-load of operation ward personell. Special programs have been carried out, for example the effect of short-term antibiotic prophylaxis. Such resolve of our data evaluation are immediately transferred to hospital practice.

04.11.04

Heterotopic autotransplantation of the ovary to prevent sequelae of ionizing radiation to the pelvis: Scheidel, P, Wendt, T G*, Hepp, H. Dept. Obestet. and Gyn. and *Dept. Radiol., Klinikum Großhadern, Ludwig-Maximilians-Univ., Munich

The nature and mode of action of ionizing radiation and its general effect on gonadal tissue have been subject of extensive investigation. In clinical conditions however, it is impossible in spite of meticulous planning of radiotherapy to preserve ovarian function in patients who will need more than 5 Gy radiation to the pelvis. Two cases are presented in which heterotopic autotransplantation of the ovary to the mid-upper abdomen was performed to prevent hormonal deficiency. In one case of a desmoid tumor the transplantation was successful with normal menstrual cycle and ovulations (progesterone). In another case, a patient with Hodgkin's disease, a negative effect of radiation could not be excluded despite a calculated maximum dose of 2.9 Gy at the site of the transplanted ovaries. When radiation is limited to the pelvis, ovarian function can be preserved safely by heterotopic autotransplantation. When radiation is extended to para-aortal nodes, radiation treatment planning can be extremely difficult especially in slim patients. In these cases explantation and replantation of the ovary will be a promising approach. This approach is currently developed in animal studies.

04.11.05

Endocrine function of autotransplanted ovaries in young women undergoing radical operation and radiotherapy for cervical cancer: Ichinoe, K, Shiina, Y, Yamada, Y. Dept. Obstet. and Gyn., Hokkaido Univ. School Med., Sapporo, Japan

In order to preserve the ovarian function in younger patients with cervical squamous carcinoma (stage Ib and II) from the damage of postoperative irradiation, autotransplantation of the ovary was carried out to the adipose tissue of the breast or of the upper lateral quadrant of the abdomen, as a position out of the radiation field. To conserve the ovarian blood circulation, ovary was transplanted with its own vessels. Seventy-five patients between 24 and 43 years of age have undergone this transplantation in the last eight years. A long-term follow-up study of the ovarian function was made in 59 patients with periodic determination of serum estradiol, progesterone, FSH and LH as well as the examination of daily changes of BBT and ovarian size. Of these cases, 57 patients (96.6%) showed a cyclic palpable swelling of the ovary and not only was there serial biphasic BBT with regular changes in the levels of serum steroids and pituitary gonadotrophins, but two of these patients have also married after the operation and are doing well. There seems to have been a long-term active function in ovaries which were autotransplanted with their own vessels to a distant place to avert the damage of postoperative irradiation, without any decrease in the five-year survival rate in these studies.

04.11.06

Dr. Nadkarni's method of intracervical total hysterectomy: Patel, U T, Patel, Y, Nadkarni, R M. K.M. School of P. G. Med. & Res., Ahmedabad, India

In certain conditions like endometriosis chronic pelvic inflammations or extensive adhesions where hysterectomy becomes a difficult problem due to fear of the damage to the surrounding structures and also of hemorrhage a surgeon has to content himself with a supravaginal hysterectomy or closing the abdomen without doing anything. In such cases intracervical hysterectomy is found of immense use. In intracervical hysterectomy after ligation of uterine vessels at the level of internal os the entire uterus is cored out of the cervical tissue without disturbing the structures around. Except for postoperative bleeding in one case out of 100 cases no complication has been noticed. The procedure has been also found useful in the management of recurrent prolapses or prolapse associated with tumors.

04.11.07

Shrinkage of uterine size: Ranney, B. Univ. of South Dakota School Med., SD, Yankton, USA

How much does uterine size diminish during and immediately after hysterectomy? Gynecologists observe perceptible, and variable, shrinkage from uterine size *in vivo*, to subsequent size in the pathology laboratory. To measure this decrease in uterine size, the thickness, breadth, and height of the corpus was measured with calipers four times: (1) as soon as the abdomen had been opened, (2) as soon as uterine arteries had been ligated, (3) as soon as the uterus was removed, and (4) after 45 minutes in fixative. Cervical diameter and length were measured twice: (1) as soon as the uterus was removed, and (2) after 45 minutes in fixative. Reduction in uterine volume varied from a low of 20% to a high of 64% in different specimens. In specimens from premenopausal women, greatest reduction occurred while arteries and pedicles were being clamped and ligated, especially in women who had uterine hypertrophy or hypermenorrhea. In postmenopausal women, greatest reduction occurred during fixation of the specimen after removal. Therefore, measurement or weight of fresh or fixed specimens bears only a diffuse and highly variable relationship to the true, *in vivo*, measurements or weights.

04.11.08

Hysterectomium: Lahodny, J. Gen. Publ. Hosp., Gmünd, Austria

It is a parametrium clamp with integrated cutting blade and attached sewing mechanism. The hysterectomium facilitates clamping cutting and sewing almost simultaneously. At the concave side of the parametrium clamp there is the blade of the scissors and at the convex exterior side there is the sewing mechanism at the end of the sewing shank which enlarges the end of the clamps by about 5 millimetres. The cutting blade and the sewing shank are fixed in the lock of the parametrium clamp. Usually the parametrium is clamped by means of the clamp. Immediately afterwards the right thumb presses the cutting blade. Without changing the position of the thumb the right forefinger presses on the ring of the sewing shank, whereby several vicryl sutures are laid and knotted. The coming off of ligatures or post-operative hemorrhages are impossible with this technique. The total procedure of clamping, cutting and sewing takes about 2 or 3 seconds. Any hysterectomy with peritoneal closure can be carried out in about ten minutes.

04.11.09

Ultra-radical surgery in the women's hospital, Univ., Basle, Switzerland: Almendral, A C, Heinzl, S. Women's Hosp., Basle, Switzerland

During the years 1970–1984, 40 pelvic eviscerations were performed at the Women's Hospital, University of Basle. The mean age of the patients was 53 years, the most frequent indication was a relapse or persistency of genital malignoma. Only in five cases, this operation was performed as primary therapy. The tumors were located as follows: 32 carcinomas of cervix and vulva; three corpus carcinomas; 3 carcinomas of the vulva and one ovarian carcinoma. One patient required the operation due to multiple fistulae after radio-therapy ("cloaca syndrome"). In 12 cases, the scheduled pelvic evisceration could not be performed, as a larger spread of the tumor was found intraoperatively. There were 25 total pelvic eviscerations, 11 anterior and four posterior operations. In 31 patients, urinary drainage was achieved through an intestinal conduit (small bowel 26, sigma five). The remaining five patients had a direct implantation of their ureters into the large bowel. A reconstruction of intestinal continuity was carried out in seven patients with a deep anastomosis between sigma and rectum. No patient died during the operation, two (5%) postoperatively of massive pulmonary emboli and peritonitis after dehiscence of the perineal wound. Considering also non-relevant complications, the post-operative rate amounted to nearly 100%. Eight patients showed no relevant post-operative complications, eight others had to be reoperated because of bleeding, ileus and/or complications due to the urinary conduit. We do have complete information on the further course. The likelihood to survive for more than five years is approximately 45 % for our patients.

04.11.10

A new surgical approach to pelvic varicosities: Rundqvist, E, Sandholm, L-E, Larsson, G. Dept. Obstet. and Gyn., Centr. Hosp., Karlskrona, Sweden

Chronic pelvic pain in women may be caused by a variety of gynecological diseases. It can even be a psychosomatic disease. It has also been demonstrated that pelvic varicosities may cause pain. Treatment of pelvic varicosities has usually consisted of ligation and resection via the transperitoneal route. Analogous with extraperitoneal resection of the spermatic vein above the inguinal ligament for treatment of varicocele of the testis one of the present authors has developed a method involving extraperitoneal resection of the left ovarian vein in women with pelvic varicosities. The operative technique consists of a left-sided McBurney incision. The aponeurosis and muscles are separated parallel to their fibers. The peritoneum is exposed and the dissection is continued retroperitoneally until the ovarian vessels are found on the left side. The ureter is carefully identified. The vessels are dissected and resected for a distance of at least five centimeters, care being taken to resect all dilated and tortuous branches. Fifteen women with chronic pelvic pain and in whom left-sided renal phlebography had demonstrated pelvic varicosities were, during an eight year period, operated upon with extraperitoneal resection of the left ovarian vein. At follow-up eight patients were completely cured and three were considerably improved, but in four women no improvement occurred. Mean period of follow-up was 5.6 years. The complication rate was low. One case of wound infection and one case with bleeding from a subcutaneous artery necessitating resuture were the only complications.

04.11.11

Lateral sling – a conservative management of uterine prolapse: Joshi, N U, Wadia B J. J J Hosp. Univ., Bombay, India

The author has worked with Prof. *V N Shirodkar* and has modified his ideas of using nylon tape to sling the uterus up. The tape is stitched posteriorly to the uterus at the junction of the uterosacrals. The sling is fixed laterally to the external oblique aponeurosis and periostium of the anterior superior iliac spine. The tape is passed extraperitoneally through the broad ligament and pelvic cellular fascia. The author has experience of over 400 operations spread over the past 15 years. The follow-up is adequate. The results show an overall cure of 80% which includes both nulliparous and parous cases.

04.11.12

The management of post-operative urinary retention: Gordon, M. DOG, Albany Med. Coll., Albany, NY, USA

Post-operative urinary retention may occur following major abdominal or vaginal gynecologic procedures. Rational management of this distressing complication requires: (1) prevention of bladder over distension post-operatively, (2) prevention and treatment of urinary tract infection, (3) evaluation of the severity of all potentially contributing factors, (4) elimination or treatment of the contributing factors, (5) prescription of appropriate medications in selected cases, (6) pre-operative evaluation of bladder function for all patients undergoing surgery for anatomical desplacements (procedentia uteri) or stress urinary incontinence, (7) pre-operative treatment and stabilization of medical and neurological complications in patients requiring major gynecologic surgery, (8) maintenance of a cheerful and confident demeanor so as to decrease the patient's anxiety, and encourage the earliest successful restoration of bladder function.

04.12.01

The association between fetal heart rate patterns and maternal posture during labor: Divon, M Y, Mushkat, Y*, Sarna, Z*, Zimmer, E Z, Vilensky, A*, Paldi, E. Depts. Obstet. & Gyn. "B" and Med. Bioengin.*, Rambam Med. Ctr, Haifa, Israel

It is well known that the position adopted by the pregnant subject can influence her cardiovascular dynamics. In particular, when a pregnant patient lies supine, the uterus may cause aortocaval compression which leads to uterine hypoperfusion. A random controlled trial was performed to compare the effects of the dorsal and the left lateral positions upon fetal well-being during labor. Fetal heart rate (FHR) and beat to beat variability (BTBV) were used as indicators of fetal health. 29 healthy parturients were studied during the first stage of labor. Contractions, FHR, and BTBV were simultaneously recorded for 20 minutes in each position, and then fed into a microcomputer for further analysis. Also recorded were maternal heart rate and blood pressure. Our findings indicate that: 1. Both systolic and diastolic blood pressure were higher in the supine position. 2. The amount of uterine work was the same in both positions. 3. BTBV was higher during uterine contractions. 4. There was no significant change in FHR between the two positions. 5. BTBV was higher in the left lateral positon, although it was significant only in a special group of the patients. Our preliminary conclusion is that left lateral posture is better for fetal well being as detected by BTBV changes during normal labor.

04.12.02

The renal handling of the acid base balance in healthy pregnant and early postpartum women: Sicińska, J, Wójcicka-Jagodzińska, J, Siekierski, B P, Szczecina, R. 2nd Dept. Obstet. and Gyn., Warsaw Med. School, Warszawa, Poland

The material consists of 135 healthy women: 50 non-pregnant, 23 in the I trimester of pregnancy, 32 in the II trim., 30 in the III trim. and 51 on the 3rd postpartum day. Biochemical tests were performed in 24-hours urine samples, namely: 1. ammonium ions concentration (NH_4^+), 2. hydrogen ions (H^+), 3. potassium and sodium concentration (K^+, Na^+). In the I trim. of pregnancy no significant differences to non-pregnant control were detectable. In the II trim. the urinary excretion of H^+ was significantly increased. In the III trim. a highly significant increase of 24 hours urinary volume, H^+, NH_4^+, K^+, and Na^+ excretion was encountered. In the third puerperal day the 24 hours urinary volume, NH_4^+ and NA^+ returned to pregestational values. Only the excretion of H^+ and K^+ maintained their high levels. In conclusion the increase of amino-acids, K^+ and Na^+ dihydrogen phosphate metabolism starts after 29th, and rise of carbonic acid metabolism in kidney tubules begins with 16th week of gestation. The significant increase of desamination in the tubules occurring in the III trim. may be linked with a high estriol concentration in this period of gestation. Estriol can be responsible for activation of glutaminase involved in ammonium production.

04.12.03

Release of β-endorphin in physical exercise in nonpregnant and pregnant women: Laatikainen, T, Rauramo, I. Dept. I and II Obstet. and Gyn., Helsinki Univ. Centr. Hosp., Helsinki, Finland

In nonpregnant women, physical exercise has been found to increase plasma concentration of immunoreactive β-endorphin. In pregnant women, plasma concentration of β-endorphin (β-E) increases greatly during labor, but no data seem to be available on the effect of physical exercise. β-E release was studied in eight nonpregnant and in eight pregnant women in their last trimester of pregnancy using a 10-min bicycle ergometer test. Plasma concentration of β-E was determined using a specific assay (*Laatikainen* et al., Clin. Chem. **31**, 134, 1985). Plasma level of β-E increased in response to exercise in seven of the eight nonpregnant and in all pregnant women. In the nonpregnant women the mean β-E level was 2.4 ± 0.7 (S. E.) pmol/l before the test, 4.3 ± 0.9 at the end of the test, and 4.3 ± 0.6 and 5.0 ± 2.0 pmol/l 15 and 30 min after the test, respectively, declining thereafter. In the pregnant women the mean β-E value was 5.1 ± 2.0 pmol/l before the test, 7.3 ± 1.7 pmol/l at the end of the test, 6.7 ± 2.0 15 min after the test, and 12.6 ± 4.1 pmol/l 60 min after the test and declining thereafter. Thus β-E release was demonstrated in response to exercise both in nonpregnant and in pregnant women. In pregnant women β-E release seems to last longer.

04.12.04

Effect of upright position on maternal circulation – a prospective study: Schneider, K T M, Weber, S, Bung, P, Fallenstein, F, Huch R, Huch, A. Dept. Obstet., Univ., Zurich, Switzerland

The compression of the pelvic vessels by the enlarged uterus late in pregnancy was demonstrated to be the cause of marked cyclic maternal heart rate accelerations when the women were standing. A longitudinal study was initiated to see when the heart rate accelerations begin to appear. We monitored noninvasively: Maternal and fetal heart rate, external tocogram, maternal blood pressure and cardiac output. The mothers were at first in the left lateral position for 10 min, then standing still for 10 min. The study comprises 40 singleton and six twin pregnancies. To date, seven singletons and two sets of twins were delivered. The following data only refer to these cases. Of the seven single pregnancies the maternal heart rate accelerations began between the 25th and the 39th week of gestation and at the 23rd week for the twin pregnancies. The amplitude of the maternal heart rate accelerations increased with gestational age from about 15 bpm at their first appearance to 23 bpm in late pregnancy. During the accelerations cardiac output decreased between 6% and 33%. Blood pressure mirrored this cyclical behavior in standing. Contractions associated with maternal heart rate accelerations occurred more frequently during standing than in the left lateral position (184 versus 57 contractions in a total of 46 recordings. 13% of these contractions were experienced subjectively in standing against 7% when the mothers were recumbent. With a delay of 16 ± 10 sec, maternal heart rate returned to normal for as long as contractions were noted. When the uterus relaxed, maternal heart rate increased again.

04.12.05

Towards a more rational study of physiology of pregnancy using contour-photography: Tympanidis, K N, Karras, G E. Mitera Maternity Hosp. and Nat. Techn. Univ., Athens, Greece
Previous studies have indicated the suitability of moiré contour-photographs in assessing local volume variations in abdomen, buttocks, breasts and thighs (*Tympanidis* and *Karras,* In: Recent advances in pathophysiological conditions in pregnancy, Elsevier, 1984). this approach is enriched when volume is combined with skinfold thickness and skin elasticity. Moiré photographs, allowing measurements at any body site, help overcome the somewhat unreliable and fragmentary character of skinfold measurements in assessing fat distribution. Finally, local volume variations, being related to skin stretching, may help furter to illuminate the changes of the mechanical properties of the collagen fibres during pregnancy. Fifteen subjects have been repeatedly photographed at various stages of pregnancy. The uncertainty in volume measurement of the abdomen has been estimated as $\pm 2\%$ at the early and $\pm 1\%$ at the late stages of pregnancy. Compared to the third month, the abdomen has been found as $1.7-2.0$ times larger in the sixth, $2.8-3.5$ in the ninth and $0.7-1.6$ 45 days post partum. The skinfold has been measured at six sites and the skin elasticity at two but no further results are currently available. It is believed, however, that the above approach allows a mor rigorous study of the physiology of pregnancy.

04.12.06

Hemodynamic characteristics of the placental circulation in relation to blood flow pulsatility in the umbilical arteris: Reuwer, P J H M, Nuyen, W C, Bruinse, H W. Dept. Obstet. and Electronics, Univ. Hosp., Utrecht, The Netherlands
Non-invasive Doppler assessment of the Pulsatility Index (PI) from umbilical arteries shows promise as a simple method for early diagnosis of placental failure. The present report discusses those hemodynamic factors which determine the PI, based on a synthesis of current knowledge of feto-placental physiology with fundamental hemodynamic physics. It is postulated that the umbilical artery PI depends directly on fetal pressure pulsatility which appears to be invariant during fetal growth. Secondly, a linear relationship is postulated between the PI and the ratio of placental capillary and arterial resistance. This ratio of resistances declines markedly with advancing pregnancy indicating that the site of predominant resistance which determines placental blood flow, migrates gradually from the capillary plexus to the arterial compartment. It is concluded that umbilical artery PI values below 1, after 28 weeks, reflect the normal reserve capacity of the functional capillary bed of the placenta. Increased PI values above 1 in the last trimester reflect a critical enhancement of placental capillary resistance which must impede blood flow to the functional chorionic villi.

04.12.07

Hair tissue mineral analysis in pregnang women: Nishijima, S, Outsuka, S, Kasahara, T, Koshino, T, Murooka, H. Dept. Obstet. and Gyn., 1st Hosp. of Nippon Med. School, Tokyo, Japan
The purpose of this study was to investiage the usefulness of hair tissue mineral analysis in pregnant women and to examine the relationship between obstetric disorders and minerals. Hair samples were obtained from 203 Japanese pregnant and puerperal women. After washing and digestion, the samples were analyzed for 23 minerals by high frequency inductively coupled argon plasma emission spectrometry and atomic absorption spectrometry. Serum minerals were analyzed by the established method. Mineral contents in food were calculated from the Standard Tables of Food Composition in Japan. The following results were obtained: (1) Hair Ca and Mg were lower and hair Na and K were higher in pregnant women than in non-pregnant women. (2) Pregnant serum Ca, Mg, P, Na, K and Zn were lower and Cu was higher than in non-pregnant cases. (3) Food Ca, Mg and Zn levels of Japanese pregnant women were lower than the standard level. (4) No significant change of hair mineral levels was obtained in cases of hyperemesis, anemia and toxemia. (5) SFD showed high As levels. It was concluded that a decrease in Ca and Mg levels was observed in Japanese pregnant women and it was suggested that the effect of living environment should be also taken into consideration in the occurrence of SFD.

04.12.08

Pregnancy related changes in the connective tissue of the uterine cervix and the uterine body: Uldbjerg, N, Ekman, G, Malmström, A, Oxlund, H, Ulmsten, U. Dept. Obstet. and Gyn., Univ., Aarhus, Denmark

Characteristics of cervical biopsies from non-pregnant/term pregnant women: hydroxyproline (μg/mg) 14.8/6.4, extractability (%) 39.4/92.8, water (%) 82.3/87.3, sulfated glycosaminoglycans (μg/mg) 0.90/0.48, "collagenase" (U/100 mg) 72/290, leukocyte elastase (μg/mg) 0.51/6.81, elastin (μg/mg) 1.1/0.4, hemoglobin (μg/mg) 1.0/19.7, albumin (μg/mg) 6.4/8.7, strength (Newton/mm^2) 2.3/0.15. As seen the contractions of all connective tissue components decrease during pregnancy. Also qualitative changes in collagen (hydroxyproline) have been described as an increase in its extractability. These observations might very well explain the decreased mechanical strength. Most probably the collagen is degraded by collagenase and leucocyte elastase. Ultrasound examinations indicate an 30% increase in cervical volume. A dramatic increase in hemoglobin suggests congestion of the organ. Plasma proteins might therefore, at least partly replace the collagen although the concentration of albumin in the organ is unchanged after delivery. Women with prolonged labor had increased hyroxyproline (8.6 μg/mg) and decreased extractability (82%). PGE$_2$ treatment decreased hydroxyproline (5.5 μg/mg) and increased "collagenase" (519 U/100 mg). The hydroxyproline concentration (μg/mg) in the uterine body was 10.5/6.6. This change might be important for the function of the muscular component, i.e. the formation of gab junctions.

04.12.09

The hormone relaxin in normal and abnormal human pregnancy: MacLennan, A H. Dept. Obstet. and Gyn., Univ., Adelaide, South Australia

Peripheral serum relaxin levels were measured in normal and abnormal human pregnancy using a homologous porcine relaxin radioimmunoassay (sensitivity 12.5 pg). In a cross sectional study of 330 normal pregnancies relaxin concentrations were found to peak around 14 weeks gestation and thereafter decline until term. Patients in labor at term had a significantly higher mean relaxin concentration compared to patients who were not in labor at this gestation. After term there was a continuing significant decline in relaxin concentrations where labor had not occurred. By the third postnatal day relaxin concentrations had fallen to the level of the non-pregnant control group. Relaxin levels were significantly higher in multiple pregnancy and in patients with pelvic pain and joint laxity during pregnancy. This is the first documented evidence of any association between the hormone relaxin and this pathology. Early studies also suggest that patients in premature labor have lower than normal relaxin concentration. The above data from normal and abnormal pregnancies is compatible with relaxin's postulated roles in the human with regards the maintenance of uterine quiescence until near term, the facilitation of uterine stromal remodelling during uterine growth and the promotion of cervical dilatation and softening in early labor.

04.13.01

Perioperative antibiotic prophylaxis in gynecology: Risks and benefits: Siekmann, U. Dept. Obstet. & Gyn., UFK Essen

In gynecological surgery the interest in antibiotic prophylaxis has been continuously developed in the last decade. Although the efficiency of prophylactic antibiotics in radical gynecological surgery meanwhile has been evaluated, several problems are still controversely especially the dose regimen (preoperative/ perioperative), the general indication in abdominal hysterectomy or the risk of adverse effects. In clinical practise the benefit of prophylactic antibiotics is differently evaluated with regard to the incidence of febrile standard morbidity or the classification of serious infections post-operatively. In an own prospective randomized study (n:100) the efficiency of a single dose of 5 g mezlocillin given prior to vaginal hysterectomy could already been demonstrated. Despite these results and similar investigations in literature short prophylactic antibiotic regimen will not prevent all kinds of post-operative infectious problems. Special risk factors (mode and duration of operation, estimated blood loss, microbiologic contamination in vaginal cuff) should be taken into account before a decision is made for the use of prophylactic antibiotics, which can never be a substitute for excellent operative management.

04.13.02

Effects of two different prophylactic antibiotic regimens on infection morbidity following vaginal hysterectomy: Mattheussens, O J A, Goormans, E, Branolte, J H*. Ziekenhuis Leyenburg, The Hague, The Netherlands, Bayer Nederland B.V., Mijdrecht, The Netherlands*

In a randomized comparative investigation in 104 patients, effects of mezlocillin and metronidazole on prophylaxis of infection following vaginal hysterectomy was studied. Infection morbidity was lower with 1 injection of 5 g mezlocillin than with 3 injections of 0,5 g metronidazole. Excess costs per patient were also lower with mezlocillin, if the shorter post-operative hospitalization period is taken into account.

04.13.03

Serum and tissue concentrations of ciprofloxacin in gynecological infections: Weißenbacher, E R, Adam, D, Gutschow, K, Lühr, H G, Schneider, A, Wachter, I. Frauenklinik, Klinikum Großhadern, LMU, München

Ciprofloxacin was taken after sensitivity testing by 40 women with gynecological infections. In two cases there was a urinary tract infection, 38 patients suffered from a soft tissue infection eg. Wound infection after hysterectomy or pelvic inflammatory disease etc. E. coli was the most frequent strain. 38 of the 40 women were clinically and 37 of 40 microbiologically cured. No serious side-effects were noticed. The highest serum levels were reached after 1–3 hours after oral administration of 100 mg ciprofloxacin. The highest tissue concentrations were found 2–5 hours after oral administration.

04.13.04

Pharmacokinetics of Ciprofloxacin (Bay 09867) in Gynecological Tissues: Gerstner, G J[1], Kronich, W[2], Dalhoff, A[2], Weuta, H[2]. 1 Dept., Stockerau Hosp., Austria, 2 Pharma Res. Ctr. Bayer AG, Wuppertal
A prospective pharmacokinetic study covering 20 patients was conducted to determine the serum (S) and genital-tract tissue (T)-concentrations of ciprofloxacin, a new broad spectrum antimicrobial agent. The quinolone compound showed outstanding antibacterial properties against gram + and especially against gram− organisms including Enterobacteria, Pseudomonas and Bacteroides sp., strains known to cause pelvic inflammatory disease (PID) or postoperative wound infections. 300 mg ciprofloxacin were administered as 15 min. i.v. infusion before operation. Samples of peripheral venous blood were obtained before (S1) and after the infusion (S2) and at the time the uterine arteries were clamped (S3). Tissue samples weighing approximately 2 g were taken from the myometrium, the Fallopian tubes and the ovaries and were stored with the serum at −20°C. Concentrations were measured biologically. The mean S2-concentration was 4.62 ± 3.02 (1.52–12.0) mg/l, the mean S3-concentration 1.26 ± 1.08 (0.34–3.44) mg/l. The mean time interval between the end of antibiotic infusion and surgical removal of the genital tissues was 40.8 ± 16.15 min. (20–67). The mean tissue-concentration in the uterus was $3.58 \pm 3,96$ (0.96–13.52) mg/g, in the tubes $2,26 \pm 1.99$ (0.12–6.11) mg/g, in the ovaries 3.5 ± 2.66 (0.6–5,81) mg/g. All tissue concentrations were higher than the simultaneous serum-concentrations. Since the MIC for most pathogenic bacteria is much less than 1 mg/l the tissue concentrations achieved are sufficient for full antibacterial activity.

04.13.05

Penetration of ciprofloxacin into female genital tract tissues following oral and intravenous administration: Goormans, E*, Kazzaz, B*, Dalhoff, A, Branolte, J***.** *Hosp. Leyenburg, The Hague; **Pharma Res. Ctr. Bayer, Wuppertal and ***Med. Dept., Bayer, Mijdrecht
Ciprofloxacin concentrations in serum, vagina, portio uteri, endometrium, myometrium parametrium, Fallopian tube, and ovary respectively were assessed following a single oral as well as intravenous administration. Samples were taken 1, 2 and 3 hours after oral administration of 500 mg and 0.5, 1 and 2 hours after intravenous injection of 100 mg. Ciprofloxacin concentrations were determined by means of the conventional cup plate agar diffusion test using E.coli 14 as test organism. In general, penetration into the extravascular space was marked. After i.v. injection the highest tissue concentrations were found after 0.5 hours. At that moment tissue levels exceeded the corresponding serum concentrations by 60% to 190%. After 1 and 2 hours tissue levels remained consistently higher than the corresponding serum concentrations. Following oral administration both serum concentrations and tissue levels reached a maximum after 2 hours and were roughly the same at that moment (ratio's for the various sites varying from 0.9 to 1.1). These tissue concentrations seem to be sufficiently high to treat most genital tract infections in women by oral administration of ciprofloxacin. This should be confirmed in clinical trials. For prophylaxis of infections during surgical interventions intravenous administration should probably be preferred.

04.13.06

The efficacy and tolerability of ciprofloxacin (CIP) in gynecological infections: Hägele, D. Marienkrankenh., Amberg, Chysky, V, Bayer AG, Med. Res., Wuppertal
23 gynecological patients, average age 24.95 (18–40) years, suffering from salpingitis (17), salpingitis and pelveoperitonitis (3), adnexitis (1), Douglas abscess (1), and vaginal abscess (1) entered into the study. Clinical efficacy and tolerability was evaluated in 21 patients. Surgical or diagnostical procedures such as pelviscopy (17 patients), abrasio (2), interruption (1) and adhesiolysis were performed prior to therapy. The most frequent pathogens isolated from vaginal or cervical swab were E.coli (8) and Staphylococcus epidermidis (8), followed by Staphylococcus aureus (2), Proteus mirabilis (1) and Streptococcus sp. (1). Two tablets containing 500 mg CIP were given at 12 hour intervals, the average daily dose being 33,14 mg/kg b.w. and the average duration of therapy 7.57 (5–11) days. Based on the microbiological evaluation and clinical results the overall response was a cure in 15 patients (71.42%), partial cure in 3 (14.28%), indeterminate in 3 (9,52%) and failure in 1 (4.7%) patients. Laboratory analysis didn't show any alterations of laboratory values. Complete ophthalmological check-up was performed in 16 patients. No alterations were reported, merely one patient complained about reduced production of tears on second day of treatment. In one patient therapy with CIP had to be discontinued on day 3 due to allergic reaction. Comparative clinical trials with lower CIP doses are needed to establish the appropriate therapeutical regimen for gynecological pelvic infections.

04.13.07

Ciprofloxacin (CF) in the treatment of patients with symptomatic and asymptomatic urinary tract infections (UTI): A comparative study of single dose application versus three days treatment: Fischbach, F, Loos, W, v. Hugo, R, Machka, K*, Graeff, H. Frauenklin. und Inst. Med. Mikrobiol. and Hyg.*, TU, München
CF shows a superior antibacterial efficacy compared to other derivates in the same substance group. It was

the purpose of this randomized study to evaluate different dose schedules of CF in gynecological patients (n = 100) with postoperative symptomatic and asymptomatic UTI. Single dose application versus 3 days treatment was evaluated. (Group I: asymptomatic UTI, single dose CF p.o. (250 mg), group II: asymptomatic UTI, CF for 3 days p.o. (100 mg, b.i.d.), group III: symptomatic UTI, single dose CF p.o. (250 mg), group IV: symptomatic UTI, CF for 3 days p.o. (100 mg, b.i.d.)). The groups were comparable concerning age, type and duration of surgical procedure and duration of post-operative bladder drainage. Excluded from the study were patients with reported CF allergy, patients treated with additional antibiotics other than CF, patients with impaired renal function and with obstructed urinary tracts. Efficacy of the treatment was judged by urine-cultures, urinalysis, leucocyte counts and clinical findings like fever or well-being of the patient. Therapy proved to be successful in over 90% of all patients studied with slightly better results in the 3 days groups. There was no alteration in BUN, creatinine, liver enzymes, coagulation parameters and red blood cell counts. It is concluded, that CF is suitable in the treatment of UTI with no significant difference between single dose application or 3 days treatment. According to these preliminary results the single dose application of ciprofloxacin can be recommended.

04.13.08

Fundamental and clinical studies on BAY o 9867: Antibacterial activity, pharmacokinetics, and clinical evaluations in obstetrics and gynecology: Cho, N, Fukunaga, K, Kunii, K, Komoriyama, K. Dept. Obstet. and Gyn., School Med., Showa Univ., Tokyo, Japan

BAY o 9867, a newly developed synthetic quinoline carboxylic acid antimicrobial agent, was studied for antimicrobial activity and pharmacokinetics in terms of absorption, excretion, tissue penetration, and placental penetration, as well as clinical effects on gyneco-obstetrical infections and adverse reactions to evaluate its usefulness in the fields of obstetrics and gynecology. The MIC for clinical isolates was determined by the standard method of Japan Society of Chemotherapy, and the concentrations of the drug were measured biologically. Clinical studies were made on gyneco-obstetrical infections. The MICs of fifteen species of clinical isolates were determined and peak level of MICs were 0.39 mcg/ml for S. aureus, 0.025 mcg/ml for E.coli, 0.05 mcg/ml for K. pneumoniae and 0.1 mcg/ml for P. aeruginosa and etc. Tissue penetration of BAY o 9867 was found to be good; the tissue levels were $0.37 \sim 1.80$ ug/g after oral administration of 200 mg and transference of the drug into umbilical cord blood and amniotic fluid were measured. Those levels exceeded the MIC_{80} values against most pathogenic organisms. When $400 \sim 600$ mg of BAY o 9867 was daily given to 61 cases of obstetrical and gynecological infection, 90.2% of clinical efficacy and 71.1% of bacteriological response were obtained with few side effects. From these findings, the usefulness of this drug in obstetrics and gynecology was suggested.

04.28.01

Ovulation detection by measurement of progesterone in saliva using a direct solid phase enzyme immunoassay: Dooley, M, Tallon, D, Fottrell, P, O'Dwyer, E. Dept. Biochem. and Obstet. & Gyn., Univ. Coll, Galway, Ireland

The purpose of this study was to evaluate the role of a novel direct enzyme immunoassay for salivary progesterone in the detection of ovulation and in the clinical management of infertile women. Saliva sampling, being non-invasive and stress free, is ideally suited for serial sampling. The enzyme immunoassay developed is a solid phase assay carried out on microtitre plates and requires no extraction steps. The sensitivity is 3.2 pmol/L. This assay has several advantages over conventional radioimmunassay techniques. During this study we compared salivary progesterone measurement against conventional methods of ovulation detection including plasma progesterone, temperature and ultrasound. The results demonstrate that follicular phase salivary progesterone levels remain below 200 pmol/L and rise to 400–800 pmol/L in the luteal phase. The clinical applications of this assay in the management of infertile women will be demonstrated by presenting a case report of a woman in whom ovulation and corpus luteal function is monitored by daily salivary progesterone measurement during untreated cycles, cycles in which ovulation is induced and in a cycle in which conception occurrs. We conclude that salivary progesterone measurement is a practical development which may have many immediate clinical and research applications.

04.28.02

Significance of prolactin (PRL) and TSH stimulation tests in women with menstrual disorders and infertility: Bohnet H G, Niemann D W. Inst. Horm. and Fertil. Disord., Hamburg

The frequency of hyperprolactinemia and hypothyroidism has been studied in women with menstrual disorders and infertility. Patients (n = 360) were subjected to a TSH test using 400 µg TRH; a PRL stimulation test was carried out during the mid-luteal phase of the menstrual cycle using 10 mg metoclopramide (*H.G. Bohnet, A.S. McNeilly*, Horm. Metab. Res. **11**, 533, 1979). Interrelations between the two tests were statistically evaluated using the co-variance selection, i.e. condesed descriptions for multidimensional data (*Wermuth* et al., Computerprograms in Biomedicine **6**, 23, 1976). Levels of significance were calculated according to Pearson's correlation coefficient. Control values for PRL and TSH were based on serum concentrations observed in conception cycles (n = 40; basal PRL $\leq$ 15, PRL maximum after MCP stimulation $\leq$ 200 ng/ml; basal TSH $\leq$ 3, TSH maximum after TRH $\leq$ 18 µU/ml). The analysis of data from the 360 patients demonstrates significant dependencies between basal and stimulated PRL (P < 0.0001) as well as between stimulated PRL and TSH (P < 0.02). There was a significant correlation of basal and stimulated

TSH (P < 0.01), but not of basal TSH and either basal or stimulated PRL and vice versa. Galactorrhea was observed in 41 of the 360 patients. Hyperprolactinemia occurred in 56%; in addition 33% had thyroid dysfunction. This disease accounted for only 17% when PRL was normal. Hypothyroidism occurred in 27% of all patients with galactorrhea. The data presented indicate that hyperprolactinemia and hypothyroidism are closely related diseases.

04.28.03
Ovarian stimulation with human gonadotrophins: Doubling of pregnancy rate with combined pure FSH and HMG: Crosignani, P G, Lombroso, G C, Caccamo, A. III Dept. Obstet. and Gyn., Univ., Milan, Italy

This study was aimed at improving current methods of ovarian stimulation with gonadotrophins. In the last two years 50 patients (24 primary amenorrhea, 20 secondary amenorrhea, six anovulations) were treated with human gonadotrophins (Pergonal, Serono, Rome) to induce ovulation and pregnancy. Follicular growth was induced by HMG in increasing doses monitored by daily E_2 radioimmunoassay. HMG was stopped and HCG (10 000 IU) administered when E_2 levels were between 500 and 1100 pg/ml. In the 83 cycles induced, ovulations occurred in 65 (78.3%) and pregnancy in ten (12%). Nineteen of these patients (12 primary, 7 secondary amenorrhea) first treated with HMG + HCG cycles were then stimulated with combined pure FSH (Serono, Rome) + HMG, in equal amounts, on the first three days of treatment. The new schedule seemed to mimic better the endocrine events in the early spontaneous cycle. In the 35 cycles induced ovulations took place in 34 (97%) and pregnancy in eight (22.8%). The significant increase in the ovulation rate (P < 0.1) and the doubling of pregnancies obtained with the second regimen appears to show a substantial improvement.

04.28.04
Eating disorders and anovulation in a private N.Y.C. practice: Weseley, A C. Lenox Hill Hosp., New York, NY, USA

A fascinating and still only partially explored aspect of anovulation is that caused by eating disorders. The aim of this retrospective study was to evaluate the types of eating disorder leading to weight loss and amenorrhea in a private N.Y.C. gynecologic practice. During the seven year study period there were 37 patients seen with eating disorders and anovulation. These disorders consisted of excessive dieting with simple weight loss (18 cases; 49%), anorexia nervosa (13 cases; 35%) and bulemia (6 cases; 16%). All but four patients have regained weight and resumed menstruating. Only seven patients (19%) who recovered are now overly concerned about their weight. Presently 22 patients (60%) who recovered are on oral contraceptives. These data clearly demonstrate that most patients with eating disorders and anovulation manage to overcome it with time. There were certain features in common in amenorrheic patients having had excessive dieting and anorexia nervosa. A sudden weight loss of 20 lbs. due to dieting suggests some degree of anorectic behavoir. In these patients there was a suppression of pituitary gonadotropins, the cause of which is yet to be established. A gynecologist is often the first to see those young women presenting with missed periods. One consequence of long intervals of amenorrhea is a prolonged hypoestrogenism which can result in osteoporosis and skeletal abnormalities. For this reason cyclic estrogen and progesterone is prescribed. Treatment in most cases of anorexia nervosa is difficult and psychologic counselling is an essential part of the management. Many problems still remain and we shall be seeing even more of these patients in years to come.

04.28.05
Immunohistochemical evidence of prolactin in human ovary: Lee, J N, Chien, D H. Dept. Obstet. and Gyn. and Path., Kaohsiung Med. Coll. Hosp., Kaohsiung, Taiwan

The hormonal regulation between prolactin and ovarian activity has been extensively studied since hyperprolactinemia has played an important role in female infertility. However, the nature of the intra-ovarian interaction between prolactin and the steroid hormones is poorly understood. Recently, immunohistochemical techniques have localised prolactin secreting activity in placenta (*Golander* et al., Science **202**, 311, 1978) and trophoblastic tumors (*Lee* et al., Gyn. Oncol. **11**, 299, 1981). The present studies were undertaken to investigate the prolactin localisation in ovarian cysts including ten cystadenomas, three dermoid cysts and one corpus luteum cyst using prolactin immunohistochemical techniques. There is a positive result shown in ovarian tissue with corpus luteum cyst.

04.28.06
Ovulation and ovarian blood flow: Makinoda, S, Nakajin, K, Koyama, T, Ichinoe, K. Dept. Obstet. and Gyn., Hokkaido Univ. School Med., Sapporo, Japan

To investigate the mechanism of ovulation, ovarian blood flow and ovarian vessel morphology were studied during the preovulatory period in rabbits induced by PMS (100 iu IM) and hCG (100 iu, IV) administration. Continuous measurement of ovarian blood flow was facilitated by the crossed-thermocouple inserted into the unilateral ovary. The ovarian blood flow change was expressed as the percentage ratio based on the dead value (= 0%) and the initial value prior to hCG administration (= 100%). Histological changes of the ovarian blood vessels were observed at intervals of every two hours after hCG administration. The ovarian blood flow increased rapidly wihin 1 h following hCG administration and high percentage increases were demonstrated during 2 h to 5 h, showing a peak value of 155.3 ± 12.7% at 3 h. The ovarian blood flow decreased gradually from 5 h to 8 h, and then increased again at 9 h and 10 h. The perifollicular and stromal vasodilatation were confirmed at 2 h, and moderate dilatation was observed during 4 h to 6 h. At 10 h just prior to ovulation, vasodilatation became most remarkable, especially at the apical vessels. These hemodynamic and histological results suggest there is congestion in ovarian blood vessels during the preovulatory period. This blood congestion may relate to a significant role in the mechanism leading to ovulation.

04.28.07
Correlation of follicle size, estradiol, LH, ultrasound and cervical score: Begum, Z, Hussain, A.
As serial radioimmunoassays (i. e. daily or alternate days) are very expensive and sometimes impossible in our country, a search for other measurements which can come close to RIA, is the aim of this study. In the hope of finding a close correlation between Graafian follicle size, urinary estradiol levels, LH levels, ultrasound endometrial changes and cervical score, a study was undertaken on 50 infertile patients. Serial assessment of the above parameters on specific days in stimulated cycles was done. The specific days for the assessment of the above values were selected based on McIntosh formula. Beginning from the twelfth day and repeated every alternate day, from the mid-point of McIntosh 95% confidence limit. As reported earlier by others, we find a close correlation between the ultrasound endometrial changes, Graafian follicle size and E2 levels. Drugs used: clomiphene citrate and HMG.

04.28.08
Contribution to diagnosis and treatment of overian follicular changes: Kliment, V, Hatvany, T, Valášek, F, Bruchač. M. Dept. Obstet. and Gyn., Fac. Med., Komensky Univ., Bratislava, Czechoslovakia
Over the period from 1958–1982 the authors tried to influence ovarial cystic follicular changes with vit. B1/thiamine Spofa inj. 100 mg/administered parenterally in a total dosage of 1000 mg. With the aim of elucidating the effect of vit. B1 treatment, experiments on infantile female rats were also carried out. Ovarial cystic changes diagnosed by palpation, sonography and endoscopy where found in 693 female patients consequently treated by the vit. B1. Hormonal cytology showed signs of hyperestrinism in all patients. The above mentioned ovarian changes disappeared after the tratment in 574 patients (82.7%) treatment failure was observed in 119 cases (17.4%). Surgery was performed in 96 patients of the latter group. Ovarian cancer was not observed. On the basis of literary data on estrogen inactivation block during vit. B1 deficiency the authors assume that deficiency of this vit. causes prolonged and increased estrogen action which in turn may cause structural and follicular changes in the ovaries. The described positive effect of vit. B1 may be the consequence of positive regulation of neurohumoral action in terms of physiological normalisation of estrogen overproduction.

04.28.09
Gonadal dysgenesis in patients with 46, XX karyotype: Millet, A, Pellicer, A, Bonilla-Musoles, F. Dept. Obstet. and Gyn., Hosp. Clin., Valencia, Spain
A primary ovarian failure was diagnosed in ten patients with primary amenorrhea after hormonal determinations and biopsy. All of the had a 46, XX karyotype. We emphasize the clinical findings in these patients and the most frequent diagnosis of this disease, probably because of the possibility of histological and hormonal (RIA) studies. Genetic and environmental factors should be involved in its etiology.

04.32.01
New drugs increasing androgen-receptor in prostate: Rehmannia eight formula: Utsugi, R, Shinkawa, T, Igarashi, M. Dept. Obstet. and Gyn., Gunma Univ. School Med., Maebashi, Japan
Effects of 22 kinds of Chinese drugs upon hypothalamo-pituitary gonadal system were investigated in immature male rats of Holtzman strain. The weights of the prostate and the seminal vesicles after 28 days oral administration were significantly increased only in the groups of Rehmannia Eight Formula (REF), Dioscorea (D) and Ginseng (G). The blood testosterone levels were significantly decreased in these three groups (REF, D, and G). Moreover, these three drugs (REF, D, and G) were confirmed to have no androgenic activity in the orchidectomized rats. Subsequently, the dihydrotestosterone (DHT) receptor in the prostate was investigated with the dextran coated charcoal method. Although the dissociation constant of DHT receptor was not significantly different, the number of binding sites of DHT receptor was significantly more increased in the REF group (34.9 ± 1.3 f mol/mg protein) than in the control (26.4 ± 1.3 f mol/mg protein). This is the world-first report on the drugs inducing the increase of DHT receptor in the prostate.

04.32.02
The influence of mesterolone on serum gonadotrophins and plasma testosterone in subfertile men with idiopathic oligospermia: Bhathena, R K, Patel, D N. N. Wadia Maternity Hosp., Bombay, India
The earlier view that mesterolone has little effect on the pituitary gonadal axis is now being questioned. Fifteen subjects, with idiophatic oligospermia, were randomly treated with 100 mg per day of mesterolone (n = 10), or placebo (n = 5), for more than three months. Serum gonadotrophins and plasma testosterone were assayed before treatment and after twelve weeks of treatment. There was a statistically significant

suppression of serum FSH ($p < 0.01$) and serum LH ($p < 0.05$) with mesterolone. Plasma testosterone was not significantly altered by mesterolone therapy. The previous view that mesterolone has little influence on gonadotrophin secretion needs to be revised.

04.32.03
Treatment of oligospermia. Comparative study of indigenous drug fortege and clomiphene citrate: Dhiraj Gada, D, Shah, C M. Gada Nursing Home, Indore, India

Four hundred and ten oligospermic men out of 1578 infertile couples were randomly treated either with Fortege or clomiphene. Of 220 cases treated with Fortege 144 had improved semenogram and 71 conceptions resulted, while of 190 cases with clomiphene 51 had improved semenogram and in 15 conception resulted. Among the cases treated with clomiphene there were 110 failures; when these were treated with Fortege 68 showed an improved semenogram and in 32 conception resulted. There were 63 failures with Fortege; when these were treated with clomiphene 14 showed and improved semenogram and in five conception resulted. Fortege showed improvement in the semenogram in 64.2%, conception in 33%, no side effects and was economical. Clomiphene showed improvement in 25.69%, conception in 7.9%, side-effects in 1.8% and was costly. With limited facilities for investigations indigenous drugs have given better results than clomiphene citrate in treatment of oligospermia.

04.32.04
Effects of long term gonadotrophic therapy on human testicular morphology: Berg, A Å, Hammar, M, Plöen, L*. Dept. Obstet. and Gyn., Univ. Hosp., Linköping and *Dept. Anat. and Histol., Fac. Vet. Med., Swedish Univ. Agr. Sci., Uppsala, Sweden

Testicular biopsy specimens were obtained from then infertile men before and during long term gonadotrophic therapy. The specimens were fixed in Bouin's fixative, sliced, stained and studied with light microscopy. Separate parts of the biopsy specimens were analyzed regarding the *in vitro* conversion of 3H-progesterone to different metabolites as a criteria of the Leydig cell stimulation by gonadotrophic hormones. In some patients the testicular progesterone conversion *in vitro* seem to be undertsimulated by gonadotrophic hormones (LH) before treatment. In these cases the Leydig cell size as well as the spermatogenic activity increased during therapy with 1500 IU hCG three times a week and the *in vitro* progesterone conversion changed towards a stimulated pattern. The therapy was in most cases combined with 75 IU hMG three times a week. In some patients the thickness of the lamina propria decreased during this therapy whereas in no case was it increased. In summary 14–35 weeks of treatment with hCG and hMG induced no detrimental effects on the testicular morphology in ten adult infertile men.

04.32.05
The effect of antibiotic treatment on semen analysis and fertility of teratozoospermic men contaminated with high background, or fecal origin bacteria: Shilon, M, Daphna, D, Lussim-Rothman, R, Bahary, C, Bartoov, B. Meir Hosp. Kfar Saba, Barilan Univ., Ramat Gan, Israel

Bacterial infection in the male genital tract may be associated with reduction in fertility potential. Two groups of suspected infertile men with positive semen cultures, one (23 patients) of high background bacteria and the other (16 patients) of enterobacteria were investigated with regard to their semen quality before and after appropriate antibiotic treatment. No differences in sperm concentration or percentage of live and motile spermatozoa in the two groups was noted; they were within the normal range. In both groups Ca^{+2} levels were high 27.8 ± 10.7 and 28.8 ± 11.8 respectively and percentage of normal form spermatozoa low 20.5 ± 15.6 and 23.8 ± 10.9 respectively. After an average of 2.6 courses of antibiotic treatment sperm morphology improved significantly (pair t test); in the high background group 36.0 ± 13.6 (P 0.01) and in the enterobacteria group 38.3 ± 10.1 (P 0.01). Head defect reduced from 54 to 40%, however only the first group was statistically significant (P 0.025). Sperm concentration and motility improved significantly only in the enterobacteria group: 151×10^6 per ejaculate to 225×10^6 per ejaculate (P 0.02) and 41.3% to 56.8% (P = 0.01) respectively. 14 pregnancies, including two abortions, (60.8%) were obtained in the high background group and eight with one abortion (50%) in the enterobacteria group. Semen quality and pregnancies improved significantly in both groups after massive antibiotic treatment.

04.32.06
Observations on sperm agglutinins in the sera and cervical mucus of unexplained cases of infertility in women: Jha, R, Mishra, J. Patna Med. Coll. Hosp., Bihar, India

The present study comprised of observations on sperm agglutinins in the sera and cervical mucus of one hundred women with unexplained sterility. The work was carried out in Patna Medical College Hospital, Patna. Eight cases out of one hundred showed positive antibody test in cervical mucus. Only five of the eight cases had positive antisperm antibody test in sera as well as in cervical mucus. On analysis of the results, the sperm agglutinins had a definite relation with advancing age and longer duration of sterility. It is apparent that the cervix is definitely a local site for antibody production and possible cause for sterility of unknown etiology.

04.32.07

The male factor in AIH treated infertile couples: Bacz, A. Inst. Obstet. and Gyn., Copernicus Univ. School Med., Cracow, Poland

A record of 80 infertile couples (infertility duration 2–15 years) who underwent AIH (split ejaculation technique, at least three consecutive cycles) in a period 1981–1983 because of male oligo- and/or astheno-spermia is presented. Seven women conceived during therapy (8.75%) and nine women became pregnant spontaneously in the next 2–18 months (11.75%). The overall pregnancy rate was 20.0%. The comparison of pregnant and non-pregnant women resulted in highly significant differences related to: duration of infertility (mean $\pm 2\,SD$ 4.9 ± 2.7 vs 6.8 ± 2.9) age (mean $\pm 2\,SD$ 28.8 ± 3.2 vs 31.3 ± 2.7), uterine factor (anatomical abnormalities, uterine surgery) 12.5% vs 23.4%, tubal factor (unilateral occlusion, adhesions, past tubal surgery with proven patency) 0.0% vs 17.2%, ovarian factor (past surgery, cystectomy, adnexec-tomy, wedge resection) 0.0% vs 25.0% and presence of at least one of the factors (12.5% vs 43.8%). The evaluation of semen in fertile and infertile males did not reveal any differences. The results point out the primary role of female disturbances in the etiology of infertility and confirm the influence of women's age and duration of infertility on the reproductive process. The low pregnancy rate and psychological problems arising during this kind of treatment show that ATH has little, if any, value in management of so-called male infertility.

04.32.08

A new device for intrauterine insemination for treatment of various causes of infertility: Makler, A, Blumen-feld, Z, DeCherney, A, Huszar, G. Infert. Inst., Rambam med. Ctr, Haifa, Israel, Yale Univ., Conn., USA

Infertility, caused by low quality of specimens, low volume or hostile cervical mucus may be treated by direct uterine insemination to increase the chance for sperm-egg union. To avoid side-effects, sperm were washed in physiologic medium, containing antibiotics, and spun at 300 g for 10 min. About 0.2 ml of the pellet was used for insemination with the aid of a special device that carries an atraumatic semi rigid plastic cannula, connected to ordinary tuberculin syringe. The cannula has a flared base to induce a sealing mechanism when the device is clamped for 10–15 min to the outer brim of the speculum by a coiled spring. Treatment was planned for up to 5–6 cycles 1–3 times every other day at the periovulatory period. During the last three years 219 women completed 5–6 cycles of Husband insemination and 72 completed 3 cycles of Donor insemination. In the AIH group pregnancy rate was 32% and 8.4% per cycle. In the AID group pregnancy rate was 49% during 3 cycles or 20.4% per cycle. Occurrence of pregnancy at any cycle of treatment for both groups was highest during the first two cycles. Abortion rate was 17%. Except for spotting and temporary mild low abdominal pain no complications such as pelvic infections occurred in more than two thousand such procedures. The simplicity, the use and the total lack of serious side-effects and the successful rate of this treatment make this technique worthwhile to try in many infertile couples. This technique is also useful for AID treatment where one specimen can be used for several women.

04.41.01

Comparison of the efficacy of ritodrine and magnesium sulfate in arresting premature labor: Tchilinguirian, N, Najem, R, Sullivan, G B, Craparo, F J. Jersey Shore Med. Ctr, Neptune, NJ, and UMDNJ, New Jersey Med. School, Newark, NJ, USA

Sixty-seven cases of premature labor (48 unruptured, 19 ruptured membranes) were treated with ritodrine or magnesium sulfate infusion supplemented with oral ritodrine in case of initial success. Both agents were found effective and safe when used with strict protocols and close medical supervision, irrespective of maternal age, parity, ethnic background and number of previous abortions. Treatment appeared more effective in the absence of significant cervical dilation and effacement and before development of pro-nounced uterine activity. When given intravenously, the drugs appeared effective both in the presence and absence of rupture of membranes. Evidence suggests that the degree of cervical dilation and effacement and the degree of uterine contractivity as measured by the "Premature Labor Units" (PLU) affected uterine response to tocolytic treatment. Close medical and laboratory surveillance showed the administration of the quoted drugs in therapeutic doses was found safe and their side-effects moderate, acceptable to patients, and manageable. The study supports clinical experience indicating that early administration is highly successful in arresting premature labor and preventing its dire consequences.

04.41.02

Calcium antagonist drugs in obstetrics: Boemi, P, Reitano, S, Platania, R, Rizzari, G. Dept. Obstet. and Gyn., Univ., Catania, Italy

From a pharmacological point of view calcium antagonists play a very important role in muscle release. They act directly on the transmembrane supply of calcium and selectively inhibit the "slow" channels. In this paper we have studied the action of calcium antagonists (prenylamine and nifedipine) administred alone or in association with beta-stimulators as stated by *Fleckenstein*. The study included 452 multigravid patients between 19 and 36 years of age with positive obstetric case history (two or more abortions or preterm deliveries or associated abortions and preterm deliveries). The scarce data obtained from the two previous studies (1979 and 1983) on the tocolytic activity in labor restrained us from furthering the study. The schedule combined the associated pharmacological treatment (calcium antagonist and beta-stimulators) with cervical suture according to *Bisset*. The results obtained demonstrated that this pharmacological association with cervical suture, administered early on in gestation is able to remove many causes of abortion, except for genetic ones. It is therefore a valid therapeutic tool in the as yet poorly defined "gestational uterine insufficiency".

04.41.03

Calcium antagonism in the control of adverse reactions during utero-inhibition: Piovano, A, Carboni, F, Casale, O, D'Angelo, A, Oses, A. Maternidad "A. Peralta Ramos" Hosp. Rivadavia, Univ., Buenos Aires, Argentina

The purpose of present paper is to evaluate the importance and differences of adverse reactions due to beta-stimulants and beta-stimulants associated with calcium antagonists in the treatment of pregnant patients with threat of premature labor. The open chance method has been used to include patients in both groups. Fixed combination doses of both drugs have been used. We evaluated, diastolic and systolic blood pressure, heart rate; PQ, QRS, and QT on maternal ECG, fetal heart rate and uterine dynamic. We also evaluated adverse reactions besides on heart areas. After evaluation of the statistical values had been observed the following conclusions were drawn: 1) During uterine inhibition the doses of uterine inhibitors used associated with calcium antagonists were significantly lower. 2) The frequency of adverse reactions was significantly higher in the group treated with beta-stimulants only. 3) Maternal ECG and fetal heart rate in both groups did not show significant changes in: fenoterol and fenoterol associated with verapamil. 4) Mean time cardiac protection is discussed.

04.41.04

Labor inhibition with B2 sympathomimetic drugs by intravenous infusion: Should it be otherwise, can it be better?: Holleboom, C A G, Merkus, J M W M, Steenhoek, A. Maria Ziekenhuis, Tilburg, The Netherlands

Premature labor resulting in premature birth makes the most important contribution to perinatal morbidity and mortality. Several methods and several drugs are used to inhibit premature labor. One of these drugs is B2 sympathomimetics. This drug is usually given by an incremental dosage scheme. From the moment complete tocolysis is reached the infusion rate is not further increased. The serum level of the B2 sympathomimetic drug will then increase far above the level which gives complete tocolysis until a steady state is reached. (Smit, 1982, Thesis University Maastricht). Side-effects which are dosage related, will increase too! We have developed an infusion scheme which started on a high intravenous dose of 2.9 y/min fenoterol (partusisten®) and then was reduced when contraction disappeared to the infusion rate which give the same steady state as the serum concentration was at the moment of complete tocolysis. The scheme was based on the half life of fenoterol of 20 minutes. The serum concentration reached at a given moment (t) by a given infusion rate® can be calculated from the equation:

$$C_t = \frac{R}{V_d K_e}(1 - e^{-k_e t}) \ (V_d = \text{distribution volume. } K_e = \text{elimination rate constant.})$$

We studied 12 patients with premature labor who were given fenoterol by intravenous infusion and took blood-samples at eight different times during the infusion period. We could find a good correlation between calculated serum concentrations and the real concentration measured in the patients serum. There were no serious side-effects and a very acceptable labor inhibition was reached with a minimum of drug administered.

04.41.05

The use of computer in monitoring materno-fetal clinico-metabolic effects induced by β-mimetics in the treatment of premature labor: Centonze, A*, Giovine, P M**, Torre, G C***, Farinini, D*, Vigliercio, G P***. Dept. Gyn. and Obstet., Hosp. S. Martino*, Genova, S. Corona***, Pietra Ligure and EDP Dept. USL 4, Finalese, Italy

There are currently increasing data concerning cardio-vascular iatrogenic lesions (pulmonary edema, angina, ischemia) in some cases induced by β-mimetics, in tocolytic treatment for pre-term labor. These drugs can also produce metabolic effects (estriol decrease, K depletion, hyperglycemia). A protocol including patient's history, clinical and laboratory data was proposed for evaluating and monitoring the β-mimetic treatment. Recently the myoglobin assay (RIA) has been introduced for discovering cardiovascular lesions. The following computer elaboration makes it possible to precodify data for easy individualisation and data uniformation from different sources. By means of these data, registered in magnetic storage medium, we produced an apt elaboration program of control factors, which is a useful method to evaluate the metabolic effects induced by β-mimetic drugs on woman and fetus.

04.41.06

Evaluation of the results in the treatment of the premature delivery with a β-mimetic (orciprenalinum sulphate): Scarpa, F, Marotta, R, Fazzi, G R, Scarpello, F, Gatto, L, Zecca, R. Dept. Obstet. and Gyn., Hosp. "M. Tamborino", Maglie (Lecce), Italy

The authors considered the effectiveness of the tocolytic therapy with β-mimetic in the treatment of premature delivery. The β-mimetic drug they used was orciprenalinum sulfate. They examined the results obtained in 90 pregnant women observed from March 1980 to March 1984 treated with orciprenalinum in dose of 5–15 mg in continuous venous infusion. After obtaining the improvement of the symptomatology they progressively reduced the dosage up to the interruption of the infused therapy. On the basis of the criteria of Richter the complete successes were 60 equal to 66.6% with P. I. of 20.25; the partial successes were 24 equal to 26.6% with P. I. of 15.1; the failures were 6 equal to 6.6% with P. I. of 3.5. The authors conclude that the therapy with orciprenalinum may be considered valid both as for the immediate block of the uterine contractile activity, and also for its inhibitory effect at a distance with results which may be considered positive on the extension of the pregnancy itself.

04.41.07

Maternal serum C-reactive protein (CRP) and the outcome of preterm labor with intact membranes: Cammu, H, Foulon, W, Amy, J J. Dept. Gyn. and Obstet., Vrije Univ., Brussel, Belgium

Forty-four women with preterm uterine contractions were studied. Criteria for treatment i. v. ritodrine were: (1) gestational age 20–36 weeks; (2) intact membranes; (3) regular contractions at a rate of at least 2/10 minutes; (4) cervical dilatation < 3 cm and (5) no signs of fetal distress on external cardio-tocography. A total as well as a differential white blood cell count and the serum CRP concentrations were serially determined. A clean caught specimen of urine was cultured. On admission, 33 women were CRP neg. and had no signs of amnionitis nor any other infection. 31 had a successful tocolysis and delivered between 37–40 weeks gestation. Two women had a p.r.o.m. within the first five days in hospital and delivered subsequently at 31 and 35 weeks gestation. Twelve women were CRP pos. In five of these, urinary tract infection was detected and subsequently treated. In one case, the elevated CRP was associated with a superficial thrombophlebitis and in an other with upper respiratory tract infection. In these seven cases of systemic infection CRP became negative under treatment and all delivered at term. In four cases an elevated CRP was found in association with subclinical chorioamnionitis proven by amniotic fluid culture or histological evidence of chorioamnionitis. These four patients were refractory to tocolysis and all delivered within the week of admission. The four patients delivered between 22–27 weeks gestation. All infants died promptly. In most cases neg. CRP reaction is correlated with succesful tocolysis. CRP may be a marker of amnionitis resulting in preterm labour refractory to tocolysis and a poor fetal outcome. When an elevated CRP is associated with systemic infection, it will become undetectable under treatment and pregnancy will further progress.

04.41.08

Echocardiographic data and systolic time intervals in normal and tocolytically treated pregnancies: Leucht, W, Olshausen, K von, Rüttgers, H, Kubli, F. Dept. Obstet. and Gyn., Univ. Heidelberg

In 1982 and 1983 at the Universitäts-Frauenklinik Heidelberg five groups of pregnant women each of 25 patients had been examined echocardiographically and systolic time intervals had been measured. The aim of the study was to prove, whether echocardiographic factors and systolic time intervals will change during normal pregnancy and what is the influence of oral long-term tocolysis with Fenoterol®. Following data had been compared in the mentioned groups of patients: blood pressure, heart rate, left ventricular electromechanical systole (QS_2), left ventricular ejection time (LVET). The ratio of pre-ejection period (PEP) and LVET was calculated. End-diastolic and end-systolic left ventricular dimension had been echocardiographically measured and fractional shortening (FS) and ejection fraction (EF) were calculated. The following groups had been examined: 1) 25 women with normal pregnancy at 20, 26, 32 and 38 weeks of gestation; 2a) 25 women at term without labor; 2b) 25 sub partu; 3a) 25 women with oral tocolytic treatment; 3b) 25 women as control-group to 3a without tocolysis. – Conclusion: The PEP/LVET ratio was elevated during normal pregnancy. No differences were found in patients with oral long-term tocolytic treatment. Oral tocolysis does not interfere with maternal cardiac function.

04.41.09

Cyclic AMP and GMP levels during normal pregnancy, threatened pre-term labor and under tocolytic treatment: Pérez Picañol, E, Gamissans Olivé, O, Rodríguez, L, Ribas, J. Dept. Obstet. and Gyn., Hosp. Clín., Univ., Barcelona, Spain

Due to the importance on the regulation of the myome-trial contractility, we determined the levels of cAMP and cGMP in the maternal plasma of 331 normal pregnant women. Twenty-seven of them presented threatening pre-term labor during the study; in ten of these 27 cases the cAMP levels were lower than normal (< −2S.D.) before initiation of clinical threatening pre-term labor. In all patients with cAMP levels lower than 10 mgr/ml, the interval between the last determination (in the absence of clinical manifestations) and the initiation of pre-term labor was shorter than 20 days. Among the patients with normal cAMP levels, only two initiated pre-term labor in the following 20 days from the last analysis. Under the tocolytic infusion the cAMP levels raised over the normal but only for a short of time (five days) unrelated to the tocolytic regime. The cGMP levels were not modified in any case. In summary, lower cAMP levels during normal pregnancy could be indicators of pre-term labor risk, but with a low predictive capacity (30%).

04.41.10

The effects of oxytocin and betamimetics on prostaglandin (PGF2a, 6-keto-PGF1a) synthesis in human pregnant myometrium *in vitro*: **Quaas, L, Hillemanns, H G, Breckwoldt, M, Zahradnik, H P.** Dept. Obstet. and Gyn., Univ. Hosp., Freiburg

The present study follows the effects of betaadrenergic agonists (orciprenaline, fenoterol) and oxytocin on the mechanical activity and prostaglandin (PG) release of superfused human pregnant myometrium. Myometrium strips freshly obtained at Cesarean sections were superfused with Tyrode solution. Oxytocin ($0.3-1.2 \times 10^{-5}$ U/ml), orciprenaline (10 ng/ml) and fenoterol (10 ng/ml) were added by an infusion pump. The effluent of the superfused myometrium was analyzed for PGF2a and 6-keto-PGF1a by specific radioimmunoassays. Both betamimetics reduced the amplitude and frequency of concentrations and myometrial PGF2a release rates were significantly decreased from $1.49 + 0.49$ (n = 12) to 0.47 ± 0.21 (n = 8) ng/min/g wet weight ($\pm$ S.D.), whereas 6-keto-PGF1a production significantly increased (3.54 ± 0.48 to 9.34 ± 0.69 ng/min/g wet wt.). Superfusion with oxytocin stimulated the frequency and amplitude of contractions according to dose. This increase in uterine contractility was associated with a significant elevation of PGF2a concentrations (1.2×10^{-5} U/ml, 3.99 ± 0.72 ng/min/g wet wt., n = 7). However, 6-keto-PGF1a production was not affected by oxytocin. Preincubation of the myometrium with indomethacin (3×10^{-5} M) abolished the effect of oxytocin. These results suggest that betamimetics diminish myometrial contractility by increased prostacyclin- and decreased PGF2a production and that oxytocin is effective in stimulating myometrial contractility of the human pregnant uterus by enhancing PGF2a formation. These *in vitro* results correlate well with *in vivo* findings.

04.42.01

Fetal and maternal oxytocin and prostaglandin levels at the onset of labor: Fuchs, F, Fuchs, A-R, Husslein, P, Rehnstrom, J V. Dept. Obstet. and Gyn., Cornell Univ. Med. Coll., New York, NY, USA

Oxycotin (OT) levels in cord blood are very high at delivery and a significant arteriovenous difference in the umbilical vessels indicates that it is of fetal origin. Fetal OT levels are high also after labor that ended in delivery by Cesarean section (CS). It is not known whether fetal OT rises as a cause or a consequence of labor. In an attempt to determine the levels at about the time of onset of labor we have measured oxytocin levels in umbilical arterial and venous plasma obtained at elective CS both before any signs of labor were present, and after uterine contractions suggested that labor had begun. Samples were obtained also from maternal peripheral vein and when possible, uterine vein. Fetal OT levels were always higher in the umbilical artery than vein and higher than maternal peripheral levels. In early labor, fetal arterial and venous OT levels were significantly higher than before labor and similar to levels observed in active labor. In preterm labor, fetal arterial OT levels were also higher than maternal peripheral levels but lower than in term labor. Uterine vein OT levels were similar to fetal umbilical vein and maternal peripheral vein levels in all situations. Uterine vein prostaglandin E, F and FM levels were not raised over maternal peripheral levels except in active labor. Thus, fetal oxytocin secretion is increased at very early stages of labor and may well be a factor in the stimulation of the uterus to contract at the onset of parturition. Since OT increases PG production in decidua, fetal OT seems to be a stimulus for uterine PG generation.

04.42.02

Role of oxytocin receptors in the initiation of human parturition: Fuchs, A-R, Fuchs, F, Husslein, P, Soloff, M S. Dept. Obstet. and Gyn., Cornell Univ. Med. Coll., New York, NY, USA, and Dept. Biochem., Med. Coll. of Ohio, Toledo, OH, USA

We have measured specific oxytocin (OT) binding to human uterine tissues obtained at various stages of gestation by Cesarean section. These binding sites present a single class of high affinity, low capacity sites that bind OT about 6 times more avidly than vasopressin. Good correlation between the number of binding sites and the physiological response indicates that they represent the biological receptor sites. OT receptors were found both in the myometrium and decidua in about the same concentrations. Fundus and corpus had about equal receptor concentrations whereas isthmus and corpus had much lower levels. Receptor concentrations increased during gestation, by 37–38 weks the concentration was about 50 times higher than in nonpregnant women. This corresponds to the increasing uterine responsiveness to oxytocin in the course of gestation. Patients in early labor, whether term or preterm, had 2–3 times higher receptor levels than patients not in labor, whereas patients with postterm pregnancies or failed inductions had low OT receptor concentrations. Uterine OT sensitivity tests performed daily during last week of gestation suggestet that the 2–3 fold rise in OT receptor levels occurs during the last 2–3 days. Measurement of plasma OT levels during induction of labor with exogenous oxytocin indicated that at term the uterus responds to levels of OT that are not significantly raised over those in term patients not in labor. Thus the rise in OT receptor concentrations in the final days of gestation sensitizes the uterus to normally circulating OT levels and causes the initiation of uterine contractions.

04.42.03

A basic study on the initiation of human parturition; Contribution of amniotic fluid and fetus to the initiation of human parturition: Takahashi, H, Maki, M. Dept. Obstet. and Gyn., Akita Univ. School Med., Akita City, Japan

In order to clarify the mechanism of initiation of human parturition, the relationship of amniotic fluid and fetus to prostaglandin synthesis was investigated. Phosphatidylinositol (PI) in amniotic fluid and phospholipase C (PLase C) activity in amniotic fluid, amnion tissue and neonatal urine were measured. The results are as follows, (1) PI in amniotic fluid began to increase from around 30 to 36 or 37 weeks of gestation, and then gradually decreased toward term. (2) PLase C activity in amniotic fluid was low before 30 weeks of gestation, but gradually increased toward term. (3) PLase C activity in $105,000 \times g$ supernate of amnion tissue homogenate was 43 fold higher than that in amniotic fluid. (4) The high PLase C activity was demonstrated in neonatal urine, which was 58 fold higher than that in amniotic fluid. (5) The molecular weight of PLase C from neonatal urine was estimated to be 33000 daltons. (6) PLase C activity in neonatal urine has enough activity to produce arachidonic acid in amniotic fluid. It was concluded that the fetus relates to the onset of labor by producing arachidonic acid in amniotic fluid resulting from the reaction between PI from the lung and PLase C from the urine.

04.42.04

A comparison of three different methods of local use of PGE$_2$ in the induction of labor in term pregnancies: Dennemark, N, De Pasquale, J F, Osmers, R, Rath, W, Griebner, D. Dept. Obstet. and Gyn., Krankenh. Am Urban, Berlin

Occasional complications, i. e. hyperstimulation and lack of fine control limit the use of locally applied PGE$_2$ in patients with unripe cervices. If these risks were reduced, could we use the method successfully in patients with ripe cervices as well? We divided patients into three groups, using identical criteria. Group A (400 pts) had 1 or 2 intracervical applications of a hospital-produced PGE$_2$ tylose gel 500 μg. Group B (200 pts) had 3–6 mg factory-produced Prostin E2 tablets inserted into the posterior vaginal fornix at 4–6 hourly intervals until labor was established. Group C (15 pts) had instillation of 1–3 mg ready-made gel into the post. fornix (Prepidil-Upjohn, for clinical trials only). Treatment A was used in patients with a pelvic score of < 5; treatments B & C were used independently of pelvic score. 13% of pts in group A showed signs of hyperstimulation, controlled by the use of i. v. Fenoterol. Hyperstimulation was not noted in any pts in the other two groups. There were no other prostaglandin-type side-effects in any of the groups. Independent of the method of management 60–70% of primiparae with a pelvic score < 5 were delivered within 24 hours. The Cesarean section rate in all three groups combined was 8%. Patients with a low pelvic score and spontaneously ruptured membranes are best treated by method A. Patients found method B the least unpleasant; because of its non-invasive nature it was also recommended for patients with ripe cervices though occasional high therapeutic doses (up to 30 mg) were needed. Will treatment C become the method of choice?

04.42.05

Therapy to ripen the uterine cervix with intravenous infusion of prostaglandin E2 before induction of labor in primigravidae: Cisternino, A, Panella, M, Ettore, G, Scollo, P, Nocera, F. 1st Obstet. and Gyn. Clin., Univ., Catania, Italy

The unripe cervix at termination of pregnancy represents a negative prognostic index due to the risks connected with protraction of pregnancy. The administration of Pg aims to increase the cervical score (pre-induction) which allows conventional methods of labor induction to be effective. To evaluate the efficacy of PgE2 intravenous infusion, a study was made of 48 primigravidae, with cervical score of 3 or less (Bishop's Index). The treatment was effected by intravenous infusion of 1 mg of PgE2 (Prostin E2 – Upjohn) in 500 ml of phys. sol. The average duration of treatment was 6 h. The results: in five cases, after an increase in cervical score, labor commenced and resulted in spontaneous delivery; in 39 cases there was an average increase of 4.5 points in the cervical score by the end of treatment; followed by amniotomy with an incidence of spontaneous delivery of 91.7%; in four cases (8.3%) Cesarean section was performed after labor failed to progress. In our study on primigravidae, the administration of PgE2 by intravenous infusion resulted in an increased cervical score in 90.8% of cases, with an incidence of spontaneous delivery of 87.5%.

04.42.06

Cervical ripening and induction of labor by single intracervical PGE$_2$-gel application: Pullè, C, Granese, D, Panama, S. Inst. Gin. and Obstet., Univ., Messina, Italy

A single endocervical application of 0.5 mg PGE$_2$ in viscous gel (prepidil) was evaluated for preinduction cervical softening in 25 patients with unripe cervix (Bishop score ≤ 5) in late third trimester of pregnancy. The prepidil gel increased the B. S. more than 3 points within 12 hours in all patients and 15 of them delivered spontaneously. The mean time from the begining of intracervical gel application in the initiation of labor (latent phase) was 4 h and 35' (Range: 1 h–11 h 10'). No maternal or fetal side-effects were observed. The authors conclude that intracervical PGE$_2$ gel application can be recommended for cervical priming and labor induction in pre- and post-term pregnancy.

04.42.07

Pre-induction priming of the uterine cervix by laminaria: Nsihijima, M, Hayashi, T, Tatsumi, H, Shimada, N, Arai, M. Dept. Obstet. and Gyn., School Med., Kitasato Univ., Kanagawa, Japan

Duration of labor is known to be more influenced by the condition of the cervix rather than the strength of uterine conctractions. Preinduction priming by laminaria tent has been used at our institution for routine elective induction to ripen the cervix. Patients are admitted to the maternity ward and pelvic score of Bishop is noted on the day before induction. Usually five laminaria tents are inserted into the cervical canal for multiparas and ten for primiparas in the afternoon of the day of admission. On the following morning the laminaria tents are removed and Bishop score is again recorded. Then artificial membrane rupture is performed which is followed by continuous infusion of oxytocics. Increase of pelvic score after priming by laminaria is from 2 to 4 points. Induction-delivery (I-D) time ranged from 187 ± 74 minutes ($M \pm SD$) for the multiparas with prepriming pelvic score of 2 points to 90 ± 35 minutes for those with 6 points. I-D time for primiparas ranged from 352 ± 57 minutes with pelvic score of 1 point to 198 ± 120 minutes with 7 points. In conclusion the use of laminaria tents has proved to be a very efficient method for preinduction priming to shorten the duration of labor especially for primiparas.

04.42.08

Prostaglandin E$_2$ intravaginally in the induction of labor – five year experience: Kalogeropoulos, A, Tsalikis, T, Stamatopoulos, P, Kalachanis, J, Mantalenakis, S. 1st Dept. Obstet. and Gyn., Aristotelian Univ., Thessaloniki, Greece

In our clinic in the last five years labor induction has been performed on a total of 1043 pregnant women with intravaginal application of PGE$_2$ tablets. Two groups of women were studied. In group I the induction of labor in 686 women with unripe cervix was induced following the preparation of the cervix the day before. In group II, 357 pregnant women with ripe cervix were included. For the cervical ripening 4 mg of PGE$_2$ tablets in primigravidas and 3 mg in multigravidas were introduced intravaginally. Then labor was induced with 3 mg of PGE$_2$ tablets in all women. Results of the study were as follows: In group I, the cervical ripening following the preparation procedure, was completed in 494 women (72%), labor was carried out in 144 (20.9%), while no significant ripening changes were observed in 48 (6.9%). The termination of labor with the second dose of 3 mg PGE$_2$, given 12 hours later, was successful in 448 women, which raised the total number of induced labors to 592 (86.2%). Failures in labor induction were limited to 17.3% (94 women). In group II of pregnant women with ripe cervix the labor with the above dose of 3 mg PGE$_2$, was successful in 324 women (successful induction rate 90.9%), while the failed inductions were limited to only 33 cases (9.9%). Uterine hypertonic contractility was noticed in 21 women (2%), among which a Cesarean section was carried out in 13 for fetal distress. No significant side-effects of PGE$_2$ tablets to the fetus and/or the mother were observed. The procedure was simple, well tolerated and efficient.

04.42.09

Prostaglandin E$_2$ gel and tablets for induction of labor in high-risk pregnancies: Segal, S, Zohav, E, Girad, A. Dept. Obstet. and Gy., Barzilai Med. Ctr, Ashkelon, Israel

High-risk pregnancies need effective induction of labor particularly in primiparas with unfavorable cervices. The use of prostaglandin E$_2$ (PGE$_2$) by intracervical gel and vaginal tablets had been shown to cause cervical ripening and uterine contractions. Induction of labor was conducted in 172 women with postmaturity, PIH, IUGR, loss of FM, diabetes, PRM and bad obstetric history. The method used was intracervical application of PGE$_2$ gel (0.5 mg) the evening before induction, followed by vaginal tablets of 3 mg, the next morning or 6 h afterwards. this study includes 55 primiparas and 117 multiparas, at 37 to 43 weeks of pregnancy with a Bishop score of ≤ 4. Intracervical PGE$_2$ gel application caused an improved cervical score in 72% of the patients and the gel & tablets created a favorable cervix for ARM, in 66%. Vaginal delivery was achieved in 162 patients (94%), while C. S. was done in 10 pts (6%). Apgar scores of $7-10$ were estimated in 96% of the newborns with only one born with a score of 3. Failed inductions occurred in 13% of the parturients and oxytocin was needed in 16% of all deliveries. Two patients developed tetany and were effectively treated with ritodrin. The indications for C. S. were fetal distress and failed induction of labor. Our conclusion was that PGE$_2$ is significantly safe and effective for induction of labor in high-risk pregnancies.

04.42.10

Effect of vaginal gel of DHA-S on human uterine cervix at term: Takahashi, T, Sakiyama, T, Kikuchi, S. 2nd Hosp. of Nippon Med. School, Kanagawa, Japan

In Xth FIGO, 1980, we reported that the reduction of cervical blood flow (CxBF) was related to the cervical ripening. We also revealed, in 1982, than an i. v. dehydroepiandrosterone sulfate (DHA-S) decreases the CxBF, that is, it ripened the insufficient cervix at term. As DHA-S elevated the estradiol level in serum, it was not clear whether its effect is direct or not. In this paper, we studied the effects of the vaginal gel of DHA-S to disclose its direct action on the cervix at term. The CxBF was measured with the hydrogen gas clearance technique in six pregnant women at term prior to the introduction of the gel. A small amount of blood was collected to determine the levels of estradiol, progesterone and DHA-S. Three hours after the introduction of 10 ml of methylhydroxyethyl cellulose (CMC) gel (7%) which contained 200 mg of DHA-S, the CxBF was measured and blood was collected again. The CxBF was reduced from 27.0 mml/min/100 g to 14.4 after the vaginal application of the gel. DHA-S level in serum was increased from 511.0 to 732.8, estradiol level slightly from 41.9 to 52.1 and progesterone was from 290.8 to 283.7. These results surely indicate that the effect of DHA-S is direct on cervix because it reduced the CxBF markedly, while the estradiol was not elevated so much as in case of i. v. injection of DHA-S.

04.42.11

The efficiency of prostaglandin E₂ vaginal suppository versus intracervical prostaglandin gel for induction of labor in patients with unfavorable Bishop score: Legarth, J, Guldbaek, E, Secher, N J. Dept. Obstet. and Gyn., Univ. of Copenhagen, Hvidovre Hosp., Hvidovre, Denmark

Two different methods for induction of labor were randomly used in 120 patients with unfavorable cervix. The patients were given either a prostaglandin vaginal suppository constaining 2.5 mg PGE₂ in a basis of Witepsol S55 (Dynamit Nobel) or an intracervical gel containing 1 mg PGE₂ in 5 g hydroxypropylmethyl cellulose. The vaginal suppository was twice as effective as the intracervical gel in relation to success rate (birth within 48 hours) as well as in relation to mean and median time interval from induction to delivery; the difference is highly significant. The number of artificial deliveries were the same in the two groups. The mean Apgar score and the fetal pH were also the same and no negative side-effects were reported in either of the groups. The induction of labor with a vaginal suppository containing 2.5 mg PGE₂ is a safe and effective method in patients with unfavorable cervix score, and it is more effective than 1 mg PGE₂ gel placed intracervically.

04.42.12

Elective induction of labor with prostin E₂ in grand multipara: Sengupta, B S, Chattopadhyay, S K, Al-Meshari, A A. Fac. Med., King Saud Univ. and Maternity and Children Hosp., Riyadh, Saudi Arabia

Studies in low parous women have shown that cervical application of prostaglandin increases cervical compliance, improves Bishop score and successfully induces labor in most cases. However, its use in grand multipara (GM) is feared for its complications. This report examines the method objectively. In a prospective controlled study, labor was electively induced in 350 grand multiparae between 37 and 42 weeks by the intracervical application of PGE₂ tablets 0.5 mg on the first day (study group). Those failed to deliver on the first day were treated further with intracervical prostaglanding 0.5 mg given every hour for a maximum total of 3 mg on the second day. Another 350 GM matched in age, parity and gestational age but went into labor spontaneously were studied as controls for comparison of labor characteristics and outcome of labor. In the study group labor was successfully induced in 329 GM (92%) of whom 310 delivered (88.57%) vaginally. Fifty GM (14.28%) delivered after 1st dose. Improvement in Bishop score was observed in 175 women (50%) and there was no change in 125 (35.72%). Two hundred and seventy-two (77.7%) delivered on the second day. The method failed in 28 GM (8%). The mean time to active labor, duration of active phase labor and total dose of prostaglandin required were determined by the Bishop score on the first as well as on the second day attempt. The mean duration of active phase labor was 5.2 ± 1.9 hours compared to 4.9 ± 2.3 hours among controls. Operative deliveries and complications in the second and third stages were twice as common in controls compared to the study group. The group profile of the intrauterine pressure chart indicating Rise-time, Fall-time, Amplitude and Montevideo Units at different stages of cervical dilatation showed significant difference only at $4-6$ cm dilatation ($p < .001$) between the two groups of women. Otherwise the characteristics of PGE₂-induced labor in GM simulate those of spontaneous labor. It is concluded that elective induction of labor in GM between 37 and 42 weeks is safe for the mother and her fetus.

04.42.13

Induction of labor with extra-amnial method: Forugh-Nassirai, G. Dept. Gyn. and Obstet., Med. School, Ghaem Mashhad, Iran

At 1976 Israel physicians carried out therapeutic abortion with extraamnial successful. We also used this technic, on the 44 cases of fetus death with success. After examination with tocography technic we proved that the uterus contractions are rhythmic but not constant and this technic is not hazardous to the fetus. We decided to use this method for induction of labor to the other cases such as post-mature pregnancy, inertia of uterus, diabetes, Rh negative situations etc., also all cases it seems necessary to terminate pregnancy at the second trimester or third trimester. 38 cases are under study during 8 months with a good result and without mortality and morbidity. – Method: For infusion of the fluid normal saline should insert a Foly or Nelaton catheter No. 16 or 18 from cervix canal to space between the uterus wall and amnion membrane of 7 cm height, fluid running should be around 15 drops per minutes and continue the infusion until the necessary dilatation is obtained.

04.79.01

Uterine malformations and reproduction: Catarivas de Ansaldo, V, Goldsman, T, Vainer, O. 1st Cathedra of Gyn., Córdoba, Argentina

According its relevance in fertility we consider six groups. Group A: Development failure in Mullerian tubes; incomplete bilateral uterine aplasia or Rokitanski syndrome is not considered because the sterility is absolute. We divide the unilateral uterine aplasia into two varieties: 1) True unicorn uterus previously accompanied by renal anomaly and 2) false unicorn uterus with solid or canalized contralateral mass. Gestation in these unicorn uteri may be normal, but when there is incomplete development they became hypoplasic uteri yielding spontaneous abortion. Group B: Junction failure of Mullerian tubes (true uterus didelphus) gestational development with no trouble. Group C: Fusion and reabsorption failure of Mullerian tubes. Generically are described as pseudo didelphus uterus and comprise numerous types: cordiform, arcuatum, subseptum, septate, bicornuate, bilocular and communicans. Reptetitive abortion are often produced and surgical treatment may restore fertility. Bret and Strassman surgical technics are used. Group D: Canalization failure of the Mullerian tubes. If it is unicavitarian, unicollis with vaginal or cervical atresia, there is sterility unless it be treated surgically. If it is bicavitarian or bicollis with cervical atresia or unilateral vaginal obstruction, may be a sterility or infertility. Group E: Growth and development failure of the muscle mass constitute hypoplasic uteri producing repetitive abortion. Group F: Cervix malformations (septi cervices or inborn dilatation) produce infertility and surgical management is recommended. It is concluded that surgical correction of an uterine malformation in an infertile female, with or without associated pathology, allows her to keep genital tract in a whole functional and gestational integrity.

04.79.02
Syndrome of "minor müllerian anomalies and oligomenorrhea": Carrasco, F, Comino-Delgado, R. Depto. Obstet. and Gyn., Univ., Valladolid, Spain
The hysterograms of 198 infertility patients were studied and classified into four groups according to the morphology of the uterus: a) Those with minor fundal anomalies and H/L ratio greater than 0.100 (H/L=ratio between the distance from the summit of the fundal convexity to the line connecting the summits of the uterine horns (H) and the length of this line (L) (52 cases)). b) Those with minor fundal anomalies and H/L ratio less than 0.100 (31 cases). c) Those with major Mullerian anomalies (24 cases). d) Those with normal uterus (91 cases). The incidence of menstrual disorders in general and oligomenorrhea-amenorrhea in particular was analysed in each of the above mentioned groups. Menstrual disorders, especially oligomenorrhea were found to be significantly more frequent in those cases with minor Mullerian anomalies and H/L ratio superior to 0.100 than in the other groups. These results confirm the new syndrome described by *Stampe-Sørensen* in 1981 with the name of "minor Mullerian anomalies and oligomenorrhea", which we propose be called "Stampe-Sørensen's syndrome".

04.79.03
Congenital atresia of the uterine cervix: Regan, L, Dewhurst, C J D. Chelsea Hosp. Women, London, UK
Adolescent girls with primary amenorrhea, pelvic pain, no visible cervix and a palpable uterine corpus require surgical exploration for both diagnosis and treatment. Experience of this rare Mullerian anomaly is necessarily limited and the two aims of management, relief of pain and preservation of reproduction potential, are frequently incompatible. Fourteen patients with cervical atresia are reported. The pelvic abnormalities were variable, and endometriosis was a frequent finding. In nine patients with a functioning uterus in place when we first saw them, four underwent hysterectomy in the first instance. In the remaining five patients a conservative procedure involving canalisation of the atretic cervix was attempted but could be accomplished in only two, the remainder requiring hysterectomy. Of these patients one developed a pelvic abscess soon after the initial operation which demanded a hysterectomy and pelvic drainage procedure. The second patient continued to menstruate for a time but the cervix is now closed; *in vitro* fertilization and embryo transfer are being considered elsewhere. Although expectant management in these patients might at first appear tempting, prompt surgical intervention following diagnosis of congenital cervical atresia is necessary if these young women are to avoid endometriosis and its complications. The choice of the primary surgical procedure depends on several variable factors, demands an individualized approach and should only be undertaken after thorough investigation and assessment of the patient.

04.79.04
Unilateral renal agenesis associated with ipsilateral blind vagina: A unique sydrome: Acien, P, Armiñana, E, Garcia-Ontiveros, E. Dept. Obstet. and Gyn., Gen. Hosp. of Elche, Univ., Alicante, Spain
We have studied 94 women with a variety of genital malformations. Twelve of these patients also had unilateral renal agenesis. All but one of these cases with renal agenesis were associated with ipsilateral blind vagina. The unique patient in whom the left renal agenesis was not linked with a blind vagina, also had a complete agenesis of all the other organs derived from the ipsilateral urogenital ridge. The clinical presentation is variable: Imperforated vagina with hematocolpos, partial reabsorption of the intervaginal septum, atretic hemicervix and blind vagina located in the upper third of the normal vagina simulating a Gartner cyst, Herlyn-Werner syndrome, and atretic hemi-uterus with blind duct parallel to perforated vagina. We have not found renal agenesis in patients with any other types of genital malformations. The obstructed vagina may have a mesonephric epithelium. Our findings support the idea that the caudal segments of the Wolffian ducts participate in the formation of the human vagina. The anomaly of one of them with lack of contact and/or opening in the urogenital sinus, would produce the blind vagina and the absence of the ureteral bud which would explain the renal agenesis.

04.79.05
Unilateral ovarian agenesis and ipsilateral agenesis of lateral end of fallopian tube. A case record and a critical analysis of the embryological origin of the fallopian tube: Chakrabarty, B K, Haldar, G. Med. Coll., Calcutta, India
A patient aged 21 years presented withe left-sided ovarian cyst. On exploration, the rt. ovary and lateral part of rt. tube were absent. Left tube was normal. Left ovarian cystectomy done for a dermoid cyst. It is presumed that developmental absence of rt. ovary has also affected the development of lateral end of

Fallopian tube of the same side. In contrast, in Mullerian agenesis although the vagina, cervix and uterus are absent, the fimbrial part of the Fallopian tubes along with the ovaries are well developed. It therefore seems possible that there are two different developmental origins of the Fallopian tube – the fimbrial and ampullary part from the surface epithelium of gonadal ridge and the medial part form the Mullerian ducts.

04.79.06
Obstetric complications of minor uterine anomalies: Stampe-Sørensen, S, Trauelsen, A G H. Dept. Obstet. and Gyn., Naestved Centr. Hosp., Copenhagen, Denmark
In two previous studies hysterosalpingography (HSG) was performed on 198 infertile women. The indentation of the fundal contour on HSG was stated and graded by the H/L ratio i. e. the relation between the height (H) of the fundal excavation and the line (L) connecting the peaks of the uterine horns. A H/L > 0.1 was found in 27 of 57 (47.4%) patients with oligomenorrhea and in 23 of 141 (16.3%) subjects with normal menstrual cycles (p < 0.001). Patients with definitely bicornuate uteri were excluded. In order to evaluate the influence of these minor abnormalities on the obstetric performance, a pregnancy history and specific data regarding pregnancy outcome were obtained from each patient by interview and review of records. Of 74 pregnancies in women with slightly abnormal uteri 21.6% were aborted spontaneously compared with 19.1% in the control group having normal contours on HSG. In women with minor Mullerian anomalies threatened abortions, premature labors and deliveries, malpresentations and retained placentas occurred in 19 of 58 (32.8%) term pregnancies. The corresponding figure in the control group was 21 of 161 (13.0%) pregnancies (p < 0.001). Cesarean section was performed in 22.4% of the former group versus 8.1% of the latter group (p < 0.005). Most oligomenorrheic women had a H/L between 0.16–0.25. In this H/L range 20.0% (6 of 30 term pregnancies) were malpresentations versus 5.3% in the control group (p < 0.005) and the aforementioned overall adverse pregnancy outcome was 43.3% versus 13.0% in the two groups (p < 0.001). A H/L < 0.13 had no influence on obstetric outcome.

04.79.07
Surgical treatment of congenital uterine malformations: Makhlouf, A M, Samaha, I M, Makhlouf, H A. Dept. Obstet. and Gyn., Ain Shams Univ., Cairo, Egypt
Developmental fusion anomalies of the uterus usually remain unsuspected until patients seek advice for dysmenorrhea, infertility or abortions. Often these anomalies cause little or no symptoms and many of these women become pregnant, in which case about 25% to 30% of them end in abortions. In such cases and whenever surgical treatment is indicated we have devised a new technique of metroplasty (FIGO Meeting 1961 – Vienna) which was developed so as to achieve unification of the uterus precluding the risks and hazards which are known to accompany many of the surgical operations currently used in the treatment of these anomalies. This paper presents 20 years experience of use of our technique in the management of the septate and bicornuate uteri, our policy for the choice of the vaginal versus the abdominal routes. The advantages and merits of our tecnique are well illustrated in the successful unification as proven radiographically and the successsful outcome of pregnancies in the treated habitual aborters. Detailed description of our techniques will be presented as well as our policy in the management of habitual abortion in relation to congenital fusion anomalies of the uterus.

04.79.08
Results of correction of Küster-Rokitansky syndrome obtain by operational method: Palčevski, S G, Popovska, S, Bogdanov, S. Clin. of Obstet. and Gyn., Med. Fac., Univ. of Skopje, Yugoslavia
In the period from 1971 to 1984, 25 patients with Küster-Rokitansky syndrome were registered in our clinic. Of these 25, 20 patients (80%) were operated on to correct absence of vagina. The McIndoe method was used. In that a perforated model of neutral glass was used. The model remained *in situ* for 15 days. In 15 cases skin transplantation was 100% successful while in five cases there appeared small granulation (ulcer) areas which were treated by silver nitrate. After treatment granulations completely disappeared in four cases, while in one case a circular stenosis on new-vagina resulted and therefore transplantation was repeated. In all cases the operation was necessary because of dyspareunia. After operation all patients have had normal sexual intercourse. Results obtained in our clinic are similar with those found in the literature.

04.79.09
Creation of an artificial vagina using a homograft of fetal skin: Luisi, M*, Giusti, G**, Luisi, V S***, Luisi, M L*. *Versilia Hosp., Via reggio, Lucca, Italy. **Inst. Clin. Obstet. and Gyn., Univ. Pisa, Italy. ***Massa C. Hosp., Massa C, Pisa, Italy
The authors describe a surgical operation in which an artificial vagina is created in order to correct congenital or acquired anomalies in the length or width of the vaginal lumen, or even the complete absence of the organ. The purpose of the operation is to create a new vagina with the following characteristics: a) a lumen of normal dimensions for the functions of the organ, without the need for postoperative expedients to maintain it; b) no prospects of further complementary surgery, especially involving risks, such as the transposition of intestinal tracts; c) no esthetic damage due to the explantation of integument of a paravulvar origin or from other parts of the body; d) valid and lasting static quality of the organ; e) adaptability of the technique not limited to congenital pathology. These characteristics are obtained by the authors through the homograft of a suitable portion of skin from a fetus expelled at the end of the fifth

month of pregnancy. The results obtained, have all been excellent. This kind of homograft demonstrates the reduced antigenic properties of fetal tissues. The new vagina thus formed assumes the anatomical and functional characteristics of a normal adult vagina in three weeks. As a result of the lack of the normal paravaginal anatomical formations, there are negative repercussions on the diastolic power of the vagina at the moment of orgasm, which, however, from the point of view of sensuality, is perfect.

04.79.10

Amnion graft for treatment of congenital absence of the vagina: Dhall, K. Dept. Obstet. and Gyn., Postgrad. Inst. Med. Educ. and Res., Chandigarh, India

A number of methods have been suggested for the surgical creation of a vagina, but none has met with wide acceptance. The present communication gives my experience with the use of amnion as an allograft and describes its advantages over other surgical procedures described in the literature. It also illustrates the process of re-epithelialization of the neo-vagina. From 1980 to 1984, 25 patients with congenital absence of vagina were seen in the gynec out-patient department of the Nehru Hospital, P.G.I., Chandigarh, India. Eight patients were selected for this procedure. Fetal membranes were obtained from the clean labor room and amnion was separated from chorion and was applied to the vaginal mould in such a way that the amnion's mesenchymal surface came in contact with the host tissue. The mould was removed on the seventh day and the patient was advised to use the mould for two weeks post-operation and use it at night only for another two weeks. She refrained from sexual activity for a total of four weeks post-operation. It was observed that when an uncontaminated mesenchymal surface is applied to the raw surfaces of the wound the amniotic membrane adheres firmly, protects the underlying granulation tissue and facilitates epithelialization. Hospital stay is considerably reduced and no postoperative dilatation is needed once normal sexual practice is started.

04.79.11

Neovaginoplasty: cilposcopical, colpocytological, histological and bacteriological aspects: Bozzini, A, Salvatore, C A, Yamashita, S A. Gyn. Clin., Univ. of São Paulo Med. School, São Paulo, Brazil

Fifteen patients with vaginal agenesis were studied to evaluate the adaptation of the skin lining the artificial vagina. The patients were aged between 15 and 32 years (average age, 23.8 years) when the operation was performed and the following propedeutical methods were performed: colposcopy, oncotic and functional colpocytology, histology, bacterioscopy and culture of the neovagina's content. The authors concluded that the adaptation of the skin in the neovagina is satisfactory from a functional view and as a possible response to hormonal stimulation.

04.79.12

Psychological sequelae of vaginal reconstruction: Ringler, M, Grünberger, W, Langer, M. Inst. Psychother. and 1st Dept. Obstet. and Gyn., Univ., Vienna, Austria

Twenty young women who had a vaginal reconstruction were interviewed one to two years after the operation. Patients age ranged from 16 to 25 years. Twelve of the patients, suffering from vaginal aplasia (Rokitansky-Küster-Hauser syndrome) were operated by Vecchiettis formation of a neovagina. All of the eight women with adreno-genital syndrome (AGS) had a reduction of the penisoid in early childhood and secondary plastic surgery for vaginal reconstruction in late adolescence. Psychological consequences were assessed by an open and standardized interview, as well as psychological tests, including Gießen test, a psychosomatic disorder inventory and a body image profile. Main importance is attributed to the general life history, the time and circumstances of the diagnosis, social support systems and its psychosexual connotations. These topics will be discussed in relation to their relevance with respect to the proper timing of the operation and counselling for the adolescent girls. If available, parents or partners were interviewed as well to assess the impact of the malformation upon family life and to enable a systemic approach to counselling.

05.14.01

Relationship between characteristics of the amniotic fluid and the status of the newborn according to fetal heart rate: Sabatino, H, Herrman, V, Barreto, M G, Pinotti, J A. Dept. Obstet. and Gyn., State Univ., Campinas, Brazil

In 3000 consecutive deliveries, we identified macroscopically the following characteristics of the amniotic fluid in labor: very light meconium (9.5%), light meconium (11.2%), heavy meconium (4.9%) and old meconium (2.4%). We observed that the newborns were statistically more depressed in presence of any type of meconium than when we had clear amniotic fluid in each group; we analyzed the repercussion of the presence of abnormal fetal heart rate (FHR) and observed that, only in the presence of very light meconium and light meconium, the incidence of depressed newborns becomes significantly higher; in the heavy and old meconium groups, this incidence does not change. We concluded that in the presence of very light and light meconium we should observe and look for abnormal FHR to interrupt labor. However, in the presence of heavy and old meconium, labor should be interrupted immediately.

05.14.02

Vernix caseosa: Immunofluorescent, histochemical and ultrastructural characteristics: Agorastos, T, Hollweg, G, Grussendorf, E I, Schwarz, C, Köhnen, M, Vlassis G, Papaloucas, A. B' Univ. Clin. Obstet. and Gyn., Univ., Thessaloniki, Greece, and Depts. Path. and Derm., Univ., Aachen

One of the most striking changes within a short time near term is the sloughing of the layer of vernix caseosa (VC) into the amniotic fluid. In attempt to explain the mechanism of the detachment of VC, especially at this stage of pregnancy, immunofluorescent, histochemical and ultrastructural examinations of VC cells have been performed. Direct immunofluorescent staining tests of frozen VC smears with fluorescein-conjugated globulin fractions of antisera to specific human serum proteins have shown that only IgG conjugate give strong positive reactions, while IgA, IgM and C_3 give relative slight positive reactions at VC cell antigen sites. Histochemistry and light microscopy was used to demonstrate the activity of acid and alkaline phosphatase in the VC cells, which show a marked increase in activity in the amniotic fluid toward term. Acid phosphatase activity was strongly present as small intracytoplasmatic granules while that of alkaline phosphatase was absolutely nonexistent. The ultrastructural morphology of the VC cells was analysed by scanning and transmission electron microscopy. Significant differences can be demonstrated in the individual surface pattern of VC corneocytes. The TEM-micrographs show irregularly flattened cells, without lamellar granules and intercellular broad lamellae. The results yield a comprehensive, three-dimensional image of the VC of a mature, normal newborn and present some of the characteristics of those tissues, whose role in the "definitive maturity" of the fetus and generally in the mechanism of initiation of labor is still unknown.

05.14.03

The significance of fetal bradycardia in obstetric behaviour: Stoimenov, G, Tchernev, T A, Ivanov, S G. Res. Inst. Gyn. and Obstet., Med. Acad., Sofia, Bulgaria

In the assessment of fetal status on a large clinical service antepartum fetal heart rate testing was used. The nonstress test was used as a routine method, while in the case of persistent nonreactivity the oxytocin test was performed. The presence of fetal bradycardia was assessed. Bradycardia was defined as a fetal heart rate at 90 bmp or a reduction in FHR of 40 bmp below baseline, for 60 seconds or greater. In a three-year period there were 45 cases of bradycardia during more than 5000 tests. Most of them were delivered the same day (36) and nine were managed in variable fashion. The incidence of fetal distress in labor with emergency delivery was one-third. Part of this group had decreased amniotic fluid volume on ultrasonic evaluation; a few cases had congenital anomalies (4) and intrauterine growth retardation (9). A reactive NST has been considered "normal" while a nonreactive NST has been considered "abnormal". The nonreactive NST followed by a negative contraction test has been considered normal although this testing should be repeated in 24 hours. The trial demonstrated that the occurrence of fetal bradycardia antepartum indicated a fetus at increased risk of developing fetal distress in labor.

05.14.04

Effect of maternal cigarette smoking on PGI2 production in newborn infants: Busacca, M, Agarossi, A, Corbella, E, Breviario, F, Dejana, E. 4th Dept. Obstet. and Gyn., Univ, Milan; Ist. M. Negri, Milan, Italy

It is well known that cigarette smoking by the mother during pregnancy can affect the fetus and newborn. It has been recently demonstrated that cigarette smoking reduces prostacyclin (PGI2) formation from umbilical endothelial cells: this reduction continues in primary cells culture even in the absence of the pathogenic factor. So smoking in pregnancy appears to induce in the fetus some modifications in the enzymes of PGI2 pathway which may persist after birth (*Busacca* et al., Am. J. Obstet. Gyn. **148**, 1127, 1984). This study was undertaken to compare the capacity in producing PGI2 of babies born to heavy smokers and non-smokers a few days after delivery. We collected blood samples 72–92 hours after delivery from two homogeneous groups of babies, respectively born to smoking or non-smoking women. Plasma was incubated with rat aortic smooth muscle cells and 6-keto-PGF1α in the supernatants was measured by a radioimmunoassay. Plasma of babies born to women who smoked in pregnancy showed significantly less capacity in stimulating PGI2 formation (2.8 ± 0.4 nmoles/10^5 cells vs 4.62 ± 0.5 in the control group: $p < 0.01$). Our preliminary data suggest a persistent damage to the endothelial cells of infants of smoking mothers: this possibility is very important for the developing child and merits further investigations.

05.14.05

Luteoma gravidarum: Cassaguerra, M A, Oliveira, H C. Serv. Gin., Hosp. Univ., Univ. Fed., Rio de Janeiro, Brazil

Luteoma gravidarum is a rare occurrence, with only 100 cases reported until 1981 in the whole world literature. The authors report a case, which is considered to be a pseudoneoplasia of the ovary, resulting from an exaggerated response of ovarian stromal cells to human chorionic gonadotropin. The authors further comment on hormonal changes that accompany the tumor and their influence upon mother and child. The patient was operated on in the 14th week of pregnancy. The tumor was bilateral; the right hand one weighing 650 g, and measuring 23 × 8 × 7 cm, and the left hand 575 g, measuring 17 × 9 × 4 cm. Operation confirmed the diagnosis previously arrived at by means of ultrasonography. The pregnancy was terminated in the 40th week by a Cesarean delivery. The child was female, without any signs of virilization. During the operation, examination of the abdominal cavity revealed normal ovaries.

05.14.06
Echocardiographic evaluation of hemodynamic response to immobilization in normotensive and hypertensive pregnancies: Skret, A, Kuźniar, J, Piela, A, Zaczek, T, Szmigiel, Z. Depts. Obstet. and Gyn. and Intern. Med., District Hosp., Rzeszow, Poland
Bed rest regimen has been reported as a constituent of many therapeutic standards in normotensive and hypertensive pregnancies. The hemodynamic effect of immobilization (5-days bed rest in left lateral recumbent position with no other treatment) was determined with the use of echocardiography in three groups of third trimester pregnant women: 1. normotensive (NT), $n = 12$, 2. pre-eclamptic (PE), $n = 7$, 3. with essential hypertension (EH), $n = 10$. In NT and EH groups bed rest evolved similar decrease in cardiac index (CI) – 8.5% and 11%, and increase in systemic vascular resistance index (SVRI) – 5% and 8%, respectively. In PE group bed rest resulted in increase of abnormally low CI by 13% and reduction of highly elevated SVRI by 14%. Concomitant plasma volume determinations (Evans blue) did not exhibit correlations with hemodynamic alterations produced by bed rest. It is concluded that 5-days bed rest reverses physiologic hyperdynamic circulatory state in normotensive and essentially hypertensive pregnancies. In pre-eclampsia immobilization tends to normalize the abnormal hemodynamic pattern and may thus have a beneficial therapeutic effect.

05.14.07
Fetal essential fatty acid deficiency and pre-eclampsia: Ogburn, P L, Turner, S, Johnson, S, Holman, R T. Brown Univ., Providence, RI, and Hormel Inst., Austin, MN, USA
It is possible that the relatively decreased percentages of arachidonic acid seen in cord sera in pre-eclampsia (PE) (Ogburn et al., Am. J. Obstet. Gyn. **148**, 5, 1984) is a result of fetal essential fatty acid deficiency. Patterns of esterified and nonesterified fatty acids were determined for cord sera from normal pregnancies and PE using gas-liquid chromatography. Six PE and six normal cord sera were measured. Essential fatty acid deficiency patterns were looked for in the nonesterified fatty acids (FFA) the triglycerides (TG), the cholesterol esters (CE), and the phospholipids (PL). Evidence of essential fatty acid deficiency (EFAD) was seen as a decrease in arachidonic acid, and an increase of oleic acid (18 : 1w9 in % total fatty acid $\pm$ S. D.):

	FFA	TG	PL	CE
PE cord	28.1 ± 2.8	36.0 ± 2.9	11.5 ± 1.4	30.0 ± 3.0
Normal cord	23.7 ± 1.2	30.6 ± 2.1	$9.5 \pm .4$	26.8 ± 2.5
p value	.01	.01	.05	NS

The fetus in a PE pregnancy has abnormal oleic acid patterns in the sera consistent with EFAD. These abnormalities may be associated with decreased prostacyclin production, IUGR, and perinatal wastage which are part of pre-eclampsia syndrome.

05.14.08
The activation of plasma inactive renin in patients with pregnancy-induced hypertension: Shibata, J Shigemitu, S, Koresawa, M, Kubo, T, Iwasaki, H. Dept. Obstet. and Gyn., Inst. Clin. Med., Univ. of Tsukuba, Ibaraki, Japan
Renin-angiotensin system is supposed to play a role in the pathogenesis of pregnancy-induced hypertension (PIH). This study has been undertaken to investigate the changes of active and inactive renin proportion in patients with PIH. Blood samples were obtained from 37 normotensive patients in th third trimester of pregnancy, six severe hypertensive and three severe proteinuric but minimal hypertensive patients. Assays were performed of plasma renin activity (PRA), total renin activity (TRA) and inactive renin activity (IRA). PRA was measured by radioimmunoassay of the angiotensin I generated. For determination of TRA, inactive renin was activated by exposing plasma to trypsin. IRA was defined s the difference between TRA and PRA. TRA did not show any significant difference in these 3 groups. PRA in hypertensive patients was 28.1 ± 7 ng/ml/hr, which was significantly higher than in normotensive patients (10.7 ± 1.9 ng/ml/hr, $p < 0.01$), whereas PRA in proteinuric patients showed lower levels. IRA in hypertensives was significantly lower than in normotensives ($p < 0.01$), but IRA in proteinuric patients showed almost same levels with normotensives. The proportion of PRA to TRA in hypertensives was 72 per cent, which was significantly higher than in normotensives (20 per cent, $p < 0.01$), but the proportion in proteinuric patients was only 7 per cent. These results suggest that the activation of inactive renin to active renin might play a possible role in the pathogenesis of PIH.

05.14.09
Enzymatic estimations of blood serum human placental lactogen (HPL) and estriol (E$_3$) levels, and fetal cardiotocography (CTG) in monitoring high-risk pregnancy: Pisarek-Miedzińska, D, Wierzbicki, A, Tas-

zycka, E, Merkel, M. Dept. Gyn. and Obstet., and Dept. Clin. Bacteriol., Med. Ctr. Postgrad. Educ., Warsaw, Poland
The authors examined 46 cases of pregnancy ranging from the 30th to the 38th week of gestation (10 patients with diabetes, six patients with EPH gestosis and ten patients with intrahepatic cholestasis). The control group comprised 20 cases of normal pregnancy at the same stage of gestation. In all subjects placental lactogen (HPL) and estriol (E_3) levels were determined twice a week by an enzymatic method with commercially available kits (Organon-Technica) while a 15 min cardiotocographic recording was performed twice a day. Enzymatic determinations of blood serum placental lactogen were found to be useful in monitoring high-risk pregnancy. Low or decreasing on consecutive determinations HPL in diabetes and cholestasis may indicate hazards to the fetus. Abnormal HPL levels appear one to three days prior to pathological CTG findings. The enzymatc determination of E_3 had no particular diagnostic value in diabetes and toxemia of pregnancy. E_3 levels above the upper limit of a normal range occur in intrahepatic cholestasis of pregnancy.

05.14.10
Pregnancy specific B1 glycoprotein and free estriol in the serum of normal, toxaemic and diabetic pregnant women during pregnancy and after delivery: Kandil, O, El-Sheikha, Z, Ahmed, A M, Soliman, A, El-Mekkawi, T. Dept. Obstet. and Gyn. and Clin. Path., Fac. Med., Al-Azhar Univ., Cairo, Egypt
The serum PSB_1G and free estriol were measured in 20 normal, 19 toxemic and 14 diabetic pregnant women. Patients were followed up during the first trimester (10–12 weeks), the 2nd trimester (20–22 weeks), the 28th week, the 32rd week, the 36th week and two weeks after delivery. Immuno-electrophoresis, single radial immuno-diffusion and radio-immunoassay were used for measurement of PSB_1G and estriol in the serum. The mean serum PSB_1G and free estriol in normal, toxemic and diabetic pregnant women showed progressive increase with the advance of pregnancy. PSB_1G was not detected when measured two weeks after delivery, while the serum free estriol was decreased. On comparing the mean serum PSB_1G and free estriol concentration in toxemic pregnant patients with that in the normal group, the toxemic group had lower mean serum PSB_1G concentration and free estriol in all the periods of pregnancy. However, diabetic pregnant women showed higher mean serum PSB_1G and free estriol concentration than normal pregnant women. A significant correlation was found between placental weight, infant weight, length, head circumference, Apgar score as well as biparietal diameter and serum PSB_1G levels at the 3rd trimester in normal, toxemic and diabetic women.

05.14.11
Influence of treatment on platelet consumption and thromboxane in pregnancy-induced hypertension: Greer, I A, Walker, J J, Calder, A A, Forbes, C D. Univ. Dept. Med. and Obstet., Roy. Infirm., Glasgow, UK
Thromboxane (TxA_2) is produced during platelet aggregation and causes further aggregation and vasoconstriction. It has been implicated in the pathophysiology of pregnancy induced hypertension (PIH), a disease characterised by vasoconstriction and platelet consumption. The aim of this study was to determine what effect treatment of PIH had on platelets and TxA_2. Labetalol treatment significantly increased platelet count in severe PIH, and maintained platelet count in patients with mild to moderate disease compared to a control group. Treatment with labetalol also significantly reduced TxA_2. It has recently become possible to measure platelet aggregation in whole blood, a more physiological method than platelet rich plasma techniques, as platelets are left in their natural milieu with red and white cells present which can themselves influence aggregation. Four adrenergic blocking agents were studied in vitro; labetalol, pindolol and propranolol inhibited aggregation in a dose-dependent manner, were synergistic with prostacyclin in inhibiting aggregation, and significantly inhibited TxA_2 production from whole blood. Atenolol had no effect on either aggregation or TxA_2 production. These studies suggest that labetalol, pindolol and propranolol can reduce platelet aggregation and TxA_2 production and may be of benefit in PIH.

05.14.12
Effect of calcium supplementation on the vascular sensitivity to angiotensin II in pregnant women: Kawasaki, K, Mastui, K, Ito, M, Ushijima, H, Maeyama, M. Dept. Obstet. and Gyn., Kumamoto Univ. Med. School, Kumamoto, Japan
The effect of calcium supplementation on the vascular sensitivity to angiotensin II (AII) was investigated in pregnant women. We administered orally 600 mg calcium L-aspartate daily to 22 pregnant women from 20 weeks of gestation to delivery. The values for the effective pressor dose of AII (EPD) in the calcium supplemented women were compared with those in 72 non-supplemented pregnant women. The vascular sensitivity was significantly decreased after calcium supplementation. The values for EPD in the calcium supplemented patients were 18.1 ± 1.2 ng/kg/min at 20 weeks of gestation, 32.2 ± 2.6 ng/kg/min at the 26th week, 41.1 ± 3.4 ng/kg/min at the 30th week and 25.9 ± 2.9 ng/kg/min at the 36th week (mean $\pm$ SEM), while those in the non-supplemented patients were 17.3 ± 1.2, 17.7 ± 1.6, 17.6 ± 1.2 and 15.0 ± 1.6 ng/kg/min, respectively. Assessment of the changes in EPD in the individual patients indicated that the percentile changes of EPD from the 20th week in the calcium supplemented patients were also significantly greater than those in 22 non-supplemented patients. The present dosage of calcium did not affect the blood chemistry and did not reduce the blood pressure. The incidence of PIH in the calcium supplemented

patients was 4.5%, which was smaller than that (21.2%) in the non-supplemented patients. Although there is no clear explanation of the mechanisms involved in such an effect of calcium, the present results do provide evidence to support the idea that oral calcium intake can prevent the onset of PIH.

05.14.13
Cellular immune response and HLA typing in patients of habitual abortion: Kandil, O, El-Tayeb, S, El Mekkawi, T, Saleh, S, Ayoub, N. Depts. Obstet. and Gyn. and Clin. Path., Fac. Med., Al-Azhar Univ., Cairo, Egypt
This work was performed in order to study the cellular immune response in 25 patients with habitual abortion without pregnancy, 25 pregnant patients with a previous history of habitual abortion and 25 patients, as non-pregnant controls. – T-lymphocyte rosette test, both active and total were done. – Mixed lymphocyte culture, one-way and two-ways were applied. – HLA-typing was done by the micro-lymphocyte toxicity test. – Histocompatibility locus antigens (HLA) frequencies was detected in 25 females with history of habitual abortion. Three hundred and thirty age matched apparently healthy unrelated persons, were studied for HLA frequencies and considered as normal control of the Egyptian citizens. There was no significant association between HLA in patients as compared with antigen frequency in control group. There is increased antigen frequency in A_3 but this increase is not significant. Significant depression of cellular immune repsonse was found in pregnant and non-pregnant patients with history of habitual abortion as compared with normal controls.

05.14.14
Studies on cellular immunity in normal pregnancy and toxemia: Matsumoto, S, Saito, H, Okamiya, H, Takahashi, M, Suzuki, M. Dept. Obstet. and Gyn., Kyorin Univ. School Med., Mitaka, Japan
Pregnancy can be regarded as allograft formation. Change in maternal immunity during pregnancy is regarded to have relation to the maintenance of pregnancy. It is further estimated that the change plays an important role in etiology of toxemia. This report presents the results of the study on changes in cellular immunity during pregnancy and that in toxemia. – Subjects and methods: The subjects of the study were: 15 healthy non-pregnant women as control, 80 women in normal pregnancy, 8 women with severe toxemia of pregnancy. The items subjected to the tests were: OKIa1, OKT3, OKT4, OKT8. The method of measurement employed was the direct immunofluorescence by flow cytometry (Spectrum III) using mono-clonal antibody. – Results: 1. In normal pregnancy the values for OKIa1+ were low, and those for OKT3+ cell showed a slight increase during the course of pregnancy. OKT4+ cell was lowest in the second trimester, whereas OKT8+ cell was highest in the same period. 2. In toxemia, OKT4+ cell was significant-ly lower (p < 0.05) and OKT8/OKT3 was significantly higher (p < 0.01) than the values for normal pregnan-cy in the third trimester. – Conclusion: In the initial stage of normal pregnancy OKIa1 and OKT3 showed a transient decrease. Decrease in cellular immunity in this period is regarded as a reasonable response, as it coincides with the time for fertilization, implantation, and placental formation. In toxemia OKT4/OKT8 was low, which is similar to the condition observed in the second trimester of normal pregnancy. It is suggested that the change in OKT4 and OKT8 may be a part of the etiology of toxemia.

05.14.15
Immunological significance of regional lymph node and decidua in the maintenance of pregnancy: Kawabata, M, Umesaki, N, Sako, H, Sugawa, T. Dept. Obstet. and Gyn., Osaka City Univ. Med. School, Osaka, Japan
The immunological mechanisms which prevent maternal rejection of the fetus has not been elucidated in detail. This study was designed to clarify the immunological mechanism at the feto-maternal interface which permits maintenance of pregnancy. Initially, we studied lymph nodes draining the uterus (DLN), namely the obturator lymph node, to determine whether the maternal immune system responded to fetal antigens at maternal-fetal frontier. DLN was found to be significantly enlarged and T-cells, especially 1a positive T-cells, were found to be increased in the immunohistological study using monoclonal antibody. T-cell mitogen response in DLN was also increased. This finding showed that the mother recognized the fetus as an allograft and actively responded to it. Therefore, a mechanism for suppression of the maternal immune response to the immunological role of decidua which lies between the fetus and mother in pregnancy was studied. Decidual tissue was obtained by miscarriage between the 6th and 10th gestational weeks. Single cell suspensions of decidua were obtained by the treatment with collagenase and DNAase. Decidua cells inhibited the mixed lymphocyte reaction (MLR). The supernatant from decidual cells cultured during 24 hours also inhibited it. In conclusion, the mechanism for maintaining the fetus throughout pregnancy might be that the decidual cell and humoral factor secreted from decidual cells suppress the maternal immune response to the fetus, even though the mother recognizes the fetus as an allograft.

05.14.16
Determination of immunologic reactions during abortion by means of monoclonal antibodies: Mallmann, P, Koenig, U D. Dept. Gyn. and Obstet., Univ., Bonn
Pregnancy must be understood as a immunological tolerance reaction between maternal immune reaction and fetal antigens. Disturbances of this probably lead to abortion. For further investigations the main

lymphocyte subpopulations T helper, T suppressor, total T and natural killer cells of 50 patients undergoing abortion and 50 age-matched pregnant women were evaluated by means of monoclonal antibodies. The coating effect of the serum on antigenic determinants of the lymphocyte membrane was determined by means of the monoclonal antibodies anti Leu 3a/3b, 11, OKT8 and 11. We were able to show a significant (p 0.05) increase of total T cells and T suppressor cells during abortion. The coating effect of the serum of patients undergoing abortion on T cell specific membrane antigens was increased (p 0.05). Thus, during abortion an increase of cellular and humoral immunosuppressive mechanisms is observed, probably as evidence for the disturbed balance between maternal immune reaction against fetal antigens and the growing immunocompetence of the fetus which may lead to an abortion.

05.14.17
Influence of autologous serum or plasma on the reduced lymphocyte alloreactivity in women with idiopathic recurrent abortions: Selvaggi, L, Lucivero, G, Iannone, A. Ist. Clin. Obstet. e Gyn. I, Clin. Med. II, Univ., Bari, Italy

Immunological mechanisms, such as changes in maternal reactivity towards paternally-derived fetal antigens or lack of maternal production of "blocking factors" might play a role in the pathogenesis of idiopathic recurrent abortions. In this regard, we have examined the influence of autologous serum or plasma on the reactivity of peripheral blood lymphocytes obtained from 36 non-pregnant women (mean age 31 years; range 21–41) with previous history of idiopathic recurrent abortions (two or more) towards alloantigens expressed by lymphocytes of their own partners or unrelated normal donors. Fifteen normal women with previous normal pregnancies were the control group. The maternal lymphocyte alloreactivity was evaluated by ^{3}H-TdR uptake in one-way mixed lymphocyte cultures. Thirty per cent of the examined patients presented a specific hyporeactivity towards their own partners' alloantigens; an additional 20% of patients were hyporeactive to alloantigens of both their partners and unrelated donors. Autologous plasma or serum did not alter significantly the maternal lymphocyte alloreactivity. The results suggest that a high proportion (up to 50%) of patients with idiopathic recurrent abortions present lymphocyte hyporeactivity towards alloantigens. This defective lymphocyte function might alter the maternal recognition of fetal antigens.

05.14.18
Use of monoclonal antibody directed to fetal red cells for immunological prenatal diagnosis: Technical approach by fluorescence activated cell sorter (FACS): Edelman, P, Villeval, J L, Edelman L, Vainchenker, W, Frydman, R, Sureau, C. Clin. Univ. Baudelocque, Paris; Inserm U. 91, Hôp. A. Béclère (Clamart), Paris, France

We have obtained monoclonal antibody (Fa6) which recognizes an antigen expressed during ontogenesis. With fluorescence labelling procedure Fa6 marks 35–50% of fetal cells whereas the recognized epitope is not present on adult erythrocytes. The method involves a double step: first after staining with double coat of fluoresceinated Ig the analyses by FACs of the labelled cells allow one to obtain routinely ratios of more than 100 of fetal versus adult erythrocytes (in high fluorescence channel). The second step, concerns the characterization of sorted erythrocytes with different ontogenic markers (FHb, I/i groups, carbonic anhydrases I) to confirm the fetal origin of these cells. Experiment use double label technic, on polylysin coated glass coverslips, with quantity of red cells as few as 3000. To evaluate the reliability of this system we have tried to isolate fetal from maternal blood after induced abortions. We have succeeded in half the cases, so that it seems necessary to improve specificity and sensitivity of the test before currently using it in normal pregnancy.

05.14.19
Study on immune cells in the decidua basalis of human pregnancy – immunohistological analysis using monoclonal antibodies: Honma, S, Sasagawa, M, Uchiyama, M, Kanazawa, K, Takeuchi, S. Dept. Obstet. and Gyn., Niigata Univ., School Med., Niigata, Japan

Distribution of immune cells in the decidua basalis was analysed by means of immunoperoxidase technique using monoclonal antibodies. Materials were obtained from pregnant uteri which were hysterectomized with medical indications at 8 to 14 gestational weeks. Monoclonal antibodies applied on consecutive frozen tissue sections were anti-Leu-1, anti-Leu2a, anti-Leu-3a, anti-Leu-10, anti-Leu-M3, anti-HLA-DR and anti-Factor VIII related antigen, which recognize pan T cells, killer/suppressor T cells, helper/inducer T cells, B cells, monocytes/macrophages, HLA-D/DR and endothelial cells, respectively. Leu-1 positive pan T cells found in a small number in the decidua were observed to include nearly equal number of Leu-2a positive cells and Leu-3a positive cells, localizing around vessels and glands. Furthermore, HLA-DR positive cells were found abundantly throughout the decidua, including a large number of Leu-M3 positive cells especially adjacent to trophoblastic cells in addition to Factor VIII related antigen positive cells and a scanty number of Leu-10 positive cells. Thus, the majority of HLA-DR positive cells were indicated to be monocytes/macrophages, which may function as "antigen presenting" cells to recognize and present fetal antigens to maternal T cells.

05.14.20

Marginal riboflavin deficiency and serum lipid peroxide levels of pregnant women: Ishihara, M, Kuroyanagi, J, Komura, S*, Ohishi, N*, Yagi, K*. Dept. Obstet. and Gyn., Aichi Med. Univ., Aichi, and *Inst. Appl. Biochem., Mitake, Gifu, Japan

We have already reported that serum lipid peroxide levels in women with toxemia during pregnancy are higher than those in women having a normal pregnancy. It is well-known that riboflavin deficiency brings about a decrease in glutathione reductase activity and, in turn, a decrease in the activity of the lipid peroxide degrading system. Accordingly, riboflavin deficiency is considered to be one factor which leads to increased serum lipid peroxide levels. Also, it has been established that pregnant women tend to be deficient in riboflavin. Therefore, the present study was undertaken to clarify the relationship between marginal riboflavin deficiency and serum lipid peroxide level during pregnancy. Serum lipid peroxide levels were determined according to *Yagi* (Biochem. Med. **15**, 212, 1976) and expressed in terms of nmol malondialdehyde/ml. Flavins were analyzed by high-performance liquid chromatography (Biochem. Int. **4**, 187, 1982). Marginal riboflavin deficiency was judged by erythrocyte glutathione reductase activity. Sixty-five subjects were arbitrarily selected from pregnant outpatients of the Aichi Medical University Hospital. An increase in the serum lipid peroxide level was found in 24 pregnant women. Among them, 17 subjects showed lower erythrocyte glutathione reductase activity, of whom 13 had decreased flavin levels in their blood.

05.14.21

The post-partum oral glucose tolerance test in the high-risk patients for diabetes – a prospective study: Kharouf, M, Charfeddine, M A, Guedri, H, Boukhris, R, Chelli, M. Ctre W. Bourguiba, Fac. Med. Tunis, Tunisie

We have carried out an oral glucose tolerance test (OGTT) with 100 g of glucose in 97 patients; the test was done in the first 72 hours after child birth and concerned 4 groups: 1. a control group: 33 women, 2. a group of women with large babies ($\geq$ 4000 g): 41 women, 3. a group of women with congenital defects: 7 women, 4. a group of women with an intrauterine death: 16 women. The results of the control group were: 0 min = 0.82 ± 0.09 g/l (ISD), 30 min = 1.42 ± 0.26 g/l, 60 min = 1.49 ± 0.26 g/l, 90 min = 1.37 ± 0.28 g/l, 120 min = 1.20 ± 0.26 g/l, 180 min = 1.02 ± 0.24 g/l. We considered that all OGTT with two or more values falling above the mean +ISD are an abnormal OGTT. According to these criteria the incidence of abnormal OGTT in the different groups is as follows: control group: 6%, large babies group: 39%, congenital defects group: 43%, intrauterine death group: 43%. We underline two points: 1. the values of the OGTT done at the onset of the post-partum period are similar to the third trimester pregnancy values reported by some authors; 2. the high incidence of abnormal OGTT in the groups of mothers who are at a high risk for diabetes.

05.14.22

Present-day results in 129 diabetic pregnancies: Somville, T A, Beck, L. Dept. Obstet. and Gyn., Univ., Düsseldorf

Obstetrical experience with 35 pregnancies in women with class A diabetes and 94 pregnancies with insulin requiring diabetes during the period 1981–1983 is presented. The perinatal mortality rate was 1.5% (identical with our overall population over the same period). Induction of labor was performed in 30%. Delivery occurred at or after 38 weeks of gestation in 80%. The frequency of spontaneous delivery rose from 26% in 1978–1980 to 36% in this period. The prevalence of Cesarean section diminished from 54% to 48%. Congenital malformations are still higher in the diabetic group (4.6%) than in the overall population (2.3%). The frequency of EPH-gestosis (23%), macrosomia (22%) and premature contractions (17%) were significantly lower than in the period 1978–1980 with respectively 48%, 38% and 27%. The intensive collaboration with diabetologists and pediatricians, the programs of education to self-control and new developments such as the use of insulin pumps in selected cases contributed to the amelioration of this high risk population.

05.14.23

Maternal complications and fetal outcome in the pregnant diabetic: Sudharsan, S, Nafeesa Beebi, A, Manime-kalai, P. Inst. Obstet. and Gyn., Madras, India

Diabetes mellitus in pregnancy poses an adverse environment for mother and baby, the ensuing complications of it being minimised with expert care by obstetrician, diabetologist and neonatologist. The present study retrospectively analyses 216 pregnant diabetics delivered over a six year period. The incidence of diabetes in pregnancy was 0.21% (*Barnes* 0.28%) with 54% prevalence in 20–29 years. 50% were para 1–2, with no increase in incidence with parity. The antenatal complications were pre-eclampsia (16–18%), hydramnios (4–7%), intrauterine death (10%), and urinary tract infection (1.9%). All intrauterine deaths occurred in unbooked cases. Spontaneous vaginal delivery occurred in 40% while 45% had Cesarean section of which 60% were elective. Pregnancy wastage comprised of 14% abortions and 10% intrauterine death. The perinatal mortality rate was 5.1%. No congenital malformations were encountered. Public awareness, improved screening methods and strict control of diabetes have reduced the maternal and perinatal complications considerably, leading to emphasis on preconceptional control of diabetes and premarital counselling for better outcome.

05.14.24
A randomized clinical trial of the insulin pump vs intensive conventional therapy in diabetic pregnancies:
Coustan, D R, Reece, E A, Sherwin, R S, Rudolf, M C J, Bates, S E, Sockin, S M, Holford, T, Tamborlane, W V. Yale and Brown Univ., New Haven, CT and Providence, RI, USA
Because pregnancy is a clinical setting in which intensive metabolic management is critical for the diabetic woman, use of the continuous insulin infusion pump has been advocated. Because the patient using the pump is generally selected on the basis of high motivation and capability, practices frequent home blood glucose monitoring, and is monitored closely by the health care team, any or all of these factors may be as important in assuring a good outcome as the pump itself. We report herein a randomized trial of pump vs intensive conventional therapy (ICT, at least two injections of mixed short- and intermediate acting insulin daily) in 22 pregnancies among 21 insulin dependent diabetic women. Both treatment groups performed home glucose monitoring approximately seven times daily. All patients were additionally studied for 24 hours in our CRC at least once each trimester. Results (mean $\pm$ S. D.):

	N	PRE-RX %HbA1	TERM %HbA1	INPT PRE-RX	GLU-MG/DL ON RX	HOME GLUC	MAGE*
PUMP	11	8.6±1.7	6.4±1.6	118±54	82±13	100±14	65±16
ICT	11	9.1±1.5	6.4±0.6	115±57	87±20	104±12	68±16

(*Mean Amplitude of Glycemic Excursions)

There were no significant differences between treatment groups for any of the above variables. Pregnancy outcomes were also similar, with hypoglycemia occurring in one neonate in each group. This study does not support the concept that pregnancy is an a priori indication for insulin pump treatment.

05.14.25
Serum glucose, insulin, and C-peptide levels after a 100-g oral glucose load in human pregnancy: Leal, M C, Orós, D, Esteva, F, Juste, G, Pérez-López, F R. Hosp. Clin. Univ., Zaragoza, Spain
The criteria recommended for diagnosis of abnormal glucose (G) tolerance in pregnancy have varied among authors. The goal of the present study was to determine G (mg/100 ml), insulin (I; μU/ml), and C-peptide (CP; ng/ml) levels after a 100-g oral G load in the first, second, and third trimester of normal pregnancies. Fasting serum G levels were normal according to *Frankel* and *Josinovich* (Diab. Care **3**, 399, 1980). The results are presented in the following table ($\bar{x} \pm$ S.E.M.).

min.	0	60	120	180
G-1	89.3±3.1	134.3±14.0	86.3± 4.8	77.1± 7.7
2	87.1±4.6	136.4±12.8	96.3± 6.5	75.4± 4.7
3	88.0±2.6	176.3±20.8	150.0±19.	104.6± 9.5
I-1	18.5±1.1	103.8±25.4	49.8± 9.9	24.6± 4.5
2	25.0±3.4	161.8±25.8	103.9±21.	36.0± 4.6
3	26.1±3.0	207.6±36.2	163.1±36.	119.1±33.3
CP-1	1.0±0.2	5.4± 0.7	3.8± 0.5	2.5± 0.4
2	1.8±0.3	9.1± 1.5	8.4± 1.4	4.7± 0.7
3	2.4±0.2	11.4± 1.8	11.1± 1.9	8.6± 1.7

It seems that serum CP levels after oral G load permit evaluation of the potential for endogenous insulin synthesis and provide information on β-cell function during pregnancy.

05.14.26
Insulin pump treatment of pregnant diabetics: Moestrup, J K, Krogh, A, Frøland, A. Gyn.-Obstet. and Med. Depts., Fredericia Hosp., Fredericia, Denmark
Fifteen consecutive diabetic women (White Class B to F) were treated by continuous subcutaneous insulin infusion. Six started treatment 14 to 4 weeks before conception, nine 8 to 17 weeks after. Metabolic control was monitored by glycosylated hemoglobin (HbA1) and patients own home measurements of blood glucose, 13 tests per day, once or twice weekly. Twelve women were delivered of normal, healthy children in weeks 35 to 39. Two weighed more than 4000 g. During pregnancy HbA1 fell from 10.0% ±1.6% (mean ±SD) to 8.4% ±1.4%. Upper normal limit for HbA1 is 8.6%. In the individual patient mean blood glucose was calculated for the last trimester on basis of home measurements. The mean blood glucose values ranged from 4.2 mmol/l to 9.8 mmol/l, median 5.95 mmol/l. The patients were treated on an outpatient basis and only confined to hospital one or two days before delivery. One patient with nephropathy and severe retinopathy gave birth to a macerated fetus in week 29. Unexplained intrauterine death occurred

in week 29 in a class B woman. Finally one patient had to be transferred to conventional treatment in week 14 for psychological reasons. The outcome of these fifteen pregnancies appears to be similar to what is seen on conventional therapy. However, pump treatment combined with frequent home measurements of blood glucose seems to normalize or nearly normalize glucose metabolism, thus improving the well-being of the patients and reducing the need for time spent in hospital.

05.14.27
The bile acids concentration in blood serum in cases cholestasis of pregnancy: Wierzbicki, A, Pisarek-Miedzińska, D, Ostrowski, J. Dept. Gyn. and Obstet. and Dept. Gastroent. Med., Ctr. Postgrad. Educ., Warsaw, Poland

The aim of our study was to investigate the value of estimation of bile acids concentration in the blood serum of pregnant women for diagnosis of cholestasis in pregnancy, and to find if there is any correlation between the bile acids concentration in blood serum and clinical state of fetus and term of delivery. Criteria of cholestasis in pregnancy were as follows: 1. Skin itching, 2. Results of laboratory tests: AP activity, GGTP, cholesterol, Fe in serum and Cu in serum, 3. HB_sAg negative, 4. total bilirubin 4 mg%, direct bilirubin, aminotransferase activity 400 U/l, 5. no clinical signs of liver cell damage, 6. retirement of clinical signs of cholestasis till 21 days post partum. Examined group: 40 pregnant women with cholestasis, control group: 40 healthy pregnant women in the III trimester of pregnancy. State of fetus was controlled by: CTG-fetus monitoring, HPL and E_3 concentration in blood serum. – Results: 1. In cases of cholestasis in pregnancy with very high level of bile acids in blood serum (average 86.05 μM/l) we observed very often signs of fetal distress resulting in the increase of CS number. 2. In our study we did not observe correlation between premature deliveries and very high level of bile acids in blood serum (average bile acids premature labor 25.16 μM/l).

05.14.28
Opioid peptides in pregnancy and labor: Evidence for pituitary and hypothalamic hypersecretion in the rat: Petraglia, F, Iughetti, L, Golinelli, S, Setti, T, Facchinetti, F, Volpe, A, Genazzani, A R. Dept. Obstet. and Gyn., Univ., Modena, Italy

Endogenous opioid peptides seem to be involved in maternal adaptation to pregnancy and parturition. Several studies have shown that plasma concentrations of beta-endorphin (B-EP), the most diffuse circulating opioid, increase in pregnant women, with a progressive trend toward the third trimester and a further increase occurs during labor, leading to values about ten times higher. It remains to be demonstrated whether this increase is only related to secretion by the placenta, which is also active in synthesizing B-EP, or is dependent on hypersecretion in the pituitary gland, the main source of plasma B-EP. We measured B-EP concentrations in plasma, anterior-pituitary (AP), neurointermediate pituitary lobe (NIL) and mediobasal hypothalamus (MBH) of pregnant (mid and late gestation) and fertile control rats, and during labor. Met-Enkephalin concentrations were also evaluated in the MBH. B-EP concentrations in plasma, AP and NIL during pregnancy were significantly higher than in controls, resulting progressive the increasing pattern in plasma and AP. Similarly while NIL concentrations remained stable at labor, plasma and AP B-EP concentrations showed a further increase at labor. In the MBH of pregnant rats the B-EP and met-enk concentrations were twice as high as in controls, markedly rising during labor. These results indicate that pregnancy and labor are characterized by elevated plasma, pituitary and hypothalamus B-EP concentrations and by high MBH met-enk content suggest that a general hyperactivity of the opioid system occurs in such conditions.

05.14.29
Thyroid function during pregnancy – measurement of free-thyroxine, free-triiodothyronine and reverse T3 levels: Nakayama, H, Ashitaka, Y, Takeuchi, Y, Mochizuki, M. Dept. Obstet. and Gyn., Kobe Univ. Hosp., Kobe, Japan

For estimating thyroid function during pregnancy, f-T4, f-T3 and r-T3 concentrations in maternal and cord sera were measured in each RIA. In cases with normal pregnancy maternal f-T4 and f-T3 levels showed a tendency to decrease during the course of pregnancy toward parturition, while r-T3 remained at 35.1 ± 10.1 ng/dl in the whole course. Twenty-nine cases with abnormal pregnancy in the third trimester (17 with IUGR, and 12 with severe toxemia) showed a lowering for maternal f-T3 ($p < 0.05$) and increasing tendency fo r-T3 ($p < 0.01$), compared to the normal cases in the same gestational age, indicating that T4 to r-T3 conversion is more dominant than T4 to T3 in cases with such abnormal pregnancies as severe toxemia and IUGR derived from maternal hypometabolism. Next, these hormone levels in cord arterial (a), cord venous (b) and maternal venous blood (c) obtained at the time of delivery in normal cases were compared. Although there was no statistical significance in f-T4 levels among these three groups, maternal f-T3 levels were significantly higher than those of cord sera ($p < 0.001$). Furthermore, r-T3 showed a tendency of (b) > (a) ($p < 0.005$), and (a) > (c) ($p < 0.001$) in the paired examination. This result might suggest that high level of fetal r-T3 is partly derived from transplacental origin, and human inner mono-deiodination could prevent the transplacental active thyroid hormones from the dam to fetus. (Supported in part by a Grant-in-Aid # 59570710 for Scientific research from the Ministry of Education, Science and Culture, Japan.)

05.14.30

The expression of renin and angiotensinogen genes in human placental tissues throughout pregnancy: Ihara, Y, Taii, S, Mori, T. Dept. Gyn. and Obstet., Kyoto Univ. Fac. Med., Kyoto, Japan

Recent studies have demonstrated that independent reninangiotensin (R-A) systems are present in some other organs than the kidney ant that they have local function in each organ. Also, in the placenta, the synthesis of renin has been suggested. We have studied the expression of renin and angiotensinogen genes in the human placental tissues throughout pregnancy and hydatidiform mole, detecting their mRNA with specific human renin and angiotensinogen complementary DNA probes (RNA hybridization analysis. Renin mRNA was detected in chorion throughout pregnancy and hydatidiform mole, but not in decidua or amnion. The concentration of renin mRNA in chorion decreased gradually throughout pregnancy, and that in hydatidiform mole was higher than that in chorion in early pregnancy ($p < 0.01$). On the contrary, total renin mRNA of the placenta increased throughout pregnancy, and at term it became about one sixth of total renin mRNA of the kidney of non-pregnant women. There was no significant difference in either the concentration of renin mRNA in chorion or total renin mRNA of the placenta between four full term healthy pregnant women and four pregnant women with toxemia. Angiotensinogen mRNA was not detected in all placental tissues or hydatidiform mole. The results imply the possibility that renin synthesized in the placenta may have some local function during pregnancy.

05.14.31

Changes in taurine levels in the blood of developing fetuses and placental transport of taurine in brush border microvillous: Moriyama, I S, Iioka, H, Kyuma, M, Amasaki, M, Ichijo, M. Dept. Obstet. and Gyn., Nara Med. Univ., Nara, Japan

In human pregnancy, maternal and umbilical blood of the 22nd and 40th weeks of pregnancy and at parturition were submitted to the analysis of total free amino-acids (FAA). The neonatal blood was also examined until the ninth day after birth. The content of FAA in the serum from the umbilical vein was higher than that from the maternal blood. However, the content of taurine kept a much higher level than the other aminoacids until term, and then it decreased to the normal level on the ninth day after birth. Placental transport of taurine was studied in isolated brush border microvillous plasma membrane vesicles by a rapid filtration technique. Brush border microvillous plasma membrane vesicles were prepared from syncytiotrophoblast of human term placenta. The specific activities of alkaline phosphatase, 5' nucleotidase and γ-GTP in the membrane preparation were enriched to $13-14$ times as high as those in the homogenate. The membrane vesicles exhibit uptake of ^{3}H-labelled taurine into an osmotically reactive intravesicular space. Taurine uptake by vesicles was stimulated specifically by an inward sodium gradient, and replacement of NaCl in the transport medium by KCl, LiCl, and choline chloride had no effect on th transport activity of the vesicles. Taurine transport is inhibited competitively by the presense of β alanine and GABA. These results indicate that transport of taurine across the placental brush border membrane is soidum dependent and carrier mediated.

05.14.32

The activities of DNA polymerases in human placenta: Ishii, A, Hayashi, M, Amemiya, A, Hamada, H. Dept. Obstet. and Gyn., St. Marianna Univ. School Med., Kawasaki; **Takayanagi, M.** Dept. Obstet. and Gyn., Toshiba Hosp., Tokyo, Japan

It has been shown that DNA polymerases play important roles in hyperplastic growth of the placenta in pregnant rats. With the purpose of elucidating the mechanisms related to placental growth, we examined changes in the enzyme activities during human pregnancy. Crude extracts of DNA polymerases (PM) were prepared from the placenta in the early (8 weeks) and late (40 weeks) stages, to measure the activities of alpha- and beta-PM, using ^{3}H-dTTP as precursor. Results obtained were: 1) The ^{3}H incorporation by crude alpha-PM was higher in the early stage than in the late stage, while that of beta-PM was not affected by the stages. 2) The distribution of PM activities in sucrose-density-gradient centrifugation also revealed a similar tendency as in crude extracts. The high activity of alpha-PM in the early stages was considered due to a rapid cell proliferation at the stage.

05.14.33

Studies on iron uptake mechanism of the human fetus from maternal serum transferrin via the placenta: Tawada, T, Nojima, M, Seida, A, Okuyama, T, Furuya, H. Dept. Obstet. and Gyn., Juntendo Univ. School Med., Tokyo, Japan

Since one-way transport of iron via the human placenta from maternal serum to the fetus has been noted, the localization of transferrin and the dynamics of iron transport mechanism in the human placental tissue were investigated. Results obtained were as follows. Peroxidase conjugated antibody methods was used for localizing transferrin at the microvillous surface of syncytiotrophoblast and the specific and reversible attachment of transferrin at this site was recognized. The villous tissue *in vitro* revealed autoradiographically that radioactive rion is taken up vigorously from ^{59}Fe-diferric transferrin and it is accumulated into hemosiderin particles neighboring the basement membrane of trophoblast cells, and colloidal gold technique revealed a pinocytosis of diferric transferrin attaching on the surface of syncytiotrophoblast into the cytoplasm and final uptake of transferrin into the lysosomes. Apotransferrin, however, was found to be neither attaching to the surface nor incorporating into the cytoplasm. These results suggest that the first phase of the placental iron transport is a specific attachment of maternal transferrin at the site of transferrin receptors of thy syncytiotrophoblast plasma membrane and the second phase is a so-called receptor mediated pinocytosis, an incorporation of transferrin bound receptors into the cytoplasm.

05.14.34
Synthesis of $1\alpha,25(OH)_2D_3$ and $24,25(OH)_2D_3$ in human fetal membranes and placenta: Tsunoda, T, Goto, M, Iida, M, Anezaki, S, Honda, T, Furuya, K, Yoshida, T, Fukui, Y. Dept. Obstet. and Gyn., Nihon Univ., School Med., Tokyo, Japan
Our previous studies have shown that during pregnancy, $1\alpha,25(OH)_2D_3$ incrases in th maternal circulation, and is also present in the fetus and the amniotic fluid though in smaller amounts. Recent studies have also suggested that vitamin D metabolism in the fetoplacental unit may take place independently from the maternal circulation. Little is known, however, about the origin, metabolism and physiological role of vitamin D_3 and its metabolites in the fetus and the amniotic fluid. Therefore, studies were designed to elucidate if the synthesis of $1\alpha,25(OH)_2D_3$ and/or $24,25(OH)_2D_3$ may occur in the human fetal membranes and placenta, and if so, in which tissues, the amnion, chorion, and/or decidua. The fetal membranes were aseptically removed at delivery and separated into the amnion and chorion. Decidua was obtained by curretage. Each tissue was cultured in RPMI medium 1640 for 48 hours, and after the addition of $(^3H\text{-}26,27)25OHD_3$ cultured for a further 24 hours. Lipids were extracted by the modified procedure of *Bligh* and *Dyer*, and chromatographed on a Sephadex LH-20 column and HPLC. the radioactivities were measured by a automatic liquid scintillation spectrometer. The conversion rates to $1\alpha,25(OH)_2D_3$ and $24,25(OH)_2D_3$ for $25OHD_3$ were 0.44%, 1.31% in the amnion 0.63%, 2.67% in chorion, 0.61%, 2.22% in decidua, and 54%, 1.34% in placenta. Our studies demonstrate that not only the decidua, but also the amnion is capable of synthesizing $1\alpha,25(OH)_2D_3$ and $24,25(OH)_2D_3$ in late pregnancy. It is, therefore, evident that the fetal membranes are participating in $1\alpha,25(OH)_2D_3$ synthesis in the fetoplacental unit.

05.14.35
Microperoxisomes in human placenta and fetal membranes: Wang, T, Schneider, J. Dept. Gyn. and Obstet., Jinan Univ., Guangzhou, China, and Dept. Gyn. and Obstet., Hannover Med. School, Hannover
The distribution of microperoxisomes in human term placenta and fetal membranes was examined by cytochemistry and electron microscopy. Catalase-positive microperoxisomes were present in placental syncytium and Langhans' cells as well as in trophoblastic cells of chorionic membrane, but they were absent from amniotic cells and maternal decidua cells. Since microperoxisomes are frequently present in tissues engaged in lipid metabolism and steroid synthesis, we propose that syncytium and Langhans' cells of human placenta and trophoblastic cells of chorionic membrane have the ability to produce steroid hormones such as estrongen and progesterone.

05.14.36
Clinical values of the intervillous blood flow for the management of pregnant women: Koresawa, M, Hiratsuku, K. Perinat. Ctr, Saiseikai Shimonoseki Gen. Hosp., Shimonoseki, Japan
The present study was designed to investigate the clinical value of the measurement of intervilllous blood flow (IBE) for evaluating the placental function. IBF was determined by ^{133}Xe clearance method in 25 pregnant women with no severe complications between 22–39 weeks of gestation. Namely, 1 mCi of ^{133}Xe was injected intravenously, and IBF was calculated by the ^{133}Xe clearance curve obtained at the placenta according to the method of *Rekonen*. Mean IBF value was 81.3 ± 7.0 ml/min/100 ml at 22 weeks gestation, and gradually decreased as the gestational age increased, reaching the nadir value of 47.9 ± 14.7 ml/min/100 ml at 34 weeks of gestation. IBF values were relatively constant between 34–40 weeks of gestation. Serial determination of IBF showed that the IBF value was significantly decreased during the uterine construction. Also, the presence of some complications such as toxemia of pregnancy was after associated with the decline of IBF values. It was concluded that the measurement of IBF may be a useful aid for monitoring the placental function in pregnant women.

05.14.37
Influence of motion activity in pregnant women on rest and post-effort values of hemodynamic factors: Poręba, R, Szulc, A, Wolnicki, J, Azis, F. IVth Clin. Obstet. and Gyn., Ist Clin. Cardiol., Silesian Med. Acad., Katowice, Poland
The relationship between motion activity in the pregnant women and cardiac output (CO) cardiac index (CI) and stroke volume (SV) estimated at rest and in submaximal exercise are still under discussion. The above-mentioned factors are estimated directly by CO_2 rebreathing method in 54 women divided into 3 groups – control, trained and non-trained pregnant women. In pregnant women a rest CO (5.33 vs 4.4, $p < 0.001$) and rest CI (3.25 vs. 2.77, $p < 0.05$) obtained higher values than in control group. We observed in trained group higher values of rest CO (5.33 vs 4.77, $p < 0.05$), exercise CO (11.79 vs 10.27, $p < 0.001$), exercise CI (6.8 vs 6.19, $p < 0.05$) and rest SV (61.4 vs 51.9, $p < 0.001$) than in non-trained pregnant women. We conclude that training has a good influence on these hemodynamic factors in pregnant women at rest and in submaxial exercise.

05.14.38

Plasma corticotrophin-releasing factor-like immunoreactvity in pregnangcy: Price, J, Campbell, E A, Halpin, D M G, Jones, M T, Taylor, R W. Dept. Obstet. and Gyn., St. Thomas' Hosp. Med. School, Londen, UK

Sasaki et al. (Abstracts, 7th International Congress of endocrinology 1984) have reported the presence of corticotrophin-releasing factor-like immunoreactivity (irCRF) in the plasma during the third trimester and in placental tissue at term. We have measured irCRF in the plasma of normotensive and pre-eclamptic patients in the second and third trimester and in arterial and venous cord blood after delivery. irCRF levels were below the detection limits (100 pg/ml) of our assay until 27 weeks of gestation when the levels increased to 100–250 pg/ml and, in some cases, reached 4000 p/ml at term. In the group of pre-eclamptics the levels tended to be higher than in normotensive controls. Following parturition, CRF fell to undetectable levels within six hurs, consistent with the circulating half-life of this peptide. However, in one patient, with an ectopic (abdominal) pregnancy, where the placenta was left *in situ*, the levels were still measurable 24 hours later. Preliminary data on CRF levels in venous and arterial cord plasma suggest a transfer of CRF to the fetus. These data are consistent with the hypothesis that this CRF-like material is of placental origin and may have some role to play in maternal and fetal physiology, including parturition.

05.14.39

Normal two dimensional echocardiographic measurement of fetal heart at weeks 16–24 of pregnancy: Bahary, C, Disegnie, E, Haimovich, L, Levi, A, David, D, Bakst, A, Saphira, H. Depts. Cardiol. and Obstet. and Gyn. "B", Sapir Med. Ctr, Kfar-Saba, Israel

Previous reports of two dimensional echocardiographic (2D echo) onitoring of the fetal heart focused mainly on the second half of pregnancy, in order to establish the normal values of the cardiac dimensions at an early period of gestation. 41 pregnant women with normal gestation were examined by 2D echo between the weeks 16–24. Measurement of the cardiac chambers, aorta and pulmonary artery were taken at each week. A gradual linear increase of cardiac dimension was observed – Mean Cardiac dimensions from week 16 to 24 were as follows: Left ventricle diastole 3 to 10 mm, systole 2 to 6 mm, right ventricle diastole 2 to 9 mm, ratio L V/R V : 1/1, left atrium diastole 4 to 10 mm, aortic root systole 2 to 5 mm, pulmonary artery systole 3 to 6 mm. these measurements may represent the basis for evaluation of cardiac anatomy in the first half of pregnancy.

05.14.40

Evaluation of estrogen metabolism in the fetoplacental unit after DHA-S injection: Sagara, Y, Okatani, Y. Dept. Obstet. and Gyn., Kochi Med. School, Kochi, Japan

To evaluate estrogen metabolism in the fetoplacental unit after dehydroepindrosterone-sulfate (DHA-S) injection, unconjugated estrone (E1), estradiol (E2), estriol (E3) and estetrol (E4) in maternal vein (MV), umbilical vein (UV), umbilical artery (UA) and amniotic fluid (AF) were measured after DHAS injection. Eighteen normal obstetrical patients (37–39W) performed elective repeat Cesarean section were injected with 100 mg of DHA-S 30–60 minutes (7 cases), 120 minutes (6 cases), 180–240 minutes (5 cases) before delivery. The injection of DHA-S resulted in a rapid marked increase of E2 levels in MV (400% of control) and E1 levels in UV (1480% of control). The increase of E1 levels in MV were slower than that of E2. The increase of E2 in UV and UA was significant, however, the values were lower than that in MV. No significant changes of E3 levels in each compartment were demonstrated. However, significant increase in E4 was observed in each compartment later than two hours after DHA-S injection. Significant correlation was found between individual MV and UV plasma E4 concentration. These results indicate that placenta secretes E1 and E2 asymmetrically to maternal and fetal circulation after DHA-S injection. Detemination of maternal E2 and E4 rise after DHA-S injection may reflect placental and fetoplacental function, however, E3 may not.

05.28.01

Salivary progesterone: a simple indicator of ovulation: Said, S, Sadek, W, Shaat, A, El Habashy, M. Dept. Obstet. and Gyn., Alexandria Univ., Alexandria, Egypt

Fifty healthy regular cycling women attending the infertility clinic were investigated for evidence of ovulation. Blood and salivary samples were obtained at the mid-luteal phase of the cycle for measurement of progesterone concentration in both fluids by the radio-immunoassay technique. An endometrial biopsy was also taken by Novak's curette on the same day. Ovulation was proved by secretory endometrium in 44 cases while, six were not ovulating. The mean serum progesterone in ovulating cases was 12.7 ng/ml and their corresponding mean salivary progesterone was 585 pgm/ml. In anovulatory cases, the mean serum and salivary progesterone levels were 1.7 ng/ml and 263.3 pgm/ml respectively. There was a positive correlation between serum and salivary progesterone values in both ovular and anovular cases. These results implies that estimation of salivary progesterone is a useful non-invasive and simple technique that can be used clinically to detect ovulation.

05.28.02

Temporal relationships between urinary, salivary and ultrasonic indices of ovulation: Sallam, H N. Dept. Obstet. and Gyn., Univ., Alexandria, Egypt

The temporal relationships between concentration changes in urinary estrone-3-glucuronide, pregnandiol-3-alpha glucuronide, L. H., salivary estradiol and progesterone were studied in 17 healthy female volunteers. The urinary metabolites were measured by specific radio-immunoassays in daily samples of early morning urine and the salivary hormones concentrations were determined by direct chemiluminescence immunoassay methods described elsewhere (*Sallam*, 1983). The results were related to the expected time of ovulation, determined by ultrasound scanning of the follicles (*Hackeloer* and *Sallam*, 1983). The results show that the peak in salivary estradiol concentration preceded that of estrone-3-glucuronide in urine (1.78 + 0.81 days compared to 1.20 + 0.55 days before the expected time of ovulation, mean + SD). A defined rise in LH concentration in urine was the most reliable index for immediate predicton of ovulation with mean (+ SD) peak-ovulation interval of I.43 + O. 89 days. The peak of estrone-3-glucuronide in urine occurred 1.20 + 0.50 days (SD) before the expected time of ovulation and a defined rise in estrone-3-glucuronide concentration was a reliable index for early predicition of ovulation for natural family planning purposes as well as for the assessment of the luteal function. the concentration of salivary progesterone peaked 6.00 + 2.24 days after ovulation.

05.28.03

Prediction and diagnosis of ovulation by cervical mucus canalisation in comparison to ultrasonic and other routine means of monitoring it: Tzafettas, J M, Papalexandrou, A, Zournatzi, V, Papameletiou, Papaloucas, A. Dept. Obstet. and Gyn., Univ. Thessaloniki, Greece

Precise timing of ovulation is of mayor significance in dealing with various infertility problems and for this purpose various methods have been used such as serial measurements of LH and estrogens and ultrasonic monitoring of the Graafian follicle. It has been demonstrated that channels are formed between the dendritic crystals of the cervical mucus when this is dried and these are estrogen dependent. In this work the canalisation phenomenon of the cervical mucus was studied in two groups of patients, one with spontaneous ovulatory cycles and the other while receiving treatment with gonadotrophins for induction of ovulation. The aim of the study was: 1) to assess the ovarian changes by means of total volume and follicular maturation as detected by ultrasonic monitoring and to compare them with the number of channels formed in the two groups of patients; 2) to evaluate the quantity of channels in relation to the ovulation, the latter having been detected by other means in routine use. The ovarian changes observed by ultrasound, showed a linear relationship with the number of channels seen in the group of patients with spontaneous ovulatory cycle, whereas in the gonadotrophin group this was noticed only when the ovarian response was satisfactory. When the mucus is dried at 50° C canalisation occurs within a few hours and this phenomenon can be a relatively simple and reliable index of clinical value in predicting and diagnosing ovulation.

05.28.04

Fertilization and pregnancy after homologous artificial insemination – EPF as a parameter?: Mesrogli, M, Maas, D H A, Tobinsky, C. Dept. Obstet. and Gyn., MHH, Hannover

To examine the incidence of early embryonic loss after AIH, we used the detection of the Early Pregnancy Factor (EPF) by the rosette inhibition test as a means of early diagnosis of human pregnancy (from 48 h after fertilization on). So far, our investigations include 38 patients (66 cycles). Artificial homologous insemination was carried out in 23 cases because of reduced sperm findings and in 15 patients with pathological cervical factors (abnormal post-coital test). In the first group, the insemination led to a recognized clinical pregnancy in every fourth case after fertilization (i. e. a wastage rate of 75% within the first two weeks of gestation). In the latter group, women became pregnant in every second cycle which was EPF-positive. In both collectives, however, every third insemination cycle resulted in a fertilization of the ovum. As early abortions are for the most part caused by chromosomal defects or by malformations, we consider positive EPF-tests which are not followed by a clinical pregnancy to be a reason for immediate chromosome studies.

05.28.05

Factors affecting outcome of artificial insemination with cryopreserved semen from men with testicular tumor on Hodgkin's disease: Scammell, G, White, N, Stedronska, J, Edmonds, D K, Hendry, W F, Joffcoate, S L. Chelsea Hosp. Women, London, UK

Testikular tumors and Hodgkin's disease not uncommonly occur in young men who later desire children. Since 1976 we have offered to these men the opportunity to bank semen. Between 1978 and 1984, 22 of these men have requested artificial insemination of their partners with the banked semen. Initially basal body temperature charts (BBT) wee used to time insemination but since 1982 measurements of luteinising hormone (LH) have been used to time ovulation and insemination. Twenty-two women were treated for between 1 and 11 cycles giving a total of 115 cycles. There were eight pregnancies, all of which occurred within 7 cycles of treatment. Of the 115 cycles, 45 were monitored with LH measurements and 70 were timed with BBTs. All but one of the pregnancies occurred in those cycles which were monitored with LH. Sperm density and motility were also important in affecting outome. No pregnancies occurred when the sperm density was <20 million/ml, or when the motility was <40% (progressing well) at the time of freezing or <30% (progressing well) post-thaw. Cryopreservation therefore has a role in the management of fertility in these men and we would advise that because of the limited quantity of semen available for insemination, methods of predicting ovulation should be as accurate as possible.

05.28.06

New aspects in AID treatment with cryosperm: Bleichrodt, W H, Mutke, H G. Munich
A significant improvement in the results of AID with cryosperm have been observed over the last three years, completing a total of 18 years in the history of this method of treatment. Results wee obtained from a total survey of 2341 cases. As well as accurate basal temperature methods, continual sonographic testing for follicle maturity (ovarian monitoring) by means of a high resolution sector-scanner (technicare) was carried out. Insufficient cycles in problem patients were treated specifically, in accordance with the collegues by whom they were referred. In this way, i. e. accurate ovulation timing, and the optimum moment for insemination could be decided. Altogether, the cumulative pregnancy rate was increased by approximately 3% from 43.5 to 46.5%, mostly in the older problematic age-group, whose menstruation disorders had to be treated. The average duration of treatment was reduced by about 1.5 insemination cycles from 9 to 7.5. A significant improvement was seen predominantly in younger women. With consistent use of currently available facilities (technical-apparatus, laborchemical, therapeutic) one can only assume that an even better result may be reached in th future by the use of AID.

05.32.01

A worldwide assessment of the today contraceptive sponge: Edelman, D A. Med. Res. Consultants, Chapel Hill, NC, USA; **McClure, D.** VLI Corp., Irvine, CA, USA
Renewed interest in barrier methods of contraception has resulted in the development of new methods, among them the "Today" vaginal contraceptive sponge. This sponge (smaller than a diaphragm) is made of polyurethane and contains 1 gram of the spermicide nonoxynol-9. Following preclinical and phase I and II clinical trials, extensive worldwide phase III trials were conducted. These multiclinic trials were conducted according to a common protocol with regularly scheduled follow-up visits and examinations. The trials included 1847 women. Significantly lower method failure rates occurred during the second year of sponge use (10.1 vs. 2.6 per 100 women). In these trials the sponge was compared with other barrier contraceptives. The results of these studies showed the one-year effectiveness rate for the sponge was similar to that of other barrier methods. No serious complications occurred in over 1000 woman-years of sponge use. The most frequently reported problem was difficulty in removing the sponge. Additional studies showed the frequency of this problem was greatly reduced after the use of several sponges. The sponge offers users several advantages over other barrier methods including its 24-hour period of effectiveness and ease of use.

05.32.02

A comparative study of the today vaginal contraceptive sponge vs neo-sampoon tablets: Borko, E. Gen. Hosp., Maribor, and Behlilovic, B. Starigrad Hlth Ctr, Belgrad, Yugoslavia
A total of 770 women were randomly allocated as follows: 390 women were assigned the Sponge and 380 women to Neo-Sampoon. The purpose of the study was to evaluate the effectiveness, safety and acceptability of the two methods. Volunteers had to be generally healthy women from 18–40 years, not pregnant or known to be infertile or sterile. Follow-up visits were at 1, 3, 6 and 12 months. Physical and pelvic examinations were included on admission, the 6 and 12 month visits. The mean ages of the Sponge and Neo-Sampoon groups were 27.8 and 26.6 years, respectively. Most were currently married with a mean parity for the Sponge group of 0.9 and 0.8 for the Neo-Sampoon group. Over 1/3 of all women had used some form of vaginal contraceptive. The Today® Contraceptive Sponge is a cup-shaped polyurethane sponge containing 1 g of nonoxynol-9. Neo-Sampoon is an effervescent contraceptive tablet containing 60 mg of menfegol. The 12-month life-table method failure rates were 5.2 ± 1.9 for the contraceptive Sponge and 7.6 ± 2.0 for the contraceptive tablet. Discomfort was reported in 16 Sponge users and in 21 tablet users. This study indicates that both the contraceptive Sponge and Neo-Sampoon foaming tablets are effective and acceptable methods of contraception in this group of Yugoslavian women.

05.32.03

Self-measurement of vaginal fluid volume: Correlation with serum hormones and assessment of the fertile period: Schumacher, G F B, Haciski, R, Holt, J A, Karrison, T, Usala, S J, Broer, K H. Dept. Obstet. and Gyn., Univ., Chicago, IL, USA
Daily self-measurements of the vaginal fluid volume by a simple volumetric aspirator yielded reliable results (at least six hours after intercourse). Using the BBT shift as reference point the evaluation of 21 presumably ovulatory cycles of nine volunteers (age 19–34) showed clearly recognizable preovulatory increases from 0.2 to 0.8 ml average. Peaks ranged from 0.4–1.8 ml occurring on days, −2, −1 and 0 in the majority of cases. A rapid decrease occurred with the BBT increase after ovulation. Studies of serum LH, E_2 and P during 12 presumably ovulatory cycles of 12 different volunteers indicated positive correlation between preovulatory increase of serum E_2 and negative correlation between postovulatory increase of serum P and BBT and vaginal fluid volume. The results lead to preliminary algorithms providing a preovulatory signal

at least 3 days before the LH peak in ten of 12 cases and a postovulatory signal at least three days after the LH peak in 11 of 12 cases. High value signals less than three days before or on the day of the LH peak were observed in 10 of 12 cases. Volumetric self-measurement of vaginal fluid volume may be a useful bioassay of estrogen activity to assess the optimal time for conception and to delineate the fertile period. (Supported by Family Health Internat. and Mothers Aid of the Chicago Lying-in Hospital.)

05.32.04
Psychosexual and pre-pregnancy counselling for the physically handicapped woman: McCullough, A M. Dept. Obstet. and Gyn., Cambridge Military Hosp., Aldershot, Hants, UK
It is recognised that the female with a severe physical disability has major problems. Her disability causes difficulties in finding a sexual partner. Often as a result of society's negative attitude she is stunted socially, emotionally, psychologically and sexually. Lack of peer group association results in poor sexual knowledge and difficulty in coping with menstruation and contraception (Ziff, S F.: The sexual concerns of the adolescent woman with cerebral palsy, Issues in Health Care of Women **3**, 55–63, 1981). It is estimated that 60% of physically handicapped patients request counselling and although facilities exist in most areas in UK their effectiveness varies from area to area (Stewart, W F R.: Sexual fulfilment for the handicapped, Brit. J. Hosp. Med. **20**, 676–680, 1978). A panel of physicians, psychiatrists, physiotherapists, psychologists and nursing staff will all be required as will supportive organisations such as the Committee on Sexual Problems of the Disabled (SPOD). Pre-pregnancy counselling should be offered for psychological and practical reasons. Many patients will require no more than reassurance that conception of a normal infant is possible and that they are able to cope with a baby. This problem may be reinforced at a specialist assessment centre where the potential mother role plays with dolls. This will help assess future practical needs and permit the doctor to be aware of potential problems during confinement, labor and puerperium. Attendance at antenatal clinics may be encouraged by the provision of transport and the roles of the community midwife and health visitor will be essential in the home. The problems of labor are poorly documented but it is suggested that for example in the case of cerebral palsy there are risks of exaggerated reflexes which may persist after delivery and in view of the postoperative complications, Cesarean section should be used for obstetric indications only (McCullough, A M.: Pregnancy in a patient with cerebral palsy, J. Obstet. and Gyn. **5**, 39, 1984). Full co-operation from all health services is required for a healthy sexual life and pregnancy in the severely disabled.

05.32.05
Sex education in Greece: Goltsiou, V, Koumandaki, Y, Koumandakis, E, Kreatsas, G, Aravantinos, D. Alexandra Maternity Hosp., Athens, Greece
The present study aims at examining Greek parents' sex eduction and their attitudes on it. The sample consists of 1000 individuals, of whom 400 are men and 600 are women. It was found that the main source of sex information for the specific group as as follows: 20.4% of the sample has been informed by their parents, 13.1% by their teachers, for 27.6% of the sample the main source was from books and 38.9% from other sources to be mentioned. Sex and level of education were not related to the source of information whereas age was found to affect it. Of the sample 80% believe that both parents themselves should act as the main source of information for their children. Also, 90% consider that the teaching of sex education should be encouraged from school, believing that the age through elementary school is the most suitable. The majority of parents believe that sex education is a very intricate issue and as such it should be taught by educators with a special background and knowledge. The implications of the above findings, concerning the Greek schools are thoroughly discussed.

05.32.06
Sexual intercourse and pregnancy. Sexual positions for preventing some obstetrical emergencies. Sites of deep dyspareunies. External version in the VIth month of pregnancy: Ionesei, G P. Dept. Gyn., D.M.Z.I., Birlad, Romania
If in a pregnant woman's history proper attention to the sexual life (frequency, date and duration of the last sexual intercourse, the partners' natural construction, etc.) is also paid, then we shall meet cases when the relationship between the sexual positions during the intercourse and the favouring of toxic pregnancy, of a disease concomitant with the pregnancy, occurrence of a metrorrhagia, abortion or premature delivery (even if the sexual intercourse was not painful) cannot be excluded. This paper is based on the fact that the space offered by the woman to the penis is a frustum of a cone orientated with the small base in the vulvar aperture and the big one in the lower abdomen, and, according to the sexual positions, the penis may be directed towards the different areas of the female lower abdomen, thus the cervix uteri, the contraindicated areas around the cervix uteri being protected and man's pressing on the pregnant woman's abdomen is avoided. Therefore, a number of sexual positions – in trimesters of pregnancy – are described, out of which the most tolerable sexual positions to be selected. With that end in view, the site of dyspareunia (vulvar aperture, vaginal duct; right, left, central, anterior and posterior deep dyspareunia) is, beforehand, specified. In the pregnant woman with transverse presentation, taking into account the weight, in the second trimester of pregnancy, of the fetal head as compared to the rest of the body, the prophylactic external version beginning with the sixth month of pregnancy is performed; but for maintaining the achieved version, proper sleep and sexual intercourse positions, according to the case, are indicated. We

mention that of 220 cases statistics all women delivered naturally. We believe that such knowledge of sexual positology, accompanied by adequate sexual tactics, are necessary during the entire sexual life, both in a state of health: at defloration, for favoring the conception, in prophylactic purposes , in some discrepancies between partners, etc., and not only in obstetrics and gynecology or andrology, but also in some deficiencies or diseases of other organs, apparatus or systems of the woman, man or both.

05.41.01

The effect of the birth-decline on maternal mortality in Sweden during the years 1780–1980: Högberg, U, Wall, S. Dept. Obstet & Gyn., Dept Soc. Med., Univ. Hosp., Umeå, Sweden

Maternal mortality declined from 900 to 6 per 100 000 live births during the period 1780–1980, while the fertility decreased from 0.5 to 1.6 children per woman. By standardization the decline in maternal mortality is analysed with respect to the changing distribution of age and parity amongst parturients. The proportion of parturients aged more than 35 decreased from 32% to 7% during the past 200 years. The shifting distribution of age contributed with almost 3% of the mortality decline between 1781–1911, and with 5% between 1911–1980. During the last 15 years, 1965–1980, however about 50% of the mortality decline has been due to decreasing maternal age. The proportion of multipara (4+) decreased from 43% to 5%, while the proportion of primipara increased from 23% to 45%. The effect of the parity factor on the mortality is the reverse, but the combined impact of age/parity neutralizes the contradictory effect of the parity factor. Age/parity remains a risk factor of increasing importance. Maternal deaths, attributable to the risk factors age and parity as measured by the so called etiologic fraction, have increased from 46% during the 19th century to 80% during the last 30 years.

05.41.02

A fourteen year survey (1971–1984) of maternal mortality at Ramakrishna Mission Seva Pratishthan: Gupta, P D, Sen Gupta, P C, Das, B N, Das, M S, Chatterjee, S K. Dept. Obstet & Gyn., Ramakrishna Mission Seva Pratishthan, Vivekanada Inst. Med. Sci., Calcutta, India

A forteen year survey (1971–1984) of maternal mortality at Ramakrishna Mission Seva Pratishthan, is reported. There was no notable change in the number of births between 1973 and 1982. There was a fall in 1984. One hundred and twenty-three maternal deaths occurred out of 80 969 births; an incidence of 1.52 per 1000 births including abortion. Maternal mortality was highest among primigravidae (37.6%) and those between 25 and 30 years of age (41.6%). Only 2.23% of women were unbooked but among the total deaths, 68 (54.4%) had emergency admission. The maternal death was highest (3.27 per 1000) in 1973 and lowes (0.34 per 1000) in 1983. The major causes were jaundice (24%), abortion (18.4%), hemorrhage (10.4%), sepsis (6.4%) and anemia (6.4%). Among the true maternal causes, abortion was the largest single group. Deaths in many of the cases were attributed to more than one cause and nearly half (over 45%) of them were due to associated factors. Infective hepatitis was the commonest cause of death during 1978 and 1979 and it was also prevalent in 1981 and 1984. The avoidable factors for all major causes of death and the possible remedies have been discussed.

05.41.03

Maternal mortality in Italy: Panella, I. Gyn. and Obstet. Dept., Univ., Catania, Italy

In Italy the maternal mortality rate has undergone a notable decrease in the past ten years (1971–1981), presenting oscillating statistical values of approximately 46 women dead per 100 000 live births in 1971, down to 17 women dead per 100 000 live births in 1981 (data from ISTAT). The index of actual maternal mortality in Italy is close to data from other European nations but is still above that of North America, corresponding to 11 per 100 000 in 1977 (data from WHO, Geneva, 1981). The most frequent causes of maternal mortality are: hypertension and eclampsia (25%); while deaths due to acute anemia and shock from hemorrhage, uterine rupture, extrauterine pregnancy, embolism from amniotic fluid, fibrinolysis and DIC are actually reduced (less than 20%). Death from infection was extremely rare (4.95%); puerperal tetanus almost disappeared (legal prophylaxis); death from uremia was also reduced to a very low level, thanks to hemodialysis. Pulmonary emboli appear in few cases in women already operated on for cardiopathy, often being discharged after delivery when puerpera at home arbitrarily suspends anticoagulant therapy.

05.41.04

Significance of prenatal intensive care in severe pre-eclampsia, eclampsia in reducing post-Cesarian section maternal morbidity and mortality: Kang, S M, Yang, M H, Woo, B H, Yu, H K, Ahn, J J. Dept. Obstet. and Gyn., Ewha Womans Univ. Hosp., Seoul, Korea

Our data based on 90 cases of severe pre-eclampsia eclampsia who underwent Cesarian section at the Ewha Womans University Hospital over a period of four years (1980 to 1983). A controlled prenatal or pre-operative intensive care with hydralazine and/or magnesium sulfate and supportive therapy was instituted on 39 cases of severe pre-eclampsia eclampsia. This study was compared with 51 cases of severe pre-eclampsia eclampsia lacking intensive care before Cesarian section. The result showed that no serious risk such as post-operative maternal mortality, postpartum eclampsia or oliguria seen in the group given the pre-operative intensive care, while 3.9% cases of postpartum eclampisa, 2% of oliguria, higher rate of wound infection (9.8% vs 5.1%) and 2% of maternal deaths were encountered in the control group lacking the controlled intensive cares for less than 24 hours (six hours on average). The prenatal or pre-operative intensive care especially for the correction of severely impaired hypertensive hepatic, renal function or thrombocytopenic microangiopathic hemolysis are essential if the postsection maternal morbidity and mortality are to be reduced.

05.41.05
Maternal mortality at Maputo Central Hospital: Songane, F F, Bergström, S. Dept. Obstet. and Gyn. (Maternidade), Eduardo Mondlane Univ., Maputo, Mozambique

A major effort was launched during the period 1/1–31/12 1984 in the biggest reference hospital in Mozambique with the intention of elucidating the main causes and characteristics of maternal mortality. During the period there occurred 11,203 deliveries, mainly high risk referrals, in the hospital. A total of 10,769 live-births and 40 maternal deaths occurred, representing a maternal mortality of 371 per 100 000 live-births. This reflects a heavy concentration of referred obstetric high risk cases. A total of 8 (20%) had severe puerperal sepsis, while 7 (18%) were eclamptics. In 24 (60%) there was a cause directly related to pregnancy and in 16 (40%) a cause indirectly related to pregnancy. During the period a total of 70 eclamptics occured, of which 7 died (10%). Maternal and child health is a high priority in Mozambique and the efforts carried out to elucidate mortality determinants in this field are given much attention. The implications of this study on the national level will be discussed.

05.41.06
Socio-economic and cultural factors in maternal mortality: Cekanski, A. IVth Dept. Obstet. and Gyn., Silesian School Med., Katowice, Poland

Retrospective evaluation of the possible influence of socio-economic and cultural factors (SECF) on maternal mortality rate among the 3.5 million population of the industrial region in Poland was undertaken. During nine years (1976–84) 147 mothers died out of the total number of 591,936 live births, i.e. maternal mortality was 25/100,000. The estimated SECF's were as follows: demographic and constitutional status, education and cultural level, environmental factors, housing conditions, occupation, income, psychological problems, nutrition and stimulants. There were 22.4% of pregnants over 35 years of age, multiparous 66%, and grand multiparous 12.9%, unmarried 4.8%. The level of education was as follows: university 10.2%, secondary 21.2%, vocational 21.2%. Housewives (miner's wives) made up 47.6%. Insufficient obstetrical care of pregnants was observed in 38.8% (less than 4 visits), and 16.3% of them have never had any obstetrical care. Living conditions were good in 67.3%, fair in 17% and poor in 6.1%. Unusual obesity was found in 12.6% of cases. 31.3% of the total number died in small municipal hospitals, 45.6% in larger district hospitals, and 21.8% in university clinics. The age over 35 years, multiparity, lack of prenatal obstetrical care, and deliveries in small hospitals may be important causative factors of maternal mortality rate. While analysing mortality rate of pregnants greater consideration should be paid to the SEC factors.

05.42.01
Major components of a rising Cesarian section rate: Poon, I M L, Woo, J S K, Ma, H K. Dept. Obstet. and Gyn., Univ., Hong Kong

The yearly incidence and indications for Cesarian section (CS) at the Hong Kong University Obstetric Hospital – Tsan Yuk – from 1969–83 were analysed along with other relevant obstetric data. The annual deliveries were around 6500. The trend of the CS rate showed a bimodal pattern. It was relatively constant at around 11% up to 1975 but reached 14.9% in 1983. The perinatal mortality rate (PMR) declined from 17.8/1000 to 6.1/1000 over the same period. Statistically significant negative correlation between these two trends was not demonstrated. The main indications for CS were labor abnormalities (LA, 36%) previous CS (30%), breech presentation (Br, 13%) and fetal distress (FD, 11%). All these contributed to the rise of CS rate from 1969–78 (4.0 to 5.2% for LA, 3.2 to 4.0% for previous CS, 1.3 to 2.0% for Br and 1.1 to 1.8% for FD). These trends were similar to those reported elsewhere. However, from 1980–83, LA and in particular cephalopelvic disproportion (CPD) and uterine dysfunction constituted the major factor in the rise of the CS rate (3.2 to 6.3%, 1.1 to 3.6% and 1.1 to 1.9% respectively) whereas CS rate for Br and FD showed only a small rise. That for previous CS remained constant. The predominant increase in CS rate for CPD is not due to a true increase in the incidence of CPD. The mean birth weight of the babies delivered by CS for CPD in 1982 (3516.0 g) was in fact significantly lower than that in 1980 (3665.2 g) (P < 0.05). As increase in diagnosis of CPD is unlikely to lower the PMR significantly, the rising CS rate at our institution does not appear to be well justified and merits a critical reappraisal.

05.42.02
Trial of labor (TOL) and previous Cesarian section: Ballas, S, Ben Shlomo, I, Zohar, S. Dept. Obstet. & Gyn., Rebecca Sieff Hosp., Sefad, Israel

Trial of labor (TOL) after Cesarian section (CS) has been a focus of much attention for the past several years. At some centers it even became the preferable mode of delivery after CS. The following is a five year experience from 1.1.79 to 30.6.84 in the management of women in a subsequent delivery after a single CS at the Obstetric Division of the Rebecca Sieff Government Hospital at Sefad. The records of 470 women on 551 deliveries were reviewed. In 359 cases women were assigned for TOL, of which 311 were delivered vaginally (86.6% of the TOL group and 56.4% of the total group). 371 of the cases studied were the immediate subsequent delivery after the primary CS. 208 of these were assigned for TOL of which 171 (82.2%) were delivered vaginally. There was no significant advantage for those who had had a vaginal delivery prior to the primary CS, to have a subsequent successful vaginal delivery. There was no maternal mortality. In one case, there was a uterine rupture though it did not cause a fetal loss. Comparison of the TOL group with the "No Trial" group revealed no perinatal death due to the mode of delivery. There was no difference in major maternal complications (fever after CS and wound complications excluded). There was no difference in neonatal complications (corrected for IUFD and death due to major malformations). The results are discussed with references to the main contributions published between 1979–1984.

05.42.03
Perinatal effects of Cesarian section in left lateral position (15°) versus supine position: Sanchez, J C, Gallo, M, Llamas, C, Torres, A, Arbues, J. Dept. Obstet. and Gyn., Hosp. Reg. "Carlos Haya", Málaga, Spain
Many authors have pointed out the fetal and maternal hazards caused by the supine hypotension vena cava-compression syndrome during Cesarian section. We have performed in a prospective and controlled study, 306 Cesarian section, with a single fetus in cephalic presentation, 139 in the lateral position with 15° deviation to the left and 167 in a supine position. 56 CS were performed for pathologic recording of FHR, 163 for arrest of labor and 87 for elective indications. We monitored 51 fetuses during Cesarian section from a scalp electrode. The anaesthesia was the same for all cases, with atropine and pentothal. We studied the following features: induction-delivery interval, incision-delivery interval, fetal heart rate, uterine contractility, tears of hysterotomy, Apgar score, acid-base status of newborn, neonatal and maternal morbidity and perinatal mortality. Our results show that the supine position during Cesarian section increased the fetal and maternal morbidity and should be substituted by the lateral position of 15–20° deviation to the left.

05.42.04
Cesarian section: A seven-year experience at a top referral hospital in Bandung, Indonesia: Rono, H, Thouw, J, Sastrawinata, S. Dept. Obstet. and Gyn., Hasan Sadikin Hosp. Padjadjaran Univ., Bandung, Indonesia
The Cesarian rates has been reported as rising in many countries in recent years. This study shows Cesarian section rates, indications, maternal and perinatal mortality at the Hasan Sadikin Hospital, Bandung, a teaching, top referral hospital. During 7 years (1978 through 1984), 2225 Cesarian section were performed out of 23,696 deliveries (9.39%). The Cesarian section rate ranged from 8.17% to 10.76%. Placenta previa, dystocia and transverse lie were the most common indications for Cesarian sections. Perinatal mortality rate ranged from 37.59% to 24.53% and maternal mortality rate between zero to 1.9%. There were 16 maternal deaths related to Cesarian section with sepsis as the major cause of death. This study does not show a definite rise in the Cesarian section rate.

05.42.05
Cesarian-section in a University clinic in Paris between 1977 and 1983: Rates and indications: Poisson-Salomon, A S, Breart, G, Cabrol, D, Chavigny, C, Maillard, F, Sureau, C. I.N.S.E.R.M.-U.149 et Clin. Baudelocque, Paris, France
Among women followed in an University clinic in 1977, 1979, 1981 and 1983. The overall Cesarian section rate was 11.5 in 1977, 17.2 in 1979, 21.1 in 1981 and 15.0 in 1983. The 9.6% increase observed between 1977 and 1981 is mainly attributable to an augmentation of primary Cesarian section between 1977 and 1979, particularly among primiparas. This does not seem to be due to sample variations. More Cesarian sections are performed in cases of hypertension, breech presentation and dystocia. A greater number of previously sectioned women explains part of the increase in the overall rate between 1979 and 1981. An other part is explained by the 18.8% increase in diagnosis of dynamic dystocia. The 6.1% diminution between 1981 and 1983 is mainly due to a decrease in Cesarian section rate among primiparas. These data show that the variations in the overall Cesarian section rate are mainly due to variations in the rate among primiparas. These variations being explained mainly by variations in attitude towards dystocia.

05.42.06
Repeated Cesarian section rate (RCSR) vs success rate in evaluating trial of labor following one previous Cesarian section: Weissman, A, Jakobi, P, Zimmer, E Z, Paldi, E Peretz, B A. Dept. Obstet. & Gyn. "B", Rambam Med. Ctr, Haifa, Israel
The main object of trial of labor (TOL) after previous Cesarian section (C/S) is to reduce the repeated Cesarian section rate (RCSR). In most studies the success rate of TOL was considered as the main index of management efficiency. The success rate relates only to patients allowed TOL, but ignores the patients who were excluded from TOL by different excluding criteria. The indication for the previous C/S determines the probability of vaginal delivery in the subsequent pregnancy. The selection itself for TOL has the greatest influence on the success rate of TOL. We critically examined our 236 patients who were excluded by us from TOL*. A decision analysis was performed to deduce if a change in our management planning might reduce our RCSR. In order to improve our vaginal delivery rate more patients could have been given

TOL, and in some oxytocin might have been used. The patients formerly excluded from TOL are poorer candidates for vaginal delivery, and according to the literature the oxytocin treated groups had a significantly lower success rate than the non-treated patients. Analysis of our data using the above assumptions showed that a reduction of our RCSR from 57% to 41% would also probably lower our present success rate from 83% to 75%. In conclusion we suggest that in assessing different management plans for TOL, the success rate should be accompanied by RCSR. A higher success rate does not necessarily indicate more vaginal deliveries or lower RCSR, the goal of TOL.

*This particular group of patients has never been presented in detail before.

05.42.07
Cesarian section in a Saudi Arabian Hospital: Badawy, A H, Lotfy M. Dr. Fakhry Hosp., Al Khobar, Saudi Arabia
A review of 425 Cesarian sections performed at a Saudi Arabian Hospital in a five-year period (1978–1982 inclusive) is made. These sections were made among 10,970 deliveries in that period. This gives a section rate of 3.9 per cent. The stillbirth rate was 13 per thousand. Emphasis is made on taking into consideration environmental factors when a Cesarian section operation is contemplated.

05.42.08
On a rational operative technique in Cesarian section with Uchida's abdominal retractor, based on over 2,000 cases: Uchida, M, Uchida, H. The Uchida Hosp., Kenroku-motomachi, Kanazawa, Japan
Cesarian section, quite a common operation, may sometimes cause some operative difficulties. 1) After fetus delivery it may be difficult to suture completely the upper and the lower incised edges which are different in thickness each other. To overcome this difficulty the location of the incision site must be carefully selected. 2) The suturing of the incised corners in the uterus tends to be incomplete because of lacerate scars and arterial injuries which are sometimes caused by untheoretical delivery of the fetal head. The way of avoiding this hazard depends on how the incised opening in the uterine wall can be utilized to its full extent, suitable for the size of the fetal head. 3) After being delivered from the uterus, the fetal head, which tends to fall into the abdominal cavity under the pubes, should be delivered smoothly through the abdominal wall. For this purpose a wide operative field should be obtained as close as possible to the pubes. In order to solve all these difficulties the author would like to introduce his operative technique based on over 2000 cases and his specially designed abdominal retractor for Cesarian section.

05.42.09
Suprapubic transverse transrecti muscles incision for obstetrical laparotomy: Horovitz, J, Maugey, B, Gonnet, J M, Fossat, G, Dubecq J P. Dept. Obstet. and Gyn., Maternité B, Hôop. Pellegrin, Bordeaux, France
The Pfannenstiel incision is the most popular lower transverse abdominal incision in France for Cesarian section, this is for cosmetic reasons. Since October 1981 we have used an incision derived from the Maylard incision which is a suprapubic transverse transrectal muscles incision. Our technique is as follows: 1) A cutaneous horizontal incision at the upper limit of the pubic hair is made. 2) The rectus sheath is opened transversely. 3) The rectus muscles are transected with a diathermy coagulating needle, the muscle bellies being subtended by scissor slip under the fascia transversalis. 4) The next step is a transvere incision of the fascia transversalis and the peritoneum. – The closure of the abdominal wound is made thus: 1) A continuous catgut suture of the parietal peritoneum. 2) Then, a continuous suture with polyglycolic acid is made on the anterior abdominal aponeurosis. A drain is left under the sheath. 3) Next, subcutaneous tissue and skin are approximated. Between October 1981 and December 1984 we performed 293 laparotomies for Cesarian section according to this procedure (including ten iterative laparotomies with the same incision). The main complications noted were two big hematomas under the aponeurosis and one eventration.

05.42.10
Myomectomy during abdominal Cesarian section: Erez, S, Benabib, M, Erez, R. Cerrahpaşa Med. Fac., Istanbul Univ. and Bakirköy Soc. Secur. Maternity Hosp., Istanbul, Turkey
A logical and simple method of myomectomy performed during Cesarian section is being presented. The risks of uterine hemorrhage and intestinal obstruction with adhesions were obviated through bilateral ligation of uterine arteries and by covering lesions of extirpated myomata with the amniotic membranes. Sixteen cases underwent this procedure with no early or late postoperative complications.

05.42.11
The subsegmentary Cesarian section: Nitzow, A, Medrea, G, Nitzow, E. Frauenklin., Wöchnerinnenheim, Augsburg
The new surgical technique proposed by the author avoids the hysterotomy, and so the uterine scar, the importance of which is well known in the obstetrical-gynecological pathology. This technique is based on the following points: 1. The bladder is dissected from the uterine segment downwards up to the point, where the anterior vaginal wall is rendered evident. 2. The incision is performed transversely on the anterior vaginal wall, at 0.5–1 cm below the lip of the uterine orifice. Through this incision the fetus with its annexes

will be extracted. 3. The new surgical technique can be used both intraperitoneally and extraperitoneally. 4. The intraperitoneal technique has been successfully used on 80 pregnant women and the extraperitoneal on 16 pregnant women. 5. The postoperative progress was normal in both the technics.

05.42.12
Perinatal mortality and Cesarian section: Wright, E A. Dept. Obstet. and Gyn., Univ., Jos, Nigeria
The experience on perinatal mortality among 757 patients who underwent Cesarian section in Jos University Teaching Hospital serving a high risk urban and rural population in a developing country is presented. During the period studied the Cesarian section rate was 4.4% and during the same period there were 69 stillbirths, 107 deaths during the first week of life giving a perinatal mortality rate of 235.2/1000. The possible factors responsible for this high rate are discussed and suggestions made to improve on this figure.

06.02.01
Occurrence of Fitz-Hugh-Curtis syndrome in acute pelvic inflammatory disease: Yasbek, L, Souza, A Z, Izzo, V M, Tomioka, E, Hegg, R. Gyn. Clin., São Paulo Univ. Med. School, São Paulo, Brazil
Bacteriology and laparoscopy were performed in 30 patients with acute pelvic inflammatory disease (PID) to identify the agents and to grade the tubal damages respectively. Two groups of patients were found: 15 patients with Neisseria Gonorrhoeae positive cultures and 15 with negative cultures from endocervix especimens four (13.3%) patients had clinical findings of Fitz-Hugh-Curtis (F-H-C) syndrome: two of N-Gonorrhoeae positive group and two of negative group. The laparoscopic findings confirmed the diagnosis of F-H-C syndrome showing fibrotic adhesions disposed like "violin strings" between visceral peritoneum and abdominal wall. The study reached the following conclusions: 1. high frequency of F-H-C syndrome among patients with acute PID, 2. normal liver function in those patients, 3. the difficulty in differential diagnosis with other disorders, mainly surgical problems.

06.02.02
Salpingitis – aspects on diagnosis and etiology: Brihmer, C, Kallings*, I, Brundin, J. Karolinska Inst., Danderyd Hosp., Danderyd, *Nat. Bacteriol. Labor., Stockholm, Sweden
Is laparoscopy compulsory for the accurate diagnosis of PID? What is the microbial etiology of PID? In order to confirm a suspected PID, laparoscopy was regularly performed together with directed oviductal culturing in 273 cases during a period of three years at Danderyd Hospital. Laparoscopic findings confirmed PID in 52%. A normal picture was found in 38% although one third of these had a cervicitis. The rest, 9%, suffered from something else. Cases of laparoscopically verified PID showed positive cervical culture in 94% as follows: Chlamydia trachomatis 50%, Bacteroides species 36%, Neisseria gonorrhoeae 23%. Abdominal culture from the fimbrial os was positive in 24%, when directed towards Chlamydia trachomatis 9%, Bacteroides species 7%, Neisseria gonorrhoeae 1%. Clinical data and laboratory tests showed no difference in the two groups. However, in the non-PID group 21% were judged as a clear case of PID by experienced gynecologists versus 30% in laparoscopically verified PID. Palpable masses were found by bimanual examination in 29% of the non-PID group versus 40% in the PID group. Serology yielded 52% positive CT in the PID group. Culture negative and serology positive were 21% i.e. CT is responsible for 48–69% of the PID cases in our region. Complications to PID: Five cases of perihepatitis of which cases three were CT positive; five cases if periappendicitis three CT positive, two were operated upon. PAD showed serositis, two cases of ileus both CT positive. Conclusion: Direct visual tubal examination is compulsory for the safe diagnosis of PID. Chlamydia trachomatis and Bacteroides species are the main cause of PID.

06.02.03
Plasma C-reactive protein levels (CRP) in diagnosis of adnexitis: Krämer, M, Schmidt-Rhode, P, Schulz, K D, Prinz, H, Sturm, G, Künzig, H J. Dept. Obstet. and Gyn., Univ., Marburg
The diagnosis of an adnexitis in a clinical workday is often difficult, since the measurement of standard laboratory parameters such as ESR, leucocytes and temperature in combination with the findings of clinical examinations shows a high percentage of false positive and negative results in patients later on checked up by laparoscopy. This study investigates the validity of simultaneous assessments of several acute-phase proteins, especially C-reative protein (CRP), for detection of genital tract infections. Quantitative determinations of CRP and other proteins were performed by means of laser nephelometric method using Behring BLN and compared to standard laboratory parameters. All patients with doubtful findings were checked up by laparoscopy. Until now about 100 patients have entered the study. Patients with established adnexitis (group 1) showed elevated values of ESR in 81%, of temperature in 55% and of leucocytes in 52% of the cases. In the same collective CRP demonstrated increased plasma concentrations in 100%. The other acute-phase proteins were positive in 88% (haptoglobin) and in 76% (orosomucoid). Patients in which we were able to exclude an acute infection disease of genital tract (group 2), in all cases CRP was found in the normal range. On the other hand we observed false positive results of ESR in 50%, of temperature in 39% and of leucocytes in 12%. Furthermore individual follows-up under antibiotic treatment will be demonstrated. In conclusion we can state, that plasma determination of CRP is a useful parameter for diagnosis and monitoring of infections of the genital tract.

06.02.04

Laparoscopic and endometrial sampling in the diagnosis of acute pelvic inflammatory disease: Heinonen, P K, Teisala, K, Punnonen, R, Aine, R, Lehtinen, M, Miettinen, A, Grönroos, P, Paavonen, J. Univ. Centr. Hosp. and Univ., Tampere, Finland

We studied the manifestations and microbiologic correlates of upper genital tract infection among 45 women with suspected pelvic inflammatory disease (PID) and 11 controls. Laparoscopy confirmed salpingitis in 30 (67%) cases, and endometrial biopsy confirmed plasma cell endometritis in 31 (69%) cases. Among the 26 cases with endometritis and salpingitis, one or more micro-organisms were isolated from the fallopian tubes of 12 (46%), and from the peritoneal cavity of nine (35%), vs. none and one (9%), respectively, among the ten cases who had neither endometritis nor salpingitis, and one (9%) and one (9%) among the 11 control women. One or more organisms were isolated from the endometrium of 22 (71%) of the 31 cases with endometritis vs. 12 (57%) of the 21 women without endometritis. Chlamydia trachomatis was the most common organism isolated from the uterine cavity (39%) or fallopian tubes (13%) of women with endometritis and salpingitis. This study demonstrates that nonpuerperal endometritis is an entity associated with PID, most likely as an intermediate stage between cervicitis and salpingitis.

06.02.05

Acute pelvic inflammatory disease. Histopathology and bacteriology of endometrium: Kesselring, G C, Tomioka, E, Souza, A Z, Czeresnia, C E, Salvatore, C A. Gyn. Clin., São Paulo Univ. Med. School, São Paulo, Brazil

The authors have studied 20 patients with acute pelvic inflammatory disease. Bacteriology and histology of endometrium were examined in the acute phase and fifteen days after antibiotic treatment. In the acute phase, aerobic germs were present in 13 (65%) patients, anaerobic in 10 (50%) and 3 (15%) patients carried Chlamydia trachomatis. After antibiotic treatment, 4 (20%) cases remained carring aerobics and 5 (25%) cases anaerobics. Chlamydia trachomatis was abolished in those positive cases. Before treatment, acute endometritis was present in 8 (40%) patients, chronic endometritis in 4 (20%) and chronic endometritis with an acute episode in 3 (15%) patients. After antibiotic treatment 1 (5%) case remained still had an acute endometritis, 5 (20%) cases chronic endometritis and one (5%) case chronic endometritis with an acute episode.

06.02.06

The effect of minocycline in acute pelvic inflammatory disease: Tomioka, E, Souza, A Z, Kesselring, G, Czeresnia, C E, Salvatore, C A. Gyn. Clin., São Paulo Univ. Med. School, São Paulo, Brazil

The microbiologic flora and the therapeutic results of minocycline were determined in 20 patients with mild or moderate acute pelvic inflammatory disease. The diagnosis was confirmed and graded by laparoscopy. All cultures were obtained from the vagina and endocervix. Chlamydia trachomatis (McCoy cells line culture), Neisseria gonorrhoeae, Ureaplasma urealyticum and Mycoplasma hominis were identified from 9 (45%), 7 (35.0%), 13 (65.0%) and 2 (10.0%) patients, respectively. Minocycline 300 mg p.o., day 1, plus 100 mg twice daily p.o., for 14 days, was the schedule selected in this trial. Control bacteriologic data were systematically obtained on the 15th day. The main results were: 1. One (5.0%) patient with Fitz-Hugh-Curtis syndrome had Neisseria gonorrhoeae recovered from endocervix. 2. Clinical improvement was observed in 19 (95.0%) patients after 72 hours treatment. 3. None of the patients showed a positive test to Neisseria gonorrhoeae on the 15th day. 4. Six (66.8%) of initial Chlamydia trachomatis positive cases were negative on the 15th day.

06.02.07

Management inflammatory pelvic disease: Czeresnia, C E, Aguiar, L, Hegg, R, Salvatore, C A. Gyn. Clin., Univ. of São Paulo Med. School, São Paulo, Brazil

Current views on the microbiological flora in acute pelvic inflammatory disease (PID) are widely divergent, partly because of epidemiologic and clinical differences in various studies. We examined 20 in-patients with symptoms and signs of PID. C. trachomatis has been isolated from the cervix in 50% of the patients, N.gonorrhoeae in 40%, U.urealyticum in 65%, and Mycoplasma sp. in 10% of them. In 17 patients analysed, three had C.trachomatis in the endometrium, and two of these did not have it in the cervix. A possible change in the aerobic and anaerobic bacteria of the cervix and vagina was observed, indicating a tendency to a more virulent flora in PID. Clinical evaluation showed no difference between the groups C.trachomatis positive and negative, N.gonorrhoeae positive and negative in relation to: the intensity of the disease; the interval between last menstrual period and the onset of symptoms; time interval between symptoms and medical care and WBC, ESR. The N.gonorrhoeae group tended to be more symptomatic. Laparoscopy had been done in 18 patients, and had shown that clinical diagnosis is not accurate in relating to PID intensity. Overall, the study indicates that in our population, C.trachomatis, N.gonorrhoeae, U.urealyticum and Mycoplasm sp. are bacteria commonly identified in acute pelvic inflammatory disease, emphasizing the need to use the antibiotics for the treatment of these etiological agents.

06.02.08

The prevalence of endocervical Neisseria gonorrhea (N. G.) and Chlamydia trachomatis (C. T.) in 60 PID patients in Amsterdam: Schoot, J T M van der, Bleker, O P. Onze Lieve Vrouwe Gasthuis, Amsterdam, The Netherlands

Sixty PID patients in hospital were examined by bacteriologic and direct immunofluorescent techniques. In 8(%) N. G. was found, in 33(%) C. T. and in 17(%) both N. G. and C. T., which means that in total 58(%) a sexually transmitted disease was found to be associated with PID. All 60 patients fulfilled at least the first four of the following diagnostic criteria: 1. history of abdominal pain, 2. lower abdominal tenderness, 3. cervical motion tenderness, 4. adnexal tenderness, 5. fever $> 100.4°$ F ($38°$ C), 6. leucocyte count $> 10.5/mm^3$, 7. elevated ESR (> 20 mm/hr). In ten patients who fulfilled only the first four criteria, 0% N. G. and 50% C. T. was found. In 50 patients who fulfilled at least five criteria 20% N. G., 20% C. T. and 10% N.G. + C. T. was found. In 25 patients who fulfilled all criteria these percentages were respectively 32%, 8% and 12%. No correlation was found between the specific etiologic agent of PID and the method of contraception. All patients were treated with a tetracyclin-metronidazol regimen, which was not adequate in only two cases associated with tetracycline resistant N. G. – Conclusions: 1. All PID patients should be examined for not only N. G. but C. T. as well. 2. The primary treatment of PID patients should aim for treatment of both N. G. and C. T. (and possible associated anaerobes). 3. The possibility of a sexually transmitted cause of PID should always be considered and examination/treatment of contacts is important. 4. Clinically mild forms of PID are more often associated with C. T., clinically severe forms with N. G.

06.02.09

Moxalactam in gynecological and obstetrical infections: Kalachanis, J, Tsalikis, T, Tambakoudis, P, Mantalenakis, S. Dept. Obstet. and Gyn., Aristotelian Univ., Agia Sophia Hosp., Thessaloniki, Greece

A therapeutic trial was made using moxalactam a broad-spectrum b-lactam antibiotic in order to evaluate the effect on the treatment of the female genital tract infections. Twenty-three patients suffering from puerperal endometritis and acute or chronic pelvic infections were treated with 4 g of moxalactam daily for five consecutive days. Speciments for culture were taken from the blood, the endometrium, uterine and vaginal discharge, pus of salpingo-ovarian abscess, from the pouch of Douglas and from the abdominal drainage. Pathogens were isolated in 18 cases (78.2%). Gram negative pathogens were found in 17 cases (73.9%) and anaerobics in 6 cases (33.3%). In two cases of infection caused by Pseudomonas aeruginosa, the pathogens were very resistant in one case and quite sensitive to the other case. Satisfactory results were obtained from the administration of moxalactam in 21 of a total 23 cases (91.3%). Failure was noticed in one case while the other one relapsed after the completion of the treatment. In three patients a slight prolongation of the prothrombin time was observed without any hemorrhagic manifestation. In two cases a slight temporary elevation of transaminases was recorded. As concluded from the study moxalactam in individual doses might be proved very effective without serious side-effects for the treatment of moderate to severe gynecological and obstetrical infections.

06.02.10

Natural defenses and their role in the prevention of gynecologic infectious diseases: Tsirulnikov, M S. Port-Royal Univ. Clin., Paris, France

Clinicians throughout the world are observing and questioning an increase of infections in the female genital tract, in particular salpingitis. This phenomenon is being observed, in spite of the fact that in all of the countries were this is occurring, women benefit from better gynecologic care and are better trained to detect early signs and symptoms. In addition, numerous diagnostic and therapeutic methods are available and widely diffused. To clarify this paradoxical situation we would like to postulate the following hypothesis: are we not overlooking the system of natural defenses? A survey of the mechanism of these anatomical, histological and biological barriers leads us to set forth the possible causes of the failure. Technological advances such as electron microscopy provide a greater understanding of the functional synergy between mucosal and ciliary cells, that assures a natural cleansing role and acts as a barrier to all types of attacks. Certain behaviours and pathologic states can diminish the effectiveness of these barriers by deteriorating the endocervical mucosa. For example: microbial, viral, mycoplasmic, Chlamidiae infections whose detection and treatment are not as simple as is often presented; local trauma (e. g. related to inappropriate obstetric manipulation) and its possible sequelae on the fibrous tissues; the continuous presence of the IUD thread in the endocervix, an ever-present foreign body which is in opposition to the physiologic closure vis-à-vis ascending infections.

06.02.11

The treatment of acute infections of the minor pelvis with particular respect to anaerobic pathogens: Stoeger, H*, Mittermayer, H**, Tews, G*. *Allgemein. Krankenh., Linz, Gyn.-Geburtshilfl. Abt.; **Inst. Mikrobiol. and Hyg., Krankenh. der Elisabethinen, Linz, Austria

Twenty menstruated Caucasian women suffering from acute infections of the pelvis were examined and treated. Predominant diseases were: pelvic peritonitis, purulent salpingitis and septic endometritis. Parameters for diagnosis were: clinical assessment, grade of inflammation, secretion of the cervix and laparoscopy. Samples for bacteriological examinations were taken from the secretion of the cervix, by laparoscopy from the Fallopian tube or from the focus of the inflammation. Cultures were assessed for the presence and/or growth of aerobic and anaerobic pathogens. Bacteria most frequently isolated were: E. coli, Streptococcus viridans and beta-hemolytic Streptococci, Staphylococci, Neisseria gonorrhoeae, Bacteriodes melanino-genicus and Gardarella vaginalis. Antibiotic therapy was given by using Ticarclav 5.2 g as short infusion t. i. d. in 100 ml aqueous solution. (Ticarclav is a combination of 5000 mg Ticarcillin plus 200 mg Clavulanic acid.) Mean duration of treatment was 5–6 days. No significant side-effects or allergic reactions were noted. With all patients symptoms were improved or clinical cure was achieved. The clinical and microbiological results are discussed.

06.02.12

Ovulation disturbances in patients with previous PID: Hamilton, C J D M, Evers, J L H, Hoogland, H J, Haan, J de. St. Annadal Hosp., Univ. of Limburg, Maastricht, The Netherlands

Failure of fertility microsurgery is usually attributed to irreversible endosalpingeal destruction, recurrent adhesion formation or progressive inflammatory disease. Ovarian dysfunction has hardly been taken into account. In order to study the late consequences of PID on ovarian function we examined a group of 25 infertile patients with, laparoscopically proven, sequelae of a previous PID. Both ultrasound and hormonal analysis were applied to investigate ovarian follicle development. A failure of the follicle to rupture, despite signs of luteinization, was observed in 52% of the patients. In the patients, who showed an unruptured follicle in one or more cycles, the occurrence rate was even 88%. The mean mid-luteal progesteron level in these aberrant cycles was significantly lower than in normal ovulatory cycles ($p < 0.01$). The length of the luteal phase was not affected. Because microsurgical adhesiolysis did not seem to influence the incidence of the ovulation disorder, causes other than pure mechanical ones must be held responsable for the failure of the follicle rupture.

06.03.01

Metabolic effects of two triphasic oral contraceptives: Gaspard, U J, Lepot, M A, Gillian D, Luyckx, A S, Buret, J, Sulon, J. Dept. Obstet. and Gyn., Univ., Liège, Belgium

The low-dose combined triphasic oral contraceptive (OC) Trigynon containing ethinylestradiol and levo-norgestrel was compared to a new triphasic OC (Trigestoden) containing the same dose of EE and a 14% smaller dose of a new progestogen, gestoden (Δ15-levonorgestrel) in a prospective randomized study conducted in two clinically and metabolically comparable groups of 19 and 12 healthy young female volunteers, respectively, for a period of 6 months. After 6 months of treatment, glucose tolerance appreciated by OGTT was unchanged while insulin levels were slightly increased under both OCs. No clinically significant change in lipid and lipoprotein plasma concentrations was recorded during treatment: triglycerides, VLDL-cholesterol, apolipoprotein AI and apolipoprotein B were slightly but significantly increased after six months of use of Trigynon, while total-, free- and LDL-cholesterol were decreased and apoB increased during Trigestoden utilization. HDL-chol was transiently but significantly increased by both OCs and the important ratios HDL chol/total chol, LDL chol/HDL chol, Apo AI/Apo B were unchanged. Total and conjugated bilirubin, ALAT and OCT levels were unchanged whereas alkaline phosphatase and ASAT were significantly decreased after six months of use of both OCs. Total and free testosterone levels were decreased by both drugs, but significantly more by Trigestoden. Levels of carrier proteins ceruloplasmin and transcortin were doubled after six months' use of both OCs. Collectively, these preliminary results indicate only very restricted metabolic repercussions and slight estrogenic dominance of both triphasic formulations studied.

06.03.02

The endometrial effect of a new triphasic oral contraceptive (SH D 415 G): Brosens, I A, Degroote, A. Univ., Leuven, Belgium

The endometrial effect of a triphasic oral contraceptive with a new progestogen (Δ15-levonorgestrel, gestoden) was investigated in 20 women. The new pill is composed of: 6 tablets of 30 y ethinyl-estradiol and 50 y gestoden, 5 tablets of 40 y ethinyl-estradiol and 70 y gestoden and 10 tablets of 30 y ethinyl-estradiol and 100 y gestoden. Twenty-five biopsies were obtained using a Novak-curette on different days of the cycle after two to ten months of treatment. The cycle control was excellent in all patients. Breakthrough bleeding and spotting occurred in respectively 1.2% and 0.6% of the cycles. The amount of endometrial tissue obtained at biopsy was scanty in all patients. Ovulation was effectively inhibited in all patients. The first series of tablets resulted in inhibition of proliferation and early secretory activity of the glandular epithelium. During the second series of tablets the endometrium remained hypoplastic, but special secretory activity was seen in the glands. During the third series of tablets glandular hypoplasia and secretory exhaustion were prominent. At the end of the cycle stromal pseudodecidualisation was seen. Sinusoid formation was not prominent. It is concluded that the new oral contraceptive has a pronounced inhibitory effect on the endometrium. It is suggested that the correlation between the excellent cycle control of this low-dose oral contraceptive and the absence of vascular sinusoid formation during the treatment should be further investigated.

06.03.03

A Canadian multi-centred clinical trial of ethinyl estradiol-norgestrel tri-phasic oral contraceptive (Triphasil):
Yuzpe, A A. Dept. Obstet. and Gyn., Univ. of Western Ontario, London, Canada
Five hundred and forty-three women were enrolled in ten participating centres. Pertinent data relative to various events are available for a total of 6383 treatment cycles. Subjects included first time oral contraceptive users, switchers from other preparations, post-abortal subjects and postpartum women. No method failure pregnancies were encountered. Breakthrough bleeding after the first three cycles of treatment in first time users was 9.9% of cycles where no tablets were missed, and double (19.6%) wen tablets were missed. When no tablets were missed, only 5.5% of the cycles had breakthrough bleeding at 24 months. Spotting among new starters occurred with equal frequency among those who missed and those who did not miss tablets (12.3% and 12.7%, respectively). After 24 months of treatment, the incidence of spotting was 3.8% of cycles when not tablets were missed and 12.2% of cycles when tablets had been missed. Two thirds of women reported no significant weight change, whereas the remaining one third complained of either a weight gain or weight loss (± 5 lb) with equal frequency. The incidence of simple headache, breast swelling and discomfort, dysmenorrhea, nausea and vomiting, GI upset and vaginal discharge was reduced in all users compared to pre-trial complaints. Acne improved in 80% of those who had this complaint prior to treatment (n = 36). The tri-phasic oral contraceptive preparation Triphasil is a well accepted, well tolerated oral contraceptive. It represents a significant reduction in the total progestin component compared to other norgestrel containing oral contraceptives.

06.03.04

Triphasic (Triquilar) oral contraceptive used in Indian women: Mehta, K, Krishnamoorthy, L, Karath, R A.
B.A.R.C. Hosp., Bombay, India
Triphasic (Triquilar) oral contraceptive pill was used in 16 cases, between the ages of 20 to 30 years and parity of one to two children, for the purpose of family planning in B.A.R.C. Hospital, Bombay, India. Triquilar has 6 dragees containing levonorgestrel 0.05 mg/ethinylestradiol 0.04 mg, 5 dragees of levonorgestrel 0.075 mg/ethinylestradiol 0.04 mg, 10 dragees of levonorgestrel 0.125 mg and ethinylestradiol 0.03 mg. In all the cases a full history was taken. Cases unsuitable for oral pills were excluded. Each case had full check-up, weight, B. P., etc., were recorded. Radio-immunological estimation of the serum levels of luteinizing hormone (LH), follicle-stimulating hormone (FSH), serum cholestrerol, (HDL) and endometrial biopsies were done in six cases. Purpose of this study is to observe and to investigate the mode of action of the triphasic pill as it is a new generation oral pill. We found it acts by inhibition of ovulation. It has the greatest contraceptive safety and fewest side-effects. This study was started on 1. 9. 1984. So far we have had no failures.

06.03.05

Comparative effects with monophasic desogestrel plus EE and triphasic levonorgestrel plus EE on lipid and carbohydrate metabolism: Kloosterboer, H J*, Wayen, R G A van**, Ende, A van der**. *Organon Sci.
Develop. Group, Oss; **Stichting Klinisch Metabool Onderzoek, Amsterdam, The Netherlands
In this comparative study one group ov 16 young healthy female volunteers received the monophasic preparation desogestrel plus EE (21 × 150/30) and a second group of 18 women received the triphasic preparation levonorgestrel plus EE (6 × 50/30; 5 × 75/40; 10 × 125/30) for six cycles. Blood samples were taken before treatment and after three and six treatment cycles. In addition to the estimation of various lipid parameters in serum (cholesterol, triglycerides, phospholipids, apolipoproteins A-1 and B, HDL-cholesterol) we separated the lipoprotein particles, e. g. VLDL, LDL and HDL subfractions, from fresh plasma in a density gradient by ultracentrifugation. Furthermore fasting glucose, fasting insulin and glycosylated proteins were estimated. Statistical differences between the groups were determined by an anlysis of covariance. HDL-cholesterol, HDL-2 cholesterol, HDL-2 phospholipids and the ratio apolipoprotein A-1 to apolipoprotein B were significantly higher in the desogestrel plus EE group than in the levonorgestrel plus EE group after three and six treatment cycles. Apolipoprotein A-1 and HDL-3 phospholipids were only higher in the desogestrel plus EE group after six treatment cycles. No differences between the group were observed for the other variables studies. In view of the inverse correlation between HDL-2 and cardiovascular disease it can be concluded that the desogestrel plus EE preparation has a favourable lipid profile.

06.03.06

Clinical and metabolic study of the triphasic oral contraceptive: Virutamasen, P, Tangkeow, P, Nitichai, Y, Tangusaha, C. Dept. Obstet. and Gyn., Fac. Med., Chulalongkorn Univ., Bangkok, Thailand
One hundred and forty healthy Thai women, mean aged 25.3 years, were recruited for clinical and metabolic study. 1288 completed cycles were evaluated of the efficacy and the clinical side-effects. The mean treatment cycles were 9.2. No pregnancy occurred during the observation period. At one year follow-up, 55.8% of the subjects had no change in body weight (± 2 kg). The most common side-effects were nausea/vomiting, headaches and irregular bleeding (5.5%). Nineteen per cent of the subjects dropped out due to medical reasons and 10.2% were lost to follow-up. An oral glucose tolerance test (OGTT 1 gm/kg/body wt) was conducted in 28 volunteers, two cases were found to be abnormal OGTT. No significant alterations of liver function tests except alkaline phosphatase which was significantly decreased.

A study of lipid metabolism was performed in twenty subjects, no significant alterations of lipoprotein fractions were found during the observation period. It was concluded that triphasic oral contraceptives was highly effective, fewer side-effects, may cause transient glucose tolerance test. No changes of lipoprotein fractions was observed.

06.03.07

Absence of lipoprotein changes during treatment with cyproterone acetate: Tikkanen, M J, Kuusi, T, Nikkilä, E A, Sipinen, S. 3rd Dept. Med., Univ., Helsinki, Finland

Previous studies have established that progestins with androgenic properties decrease serum HDL cholesterol. The lipid metabolic effects of an antiandrogenic progestin, cyproterone acetate (CA) was studied in 13 menstruating women. CA (5 mg/day) was administered on days 15–28 of the cycle. Laboratory examinations were carried out before treatment and on day 28. Cholesterol values (mmol/l) in the HDL fraction did not change:

	HDL	HDL-2	HDL-3
Pretreatnebt	1.63 ± 0.43	1.03 ± 0.43	0.60 ± 0.28
Cyproterone	1.59 ± 0.35	0.94 ± 0.33	0.65 ± 0.16

Postheparin plasma hepatic lipase is increased by androgen and is therefore a sensitive indicator of progestin androgenicity (*M. J. Tikkanen* et al., Atherosclerosis **40**, 365, 1981). Pretreatment hepatic lipase activity ($15.9 \pm 3.5 \mu$mol FFA/h per ml) did not differ from the posttreatment value (16.1 ± 5.1). Nor did CA treatment cause any changes in total serum cholesterol, triglycerides, very low density or low density lipoproteins. Thus therapy with CA 5 mg/day was not associated with any lipoprotein alterations. The absence of HDL cholesterol lowering, and the lack of hepatic lipase stimulation by CA both reflect the nonandrogenic properties of this progestin.

06.03.08

Effects on serum lipoproteins of cyproterone acetate (CPA) administered alone and in combination with ethinyl estradiol (EE): Lindberg, U-B, Crona, N, Enk, L, Samsioe, G, Silfverstolpe, G. Dept. Obstet. and Gyn., Sahlgren's Hosp., Univ., Göteborg, Sweden

CPA is a 17-hydroxyprogesterone derivative, with certain anti-androgenic effects, which have been successfully exploited clinically. Young oophorectomized women (n = 21) have been engaged in a study with the following design: after four weeks without any medications all patients were given CPA orally 2 mg/day for four weeks. After this period nine patients were given 35 μg of EE and the other 12 patients were given 50 μg of EE added to their CPA dose for 12 weeks after which time there was a cross-over. Before treatment and after each period total and free cholesterol (TC, FC), phospholipids (PL) and triglycerides (TG) were analysed in serum and in the ultracentrifugally isolated lipoprotein fractions, very low-density lipoproteins (VLDL), low-density lipoproteins (LDL) and high-density lipoproteins (HDL). CPA, when administered alone did not influence the lipid components within VLDL or LDL, but there was a modest decrease in the free cholesterol and phospholipid content of HDL. The modest decrease in HDL lipids induced by CPA is not a common finding after the administration of low oral doses of 17-hydroxy-progesterone derivatives. The overall impression, however, is that CPA is rather inert in its effect on lipoprotein metabolism in this low dose. The two studied EE – CPA regimens surprisingly did not induce effects on lipoprotein lipids typical of estrogen dominated oral contraceptives.

06.03.09

Ultrasonographic and biochemical investigations under long-term therapy with cyproterone acatate (CA): Kaiser, E, Gruner, H-J. Dept. Gyn. Endocr. and Gastroent., Dtsch. Klin. Diagn., Wiesbaden

Since the introduction of oral contraceptives, there has been a drastic rise of benign and malignant liver tumors. Besides hormonal contraception, treatment of endometriosis, mastophathy and premenstrual syndrome, a long-term therapy in androgenization might also induce liver tumors. 77 patients with moderately severe to severe androgenization manifestions and raised levels of androgens in the blood had been treated over three to eleven years with continuous or reverse cyclic treatment with 100 mg CA. Besides determination of the androgens testosterone, DHEA-S and androstendione, the liver and lipid metabolism parameters were determined and ultrasonography of the liver was carried out. Whereas the biochemical parameters under long-term CA therapy undergo pathological alterations which were reversible only in occasional cases, a moderate fatty degeneration of the liver parenchyma but no liver tumors could be demonstrated ultrasonographically.

06.03.10

Evaluation of the efficacy of a new oral contraceptive drug in hyperandrogenic women: Cagnazzo, G, Fanizza, G, Caradonna, G. 1st Obstet. and Gyn. Clin., Univ. Bari, Italy

A longitudinal study has been carried out on 50 women, age between 15 and 34 years, all of them with signs of hyperandrogenism (acne, seborrhea, hirsutism). Before the treatment, the patients had a gynecological examination, pelvic ultrasonography, vaginal cytology and FSH, LH, PRL, E2, P, T DEAS, cortisol, androstenedione, SHBG, albumin, E1, R.I.A. All the women were treated, in a double-blind study for 21 days of nine consecutive cycles, with 0.035 mg E.E. + 2 mg C.P.A. and 0.05 mg E.E. + 2 mg C.P.A. Follow-up examinations were made after 3, 6, 9 months of treatment. The results showed that both combinations were effective in treating the signs of hyperandrogenism. The pill containing a smaller amount of estrogens (0.035 mg) gave fewer side-effects such as nausea, breast tension, weight gain. Both the combinations proved effective in contraception; no pregnancy was recorded during the treatment period.

06.03.11

Neo-Eunomin, a new hormonal contraceptive in women with androgenization of the skin: Beckmann, R, Kaiser, E, Durra, S. Dept. Clin. Res., Grünenthal GmbH, Aachen and Gyn. Endocr., Dtsch. Klin. Diagn., Wiesbaden

The positive experience in the treatment of androgenization already obtained with the sequential preparation Eunomin gave rise to the development of Neo-Eunomin. By administration of the antiandrogenically active progestagen chlormadinone acetate in two dose levels over the entire cycle and a reduction of the estrogen dose, this preparation has become even more effective. The effect of Neo-Eunomin on androgenization was investigated in a long-term trial covering 165 patients over 3379 cycles. Acne, seborrhea and alopecia showed clear improvement after a maximum of six months of treatment, and in many cases a cure was achieved after 12 months of therapy. In the treatment of hirsutism the drug was less effective. In a further study Neo-Eunomin was compared with a contraceptive containing a nor-testosterone derivative (Conceplan 21). Neo-Eunomin convincingly showed greater efficacy in the treatment of androgenization of the skin than the comparable preparation.

06.04.01

Comparison of cyclophosphamide and cisplatin versus hexamethylmelamine, cyclophosphamide, doxorubicin, cisplatin in combination as initial chemotherapy for stage III and IV ovarian carcinomas: Malkasian, G D, Edmonson, J H, Podratz, K C, Jefferies, J A, Fleming, T R, et al. North Centr. Ca Treatm. Group and Mayo Clin., Rochester, MN, USA

Among 187 women with stage III and IV ovarian carcinoma who participated in this comparative clinical trial, 182 were eligible for analysis. Of these, 89 received monthly treatment with CP (cyclophosphamide 1 g/m^2 plus cisplatin 60 mg/m^2) and 93 received HCAP (hexamethylmelamine 150 mg/m^2 × 7 cyclophosphamide 400 mg/m^2, doxorubicin 30 mg/m^2, and cisplatin 60 mg/m^2). All treatment was administered i. v. on day one of each monthly treatment cycle except oral hexamethylmelamine on days 2–8. With median follow-up time of 17.5 months survival curves for the two treatment groups were almost identical, as were their times to progression (estimated median survival 24 months – *Kaplan-Meier*). Women under 50 were surviving longer than older women (p = .03). Those with well differentiated tumors survived longer than patients whose tumors were moderately or poorly differentiated (p = .04). Fully ambulatory patients survived longer than those with some impairment of activity (p = .02). Extent of residual disease (p = .005) also was predictive of survival. Women with serous adenocarcinomas have survived longer than those with the less common histologic types considered together (p = .0005). Results of post-treatment laparotomies have been equal for the two treatment groups according to a preliminary analysis. Toxic effects of the two regimens have been similar except for more frequent, more severe, and earlier neurotoxicity among HCAP treated patients. CP has the better therapeutic index.

06.04.02

Treatment of relapsing ovarian cancer patients with combined recombinant human interferon α_2 and doxorubicin: Welander, C E, Homesley, H D, Spiegel, R J. Bowman Gray School Med., Wake Forest Univ., Winston-Salem, NC, USA

Although responses of advanced ovarian cancer patients have improved with cisplatin containing chemotherapy regimens, response duration and median survival remain < 2 yrs., with cures seen only rarely. No clearly superior regimen of salvage therapy for relapsing patients has been identified. *In vitro* data (Proc. ASCO **2**, 42, 1983) and human tumor xenograft studies (Can. Res. **44**, 904, 1984) have shown increased cytotoxic activity when recombinant human interferon α_2 (rIFNα_2) (Schering Corp.) is tested in combination with doxorubicin (DOX). Based upon this laboratory observation, a clinical trial has been initiated using combined rIFNα_2 and DOX, administered to patients with recurrent ovarian carcinoma who have failed primary therapy. They receive 10 mil IU/m^2 IM followed by 10 mil IU/m^2 i. v. over 30 min. A two-hour i. v. infusion of DOX follows. Three induction treatments are given one week apart. Two weeks later response evaluation is done, adding maintenance therapy every two weeks for patients showing stabel disease or any degree of clinical response. Twenty evaluable patients have been treated with this regimen, with partial responses seen in 6/20 and a complete clinical response in 1/20 (total responders 7/20, 35%). The regimen is well tolerated with minimal hematologic toxicity and no cardiac toxicity. The observed clinical efficacy is being studied further.

06.04.03

Cis-DDP and hexamethylmelamine (HMM) chemotherapy in advanced ovarian cancer refractory to initial chemotherapy: Meerpohl, H G. Pohl, J. Dept. Obstet. and Gyn., Univ., Freiburg

Second-line chemotherapy-regimens containing cis-DDP have recently been shown to have substantial activity also in heavily pretreated ovarian cancer patients. In the present phase II study 16 patients with measurable or evaluable epithelial ovarian cancer FIGO stage III or IV were included. All patients had received prior chemotherapy including alkylating agents, adriamycin and vincristine. Four patients had received induction chemotherapy with CP (1) or CAP (3). None had received radiotherapy. The regimen consisted of cis-DDP (75 mg/m^2) on day 1 and HMM (200 mg/m^2 p. os) on day 4--17. Dose modification depended on hematologic toxicity. In one patient a complete remission (CR) was observed lasting more than 17 months. Two patients had partial response (7 and 12 months) and four patients stable disease. Nine patients had progressive disease. The average duration of response was 8.1 months. Sixty-six courses of therapy were associated with serious toxic side-effects in eight instances. GI-toxicity was not included. These results indicate, that cis-DDP/HMM is a toxic regimen with modest activity in patients with previously treated advanced ovarian cancer. New approaches will be necessary to improve the poor prognosis of these patients.

06.04.04

Treatment of advanced ovarian carcinoma with cisplatin (DDP), cyclophosphamide (CPM), and adriamycin (AD) associated with medroxyprogesterone acetate (MPA): Pérez-López, F R. Dept. Obstet. and Gyn., Univ. of Zaragoza Fac. Med., Zaragoza, Spain

Women with advanced irremovable bulky and histologically proved ovarian cancer were treated with DDP (50 mg/m^2), CPM (500 mg/m^2), and AD (50 mg/m^2), administered on day 1 every four weeks intravenously for eight cycles. The patients also received 1000 mg MPA i. m. daily/30 days, and later the same dose twice weekly to complete one year. Eligibility was restricted to FIGO stage III or IV with unresectable residual masses at the start of chemotherapy, and a very low Karnofsky performance status (KPS) (mostly 10–20%). All patients were to exhibit normal BUN and creatinine, and normal leucocyte and platelet counts. AD was eliminated if ECG abnormalities were present. Complete (disappearance of all measurable lesions) and partial (50% or more reduction of all measurable lesions) responses occurred in all women, and KPS increased to 80–100%. Removal of residual tumor at a second laparotomy was possible in some cases. Toxicity of the regimen was mild to moderate and there were minor side-effects related to MPA. It can be concluded that the treatment substantially improves the rate of objective response as well as the quality of these responses.

06.04.05

Cisplatin, adriamycin, cyclophosphamide (PAC) or fluorouracil, adriamycin, cyclophosphamide (FAC) in ovarian cancer (randomized cooperative Berlin trial): Mayr, A C, Imholz, G, Schmoranz, W, Grüneisen, A, Hindenburg, H J, Karger, N, Maassen, V, Pschyrembel, I, Suchy, B R. Ovarian Tumor Study Group, Tumorzentrum, Berlin

From 07/80 to 01/84 the response to PAC (P-60 mg/m^2 + A-30 mg/m^2 + C-300 mg/m^2 q 21 d × 10 cycles) or FAC (F-500 mg/m^2 + A-50 mg/m^2 + C-500 mg/m^2 q 21 d × 10 cycles) was evaluated by randomized trial. 113 of 128 patients collected were evaluable.

		PAC (n)	FAC (n)
FIGO	II	9	10
	III	41	43
	IV	4	6
BSOHO	compl.	30	32
	incompl.	13	21
Biopsy only		11	6
PD-free	12 Mo	77%	54%
survival	24 Mo	50%	27%
Overall	12 Mo	87%	82%
survival	24 Mo	66%	56%

Stage, age and surgical extension with bilateral salpingo-oophoro-hystero-omentectomy (BSOHO) was balanced. Early progressive disease (PD) within six months of the start of treatment was found in 29% on FAC and 13% on PAC. The short time to relapse on FAC is influenced by crossover to PAC regarding overall survival. By trend PAC is superior to FAC.

06.04.06

The treatment of ovarian cancer with malignant pleural effusion and metastatic liver cyst: Soh, E*, (Ronghuei Tzeng), Ishihara, T*, Wagatsuma, T**. Dept. Gyn. and Obstet., Toranomon Hospital*, Nat. Med. Ctr Hosp.**, Tokyo, Japan

Pleural effusion is a commom complication of ovarian cancer, and poses a considerable problem in management. Despite the variety of methods tried, cinical effectiveness is entirely unsatisfactory. Whereas, metastatic liver cyst in ovarian cancer is rare, and can be fatal due to a sudden spontaneous rupture. Some pleural effusions were controlled by systemic chemotherapy alone. However, in ovarian cancer, pleural effusions were not palliated unless tube thoracostomy with local instillation of anticancer agent was utilized. The report presents our experience with a simple bedside technique for controlling maglignant pleural effusion and with metastatic liver cyst in ovarian cancer: (1) a tube thoracostomy drainage with continuous mild suction for pleural effusion, (2) for the liver cyst, under ultrasound guided percutaneous transhepatic cholangiodrainage (PTCD), (3) subsequent instillation of adriamycin combined with OK 432. Twelve ovarian cancer patients with pleural effusion and two cases with ovarian cancer with metastatic liver cyst were treated. The systemic chemotherapy consists of administration of cisplatin and adriamycin. The procedure successfully prevented recurrence of both pleural effusion and liver cyst. Only moderate nausea and fever were notice as untoward effect of anticancer agents. It can be conluded that this approach could be recommended for the series of ovarian cancer.

06.04.07

A prospective randomized study of 160 ovarian cancer patients stage III and IV: Sevelda, P, Salzer, H, Gitsch, E, Dittrich, C, Karrer, K. Aust. Collabor. Ovarian Ca Study Group, I. Dept. Gyn. and Obstet., Univ. Vienna, Austria

A new sequential polychemotherapy called "changing-scheme" comprises A/P as first part, V/C as second one, and HD-MTX as third one with monthly administration intervals between the three successive parts, and has been compared to the Parker-scheme (A/C) and the Bruckner-scheme (A/P). To get comparable results all prognostic factors of ovarian cancer were equally distributed in the therapy groups by a special computer randomization. Survival of women with minimal residual postoperative tumor mass ($< 2\,cm^3$) was significantly longer ($p < 0.01$) than that of patients with macroscopic residual disease ($> 2\,cm^3$), irrespective of the choice of postoperative chemotherapy. Patients with highly differentiated tumors had longer survival ($p < 0.01$) than those with tumors of low differentiation, independent of postoperative chemotherapy. Remission rates of the different chemotherapies were 89% for the changing-scheme, 78% for the A/C-regimen, and 83% for the A/P-regimen. The remission duration and mean survival time of patients under the changing-scheme showed an advantage for, but no substantial difference in favour of the new therapy protocol for an unselected group of women. In particular, the subgroups of women with highly differentiated tumors and with liver metastases seem to profit from the new therapy.

06.04.08

Clinical evaluation of FCAP chemotherapy for ovarian cancer: Kanazawa, K, Yuzawa, H, Honma, S, Takakuwa, K, Takeuchi, S. Dept. Obstet. and Gyn., Niigata Univ., School Med., Niigata, Japan

For the purpose of clinical analysis of four drug regimen FCAP, treatment with the combination was performed in 65 patients with malignant common epithelial tumor of the ovary. FIGO stage was Stage I in 14 cases, II in six, III in 28, IV in four and recurrence in 13. Operation prior to chemotherapy was done in 48 cases. Tumor was removed completely in 21 cases but not in 27. Second look operation after or during chemotherapy was done in 29 cases. FCAP was administered with the following schedule: F (5-fluorouracil) $350\,mg/m^2$, i. v., day 1–5, C (cyclophosphamide) $350\,mg/m^2$, i. v., day 1, A (adriamycin) $40\,mg/m^2$, i. v., day 1 and P (cisplatin) $50\,mg/m^2$, i. v., day 1. Number of courses of FCAP given was from 1 to 10 (mean 4.5) per one case. Response rate in 32 cases in whom response criterion of ECOG-WHO was available was 75.0% (complete response 28.1% and partial response 46.9%). Although the majority of patients experienced gastrointestinal disturbance, myelosuppression, fever and alopecia to various extent, none of them died from these adverse effects. Survival rate was significantly improved compared with that in the historical control group which was roughly homogeneous with the present study group in prognostic background. Thus, FCAP was evaluated to be an active chemotherapeutic combination in the management of ovarian cancer.

06.04.09

Trial of intraperitoneal chemotherapeutic perfusion method in the treatment of ovarian malignancies: Hirabayashi, K, Okada, E. Dept. Obstet. and Gyn., Fukuyama Nat. Hosp., Hiroshima, Japan

We have tried this method for killing the tumor cells which are prone to remain in the abdominal cavity after debulking operation, to evaluate its usefulness and to study the indication This method is as follows: 1) After the tumor is extirpated as much as possible, two silicone drains are inserted into the abdominal cavity through abdominal wall. 2) On the first and seventh postoperative day, the cocktail of various anti-cancer drugs (10–20 mg MMC, 3–5 mg CQ, 300 mg CPM and 300 mg 5-FU dissolved in 300 ml of normal saline) is given by one shot through a drain. 3) The cocktail is made to act on tumor cells for 30 minutes, and is then washed out with 2–3 l of normal saline. In the 57 cases who were treated by this method, three-year survival rate and disorders were examined and compared with those of 74 control cases.

Three-year survival rates after the treatment by this method were 95.5% (21/22) in stage I, 76.9% (10/13) in stage II, 23.5% (4/17) in stage III and 0.0% (0/5) in stage IV. Among ten surviving cases in stage II, two cases had relapse later, and among the four surviving cases in stage III, one died of cancer seven years after. No severe side effects were observed in any of the cases. When these rates were compared with those of the 74 control cases, significant improvement was seen in the rates in stage I and II. From the above results, it has been concluded that this method would be indicated for postoperative adjuvant therapy of cases with ovarian malignancies in stage I or II who have no remaining cancer as a mass but may have remaining tumor cells.

06.04.10
A phase II study of doxorubicin combined with cisplatin in advanced ovarian cancer: Skjaerris, J, Tropé, C, Simonsen, E, Horváth, G, Clase, L. Dept. Oncol., Gyn., Sect. Univ. Hosp., Lund, Sweden
Introduction: In our clinic we have used doxorubicin (DX) + melphalan as standard treatment in advanced ovarian cancer. Because of the promising results with the combination DX + cisplatin (P) with a response rate of 80%, we decided to change our standard regimen to DX + P. – Method: 41 patients with advanced ovarian cancer previously not treated with chemotherapy have been treated with DX (50 mg/m^2) + P (50 mg/m^2) with hyperhydration, day 1 q 4 w. Stage at start of treatment according to FIGO 80% (33) st III, 20% (8) st IV. Histology: serous 63% (26), mucinous 5% (2), undiff 2% (1), mesonefroid 7% (3), endometroid 22% (9). Differentiation: well 7% (3), moderately 24% (10), poorly 69% (28). – Results: The overall response rate was 63% (26). In stage III 67% /22); of these CR 21% (7), PR 46% (15), SD 18% (6), PD 15% (5). In stage IV resp. 50% (4), CR 25% (2), PR 25% (2), SD 50% (4). Median duration of response for stage III CR 5+ (2+,9+), PR 4+ (1.13+), SD 2.5+ (1.11). For stage IV CR 5+, 9, PR 4.8, SD 3.5+ (2,8+). Median survival for stage III CR 9+ (7+, 13+), PR 7+ (5+, 17+), SD 9+ (3+,16), PD 4 (3,6). For stage IV CR 6+,24+, PR 12,12+, SD 8.5+ (6+,9+). – Discussion: The response rate of DX + P compares favorably with DX + melphalan – though the very promising results of other studies have not been confirmed. No serious neurotoxicity, renal toxicity or bone marrow toxicity occurred. However, one patient developed myocardial infarction, but is still in remission.

06.04.11
Role of external irradiation after cisplatin-therapy of advanced ovarian carcinoma: Maseela, T. Inst. Radio-Oncol., MHH, Hannover
In the period between 1982 and 1984, forty patients with carcinoma of the ovaries were subjected to abdominopelvic irradiation to provide a survival benefit after surgery and polychemotherapy. The age-distribution ranged from 28 to 75 years, with a cumulation between 40 and 60. In 60% of the patients primary surgery was BSOHO and in 40% it was palliative resection or biopsy. The histological finding in over 50% was serous, papillary cystadeno-carcinoma. In 22 cases postoperative chemotherapy with cispla-tincombinations was conducted; medium range = 8 cycles. The tumor-staging in 16 cases was FIGO-III and 6 cases had FIGO-IV. Before radiotherapy, CT-scan was performed in 18 cases and second-look laparotomy in 20 cases to evaluate the response to chemotherapy. An open-field irradiation of the abdomen and pelvis was conducted in 20 fractions over eight weeks. Alimentary side-effects remained within minimal levels. No leukemogenic effect has been noted; neither was any enhancement of the dose-limiting toxicity of aggressive chemotherapy observed. In a follow-up study of maximal 36 months after cessation of radiotherapy, 70% of the patients were in complete or partial remission without symptoms, and 10% DOD despite multimodal treatment.

06.04.12
Whole-abdominal radiation (WR) in ovarian carcinoma after surgical cytoreduction $\pm$ chemotherapy and second-look operation: Dreher, E, Greiner, R, Goldhirsch, A. Depts. Gyn., Oncol and Radiat. Ther., and Ludwig Inst. Ca Res., Univ., Bern, Switzerland
From September 1979 to December 1984, WR was performed in 86 patients (pts), in 53 of them by the moving strip technique and in 33 by the open field technique. The WR consisted of 30 Gy $\pm$ 14 Gy to the pelvis. WR was given after surgery alone to 31 pts (non-serous tumors FIGO Stage I Grade 1–3 or serous FIGO Stage I–II Grade 1–2). 24/31 (77%) were without evidence of disease. 55 pts with higher stage and/or grade received WR after first operation, chemotherapy (CT = in 80% a platinum combination) and a II-look operation. 35/55 (64%) were in complete remission (CR) at WR start. Thrombocytopenia was the radiation-limiting toxicity for WR. Moving strip WR had to be stopped or delayed in 85% of pts with previous CT and in 50% of pts without previous CT. Pts treated by the open field technique had a better tolerance: it was necessary in only 15% of the CT-pretreated and 10% of the non-pretreated pts to interrupt WR. At a median observation time of 24+ months (range 12–41 mos) there was no evidence of disease progression in 50/59 (85%) of the pts who had been free of disease after operation, either primary or II-look. 9/14 (64%) partial responders (PR) to a non-platinum-containing CT remained asymptomatic after WR, while only 1/13 (8%) of the PR to a platinum-containing CT remained asymptomatic after WR. WR does not seem to be indicated in pts with PR after a platinum-containing CT. Further follow-up is needed to confirm these preliminary observations.

06.04.13

Comparison of treatment results and side-effects of PAC and PEC regimens on patients with advanced ovarian cancer in randomised prospective study: Hernádi, Z, Lampé, L G, Juhász, B. Clin. Obstet. and Gyn., Univ., Debrecen, Hungary

As the majority of other and new combinations has proved to be less efficacious than the PAC combination we use at our center this combination instead of cyclophosphamide monotherapy as the standard for comparison. The drug 4-epi-doxorubicin has activity similar to that of doxorubicin at a lower level of toxic, first of all cardiotoxic, side-effects. This drug was also combined with cyclophosphamide and cis-DDP. Out of patients randomised to the PAC and PEC arms 14 identical in respect of most relevant prognostic factors were matched and selected for the final analysis. The main issue in this study was to evaluate and compare the objective response rate achieved and side-effects caused in the two arms. The objective response rate was established on basis of tumor measurements with ultrasound and of findings at second-look operations. Using the epirubicin containing regimen we managed to reach the same objective response rate (78,6%) as in case of the doxorubicin containing regimen, and it could be achieved at a lower level of toxicity. This study represents a part of the activity of the South Eastern Study Group on Epirubicin.

06.06.01

Malignancy grading of squamous cell carcinoma of the uterine cervix. A critical review: Stendahl, U. Dept. Gyn. and Oncol., Univ. Hosp., Umeå, Sweden

A histopathologic malignancy grading system (MGS) for prognosis in squamous cell carcinoma was modified for carcinoma of the uterine cervix. The MGS embodies 8 factors. Structure, mode of invasion, nuclear polymorphism and mitosis representing the tumor cell pupulation, and mode of, stage of invasion, vascular invasion and lymphoplasmocytic response representing the tumor host relationship. Each factor was graded from 1 to 3 points with a total score of 8 to 24 points. Studies on retrospective material were promising as regards the capacity of the MGS to predict individual patients. By means of AID-analyses it was possible to divide the patients into low and high point groups with corresponding mortality rates. Studies of intra- and interobserver reproductibility showed a considerable variation, mainly between pathologists and consequently further standardization of the factors was mode. Still a considerable gliding in assessement remained between observers. Single factors such as differentation into cell type, nuclear polymorphism and frequency of mitosis had little prognostic value which disappeared in the regression analyses. The results attract attention to the use of these parameters in clinical practice to evaluate tumor malignancy, the definitions of the factors and the possibilities of improved methods. Considering the latter, single cell, and flow cytometric DNA measurement are now being used and at the same time providing new features such as S-phase rate and multiple stemlines. If a prognostic factor affects the survival of the patient during a limited period of time, prospective studies should be preferred. Vascular invasion and lymphoplasmocytic response contained most prognostic information. There are both qualitative and quantitative difficulties to assess. By using a monoclonal antibody technique it is now possible to stain the endothelial cells of the vessels. This approach can also be used to separate T and B lymphocyts and for the identification of plasma cell globulins. Equidistant steps were used in the grading. Computer aided changing of the intervals did not affect results. Multifactorial collecting of prognostic information is necessary in the absence of a valid single predictor. All comparison mode with predictors such as clinical staging, treatment, age, monofactorial histopathological classifications were based on retrospective material. A randomized study is now running with adjuvant chemotherapy to high risk patients selected according to the MGS and clinical staging. In another prospective study flow cytometric data are included in the selecting of patients for therapy. Thus, not only the way of selecting high risk patients but the design of cytostatic therapy will decide if this is a recommendable way.

06.06.02

Stimulation of ureteral motility after radical surgery of cervical carcinoma: Philipp, K. 1st Dept. Gyn. and Obstet., Univ., Vienna, Austria

The principal disadvantage of extended radical abdominal surgery for cervical carcinoma of the uterus against other surgical techniques is that it is associated with a higher incidence of urological complications. At the first Department of Gynecology and Obstetrics, Vienna University Medical School main emphasis of postoperative prophylaxis is the stimulation of ureteric activity by distigmine bromide and hexoprenalin. Distigmine bromide stimulates the prevesical part of the ureter and increases the number of urinary excretions into the bladder. Hexoprenalin is a betamimetic substance which increases both local blood flow and the number of ureteric contractions. The increase of the ureteric activity is documented by urokineto-grams. In a prospective study after administration of ^{99m}Tc-MDP urine transport within the ureter is documented with a gamma scintillation camera by functional waytime-matrices. The results show an increase of ureteric contractions after administration of distigmine bromide from 7.7 to 13.0 within six minutes and from 8.1 to 13.0 after hexoprenalin. In a control group there was no change in the frequency of the ureteral contractions.

06.06.03
Intraoperative control of lymphadenectomy: Kolstad, P. Norsk Hydro's Inst. Ca Res., Norweg. Radium Hosp., Oslo, Norway

In 1970–1973 300 cases of servical cancer Stage Ib and II were treated with radium followed six weeks later by radical hysterectomy and pelvic lymphadenectomy. Lymphography was performed during the first hospital admission. New pictures were taken immediately before and during the operation to assure a near complete lymphadenectomy. A total of 9187 nodes were removed, 770 of which were found with the aid of the radiograms. Of these 770 nodes 21 contained metastases. the majority of the lymph nodes removed (98.9%) contained contrast medium. Of 209 nodes with metastases 15.9% did not contain contrast. A decrease in the average number of remaining nodes from 3.4 per patient in the first 100 operations to 1.6 per patient in the last 100 patients was noted. Follow-up at 5 and 10 years showed a survival rate of 86% and 83%, respectively. If none or 1–3 nodes were left behind the 5 and 10 year survival rate was 90% and 88%. If 4 or more node were left behind the corresponding figures for 5 and 10 year survival were 77% and 74%. The patients with metastases (25.1%) received postoperative irradiation. Their 5 and 10 year survival was 63% and 58%, respectively. In 47 cases (15.7%) no remaining nodes could be seen in the intraoperative radiograms. In another 40 cases lymphadenectomy became complete with the aid of the intraoperative radiograms, giving a total of 87 (29%) complete lymphadenectomies.

06.06.04
Intraoperative control of pelvic lymphadenectomy by radioisotope labelling: Gitsch, E. 1st Dept. Gyn. and Obstet., Univ., Vienna, Austria

Involvement of the lymph nodes should invariably be expected to be present in stage Ib and II cases of cervical carcinoma. Lymphadenectomy therefore should be as radical as possible. For this purpose the radionuclide controlled radical surgery of cervical carcinoma was established at the First Department of Gynecology and Obstetrics, Vienna University Medical School. Lymphadenectomy is performed with prior radionuclide labelling of the pelvic lymph nodes. Intraoperatively the patient is placed on a gamma scintillation camera converted to serve as an operating table, which allows us to monitor the progress of lymphadenectomy. Between 1970 and 1978 in 203 cases intraoperative control of pelvic lymphadenectomy was performed. The increase in the rate of complete lymphadenectomy was associated with a decrease of 5-year-recurrence mortality from 15.8% to 2.8% in stage Ib cases and from 43.5% to 22.2% in stage II cases. Patients undergoing incomplete lymphadenectomy have a poorer prognosis than those with complete lymph node removal.

06.06.05
The role of surgery in the management of cervical cancer: Barber, H R K. Dept. Obstet. and Gyn., Lenox Hill Hosp., New York City, NY, USA

In 1939, *Joseph V. Meigs* reintroduced a radical surgical approach to carcinoma of the cervix. Although he selected his cases for surgery during the early years of his program, *J. V. Meigs* proved that surgery could be carried out with a low morbidity and mortality. *Brunschwig* expanded the scope of the operation and operated on "all comers" with selection held to a minimum while reporting a low morbidity and mortality. It is generally accepted that when the patient is under 65 years of age with a Stage I or IIa, radical hysterectomy and pelvic lymph node dissection is usually chosen. The rationale and indications for radical surgery will be presented and the nine different operations employed will be presented. The management of the fresh cases and recurrent carcinomas of the cervix has been established with the indications and contraindications clearly identified.

06.06.06
Prognosis and lymph node metastasis of uterine cervical cancer patients: Sonoda, T, Kasamatsu, T, Matsumoto, Y, Kishi, K. Nat. Ca Ctr Hosp., Tokyo, Japan

Eight hundred and twenty-eight patients with uterine cervical cancer who were operated on in our hospital from June 1962 to December 1975, were analysed as to their pathology of surgical specimen and prognosis. The results were summarised as follows: (1) The five-year survival rate of negative lymph node group and that of positive lymph node group were 88.9% and 57.7%, respectively. (2) Depth of invasion, vaginal and parametrial infiltration, and vessel invasion of the primary lesion presumably influenced lymph node metastasis. (3) The incidence and extent of these pathological findings were probably related with the histological typing of the primary lesion, which were in this analysis classified into three groups, namely keratinizing, and non-keratinizing squamous cell carcinoma, and adenocarcinoma.

Prognosis – 5-year survival rate (No. of the cases)

histologic type	lymph node negative	lymph node positive
keratinizing	89.7% (291)	64.2% (95)
non-keratinizing	90.7% (302)	53.3% (45)
adenocarcinoma	77.6% (67)	42.9% (28)

Parametrial and lymph (lv) – blood (bv) vessel involvement

	lymph node negative			lymph node positive		
	ker.	non-ker.	adeno.	ker.	non-ker.	adeno
parametrium (−)	263	282	61	56	35	18
parametrium (+)	29	20	6	38	10	10
lv (−) bv (−)	35	20	7	11	8	5
lv (+) bv (−)	28	19	4	33	23	8
lv (−) bv (+)	1	–	1	1	1	–
lv (+) bv (+)	5	12	1	13	7	3

Depth of invasion and vaginal involvement; omitted

06.06.07
"Mitra operation" for cancer of the cervix: Roy Chowdhury, N N. Eden Hosp., Med. Coll., Calcutta, India
This is a review of a personal series of 500 cases of carcinoma of the cervix of various stages treated by the Mitra technique from Januar, 1963 to July, 1983 both in hospital and private services. This operation consists of bilateral extra-peritoneal pelvic lymphadenectomy followed in the same sitting by radical vaginal hysterectomy with massive removal of parametrial, paracervical, paravaginal and vaginal tissues. Postoperative telecobalt therapy was administered in those cases only where paracervical and pelvic lymph nodes showed evidence of metastasis. Five-year end-results: Distribution of 500 cases according to clinical staging was as follows: Stage I: 104 (20.8%), Stage II: 368 (71.6%), Stage III: 28 (5.6%). Lymph nodes metastases were – Stages I, II and III combined: 156 (31.20%). Stage I: 18 (17.30%), Stage II: 120 (12.61%) and Stage III: 18 (64.28%). Five-year end-results of 264 cases were critically analysed according to clinical staging – Stage I: 77.90%, Stage II: 51.90% and Stage III: 40.00%. Prognosis in cases with gland metastases is definitely unfavorable. 34.28% five-year salvage rate being in the lymph node metastatic group in comparison to 72.30% in the nonmetastatic group. With negligible risk of bladder, ureteric or rectal injury, and secondary fistuale and greater possibility of removal of parametrial tissue this technique is ideally suited even for poor surgical risk patients.

06.06.08
Wertheim radical hysterectomy. Surgical complications, accuracy of clinical staging and value of lymphangiography in cervical carcinoma: Kajanoja, P, Räisänen, I, Lehtovirta, P. 2nd Dept. Obstet. and Gyn., Univ. Centr. Hosp., Helsinki, Finland
Wertheim radical hysterectomy combined with pelvis lymphadenectomy was performed on 132 women of whom 120 had cervical carcinoma from Stage IA to early IIB and 12 had endometrial carcinoma Stage II. None of the patients died during their stay in hospital. The left ureter was accidently transected in two patients and both were corrected immediately. Wound complications occurred in 16 patients (12%). The high incidence of wound complications is probably partly related to the low-dose heparin prophylaxis. The initial clinical staging was found to be correct in 85% of the cases. Ten cases of early Stage IIB, none of whom had parametrial invasion were overstaged. The predictive value of lymphangiography was low, 14% in histologically positive cases. Lymphangiography proved to be only of value in facilitating complete lymph node dissection. Intraoperative lymphangiographic control revealed radiopositive nodes and lead to further dissection in 30 patients (24%).

06.06.09
Analysis of factors contributing to treatment failures in surgically staged cervical cancer cases: Park, T K, Lee, K G. Dept. Obstet. and Gyn., Yonsei Univ. Coll. Med., Seoul, Korea
One hundred and seventy-four surgically staged cervical cancer patients were followed and treatment failures were analysed with prognostic factor guidelines. According to the surgical stage the 5-YCFR (year cumulative failure rate) for Stage 1b was 7.7% and for Stage II 44.2%. The 5-YCFR for histologic cell types were as follows: large cell nonkeratinizing 10.7%, large cell keratinizing 15.5%, and adenocarcinoma 36.5%. The 3.5-YCFR for small cell was 60%. The failure rates increased proportionately with the size of the lesion. Those lesions ≧4 cm in diameter had a 3.5-YCFR of 42.7%. The failure rates increased proportionately with the depth of invasion into the stroma of the cervix. Depth of invasion ≧10 mm resulted in a 5-YCFR of 37.7%. Lymph vessel invasion and blood vessel invasion of the stroma of the cervix resulted in a greater than two-fold and five-fold respectively increase in the failure rates as compared to those cases with no invasion. Absent lymph node metastases resulted only in a 10% 5-YCFR while macroscopically visible lymph node metastases resulted in a 87.5% 30-month failure rate and microscopically visible lymph node metastases only resulted in a 25% 5-YCFR. Failure rates according to lymph node morphology were as follows: lymphocyte predominant 8.4% (5-YCFR), germinal center predominant 10.3% (5-YCFR), and lymphocyte depletion 33.3% (54-month cumulative failure rates).

06.06.10

The postoperative classification for uterine cervical cancer and its clinical application: Noguchi, H, Shiozawa, I, Yamazaki, T, Shiozawa, K, Iwai, S, Fukuta, T. Dept. Obstet. and Gyn., Shinshu Univ. School Med., Matsumoto, Japan; and Baltzer, J, Lohe, K, Kürzl, R, Zander, J. 1st Frauenklin., Univ., Munich

Our postoperative classification for uterine cervical cancer has been made in consideration of the spacial spread of cancer and biological malignancy of 120 cases which were treated with radical hysterectomy and pelvic lymphadenectomy. This classification corresponds extremely well to prognosis. The 5-year survival of the cases with prognostic index (P. I.) 9 or less was 96.1%, while those with P. I. above 10 showed 31.8%. In our clinic, postoperative irradiation and/or chemotherapy would be selected based on this classification. Namely, only the cases with P. I. 6 or more have pelvic irradiation after surgery, and chemotherapy should be given to the patients with positive lymph node metastasis or L type of CPL classification. When comparing the outcome of the cases before and after using this clinically, the prognosis of the cases with high P. I. or classed as advanced clearly improved. To certify the reliability of this classification, we applied it to the surgical specimens in Munich University. Results of 230 cases showed the same tendency. From these data, this classification may be important for individualization of postoperative treatment and for prognostic factor.

06.06.11

Role of surgery in the treatment of primary invasive cervical cancer: Cavagnini, A, Bianchi, U A, Sartori, E, Schreiber, C, Gastaldi, A. Dept. Obstet. and Gyn., Univ., Brescia, Italy

From 1965 to 1977, 995 pts affected by primary cervical cancer were treated according to the following guidelines: 1) Stage IB and IIA: low-risk pts, small and moderate tumors: radical hysterectomy; large tumors: intracavitary (i.c.) radium followed by radical hysterectomy. Postoperative ^{60}Co in cases of adverse pathological factors. In all other conditions Rxtherapy alone. Complete Rxtherapy followed by extrafascial hysterectomy and pelvic lymphadenectomy in barrel shaped or large infiltrative tumors. 2) Stage IIB: a) exclusive Rxtherapy in most cases, b) Rxtherapy followed by total hysterectomy and pelvic lymphadenectomy, c) radical hysterectomy + T.C.T. in cases with medial parametrial involvement (only at the beginning of our experience). 3) Stage III and IV: exclusive Rxtherapy. Only in very few selected cases primary exenteration. The results are expressed in term of five year crude survival rates (5-yr-surv.). Some remarks should be outlined. Stage IB: 39.3% of the pts underwent primary radical surgery and 34.9% of these were postop. treated with ^{60}Co teletherapy. The 95.9% 5-yr-surv. for the pts who received radical surgical treatment alone stresses the validity of the selection criteria. In the positive pelvic nodes cases, postop. ^{60}Co treated, 67.9% 5-yr-surv. has been achieved. Stage IIA: 93.3% 5-yr-surv. with radical hysterectomy alone, and 76.5% with postop. ^{60}Co, 74% and 64.3% with preop. radium respectively. Disappointing results were obtained with the program "^{60}Co + i.c. radium + total hysterectomy and pelvic lymphadenectomy" – 31% 5-yr-surv. – mainly for adverse selection of cases. Stage IIB the removal of the uterus after a complete Rxtherapy has allowed 63.3% 5-yr-surv. Moreover the cost of this treatment is high: 41.9% moderate and severe complications. The good result with primary radical surgery makes the surgical approach the treatment of choice in most stage IB and IIA.

06.06.12

Perioperative morbidity after extended hysterectomy (Wertheim-Meigs) including lymphadenectomy: Almendral, A C, Heinzl, S, Hendry, M. Women's Hosp., Univ., Basle, Switzerland

During the years 1970–1983, 203 extended hysterectomies (Wertheim-Meigs) – including pelvic lymphadenectomy – were performed. Since 1978, resection of para-aortic lymph nodes has been obligatory. The mean age of the patients was 50 with a standard deviation of ±11.3 years. The operation was performed in 227±63 minutes with an average blood loss of 1509±1171 ml. Intraoperatively there was an accidental occurrence of the following lesions: large vessels – 22; urinary tract – 12; nerves – 3 and intestines – 1. There were no intra- or postoperative deaths. Patients were in hospital for 22.3±9.4 days. The incidence of fistulae was 1.9%. During the past six years we have been able to decrease significantly operating time, blood loss, number of intraoperative lesions, incidence of fistulae and length of hospital stay. Possible causes for this marked decrease in morbidity are under discussion.

06.06.13

Surgical criteria of cervical carcinoma: Goldsman, T, Vainer, O, Catarivas de Ansaldo, V. 1st Cath. Gyn., Nat. Univ., Córdoba, Argentina

Most significant progress in the last 20 years is fundamentally the "individualization" of the treatment. Improving of surgical management gives advantages for surgical stages, as follows: 1) It allows the exploring of the lesion at primary source level, likewise, its possible spreading. 2) It allows one to perform lymphadenectomy. 3) It allows conservation of ovaries. 4) A short vagina is kept but with normal features. 5) Chromosomic genetic damage is avoided. 6) Central focus is eliminated so avoiding central recurrence. 7) It allows exploring lumboaortic lymph node chain. 8) Radium necrosis is avoided. 9) "Resistance" factor is not present as may be observed in radiotherapy. We divide cervical carcinomas according surgical criteria, as follows: 1. Primary selective surgical: A) stage Ia, B) stage Ib, C) stage IIa, D) post-conus occult carcinoma (Ia and Ib), E) stump carcinoma, F) associated genital pathology. 2. Absolute no surgical: A) simple total post-hysterectomy occult carcinoma, B) advanced stages (hydronephrosis, limb edema, compression pain from sacral plexus), C) medical contraindications. 3. Transient or relative no surgical: tumors which require previous radiotherapy: A) blowing cervix, barrel or endophytic carcinoma, B) exophytic carcinoma with wide vegetative mass. 4. Special group: tumors which require surgical management combined with radiotherapy: A) adenocarcinoma previously treated with radiotherapy, B) radiotherapy resistance, C) incomplete or insufficient radiotherapy, D) intraoperative tumor rupture, E) close section line or in contact with the tumoral mass, F) resistance or recurrence after radiotherapy. In the last 12 years we have performed 162 coni; 174 Wertheim-Meigs; six extrafascial hysterectomies; 12 abdominal hysterectomies; three vaginal hysterectomies with haft; three amputations.

06.06.14
Interstitial lymphoscintigraphy in cervical cancer: Vainer, O, Goldsman, T, Catariva de Ansaldo, V. 1st Cath. Gyn., Nat. Univ., Córdoba, Argentina
Both therapeutic success and prognosis and consequently survival of patients who suffer from this disease, depend on the spread of the disease to pelvic and lumboaortic nodes. Therefore it is essential to know the degree of dissemination of the processs as a step previous to the treatment. The frequency of nodular metastases varies according to the clinical state, the vascular invasion of the tumor, its size, location and histological structure and finally to the presence of stromal reaction. Lymphoscintigraphy consists in obtaining a gammagraphic image resulting from the uptake and concentration of radioactive colloid when injected via interstitial bipodal. We used colloidal 99 technetinum, pure gamma emitters; thus we obtain images within 24 and 28 hours with camera gamma apex 400. We studied 44 patients with cervical cancer. Stages Ib: 32; stages II: 6; stages III: 6. Images were classified into: 1) images of complete uptake (probably normal), 2) images of doubtful interpretation (the uptake is diminished or is missing due to scarce progression of the contrast substance or by micro-metastasis, 3) abnormal images due to a) delay in the progress towards the nodes, b) partial interruption or complete lack of images in the nodular chain, c) asymmetry in the size and or activity in nodular areas, d) enlargement of a nodular group confined with lack of image in the underlying group, e) complete absence of liver radioactivity, f) deviaton of lymphatic chain. The technique is simple, harmless and easily repeated; there is good tolerance to it and it brings about functional and morphological information. It is the complement and supplement of other diagnostic techniques; we can see areas that cannot be visualized by lymphography.

06.07.01
Decrease of nosocomial infections during a seven-year surveillance program: Hirsch, H A, Niehues, U, Decker, K. Dept. Obstet. and Gyn., Univ., Tübingen
From April 1976 to March 1983 a total of 47,551 obstetrical and gynecological patients were continuously monitored for nosocomial infections according to criteria established by Centers for Disease Control, Atlanta, Georgia, USA. The highest infection rate occurred after major surgery (40.5%), followed by Cesarean section (16.1%). The lowest infection rate was found after vaginal deliveries (2.0%), in prepartum patients (1.9%) and after minor surgery (0.5%). Bacteriurias were the most frequent type of infection: 67% and 59% of all infections in 1976 and 1983, respectively. In the seven-year period, the global rate of nosocomial infections decreased from 16.8% to 4.8%. The decrease was most pronounced in bacteriurias (from 11.3% to 2.8%) and in standard febrile morbidity (from 8.5% to 1.6%). A significant reduction of infections was also demonstrated when the major operative procedures were assessed individually. In radical hysterectomies, total abdominal hysterectomies, and in vaginal hysterectomies with colporrhaphy the total rate of infections was about halved. Though, during the seven-year period, our anti-infection policy was repeatedly scrutinized and improved no major changes like prophylactic antibiotics were instituted. The decrease of infections was interpreted mainly as a result of the surveillance program.

06.07.02
Postvaginal surgery ultrasonic assessment of residual urine: Tohar, M, Abramovicz, J, Bahary, C. Dept. Obstet. and Gyn. "B", Meir Hosp., Kfar Saba, Israel
A bedside method is described to assess residual urine volume by Real-Time ultrasound after vaginal operations. We assumed that the post-hysterectomy bladder containing urine is not being compressed any longer between the pubic bone and the uterus and has a regular ellipsoid shape. We thus used the formula:

$$volume = \frac{3}{4} \times \pi \times \frac{AP}{2} \times \frac{SI}{2} \times \frac{T}{2}$$

where SI and T are respectively the antero-posterior supero-inferior and transverse diameters of the bladder. Used in 80 patients (100 measurements) this method proved accurate enough to avoid using a catheter for measuring the residual urine, thus greatly reducing one of the main postoperative complications: urinary tract infection.

06.07.03
Post-hysterectomy adnexal inflammatory disease: Hewson, A D. Royal Newcastle Hosp., Newcastle, Australia
A study of 96 pre-menopausal patients who had had a hysterectomy performed, in whom the adnexa were conserved and who subsequently presented with adnexal disease in subsequent years. The most common

symptom complex included pelvic pain, various urinary symptoms, dyspareunia and vaginal discharge. A common feature was the failure of many practitioners to recognise the significance and etiology of this symptom complex leading to long delays before the patient received definitive surgical treatment. Cure was always effected by removal of the residual diseased adnexa plus suitable hormone replacement therapy. The technical reasons for this syndrome being more common after vaginal hysterectomy are noted: and specific suggestions made as to how this unpleasant late complication of pre-menopausal hysterectomy may be avoided: specifically by routine removal of the Fallopian tube at hysterectomy or alternatively utilisation of an operative technique to minimise the development of a tubal fistula during vaginal vault closure.

06.07.04

Surgical complications in gynecological patients with associated diseases: Jurukovski, J, Naumov, J, Adamova, G, Boškovski, R. Dept. Obstet. and Gyn., Univ., Skopje, Yugoslavia

In order to evaluate the surgical risk in gynecological patients who carry related associated diseases all hospital records of such patients have being subjected to major gynecological surgery at the Department in 1971–1975 and 1979–1981 were reviewed and the results achieved compared. A total of 402 such patients were found in first and 498 in the second period searched. Nine deaths occurred in the whole series (1%), seven (1.74%) in the first and two (0.4%) in the second study period. Out of total 900 patients operated upon, 285 had severe anemia, 149 serious cardiac disease (CD), 186 long-standing hypertensive disease (HD), 67 respiratory disease (RD), 49 chronic thrombophlebitis, 25 diabetes mellitus, 34 gross obesity, but 48 were combined HD + CD, 13 HD + RD, 10 CD + RD and 34 had more than two types of associated diseases. Intraoperative complications occurred in 1.7% of the patients in the whole series, 3.2% in the first and 0.4% in the second study period. Corresponding figures for the postoperative complications were 19.2%, 33.1% and 7.6%. It was shown that overall incidence rate of surgical complications, both intra- and postoperative, were significantly reduced after team work, interdisciplinary approach and improved pre-operative care were established at the Department.

06.07.05

Complications after vaginal surgical procedures in 593 patients: Celestino, C A, Souza, A Z, Salvatore, C A. Gyn. Clin., Univ. of São Paulo Med. School, São Paulo, Brazil

Between 1972–1982, 593 patients with partial uterovaginal prolapse, cystocele, rectocele and perineal lacerations underwent conservative vaginal surgery at the Gynecologic Clinic of São Paulo University Medical School. None of them had pelvic malignancy, stress urinary incontinence or chronic pelvic infection. The frequency of surgical complications was analysed intrasurgically, early and late post-operatively. 1. Intrasurgical – The frequency of complications was 3.7%. In 13 (2.2%) cases, the blood loss was more than 300 ml. 2. The complications during the first 30 days postoperative whose etiology started in the genital system were observed in 86 (14.4%) cases. More frequently we found 6.9% of urinary retention, 3.4% of symptomatic urinary infection and 1.1% of moderate blood loss. 3. The complications in the first month unrelated to the genital system occurred in 1.2% cases. Only one (septicemia) could be related to the surgical procedure. 4. The total frequency of late complications, i. e., 30 days after the operation was 4.3%. Nine (1.5%) had stress urinary incontinence. Four (0.7%) had dyspareunia and four (0.7%) vaginal introitus stenosis. There was no mortality in this series.

06.07.06

Early and late effects of subtotal and total hysterectomy on bladder function: Lalos, O, Bjerle, P. Dept. Obstet. and Gyn., and Dept. Clin. Physiol., Univ. Hosp., Umeå, Sweden

Subtotal hysterectomy has been considered as superior to total as regards postoperative disorders of micturition (*Kilkku* et al., Maturitas 3, 197–204, 1981). The aim of present study was to evaluate and compare the effects of subtotal and total hysterectomy on bladder wall mechanics and micturition. Twenty-two women who were going to undergo hysterectomy were divided at random into two groups: One group (n = 11) for subtotal and another (n = 11) for total hysterectomy. Before, six weeks and six months after the operation micturition habits were documented and urodynamic investigation was performed. Six weeks after hysterectomy the number of daytime micturitions decreased and the urethral conductance increased in the entire patient series. Bladder volume, bladder compliance, maximum flow rate, intravesical pressure at maximum flow and residual urine did not change. Six months after the operation no changes of the urodynamic parameters were found compared with the pre-operative investigation. The two operative methods did not differ with respect to pre- and postoperative changes (early and late) of micturition habits and urodynamics. None of the methods caused any deterioration of the bladder function.

06.07.07

Paralysies crurales post-opératoires en chirurgie gynécologique: Cognat, M, Brinnel, H. Serv. Gyn.-Androl., Hôp. Saint-Joseph, Lyon, France

Les paralysies crurales post-opératoires en chirurgie gynécologique par voie abdominale représentent une complication rare. Dans notre observation une telle paralysie a été observée après une intervention de salpingoplastie micro-chirurgicale. Parmi les causes évoquées, la compression nerveuse per-opératoire du nerf crural par l'écarteur auto-statique est la plus évidente, elle est confirmée par notre observation personnelle (utilisation de l'écarteur O'Connor, O'Sullivan). Le type d'incision et la mauvaise adaptation de l'écarteur à la morphologie pelvienne augmentent le risque. La chirurgie tubaire utilisant la méthode micro-chirurgicale augmente aussi un peu le risque du fait de l'allongement du temps opératoire et de l'appui prolongé des avant-bras de l'opérateur et des aides sur le champ opératoire. L'évolution de la paralysie crurale post-opératoire est en général favorable.

06.07.08
Necrotizing fasciitis: Oliveira, H C, Cassaguerra, M A. Serv. Gin., Hosp. Univ., Univ. Fed., Rio de Janeiro, Brazil
Necrotizing fasciitis is a severe infection resulting in extensive tissue destruction in the skin, subcutaneous connective tissue and fascia. Affected areas show edema, color changes, generally with a central ecchymosis, with signs of circulatory disturbance. The patient is toxemic, with raised temperature, oliguria, tachycardia, hypotension, mental confusion and appears severely ill. It is a necrotizing infection due to a progressive synergistic bacterial association between aerobic and anaerobic organisms. Surgical treatment must be initiated as soon as possible for if a wide resection two centimeters away from the margin of the necrotized area is not performed, antibiotic therapy alone is useless. General care must be strict as in any serious case and therapy should be conducted preferably in a spirit of interdisciplinary cooperation. Culture of the exudate and hemoculture should be carried out in every case, but the initial measure should be intravenous crystalline penicillin – 3 to 5 million units every 3 h, gentamycin – 1 mg/kg every 8 h by intramuscular injection and chloramphenicol 2 g every 6 h or metronidazol 500 mg every 8 h intravenous route. The wound must be washed three times a day with saline and iodopovidine solution. Application of sugar has shown itself useful in promoting healing.

06.07.09
Ruptured uterus, a dangerous sequel of childbirth: Taher, M, Elkady, A, Wahba, A, Bayomy, H, Elantably, M. Dept. Obstet. and Gyn., Bolak El Dakror Hosp., Guiza, Egypt
Ruptured uterus is a grave obstetric complication; it is associated with high maternal mortality, increased perinatal mortality and loss of future fertility as hysterectomy is inevitable in many cases. This study reviews the incidence, causes, and other associated factors leading to ruptured uterus, in order to define problem areas and propose preventive measures. 56 cases of ruptured uterus were recorded in 16,597 deliveries between the years 1979–1983, those 56 cases were retrospectively analysed in relation to etiology, age, parity, maternal mortality, perinatal mortality and management. Some of the results were compared with other authors from different countries. The incidence in our series was 0.34%. Spontaneous accounted for 55.35% of cases, while traumatic rupture occurred in 44.65% of cases. 3.57% of cases occurred below 20 years, 46.43% occurred in the age group 21–30 years, 46.43% occurred in the age group 31-40 years, and 3.57% above 40 years. The incidence was high in the high parity group, 38 cases (67.86%) had 4 or more previous deliveries. Maternal mortality in our series was 10.71%, perinatal mortality was 89.28%. 43 cases (76.79%) were treated by supravaginal hysterectomy, 11 cases (19.46%) by repair and sterilisation and two cases (3.57%) by repair without sterilisation. Two cases developed vesicovaginal fistulae due to the surgical procedures, one case cured spontaneously after conservative management and the other underwent a successful surgical repair. To conclude, the following recommendations are proposed: proper antenatal and intrapartum care, prohibition of dispensing drugs without medical prescription to prevent oxytocic abuse by paramedics, hospital delivery for high risk groups and lastly training and upgrading midwives and TBAs who attend to the majority of deliveries in Egypt.

06.08.01
Intrapartum management of insulin-dependent diabetes mellitus (IDDM) patients by continuous intravenous insulin infusion and subcutaneous insulin infusion pump: Feldberg, D, Goldman, J, Dicker, D, Samuel, N, Karp, M. Dept. Obstet. and Gyn., Golda Meir Med. Ctr., Petah-Tiqva, Israel
Strict glycemic control is essential in insulin-dependent diabetic parturients. The management in active labor was compared in three groups of women (1975–1984). Group I – 37 diabetic parturients managed by continuous i.v. insulin infusion during labor. Group II – 14 severe diabetic parturients managed by subcutaneous insulin infusion pump during labor and delivery. Group III – 20 non-diabetic, matched women in labor. Maternal glycemic control was evaluated during labor, and the hydration status and urinary output were measured. Fetal and neonatal well-being were noted. Mean blood glucose was 126 ± 21 mg% and 101 ± 12 mg% in groups I and II, respectively. Mean i.v. insulin dosage was 1.1 ± 0.3 and 0.8 ± 0.1 units/h, respectively. The indication in six of 14 parturients delivered by C/S, in the group I, and in one of five in group II was acute fetal distress. Mean birth weight of the babies was 3501 ± 15 g and 3120 ± 69 g, respectively, and neonatal hypoglycemia developed in 16% in the first and in none of the second group. No congenital malformations occurred in either group. Our results indicate that the subcutaneous insulin infusion pump is preferable to the continuous intravenous insulin infusion for a better glycemic control and prevention of neonatal complications.

06.08.02

The management of insulin-dependent diabetes mellitus in pregnancy by self blood glucose monitoring versus subcutaneous insulin infusion pump. A critical re-evaluation: Goldman, J, Karp, M, Feldberg, D, Dicker, D, Samuel, N. Dept. Obstet. and Gyn., Golda Meir Med. Ctr. (Hasharon), Petah-Tiqva, Israel

The importance of strict diabetic control in pregnant insulin-dependent patients is well-documented. The management in pregnancy of two groups of diabetics and a control group was compared (1975–1984). Group I – 35 pregnant diabetic women managed by SBGM. Group II – 16 pregnant, severely diabetic, highly selected patients managed by means of SIIP. Group III – 20 non-diabetic pregnant women – the control group. Parameters for diabetic control were mean blood glucose, glycosylated Hb, M value, MAGE and C-peptide. Mean blood glucose was 118 ± 18 mg% in group I and 102 ± 12 mg% in women of group II. Four patients (11.5%) developed PIH in the first, and four (25%) in the second group. Twelve women (34.2%) and six (37.5%), respectively were delivered by Cesarian section. Mean birth weight of the babies was 3431 ± 176 g and 3216 ± 161 g, respectively and four neonates (11.4%) developed hypoglycemia in the first and none in the second group. No congenital malformations occurred in babies of all groups. Our results do not reflect a marked difference in maternal complications in patients managed by SBGM vs. SIIP. While both methods are considered an excellent means of management of pregnant diabetic women, considering the deficiencies of SIIP and the similar good results with SBGM, the latter is preferred by most patients.

06.08.03

A conservative policy in the management of diabetes in pregnancy: Stronge, J M, Foley, M E, Drury, M I. Nat. Maternity Hosp., Dublin, Ireland

Since January 1st 1979, the policy of routine delivery at 39 weeks gestation in diabetic women was abandoned. Diabetes itself was no longer considered a sufficient indication to interrupt the course of pregnancy. Elective delivery was performed only when there was a clear medical indication, for example, hypertension and proteinuria or hydramnios or fetal macrosomia. After 40 weeks, labor was induced for social reasons if the conditions were favorable for vaginal delivery. Between 1st January, 1979 and December 31st 1984, a total of 181 infants weighing 500 grams or more were born to 181 mothers. All but four were insulin dependent. Gestational diabetics were excluded. There were ten perinatal deaths, a rate of 55 per thousand. Four deaths were due to malformationa and none occurred after 38 weeks gestation. The malformation rate was 6% and other significant morbidity occurred in 10% of infants. The rate of Cesarean section was 20% and the rate of forceps delivery was 15%. Spontaneous onset of labor occurred in 40% of mothers. These results show that a conservative policy to the timing of delivery reduces the need for operative intervention. Provided there is strict control of the diabetes, this can be achieved without an increase in perinatal morbidity or mortality.

06.08.04

Fetal outcome in diabetic pregnants under intensive outdoor care: Rost, I, Bali, C, Fuchs, G, Irsigler, K, Leodolter S. Gyn.-Geburtshilfl. Abt., Krankenh. Stadt Wien, Lainz, Austria

From 1980 to 1983 we cared for 106 insulin-dependent pregnants. Throughout recent years we have tried to lower the malformation rate by already reaching normoglycemia before conception and by very strict metabolic control during the whole pregnancy. We found the following complications in these pregnancies: gestosis (12.8%), tocolytic therapy (19.4%), cerclage due to cervix insufficiency (6.6%). In all White-classes the delivery averaged in the 38th week, (53% spontanous births, 39 Cesarean sections, 8% vacuum extractions). Perinatal mortality was 9.4%, seven babies showed malformation. We were able to lower the malformation rate from 9.6% – as published in the year 1980 – to 6.6%. The hospital stay was reduced to a minimum by self monitoring and by accurate obstetrical care.

06.08.05

Routine prenatal screening for diabetes mellitus: Frishmuth, G J, Iddenden, D A, Emini, J C. Dept. Obstet. and Gyn., Presbyt.-Univ. of Pennsylvania Med. Ctr., Philadelphia, PA, USA

For some time it has been accepted that certain high risk groups of pregnant women should be screened for diabetes mellitus during pregnancy. There has been considerable debate over the screening test that should be used and there has also been considerable disagreement over whether such screening tests should be applied to the pregnant population as a whole. We present data gathered over three years during which time all patients in our obstetric practice were screened for diabetes mellitus at 28 weeks of pregnancy with blood glucose measurement one hour following a 50 gram oral load of glucose. Based on our findings, we recommend that this test be instituted on a routine basis as a screening test for all pregnant women.

06.08.06

Antenatal cardiotocography for surveillance of diabetic pregnancies: Olofsson, P, Sjöberg, N-O, Solum, T. Dept. Obstet. and Gyn., Univ. Hosp., Lund, Sweden

The reliability of the nonstress test (NST) and oxytocin challenge test (OCT) in diabetic pregnancy has been questioned due to isolated cases of poor fetal outcome following normal tests. This study is an evaluation of the tests and a comparison between them. – Material and methods: From about the 30th gestational week, NST was performed 1–2 times weekly in out-patients and daily in in-patients. OCT was routinely performed in week 38. 99 pregnant diabetics were monitored with altogether 2672 NSTs. 61 women were also monitored with altogether 90 OCTs. The tests were classified normal, suspect, slight, or severe pathological. The predictive values of the tests were calculated in relation to different variables of fetal outcome. – Results: When performed ≤ 2 days antepartum, the normal NST predicted a normal 1-min Apgar score in 92%, and at 5 and 10 min in 99%. Including "worst ever" NSTs, the figures improved to 100%. The baby's first cry within 1 min postpartum was predicted in 96%, and normal intrapartum cardiotocograms, normal pulmonary function, and normal metabolic balance, in about 80%. The perinatal mortality was 1%. No statistically significant differences were found between the NST and OCT. – Conclusions: NST performed according to our program has shown to be a good predictor of normality in diabetic pregnancy and is thus highly reliable in fetal surveillance. The OCT does not favour the NST for routine surveillance.

06.08.07
Relationship between glucose levels and fetal insulin secretion in the fetus: Fujino, Y, Shimura, K, Miyazaki, A, Ogita, S, Sugawa, T. Dept. Obstet. and Gyn., Osaka City Univ. Med. School, Osaka, Japan
Transplacental supply of the nutrients and fetal anabolic ability may be the essential factors of fetal growth, though the details remain obscure. To clarify the effect of feto-maternal glucose environment on the fetal insulin response and subsequent growth, glycosylated protein (GP) levels and C-peptide (CPR) levels in amniotic fluid as the indices for fetal glucose levels and insulin secreting ability were measured respectively. As pregnancy progresses, GP increased gradually and showed a peak around 33th to 35th gestational week, while CPR showed a peak at 36th to 37th gestational week. Active alimentary area (AAA) calculated from oral glucose tolerance test curve over 80 mg/dl for 120 min., as an indicator of the maternal glucose metabolism, was correlated with GP and CPR levels in amniotic fluid, and these were correlated with fetal growth closely. On the other hand, insulin accelerated transplacental nutrients transport ensured using *in vitro* experimental system. Above the experimental results, it was considered that fetal insulin plays an important role on the growth of fetus.

06.08.08
Maternal glucose tolerance test after birth of a large baby: Ogata, E, Takahashi, T, Iwasaki, K, Uetake M, Saito, M, Kikuchi, S. 2nd Hosp. of Nippon Med. School, Kanagwa, Japan
The glucose amount used in oral glucose tolerance test (OGTT) was either 50 g or 100 g, but today 75 g is recommended by WHO (March, 1980). In Japan, for the diagnosis of impaired glucose tolerance (IGT), a criterion, different from WHO's, is employed and few studies with 75 g OGTT have been reported on puerperal women. Maternal carbohydrate intolerance (CI) is closely related with the birth of an excessively large infant (LI), and once a mother has LI, she is classified into group of potential abnormality of glucose tolerance (PAGT). In Japan, an infant with the weight of more than 4.0 kg is generally taken as LI, but the ground of its definition is not clear. In the present study, 75 g OGTT has been performed on more than 150 women who had LI (more than 3750 g at birth). As the result, CI, that is, DM and PAGT in Japanese criteria, was found in one fourth of them within the initial six months after birth of LI, it is quite liable for her to have another LI in her successive pregnancy, which would aggravate her CI. For the purpose of prevention of DM, it is necessary and also effective to check CI within 6 months after birth of LI and follow closely especially the cases with IGT.

06.08.09
The advantage of using an insulin infusion system on diabetic pregnants: Fuchs, G, Bali, C, Kritz, H, Rost, I, Irsigler, K, Leodolter, S. Gyn.-Geburtshilf. Abt., Krankenh. Stadt Wien, Lainz, Austria
If it is not possible to reach normoglycemia by injecting insulin s.c. 3 or 4 times a day the use of an insulin infusions system is indicated also in pregnant diabetics and even better already starting before conception. From the year 1981 to 1983 we cared for 12 diabetic pregnants using insulin infusions systems. We computed the MBG-level and the mean insulin need under this treatment. To find the use of insulin infusion systems we compared the HbA_1 before and under this therapy. We found the MBG-level – averaged over all patients – being 117.32 mg% and an insulin need of 56.7 U. HbA_1 under conventional therapy was 9.17% but it was lowered to 6.35% by using an insulin infusion system. This result shows the advantage of this new way of treating insulin-dependent pregnant women.

06.08.10
Amniotic fluid C-peptide and cortisol interrelationship in diabetic and intrauterine growth retarded pregnancies: Lunell, N O, Pschera, H, Persson, B. Dept. Obstet. and Gyn., Huddinge Univ. Hosp., and Dept. Pediat., St Görans Hosp., Karolinska Inst., Stockholm, Sweden
Amniotic fluid (AF) C-peptide-cortisol interrelation was studied in 26 pregnancies complicated by diabetes and in 11 intrauterine growth retarded pregnancies (IUGR). C-peptide in AF reflects the production of fetal insulin. To determine total amounts of fetal C-peptide and cortisol produced AF volume was determined by PAH-dilution technique. Type I diabetic women had significantly higher AF C-peptide concentration and content (AF × conc) than normal controls. The corresponding values were significantly lower in mothers with IUGR compared to controls. The C-peptide/cortisol ratio was lowest in the IUGR group indicating a possible reduced insulin effectiveness due to the elevated cortisol levels. The opposite

finding of an increased C-peptide/cortisol ration in type I diabetics could favor a state of functional hyperinsulinism. Both cortisol and C-peptide contents were significantly interrelated in both control women and women with gestational or type I diabetes. The lack of correlation in IUGR pregnancies reflects the inability of the IUGR fetus to increase insulin secretion to an appropriate level of anabolic activity.

06.08.11
Studies on diagnostic criteria for the gestational diabetes by 75 g oral glucose tolerance test: Hamada, T, Yoshimatsu, K, Ooshima, T, Kubo, N, Tetsuo, M, Kato, T. Dept. Obstet. and Gyn., Kurume Univ., Fukuoka, Japan

A 75 g glucose tolerance test (75 g GTT) has been performed in 338 pregnant women at 28–40 weeks of gestation, without being complicated by potential abnormal glucose tolerance, glycemia and pre-eclampsia. The mean venous plasma glucose concentrations at fasting, one and two hours after glucose administrations were 85.7 ± 7 mg/dl, 128 ± 27 mg/dl, 109 ± 19 mg/dl, respectively. It was noted that the incidence of morbidity of neonates born to mothers in whom there was abnormal glucose tolerance, was statistically higher than those mothers with normal carbohydrate metabolism. The criteria considered suitable for gestational diabetes consisted of any two or more the following values being exceeded: fasting 100 mg/dl, one hour 180 mg/dl, and two hours 150 mg/dl. Many more detailed problems will be discussed.

06.08.12
Improvement of glycaemic control in diabetic pregnant women by guar administration: Arbues, J, Maldonado, J, Rosas, F, Campillo J E. Dept. Obstet. Gyn., Fac. Med., Badajoz, Spain

The importance of maintaining good glucose control in diabetic pregnancy is unquestioned, but the achievement of an acceptable and safe compromise between hyper- and hypoglycemia, especially in insulin-dependent diabetes, is in most cases a difficult task. Since it has been shown that high-fibre diets have great potential in reducing the mean amplitude of glycemic excursions in diabetes, we have studied the effect of guar fiber administration in diabetic pregnant women. Blood glucose levels (glucose oxidase) during a 24 hr period were measured in 24 non-diabetic (N D); 23 non insulin-dependent diabetic (N I D D) and 19 insulin-dependent diabetic (I D D) in-patient pregnant women, both without guar and after a week of 15 g guar supplementation (Fibroguar, Jorba, Spain) at breakfast, lunch and dinner. Results were statistically evaluated by the paired Manova test. Guar supplementation siginificantly reduced blood glucose levels after meals both in N D and diabetic women, such an effect being especially important in I D D pregnant women. The overnight (3 hr a.m.) blood glucose levels (mean $\pm$ S D) after guar were slightly, but significantly (P < 0.01) increased in both I D $-(128.74 \pm 30.32$ versus $135.68 \pm 18.67)$ and N I D $-(85.61 \pm 7.04$ versus $95.48 \pm 6.73)$ diabetic women. In conclusion, guar administration improves blood glucose control in diabetic pregnant women. In I D D women conventional therapy can be intensified without the swings which predispose to hypoglycemia, especially overnight.

06.08.13
Lipid metabolism in normal and diabetic pregnancy: Saiz Marti, A. Tocol. Dept., Municip. Hosp., Xativa, Spain

A study of the oral glucose tolerance test (OGTT) and the serum lipids in 100 pregnant women selected for potential diabetes (Family, Medical and Obstetrical history) and in normal pregnancy was made in the third trimester and 8 weeks postpartum. In normal pregnancy, a decrease of the fatty acids (NEFA) and α-lipoproteins was observed. In addition, the patients had statistically significant decrease in triglycerides, cholesterol and pre-β-lipoproteins in the postpartum period. In pregnant women with potential diabetes, an increase of plasma NEFA, triglycerides, total lipids and α-lipoproteins was observed. Compared to controls of non-diabetic nulliparous women the concentrations of NEFA, triglycerides, total lipids and cholesterol were higher. In non-pregnant diabetic women in the postpartum period, an increase of NEFA, triglycerides, pre-β-lipoproteins and a decrease of α-lipoproteins were observed in comparison with a homogenous group but with normal OGTT and other groups without a diabetic history. These results demonstrate the importance of determining the free fatty acids and total triglycerides in early diagnosis of prediabetic patients.

06.08.14
Diabetes mellitus in pregnancy – a 6-years study in Singapore: Ng, C, Kek, L P, Lee, K O, Yeo, P, Joseph, R, Cheah, J S, Tan, K L. Dept. Obstet. and Gyn., Kandang Kerbau Hosp., Nat. Univ., Singapore

From 1978 to 1984, 502 pregnant women with diabetes were managed with a standardised regime. During this period the department delivered 50,802 women. The incidence of diabetes was 0,99% or 1 in 101 pregnancies. All "high risk" mothers were screened at booking with a 50 g oral glucose tolerance test. There were 68 established diabetics and 434 women diagnosed as diabetes in pregnancy. Treatment was instituted with diet, or diet and Insulin. HbA1c estimation and home glucose monitoring for 24 hour sugar profiles were done to control the diabetes. There were no maternal deaths. There were 21 babies with congenital malformations (4.2%), mostly of minor nature. The mean birthweight of the diabetic babies above 36 weeks' gestation (3200.4 g) was only 27.3 g more than the general population at the same gestation (3173.1 g) and was not statistically significant. 24 babies weighed less than 2 kg and 33 above 4 kg. Only 18 babies had Apgar score of less than 7 at 5 minutes. 129 mothers were still diabetic at 6 weeks after delivery. 37.5% of women had Cesarean section (elective or emergency). The postpartum maternal complication rate was 4.6%. The associated obstetric complications were hypertensive disease in pregnancy, urinary tract infection and polyhydramnios. Perinatal mortality rate was 1.99%.

06.09.01

Cell-mediated immunity and immunotherapy in trophoblastic tumors: Kawagoe, K, Kawana, T*, Mizuno, M*. Ibaraki Prefect. Centr. Hosp., Japan; *Univ., Tokyo, Japan
The relationship between the clinical course of trophoblastic tumor and the status of cell-mediated immunity of the patient was studied in seven cases of trophoblastic tumors. The status of cell-mediated immunity was also measured in 15 cases of trophoblastic disease in remission. The PPD skin reaction and phytomitogen blastogenesis of lymphocyte (PHA reaction) were used as parameters of cell-mediated immunity. In most cases, both PPD and PHA reactions showed a similar tendency. In cases other than choriocarcinoma, the cell-mediated immunity retained good status, in which PPD reaction could be improved easily with the use of BCG. Contrarily, the cell-mediated immunity of choriocarcinoma changed remarkably in the clinical course. In cases with a good prognosis, the cellular immunity was improved at the time of remission. However, in a fatal case, PHA reaction remained at a low level all through the course. Judging from the urinary HCG level, chemotherapy with immunopotentiators obviously effective in the treatment of trophoblastic tumors, especially in a case of choriocarcinoma. In a remission state, PHA reaction was at a high level except for two cases of choriocarcinoma. It can be said that from the standpoint of cell-mediated immunity, choriocarcinoma is different from other trophoblastic tumors in character. In choriocarcinoma, PHA reaction can provide valuable information on the propriety of the treatment and on prognosis. As for choriocarcinoma with poor cellular immunity, the patient should be treated actively by immunopotentiators even if in a state of remission.

06.09.02

T-cell subpopulations and natural killer cell activity in gestational trophoblastic neoplasia: Ho, P C, Lawton, J W M, Wong, L C, Ma, H K. Dept. Obstet. & Gyn., and Dept Path., Univ., Hong Kong
The lymphocyte counts, the percentage of T-cells, helper T-cells and suppressor T-cells were measured in 24 patients with persistent gestational trophoblastic neoplasia (GTN) and 27 normal controls. Natural killer cell activity was also assayed in 16 patients with GTN and 16 normal controls. The percentage of T-cells was measured by the E-rosette method; the percentage of helper T-cells and suppressor T-cells was measured by using the monoclonal antibodies OKT4 and OKT8; the natural killer cell acitivity was assayed by studying the effect of the lymphocytes on a cell line (K562) labelled with radioactive chromium-51. The lymphocyte counts and T-cell counts in patients with GTN were significantly lower than those of normal controls but there was no significant difference in the percentage of helper T-cells and suppressor T-cells and natural killer cell activity. In patients with GTN, there was no significant difference in all these features between the low risk group and the high risk group. The measurement of T-cell subpopulations and natural killer activity is of little value in the prediction of response to chemotherapy in patients with GTN.

06.09.03

Clinic correlation and auxiliary technics in the analysis of a series of 62 trophoblastic diseases from 1968 to 1984: Masi, C, Ellena, A, Musacchio, R, Mahieu, E. Oncol. Nat. Inst. and "J.B. Iturraspe" Hosp., Santa Fé, Argentina
The diagnoses was based in the clinical state, histopathology and quantitative titration curve of HCG by immunological, biological and radio-immunoassay technics and diagnosis by image. We consider HCG quantisation as a fundamental auxiliary method. The values found in graphs in the diagnostic stage were between a range that oscillates: HCG immunologic till 3000 to 4,300.000 UI/24 h and HCG sub-unit beta till 2500 to 460,000 mU/ml. During the following 18 months after the chemotherapy we made determinations by biological methods, weight uterus rat (*Klinefelter* modified by *Delfs* with hypophysis bridled), to obtain lower values to 5 UR/24 h and in the last years by radio-immunoassay sub-unit beta accepting values lower than 5 MU/ml. – Conclusion: 1. Early diagnosis by clinic and auxiliary technics. 2. Clinic and histological evaluations of type and extension of the disease. 3. Adequate therapeutic (chemotherapy). 4. Following up for 18 months by means of tumoral assay muster.

06.09.04

Hysteroscopy in the diagnosis and treatment of choriocarcinoma: De Prins, F*, Herendael B J van***, Van der Past, H**, Stuyven, G***. *Jan Palfijn Gen. Hosp., OCMW, Antwerp; **Gynecologist, Turnhout, Belgium; ***Gynecologist, Herentals, Belgium
In two cases of choriocarcinoma routine biochemistry was performed after suspicion of choriocarcinoma. Dilatation and curettage in both cases revealed aspecific inflammation and retention products. The HCG however remained high. HCG Beta subunits remained positive, because of lack of diagnosis and continuous bleeding, hysteroscopy was performed. In both patients abnormal tissue was located. In the first patient hysteroscopic directed biopsy was performed. In the second patient hysteroscopic directed curettage with subsequent hysteroscopic control was performed as the lesion was quite extensive. Both pathology reports confirmed the visual diagnosis of choriocarcinoma. In the first patient as the lesion was small the titers of Beta HCG fell rapidly. In the second patient chemotherapy was necessary. In conclusion the

authors feel that hysteroscopy has a place in the diagnosis and treatment of choriocarcinoma so as to evaluate implantation and the extent of the lesions.

06.09.05
Aspects of management of gestational trophoblastic disease (GTD): Bloch, B. Univ. of Cape Town & Groote Schuur Hosp., Cape Town, South Africa

As a regional referral centre for a large area of Southern Africa, experience at Groote Schuur Hospital has, over the past three years, involved the care of 80 patients with non-metastatic GTD and 55 with metastatic GTD. The following aspects will be discussed: 1. Epidemiology in South Africa. 2. Hormonal contraception following non-metastatic GTD with particular reference to depo-medroxyprogesterone acetate (Depot Provera). 3. The management of catastrophic vaginal bleeding by selective embolisation.

06.09.06
Pregnancies after chemotherapy of gestational trophoblastic neoplasm: Tscherne, G. Dept. Gyn. and Obstet., Univ,. Graz, Austria

Since the introduction of chemotherapy for treatment of gestational trophoblastic neoplasm, conservative management of this disease has become possible. This is a great advance, especially for young women, as fertility may be maintained. During the last 12 years 31 patients with gestational trophoblastic neoplasm were treated at the gynecological department of Graz University. This is a high number for a central European region. 21 women had chemotherapy only, 11 of them later became pregnant. Eight of these were classified as low risk-, three as high risk-patients. They were treated with methotrexate as monotherapy, one to three courses were administered. In all the cases the reaction to the medication was very good. The interval between the end of treatment and the onset of pregnancy was at least one year. In one case pregnancy ended by missed abortion, in another pregnancy was interrupted intentionally. Nine women had 12 pregnancies, delivering 13 children, including one premature twin birth; all the others came to term. One child suffers from coeliac disease. All the other 12 children showed no abnormalities at all, physical and intellectual development was normal; the oldest child is now 11. This observation agrees with reports about pregnancies after chemotherapy of gestational trophoblastic neoplasm.

06.09.07
Moderate-dose MTX regimen in chemotherapy of gestational choriocarcinoma: Kobayashi, O, Shirotake, S, Matsui, H, Sekiya, S, Takamizawa, H. Dept. Obstet. and Gyn., Chiba Univ., School Med., Chiba, Japan

A high cure rate has been achieved in gestational trophoblastic tumors with chemotherapy. But MAC (methotrexate, Actinomycin D, cyclophosphamide) resistant cases, the therapeutic results have been unsatisfactory. In order to improve the prognosis of MAC resistant choriocarcinoma, we studied cell growth, ^{3}H-deoxy-uridine uptake and dihydrofolate reductase activity in HM cells, drug resistant choriocarcinoma cell lines, treated with various concentrations of MTX and Act-D. Based on these results and serum MTX concentrations (administered to 0.4 mg/kg to 9 mg/kg), we treated choriocarcinoma patients with moderate-dose MTX regimen (MOA). MOA protocols were as follows. Day 1: MTX, 150 mg bolus, 300 mg drip infusion for 4 hours. Oncovin 2 mg bolus. Act-D 0.5 mg bolus. Day 2–5: Act-D 0.5 mg bolus. Citrovorum factor administered intramuscularly (Day 2–3) 15 mg every 12 hours, three times. MAC was administered as the primary treatment to 39 choriocarcinoma patients. Twenty-eight (71.8%) patients attained complete remission, but eight (28.6%) patients had recurrences. We administered MAC to these recurrent cases. Only one patient attained complete remission. We administered MOA protocol in five choriocarcinoma patients including two recurrent cases whose remission was not successful with MAC. All five patients attained complete remission with MOA. We considered MOA more effective than MAC to treat gestational choriocarcinoma.

06.09.08
Effects of EMA regimen in patients with trophoblastic disease: Kim, D K, Kang, B C, Lee, J W, Namkoong, S E, Kim, S J. Dept. Obstet. & Gyn., Cath. Med. Coll., Seoul, Korea

The effects of EMA (ectoposide, methotrexate, folinic acid and actinomycin-D) regimen were investigated by comparing the initial response after the first course and the ultimate remission rate after variable courses of treatment in 27 subjects classified as medium risk group of trophoblastic disease with those of 105 subjects treated by combination therapy (methotrexate and actinomycin-D). 1. In the group treated with EMA regimen 74.1% (20/27) of "response" (log-fall of hCG) and 18.4% (5/27) of "improvement" (half-fall of hCG), totally 92.5% (25/27) of patients showed meaningful response, while in the group treated with combination therapy 32.4% (34/105) of "response" and 41.9% (44/105) of "improvement" totally 74.3% of patients showed meaningful response after the first course of the both regimens. 2. The ultimate remission rates were 100% (27/27) and 88/6% (93/105) in the groups of EMA regimen and combined therapy respectively with the same mean number of courses treated (5.8) 3. For the life threatening toxicities the EMA regimen revealed only 11.1% (3/27) of hepatotoxicity, whereas the combination therapy caused 8.6% (9/105) of leucopenia, 10.5% (11/105) of thrombocytopenia, 13.3% (14/105) of hepatotoxicity and 13.3% (14/105) of mucosal destruction. It is then concluded that the group of EMA regimen proved much more significantly effective than the usual combination therapy.

06.09.09

**Pathologic findings of hysterectomized trophoblastic neoplasms: Sutoto*, Saryadi **. *Dept. Obstet. & Gyn.,
Dept. Path., Diponegoro Univ., Semarang, Indonesia
Hysterectomy is still one of our most important alternatives in the management of gestational trophoblastic
neoplasms, because of: too expensive chemotherapy, constraints from attending follow-ups, patients want
to be sterilized, clues indicating that older patients suffer more malignant degenerations of the disease. Our
pathologic examinations were based after Tjokronegoro S. classification (1955). In the course of five years
since 1980, we got 316 cases of clinical hydatidiform moles. After evacuation, we found three cases (1.4%)
Choriocarcinomas from curettings consists of two villous and one nonvillous type, and 20 patients had
"coin lesions/s" on their chest X rays (5.4%). Follow-up yielded another nine cases (2.8%) clinical
choriocarc. (Ratnam); gave a total of 9.6% cases of malignant degeneration of H.M. which required either
chemotherapy or operation. During this period there were 48 hysterectomies performed, seven of these
were by indications, such as: bleeding (3), positive curettage finding (3), clinical choriocarc. (1); yielded 3
villous and 3 nonvillous choriocarc., but one case did not show any evidence of malignant trophoblastic
neoplasma (indication: bleeding). The other 41 patients wanted to be sterilized, with no clue of trophb.
activities. Pathologic findings of these uteri: 30 villous (73.3%), five nonvillous Ch.carc (12.2%), two
H.M.tissues and four with no trophoblastic tissue found; gave a total of 85.5% cases of malignancies. This
significant discrepancy between M.D. on removed uterus and "follow-up"makes us wonder whether
immunology plays an important role in these spontaneous regressions.

06.09.10

**Non metastatic gestational trophoblastic disease including intensive cases, therapy by chemotherapeutic
agents: Suer, S. Dept. Gyn. and Obstet., Ankara Hosp., Ankara, Turkey**
19 patients were admitted to the Ankara Hosp. with the diagnosis of gestational trophoblastic disease
(GTD), and they have been separated, non metastatic cases, including invasive ones, and treated by
chemotherapy, with single, double, or triple agent applications (methotrexate, Actinomycin D, cytoxan).
Only one case have been got triple application. They have been followed up strongly and frequently by
physical examination, chest x-ray, all laboratory analysis, laboratory investigations for chemotherapeutic
toxicities and especially B-HCG, weekly intervals. Of 19 patients, nine had methotrexate (five days) for
prophylactic reason, and invasive cases, for therapy. 4 of them were invasive which had one cure of
methotrexate or more, single or double and one triple treatment. Ten patients were mole hydatidiform and
no prophylactic chemotherapeutic therapy applied. One patient in prophylactic group and 3 patients in non
prophylactic group showed recurrence in one year. They all got 100% remission by chemotherapy. In our
understanding of the results we got, surgical intervention is not necessary in the treatment of NMTD, and
surgical operations may be harmfull and bears operative risks.

06.09.11

**Rare types of choriocarcinoma: Kanthamani, C R, Selvakumari, Devambigai. Dept. Obstet. and Gyn.,
Madras Med. Coll., Madras, India**
The incidence of choriocarcinoma in the uterus primary varies from 1 in 5000 to 30,000 pregnancies.
Ovarian primary carcinoma is in the range of 1 : 392.000,000 and non-gestational ovarian choriocarcinoma
is still rarer. It is described in ovarian teratoma or embryonal rests. A primary tubal choriocarcinoma is
also a rare entity described by *Segal* and *Garcie* and others. Two rare cases, one – a non gestational ovarian
choriocarcinoma and another tubal choriocarcinoma – are reported for their rarity. A 25-year-old woman
who had two children, the younger 18 months old, was admitted after four months amenorrhea with acute
pain, vomiting and mass in the abdomen. At laparotomy the right ovary was the seat of multiple cysts in
one portion and friable placenta-like tissue in the other. Uterus was normal and the other ovary had a lutein
cyst. On histopathological examination the uterus showed proliferative endometrium. The tumor showed
a non-gestational ovarian choriocarcinoma. The second patient was a 22-year-old woman who had one
child two years old and three spontaneous abortions. She came with a history of nine months amenorrhea,
vomiting, pain and a mass in the abdomen. Clinically a tumor of varying consistency was felt close to the
uterus which was just bulky and another fairly mobile multiloculated tumor was felt high up on the right
side. At laparotomy the right ovary showed a multicystic tumor. The right tube was normal, the uterus was
just bulky and the lateral half of the left tube was dilated and adherent to a multicystic ovary with a friable
placenta-like mass, adherent to the cystic tumor, tube, back of uterus, omentum and pouch of Douglas.
The histopathological examination report was choriocarcinoma with tubal pregnancy.

06.09.12.

**Choriocarcinoma following ectopic pregnancy. Case report – two cases: Revathi, S. Govern. Rajaji Hosp.,
Madurai, Tamilnadu, India**
Two rare cases of choriocarcinoma following ruptured tubal gestation are presented here. – Case No. 1)
19-year-old primigravida underwent left salpingectomy for ruptured tubal gestation. P.O. period was
uneventful. Exactly three months after she came in with hemoptysis and bleeding p.v. X-ray chest showed
cannon-ball secondaries. Gravindex was 1 in 400 positive. Sonar revealed uterus filled with soft mass and
right ovary cystic (8 cm). – Case No. 2) 35-year-old para-1, was operated on for ruptured tubal pregnancy
and two weeks later she developed suburethral nodule, which was proved to be secondary choriocarcinoma.

She developed hemiplegia after a month due to cerebral secondaries. Combination chemotherapy was given to both. Case No. 1 survived for one year and case No. 2 for five months. These two cases are presented for their rarity.

06.10.01

Early management of C.I.N. with CO₂-laser: Meandzija, M. Dept. Obstet. and Gyn., Univ., Bern, Switzerland

Four hundred and fifty-two patients have been treated for C.I.N. grade one, two and three, using the technique of volume destruction or the excision of the transformation zone and its glandular part with CO_2-laser. The average age was 27.7 years and the average time of the follow-up 18 months. The overall success rate at the twelve months follow-up control was 98.78%. 9.27% patients needed repeated treatments to achieve complete disease eradication. In two cases a hysterectomy had to be perfomed for persistence of the disease. Laser procedures were performed throughout, under local or general anesthesia. We observed fewer postoperative complications, a better healing of the wound and a shorter hospital stay in the laser-treated group than among controls. Laser is a safe, easy to perform, reliable and ideal mode of therapy for the C.I.N. In addition, it contributes to lower medical costs by reducing the duration of the stay in hospital.

06.10.02

The treatment of cervical intra-epithelial neoplasia using the carbon dioxide laser: Paldi, E, Friedman, M, Peretz, B A. Dept. Obstet. & Gyn. "B", Rambam Med. Ctr., Haifa, Israel

Recently laser surgery has been shown to be very effective for all grades of cervical intra-epithelial neoplasia (CIN) and has been observed to provoke few complications. The presented study group consisted of 116 selected patients with varying degrees of CIN, which was treated with the Coherent Radiation model 400 CO_2 surgical laser in the outpatient colposcopy clinic. These women were referred to the clinic for investigation of an abnormal pap smear. They ranged in age from 17 to 41 years. The CO_2 laser beam was focused at 400 mm delivering a treatment spot approximately 1.5 mm in diameter. All treatments were carried out with a continuous beam at a power density of 700 to 1000 W/cm^2. The whole transformation zone was ablated and the tissue was evaporated to a consistent depth of 7 mm. In this study 104 of the 116 patients were cured after one laser treatment (89.8%). The 12 women who had persistent abnormal cytologic findings seven months after treatment were either retreated with the CO_2 laser or had cone biopsies. Of the patients with CIN in whom primary treatment failed, eight (6.8%) had CIN III and four (3.4%) had CIN II. In all patients with CIN I the primary CO_2 laser treatment was sufficient.

06.10.03

Treatment of cervical dysplasia with bromocriptine: Donath, E M, Schindler, A E. Dept. Gyn. and Obstet., Univ., Tübingen

The clinical experience of Guthrie and the experiments of Forsberg on ovariectomized mice point to a possible effect of bromocriptine on cervical neoplasia. Therefore, we have done a pilot clinical study in women in whom we wished to avoid surgery for cervical dysplasia. So far twenty-four women (average age of 32) with persistent intraepithelial neoplasia (mean observation time 13 months) were studied. Before therapy the lesions found were CIN I in twelve patients, CIN II in eleven and CIN III in one. The treated women took bromocriptine 2 × 2.5 mg daily for between 3–8 months. In twelve women we observed complete remission, twice partial remission and in ten cases a persistence or progression of the lesions. The results suggest that therapy with bromocriptine might be an alternative treatment for cervical dysplasia. Further investigations by randomized studies are necessary.

06.10.04

Basis for an integrated CIN therapy: Dexeus, S, Labastida, R, Manubens, M. Inst. Dexeus, Dept. Obstet. and Gyn., Barcelona, España

During the last few years, there has been a considerable increase in CIN destructive local treatment (DLT). The authors propose the use of colposcopy, NOT specifically to extend the indications for D.L.T. but to reduce this to its strictest limits, avoiding useless of insufficient treatment. The recommended colposcopy, defined as dynamic involves the whole of the lesion in question. A differential diagnosis is established between the different ectopia repair processes. The use of microcolpohysteroscopy allows a better knowledge of cervical pathology as it is possible to view the endocervix. The different methods of treatment for cervical pathology analysed, proposing cryocoagulation in the CIN II which provides a 98% success rate. Conisation is almost completely abolished as a diagnostic method. The percentage of lesion persistence after the former treatment being 2%. The different records of treatment are summarised, being based on the use of cytology, colposcopy, microcolpohysteroscopy and directed biopsy.

06.10.05

Endocervical curettage, portio biopsy and diathermy in the treatment of cervical intra-epithelial neoplasia. A long-term follow-up: Claesson, U, Tronstad, S-E. Dept. Gyn. & Obstet., Centr. Hosp., Skövde, Sweden

The aim of this study was to determine whether diathermy on the portio in connection with diagnostic cervical curettage and portio biopsy resulted in better healing of CIN, compared to treatment without diathermy. – Patients and methods: In a prospective study performed in 1979–81, 310 patients with cytological atypia were found and treated by portio biopsy and endocervical curettage. After randomisation, portio diathermy was added in half of the patients. 247 patients had CIN, the distribution being CIN I 32%, CIN II 32% and CIN III 36%. One case of invasive cancer was discovered. 62 patients had benign histology. The treatment was given under full anesthesia on an out-patient basis. The cervical canal was not treated with diathermy. All patients were followed up with cytological controls. The mean period of observation was 46 months. – Results: Altogether 158 of the 247 patients healed during the time of observation (64%). In the diathermy group 100 patients (74%) healed, compared to 58 patients (52%) in the group not subjected to diathermy (p < 0.001). 50% of the relapses occurred within three months. The rate of complications did no differ. Of the 62 patients with primarily benign histopathology, 26% later showed CIN. – Conclusions: The treatment of CIN was significantly improved when diathermy was added. This conservative regimen depends upon effective patient follow-up. Patients with cytological atypia and primarily showing benign histopathology should also be followed up.

06.10.06
Endocervical curettage: Does it contribute to the management of patients with abnormal cervical cytology: Oyer, R, Hanjani, P. Temple Univ. Hosp., Philadelphia, PA, USA
Routine endocervical curettage has been advocated in the colposcopic evaluation of patient with abnormal cervical cytology. To assess the usefulness of this procedure, we reviewed the records of 518 patients referred to the Colposcopy Clinic with abnormal pap smears. The data were reviewed retrospectively in 411 patients and collected prospectively in 107 patients. Dysplasia was present in 1.4% of ECC specimens obtained in patients with conclusive colposcopic examinations, and in 24.6% of specimens in patients with inconclusive examinations. Invasive cancer was not detected in any ECC specimen. Eighty patients with inconclusive colposcopic examinations underwent conization of the cervix; in this group, the final pathologic diagnosis was CIN III in 51.2%, microinvasive cancer in 2.5%, and invasive cancer in 1.2%. In patients with conclusive colposcopic examinations, the final pathologic diagnosis was CIN III in 17.2%, and no cases of microinvasive or invasive cancer were present. When the colposcopic examination is conclusive, the incidence of positive ECC is too low to warrant performing ECC in all patients. ECC rarely yields a diagnosis of invasive cancer; its routine use would seldom replace the need for cervical conization in patients with inconclusive colposcopic examination.

06.10.07
Recurrence rate of cervical carcinoma *in situ*: **Szalmay, G, Haller, U.** Dept. Gyn. and Obstet., Kantonsspit., St. Gallen, Switzerland
One thousand and twenty-two cases stage 0 of carcinoma of the cervix (F.I.G.O.) were examined between two and 15 years after the primary therapy at the occurrence of recurrence and persistence of the cervical intra-epithelial neoplasia (CIN). In all 114 patients were treated by laser vaporisation, 76 patients by cryosurgery, 448 patients by cervical conization, 384 cases by hysterectomy. The persistence rate is 7.5% and depends on the method of primary therapy. The recurrence rate is around 3.13% and includes also invasive carcinomas. The recurrence does not depend on the primary therapy. The exact schedule of the therapy procedure and time period between treatment and the recurrence will be described.

06.10.08
The value of microcolposcopy in the management of cervical intra-epithelial neoplasia (CIN): Vancaillie, T, Bonk, U, Schmidt, E H, Beller, F K. Frauenklin., Diakonissenanst., Bremen, and U.F.K., Münster
Women presenting with postcoital bleeding (PCB, n = 5) or with an abnormal cervical smear (n = 21) underwent a microcolposcopy with the instrument developed by *Hamou* (Storz & Co). The result was communicated to the pathologist. A cone-biopsy or a hysterectomy followed. In 23 cases (88.5%) both the presence and the degree of CIN were confirmed. In four of them a single small focus was spotted. The pathologist diagnosed once a basal cell hyperplasia and twice an acute cervicitis. The latter represents the false positive incidence in this study (7.7%). There was no false negative case. Two patients with PCB and negative smear, proved to have CIN. In conclusion, microcolposcopy is very accurate as a diagnostic tool, by the absence of false negative results. Its major contribution is the precise localization of small foci of dysplasia. As a cone-biopsy is routinely cut up every 2 mm, a false negative outcome is a real danger. This calls for the need of a biopsy, directed through the microcolposcope, a method which has been developed by the author. The microcolposcopist does not stand in for the pathologist, but provides him with the selected material he needs, whatever the size of the lesion may be, so that one can state that microcolposcopy contributes to the diagnosis of CIN in the very early stages.

06.11.01
The fate of serum prolactin in surgically castrated women: Idil, H M, Aksu, M F. Cerrahpaşa Fac. Med., Dept. Obstet. and Gyn., Univ., Istanbul, Turkey
The endogenous relationship between the prolactin (PRL) and estradiol (E2) is partially well known, because of limited human research. Twenty-one normal (group I) and nine menopausal women (group II) comprise this study. Cases were underwent operation for benign causes. Serum estradiol and prolactin

levels were assayed before the operation. In both groups probably due to stress factors prolactin levels are high. Blood for serum PRL and E2 obtained at 0, 1, 4, 12, 18 hours and 4, 6, 30 days. One hour after removal of the ovaries PRL levels rises 3 to 4 fold in all cases, then decreases gradually in 48 hours and keeps same level until 30 days. Serum E2 levels in group I decreases rapidly, after the operation. No change was found in the second group. No significant relations have been observed between the prolactin and estradiol levels after the removal of the ovaries, in both groups, this finding suggests to us that this matter on this field needs more *in vivo* human experiments.

06.11.02

Endocrine and histopathological studies in uterine postmenopausal bleeding: Bayad, M A, Abdalla, M I, Ghoneim, M A, Shafeek, M A, Ibrahim, I I. Reprod. Endocr. Res. Unit, Dept. Obstet. and Gyn., Cairo Univ., Cairo, Egypt

Serum levels of FSH, LH, estrone, estradiol, progesterone, testosterone and androstenedione were estimated by radioimmunoassay procedures in 44 patients with uterine postmenopausal bleeding. Determined levels were interpreted according to the histopathological change of endometrium diagnosed in all patients by fractional curettage. Fifty healthy postmenopausal women were the control group. They had the same specifications as the patient group and were subjected to similar studies during management of minor gynecologial lesions e. g. repair. Endometrial specimens from patients showed atrophic changes (48.89%), adenomatous hyperplasia (22.22%), proliferative endometrium (15.56%) and adenocarcinoma (11.11%), while the control had atrophic endometrium (84.31%) and cystic glandular dilatation with atrophic stroma (15.69%). Endocrine disturbance in patients was shown by significant decrease in overall mean $\pm$ SE FSH value compared with control (30.77 $\pm$ 2.47 and 40.27 $\pm$ 1.87 miu/ml, respectively). Patients with adenomatous hyperplasia demonstrated significantly lower FSH and LH, and higher estradiol levels compared with control (17.22 $\pm$ 3.98, 24.84 $\pm$ 6.45 miu/ml and 42.02 $\pm$ 10.95 pg/ml, respectively). Their FSH $\pm$ SE values were significantly lower in comparison with patients with atrophic or proliferative endometrial changes (17.22 $\pm$ 3.98, 30.81 $\pm$ 3.59 and 31.22 $\pm$ 4.38 miu/ml, respectively). No significant differences were demonstrated in other estimated hormones.

06.11.03

Psychogenic and endocrine status after hysterectomy and bilateral oophorectomy: Gökmen, O, Durmuş, Z, Dündar, G. Ankara Maternity Hosp., Ankara, Turkey

The symptomatic and endocrine changes and depression following hysterectomy and bilateral oophorectomy have been studied in 49 women. Three blood samples were obtained on the day before operation, at seven days and at eight weeks after operation. Serum was separated and stored frozen at $-20°$ C. FSH, LH, estradiol, prolactin and testosterone were measured in each sample by radioimmunoassay methods. The occurrence of vasomotor symptoms was evaluated as objectively as possible. Hot blushes were detected in 61 and 83.6 per cent respectively at 7th and 60th day after operation. For checking the incidence of depression all patients were given Zung's SDS self rating scale the day before operation and again at eight weeks postoperatively. Pre-operatively 17.5 per cent patients were depressed whereas 19.25 per cent were depressed postoperatively. The difference was not statistically significant. It is concluded that the idea of a posthysterectomy depression is misleading. There was no correlation between depression, vasomotor symptoms and plasma hormonal levels. Plasma estradiol levels at 7th day and 60th day postoperatively were 83.6%, 80.8% respectively below the values before operation. The difference was statistically significant (p < 0.01). Plasma testosterone levels showed slight decline after operation, but the difference was not significant. There was a rise in FSH and LH after operation. At seventh day after operation FSH level was 5.8, LH level was 4.6 times the respective pre-operative values. The rises were significant (p < 0.01). Plasma prolactin levels had showed an incline at seven days after operation. The difference was significant (p < 0.01). The values at 60th day after operation were similar to those on the seventh day.

06.11.04

Study on response to corticotropin-releasing factor (CRF) in climacteric women: Ui, K, Makino, T, Sugahara, M, Kobayashi, J, Yanagida, R, Iizuka, R. Dept. Obstet. and Gyn., Keio Univ. School Med., Tokyo, Japan

Corticotropin-releasing factor (CRF) was administered to eight normal and 11 climacteric women. The alteration of serum ACTH and LPH were analyzed. In follicular phase serum levels of ACTH showed low basal level (2 pg/ml) and rose significantly 13.3 times 30 min after 50 μg of CRF administration. In luteal phase ACTH levels showed higher basal levels than those of follicular phase and increase 2.9 times at 15 min and the basal levels of LPH were also slightly higher than those of follicular phase. The basal levels of serum ACTH as well as LPH in climacteric subjects were higher than those in normal women. The responses to CRF in climacteric subjects were divided into three different patterns. The first group with CMI of type III–IV and median Kupperman index of 22 indicated low basal ACTH levels and no responses to CRF administration. LPH showed also no significant responses. The second group with CMI of type III and median Kupperman index of 19.7 rose to approximately 3.7 times at 30 min as compared to the basal level and LPH showed only 1.23 times increase than the basal level. The last group with CMI of type I–II and Kupperman index of 14 had high basal ACTH and LPH levels and showed two peaks by CRF administration. Our animal study also indicated that CRF content in the hypothalamus of the postovariectomized rats were significantly higher than those of intact control female rats. These data suggest that combination of CRF tests with YG and CMI questionnaire can be a useful method for analysing different types of climacteric women.

06.11.05

Induction of sex hormone binding globulin (SHBG) by estrogens and growth hormone: Schoultz, B von, Fröhlander, N. Dept. Obstet. and Gyn., Univ. Hosp., Umeå, Sweden

The synthesis of SHBG within the liver is currently believed to reflect the estrogen/androgen balance but recent observations are at variance with this concept. While during oral estrogen therapy SHBG serum levels increase in a dose-dependent manner and have been suggested as a marker of estrogenicity there is little effect of parenteral treatment even with high doses of estrogen. Furthermore SHBG levels do not vary significantly during the menstrual cycle and are not affected by menopause or by orchidectomy in men with prostatic cancer. The liver is a main target organ for growth hormone and animal experiments indicate that this pituitary factor is important for liver protein synthesis. In 30 postmenopausal women a dose dependent increase of growth hormone and SHBG serum levels was recorded during oral estrogen replacement therapy with $10\,\mu g$ of ethinyl estradiol daily. The sequential addition of tamoxifen 10 mg twice daily normalized the serum concentrations and percutaneous therapy with equipotent amounts of estrogen had no apparent effects. In a pilot study of seven women taking no estrogens, treatment with growth hormone (4 IU twice daily) for four days was found to increase mean SHBG levels from 62 nM before treatment to 79 nM after 9–12 days ($p < 0.05$). Growth hormone may be important for the regulation of "steroid sensitive" liver protein synthesis.

06.11.06

Changes in skin collagen content with estrogen therapy: Tapp, A, Brincat, M, Versi, E, Moniz, C F, Studd, J W W. Dulwich Hosp., Menopause Clin. and Urodynamic Unit, King's Coll. Hosp., London, UK

Brincat et al. (Brit. med. J. **287**, 1337, 1983; Brit. J. Obstet. Gyn. 1985) showed that the skin collagen content in postmenopausal women receiving estradiol 50 mg and testosterone 100 mg for 2 to 10 years was higher than in an untreated group of age-matched postmenopausal controls. Skin collagen and skin thickness declines after the menopause and this can be prevented with sex hormones. Postmenopausal women who had never been treated with hormones were recruited and split into four groups. The first (16) received estradiol gel (E) (Besins, Paris) 1.5 mg daily. The second (22), estradiol 50 mg (E50), the third (20), estradiol 50 mg and testosterone 100 mg (E50 + T100) and the fourth (20), estradiol 100 mg (E100) implants (Organon, UK). Full thickness 3 mm skin biopsies were taken from the lateral aspect of the right thigh at 0, 3, 6 months and in the case of the estradiol gel group skin biopsies were also taken from the abdomen and collagen content estimated. Thigh skin collagen increased significantly ($p < 0.001$) in both the estrogel and the implant treated groups. In each treatment group, the change in skin collagen content was inversely correlated with the original thigh skin collagen of the women ($r = 0.72$, E; $r = -0.62$, E50; $r = -0.83$, E50 + T100; $r = 0.84$, E100). All correlations were highly significant. In conclusion it can be stated that skin collagen increased to an optimum premenopausal level in postmenopausal women who are treated with estrogen and testosterone.

06.11.07

The relationship of skin collagen and skin thickness to postmenopausal osteoporosis: Brincat, M, Kabalan, S, O'Dowd, T, Versi, E, Studd, J W W. Dulwich Hosp., Menopause Clin. and Urodynamic Unit, King's Coll. Hosp., London, UK

Brincat et al. (Brit. med. J. **287**, 1337, 1983) has shown that skin collagen content in postmenopausal women receiving estradiol and testosterone implants for 2 to 10 years was higher than in an untreated group of age matched postmenopausal controls. In this study 144 untreated postmenopausal women were recruited and collagen assayed from 3 mm skin biopsies from the lateral aspects of the thigh. Forearm skin thickness (ST) was measured using a radiological method and a hand Metacarpal Index (MI) was taken at the same time. The Bone Mineral Content (BMC) at 8 cm up the forearm was estimated. All four parameters from these cross-sectional data showed highly significant correlations when compared with menopausal age (MA) (SC vs MA, ST vs MA, MI vs MA, BMC vs MA, all $p < 0.0001$). MI and BMC also had highly significant correlations with actual chronological age. SC, ST and MI all had highly significant correlations ($p < 0.0001$) with each other, while BMC correlated significantly ($p < 0.001$) with MI. It is suggested that SC, ST, MI and BMC all decline after the menopause and this decline is due to hypoestrogenism. It is also suggested that SC and ST are representative of the connective tissue element of bone and their decline indicates a general susceptibility of connective tissue to hypoestrogenism. Both the connective tissue and the BMC play a part in the decline of bone mass after the menopause. By using a combination of these simple tests a more effective cheap mass screening technique for picking out those women at risk of developing postmenopausal osteoporosis can be developed.

06.11.08

Cigarette smoking, serum estrogens, and bone loss in early postmenopausal women during hormone replacement therapy: Jensen, J, Christiansen, C, Rødbro, P. Dept. Clin. Chem., Glostrup Hosp., Univ., Copenhagen, Denmark

In order to elucidate the effect of smoking on estrogen metabolism, we examined 136 postmenopausal women treated for one year with three different doses of combined estrogen-gestagen or placebo. The women were grouped according to smoking habits, and the serum levels of estrone (E_1) and estradiol (E_2) were measured before and after treatment. The results demonstrated reduced levels of both estrogens in smokers compared to non-smokers in all three dosage groups. This reduction was most pronounced in the high dose group (4 mg E_2) were the serum levels of E_1 and E_2 in smokers were only 50% of those in non-smokers ($p < 0.001$ and $p < 0.05$, respectively). In contrast, no significant changes could be demonstrated in the corresponding placebo groups. Moreover, it was possible to demonstrate significant inverse correlations between the number of cigarettes smoked daily and the change in serum E_1 and E_2, respectively ($p < 0.001$). The present study suggests that an increased hepatic metabolism of estrogens results in a lower estrogenity among postmenopausal smokers, leading to an increased risk of developing osteoporosis.

06.11.09
Regional variations in bone density with comparison to total body calcium in the early postmenopause: Padwick, M L, Whitehead, M I, Stevenson, J C. Dept. Obstet. and Gyn., King's Coll. Hosp., London, UK

Measurement of vertebral bone density (BD) by quantitative CT scanning offers an accurate assessment of axial trabecular bone. To evaluate the use of other bone measurements in predicting vertebral bone mass, we have measured vertebral trabecular BD in early postmenopausal women and compared the results with measurements of forearm BD, and total body calcium. Vertebral trabecular BD was measured in three lumbar vertebrae ($L_2 - L_4$) by quantitative CT scanning. Forearm trabecular BD was measured at the distal radius and cortical BD at the mid-shaft radius by an Isotom CT scanner. Total body calcium (TBCa) was measured by neutron activation analysis. There were close correlations between TBCa and forearm trabecular ($r = 0.87$) and cortical ($r = 0.82$) BD. Vertebral trabecular BD correlated more closely with a ratio of measured/predicted TBCa ($r = 0.69$). There was no significant correlation between vertebral trabecular BD and forearm trabecular or cortical BD. Our results demonstrate that in normal women in the early postmenopause, vertebral trabecular BD is probably determind mainly by age and years postmenopause, whereas forearm BD is much more dependent on body size. It appears essential to perform regional bone mass determinations if rates of bone loss and effect of preventive therapies for osteoporosis are to be assessed.

06.11.10
The effect of estrogen/cyproterone acetate treatment on postmenopausal bone loss: Riis, B, Jensen, J, Gotfredsen, A, Christiansen, C. Dept. Clin. Chem., Glostrup Hosp., Univ., Copenhagen, Denmark

Our group has recently demonstrated that estrogen/gestagen therapy is the optimal prophylactic treatment of postmenopausal bone loss. In contrast to gestagens, cyproterone acetate, a progestional compound, has been shown to have a positive effect on lipid metabolism. In order to examine the effect of estrogen/cyproterone acetate (E/C) treatment on postmenopausal bone loss, 80 healthy early postmenopausal women participated in a double-blind controlled therapeutic trial for two years. After an initial examination the women were allocated to treatment with E/C or placebo. Thereafter the participants were examined every third month. 68 women completed the study. In the placebo group the total body bone mineral and the lumbar bone mineral (measured by dual photon absorptiometry) and the forearm bone mineral (measured by single photon absorptiometry) decreased significantly. Contrary, the E/C treatment prevented bone loss. In the E/C group, estimates of bone resorption (fasting urinary calcium and hydroxyproline) and estimate of bone formation (serum alkaline phosphatase) showed a highly significantly decrease, whereas these figures were unchanged in the placebo group. Our findings demonstrate that estrogen/cyproterone acetate is effective as a prophylacticum of postmenopausal bone loss.

06.11.11
Local and systemic effects after the intravaginal administration of estrogens (Promestrien) in menopausal women: Pálácios, S J, Uribe, L, Fernandez Villoria, E. Dept. Obstet. and Gyn., F.J.D., U.A.M., Madrid, Spain

A study of forty menopausal women studied in our department, presenting dyspareunia and/or vaginal dryness, is presented. Blood samples of FSH, LH, estradiol and vaginal biopsy and endometrial histology were taken. All these studies were repeated after forty days of daily intravaginal administration of ten mg of Promestrien in gynecological pills (ovules). – Conclusion: Statistically, there are neither variations in the plasma levels of gonadotrophins nor of estradiol. There are no variations of endometrial histology; but an important clinical improvement and vaginal trophism is observed.

06.11.12
The vaginal absorption of estriol and dienestrol in post-menopausal women: Widholm, O, Vartiainen, E, Stenman, U-H, Wahlström, T. Helsinki Univ. Women's Hosp., Helsinki, Finland

Eighty-seven post-menopausal women, mean age round 60 years with clinical signs of atrophic vaginitis, were treated with estriol pessaries 0.5 mg Ortho-Gynest (33), estriol ointment Ortho-Gynest (21) and dienestrol 0.5 mg pessaries (33). During the first treatment week the drugs were administered twice a day vaginally and during the following three weeks one dose (0.5 mg) twice a week. Menopausal symptoms were assessed and blood levels of E_2, E_3, LH and SHBG were followed prior to the treatment, after one week and after four weeks. The blood samples were taken eight hours after the last administration of the drug. Pap smears and endometrium biopsies were taken before and at the end of the treatment. The cure rate of atrophic vaginitis and dysuria was after four weeks of treatment round 80% in all groups. Prior to treatment 54 patients representing three different treatment groups had an atrophic endometrium. After four weeks a slight or moderate estrogen effect was seen in round 80% in both the estriol groups and in the dienestrol group. A slight decrease of the FSH levels was seen during the treatment with estriol ointment. All the other hormone analyses showed no significant changes during the observation time.

06.12.01

Fetal umbilical velocity wave ratio in hypertensive women: Cohen, H, Bessis, R, Doumerc, S, Crenn, C, Frydman, R. France

One hundred and forty-eight determinations of umbilical artery velocity waves were performed on women with pregnancy hypertension between the 20th and 40th weeks gestation. A spectrum analyser pulsed Doppler combined with a B-scan was used for this study. The resistance index (R.I.) of Doppler flow signals is used to study flow resistance of the placental villous circulation. The R.I. can be characterized with the ratio: $\frac{A-D}{A}$, with A, maximum systole amplitude, A, D, end diastole amplitude. The R.I. decreased during the pregnancies with hypertension disorders similarly to normal pregnancies. In case of hypertension, the R.I. of small-for-date fetuses was significantly higher compared with the one of normal-for-date fetuses. Rapid changes of the R.I. (decrease) were observed at the beginning of the hypertension treatment and on the other hand, an increase was noticed in case of sudden severe pre-eclampsia or fetal compromise. An attempt to correlate the values of the resistance index with the placental histology was performed. The data suggested that repetitive evaluation of umbilical artery velocity waveform is an important method of fetal management during toxemia of pregnancy. The changes of R.I. occurred earlier than the other classical patterns.

06.12.02

Blood and plasma viscosity and blood fibrinogen values in EPH gestosis: Küçükoğlu, F, Deniz, Y, Egeci, Y, Narter, I, Tükel, S. Istanbul, Turkey

Blood and plasma viscosity, blood fibrinogen and hematocrit values were investigated in 46 pregnant and 10 nonpregnant patients. Of the 46 pregnant patients 25 had toxemia of pregnancy. Blood and plasma viscosities and hematocrit values were found to be significantly higher in pre-eclamptic patients when compared with those obtained from normal pregnant patients. Blood fibrinogen levels were also somewhat higher in pre-eclamptic patients (607 mg vs 551 mg), but these findings were not significant. Significantly higher values for plasma and blood viscosity and blood fibrinogen levels were obtained in pre-eclamptic patients when compared with those of nonpregnant women, but no differences were found in hematocrit values between these two groups. Intrauterine growth retardation was found to be more frequent in pregnant patients who developed high plasma viscosity and elevated fibrinogen values.

06.12.03

Blood volume's expansion and fetal growth: Grella, P V, Lenardo, L di. Clin., Ostet. and Gyn., Univ., Padova, Italy

Expansion of the blood volume in the pregnant woman assures an adequate placental perfusion which is absolutely necessary for optimum fetal growth; a reduction of this volume often carries with it a fetal growth retardation. This research aims at evaluating whether the fetal growth rate may be improved by dextran infusion, a plasma expander. Our study was carried out on 39 pregnant women: of these 23 had an AGA fetus and 16 had a SGA fetus. During the dextran therapy period (which lasted one week), we measured daily: bodyweight, diuresis, blood pressure, total estriol, HPL, fibrinogen, and hematocrit; fetal growth was monitored by ultrasound before and after the therapy. The results point out that the dextran infusion increases the body fluids and particularly the plasma volume. This was substantiated by the weight, diuresis and hematocrit variations. The hemodilution is a favorable factor in relation to fetal growth since it increases its rate, in a statistically very significant way, mainly in SGA fetuses.

06.12.04

The rheological properties of blood in pre-eclampsia (PIH): Heilmann, L, Siekmann, U. Dept. Obstet. and Gyn., Univ., Essen

The diagnosis of PIH is based on the development of hypertension with proteinuria and/or edema after the 20th week of gestation. Arterial blood pressure is controlled by various factors including cardiac output, peripheral resistance, elasticity of blood vessels, and rheological properties of blood. – Patients: Twenty nonpregnant women were compared with 120 pregnant patients. The third group consists of 70 pregnant women with PIH. Forty of them were treated with hypervolemic hemodilution of hydroxyethyl starch (HAES 10%, MW 200,000). – Results: The rate of aggregation was significantly different between patients with PIH and normal ones. Hematocrit values increased in patients with PIH. Erythrocyte deformability was decreased in pre-eclamptic women and we found an increased water content. Red cell fragility was not statistically different to the results of normal pregnancy. After infusion of HAES hematocrit and red cell aggregation were decreased. In PIH we found a hemoconcentration as a result of lower plasma volume. It is possible that these hemorheological abnormalities interfere with placental perfusion. Hemodilution causes an improvement of uteroplacental blood flow. – Methods: Erythrocyte deformability, white cell deformability, red cell aggregation, serum osmolality, colloid osmotic pressure, plasma viscosity, erythrocyte fragility, water and sodium content of erythrocytes.

06.12.05

Increased arterial adrenaline highly correlated to blood pressure and *in vivo* platelet function in pre-eclampsia: Øian, P, Maltau, J M, Kjeldsen, S E, Eide, I, Lande, K, Gjesdal, K. Dept. Obstet and Gyn., Univ., Tromsø, and Dept. Med., Ullevål Hosp., Univ., Oslo, Norway

Compared to normotensive pregnant (BP $113 \pm 3/67 \pm 3$ mm Hg, n = 13), patients with severe pre-eclampsia (BP $170 \pm 4/111 \pm 4$ mm Hg, n = 13) had increased arterial adrenaline (125 ± 24 vs 43 ± 5 pg/ml, p < 0.001), peripheral venous adrenaline (67 ± 10 vs 37 ± 6 pg/ml, p < 0.01) and arterial-venous difference of adrenaline (58 ± 17 vs 6 ± 2 pg/ml, p < 0.001) concomitant with increased heart rate (89 ± 2 vs 81 ± 2 beats/min, p < 0.01) and venous concentration of the *in vivo* platelet release product beta-thromboglobulin (93 ± 12 vs 35 ± 4 ng/ml, p < 0.001). In the pre-eclamptic group, arterial adrenaline correlated with mean arterial blood pressure (r = 0.89, p < 0.001), heart rate (r = 0.78, p < 0.01) and beta-thromboglobulin (r = 0.82, p < 0.001). In the normotensive group, no correlation appeared between arterial adrenaline vs blood pressure or heart rate, only vs beta-thromboglobulin (r = 0.76, p < 0.01). Arterial noradrenaline and venous catecholamines showed less linear relationships to blood pressure, heart rate and beta-thromboglobulin than did arterial adrenaline. According to our results sympathetic adrenal tone is increased in pre-eclampsia. Adrenaline released into arterial and later mixed caval blood relates directly and to a high degree to blood pressure, heart rate and *in vivo* platelet function and may play a central role in the pathogenesis of the high blood pressure and the activation of the coagulation system in this disease.

06.12.06

The HELLP syndrome – part of EPH toxemia?: Goecke, C, Heyes, H. Dept. Obstet. and Gyn., Luisenhosp., Aachen

The HELLP syndrome includes hemolysis (H), elevated liver enzymes (EL), low platelet counts (LP) in addition to epigastric or right upper quadrant pain in combination with EPH toxemia. Seven cases with this syndrome are presented with description of diagnosis and management. In all cases pain and tenderness in the epigastric region associated with nausea and vomiting were the major findings leading to early diagnosis of HELLP syndrome. The treatment was prompt termination of the pregnancy by Cesarean section regardless of fetal maturity. The liver was always pale or white, hard and mostly with subcapsular hemorrhages. Signs of microangiopathic hemolytic anemia (schistocytes in the peripheral blood) and disseminated intravascular coagulation were present to a varying degree in all patients. Therefore, the administration of fresh frozen plasma is important. The recognition of this syndrome with early treatment prevents maternal and neonatal death.

06.12.07

Plasmatic serotonin concentrations in smoking women, fetuses and newborns: Natale, N, Busacca, M, Coletta, P, Paolino, G, Gementi, P. Clin. Obstet. and Gyn. IV; Hosp. S. Giuseppe, Milano, Italy

Infants from smoking mothers present low weight and high morbidity, which can be related to the vasoconstriction and the consequent low placental perfusion induced from maternal plasma serotonin release. We studied by HPLC-method the concentrations of serotonin in plasma through pregnancy and delivery up the fourth day of newborn's life in smokers (group A) and non-smokers (group B). Serotonin increases through pregnancy in smokers, according a week-related linear progression (p < 0.001). This increase is always significantly higher than in non-smokers. At delivery serotonin reaches a peak in both groups, still significantly different. Fetal cord blood serotonin approaches maternal levels with statistical difference between group A and group B. Serotonin clearance in the newborn is very high during the first four days, so that plasma values fall in both group of infants (p < 0.001). We can confirm previous reports that serotonin increases in smokers and passes through placental barrier. The newborn excretes maternal serotonin during the first four days of life. The persistence of high levels of serotonin in newborns of smoking mothers might be the consequence of the stimulation of serotonin producer fetal cells through pregnancy.

	1°trim	2°trim	3°trim	deliv.	cord	newb
smokers	3.82	5.59	9.46	20.11	19.7	4.60
non-smokers	2.88	3.02	4.02	13.92	13.5	3.53

Serotonin values are expressed in ng/ml of plasma.

06.12.08

The influence of maternal hypertension upon fetus and newborn: Bogdanov, N, Koleva, J. Dept. Obstet. and Gyn., Med. Acad., 3rd Municip. Hosp., Sofia, Bulgaria

Retrospective evaluation was applied to 472 pregnancies of women with hypertension for the period between 1975–1983. The birth record in that period amounted to 18,242. Hypertension was recorded from 2.59 per cent of the deliveries. 2.33% (n = 11) of the observed pregnant women with hypertension had spontaneous abortion, 13.98% (n = 66) had premature labor and 83.68% (n = 395) were labor on term. The dystrophic infants were found in 8.05% (n = 38), intrauterine death in 7.41% (n = 35) and depressive new-born infants in 18.0% (n = 85). The perinatal mortality was 82.63‰ (n = 39). The analysis of premature deliveries in pregnant women with hypertension revealed that impairment of the fetus (dystrophy and intrauterine death) was found most frequently, 34.84% (n = 23) and 59.09% (n = 39), respectively. Maternal hypertension influenced unfavorably the fetal growth and the state of the newborn more often in the second trimester.

06.12.09

Hormonal milieu in severe pregnancy toxemia before and after treatment: Lichtenberg, R v., García, C E, Santos, J, Valdes, M E, Marcushamer, B. Hosp. "Luis Castelazo-Ayala", IMSS, México, D.F.

There have been no reports on regards to the modifications of the hormonal milieu with treatment of severe pregnancy toxemic patients. We have studied ten patients with severe toxemia who were admitted to the intensive care unit and measured their circulating levels of cortisol, estradiol, estriol, progesterone, thyroid hormones, TSH, prolactin, HCG B subunit, growth hormone, chorionic somatomammotropin, insulin, aldosterone, renin, prostaglandins E and $F_{2\alpha}$. After eight hours of treatment these hormonal levels were again measured. Pregnancy was interrupted by a Cesarean section, during which a sample of cord blood and amniotic fluid was taken and the same hormonal determinations were undertaken. Tests for fetal pulmonary maturity were also done in the amniotic fluid. The hormonal determinations were repeated 72 hours after termination of pregnancy. The hormonal values were compared to normal standards for the same gestational age. When the hemodynamic conditions were normalised during treatment, we found modifications in the stress hormones: cortisol, growth hormone, prolactin as well as insulin, aldosterone and renin.

06.12.10

Serum and amniotic fluid prolactin level in ante-partum eclampsia: Abdulah, S A, Shaaban, M M, Ghaneimah, S A, Hammad, W A, Sayed, E H, Abdel-Aleem, A M. Depts. Obstet./Gyn. and Biochem., Univ., Assiut, Egypt

Prolactin levels in the maternal plasma and amniotic fluid of 38 patients with ante-partum eclampsia were measured and the levels were compared with those of 132 normal healthy pregnant women. Mean serum PRL levels in the patients were significantly higher than those of the controls of the corresponding gestational weeks (p < 0.001). The difference from normal was particularly marked in eclampsia that occurred before 34 weeks; the mean levels were four times higher than normal controls. The amniotic fluid PRL concentrations in eclampsia were lower than the corresponding normal pregnancy levels especially in the late third trimester.

06.12.11

Main causes of coma and/or convulsions in pregnancy in Maputo, Mozambique: Ching, C Y P, Songane, F F, Bergström, S, Povey, G. Dept. Obstet. and Gyn. (Maternidade), Eduardo Mondlande Univ., Maputo, Mozambique

A detailed inquiry was carried out in all pregnant women entering the Maputo Central Hospital with coma and/or convulsions during the period 1/1–31/12 1984. A total of 91 such women entered, among whom 17 died (18%). The number of deliveries was 11,203, mainly women at high obstetric risk. The majority of all cases with coma/convulsions suffered from eclampsia (76%), followed by cerebral malaria (6%) and meningitis (5%). An analysis of the eclampsia subgroup shows a predominance of nulliparas (67%), about three times the frequency encountered in the general pregnant population. Half of the eclamptics (54%) were below 20 years of age. Maternal eclamptic deaths occurred in 8/69 (12%) cases. Living children were born to 75% of the eclamptics. Puerperal eclamptics constituted 31% of all. Over half (54%) of eclamptic women had attended an antenatal clinic more than three times. As far as climatic conditions are concerned a clear concentration to the cold period was noted, resulting in monthly totals of 14% in June, 17% in July and 11% in August, giving 42% of eclamptic incidents during this three month period. Policy implications of the findings in this study will be discussed.

06.13.01

Bromocriptine treatment of fibrocystic breast disease, a survey: Dogliotti, L, Orlandi, F, Torta, M. Pat. Med. D, Univ., Torino, Italy

Rational endocrine protocols for the management of fibrocystic breast disease (FCD) have been recently proposed in the light of better knowledge of its pathophysiology and biochemistry. Prolactin (PRL), along with sex steroids, is now assigned a leading part in the hormonal connection with FCD. Consequently, hypoprolactinemic treatment, through restoration of altered dopaminergic tone, enhancement of progesterone secretion and modulation of steroid hormone receptor activity at the breast level, has been gaining interest in treating some forms of benign breast disease. Bromocriptine is the drug of choice for suppression of PRL and its efficacy in severe breast pain and premenstrual tension has been demonstrated in numerous open and controlled studies. Bromocriptine is also effective against FCD: we reported, first, subjective and objective success in nearly all of 23 patients treated with bromocriptine 7.5 mg/day × 3 months and soon after we confirmed these data in a sequential study, comparing it with methergoline (1979). Thereafter our series of patients increased up to 200 with a mean response rate of 80%. Extensive work related to this topic has been carried out in Europe in recent years: the reported results (more than 1200 pt. evaluated, with a response rate of 70 up to 86%) are very similar and lead us to consider bromocriptine, also in the light of the paucity of side-effects, a drug of choice in symptomatic FCD.

06.13.02

Unique aspects of the biochemistry of human breast cyst fluid: Bradlow, H L[1], Fleisher, M[2], Schwartz, M K[2], Breed, C[3]. [1]Rockefeller Univ., [2]Memo. Sloan-Kettering Ca Ctr, and [3]Doctors Hosp., New York, NY, USA

Studies on the biochemistry of breast cyst fluid have demonstrated the presence of a remarkably diverse variety of compounds and elements at frequently extraordinary levels. The substances present ranged from proteins like GCDP-15, β-HCG, CEA reactive material, relaxin and α-fetoprotein. A variety of enzymes including lactic dehydrogenase (LDH), phosphohexose isomerase (PHI), γ-glutamyltranspeptidase, α-amylase and β-glucuronidase are elevated as well as steroid hormone metabolites including dehydro-isoandrosterone, androsterone and their sulfates, the corresponding diol monosulfates, and estradiol, estrone and estriol sulfates but not the parent steroids like testosterone, cortisol and progesterone. A characteristic of most of these substances is that they are present at levels greatly in excess of plasma levels and in many cases where they are totally absent from the plasma. This broad array of biological substances can be arranged in ordered pattern using the ionic composition as a sorting index into two classes of breast cysts; one characterized by plasma-like levels of Na^+, K^+, Cl^- (Na 100–150 meq/l, K 5–20 meq/l, and Cl 60–100 meq/l), high levels of LDH, PHI and CEA reactive material and low levels of steroids, hPRL, relaxin and β-HCG while the other grouping is characterized by the reverse levels of Na^+ and K^+ (Na < 50 meq/l, K > 100 meq/l), almost undetectible levels of Cl^- < 10 meq/l and a major anion gap contains low levels of LDH, PHI and CEA reactive material, elevated levels of steroids, hPRL, β-HCG and relaxin. In addition this later class appears to be associated with an increased risk for breast cancer.

06.13.03

Abnormalities of prolactin secretion in patients with fibrocystic breast disease: Angeli, A, Faggiuolo, R, Berruti, A. Pat. Med. D, Univ., Torino, Italy

The role of prolactin (PRL) in the pathophysiology of fibrocystic breast disease (FCD) has been re-evaluated in the light of experimental studies and of the effectiveness of bromocriptine therapy. Plasma PRL levels measured on single blood samples in diverse groups of patients with FCD were comparable to controls, but the circadian-adjusted mean obtainable with proper sampling protocols was mostly higher than normal due to enhanced nocturnal peak. Significant abnormalities of the PRL response to TRH stimulation and dopaminergic inhibition were found in cases diagnosed as having FCD or presenting with cyclical mastalgia and nodular breast disease. We evaluated plasma PRL dynamics after acute TRH or domperidone injection in the follicular phase of the menstrual cycle in selected patients with FCD and in age-matched controls. Baseline levels of PRL, TSH, total and free T_4, total and free T_3, and 17β-estradiol were in the normal range. TSH response to TRH (200 μg i. v.) was superimposable in both groups. PRL response, however, was significantly higher in patients (net increase, p < 0.001; per cent increase, p < 0.001; integrated area of response, p < 0.01). On the other hand, PRL profile after i. v. injection of 0.5 or 4 mg domperidone (both doses did elicit an apparently maximal release from lactotropes) was similar in patients and controls. The significance of increased PRL release after submaximal stimulation in patients with FCD is unclear; in our series this feature appeared independent of actual or previous estrogen dominance. Whatever mechanism are involved, abnormalities in the control of PRL secretion also the deserve consideration better to define those patients who are candidates for bromocriptine therapy.

06.13.04

Significance of serum prolactin levels in the management of benign breast diseases: Peters, F. Dept. Obstet. and Gyn., Univ., Freiburg

Fibrocystic breast disease (FCD) may be complicated by cyclical mastodynia (CM) or by nonpuerperal inflammatory mastitis (npM). This study deals with diagnostic value of serum prolactin (PRL) levels and therapeutical significance of PRL lowering by dopamine agonists (DA) in FCD. Patients with CM exhibited slightly elevated basal PRL levels, stimulation by thyrotropin-releasing hormone (TRH), however, revealed significantly higher PRL responses in patients than in healthy controls. The efficiency of treatment of CM with DA in patients with elevated basal values (> 15 ng/ml) was positively correlated to the height of the PRL levels, while no correlation was found in patients with normal PRL levels. Patients with higher TRH-induced PRL responses derived more benefit from DA treatment than women with normal responses. In npM 37 of 82 patients exhibited elevated PRL levels, 13 had prolactinomas. In cases with no suspicion of an abscess, DA were quite as safe as antibiotics in treating acute inflammation. Long-term DA administration could prevent recurring inflammation. These data indicate that CM coincides with increased PRL secretion. NpM may be indicative of hyperprolactinemia. Therefore, PRL inhibition by DA represents a meaningful therapeutical approach for these complications of FCD.

06.13.05
Double-blind of bromocriptine, diuretic and placebo for patients with mastalgia: Russell, I S, Collins, J P.
Breast Serv., Royal Melbourne Hosp., Melbourne, Australia
A double-blind three arm parallel study was conducted to compare the efficacy of bromocriptine, a diuretic and a placebo for the treatment of patients with mastalgia who had no demonstrable breast lesion. 100 patients with severe mastalgia, some of whom had been treated before, were entered into the study. 73 patients had cyclical mastalgia and 23 suffered continuous, non cyclical, pain. After 4 months the patients and clinicians separately assessed response to treatment. This will be reported in relation to patients age, menopausal status, response to previous treatment and prolactin levels.

06.13.06
Treatment of benign breast disease by progesterone and progestins: Sitruk-Ware, R, Kuttenn, F, Contesso, G, Sterkers, N, Mauvais-Jarvis, P. Dept. Reprod. Endocr., Hôp. Necker, Paris, France
Until recent years the definition of benign breast disease (BBD) has often been restricted to chronic fibrocystic disease (FCD). The recent data on the presence of specific receptors for estradiol and progesterone (P) in normal and pathologic breast tissue definitely allows one to consider the human breast as hormone-dependent. The present study was carried out with the aim of correcting the P insufficiency found in 380 women with various BBD and an hormonal profile of inadequate luteal phase or anovulation. Thus P supplementation was given by combination of a sequential administration of an oral progestin-Lynestrol (LYN)- and of percutaneous P applied daily on the breast. The best results have been obtained in mastodynia (96%) in increased nodularity (85%) and in recent fibroadenomas. The hormonal treatment was found to be more effective in the case of recent lesions where edema is the predominant factor and when glandular hyperplasia is the most constant histologic finding (increased nodularity). By contrast, the long-standing lesions FCD where fibrosis is the main histologic component were insensitive to this treatment. In order to provide more information about the progestin action on breast tissue, biochemical and pathological studies were performed in patients under treatment. *In vitro* experiments showed a potent antiestrogenic effect of progestins on receptor kinetics and cell proliferation. Pathological findings indicate that LYN does not increase the mitotic activity of mammary cells from a morphological viewpoint. It is suggested that BBD should be treated early before the development of irreversible sclerosis and for a long time, especially in the cases with other risk factors for breast cancer.

06.13.07
Surgeon's view of fibrocystic breast disease: Mansel, R E. Univ. Dept. Surg., Univ. of Wales Coll. Med., Cardiff, UK
The term fibrocystic disease includes a wide spectrum of breast conditions that are often confused both clinically and pathologically. The borderline between normality and disease is blurred and the confusion is perpetuated by a plethora of ill-defined descriptive terms. The pathology can be subdivided into variations of development and involution; duct ectasia and its associated inflammatory states and neoplasia. Clinically, benign breast disease (BBD) presents as painful nodularity; lump; nipple discharge, and inflammation. The clinical presentations do not predict the histopathological findings on biopsy as any of the histological changes ascribed to BBD may be seen in a totally asymptomatic breast examined post mortem. The surgical approaches are straightforward: dominant lumps should be biopsied; cysts should be aspirated and persistent nipple discharge of inflammation treated by duct excision. Pain and nodularity is treated by exclusion of cancer and reassurance in the first instance. Severe and persistent mastalgia can be treated by modern anti-hormone drugs with good results. Finally, pathologists should define the subgroups of proliferative BBD with great care, as the risk of subsequent breast cancer has been shown to be associated with those lesions demonstrating atypia.

06.28.01
Blepharophimosis, ptosis, epicanthus inversus, and primary ovarian failure: Graf, M[1], Distler, W[1], Koldovsky, U[1], Schnuerch, H G[1], Majewski, F[2]. [1]Dept. Obstet. and Gyn., [2]Dept. Hum. Genet., Univ., Düsseldorf
Combined blepharophimosis, ptosis, and epicanthus inversus (BPEI) present a rare syndrome with autosomal dominant transmission. Two different types of the syndrome are described. Type I is associated with infertility in affected females (Am. J. hum. Genet. **35**, 1020, 1983). Although the ocular disorder has been reported in more than a hundred cases in the literature, little is known about the etiology of infertility in those patients. In this case report we were able to follow the development of primary ovarian failure in a 28-year-old woman with BPEI right from the beginning. Repeatedly we determined peripheral hormone levels of LH, FSH, prolactin, estradiol, DHEAS and testosterone within a two-year period. During this observation basal levels of gonadotropins increased. The menstrual cycles became more and more irregular. Morphologic examination of ovarian tissue obtained by wedge resection revealed no signs of follicular maturation. The occurrence of corpora albicantia gave evidence of ovulations during earlier life time. Later

on, the serum was investigated for specific antibodies against ovarian tissue by using indirect immunofluorescence methods. So far we could find no indication for an immunologic etiology of the ovarian failure associated with BPEI syndrome. We conclude that primary ovarian failure can be the cause of infertility in women with BPEI syndrome and it can also develop during later life. Therefore serum hormone levels should be evaluated whenever this ocular disorder is diagnosed in females.

06.28.02

Clinical and cytogenetic findings in 83 patients with primary amenorrhea: Bonilla-Musoles, F, Millet, A, Pellicer, A. Dept. Obstet. and Gyn., Hosp. Clin., Valencia, Spain

The new cytogenetic techniques have contributed to the gynecologist's knowledge about chromosomal alterations in the clinical setting. This is a study of 83 patients with primary amenorrhea. Twenty-three patients presented chromosomal anomalies, nine with a chromosomal constitution 45,X; two mosaicisms 46,XX/45,X; two isochromosomes 46,Xi(Xq) and one mosaicism with isochromosome 46,XX/46,Xi (Xq); four with karyotype 46,XY; one mosaicism 45,X/46,XY and other 45,X/46,XY/47/XYY and three polymorphisms. The clinical findings are described and the possibility of malignant gonadal changes in XY patients and XY mosaicisms.

06.28.03

Primary ovarian failure and somatic anomalies with various chromosomal complements: Blažek, L, Grizelj, V, Poje, Z, Kaić, Z, Škrinjaric, I. Gen. Hosp. "Kajfeš", Zagreb Univ. Med. School, Stomat. Fac., Zagreb, Yugoslavia

Forty-six patients with primary ovarian failure were evaluated in order to determine possible connections between gonadal dysgenesis and somatic anomalies. In addition to detailed clinical, hormonal and cytogenetic studies, an examination of gnatho-facial system and palmar dermatoglyphs was done. According to their karyotypes all of the patients were divided into two major groups: (i) chromosome competent ovarian failure (CCOF), 46,XX in 23 patients and (ii) chromosome incompetent ovarian failure (CIOF) in 23 patients, out of which 10 with 45,X, ten with mosaicism and three with X chromosome structural abnormalities. The CCOF patients were of mean age 19.8 and 159.9 cm tall. The CIOF patients were of mean age 16.9 and 146 cm tall, hence much shorter. Somatic anomalies were found in 17% of CCOF patients, but as much as 96% of CIOF patients. Orthodontic anomalies, morphological tooth malformations and palmar dermatoglyph disorders were also found in both groups, predominantly in CIOF patients. The present data suggest that the patients with gonadal dysgenesis and various chromosomal abnormalities are likely to develop numerous somatic anomalies.

06.28.04

Clinical profile of 32 cases of primary amenorrhea: Chandravati. Dept. Obstet. and Gyn., King George Med. Coll., Lucknow, India

Primary amenorrhea is a symptom of many etiologically heterogeneous disorders. High incidence of illiteracy and ignorance in our population has made it an important social problem. Thirty-two cases of primary amenorrhea admitted in Queen Mary Hospital, Lucknow/India were evaluated by clinical examination, diagnostic laparoscopy, chromosomal and hormonal studies. The results showed Mullerian duct anomaly in 65.6% cases, gonadal dysgenesis in 9.4%, uterine hypoplasia in 9.4% cases. One patient showed hypogonadotrophin hypogonadism, one premature ovarian failure and one Turner syndrome, one polycystic ovarian failure and two cases had genital tuberculosis. The study indicates that on clinical examination if the uterus is absent, further investigations are not required except for academic interest. But if the uterus is present, extensive investigation should be done to reach a definitive diagnosis. In cases who are incurable in terms of menstruation and reproduction, counselling of patients is required.

06.28.05

Naloxon-induced gonadotropin alterations in amenorrheic women: Egarter, C, Huber, J, Schurz, B, Spona, J. 1st Dept. Obstet. and Gyn., Univ., Vienna, Austria

In 51 amenorrheic patients the pituitary reactivity was investigated by way of a GNRH stimulation test. At the same time, the opiate antagonist naloxon was infused into all of these women in the frame of a further test. In seven of the 51 women a significant increase of luteinising hormone was encountered, as compared to the basal values. On comparing the pituitary kinetics of these seven patients, only an insufficient or missing gonadotropin release is observed after the second bolus, which immediately follows the first GNRH-bolus. This seems to confirm the theory that endorphins mainly influence the gonadotropin storage capacity. Where the influence has been definitely assessed, the second pool is missing.

06.28.06

TRH-test in diagnostic undefined secondary amenorrhea: Schurz, B, Huber, J, Lopez-Zepeta, M A, Metka, M, Spona, J. 1st Dept. Gyn. and Obstet., Univ., Vienna, Austria

In 50 secondary amenorrheic patients the TRH-test was performed during an untreated period. Normal results were found 26 times; in 24 patients a hypothyroid reaction type was confirmed. These results seem to prove the interaction between thyroid and sex hormones. After a short period of thyroxin treatment normal menses started in five cases. Three times a hypergonadotropic amenorrhea corresponding to WHO

III was confirmed in correlation with a hypothyroid reaction type. After thyroxin treatment there was a normalisation of the gonadotropins and subsequently ovulation was observed after clomifen treatment. Further results: Five hypothyroid patients showed hirsutism with normal values for androgens. In two cases thyroxin treatment significantly reduced complaints such as abnormal hair growth.

06.28.07
Effects of gynecologic operation on biogenic amines determined by gas chromatography mass spectrometry: Ikeda, H, Yoshizawa, H, Kuwabara, S. Dept. Obstet. and Gyn., Kanazawa Med. Univ., Uchinada, Ishikawa, Japan
This paper aimed at determining urinary biogenic amines in relation to vasomotor symptoms after oophorectomy and adrenal response to operative stress. Eight patients, aged 35 to 50 years, each with myoma uteri combined with an ovarian tumor were examined to determine adrenaline (A), noradrenaline (NA) and dopamine (DA) by gas chromatography mass spectrometry (GC-MS). All patients were operated on under lumbar epidural analgesia and grouped into the hysterectomy only, the hysterectomy with unilateral oophorectomy and the hysterectomy with bilateral oophorectomy. In patients who still had both ovaries, mean urinary A, NA and DA were decreased from 90.2 ± 79.3, 204.7 ± 169.6 and $152.6 \pm 101.1 \mu g/day$ for 1–5 days after operation to 47.8 ± 61.1, 109.9 ± 62.7, and $111.9 \pm 33.2 \mu g/day$ two weeks later. Those patients following unilateral oophorectomy showed decrease of A, NA and DA from 116.9 ± 227.3, 173.8 ± 145.2 and $272.4 \pm 230.7 \mu g/day$ for early days after operation to 27.5 ± 15.0, 72.2 ± 40.2 and $98.8 \pm 88.0 \mu g/day$ two weeks later. Following bilateral oophorectomy, both A and NA were decreased from 50.0 ± 27.7 and $125.3 \pm 64.5 \mu g/day$ of early stage to 21.6 ± 10.3 and $82.6 \pm 46.5 \mu g/day$ two weeks later. But DA increased significantly from $273.7 \pm 207.4 \mu g/day$ of early days to $750 \pm 640.2 \mu g/day$ two weeks later. From above results it is suggested that both A and NA responded to operative stress at an early stage postoperatively and recovered within two weeks, and that marked increase of DA following bilateral oophorectomy might be one of important factors responsible for initiating vasomotor symptoms.

06.28.08
Ovarian failure phenomena after hysterectomy: Lehmann-Willenbrock, E, Riedel, H-H, Semm, K. Dept. Obstet. and Gyn., Univ., Kiel
As early as 1889 and 1896 *Glaevecke* and *Mond* suggested that not only castration, but also simple hysterectomy leaving both ovaries in place may be a cause for ovarian failure phenomena and menopausal symptoms. Out of 14 women hysterectomized with ovaries left intact, only four had no such complaints. These results were affirmed in 1899 by *Werth* and by *Sessums* and *Murphy* in 1932. In 1983 and 1984 *Riedel* and *Semm* were able to find similar failure phenomena in sterilised patients. With more than 200 women under 40 years of age having been hysterectomized for different reasons in the gynecological clinic of the University of Kiel, we conducted a follow-up investigation with respect to the prevalence of ovarian failure phenomena. In addition, serum levels of E_2, progesteron, FSH and LH were measured in a specially selected subgroup of these women, and comparisons with the follow-up data were made.

06.28.09
Recovery of ovarian function after laparoscopically treated torsion of the adnexa: A case report: Bähner, U, Vancaillie, T, Schmidt, E H. Frauenklin., Diakonissenanst., Bremen
A 19 year old girl admitted to our hospital as an emergency, presented with acute lower abdominal pain. Laboratory findings excluded pregnancy and acute infectious disease. By ultrasonography, a pelvic mass, merely cystic and tender by pelvic examination, was detected at the left side of the uterus. A diagnostic laparoscopy revealed the presence of an ovarian cyst, the entire adnexa being twisted around the ligamentum ovarii proprii and the isthmus tubae. Both oviduct and ovary were extremely congested. Laparoscopic surgery was initiated by excision of $2 cm^2$ of the cyst. The ovary and oviduct were then brought back in their anatomical position and to prevent recurrence, the ligamentum ovarii proprii was shortened with a single suture. In the postoperative period, a transient elevation in BSR was noted and the involution of the pelvic mass could be monitored by serial ultrasound examinations. The second look laparoscopy, three months later showed the left ovary of about two thirds the volume of the right ovary, bearing a follicular cyst. The oviduct was stenosed at the site of the torsion, but the ampulla was fully healed. In conclusion, laparoscopic surgery does not only reduce to the strict minimum the traumatic insult, but it is at the same time the very item, which offers the best opportunity for spontaneous healing.

06.28.10
Effect of prostaglandin inhibition on the mechanism of ovulation: The production of luteinized unruptured follicles: Killick, S R, Elstein, M. Univ., Manchester, UK
Serial ultrasonographic measurements of the mean diameter of the dominant follicle were made throughout the follicular phase in 12 ovulating volunteers in whom ovulation was stimulated by the administration of human chorionic gonadotrophin (HCG) as soon as the follicle became 18 mm in diameter. The time of the appearance of ultrasonographic evidence of follicle wall rupture was noted. Prostaglandin synthetase inhibitors either azapropazone or indomethacin, were administered during the late follicular phase to see if they had an effect on this process. Serum assays of estradiol and progesterone were made at specific points in each cycle. The incidence of a luteinised unruptured follicle (LUF) was increased in treatment

cycles over that seen in controls (LUF being defined as occurring in a cycle where the follicle is still intact 72 hours after HCG administration in the presence of serum levels of progesterone normally indicative of ovulation). Indomethacin seemed particularly effective in inducing this change and there appeared to be a carry-over effect to the next cycle but only when the same ovary ovulated for two months in succession. Hormone levels were unaltered by prostaglandin inhibition even when follicle rupture was prevented.

06.28.11
Gonadotropin kinetic in 22 amenorrheic patients: Huber, J, Schurz, B, Metka, M, Spona, J. 1st Dept. Obstet. and Gyn., Univ., Vienna, Austria
A modified gonadotropin-releasing test was performed in 22 amenorrheic (gestagen- and clomifen-non-reactive) patients. The first part of the test includes two bolus injections of $50\,\mu g$ gonadotropin releasing hormone (GNRH) at an interval of 90 minutes. Blood samples were drawn every 15 minutes. The role of the second bolus was to show a short time priming effect of GNRH. After the last blood sample a conjugated estrogen was given to the patients. The reason for this procedure was the hypophysis priming effect of estrogen. The third releasing test was done 72 hours later: GNRH was given as an infusion for about three hours to watch the long-time priming effect of GNRH. – Results: Six patients already showed a normal hypophyseal reaction after the first bolus. No response was observed in four women. An estrogen priming effect was found six times, a GNRH short time priming in five patients. These results confirmed the usefulness of an GNRH stimulation test.

06.32.01
A simplified quick semi-quantitative determination for urinary estrogen in non-pregnant female: Kamata, S[1], Kubota, T[1], Otsuka, H[2], Nishi, N[1], Saito, M[1]. Dept. Obstet. and Gyn., Tokyo Med. and Dent. Univ., School Med., Tokyo[1], and Tokyo Metrop. Hosp., Fuchu, Tokyo[2], Japan
Although various urinary estrogen determinations, such as RIA, EIA and gas chromatography etc., are available, they all require complicated procedures and take too much time. In this paper, a simplified quick semi-quantitative determination for urinary estrogen in non-pregnant female by utilizing Amberlite XAD-2 and latex hemagglutination inhibition reaction (LAIR) which we have developed recently, is reported. – Methods: 20 ml of urine added to 10 ml of XAD-2 suspension in 100 ml container was stirred for three minutes by the magnetic stirrer. The supernatant fraction was discarded followed by washing with 50 ml of destilled water, and then 20 ml of ethyl alcohol was added to the deposit and stirred for another three minutes. The supernatant alcohol fraction was evaporated to dryness by rotary evaporator, and the residue was dissolved in 2 ml of buffer solution. The specimen was semi-quantitated by LAIR of which the sensitivity was 100 ng/ml and the reaction time was two minutes. – Results: The sensitivity of this method was 10 ng/ml. Interassay variation was 10% and intra-assay variation was 7%. There was a highly significant correlation between this method and RIA. – Conclusion: This method was very prompt and simplified, and therefore, it could be well applied for the monitoring of follicular maturation in HMG-HCG therapy and IVF-ET.

06.32.02
Automatic direct assay system for measurement of sex steroid hormones in serum using high performance liquid chromatography: Suzuki, Y, Hayashi, N, Noma, J, Sekiba, K. Dept. Obstet. and Gyn., Okayama Univ. Med. School and Okayama Municip. Hosp., Okayama, Japan
In clinical practice, it is important to obtain the results of sex steroid measurement rapidly. In this study, an automatic direct assay system for the simultaneous measurement of estradiol (E2), estrone (E1), testosterone (T), 17α-hydroxyprogesterone (17-OHP), 20α-hydroxyprogesterone (20-OHP) and proges-terone (P) in serum was investigated using a high performance liquid chromatograph with both an electrochemical detector (ECD) and an ultraviolet spectrometric detector (UVD). This system was orga-nized with two pumping units for pretreatment and analysis. Sex steroids in a sample were first absorbed onto a pretreatment column (dimethyl octyl silane-silica column). After washing the column with water followed by a 20% acetonitrile solution, it was incorporated into the analytical unit (an octa decyl silane-silica column and an eluent of acetonitrile-phosphate buffer solution [5/6, v/v]). E1 and E2 were measured with an ECD (+1.0 V vs. Ag/AgCl); P, 17-OHP, 20-OHP and T with a UVD (242 nm). The pretreatment column was re-incorporated into the pretreatment unit to clean up after the elution of steroids. The steroids could be measured in 1 hour at the level of about 100 pg/ml for E1 and E2, and 1–3 ng/ml for other steroids. The recovery rates, reproducibility and calibration lines were excellent. The correlation of measurements with this method to radioimmunoassay was significant (ex. E2; r=0.77 p < 0.001). Sex steroids could be measured rapidly on every occasion. Moreover, by only exchanging the eluent, estriol in maternal serum could be measured.

06.32.03
Pulsatile LH secretion in the human follicular phase: Kiesel, L, Rabe, T, Schweizer, M, Hartmann, A, Runnebaum, B. Dept. Obstet. and Gyn., Div. Gyn. Endocr., Univ. Women's Hosp., Heidelberg
The 24 hour pulsatile pattern of LH has been studied during various periods of the human follicular phase (FP). In female volunteers (n=35) venous blood samples have been collected in the early (EFP, n=21), mid (MFP, n=7) or late phase (LFP, n=7) of their follicular phase (day 3–4, 7–8, 11–12 of cycle) every

10 minutes for 24 hours. Serum LH were measured by radioimmunoassay and analysed by a specially developed computer program. Mean pulse number of LH increased from 8.4 pulses/24 h in the EFP to 9/24 h in the MFP and 9.4/24 h in the LFP. The velocity of LH increase (increase from the nadir up to the maximum of the pulse) has been divided into four types A–D (10–40 min). Using this classification 41% of all pulses (254) could be found to be of type B (20 min), 35% of type A and 17% were of type C, whereas type D pulses occurred only in 7% of all LH pulses. LH pulses according to the size of the amplitude (grade I–VI); starting from amplitude up to 30% of the basal value (grade I) up to more than 70% (grade VI). It could be shown that 27% of all pulses (254) showed an amplitude higher than 70% of basal value (grade VI), 22% higher than 20% of basal value (grade II). The examination of combined both pulse characteristics (grade and type) revealed that the largest group was that with grade VI/type B pulses. The mean pulse amplitude increased during the FP from 0.9 ng/ml (EFP) to 1.2 ng/ml (MFP) to 1.8 ng/ml (LFP). The mean serum LH shifted from 1.62 ng/ml in the EFP to 2.56 ng/ml in the MFP and to 4.50 ng/ml in the LFP. The estimated LH half-life was about 100 minutes. The pulsatile LH secretion increased in amplitude and frequency during the course of the follicular phase. This pattern was investigated together with other serum peptide and steroid hormones as a criterion for follicle function and selection.

06.32.04

Plasma testosterone levels in infertile women: Mukherji, M, Singh, L, Chowdhury, S R, Agarwal, N, Chandra, H. Dept. Obstet. and Gyn., King's Med. Coll. and Centr. Drug Res. Inst., Lucknow, U. P., India
Plasma testosterone levels were measured by specific radioimmunoassay method in 59 infertile married women and compared with those of normal fertile women (8). Male partners were normal on clinical and semen investigations. The infertility in these women was diagnosed as being associated with ovulatory menstrual cycles (29), anovulatory menstrual cycles (19), primary amenorrhea (3) and secondary amenorrhea (8). Four ml of blood were collected by venipuncture in heparinised test-tubes between 10 and 11 a. m. plasma, thus obtained was kept at −20° C till analysis. The testosterone levels were found to be relatively higher in women with primary amenorrhea (3.68 ± 1.43 nmol/l), secondary amenorrhea (1.81 ± 0.36 nmol/l) and 2.50 ± 0.31 nmol/l in women having ovulatory cycles as compared to 1.57 ± 0.12 nmol/l in normal fertile women.

06.32.05

Thyroid profile in infertile women: Singh, L, Mukherji, M, Verma, K D, Khare, R. King's Med. Coll., Lucknow, U.P., India
Forty-seven infertile and ten healthy fertile women were studied. Apart from clinical evaluation, their thyroid profile (T_3, T_4, radio-active iodine uptake, serum cholesterol and thyroid scan) were studied. Other reproductive hormones including FSH, LH, prolactin, estradiol, progesterone and testosterone were estimated by radioimmunoassay to find out the integrity of pituitary thyroid-gonadal axis. Out of 47 fertile women, 19.2% were hypothyroid, 23.4% hyperthyroid and 57.4% were euthyroid patients. Patients with hypothyroidism and hyperthyroidism had delayed menarche in 22% and 36.3%, respectively. Menstrual irregularities were present in 72.5% of patients. Anovulatory cycles were present in 78% of hypothyroid and 64% hyperthyroid patients. 57% of hyperthyroid and 60% hyperthyroid patients had high gonadotrophins in contrast to the postulated depression of pituitary function in hypothyroid patients. Hyperprolactenemia and anovulatory cycles were present in 57% of hypothyroid patients. Infertility due to estrogen deficiency state was not found in present series. Patients with thyrotoxicosis showed significantly high plasma testosterone levels. Both hypothyroid and hyperthyroid states can cause anovulation due to disturbed pituitary-thyroid-gonadal axis and hence infertility.

06.32.06

Superovulation of habitual aborts with subtle luteal phase deficiency: Muechler, E K, Huang, K E, Zongrone, J. Dept. Obstet. and Gyn., Univ. of Rochester School Med. and Dent., Rochester, NY, USA
Five habitual aborters without a known organic cause of their pregnancy losses were studied in detail by serial blood sampling for immunoreactive estrogen, progesterone, FSH, LH and FSH/LH ratio. All patients had premenstrual spotting regularly. Luteal phase progesterone on the sixth postovulatory day was significantly lower (11.8 ± 1.2 ng/ml, mean ± SEM) than in control patients (20.8 ± 3.5 ng/ml, mean ± SEM). Results of immunoreactive estrogen, FSH, LH, and FSH/LH ratio did not reveal a discernable pattern of deviation from normal. Indirect immunofluorescence of blood samples from all habitual aborters showed evidence of autoimmunity in three of five patients without clinical symptoms of autoimmune disease. It is postulated that luteal phase abnormalities and chemical evidence of autoimmunity may be linked in habitual aborters. Treatment by superovulation produced at least one living child in each couple. This result suggests that treatment with superovulation may be the treatment of choice for habitual aborters with a subtle luteal phase deficiency.

06.32.07

Follicular phase treatment of luteal phase defect with follicle-stimulating hormone in infertile women: Huang, K E, Muechler, E K, Bonfiglio, T. Dept. Obstet. and Gyn., Univ. of Rochester School Med. and Dent., Rochester, NY, USA
Fifteen infertile women diagnosed by endometrial dating to have a luteal phase defect were treated with

human pituitary follicle-stimulating hormone (hFSH) for 45 cycles. Human follicle-stimulating hormone was given IM in a dose of 50 IU/day (group 1) for 35 cycles and 100 IU/day (group 2) for ten cycles from either the third or fifth day of the cycle for five days. Plasma estrogen was measured daily during drug injection. Plasma progesterone was measured on the 4th, 7th and 10th days after ovulation by basal body temperature during 11 pretreatment control cycles and 39 treatment cycles. Endometrial biopsies were performed on the 7th day after ovulation. The daily estrogen levels increased gradually during hFSH treatment. There was no significant difference between the two dosage groups. The mean progesterone levels were: 1) significantly ($p < .02$) greater in the treatment cycles than in the control cycles, 2) significantly ($p < .05$) greater in the pregnancy cycles than in the non-pregnancy cycles, 3) significantly ($p < .01$) greater in the cycles with normal endometrial dating than in the cycles with abnormal endometrial dating after treatment and 4) significantly ($p < .05$) greater in group 1 than in group 2. After treatment the endometrial biopsy specimens were improved to normal in 20 of 38 cycles. Five patients became pregnant during the treatment. The authors have concluded that hFSH may be useful in treatment of luteal phase defect.

06.32.08

The efficiency of lisuride in hyperprolactinemic luteal phase defect: Aksu, M F. Dept. Obstet. and Gyn., Cerrahpaşa Fac. Med., Univ., Istanbul, Turkey

The effect of lisuride-hydrogen maleate on luteal function in hyperprolactinemic infertile women was studied. Endometrial biopsies were performed in thirty-seven women, immediately prior to menstruation. The pretreatment diagnosis of luteal phase defect was made short luteal phase – luteal phase less than eight days – in fifteen women. The remaining twenty-two were diagnosed as luteal phase inadaquacy – luteal phase more than ten days – mean prolactin levels measured $650 \pm 25\ \mu U/ml$ (normal 25–450, $\mu U/ml$) in both groups prior to treatment. Lisuride (Dopergine) highly active dopamine agonist, 10–30 times more potent as a prolactin lowering substance than bromocriptine. Lisuride 0.2 mg daily given to both group for six months. In short luteal phase cases 25% and the other group 35% pregnancy detected. 10% abortions occurred. Well tolerance and simple side-effects (ten times less) were found with lisuride to compare to our previous study with the other dopaminergic agents. As a result lisuride is an efficient drug and should be added to armementarium for the treatment of the defective luteal phase with hyperprolactinemia.

06.32.09

The diagnosis of luteal phase defect (LPD) with more parameters: Chryssikopoulos, A, Liapis, A, Grigoriou, O, Arnoyannaki, N. 2nd Dept. Obstet. and Gyn., Univ. of Athens, Aretaion Hosp., Athens, Greece

A total of 149 women with LPD have been studied. The criterial of LPD were supported by following parameters: 1. The length of the curve of BBT in the second phase was less than 11 days. 2. Serum progesterone levels (P), less than 10 ng/ml in mid-luteal phase or mean P value less than 15 ng/ml. 3. An over two days out-of-phase endometrium according to biopsy. These women were divided into 4 groups. The first group included women with LPD caused by hyperprolactinemia (n = 35, 23.5%). The second group was composed of women with LPD (n = 79, 53.0%). The third group was consisted of women with second amenorrhea and LPD caused by clomiphen citrate (CC) (n = 20, 13.5%) administration and the fourth group with oligomenorrhea and LPD caused by CC (n = 15, 10.0%). We have concluded the following: 1. The duration of the second phase was 9.5 ± 1.6, 9.4 ± 1.9, 9.4 ± 1.7 and 9.8 ± 1.7, respectively. 2. Out-of-phase endometrium were 4.1 ± 1.1, 3.9 ± 1.2, 4.1 ± 1.1 and 4.0 ± 1.1. 3. Mean P levels were 9.9 ± 2.0, 10.9 ± 3.1, 10.4 ± 2.9 and 11.7 ± 3.5. No statistically significancy difference was found. Although the mean values of all parameters were related to the generally accepted characteristics of LPD, after studying each separate case, we concluded that in a great percentage at least one parameter was not in accordance with LPD criteria. The three parameters were presents in 38.25%. A necessary requirement to characterize a menstrual cycle as LPD is that, at least two parameters must be present.

06.32.10

Study on pathogenesis and treatment of normoprolactinemic galactorrhea syndrome: Aisaka, K, Yoshida, K, Ando, S, Kokubo, K, Mori, H*. Dept. Obstet. and Gyn., San-ikukai Hosp., Tokyo, *Oita Med. Coll., Oita, Japan

To investigate the pathogenesis of the normoprolactinemic galactorrhea syndrome, the response of prolactin secretion to TRH administration and the circadian profile of serum prolactin levels were measured in seven women with galactorrhea whose resting levels of serum prolactin were lower than 25 ng/ml. Bromocriptine (5 mg/day) was administered for 30 days and mid-luteal serum estradiol and progesterone levels for the indicators of the luteal function were also measured before and after the administration. The response of prolactin secretion increased significantly at 30, 60, 90 and 120 min. After TRH administration compared to those of the control ($p < 0.05-0.005$). The circadian profile of serum prolactin showed significantly higher levels from 22 to 6 o'clock compared to those of the control ($p < 0.01-0.05$) and serum prolactin levels of these patients tended to be over 25 ng/ml during the nocturnal period. By the administration of bromocriptine, serum prolactin levels of the patients decreased conspicuously, and the nocturnal surges of prolactin also suppressed. Serum estradiol and progesterone levels in the mid-luteal phase improved significantly by the administration of bromocriptine ($p < 0.01-0.05$), and galactorrhea was also disappeared. These facts suggested that the normoprolactinemic galactorrhea syndrome might be caused by the transient occulted hyperprolactinemia and the treatment with bromocriptine was useful not only for the suppression of galactorrhea but also for the improvement of the luteal function in these patients.

06.32.11

Luteal phase defects: Popovska, S, Lazarevski, M. Div. Endocr., Dept. Obstet. and Gyn., Univ., Skopje, Yugoslavia

The diagnosis and etiology in 108 cases with luteal phase defects are discussed from the clinical viewpoint. Endometrial biopsy was performed to 108 cases of infertility with abbreviated thermal shift on the basal body temperature chart, and suboptimal plasma progesterone levels. Insufficient stimulation of the ovary by insufficient hypothalamic-pituitary activity was found in 60%, inappropriate gonadotropin secretion due to elevated plasma androgens in 25%, permanent hyperprolactinemia in 5% and transient hyperprolactinemia in 10% of cases with luteal phase defects. The authors conclude that luteal phase defects can be considered as a deficiency state, produced by a variety of factors, leading to infertility and requiring etiologic treatment.

06.32.12

The luteal phase of *in vitro* fertilization (IVF) cycles – role of exogenous human chorionic gonadotropin (hCG): Wisanto, A, Devroey, P, Naaktgeboren, N, Traey, E, Steirteghem, A van. Dept. Gyn., Androl. and Obstet./RIA and IVF Labor., Vrije Univ., Brussel, Belgium

To determine whether administration of hCG during the second half of the IVF cycles could influence the luteal phase and increase the pregnancy rates, we randomly divided 76 patients who had embryo replacement after IVF into two groups: Group A (n=33) received 1500 IU hCG i. m. on day +3, +6 and +9 after spontaneous LH surge or after i. m. administration of 10,000 IU hCG to induce ovulation. Group B (n=43) received no additional hCG during the luteal phase. The luteal phase was assessed by recording its duration and by the determination of serum concentrations of progesterone (P) and 17β-estradiol (E_2) every other day. The length of the luteal phase was longer in group A (17.1 ± 1.9 days) than in group B (13.9 ± 1.6 days), $p < 0.01$. In all non-fertile cycles, serum P and E_2 were similar during the first seven days of the luteal phase. Afterwards, serum P and E_2 concentrations were higher in group A. The same pattern was observed in fertile cycles, except that serum P concentrations were higher than in the non-fertile cycles. Although these facts may point to a beneficial effect of hCG administration, pregnancy rate was not higher in group A (5/33) than in group B (7/43). Further study using another dose and timing of hCG administration is in progress.

06.41.01

Admission test – a fetal heart rate screening test in low-risk pregnancies: Arulkumaran, S, Ingemarsson, I, Ingemarsson, E, Tamby-Raja, R L, Ratnam, S S. Univ. Dept. Obstet. and Gyn., Kandang Kerbau Hosp., Singapore

This study examines the hypothesis that the Admission Test (AT) – an electronic fetal heart rate trace for 20 minutes just after admission patients in labor – could serve as a screening test for fetal distress and missed high-risk pregnancies and reduce the need for continuous monitoring in low-risk patients (*E. Ingemarsson*, Acta obstet. gyn. scand., Suppl. 99, 1981). 130 patients were, after an AT, monitored by intermittent auscultation, scalp pH:s at a cervical dilatation of 5 and 10 cm and cord artery pH but not by electronic monitors. The result of the AT was concealed to the investigators. If AT was reactive (112 patients, 86.2%) the risk for fetal hypoxia was low. Only one baby showed intrauterine asphyxia and another two had low Apgar score (< 7) at 1 min. The other 109 babies had normal Apgar scores and a normal cord artery pH (≥ 7.15). Of nine patients (6.2%) with equivocal AT one had intrauterine asphyxia (forces delivery) and another low Apgar score at 1 min. Another nine patients (6.2%) had ominous AT and out of these three had intrauterine asphyxia with low scalp pH, cord pH and Apgar score at 1 min – one forceps delivery, two Cesarean sections (both babies intrauterine growth retarded). The results are promising. Four out of five patients with intrauterine asphyxia had an equivocal or ominous AT. With a reactive AT the risk for fetal hypoxia later in labor seems to be low.

06.41.02

The predictive value of fetal breathing movements in the outcome of premature labor: Grunstein, S, Ellenbogen, A, Anderman, S, Jaschevatzky, O A. Dept. Obstet. and Gyn., Hillel-Yaffe Memo. Hosp., Hadera, Israel

PGE_2 causes arrest of fetal breathing movements (FBM) in sheep and other laboratory animals, as well as in human neonates treated to maintain the patency of ductus arteriosus, who developed, as a complication, intermittent neonatal apnoea. There is reduction or cessation of FBM in women before the onset of established labor. It also has been reported that it is possible to diagnose false or true premature contractions by ultrasound scanning of FBM. Two groups of women, presenting with uterine contractions before the 34th gestational week were investigated. External tocometry was performed for objective determination of uterine contractions. The first group consisted of 18 patients, treated by tocolytics after the ultrasound scanning showed absence of FBM. The second group comprised 11 patients with FBM present, who were observed only. Nine patients of the first group delivered within one week, while of the second group no patient delivered, all of them being discharged. In cases of premature contractions the presence of FBM seems to indicate that pregnancy will continue, while absence of FBM foreshadows early delivery.

06.41.03
Fetal quiet-activity cycle: Echographic determination of behavioral states: Romanini, C, Moneta, E*, Dell'Acqua, S*, Arduini, D*, Giorlandino, C, Rizzo, G*, Tranquilli, A L, Valensise, H. Clin. Obstet. and Gyn., Univ. Ancona; Ist. Clin. Obstet. and Gyn, Univ. Catt., Roma*, Italy
The existence of fetal quiet-activity cycle has been demonstrated by the use of cardiotocographic recordings for long periods. The "active" phase shows FHR variability greater than 10 bpm, presence of FAD (15 bpm per 15 sec) and fetal movements, and is usually followed by the "quiet" phase, in which FHR recording shows FHR variability smaller than 10 bpm, absence of both FAD and fetal movements. The length of both phases has been widely investigated in our previous reports (activity = 52.53 min, quiet = 21.42 min, total cycle = 72.75 min, mean) (1). In this report the echographic evaluation is added for the assessment of a fetal "state". 27 healthy pregnant women, between 38 and 40 weeks of gestation, underwent simultaneous cardiotocographic and echographic investigation. Using two real-time scanners for the observation of fetal head and body, fetal eye movements (FEM), breathing movements (FBM), and micturition have been analysed. During the "active" cardiotocographic phase: FEM are 87.2% REM, 7.2% IEM, 3.3% absent; FBM are 42.3% present, 57.7% absent; bladder volume is 74.2% decreased, 23.1% increased. In the "quiet" cardiotocographic phase: FEM are 0% REM, 6.1% IEM, 92.3% absent; FBM are 7.6% present, 92.2% absent; bladder volume is 10.2% decreased, 88.0% increased. These data support the assumption that FEM is one of the most important features to be considered, together with gross movements and heart rate variations, for the correct assessment of fetal behavioral states. This allows the identification of different stages from quiet to active (1F to 4F). No adequate accuracy seems to come out from the use of FBM and micturition, though in 66% of our observations this occurred during the change from the quiet to the active state. – (1) *Romani C*. et al.: Assessment of fetal cyclic behaviour by mean of FHR recording. Ann. Ostet. Ginec. **104**, 408, 1983.

06.41.04
A computer analysis of short-term ultradian rhythms in human fetal heart rate: Hoffman, H J, Denman, D I, Dawson, A J, Dalton K J. Dept. Obstet. and Gyn., Univ., Cambridge, UK; Univ. of Wales Coll. Med., Cardiff, UK; Nat. Inst. Child Hlth & Hum. Develop., N.I.H., USA
As part of a study into the response of the fetal cardiovascular system to maternal hypertension and diabetes, we used *Dalton* et al.'s computerised system of fetal heart rate monitoring (*Teleplot*, 1984) to make over 1600 recordings from 11 weeks to term on over 300 normal and abnormal human pregnancies. Of these recordings 190 had fail times of 100% or less, and we transferred these into the N.I.H.'s IBM 3081K computer for time series analysis using BMDP and SAS statistical software. We were particularly interested in conducting a pilot study to determine whether those oscillations visibly present in fetal heart rate recordings are in fact highly organised, in reflection of underlying fetal rhythms, or whether they are entirely random and haphazard. We found that the human fetal heart does indeed exhibit several specific short-term rhythmical oscillations of rate, and that these rhythms can be measured objectively in terms of their frequency, amplitude and phase. We also showed that standard techniques of time series analysis (such as spectral analysis, digital filtering and complex demodulation) can be usefully applied to conventional fetal heart rate recordings in order to investigate these rhythms. Such rhythms can be present more or less consistently for long periods of time, and whenever they disappear they may later reappear and lock back into phase again with a previous oscillation. Any particular oscillation rhythm is not necessarily immutable in character, but rather it may undergo amplitude change, phase shift, and even frequency shift.

06.41.05
Heart rate variability during antenatal and neonatal periods: Tsuji, M, Ohno, Y, Yamamoto, T, Okada, H. Dept. Obstet. and Gyn., Kyoto Prefect. Univ. Med., Kyoto, Japan
The present study was designed to analyse the fetal-neonatal heart rate variability using a new STV index. Fetal heart rates were recorded by abdominal fetal ECG monitors in 71 normal pregnant women between 20 and 42 weeks gestation. Neonatal heart rates were recorded in 26 mature neonates between days 4 and 6 of life. R-R intervals less than 300 msec and more than 550 msec were judged as errors and were excluded from the results. The maximum difference in successive R-R intervals accepted was 40 msec. The mean and S. D. of R-R intervals, the mean of absolute beat to beat difference (ABB) and the proportion of ABB below 1 msec and 2 msec (1 msec%, 2 msec%) were calculated by minicomputer. There was significant negative correlation between the mean of ABB and the 2 msec%, and the influence of the errors on the 2 msec% was less than that on the mean of ABB. The 2 msec% decreased in parallel with advancing gestation until 35 gestational weeks and showed a broad distribution thereafter. But in the neonate, the 2 msec% decreased significantly. Various behavioral states in fetus and neonate had effects on the 2 msec%. In the fetus the 2 msec% in the resting phase was higher than that in the active phase. In the neonate the 2 msec% during active sleep was higher than that during quiet sleep. Discriminant analysis was performed for each behavioral state by applying heart rate parameters. The resulting function gave percentages of

correct classification of 80–85% for each state. The 2 msec% was found to be a reliable index of STV assessment.

06.41.06
Intrapartum fetal activity: Yarkoni, S, Hobbins, J C. Yale Univ. School Med., Dept. Obstet. and Gyn., New Haven, CT, USA
The purpose of this study was to evaluate fetal movements (FM) and fetal breathing movements (FBM) during active labor in uncomplicated pregnancies and normal deliveries. Using real time ultrasound, the incidence of FM and FBM were measured in 18 fetuses during normal labor at term. The results were correlated with the simultaneous fetal heart rate (FHR) changes and with the postpartum cord blood pH and Apgar score. Recordings were made for one hour on every patient. The percentage incidence (PI) of FM (the percentage of the observation time in which fetal movements were observed) was 19.5 per cent (range: 10.1–28.6 per cent), and the PI of FBM was 8.5 per cent (range: 0–27 per cent). All FM were associated with FHR accelerations, stronger movements were associated with higher FHR accelerations. No FHR accelerations were observed with FBM unless accompanied by fetal movement. The lowest PI of total fetal activity (TFA, i.e. FM plus FBM) observed in fetuses with good outcome (cord blood pH of > 7.25 and Apgar score of ≥ 7) was 12.1 per cent. Fetal movements tended to decrease as labor progressed, while FBM was not affected by the stage of labor. Fetuses under the influence of narcotic drugs showed a lower PI of FM and FBM. These findings indicate that the normal fetus continues with its "routine" activities during labor. These fetal activities may prove to be helpful in the intrapartum assessment of fetal well-being.

06.41.07
Evaluation of fetal well-being during the third trimester of pregnancy: Salamalekis, E, Loghis, C, Kassanos, D, Kilbassanis, H, Zourlas, P. 2nd Dept. Obstet. and Gyn., Univ. of Athens, Areteion Hosp., Athens, Greece
The purpose of this study is the simultaneous evaluation of the value of many parameters for the estimation of fetal well-being. In 48 women who had been admitted in our clinic with pathological conditions during pregnancy (i.e. prolonged pregnancy, toxemia, diabetes), hormonal assays, ultrasonograms and cardiotocograms were performed. Eleven of these patients were found by ultrasonograms to have grade III placentas. Out of 66 non-stress tests 54 were reactive and 12 were non-reactive. In these 12 cases oxycotin challenge tests were performed. Seven of these tests were negative and five were positive. In all cases an evaluation of the way of delivery, the weight of the newborns, the condition of the placentas and the amount and condition of the amniotic fluid was made.

06.41.08
Role of acceleration: Fetal movement ratio on fetal well-being: Matsuoka, R, Mori, H, Kigawa, T. Dept. Obstet. and Gyn., Oita Med. Coll., Oita, Japan
The non-stress test (NST) was used as the primary tool in the management of 56 pregnancies. An objective method for interpreting the NST is obtained by dividing the total number of fetal heart rate accelerations associated with fetal movements by the total number of fetal movements. This is expressed as a percentage called the acceleration: fetal movement ratio (AFMR). Accelerations were defined as excursion of the fetal heart rate rising to 15 beats per minute or more above the base line and lasting a minimum of 15 seconds. Fetal movements were recorded as perceived by mother. AFMR in normal pregnancies significantly increased with the gestational age ($Y = 2.83X-44.42$, $r = 0.4114$, $p < 0.005$, Y:AFMR, X:gestational week). In severe toxemia cases, AFMR was significantly low compared with that of normal pregnancies ($p < 0.05$). Moreover, an idiopathic thrombocytopenic purpura case expressed 0% AFMR and resulted in intrauterine fetal death. In diabetic cases with intrauterine growth retardation, AFMR tended to be lower. AFMR in normal pregnancy correlates with the fetal growth, and if AFMR is kept at a low level, the fetus is diagnosed as being possibly at poor risk for the growth.

06.41.09
Does triamcinolone induce changes in fetal behavioral states?: Arduini, D, Rizzo, G, Parlati, E, Valensise, H*, Dell'Acqua, S, Romanini, C*. Dept. Obstet. and Gyn., Univ. Catt. S. Cuore, Rome, and *Univ., Ancona, Italy
Recent cardiotocographic and ultrasound investigations have evidenced the existence of different fetal behavioral states and their possible circadian pattern. In our previous study (submitted for publication) we demonstrated that maternal plasma cortisol (F) and adrenocorticotrophic hormone (ACTH) circadian variations may significantly interrelate with these fetal states, even though the mechanisms regulating these interrelationships require further investigations. In order to verify whether maternal adrenal activity suppression may induce effects on fetal behaviour, triamcinolone (Kenacort, Squibb) was administered to five healthy pregnant women at 35 weeks gestation. Five patients at the same gestational age were used as controls. Fetal heart rate and fetal movements were recorded continuously for 24 hours by means of cardiotocography. F, ACTH, unconjugated estriol (E_3) and 17β-estradiol (E_2), were measured every two hours in maternal peripheral plasma using radioimmunoassay technics. Our results have shown a significant decrease of fetal rest phases and a lack of circadian variations of fetal behavioral states in the treated

group as compared with the control. The hormonal patterns and their possible interrelationships in the two groups of patients are then discussed.

06.41.10
The effect of pethidine on the fetal heart rate response to vibroacoustic stimulation: Zeevi, D, Simon, A, Evron, S, Ohel, G, Sadovsky, E. Dept. Obstet. and Gyn., Hadassah Univ. Hosp., Jerusalem, Israel

Pethidine given in labor is known to have a depressive effect on the neonate and in some cases induces abnormal fetal heart rate (FHR) patterns. As FHR accelerations, in response to vibroacoustic stimulation have been shown to correlate with fetal well-being, we decided to evaluate the effect of pethidine on the FHR response to such stimulation. Thirty randomly selected parturients were studied. Ten had pethidine analgesia, given as 50 mg i.v. bolus during uterine contraction. The remainder had either segmental epidural analgesia or no analgesia at all. The FHR response to the vibroacoustic stimulation (Electrolarynx; battery powered noise source; audible sound 750 to 1000 Hz, vibrations 110–200 Hz; 110 dB) was tested before analgesia was given and every 15 minutes for two hours thereafter. The degree of tachycardic response in the pethidine group was noted to decrease by 30% to 50% in all cases, starting 15 minutes following its administration. This response differed significantly compared to the other groups of parturients who showed no change in FHR response with time. – Conclusion: The fetus does respond to vibroacoustic stimulation following pethidine administration. Nevertheless, pethidine-induced fetal depression may be anticipated even in those cases which following its administration demonstrate a normal FHR pattern.

06.41.11
The effect of maternal hyperoxygenation on fetal blood gas values during mid-pregnancy: Castle, B, MacKenzie, Z, Johnson, P. Nuffield Dept. Obstet. and Gyn., John Radcliffe Hosp., Oxford, UK

The administration of oxygen to the mother prior to elective Cesarean section or for suspected fetal distress has been found to have some benefit to the fetus. Fetal hyperoxia has not been observed so that the harmful effects of oxygen have not had to be considered. At present no information exists for such therapy during mid-pregnancy. At 17–22 weeks gestation, pure samples of fetal blood have been aspirated at fetoscopy under local anesthetic from the umbilical vein and/or umbilical artery in 17 patients scheduled for therapeutic abortion before and after the administration of 100% oxygen at 8 litres/minute to the mother. The mean values before and after maternal oxygenation are shown in the table.

| | Fetal artery | | Fetal vein | |
	Pre O_2	Post O_2	Pre O_2	Post O_2
pH	7.32	7.26	7.36	7.36
pCO_2	45	48	38	36
pO_2	20	37	40	68
BE	3.3	5.5	3.3	4.5
% O_2 Sat.	28	37	70	89

With the exception of pH, all values in the umbilical vein were significantly altered by oxygenation while only pH was significantly reduced in the umbilical artery. It appears that with oxygen administration to the mother fetal umbilical venous pO_2 during mid-pregnancy can approach adult arterial values and the fetal arterial pH falls. While the factors causing these changes are not known, the administration of oxygen to the midtrimester fetus would not seem to be justified. With the advent of intrauterine fetal surgery these findings may be important.

06.41.12
Acute changes in the fetal circulation after maternal smoking: Sindberg-Eriksen, P, Marsal, K. Dept. Obstet. and Gyn., Univ. Hosp., Malmø, Sweden

It is a question if the acute fetal response to maternal smoking is a pure adrenergic/nicotine action as seen in adults or the fetal response is due to a compromised placental circulation. The present study tries to elucidate this problem. – Method: Ten normal pregnant women in the last trimester were included. The study was randomised to two days of investigation with the women smoking a cigarette only the one day. The study period included a 15 min control time followed by a 45 min registration period after smoking. The velocity wave form and the mean blood flow were measured in the fetal thoracic aorta using a 3.5 MHz real-time scanner combined with a 2.0 MHz pulsed Doppler. – Results: The fetal heart rate rose from 138 beats/min to 165 beats/min within the first 20 min after smoking. The systolic part and the Pulsatility Index (PI) of the velocity wave form remained unchanged during the study period. The volume blood flow increased by 21% during the first 20 min after smoking as characterized by an increase in the diastolic blood velocity and an enhanced aortic diameter. Furthermore, the rising slope of the velocity wave form increased by 13% within the first 15 min after smoking. – Conclusion: The increase in the rising slope compared with the unchanged PI points to an increased myocardial contractility. This, together with the enhanced volume blood flow found, are compatible with an increased adrenergic tone in the fetus during and after maternal smoking.

06.41.13

The effect of abdominal decompression on the fetus: Ugianskytė, S, Puodžius, S. Med. Inst., Kaunas, Lithuania, USSR

Among the methods enhancing utero-placental blood flow is abdominal decompression (AD), that is reduction of the intra-abdominal pressure by decrease of the atmospheric pressure on the abdomen. The aim of our study was to define the influence of AD on the human fetus. Electronic fetal monitoring, daily fetal movement recording and urinary estriol values were used for fetal state estimation. Fetal heart rate baseline variability increased in 45.3% cases, was not altered in 47.5% and decreased in 5.5% cases following AD. A marked decrease in silent and narrowed undulatory patterns was noticed: from 23.7% to 9.0% and from 43.3% to 25.0%, respectively. Undulatory patterns were most common after AD (66.0%). Quantity of fetal movement increased from 7.5 (1–14) to 15.5 (1–30) during ten minutes time interval. In 75.0% of the cases estriol values showed a slight increase and in the remainder no change was found. We suppose AD improves fetal state.

06.41.14

Evaluation of fetal well-being by non-stress test in normal pregnancy and high risk pregnancy: Saxena, K, Prabha, Malhotra, N. Dept. Obstet. and Gyn., J.N. Med. Coll., Aligarh, India

Accurate evaluation of fetal well-being in the antenatal period is essential in the management of high risk pregnancy which frequently requires termination, to save the fetus from unfavorable environment. In the present study NST was done in a total of 200 cases out of which 100 cases were of normal pregnancy and 100 of high risk group. In our study NST was reactive in 96% in the normal group and 71% in the high risk group. It was nonreactive in 4% of normal group and 29% in high risk group. In babies born with reactive NST good Apgar score was seen at 1 and 5 m in both normal and high risk groups while babies born with nonreactive NST had low Apgar score at 1 m and good score at 5 m showing hypoxia. At 1 m it was 25% in normal group and 31% in high risk group which improved at 5 m: 100% in normal and 82.7% in high risk group. The incidence of meconium staining was found to be higher in cases showing nonreactive NST in both groups. It was observed that incidence of Cesarean section was higher in cases showing nonreactive NST, 50% in normal group and 69% in high risk group. The incidence of perinatal mortality was higher in high risk group (5%), than normal group (1%). The predictive value of reactive NST is more than nonreactive NST. To conclude NST is a reliable screening index and a help in reducing perinatal mortality.

06.42.01

The management of term breech deliveries by Bracht's maneuver: Pavert, R L van de*, Bennebroek Gravenhorst, J*, Bouwhuis-Hoogerwerf, M L**. *Dept. Obstet and Gyn; **Dept. Med. Statist., Univ. Hosp., Leiden, The Netherlands

In a retrospective study over the period 1974–1982 perinatal mortality and morbidity of singleton infants born at term in breech position were studied (244). A group of 263 infants born spontaneously in vertex position served as a control group. The control group was matched for age and parity. All infants were born after an uncomplicated pregnancy of 37 weeks and had a birthweight of 2500 g or more. The number of vaginally delivered children in the breech group was 186/244 (76.2%). Bracht's maneuver, secondary extractions and primary extractions were performed in respectively 76.3%, 21.5% and 2.1% of the deliveries. The number of abdominally delivered breech presentations was 58/244 (23.8%). Birth trauma occurred in six (3.2%) of the vaginally and in two (3.4%) of the abdominally born children. In the control group no trauma occurred. Corrected neonatal mortality rate was 1/186 (0.5%) in the vaginally delivered breech presentations. Among the abdominally delivered infants in the breech group and in the controls no mortality occurred. An A. S. (5) > 7 occurred in 172 (94.5%) of the vaginally delivered breeches and in 49 (90.7%) of the abdominally delivered infants in breech position. In the control group an A. S. (5) > 7 occurred in 97.7%. Congenital malformations were detected in 11.9% of the deliveries in the breech group and in 1.1% of the controls. As a result of the study, it is suggested that breech deliveries can be safely managed by Bracht's maneuver in well selected patients.

06.42.02

Vaginal versus abdominal delivery in breech presentation: A prospective comparative study: De Leeuw, J P*, Derom, R**, De Haan, J*, Thiery, M**, Martens, G**. Dept. Obstet. and Gyn., State Univ. of Limburg, Maastricht*, The Netherlands; and State Univ., Gent**, Belgium

The management of breech delivery remains controversial and increasing numbers of Cesarean sections are performed in an attempt to reduce perinatal mortality and morbidity. In order to clarify the use of abdominal delivery for this indication, a prospective breech management study at two university hospitals (Gent and Maastricht) was started in 1984. Perinatal morbidity was assessed by Apgar scoring, cord blood analysis, general and neurological examinations, including intracranial sonography. The incidence of Cesarean section reached 31% in Gent and 33% in Maastricht. No statistically significant differences in mortality and morbidity could be demonstrated among full term babies (gestational age > 37 weeks, birthweight ≥ 2500 g), either between groups (vaginal vs abdominal delivery) or hospitals with one exception: The Maastricht vaginal delivery group showed a statistically significant lower umbilical artery pH (7.26 vs 7.22) than its abdominal delivery counterpart. The number of cases involving low-birthweight infants is still too small for meaningful statistical analysis. Additional cases of breech delivery will be entered in the study and further neurological investigations will be performed at the age of one year. At that stage, data analysis may reveal for which birthweight group and/or gestational age, a vaginal delivery is acceptable on consequently preferable. The study provides an excellent opportunity to perform an external medical audit.

06.42.03
External turning from breech into a head presentation near term: Retzke, U, Ketscher, K-D, Kindt, J. Dept. Obstet. and Gyn., Main-Hosp., Suhl, GDR

The external turning of fetus from breech into a head presentation is one of the methods to avoid maternal and fetal risk by Cesarean section and by vaginal delivery. As a supposition, we see a technique which is undangerous for mother and fetus. Our procedure corresponds in many points a practice, which is published by *B. Westin* (1979). The sober patient is positioned head down on the side of fetus' small parts. Then an intravenous infusion is given over 30 min with $2 \mu g$ terbutaline/min. The turning is performed in many single and little steps. It needs time, a soft hand and the readiness of the Cesarean section. In 201 patients with breech presentation there was the indication with fulfilled suppositions for such a turning. The success-rate was 50%. In no case there was a complication. The turning of breech-presentation is recommended.

06.42.04
Tocolysis and external cephalic version for breech presentation: Yanagita, T. Dept. Obstet. and Gyn., Osaka Welfare Pension Hosp., Osaka, Japan

It is well known that breech presentation (BP) delivery always has high mortality and high morbidity. We have been trying to use tocolysis and external cephalic version (ECV) in a new conception as one of lots of countermeasures for it. From August 1979 to the end of 1984, there were 3031 deliveries including 127 BPs (4.2%) over 36 weeks of gestation. The cases with complications such as uterine malformation, fetal anomaly, cephalopelvic disproportion, twin, hypertension etc. were excluded. It has been thought natural version is very rare and ECV is very difficult over 36 weeks of pregnancy. We dare perform ECV at this stage, because if something troublesome had happened, we can avoid premature delivery by Cesarean section. 114 patients were receiving infusion of tocolytic agent (terbutaline) for about a week before the performance of ECV. Nine cases converted to vertex presentation (VP) naturally with only tocolysis. ECV was performed on another 105 cases under the supervision of cardiotocograph and real time B-scan without anesthesia. We succeeded in ECV of 83 cases. So 92 cases (80.7%) converted from BP to VP with tocolysis or ECV under tocolysis. Marked deceleration of fetal heart rate was seen in one case. Immediate Cesarean section delivered the infant safely. We could decrease the number of BP up to 19.3%.

06.42.05
Twin deliveries in Sweden 1973–81: The value of an increasing Cesarean section rate: Rydhström, H, Ohrlander, S. Dept. Obstet. and Gyn., Univ. Hosp., Lund, Sweden

The number of twin deliveries in Sweden between 1973 and 1981 was 7714. The twin Cesarean section rate during the period increased from 8.7% to 41.2%. During the same period the twin perinatal mortality fell from 9.1% to 3.8%. The perinatal mortality in twins delivered vaginally decreased from 9.2% to 2.8%. Twins delivered by the abdominal route showed a decreasing perinatal mortality up to 1975: thereafter extended indications for Cesarean section in the lower weight-groups caused a rise in the perinatal mortality in twins delivered abdominally from 2.4% in 1975 to 7.4% in 1977. However, an expected concomitant decrease in the perinatal mortality in twins delivered vaginally did not appear. The death-ratio of twins/ singletons according to birthweight during the period increased in the weight-group < 1000 g. In the other weight-groups no consistent changes took place. During this period the Cesarean section rate in twins as compared to singletons increased almost fourfold. The Cesarean section rate was compared to the perinatal mortality in each of the 24 provinces in Sweden during 1973–76 and 1977–81 respectively. No obvious correlation between these two variables could be traced in either period. Our study lends further support to the opinion that the declining perinatal mortality in twins seen during the last decade has no direct correlation to an ever-increasing Cesarean section rate.

06.42.06
Bed rest and perinatal outcome in twin pregnancies: Gandhi, J A, Soper, R. Metrop. Hosp. Ctr, New York Med. Coll., Scarsdale, NY, USA

Intensive antepartum care in twin pregnancies has shown to be of utmost importance in the ultimate survival and overall perinatal outcome in twin pregnancies. However, the role of in-patient bed rest in promotion of increased fetal age and growth is still widely debated in the modern times of increasing hospital costs. A prospective program of intensive twin care was begun at our institution in 1980, which included reduced maternal activity and bed rest. Bed rest in hospital was offered to all mothers between 28 and 34 weeks of pregnancy. Among a total of 95 patients in the study group, 53% were never admitted (group A), 10.5% stayed in hospital for less than 10 days (group B), and 36.5% for over 11 days (group

C). Total neonatal weights of both infants were 4786 g, 4417 g, and 4826 g in groups A, B, and C and the gestational ages of infants at birth were 35.8, 35, and 36.7 weeks, respectively. Overall perinatal mortality in the appropriately hospitalized (group C) was 3%. Where as it was 10% in those either not hospitalized at all or inadequately hospitalized (groups A and B). Maternal complications generally associated with increased perinatal loss were 18% in group A, 16% in A and B. The difference was not statistically significant. It is our belief that bed rest for multiple gestations is an important component of intensive antepartum care for this entity most commonly associated with low birth weight and prematurity. In-patient bed rest is desirable, having a minimal gain over home bed rest when only gestational age and birthweight are taken into account. However, overall perinatal mortality is greatly reduced in those under intensive prenatal care including bed rest in hospital.

06.42.07

Factors affecting the management of twin delivery: Mueller-Heubach, E, Heckman, L, Tyndall, C. Dept. Obstet. and Gyn., Univ. of Pittsburgh School Med., Magee-Womens Hosp., Pittsburgh, PA, USA

Optimal management of twin delivery is uncertain due to the many variables affecting perinatal outcome, thus requiring very large patient series to assess the role of these variables. We reviewed 915 consecutive twin deliveries which occurred between 1970 and 1981 at our institution. There were 1789 liveborns and 41 stillborns. The incidence of birth asphyxia (AX) was $207/1789 = 11.3\%$ (6.9% moderate, 4.4% severe). Moderate and severe AX was defined as the need for positive pressure ventilation with oxygen for < or > one minute. We have previously shown that this definition of AX is a better predictor of developmental outcome than the 5 minute Apgar score. The Cesarean section rate was 26.8%, twelve sections were done for delivery of the second twin only. Overall AX incidence was not different in vaginal deliveries (VD) versus Cesarean sections (CS). AX risk was higher for twin B than twin A with VD but the same with CS. Gestational age was a far more important AX predictor than route of delivery. Even with breech-breech deliveries, there was no difference in AX risk between VD (13/92) and CS (10/92); however, the AX risk was higher than with vertex-vertex deliveries ($p < 0.01$). This largest series of twin deliveries from a single institution does not support the current trend towards abdominal delivery of twin pregnancies.

06.42.08

Simultaneous recording of fetal body and breathing movements in twin pregnancies: Goldstein, I, Zimmer, E Z, Peretz, B A, Paldi, E. Dept. Obstet. and Gyn. "B", Rambam Med. Ctr, Haifa, Israel

Twin pregnancy is associated with increased perinatal mortality and morbidity. Recently more emphasis has been placed on detailed ultrasonic evaluation of these pregnancies and a slowing down of BPD and abdominal circumference was noted in the third trimester. It is known that the heart rate differs between these fetuses but there is not much knowledge on fetal behaviour in these pregnancies. Twelve patients with twin pregnancies at 34–37 weeks of gestation were included in the study. Each patient was scanned for 40 min and a simultaneous recording of fetal breathing movements and body movements in both fetuses was performed. All recordings were performed in the evening, at least two hours after the last meal. The number and duration of both types of movements were coded and analysed in order to compare total activity as well as the coincidence of simultaneous activity of both fetuses. Our results will be discussed.

06.42.09

Decline of perinatal mortality in twin pregnancies in 1970–81 in Turku, Finland: Erkkola, R, Kero, P. Dept. Obstet. and Gyn. and Pediat., Univ. Centr. Hosp., Turku, Finland

Altogether, 476 twin pregnancies were delivered at our institution between 1970–81. When four consecutive 3-year periods were compared, the perinatal mortality in twin pregnancies with babies of 500 g or more decreased from 10.1 to 3.6 per thousand. The perinatal mortality of A-twins was 6.3 and that of B-twins was 8.0 per thousand throughout the period. The duration of pregnancy at birth was unchanged, being 34.8 weeks and so was the combined weight of twins being 4883 g in the first 3-year period and 5050 g in the last period. The increase of hospital stay or sick leave did not affect significantly the weight of twins. The week of detection of twins decreased from 33 weeks in the beginning of the study period to 27 weeks in 1979–81. Cesarean section rate in twin pregnancies increased from 13 per cent to 49 per cent, when consecutive 3-year periods were compared. A particular risk group of twins was detected; when the weight difference between twins was more than 25 per cent, the risk of intrauterine death was sixfold when compared to twin pregnancies with more equal growth.

06.42.10

Twin cervical pregnancy presenting as abortion: A case report: Lemnete, I, Sihota, S, Peltecu, G, Bedivan, M, Iliescu, D. Dept. Obstet. and Gyn., "Filantropia" Hosp., Bucharest, Romania

We present a personal case of twin cervical pregnancy, diagnosis established by anatomopathologic examination. The diagnosis and the treatment of this uncommon form of ectopic gestation is discussed. Cervical pregnancy was clinically confused with abortion, the clinical aspect being dominated by hemorrhagic shock. Diagnosis was suspected during operation and the confirmation was performed by histopathologic examination. We used *Rubin's* rules for diagnosis of cervical pregnancy. The management consisted in uterine curettage, initially performed because of the confusion with abortion. Then, we performed total hysterectomy, the only method which we recommend in this situation. We show unusual aspects of our case report – twin cervical pregnancy – which have not been reported in the literature up to now.

06.79.01

Morphological findings in normal uterus: Tortajada, M, Pellicer, A, Plasencia, J. Dept. Obstet. and Gyn., Univ. School Med., Valencia, Spain

The purpose of this work was to evaluate the morphology of the theoretically "normal" uterus, because they correspond to women who have had three or more pregnancies and asked in our clinic because they wished for sterilization. All 440 women evaluated were subjected to a laparoscopy and electrocoagulation of both tubes or minilaparotomy and Pomeroy post-partum. Three to six months after the procedure a control HSG was performed and the morphology of these uteri evaluated and compared with 50 patients who entered our infertility clinic because of repeated abortion. Only 252 uteri (57.3%) presented a "normal" morphology, having a 2.7% of uterine malformations and other anomalies which, in an infertile population could be easily classified as an abnormal uterus. The difference in morphological findings between the normal population and the infertile group were not statistically significant.

06.79.02

Fractional uterine curettage: Barros, R D, Bastos, A C. Dept. Obstet. and Gyn., Med. School of Jundiai, São Paulo, Brazil

The importance of fractional uterine curettage as a gynecological examination recourse is emphasized. The technique employed in 350 patients is described. It was the most frequent procedure among the patients with a clinical diagnosis of functional disorders of menstruation and myoma of the uterus, aged between 40 and 49. The anatomo-pathologic diagnosis of the specimens obtained are presented. Two cases of endocervical carcinoma (0.58%) and 4 cases of endometrial carcinoma (1.14%) were found. Of the patients submitted to this technique 39 had post-menopausal bleeding and four of the six cases of carcinoma were detected among them. The fractional uterine curettage allows one to find out accurately the origin of the malignant lesion when it is present.

06.79.03

A new method for out-patient diagnostic curettage ("Abradul"): Gerretsen, G, Velde, J te. Dept. Gyn. and Path., Leyenburg Teach. Hosp., The Hague, The Netherlands

Of 61 patients prior to hysterectomy an endometrial sample was obtained by a simple plastic device the "Abradul". The shape of the endometrial sampler and the way it is handled mimics the contraceptive IUD, in that a round loop instead of a T-figure is inserted in the uterine cavity. Histological evaluation of the tissue samples was performed blindly. Afterwards the findings were compared with the pathology report on the hysterectomy specimens. The disorders found were grouped according to: atrophy (14), hormonal changes (35), inflammation (4), carcinoma and/or severe endometrial atypia (5), and moderate atypia of the endometrium (3). A good correlation was found in 56 out of the 61 curettings (92%). The unsatisfactory results were due to sample error in one case (2%) and inadequate material in four cases (6%). Inadequate material was found in three out of 13 cases of atrophy and in one case out of 35 of hormonal changes; the later being due to non-optimal handling of the device during scraping by which endometrium was obtained from the lower uterine segment only. The missed diagnosis by sample error was related to an endometritis of the deeper layers of the endometrium. It has to be stressed that all the carcinomas and the atypical lesions were diagnosed by "Abradul" curettage. – Conclusion: This new technique with the "Abradul" seems superior to a conventional D & C in respect to its easy handling and great convenience to the patient.

06.79.04

Endometrial biopsy with "Abradul" – an alternative to dilatation and curettage: Calder, A A, Serle, E, Govan, A D T. Univ. Dept. Obstet. and Gyn., Glasgow Roy. Infirm., Glasgow, Scotland

"Abradul" is a device designed to obtain tissue from the cavity of the uterus for diagnostic purposes. It consists of a simple collapsable plastic ring which is introduced to the uterus much in the manner of an intrauterine contraceptive device. This allows tissue to be removed for histological evaluation without the need for general anesthesia. We have conducted a study to evaluate the efficiency of this device in comparison with formal cervical dilatation and curettage under general anesthesia. 213 patients were studied using the device, all of whom subsequently underwent additional formal diagnostic curettage under anesthesia. In 50 cases (23%) no tissue was retrieved with either method (the majority of these were cases presenting with postmenopausal bleeding). In the remaining 163 cases "Abradul" was successful in 136 and dilatation and curettage in 152. The same diagnosis was reached in 95% of the patients in whom both methods yielded tissue suitable for histological evaluation. In both cases of endometrial carcinoma in the study "Abradul" successfully yielded diagnostic tissue. Among 87 patients who had "Abradul" performed without anesthesia and in whom a record of pain experience was made, 77% experienced no pain or mild discomfort only. The "Abradul" device would seem to provide a simple and effective alternative to dilatation and curettage in selected clinical circumstances.

06.79.05

The Mi-Mark endometrial sampler in routine practice: Uvebrant, M, Mattsson, L Å, Bergström, H. Dept. Obstet. and Gyn., East Hosp., Univ., Göteborg, Sweden

D & C is mainly performed to diagnose endometrial malignancy. Other methods used without anesthesia have proven good acceptance and reasonable diagnostic accuracy in specially designed studies. However, when introduced into routine practice, the outcome may be different. This study evaluates the use of Mi-Mark as primary method at a department with twenty-eight gynecologists. Exception from the routine could be done for special reasons. A secondary D & C was performed if the Mi-Mark specimen was too scanty for diagnosis, if malignancy was suspected or if symptoms recurred. The experience of 376 patients is presented. – Results: Mi-Mark was primarily used in 54% of the cases. The main reasons to exclude Mi-Mark were "need for exploration under general anesthesia" (21%) and "narrow cervical canal" (7%). Five per cent of the patients refused sampling without anesthesia. Severe discomfort was reported by 11%. In 10% of premenopausal women the specimens were too scanty for histopathological diagnosis. In women over 60 years of age as many as 60% of the specimens were not suitable for evaluation, which unfortunately did not exclude malignancy, although atrophy was the main reason. In this age-group 15% of the Mi-Mark or D & C samples were "not benign". The corresponding figure for remaining postmenopausal women was 6%. – Conclusion: This study indicates that severe discomfort may be a problem when Mi-Mark is introduced in routine practice. The method is not relevant for women over 60 years of age. If this age-group was excluded the Mi-Mark method reduced the number of D & C by 46%. No primarily undetected malignancies were found during a six month follow-up.

06.79.06

Endometrial abnormalities diagnosed by the gynoscann technique: Magalhães Costa, M, Einhorn, N, Nasiell, M, Roger, V. Dept. Gyn. and Oncol., Radiumhemmet, Karolinska Hosp., Stockholm, Sweden

A simple technique for screening the endometrium is a desirable complement to gynecological examination. Ninety-four patients underwent cytologic sampling by the Gynoscann technique immediately before fractionated curettage. Ninety-six per cent of the cytological samples were adequate for cytologic diagnosis and 96% of the curettage specimens for the histology. There was a correct correlation between cytology and histology in 84% of the cases. Among the 26 cases of endometrial carcinoma, 21 (80%) were correctly diagnosed by the cytology. There were no false positives for carcinoma. Atypical hyperplastic endometrium was found in two cases by curettage and correctly correlated with cytology in one case. Sensitivity for endometrial carcinoma was 80% and specificity 100%. We concluded that Gynoscann is safe, easy, and it was shown to be reliable for the diagnosis as well as screening of endometrial carcinoma, but it deserves further evaluation including a larger series of patients and with the increasing experience of the cytologists in the diagnosis of the endometrial abnormalities.

06.79.07

Resumption of menstruation after curettage in non-pregnant women: Hany, A, Rizk, M, Toppozada, M. Dept. Obstet. and Gyn., Univ., Alexandria, Egypt

Resumption of menstruation after curettage was studied in 30 regularly cyclic women. Curettage was performed on day 10 of the cycle in 15 cases and on day 20 of the cycle in other 15 cases. Menstruation occurred approximately within the expected date of the next menses in both groups. The hormonal profile did not point to any alteration secondary to curettage.

06.79.08

Diagnosis of occult female genital tuberculosis: Salem, H T, Aboloyoun, E M, Farid, A, El-Timawy, A A, Abdallah, N M. Dept. Obstet. and Gyn., Bacteriol. and Path., Fac. Med., Univ., Assiut, Egypt

Fifty infertile patients were recruited for the possibility of having genital tuberculosis on the basis of: unexplained infertility, chronic pelvic pain, or suspicious hysterosalpingograms. Endometrial curettings were obtained for histopathological examination and for culture on Löwenstein medium. Laparoscopy was done and peritoneal fluid samples were aspirated for culture. Diagnosis of tuberculosis was positive in 72% of peritoneal fluid samples; 55% endometrial fluid cultures and in 20% after histopathological examination of the endometrium. No typical laparosocopic findings of genital tuberculosis were detected in all subjects. Culture of peritoneal fluid aspirate obtained at laparoscopy could be of great diagnostic value in detecting occult pelvic tuberculosis.

07.02.01

Second-look laparoscopy after operation for infertility: Freude, G, Leodolter, S. Ludwig-Boltzmann-Inst. Erforsch. u. Behandl. weibl. Sterilität, Krankenh. Stadt Wien, Lainz, Austria

Forty-seven patients underwent second-look laparoscopy following pelvic surgery for infertility. 29 of these patients had been operated on by microsurgical technique and 18 of them by "conventional" technique (without using a microscope). In almost all cases dextran 40, 250 cm³, and 250 mg prednisolon were left in the peritoneal cavity to minimize the adhesions postoperatively. In many cases the great omentum was resected to prevent adhesions of the omentum. The aim of second-look laparoscopy treatment was a) to evaluate the surgical technique controlling the results by additionally performing chromo pertubation, b) to enhance the primary surgical results by lysis of postoperative adhesions. To classify the adhesions we used a score from 0 to III. This score was related to four different intervals from pelvic surgery to second-look laparoscopy (up to three months, 3–6 months, 6–12 months, after 12 months). Our results show an increase of density and vascularisation of adhesions as the interval from pelvic surgery to second-look laparoscopy is extended. An efficient and unbloody lysis becomes more and more difficult in these cases. Our suggestion is that the optimal timing for performing second-look laparoscopy should be 8–12 weeks after a major operation.

07.02.02

Psychological problems in patients seeking tubal re-anastomosis: Palaniappan, B. Dept. Obstet. and Gyn., Kilpauk Med. Coll., Univ., Madras, India

Previous works on psychological studies in many centers are mostly on women seeking tubal sterilisations. This paper deals with such problems in 30 mothers seeking tubal re-anastomosis (TRA). The main reasons for seeking TRA are: loss of the only child or all children, half-hearted acceptance of sterilisation previously, a desire to increase the family especially male children, poor pre-operative information, guilt feeling. There are a few examples where the patients were faced with the husband's threat to take another wife. Most of the women who had successful pregnancies were jubilant and satisfied. One group, who had not conceived, insisted on further treatment or surgery becoming hysterics. Another ones who have had successful pregnancies are not consistently happy due to repeated child births. The interesting group is that of mothers who have not conceived but are quite satisfied that they have done their best – the Indian Philosophy of "Action is your duty; Fruit is not your concern". There were cases of depressives, introverts and masochists. The implications of tubal ligation should be fully explained to mothers before operation. When they seek TRA they must be taken up with sympathy and care because TRA affords in many cases not only desired results but tremondous satisfaction, security and psychological relief.

07.02.03

Clinical results of microsurgical tuboplasty: Song, C H. Dept. Obstet. and Gyn., Yonsei Univ. Coll. Med., Seoul, Korea

This is the review of the clinical results of infertility microsurgery. From January 1981 through July 1984 microsurgical tuboplasty was carried out in 152 patients. Seventy-five patients underwent reversal of tubal sterilization and 77 patients underwent reconstructive surgery of postinflammatory tubal damage, 22 patients salpingolysis, 12 patients fimbrioplasty, 31 patients salpingostomy, seven patients tubal reanastomosis and five patients uterotubal implantation. Among the patients who underwent reversal of tubal sterilization intrauterine pregnancy occurred in 48 patients and ectopic pregnancy in three patients. The factors influencing the outcome of tubal reversal were reviewed. Type of sterilization, site of reanastomosis and postreversal tubal length influenced the outcome but the interval from sterilization to reversal and age of patients did not. Among the patients who underwent reconstructive surgery of postinflammatory tubal damage, intrauterine pregnancy occurred in 30 patients and ectopic pregnancy in five patients.

07.02.04

Injectible iodine for prophylactic adhesiolysis in 30 cases of tubal microsurgery: Kanthamani, C R, Mohanalakshmi, T K, Jaya, S, Gajaraj, J, Shanthini, M, Revathy, T G. Governm. Kasturba Gandhi Hosp. Women and Children, Madras, India

Thirty cases of tubal microsurgery for both recanalisation of the oviduct for reversal of sterilization and the reconstruction for infertility were given injectible iodine postoperatively 200 mg deep i. m. into the gluteal region weekly for 20 injections to study whether the iodine prevents postoperative adhesions in the area of operation on the tubes, the ovaries and pelvic peritoneum. Ten cases were treated postoperatively without Entodon as case controls. The above 40 cases were investigated with a second-look laparoscopy after three months and it was found that iodine does prevent adhesions where pre-operatively grade-II adhesions of Hulka were present. Successes of prophylactic adhesiolysis in cases of tubal microsurgery (75%) are being discussed in this paper.

07.02.05

Forty cases of tubal microsurgery: Mohanalakshmi, T K, Kanthamani, C R, Selvakumari, Devambigai, Nalini, Jaya, S, Gajaraj, J, Shanthini, M, Revathy, T G. Governm. Kasturba Gandhi Hosp. Women and Children, Madras, India

As the conventional methods of tuboplasty for recanalisation and for infertility are not as successful as microsurgery, a research study was conducted at Government Kasturba Gandhi Hospital for Women and Children, Madras, from March 1982 to December 1984, and the cases were analysed. There were 40 cases of tuboplasty done during the above period, of which 30 cases (75%) were for recanalisation and ten cases (25%) were for tubal block in infertility. Out of 30 cases of reversal there were four pregnancies, of which one was ectopic and remaining three were intrauterine pregnancies with livebirths. Of the ten cases of reconstructive tuboplasty for infertility there were three intrauterine pregnancies with livebirths and one abortion. The percentage of adhesions was 40 (group I to group II) in both infertility and reversal. Follow-up by hystero-salpingography and second-look laparoscopy after three months showed patency without alteration.

07.02.06

New approaches using tissue adhesives for microsurgery: Osada, H, Fujii, T K, Tsubata, K, Takagi, S. Dept. Obstet. and Gyn., Nihon Univ. School Med., Tokyo, Japan

The tubal factors involved in female infertility are said to be 30–50%, and a method to bypass the tubes is *in vitro* fertilization and embryo transfer, which is presently being used internationally. However, the success rate for IVF & ET remains less than 10%. Another method for the treatment of tubal infertility is microsurgery, with the aim of attaining conception through normal sexual activity has been said to have a success rate as high as 30–50%. Thus, we believe that tubal reconstruction by microsurgery with its higher potential success rate should be attempted, leaving IVF & ET for those cases where the tubes are so damaged as to not warrant microsurgical intervention. In Japan, a high percentage of tubal infertility is due to inflammation, endometriosis etc., in contrast to areas where the major cause is tubal ligation. Thus, in Japan, tubal reconstruction is complicated by a high percentage of inflammatory adhesion, which require adequate preparation to prevent the formation of post-surgical adhesions. Our method to prevent those post-surgical adhesions is to use a fibrinogen thrombin adhesive system, together with peritoneal transplantation to cover damaged tubal areas. Using the techniques stated above, we have achieved acceptable results and so wish to report our findings.

07.02.07

Reversal of female sterilization using the Filshie Clip: Filshie, G M. Queens Med. Ctr., Nottingham, UK

The Filshie Clip for female sterilization has been used in over 200,000 patients worldwide. In Nottingham over 2000 Clips have been applied (including prototypes). The overall failure rate in Nottingham is approximately 2/1000. Of the first 15 reversal operations performed after counselling one patient had the operation reversed because she did not feel a complete woman; the other 14 had their operations reversed because of re-marriage. Patients were unselected and no patient had refused the operation. There was no pre-operative laparoscopic assessment of the Fallopian tubes but a sperm count was performed if the new partner had not proved his fertility. All cases were operated upon using microsurgical techniques. Anasto-mosis was performed using nylon sutures ranging from 6.0 to 8.0. Splints were normally employed. Of the 15 patients reversed, 12 patients had a total of 18 intrauterine pregnancies. Of these, two miscarried, two had a termination of pregnancy and the other pregnancies achieved a livebirth. No ectopic pregnancies occurred. Histology of the Fallopian tubes revealed normal, healthy tissue present beyond 1.5 mm from the clipped part of the tube.

07.02.08

Tubo-ovarian microsurgery: Khandwala, S D. Khandwala's Hosp., Bombay, India

This paper reports on 61 cases of tubo-ovarian microsurgery done by standard microsurgical technique, the modification being the position of the surgeon in the center between the spread-eagled legs of the patient. Of the 54 (88.5%) cases of tubal microsurgery, 16 (29.6%) were reversal of sterilization and 38 (70.4%) were of infertility tubal block. Of the 16 reversal of sterilization cases, 12 (75%) were Pomeroy's cases requiring ampullo-ampullary anastomosis in six (37.5%) cases and ampullo-isthmic in six (37.5%) cases. There were four (25%) cases of silastic ring reversal requiring isthmo-isthmic anastomosis. 38 infertility cases with tubal block at different levels required anastomosis such as isthmo-intramural in one case (2.6%), isthmo-isthmic in three cases (7.9%), ampullo-intramural in seven cases (18.4%), ampullo-isthmic in seven cases (18.4%), ampullo-ampullary in six cases (15.9%), salpingostomy in seven cases (18.4%) and fimbrioplasty in seven cases (18.4%). There were seven (11.5%) cases of ovarian microsurgery, six (85.7%) for endometriosis and one (14.3%) for polycystic ovary. Pelvic adhesiolysis was necessary in 30 (49.2%) cases – which was extensive in 11 (36.7%) and only salpingo-ovariolysis in 19 (63.3%) cases. The pregnancy rate was 62.5% for reversal of sterilization (10 of 16), 31.6% for infertility cases (12 of 38) and 57.1% for ovarian microsurgery (4 of 7). This corresponds to the average pregnancy rates reported by various workers viz 65% for reversal of sterilization and 38.3% for infertility cases.

07.02.09

Vascular anastomosis and microsurgery for tubal sterility: Kanemaki, Y, Yasui, F. Carnegie Hosp. Obstet. and Gyn., Shizuoka, Japan

Stress was made of the constant practice of vascular anastomosis on animals for improvement of the results of operation on tubal sterility. With 10-0 nylon thread used for tubal end-to-end anastomosis and tubal opening, the rate of pregnancy is improved. Thus, practice is made with 11-0 and 12-0 threads used on 1.0–1.5 mm diameter arteries of animal. Vascular anastomosis with 12-0 thread is a particularly difficult operation, and a case of such operation is reported. Once vascular anastomosis is made successfully with one 10-0 thread, tubal end-to-end anastomosis with 10-0 thread is now a complete operation, to say nothing of post-Madlener (tubal sterilization) tubal end-to-end anastomosis. The most difficult operations are end-to-end anastomosis of interstitial occlusion and tubal edema after operation of chocolate cystoma. Microsurgery for tubal sterility was conducted of 517 cases from August 1974 to December 1984, with 167 (33%) pregnancies presently (including conceptions and extrauterine pregnancies). 1) Post-Madlener end-to-end anastomosis, 25 cases with 16 pregnancies (64%); 2) Interstitial occlusion, 126 cases with 40 pregnancies (32%); 3) End-to-end anastomosis + opening, 66 cases with 25 pregnancies (38%); and 4) Opening only, 300 cases with 86 pregnancies (29%). If these cases are followed up for two more years, the results will be improved further.

07.13.01

Oral contraception and lipoprotein metabolism: Nikkila, E A. 3rd Dept. Med., Univ., Helsinki, Finland

Both estrogenic hormones and progestins influence plasma lipoprotein levels. These changes may be reflected as an accelerated atherogenesis and increased risk of premature arterial disease. Estrogens stimulate the synthesis of very-low-density (VLDL) triglycerides without affecting their removal. The concentration of VLDL particles tends to rise and may even lead to hypertriglyceridemia. On the other hand, estrogens increase the number of (hepatic?) low-density-lipoprotein (LDL) receptors and reduce plasma LDL levels. A third effect is suppression of hepatic lipase activity, an enzyme responsible for removal of high-density-lipoproteins (HDL). This results as an increase of HDL. The progestins with androgenic activity inhibit the synthesis of VLDL and decrease the plasma VLDL levels. They are, however, powerful inducers of hepatic lipase the activity of which rises 2–3 fold. Simultaneously the concentration of HDL-2 is dramatically reduced while HDL-3 is less influenced. In contrast, weakly androgenic progestins like medroxyprogesterone acetate and desogestrel do not influence hepatic lipase and they also have little effect on HDL levels. The estrogens are not able to counteract the induction of hepatic lipase by androgenic progestins.

07.13.02

Progestogen dose in oral contraceptives: Bergink, E W, Jager, E de. Sci. Develop. Group, Organon Int. BV, Oss, The Netherlands

The broad spectrum of activities of progestagens makes it difficult to establish the ideal dose of progestogen in oral contraceptives. The emphasis given to the safety issue has led to recommend lower and lower doses of progestogen. However, not only the dose and progestagional potency of the progestogen but also the additional hormonal properties are important for the safety aspects. For instance, our present results show that the effect of progestogens on lipid metabolism depends on additional synandrogenic or anti-androgenic properties. There is also the possible risk of an overemphasis of the safety aspect at the cost of reliability, cycle control and health benefits. Present experience with the progestogen desogestrel in monophasic, and multiphasic combinations show that for each regimen and for each estrogen dose, a critical dose of the progestogen is needed for proper efficacy and cycle control.

07.13.03

Effects of gestagens on pituitary and CNS concentrations of opioid peptides: Genazzani, A R, Petraglia, F, Bergamaschi, M, Di Meo, G, Genazzani, A D, Facchinetti, F, Volpe, A. Dept. Obstet. and Gyn., Univ., Modena, Italy

Sex steroids influence central functions affecting the activity of classical neurotransmitters, probably through the changes induced in the turnover of the newly identified neuropeptides, which seem to play the function of neuromodulators. On this basis we compared the effects of various estrogens and gestagens on the hypothalamic and pituitary concentrations of beta-endorphin (B-EP) and met-enkephalin (met-enk) in Sprague-Dawley ovariectomized rats. Estradiol benzoate, progesterone, desogestrel, medroxyprogesterone acetate, cyproterone acetate, ORG OD 14 were administered at different doses for 14 days starting three weeks after castration. The rats were killed by decapitation, the mediobasal hypothalamus (MBH), the anterior (AP) and the neurointermediate (NIL) pituitary lobes were removed and homogenated with acetic acid. The peptide concentrations were measured by RIA. The estradiol benzoate and ORG OD 14 showed a positive effect on the B-EP and met-enk concentrations in both tissues, while gestagens reduce the met-enk concentrations in the MBH and differently counteract the effects of estradiol benzoate. These results indicate that gonadal steroids influence the central opioid tonus and as a consequence interfere in the CNS functions. In fact opioid peptides play a role in the modulation of pain perception, mood and behavioral changes, thermoregulatory and neuroendocrine activities. The same treatments performed in postmenopausal and castrated women increase the circulating levels of B-EP and improve the LH responsiveness to the opiate antagonist naloxone, demonstrating their efficacy in humans to modulate CNS opioid tonus and AP B-EP secretion.

07.13.04

New frontiers in progestogen research: Potts, M. Family Hlth Int., Research Triangle Park, NC, USA

A gap exists between the consumer perception of hormonal contraceptives and the epidemiological and clinical experience of their use. Combined contraceptives have been intensively studied for more than a quarter of a century. Among younger women, the protective effect of the pill provides against reproductive cancers more than outweighs adverse effects on the cardiovascular system. However, use of combined oral contraceptives in developed countries has declined in the past decade. Progestogen-only contraceptives are an important choice for older women and women who are breast-feeding, but are often completely overlooked. Injectable progestogens have proved uniquely effective reversal methods of contraception but broadly reassuring observations from human use are in conflict with adverse findings from animal experiments and remain limited. It is suggested that consumer perceptions of progestogen containing contraceptives will eventually catch up with clinical and epidemiological reality. New progestogens are proving important and more should be sought. New formulations of existing progestogens are likely to be introduced. It is suggested that the greatest use of progestogen containing steroids is still to come and that this method will be with us long into the twenty-first century.

07.41.01
Techniques for fabrication of a custom-fitted, valved, cervical cap (contracap): Goepp, R A. Univ. of Chicago Pritzker School Med., Freese, UE, Univ. Hlth Sci.-Chicago Med. School, Chicago, IL, USA
The Contracap is a barrier device that covers the entire surface of the cervix and prevents the ascent of sperm into the endocervical canal. Since the Contracap is custom-fitted to the individual cervix, it is designed to stay in place up to one year, and needs to be removed only for medical indications. The purposes of this videotape presentation are: (1) to demonstrate a non-invasive procedure for obtaining an accurate impression of the cervix, (2) to show the vacuform process used to fabricate the Contracap, and (3) to describe briefly proper techniques for the placement of the Contracap onto the cervix. As an instruction and training aid, this videotape will facilitate an organized and safe system of impression taking and cap placement for the use of the Contracap as a contraceptive device.

07.41.02
Implant therapy for the climacteric syndrome: Studd, J W W, Brincat, M. Dulwich Menopause Clin., London, UK
The symptoms of the climacteric syndrome and the different routes of estrogen therapy are discussed. The biochemical changes following percutaneous implantation of estradiol 50 mg and testosterone 100 mg as well as a placebo controlled study of symptomatic response are shown. The technique is a simple outpatient procedure performed under local anesthesia. The importance of skin collagen, skin thickness and metacarpal index before and after implant therapy has been studied and the relationship of loss of collagen to the etiology of postmenopausal osteoporosis demonstrated. A cheap x-ray screening test for osteoporosis has been devised. This utilises skin thickness and metacarpal index as a normogram to indicate the women who are particularly at risk from postmenopausal bone loss.

07.41.03
Hysteroscopy for intrauterine diagnosis and treatment: Wamsteker, K, Pas, H v.d. Mariastichting Haarlem, VZW Jan Palfijn, The Netherlands
The instrumentation and method of hysteroscopy with dextran – and CO_2 distension of the uterine cavity will be demonstrated. Intrauterine disorders will be demonstrated and the technique of performing surgical procedures in the uterine cavity will be showed. Hysteroscopy will be presented as a routine out-patient procedure for intrauterine diagnosis with CO_2 distension and a surgical procedure for treatment of intrauterine disorders with dextran distension.

07.41.04
Endoscopic alternatives: Laparoscopy: Wolfe, W M. Dept. Obstet. and Gyn., Univ. of Louisville School Med., Louisville, KY, USA
Literature on laparoscopy is voluminous and worldwide in scope. Many instruments, methods, and procedures have been described, some of which may merit adoption as fundamental procedures. At the University of Louisville we have attempted to review these procedures and to select basic procedures which widen the safe application of laparoscopy as a diagnostic and therapeutic tool. Conditions which were in the past considered contraindications to laparoscopy can be circumvented by the selection of the alternative technique which makes safe laparoscopy available to these patients. In addition, it is our goal to teach these fundamental alternatives to our residents. It is expected that this should extend their use of laparoscopy, particularly for diagnostic purposes and ultimately for therapeutic purposes. This videotape reviews the alternative techniques taught in our Dept. of OB/GYN to all residents.

07.42.01
Management of tubal disease in human infertility: Kawakami, S, Morisada, M, Iizuka, R. Dept. Obstet. and Gyn., School Med., Keio Univ., Tokyo, Japan
We will display our movie picture to introduce our recently developed diagnostic and standardized methods for the treatment of disturbed Fallopian tubes at our University Clinic. The contents of this movie picture are divided under seven heads, i.e., 1) Diagnosis of patency of oviducts by use of kymographic hysterosalpingography. 2) Observation of endosalpinx by tubaloscope. 3) Successful pregnancy rates after macro- and microsurgery for occluded tubes. 4) Microsurgery technique for occluded tubes. 5) Newly developed Silikon Hood on purpose to prevent any postoperative re-adhesion. 6) Effects of estrogens on endosalpinx. 7) Early Pregnancy Factor (EPF); possible diagnostic method to detect any hindrance in fertilization and/or implantation.

07.42.02

Microsurgery and ectopic tubal pregnancy: Tran, D K. Hôp. Annexe Républ. Univ., Nice, France
The early diagnosis of ectopic pregnancy makes possible the conservative microsurgery in an emergency. We use conservative surgery in 80% of 149 patients between 1978 and 1983. We use specially the salpingotomy-suture. Hemostasis is obtained by ornithine-8-vasopressin which is injected into the mesosalpinx. The pedicle of the ectopic pregnancy is present in the proximal segment of the oviduct in 75% of these patients. We found a pathologic proximal segment in 44 cases. In these cases, in the second time, we use Danazol and we obtain much success. When the Danazol is not efficient, a microsurgical technique is indicated: the isthmo-ostial reimplantation.

07.42.03

The abdominal radical operation for cancer of the cervix (Magara's method): Araki, T, Katoh, S, Senda, T, Kaneko, K, Yamada, T, Yamada, K. Dept. Obstet. and Gyn., Nippon Med. School, Tokyo, Japan
The abdominal radical operation for cancer of the cervix (Magara's method) can be performed easily and systematically even by beginners, based upon the unique operative procedures refering to the topographic anatomy of the pelvic cavities, including the blood vessels, especially veins, lymph nodes, ligaments, nerves and muscles, etc. The film shows the operative technique performed by Magara's staff members, particularly being characterized by the exposure of the pelvic cavities, removal of the regional lymph nodes and the management of the cardinal ligament, which minimizes the intraoperative bleeding and postoperative urinary fistula formation.

07.42.04

Future surgical incontinence and descensus therapy: Lahodny, J. Gen. Publ. Hosp., Gmünd, Austria
The film shows the peripheral bladder denervation by separation of the pelvic plexus from the exterior bladder wall. After the separation of the bladder and levator ani muscle follows the presentation of the endopelvic fascia (pubourethral ligaments). These ligaments loosely hold the urethra at the symphysis as a short arm sling plastic. Thereby the interior levator ani muscle side is exposed, so that now the hernia of the hiatus genitalis is eliminated by bringing together of the exposed levator parts in the midline. Peripheral bladder denervation, short arm sling plastic and ventral levator plastic repair, can cure urgency incontinence, stress incontinence and descensus. The results by far surpass the conventional methods.

07.79.01

Vasopressin levels in female plasma during the menstrual cycle: Pinku, A, Katz, M, Leiberman, J R, Glick, S. Div. Obstet. and Gyn., Fac. Med. Sci., Ben Gurion Univ. of the Negev, Beer-Sheba, Israel
The symptoms of irritability, headache, transient weight gain and discomfort from which women tend to suffer prior to, and during their menstrual period are known as perimenstrual syndrome. The rise in estrogen and effect of menoxines, produced by menstruating endometrium, were in the past thought to be the cause of most complaints. In the present study vasopressin levels in serum of eight healthy young women, with regular menstrual period, where measured daily through the entire menstrual cycle. A.D.H. levels were ascertained by radioimmunoassay. A total of 172 measurements was done, an average of 22 per patient. The mean vasopressin level during day 26 to 6 of menstrual cycle (perimenstrual period) was 1.697 pg/ml, and during the days from 7 to 26 of the cycle – 0.941 pg/ml. The difference in vasopressin levels between the two periods was statistically significant – $p < 0.0025$. Although the rise in vasopressin during the perimenstrual period was significant, the role it has in cusing some of the symptoms of perimenstrual syndrome is to be further investigated. It is of interest that in the single case in which vasopressin remained at stable levels throughout the menstrual cycle, no signs or symptoms of perimenstrual syndrome were observed.

07.79.02

Changes in transcapillary fluid dynamics – a possible explanation of fluid retention in the premenstrual phase?: Tollan, A, Øian, P, Maltau, J M. Dept. Obstet. and Gyn., Univ., Tromsø, Norway
The aim of the present study was to examine the interstitial fluid balance during the menstrual cycle. Many women experience edema in the extremities and weight gain during the premenstrual phase, symptoms which are aggravated in the premenstrual syndrome (PMS). New methods have made it possible to study the transcapillary fluid dynamics by measuring interstitial fluid colloid osmotic pressure, COPi (wick-method), and interstitial hydrostatic pressure, Pi (wick-in-needle method). Net transcapillary fluid transport can be described by the Starling equation: $F = CFC [(PC - Pi) - \sigma(COPp - COPi)]$ where CFC is the capillary filtration coefficient, σ the reflection coefficient for plasma proteins, Pc the capillary hydrostatic pressure and COPp the colloid osmotic pressure in plasma. Ten women without PMS and with regular menstrual cycles volunteered for the study. The procedures were carried out early in the follicular phase, day 2–5 (mean 3.8), and late in the luteal phase, day 23–28 (mean 25.5). COPi and Pi were measured both on thorax and ankle. There was a significant reduction of the COPi-ankle, and also a significant weight gain. Foot-volumetry showed an increase, but the changes did not reach significance. COPp, COPi-thorax and Pi-thorax and ankle did not show any significant differences. – Conclusion: In the late luteal phase there is a significant reduction of the COPi-ankle and increased body weight. These findings may be due to changes in the Pc or in the CFC.

07.79.03

Vasotocin analogs which competetively inhibit vasopressin stimulated uterine activity in healthy women: Åkerlund, M, Hauksson, A, Melin, P, Trojnar, J. Dept. Obstet. and Gyn., Univ. of Lund and Ferring Pharmaceuticals, Malmö, Sweden

1-deamino-2-D-Tyr (OEt)-4-Val-8-Orn-vasotocin (dE-VVT), 1-deamino-2-D-Tyr(OEt)-4-Thr-8-Orn-vasotocin (dE-TVT) and 1-deamino-2-D-Tyr(OEt)-oxytocin (dE-OXY) were compared as to their inhibitory effects on vasopressin induced uterine activity in healthy women. At menstruation, during recording of intrauterine pressure (18 recording sessions in 11 women), an intravenous infusion of lysine vasopressin (LVP, 1 ng/min/kg/body weight) was given, which induced an increase of the uterine activity and dysmenorrhea-like symptoms. Intravenous injections of all analogs (10 μg/kg/body weight) caused relief of symptoms and an inhibition of uterine activity, dE-TVT being the most effective one followed in order by dE-VVT and dE-OXY. With dE-TVT an almost complete inhibition of contractions was seen during the first 10 min after injection, and the effect lasted 40–50 min. An agonistic effect on the spontaneous uterine activity was only seen with dE-OXY. The marked, selective and comparatively long-lasting inhibitory effect of dE-TVT should encourage further studies of its therapeutic effect in primary dysmenorrhea, where an increased VP-secretion could be an important etiological factor. Studies should also be performed in premature labor, where an increased concentration of oxytocin receptors in the myometrium has been demonstrated.

07.79.04

An objective evaluation of the efficacy of ibuprofen in the treatment of primary dysmenorrhea: Milsom, I, Andersch, B. Dept. Obstet. and Gyn., Univ. of Göteborg, East Hosp., Göteborg, Sweden

The development of the catheter-tip microtransducer for intrauterine pressure (IUP) recording has made objective evaluation of dysmenorrhea therapy possible. In the present study the effect of oral administration of ibuprofen (400 mg), naproxen-sodium (250 mg) and paracetamol (500 mg) on the IUP and menstrual pain of 12 dysmenorrheic women was evaluated using a microtransducer catheter technique. In addition IUP, pain severity and serum concentrations of ibuprofen were recorded in a patient suffering from primary dysmenorrhea for a period of 10 h after oral administration of ibuprofen (400 mg). Ibuprofen in a single oral dose of 400 mg significantly (p < 0.05) reduced resting pressure, active pressure, the frequency of the pressure cycles and the area under the curve. The decrease in IUP was associated with a significant (p < 0.01) reduction in pain intensity. No significant changes in IUP or pain score were recorded for the patients who received paracetamol or naproxen-sodium in the dosages indicated. Maximum serum concentration of ibuprofen (37.4μg/ml^{-1}) was achieved 1 h after oral administration (400 mg). The terminal half-life of ibuprofen in serum was approximately 2 h. Despite low concentrations of ibuprofen 4 h after medication IUP never regained the level recorded before medication during the 10 h observation period.

07.79.05

Efficacy and toleration of piroxicam in the treatment of 298 patients with primary dysmenorrhea: Bagnoli, V R, Fonseca, A M, Bastos, A C, Halbe, H W, Salvatore, C A. Gyn. Clin., Univ. of São Paulo Med. School, São Paulo, Brazil

To evaluate the efficacy and toleration of Piroxicam in the treatment of primary dysmenorrhea 298 patients, referred for very severe to moderate pain due to primary dysmenorrhea, were studied. In this open non-comparative multicenter study, all the patients with primary dysmenorrhea were observed during 4 consecutive menstrual cycles, one as baseline and three with active drug treatment. The treatment with Piroxicam consisted of the use of 2 capsules (40 mg) as a single dose after the beginning of pain or menstrual period, followed by 1 capsule (20 mg) after lunch on the 3rd and 4th days. From the 298 patients included in this study, 269 (90.3%) completed 4 menstrual cycles, but 19 (6.4%) dropped out voluntarily, eight (2.9%) were excluded from the study due to adverse reactions, and two (0.4%) due to therapeutic failure. Regarding medical evaluation, the therapeutic results were considered as excellent and good in 230 (85.5%) of the treated patients; concerning patients self-evaluation, 261 (97.0%) considered themselves as asymptomatic or better. Adverse reactions occurred in 54 (19.5%) patients, however, only eight (2.9%) patients were excluded from the study due to adverse reactions. Considering the results obtained, the severity of pain in the patients included in this study, the criteria of including only patients who were not responsive to conventional analgesic drugs, consequently excluding patients responsive to placebo, it is concluded that Piroxicam is a highly efficient drug, presenting good toleration in the treatment of primary dysmenorrhea.

07.79.06

Contraception and dysmenorrhea: Schellen, T M C M. Med. Res. Bureau, Nijmegen, The Netherlands

For several reasons there are many more menstrual cycles than 50 years ago. There are also more ovulations and as a consequence more cycles with dysmenorrhea. The introduction of the so-called subfifties demonstrated clearly that these pills are less effective in suppressing a pre-existing dysmenorrhea. The evidence that an IUD may increase the PGE concentration of the human endometrium may account for the fact that dysmenorrhea is often seen after insertion of an IUD. However, the exact etiology of the increase of menstrual pain secondary to an IUD-insertion is not fully known. According to *Kurz* (1981) more attention should be paid to 'tailor-made' IUD's in order to prevent side-effects such as dysmenorrhea and menorrhagia. In our study we included 202 women using the pill and 40 women using an IUD. The results with respect to dysmenorrhea are dealt with. It will be shown that dysmenorrhoic women asking for the pill should preferably use an OC with a progestagenic profile. Women asking for an IUD should preferably be given a fitted model. Should dysmenorrhea occur in women using the pill or an IUD, or should an existing dysmenorrhea get worse, a prostaglandin-synthetase inhibitor is recommended.

07.79.07

Therapeutic amenorrhea in mentally deeply retarded women caused by irradiation of the endometrium with high dose-rate afterloading unit: Salmi, T, Grönroos, M. Dept. Obstet. and Gyn., Turku Univ. Centr. Hosp., Turku, Finland

Therapeutic amenorrhea is often indicated in mentally deeply retarded women, who have restlessness and increasing amount of epileptic seizures before and during menstruation and for whom personal hygiene during the bleeding is difficult. Therapeutic amenorrhea has usually been caused by continuous progestin therapy. With this treatment, anyhow, some patients have break-through bleedings and also the costs of the treatment continued for years must be taken into account. As an alternative to the progestin treatment high dose-rate afterloading Cathetron unit has been used since 1969 in the Department of Obstetrics and Gynecology of the University Central Hospital of Turku. Altogether 39 mentally retarded patients have been treated. The mean dose to the endometrium was 13.6 Gy (range 10.0–15.0 Gy). After the first treatment, menstruation ceased in 54% and after the second treatment in 95% of the patients. All the patients recovered without complications. It can be stated that irradiation of the endometrium with a quick and effective method of high dose-rate afterloading unit is a good alternative to conservative progestin treatment in causing therapeutic amenorrhea in mentally deeply retarded women. It can also be used in the treatment of functional uterine bleedings in patients who have contraindications to operation. In most of the cases no decrease in the ovarian secretory function has been found.

08.02.01

Chlamydial infections in the female genital tract: Hoyme, U B, Donath, E-M, Schrage, R, Bäumler, C. Univ.-Frauenklin., Tübingen

The prevalence of Chlamydia trachomatis (C.t.) in the female genital tract was evaluated by means of a tissue culture method. In 269 gynecologically healthy women seen in our out-patient department for cancer screening the rate was 3.3%. The prevalence in 367 pregnant women was 5.4%, however, none of 294 amniotic fluid specimens obtained by amniocentesis was found to contain C.t. A prevalence of 11.8% was found in 315 women complaining of vaginal discharge. In a 2 to 22 month follow-up of women with abnormal cervical cytology C.t. was seen in 19.6% of women with recurrence to normal cytologic pattern, however, in 10.8% of 65 patients with persistence or progression (p < 0.025). 18.8% of 85 patients with laparoscopically verified salpingitis had positive chlamydial cultures from tubal specimens obtained by means of a new laparoscopic instrument. In 250 patients with tubal infertility a prevalence of 4.4% was found, however, none of 122 women laparoscoped of other reasons harboured C.t.

08.02.02

Cytology in cervicitis infection by chlamydia: Yamashita, S A, Fonseca, A, Tomioka, E, Souza, A Z, Salvatore, C A. Gyn. Clin., Univ. of São Paulo Med. School, São Paulo, Brazil

Colposcopic findings were observed in fifteen patients that had mucopurulent cervicitis caused by Chlamydia trachomatis, confirmed by culture in McCoy cells line and identified by indirect immunofluorescence. At the first visit, after endocervical swabs for culture of Chlamydia trachomatis had been done, the patients were submitted to colposcopic examination. The control group consisted of thirty patients with the same clinical features but which had negative culture for this agent. We found a high incidence of atypical transformation zone in the Chlamydial positive group.

08.02.03

Chlamydial and mycoplasmic infections in ambulatory patients: Garozzo, G, Montoneri, C, Garofalo, A, Granà, G, Caruso, M, Gulisano, A S. Gyn. and Obstet. Dept., Univ., Catania, Italy

chlamydia trachomatis (C.t.) and mycoplasma infection associated with other pathogenic agents and cervical pathology have been studied in 167 women, aged between 18 and 69 years, who were followed in this project. C.t. was found in 57 women (35.18%) and mycoplasma in 30 women (18.4%). Neither the chlamydia nor the Mycoplasma were found in 83 women (46.31%). In about 50% of the patients C.t. was associated with other pathogenic agents and/or with cervical pathology. Mycoplasma was found to be associated with aspecific pathogenic agents only in 6.66% of women and with cervical pathology in 86.66%. C.t. was associated with mycoplasma only in eight patients. When neither C.t. nor mycoplasma were present, an aspecific cervico-vaginitis was found in 36.06% of women, specific cervico-vaginitis in 13.95%, cervical pathology in 44.25%.

08.02.04

Laparoscopic diagnosis of chlamydial infection in infertile couples: Rousseau, S, Gattereau, D, Bolte, E, Kurstak, C, Phaneuf, D, Morrisset, R. Hôp. Sainte-Justine, Montréal, Qué., Canada

At our infertility clinic 49 patients underwent laparoscopy to determine prevalence of disseminated pseudo-bullous lesions of the peritoneum, excess of gelatinous liquid and peritubular and periovarian adhesions, features indicative of chlamydia infection. Cultures of peritoneal cavity, cervix and the male partner's urethra, 28 of 49 (57.2%) were positive for Chlamydia trachomatis, 17 from the peritoneum and 11 from genitalia. Streptococcus β-haemolyticus and Ureoplasma were also grown usually when severe tuboperitoneal lesions were present. It is therefore not unusual to recover Chlamydia in investigation of infertility even in the absence of tubal obstruction. The signs described by Dr. *J.H. Suchet* should be borne in mind and a search for pathogens in both sexual partners be done.

08.02.05
Efficacy of single-dose 10% clotrimazole vaginal cream versus fourteen-days treatment with 2% miconazole vaginal cream in patients with vulvo-vaginal candidosis: Loendersloot, E W, Van Kempen, P J H, Branolte, J H*, Barthel, P J*. Pieter Pauw Hosp., Wageningen, *Bayer Nederland B.V., Mijdrecht, The Netherlands

Candida infections are the most frequent cause of vulvo-vaginitis. The results of a single-dose treatment with a vaginal tablet containing 500 mg clotrimazole are very good. Some patients, however, prefer the application of a cream to a vaginal tablet and especially in the presence of a vulvar infection a cream may have definite advantages. In a preceding open study performed in two centers a single-dose treatment with 5 g 10% clotrimazole cream was used in 143 patients with vulvo-vaginal candidosis. Mycological cure was achieved in 94% of the evaluable patients after one week and 90% after four weeks. We can now report about a comparative study between a single-dose treatment with 10% clotrimazole cream and a fourteen-days treatment with 2% miconazole cream in 102 patients with vulvo-vaginal candidosis. No statistical differences could be found in the cure rates of the two groups of patients. With both formulations in the comparative study cure rates were a bit lower than in the open study. It can be concluded that single-dose treatment with 10% clotrimazole cream provides good results in vulvo-vaginal candidosis. In view of the problem of patient compliance single-dose treatment with 10% clotrimazole cream must be preferred to fourteen-days treatment with 2% miconazole cream.

08.02.06
Terconazole – a new efficient antifungal imidazole derivative: Kjaeldgaard, A. Dept. Obstet. and Gyn., Karolinska Inst., Huddinge Univ. Hosp., Stockholm, Sweden

Following the introduction of the antifungal imidazole derivatives, the treatment period of vaginal candidiasis has been continuously reduced during the last decade. The aim of the present comparative randomized double-blind study was to evaluate the clinical efficiency of one-day and three-day treatment with a new antifungal drug, terconazole, which was compared to clotrimazole. Sixty women, aged 14–47 years and suffering from vaginal candidiasis confirmed by direct microscopy and positive culture on Nickerson's medium, were included in the study after their informed consent. All patients were followed one and four weeks after treatment with three vaginal tablets containing either 200 mg clotrimazole, 80 mg terconazole or 240 mg terconazole the first day and pacebo the next two days. The randomized treatment groups were comparable with respect to age, use of oral contraceptives and factors predisposing to candidiasis. No significant differences in initial relief and symptomatic cure rates were demonstrated between the treatment groups. However, significantly higher (p < 0.03) mycological cure rate (94%) was demonstrated in patients treated with the 3-day terconazole regimen. Whereas, the mycological recurrence rates in the other two treatment groups were high (about 35%) because of high frequency of symptomatic and mycological failure in patients with antifungal treatment within the last six months. Thus, 3-day treatment with terconazole seems to be a highly efficient therapy of vaginal candidiasis, and the single vaginal tablet may be a valuable therapeutic alternative in the treatment of patients without factors predisposing to recurrence.

08.02.07
Soluble antigen fluorescent antibody test for diagnosis of genital tuberculosis. – A preliminary report: Takkar, D, Kiran, U, Raj, M, Bhatnagar, A, Shrinivas, Bhargava, V L, Prakash, P. Dept. Obstet. and Gyn., and Dept. of Microbiol., All India Inst. Med. Sci., New Delhi, India

Soluble antigen fluorescent antibody test (SAFA) was carried out in fifty-five women who had clinical evidence of pelvic inflammatory disease. Twenty-three women showed a strong positive reaction and in them corrected correlation with documented tuberculosis was 100%. Twelve showed weak positive response of tuberculosis was 77.7%. However, in twenty women who showed a negative response to SAFA, two women had evidence of treated tuberculosis (11.1% false negative response). However, this could be explained on the basis of quiescent phase of the disease in both of them. (This study is supported by the grant from the Research Fund of All India Institute of Medical Sciences, New Delhi – 110029 – India.)

08.02.08
Treatment of genital mycoplasmosis: Gregoriou, O, Kalabocas, E, Papadias, C, Konidaris, S, Zourlas, P A. 2nd Dept. Obstet. and Gyn., Univ. of Athens, Areteion Hosp., Athens, Greece

Presence of asymptomatic mycoplasmas in the genital tract play a role in spontaneous abortion, prematurity and perinatal morbidity and mortality. Seventy-eight women with histories of pregnancy wastage were cultured for mycoplasmas. Forty-eight women who were mycoplasma positive in the vaginal mucus were treated prospectively for 52 pregnancies with one of three antibiotics regimens: 1) doxycycline HCl per os with oxytetracycline vaginal suppositories prior to conception only, 2) erythromycin stearate per os with oxytetracycline vaginal suppositories only during pregnancy, 3) doxycycline HCl per os with oxytetracycline vaginal suppositories before pregnancy plus erythromycin stearate and oxytetracycline vaginal suppositories during pregnancy. The pregnancy loss rate was significantly reduced from 91.6% to 46.6% among those treated with doxycycline HCl and oxytetracycline prior to conception and less than 15% among those treated with erythromycin stearate and oxytetracycline during pregnancy and doxycycline HCl with oxytetracycline before pregnancy plus erythromycin stearate and oxytetracycline during pregnancy. The reduction in pregnancy loss rate was independent of maternal age, the number of previous abortions and the gestational age of abortion.

08.04.01
Second-look laparotomy in stage III and IV ovarian carcinoma: Podratz, K, Malkasian, G, Hilton, J, Williams, T, Lee, R, Stanhope, C R. Mayo Clin., Rochester, MN, USA

During the period 1977 through 1983, second-look laparotomies (SLL) were performed to assess persistence of ovarian carcinoma in 106 patients originally presenting with stage III or IV disease. Following initial tumor reductive surgery, all patients received postoperative adjunctive chemotherapy consisting predominantly of multi-agent cyclophosphamide/platinum based regimens for a median of 12 months prior to re-exploration. No surgical or histologic evidence of disease (negative SLL) was detected in 40 patients (38%) and was associated with a three-year survivorship of 83%. In contrast, only 31% of the 66 patients with documentable disease (positive SLL) were alive at three years. Peritoneal cytology at SLL (negative 76% three-year survival; positive 22%) and size of residual tumor at completion of the SLL (83, 44, 25, and 19% three-year survival for no residual, microscopic, macroscopic ≤ 5 mm, and macroscopic > 5 mm, respectively) were highly predictive of extended longevity. Subsequent recurrences were observed in 13 patients (32%) declared disease free at SLL between 6.5–45 months (median 16.5 months) after re-exploration. Residual tumor size exceeding 2 cm and/or Broder's grade 4 histology at initial operation were identifiable risk factors in 69% of those patients demonstrating recurrences after negative SLL. Hence, there appears to be an identifiable subset of patients having negative SLL that might potentially benefit from postre-exploration adjunctive therapy.

08.04.02
Results of second-look laparotomy in stage III and IV ovarian cancer: Hanke, J, Kaufmann, M, Schmid, H, Kubli, F. Dept. Obstet. and Gyn., Univ. Hosp., Heidelberg

Between 1979 and 1984 patients (pts.) with ovarian cancer stage III and IV were treated with combination chemotherapy containing cisplatinum. All the pts. had an initial laparotomy performed for tumor reduction, staging and histological classification. On 35 pts. a second-look laparotomy (SLL) was done after a mean interval of 9 months and a mean of 8 chemotherapy cycles. 23 of these pts. were primarily assessed as stage III disease; 12 cases had stage IV disease; two with metastases in the lung or pleura, 10 with liver metastases. The findings at SLL showed macroscopic tumor lesions in 14 pts., microscopic disease was found in 7, and 14 pts. were histologically negative in all biopsies taken. Of 18 pts. with gross residual disease (> 2 cm) after initial surgery 14 still had macroscopic tumor lesions at SLL. In the other group of 17 pts. with minor residual disease (< 2 cm) prior to chemotherapy, 7 had microscopic disease only and 10 were histologically negative. All 14 pts. who were histologically free of disease at SLL are alive with a median follow-up of 24 months; only one of them has had recurrent disease so far. Ten pts. have died, all of them had macroscopic or microscopic disease at SLL. Disease volume at the onset of chemotherapy was found to correlate well with clinical response as well as surgical and histological findings at SLL and appears to be the most important prognostic factor.

08.04.03
Second-look operation of ovarian malignancy: Yasuda, M, Nakabayashi, Y, Obata, I, Terashima, Y, Hachiya, S. Dept. Obstet. and Gyn., Jikei Univ. School Med., Tokyo, Japan

Second-look operation (S.L.O.) has been carried out as one part of a randomised therapy. The number of subjects were 43 common epithelial and 50 of germinal origin tumors, totalling 93 cases. The objects of S.L.O. were concentrated on removal of persisting tumor in 83 cases and evaluation of therapeutic effects in 20 cases. – Conclusion: 1. The average 5-year survival rate was 43% in S.L.O. group, while it was 18% in a control advanced carcinoma group. 2. The mean survival periods of the S.L.O. group were 20.7 months of epithelial tumor and 31.0 months of germinal tumor respectively. Comparatively, control advanced carcinoma group showed 14.3 months and 10.6 months for each tumor group. 3. The complete removal of the tumor was found possible in 19 cases receiving postoperative therapy, out of 44 cases which had initial incomplete surgery. This suggests the importance of postoperative therapy. 4. The sites of recurrence found at the S.L.O. were 29 cases of intra-abdominal, 21 cases of intrapelvic, 17 cases of lymph nodes and three other locations. Results obtained indicate that the following are important factors at the S.L.O: (1) initial complete surgery, (2) determination of staging by multiple biopsies and cytological examination. (3) Optimal interval between initial surgery and S.L.O. is about one year.

08.04.04.

Second-look laparotomy in the management of epithelial carcinoma of the ovary: Fotiou, S, Tserkezoglou, A, **Fakas, G, Aravantinos, D.** Univ. Maternity Hosp., Alexandra, Athens, Greece

A total of 42 patients underwent second-look laparotomy in the course of their management for ovarian carcinoma, in order to evaluate the disease status and possibly stop treatment. All patients had been primarily operated on and subsequently treated with chemotherapy for a period of 12–16 months. A thorough clinical and laboratory (CT scan included) investigation revealed no sign of disease before the re-operation. According to the initial staging most patients belonged to stage III (76%), while the rest were as follows: stage I 10%, stage II 7% and stage IV 7%. Second-look operations were performed according to a specific protocol including: meticulous inspection and palpation, cytological samples and multiple biopsies. Gross disease was identified during laparotomy in 12 cases (28.5%). At another eight patients (19%), thought to be disease free at laparotomy, microscopic examinations were found positive. Finally in 22 cases (52.5%) there was no evidence of disease. It was remarkable that a positive cytologic examination was the only sign of disease in four cases. The observation period ranged from 4 to 30 months. During this time two "negative" patients suffered recurrence and died 7 and 19 months after the operation.

08.04.05

A prospective randomized study to assess the survival benefit of second-look laparotomy and subsequent management in epithelial ovarian cancer: Luesley, D M, Chan, K K, Jordan, J A, Lawton, F, Blackledge, G R. Dept. Obstet. & Gyn. and Med., Univ., Birmingham, UK

Many studies have suggested a role for second-look laparotomy (2LL) in the management of ovarian cancer (OC), yet the survival benefit remains unproven. A prospective study of patients with macroscopic residual OC after primary staging and debulking surgery has been performed. Patients were randomized at the time of diagnosis to one of three arms of treatment. All received primary chemotherapy with five courses of cis-platinum (100 mg/M^2), in arm X this was followed by 2LL then cyclical oral chlorambucil, in arm Y by chlorambucil only and in arm Z by 2LL followed by total abdominal and pelvic irradiation. The study has a median follow-up of 24 months. There are 46 patients in X, 45 in Y and 45 in Z. The overall median survival is 18 m and there are no significant differences in survival between the three treatment arms. Partial responders (PR) to DDP not having a 2LL have a similar survival to PRs undergoing cytoreduction at 2LL. Patients with no clinical evidence of disease after DDP had similar survivals in arms X and Y although disease was found and resected in a proportion of the former. Within the context of this study neither 2LL nor the choice of subsequent management were shown to influence survival.

08.04.07

Ovarian tumors of borderline malignancy: An analysis of 53 cases from the University Women's Hospital Zurich/Switzerland (1970–1982): Ziogas, W, Kunz, J, Genton, C Y*, Schreiner, W E. Univ. Women's Hosp., and *Inst. Path., Zurich, Switzerland

At the Clinic of Gynecology of the University Women's Hospital of Zurich, 53 serous (24) and mucinous (29) borderline tumors of the ovary were observed from 1970 through 1982, thus representing 4.3% of all benign and malignant ovarian neoplasms seen at this institution during the same period of time. The most common subjective symptoms were abdominal enlargement and indefinite abdominal pain. A pelvic mass was clinically present in 80% of patients. The average age at diagnosis was 57 years (24–82 years), 70% of the patients being older than 50 years. More than half (60%) of the tumors were larger than 20 cm at diagnosis, only 6% measured 5 cm or less. Every fifth patient presented with ascites; a pleural effusion was never observed. 12.5% of the serous and 13.8% of the mucinous tumors were bilateral, a finding which did not influence the prognosis. Adhesions to surrounding organs were found in 12.5% of the serous but in none of the mucinous tumors. In a single case of serous tumor omental metastases were present. Histological diagnosis at frozen section examination as well as age of patient and/or wish to preserve fertility determined the extent of the primary operation. In patients over 45 years of age, the operation consisted as a rule in bilateral salpingo-oophorectomy and total hysterectomy. Patients under the age of 40 who wished to preserve their fertility were if ever possible treated by unilateral salpingo-oophorectomy only. During the average observation period of 3.6 years (1–12 years), a recurrence was observed in 7% of the mucinous but in none of the serous tumors.

08.04.07

Impact of surgery on prognosis in ovarian cancer (results of the cooperative Berlin trial): Imholz, G, Mayr, A C, Schmoranz, W, Grüneisen, A, Hindenburg, H J, Karger, N, Maassen, V, Pschyrembel, I, Scholtes, G. Ovarian Ca Study Group, Tumorzentrum, Berlin

Seventy women with epithelial cancer, not previously treated were included in the cooperative therapeutic trial. From a total of 165 patients, 15 could not be assessed, 37 had stage I to IIA. Of patients with stage II B–IV, 113 were followed for a median observation time of 20 months (range 6–46 months). In 34 pts. incomplete bilateral salpingo-oophorectomy + hystero-omentectomy (BSOHO) and in 62 pts. complete BSOHO was performed initially. In 17 pts. only a biopsy was taken.

	compl. BSOHO	incompl.	Biopsy only
PD free survival 12 Mo	80	47	47
24 Mo	51	18	17
Overall survival 12 Mo	92	75	64
24 Mo	77	41	41

After 6 months without relapse a second-look procedure (SL) was recommended. In 1981/82 40% of the pts. got a SL, while in 1983/84 72% got a SL. Of 22 women with completion of initially incomplete BSOHO 8 died, and SL 9 of 17 women have died up to now. Primary complete BSOHO or completion at SL is recommended.

08.04.08
Resection of a giant ovarian cyst with immediate reconstruction of the abdominal wall: Fozzard, C E. Royal Cornwall Hosp. – Freliske, Truro, Cornwall, UK
Removal of an 89 kg benign, giant ovarian cyst and reconstruction of the abdominal wall is described. A 59-year-old woman, virtually immobile, presented with a cyst of 10 years duration; abdominal girth 170 cm, after five days pre-operative drainage of 55 litres, the cyst was removed intact in two hours without damage to the bladder, ureters or intestine. Reconstruction of the abdominal wall took three hours and is discussed. Postoperative intensive care supervision is outlined. The patient walked unaided out of hospital on the 15th day. Follow-up shows normal muscle tone, posture and full mobility of the patient.

08.06.01
Bacterial spectrum of gynecological infections and therapy: Petersen, E E. Univ.-Frauenklin., Freiburg/Br.
It has repeatedly been shown in many studies that various aerobic as well as anaerobic bacteria can be isolated from the site of gynecological infections. Increasing improvements in the cultivation and identification of anaerobic bacteria have led to these bacteria being detected more and more often in gynecological infections, indeed in some cases they have even been found to be the predominant bacteria. – However, anaerobic bacteria are also being increasingly detected in females with no complaints and in females with a bacterial vaginal disorder. Whereas the detection of pathogenic bacteria such as Neisseria gonorrhoeae and Staphylococcus aureus, as well as of certain Enterobacteriaceae has resulted in their being recognised as causing disease since they are found only relatively rarely in the healthy vagina, it has so far been difficult to interpret the detection of the more common Anaerobes such as the various Bacteroides sp., Peptococcus, Peptostreptococcus sp., Veillonella etc. It would seem that anaerobes can particularly be considered as infective agents when they are already present in very large numbers before surgery. Synergism with other anaerobic bacteria and even with aerobic bacteria plays an important role here. In a prospective study from the field of obstetrics we have now shown that females with very high counts of facultatively pathogenic bacteria in the vagina – where incidentally the anaerobes were by far the most common – run a risk of infection more than 10 times greater than that of femals with Lactobacilli. – The therapy of gynecological infections should cover approximately the expected bacterial spectrum. Matching the therapy solely to individual detected bacteria in gynecology seems questionable and possibly dangerous. Priority should be given to preparations with activity also in the anaerobic range, or if necessary the therapy must be combined with an anaerobically active preparation. In the early stage of infection or if the infection is fairly mild, therapeutic responses can also be achieved – because of the synergism between the different bacteria – with preparations that do not cover all possible bacteria.

08.06.02
Significance of pharmacokinetic properties for clinical use of newer cephalosporins: Lode, H, Höffken, G, Kemmerich, B, Hampel, B, Koeppe, B, Borner, K. Med. Klin. u. Poliklin., Klinikum Steglitz, FU, Berlin
Rational evaluation of a chemotherapeutic substance is based upon various factors: physico-chemical properties, antibacterial activity, pharmacokinetics, clinical efficacy, tolerance and cost. Pharmacokinetic parameters give indication of release, resorption, distribution, protein fixation, metabolism, and elimination of a pharmacon. Between the cephalosporins currently on the market there are considerable pharmacokinetic differences which may also have clinical relevance. According to a modified classification by *Stoeckel* (1982) there are four different groups of cephalosporins, which differ mainly as to their protein binding, elimination half-life and mechanisms of renal excretion. The biological half-life of most cephalosporins varies from 1 to 2.5 hours, with the exception of cefotetan (3–4 h) and ceftriaxon (7–8 h) where half-life is clearly longer. Whereas pharmacokinetic behaviour of ceftriaxon follows a non-linear curve due to very high protein binding of the compound, it is linear with cefotetan, where a twice daily dosage appears to be optimal. Because of its high antibacterial activity against Enterobacteriae and Anaerobes and due to its advantageous pharmacokinetic properties, cefotetan may be considered an excellent cephalosporin for the treatment of gynecological infections, with a relatively low dose of 2 g b.i.d. – Lit.: *Stoeckel, U.* (1982) Pharmakokinetik parenteraler Cephalosporine in Prüfphase III. FAC 1: 104–114.

08.06.03

The placental pharmacokinetics of cefotetan using an *in vitro* perfusion model: Wachter, I, Weissenbacher, E R, Gutschow, K, Schneider, A, Adam, A, Tischler, A, Drexel, R. Frauenklin., Klinikum Großhadern, München

Using the *in vitro* placental perfusion model developed by *Leichtweiß* and *Schneider* 14 placentas were perfused with cefotetan within 1–40 minutes postpartum. Using a single injection of 10 mg/1 ml cefotetan, 5 placentas were tested in both materno-fetal and feto-maternal directions. 9 placentas were continually perfused with a concentration of 10 mg/100 ml cefotetan. Samples were taken simultaneously at regular intervals from the maternal and fetal veins. The cefotetan concentrations were determined by microbiological assay methods. Using the infusions method the concentrations of cefotetan in maternal tissue reached 64.3 mcg/ml after 5 minutes, 2 minutes later a plateau of 16.3 mcg/nl was reached and on the fetal side 1 minute later the concentration reached 3 mcg/ml. Increasing the concentration led to similar but higher levels being determined. Using the single injection technique 2 minutes later on the maternal side a concentration of 334.5 mcg/ml was reached. The concentrations of the fetal side demonstrated a time lag of 1 minute. Levels were also determined following single injection in the other direction (feto-maternal).

06.06.04

The role of cephalosporins in gynecological and obstetric infections: Lang, E. Univ.-Frauenklin., Erlangen

Ever since their introduction into therapy, cephalosporins, have been widely used for the treatment of infections in gynecology and obstetrics. This is especially true for the USA, where cephalotin seemed to prove effective in prophylaxis in vaginal hysterectomy. Only when the importance of anaerobic pathogens in gynecological and obstetrical infections became more and more evident the situation changed in favor of more suitable antibiotics or combination therapy respectively. By the development of new cephalosporins with high β-lactamase stability it was possible to fill in this gap. At present some newer cephalosporins meet all requirements that are made on an antibiotic for efficacy in gynecological and obstetrical infections: good activity against important pathogens (with some exceptions in obstetrics), good tissue penetration, good tolerance and easy administration. Good antibacterial activity, advantageous pharmacokinetic properties and good tolerance make some newer cephalosporins to drugs of first choice in gynecological and obstetrical infections.

08.06.05

Cefotetan versus cefotaxim/metronidazole in GYNOB infections: Weissenbacher, E R, Gutschow, K, Adam, D, Wachter, I, Schneider, A. Frauenklin., Klinikum Großhadern, München

25 patients were treated with 2 × 2 g cefotetan i. v. for 7 days. A further 25 patients received 3 × 2 g cefotaxim together with 2 × 500 g metronidazole i. v. for 7 days. The commonest strains isolated were E. coli and Enterococci. The most common infections found were urinary tract infections, pelvic inflammatory disease, soft tissue infection etc. There were so significant differences between the two groups with respect to the bacterial elimination rate and the clinical rate of recovery. One possible explanation is that the infections were seldom caused by anaerobic bacteria alone.

08.07.01

Ultrasound examination of the breast in symptomatic patients: Results of an integrated breast clinic: Honkomp, C C, Pfeiffer, K H, Kieback, D G, Pläcking, C. Univ.-Frauenklin., Tübingen

Up to the present, 500 ultrasound examinations of the breast have been performed in addition to the established routine diagnostic procedures in an integrated gynecologic/radiologic breast clinic at the Univ.-Frauenklinik Tübingen. These examinations were performed with Compound- (4 MHz) and Real-time (3 MHz) techniques on 471 female patients with symptoms of breast disease. In 348 patients, pathologic sonographic findings were observed. In 180 cases, the diagnosis by ultrasound was reexamined by aspiration cytology of the cystic tumors and by histologic examination of the solid tumors. The diagnosis suspected by ultrasonography was reconfirmed in 96% of the cystic findings, 90% of the mastopathic changes, 83% of the carcinomas and 77% of the fibroadenomas. Since the recent introduction of a 5-MHz-transducer, the ultrasound examination led to the primary diagnosis of cancer in a remarkable number of cases, while radiologic techniques were non-contributing. The additional use of ultrasound techniques for the evaluation of the breast resulted in 90% overall correct positive diagnoses and improved the detection and differentiation of benign and malignant breast disease.

08.07.02

Mammographic diagnostic problems, indications and results in 335 patients with subcutaneous mastectomy (SCM): Arabin, B, Fournier, D v., Müller, A, Kubli, F. Univ.-Frauenklin., Heidelberg

From 1974–1982 we performed a SCM in 335 patients. The mammograms of 265 patients were analysed retrospectively and compared to the final histology in order to redefine mainly the radiological indications. The radiological criteria: dysplasia, difficult interpretation and macrocystic disease were significantly increased when we found a non-invasive or invasive cancer in the tissue of the SCM. We found no correlation between the radiological pattern according to *Wolfe* and the rate of cancer. The typical criteria of malignancy could be analysed less frequently in this study group because of the selection of patients with mammograms which were difficult to interpret. Concerning the indications we differentiated between three groups of patients: In patients with contralateral carcinoma and difficult to interprete mammograms the indication for the SCM was justified by the rate of carcinoma (4/18). In patients with only clinical and/or radiological indication the SCM was not justified in patients with "benign" mammograms (the rate of carcinoma was only 1/73), whereas in cases with difficult to interprete mammograms the rate was 12/58. No case of confirmed cancer showed signs of malignancy prospectively or retrospectively. In patients with pre-operative biopsy – leading to the indication for SCM – we found in eight cases an invasive carcinoma though the biopsy had only shown atypical or non-invasive tissue. – Conclusion: In patients with "benign" mammography there is no indication for the SCM. In patients with mammograms difficult to interprete, all diagnostic procedures should be evaluated before performing a SCM which is still "the last step in the diagnostic scale".

08.07.03
The use of ultrasound in the diagnosis of breast disease: Gyr, T, Stucki, D, Hendry, M, Koudelka, G, Rageth, C, Tschumi, P. Dept. Obstet. and Gyn., Univ., Basle, Switzerland
The purpose of this study was to determine the benefit of ultrasonic examination in our out-patient breast clinic. Over 14 months starting January 1984, 2600 examinations because of signs suggesting breast disease were performed. The procedure included clinical examination, plate thermography and upon special indication mammography, sonography, telethermography and fine needle aspiration. 2256 ultrasonic examinations with a 6 MHz handheld transducer were performed. 1233 examinations revealed no specific findings. Of this group, 16 patients underwent biopsy. Histological diagnosis revealed two carcinomas. 609 cystic lesions were found with ultrasound, four of which were operated, two carcinomas were diagnosed. Of 414 solid breast lesions sonographically identified, 114 were operated; 39 were invasive carcinomas. Of 884 x-ray mammograms 727 showed no signs of malignancy. 20 of the patients underwent biopsy; carcinoma was found in two cases. Of the 157 patients with questionable or suspect findings on x-ray, 64 underwent biopsy; 41 had carcinomas. Fine needle aspiration was mainly of diagnostic value if malignant cells were found. Thermography, however, was of little diagnostic use. Sonography proved to be an excellent complementary diagnostic tool. With the help of ultrasound two carcinomas not recognized on x-ray were diagnosed. Two invasive and two *in situ* carcinomas otherwise suspected were not identified with ultrasound. The decision to perform biopsy was facilitated by ultrasound and this technique helped to prevent unnecessary surgery.

08.07.04
Breast aspiration cytology as a screening procedure of breast lesions in gynecologic practice: Hindle, W H, Navin, J J. Dept. Gyn. and Cytopath., Straub Clin. and Hosp., Inc., Honolulu, HI, USA
Breast aspiration cytology as a diagnostic procedure is well known in Europe, but little utilized clinically in the United States. At the Straub Clinic, breast aspiration cytology is used as a screening procedure for breast lesions. 1787 aspirations have proved the reliability, simplicity, and cost-effectiveness of breast aspiration cytology as a screening adjunct in the clinician's office. Evaluation is carried out by palpation and mammography in addition to aspiration cytology. The use of all three modalities approaches 99% accuracy. Definitive open biopsies are done as indicated. A histologic diagnosis of benign and malignant lesions is made cytologically and confirmed by subsequent biopsies. Approximately 4% of these screening breast aspirations proved to have carcinoma. This technique is easily learned. The equipment required is readily available in the office of any gynecologist who does Papanicolaou smears of the cervix. Office aspiration cytology examination for breast lesions is efficient, cost-effective and cytologically accurate.

08.08.01
Excessive weight gain during pregnancy – a possible first step to obesity: Nyirjesy, I, Nyirjesy, P. Georgetown Univ., Washington, DC, USA
Several studies have indicated a favorable relationship between adequate weight gain during pregnancy and reduced low birthweight incidence. Because of these observations, good prenatal nutrition is emphasized and possible side-effects of excessive weight gain tend to be minimized in most American institutions. It has been reported that the mean postpregnancy weight loss is 8.2 kg at six weeks, but few data are available about the longer term persistence of weight accumulated during pregnancy. The net weight gain, defined as the difference in pre-pregnancy weight and the weight between 6 and 12 months postpartum, has been determined in 108 consecutive private patients and correlated to their weight gain during pregnancy. The mean weight gain in pregnancy was 25.19 lbs (11.58 kg). The mean net weight gain was −2.47 lbs (−1.12 kg) in patients with a weight gain of less than 25 lbs (11.36 kg), 1.23 lbs (0.559 kg) in those who gained 26 to 30 lbs (11.8 to 13.5 kg) and 4.46 lbs (2.02 kg) in patients who gained over 30 lbs (13.6 kg). Twenty-eight (25.9%) of the patients had a net weight gain of over 5 lbs (2.27 kg); in 11 (10.2%) of these, the gain exceeded 10 lbs (4.54 kg). Over 2/3 of the patients (19/28) with a high net weight increment gained over 30 lbs (13.6 kg) during their pregnancy (p < .0001). Weight gain over 30 lbs (13.6 kg) increases the number of excessively large infants, of prolonged labors and of operative deliveries. Preliminary data indicate that its effect on net weight gain is cumulative in successive pregnancies and it is believed that it can lead to obesity.

08.08.02

Intrauterine growth retardation, diet and maternal zinc depletion: James, C E, Simmer, K, Iles, C A, Thompson, R P H. Depts. Obstet. and Gastroent., St. Thomas's Hosp., London, UK

To identify factors associated with intrauterine growth retardation (IUGR) the smoking habits, socio-economic class, anthropometric measurements, diet and zinc status of 118 mothers were investigated 24–48 hours after delivery. Sixty-seven mothers had babies whose size was appropriate for gestational age (AGA) and 51 mothers had babies which were small for gestational age (SGA) as defined by obstetric and pediatric criteria. Lower social class (IV–VI) and maternal smoking were significantly associated with IUGR ($p < 0.001$ and $p < 0.02$, respectively). A typical seven day dietary survey for the last trimester of pregnancy showed daily zinc intake to be lower in mothers with SGA babies (11.3 ± 0.5, $n = 28$, v 13.0 ± 0.6 mg, $n = 29$, means $\pm$ SEM $p < 0.05$). Carbohydrate, fat, essential fatty acids and energy intake were not significantly different. In 75 mothers, polymorphonuclear (PMN), mononuclear (MN) and plasma zinc concentrations were measured. There was a highly significant difference in both PMN and MN zinc concentrations between the mothers of AGA and SGA babies (77.3 ± 3.8, $n = 42$ v 61.1 ± 2.1 µg/10^{10} PMN $n = 33$, $p < 0.001$; 87.2 ± 9.0, $n = 34$ v 140.7 ± 5.9 µg/10^{10} MN, $n = 34$ $p < 0.001$). Plasma zinc levels did not correlate with the leucocyte values and reduced levels of plasma zinc were not associated with IUGR. This corroborates previous work which showed that PMN zinc measurement is a better guide to tissue zinc status. In this study a low PMN zinc level in conjunction with the smoking history had an 85% sensitivity in detection of IUGR. We conclude that maternal tissue zinc depletion is strongly associated with IUGR and suggest that dietary zinc depletion may be an important etiological factor.

08.08.03

Lipids, lipoproteins, placental hormones and insulin during normal pregnancy: Schweditsch, M O*, Desoye, G*, Kostner, G M**, Pfeiffer, K H***, Zechner, R**. *Dept. Obstet. Gyn., **Inst. Med. Biochem., ***Inst. Physiol., Univ., Graz, Austria

Forty-two women with normal pregnancy were studied, beginning at the first weeks of pregnancy and at three to five weekly intervals until delivery. Plasma levels of phospholipids (PL), total and free cholesterol (TC, FC), HDL- and LDL-cholesterol, triglycerides (TG), apolipoproteins AI, AII, B and lipoprotein a (Lpa) were measured. HCG, hPL, insulin, progesteron and estradiol were also recorded. Until term TG increased 300%, PL 50%, TC 62%, FC 260%, LDL-C 80% and HDL-C 30%. Apo AI rose until the 22nd week, Apo AII showed minor variations and Apo B reached a maximum at the 30th week of pregnancy. Lpa levels rose steadily until the 19th week of pregnancy and declined thereafter. The gradual fall of the ratio AI/B is of interest. Beginning at the 22nd week of pregnancy insulin levels increased continuously, the placental hormones showed the known variations. The results indicate: 1) regulatory effects of placental hormones and insulin on apolipoprotein composition and lipoprotein metabolism, 2) independence of the metabolic control of plasma Lpa, 3) the hyperlipidemia of pregnancy could in itself function as an arteriosclerotic risk factor.

08.08.04

Arm circumference for nutritional assessment of Mozambican gravidae: Liljestrand, J, Bergström, S. Dept. Obstet. and Gyn., Univ., Uppsala, Sweden

Primary health workers in developing countries are not always able to use the prepregnancy weight/height or pregnancy weight gain for assessing nutritional status of pregnant women. The mid-upper-arm circumference has had some use in Latin America and India for nutritional screening of gravidae but we found no such references from Africa. In seven of Mozambique's ten provinces 833 pregnant women were examined, mainly at community level in rural areas. Gestational age was noted, and weight, height, mid-upper-arm circumference, triceps skinfold thickness and symphysis-fundus distance measured. Average monthly weight gain, as calculated from a regression line in a plot of gestational age versus weight, was 0.8 kg. Non-pregnant weight was estimated for each woman by subtracting 0.8 kg $\times$ months of pregnancy from her actual weight. When comparing arm circumference with estimated non-pregnant weight for height (WFH), it was found that arm circumference was useful in detecting women with low WFH. An arm circumference below 25 cm had a sensitivity of 75% in detecting women with WFH below 85% of standard, and a specificity of 85%. The predictive value of an arm circumference below 25 cm was 46% as regards WFH below 85% of standard. Arm circumference was strongly correlated to arm muscle circumference as calculated from skinfold thickness and arm circumference. It is concluded that the mid-upper-arm circumference is quite useful in detecting malnutrition or wasting (for instance because of T. B.) in pregnant women. In Mozambique, a measurement below 25 cm is a warning of, and below 23 cm strong evidence of malnutrition.

08.08.05

Metabolic effects of high and low fiber diets in pregnant women and non-pregnant women: Fraser, R B, Ford, F A, Lawrence, G F. Univ. Dept. Obstet. and Gyn., Sheffield, UK

Previous studies have suggested that glucose homeostasis deteriorates in pregnancy despite an increased secretion of insulin, and that normal pregnancy is associated with net maternal fat storage despite increased lipolysis in late gestation. We have examined these paradoxes in a crossover study of low dietary fiber (1830 kcal 41% CHO 39% fat 20% protein 10 g fiber) and high dietary fiber (1820 kcal 40% CHO 38.5%

fat 21.5% protein 52 g fiber) diets in normal weight non-pregnant women, and women in the third trimester of pregnancy. Diurnal profiles of plasma glucose, insulin, βOH butyrate, glycerol and lactate were obtained. On both diets there was a significant improvement of glucose homeostasis in pregnancy throughout the diurnal profile. On the low fiber diet there were significant rises in βOH butyrate and glycerol levels, in pregnancy, but this effect was abolished by the high fiber diet. These results suggest that (a) late pregnancy is a state of improved glucose homeostasis and (b) increased preprandial lipolysis in late pregnancy may be an abnormality induced by a low fiber "Western" diet.

08.08.06
Eight essential major and trace elements in maternal and umbilical cord blood, and placental tissue: Chen, S, Mori, H, Kigawa, T. Dept. Obstet. and Gyn., Oita Med. Coll., Oita, Japan
In order to investigate the feto-maternal interrelation of the essential major and trace elements, Na, K, Mg, Ca, P, Fe, Cu, and Zn were determined in the maternal and umbilical cord blood and placental tissue from 102 pregnant Japanese women during 1982 and 1984. The placenta was irrigated with physiological saline containing heparin via an intra-arterial catheter to remove the blood as completely as possible. The samples were digested and heated by 14 N nitric acid in 140 °C for 4 hours and determined simultaneously by Inductively Coupled Plasma Emission Spectrometer for the eight elements. Concentration of K, P, Fe ($p < 0.001$) and Mg ($p < 0.05$) were significantly higher in cord blood than in maternal blood, whereas Na, Cu, and Zn were significant lower ($p < 0.001$) in cord blood than in maternal blood and Ca showed no gradient. Although Zn and Cu have been regarded as very important nutritional factors during fetal and neonatal growth, our data indicated that these elements in cord blood are 40% less than those in the maternal blood level. Significant positive correlation were observed between maternal blood and cord blood on K, Mg, Ca, Fe, and Zn. The ratios of the mean concentration of elements in placenta to that in maternal blood are Na: 1.07, K: 0.28, Mg: 1.33, Ca: 8.11, P: 3.86, Fe: 0.06, Cu: 0.24, Zn: 1.09. These findings may indicate the variety of feto-maternal relationship of the essential elements, and the different transfer mechanism for elements through the placenta.

08.08.07
Maternal plasma zinc and normal and abnormal fetal growth: Jenkins, D M, Fehily, D, Cremin, F, Flynn, A. Dept. Obstet. and Gyn., Nutrition, Univ. Coll., Cork, Ireland
The relationship of maternal and fetal tissue and plasma zinc to fetal growth is the subject of intense current interest. Results are apparently contradictory (*Meadows, W. J., Ruse, W.* et al. Lancet **39**, 879–887, 1981; *Metcoff, J., Costiloe, J. P.* et al. Amer. J. clin. Nutr., **34**, 708–721, 1981). We report evidence suggesting a normal maternal adaptation to fetal demands for zinc involving transfer of plasma zinc from the less available α_2-macroglobulin form to the loosely bound more available albumin bound form during pregnancy. We also report an inverse relationship between maternal plasma albumin bound zinc and measures of fetal growth including mid arm circumference and ponderal index. We will propose mechanisms to explain this inverse relationship.

08.08.08
The course of pregnancy and its risk for the fetus in obese women: Karoblienė, L. Med. Inst., Kaunas, Lithuania, USSR
Approximately 15% of pregnant women are obese. In cases of obesity adaptive and regulating mechanisms of organism and neurohumoral correlation are deranged. All this disturbs normal functioning of mother-placenta-fetus system. We have investigated 1352 obese pregnant women. To ascertain the degree of obesity we followed *Broka* formula and *Jegorov* classification. According to our data pregnancy toxemia in obese women was four times as frequent as in controls. Nonreactive nonstress test while electronic fetal monitoring was found in 60% of cases. 30% of the fetuses showed a positive oxytocin challenge test. 13% of obese women were delivered by emergency Cesarean section because of fetal distress. Post term delivery was more frequent in obese women (18%) than in those of normal weight (10%). Obese women showed excessive hemorrhage in the placental period. In conclusion, obesity is a risk factor not only for fetus but also for mother.

08.08.09
Assessment of immune status of malnourished pregnant females: Kala, S. India
In this study, assessment of the immune status of 46 malnourished pregnant females was done and results were compared with 44 healthy pregnant females. Lymphocyte subpopulation studies were done along with other hematological and biochemical investigations to assess the malnutrition. The incidence of anemia during pregnancy was 51.1 per cent. Malnutrition increased with the advance of pregnancy i.e. in first trimester 40%, second trimester 66.6% and in third trimester 66.6%. Lymphocyte subpopulation studies showed a significant depression of total T cell and active T cell ($p < .001$) with significant rise of B cell level ($p < .001$) which reverted back to normal in third trimester. Malnourished pregnant females showed a greater depression of cell mediated immunity (CMI) in all trimesters as compared to normal pregnant females.

08.09.01

Hyperplasia of the human endometrium: A light and electron microscopic study: Kyparissi, M, Klearchou, N, Vakiani, M, Papathanasiou, K, Mantalenakis, S. 1st Dept. Obstet. and Gyn., Aristotelian Univ., Thessaloniki, Greece

Samples of hyperplastic endometrium from 80 patients were studied by light microscopy. Fifteen of these cases were also examined ultrastructurally. The material was obtained by endometrial curettage, followed by hysterectomy in the half of the cases. The rest of the patients were treated conservatively. In some cases the patients were re-examined and a diagnostic curettage carried out. The samples were diagnosed histopathologically as glandular cystic hyperplasia, adenomatous hyperplasia and atypical adenomatous hyperplasia of the endometrium. Some of the most striking ultrastructural features of adenomatous hyperplastic endometrium were the prominent and enlarged rough endoplasmic reticulum (RER) closely associated with mitochondria and nucleus, a network of microfilaments found mainly perinuclear and nuclear membrane infoldings. The significance of the histopathological findings, as related to their importance for the treatment of the patient is briefly discussed.

08.09.02

Endometrial hyperplasia: Ruf, H, Blanc, B, Conte, M, Charpin, C. Maternité de la Belle de Mai 23, Marseille, France

Analysing 81 cases of endometrial hyperplasia, the authors provide the specific ground on which these hyperplasias arise and the action of endogenous and exogenous estrogens. They distinguish between the different forms of hyperplasia of the endometrium. Working on the basis of *Hendrickson* and *Kempson's* classification, severe atypical hyperplasias should be dissociated from other atypical forms by reason of their frequent association with endometrial carcinoma, on the one hand, and the risk of degeneration of this kind of lesion, on the other. Finally, they propose a therapeutic approach adapted to the anatomo-pathological response and the age of the patient. Epidemiological investigation, diagnosis and treatment of hyperplasia comes within the field of prophylaxis of the endometrial adenocarcinoma. The study of this high-risk population appears, at all events, to prove this.

08.09.03

Office use of the endometrial biopsy: Speir, B R. Univ. of South Alabama Coll. Med., Mobile, AL, USA

Study was done to assess the various uses of the endometrial biopsy in the practice of gynecology and to determine the accuracy of diagnoses obtained. One thousand endometrial biopsies were done in the office by the investigator. Indications for the biopsy and correlation with cytology and surgical pathology are included in the study. Among the indications for biopsy are: biopsies done prior to initiation of estrogen replacement therapy, peri- and post-menopausal bleeding, dysfunctional uterine bleeding, infertility work-ups, post-partum bleeding and women having regular menses after expected menopausal age. Correlation of biopsy, cytology and any subsequent surgical pathology are reported. No endometrial carcinoma was found at D & C and/or hysterectomy which had not been diagnosed in the office. No patient taking exogenous estrogen who was followed with annual endometrial biopsy developed endometrial carcinoma. Biopsy was "curative" in 75% of patients with dysfunctional bleeding. Investigator feels that the endometrial biopsy is a simple, inexpensive diagnostic test which is often under-utilized in office practice.

08.09.04

The anatomical basis of aspiration cytology of the endometrium – a contribution ot the discussion of the problems of the early diagnosis of carcinoma of the endometrium and its precursors: Anastasiadis, G P, Lolis, E D V, Lüdinghausen, M. Dept. Obstet. and Gyn., Univ., Ioannina, Greece

In 300 patients from age 38 to 83 aspiration cytology of the endometrium was carried out and compared to microscopic findings of the surface of the endometrium after hysterectomy. The samples were obtained from women with post-menopausal and pre-menopausal bleeding and from women without bleeding prior to hysterectomy for various indications. In 4.9% of the cases adenocarcinoma of the endometrium was detected, and in 4.2% of the cases precancerous lesions such as adenomatous or atypical glandular hyperplasia of the endometrium and of the endocervix were observed. In a third of all the cases there was an important difference between the grade of Papanicolaou and the histologic findings, which will be discussed.

08.09.05

Long-term follow-up study using the Mi-Mark technique in the diagnosis of endometrial cancer: Kloster-Jensen, A, Tronstad, S-E. Dept. Gyn. and Obstet., Centr. Hosp., Skövde, Sweden

A previous study has shown the patient acceptance and diagnostic reliability of Mi-Mark for histological examination (1). In this prospective controlled study, the Mi-Mark technique was used for routine clinical diagnosis of endometrial cancer. – Method: Vaginal smears and Mi-Mark biopsy were performed without analgesia. A few patients with cervical stenosis were excluded. Only when biopsy material was inadequate for diagnosis or showed malignancy were the patients referred for conventional curettage. Routine control including a new Mi-Mark biopsy six months later was added during 1979–1980. – Patients: From 1979 till 1982, 275 patients were examined by primary Mi-Mark biopsy; 137 of these were also subjected to control Mi-Mark biopsy. Mean age of the patients: 55 years. Length of observation 2.5–6 years. – Results: Of the 275 primary Mi-Mark biopsies, 216 were benign, 14 specimens were malignant or atypical and 45 specimens (16%) inadequate for diagnosis. In the latter group, two endometrial cancers were discovered by additional diagnostic methods. In the group of 14 atypical/malignant specimens there were verified nine endometrial cancers, three cases of adenomatous hyperplasia and one CIN. By the vaginal smear method, three cases of CIN could be diagnosed. No further malignancies could be detected at the control Mi-Mark biopsy. Control examination was therefore discontinued later on in asymptomatic patients. – Conclusions: With adequate sampling material, the simple Mi-Mark endometrial biopsy is an efficient method for routine diagnosis of endometrial cancer. – (1) Acta obstet. gyn. scand., Suppl **93**, 1981.

08.09.06

The correlation of estradiol and progesterone receptor concentration to relapse in endometrial carcinoma patients: Lindahl, B, Alm, P, Fernö, M, Grundsell, H, Norgren, A, Tropé, C. Dept. Obstet./Gyn., Path. and Oncol., Univ. Hosp., Lund, Sweden

The 5-year survival rate of patients with well and moderately differentiated stage I–II endometrial carcinomas is around 90%, whereas that of the poorly differentiated ones is only about 70%. At present there is difficulty in selecting patients most likely to benefit from additional chemotherapy. This study measured the E_2 and P receptor concentrations in endometrial carcinomas and correlated these with staging, histologic grading, degree of myometrial invasion and relapse. The concentrations of E_2 receptors were assayed with isoelectric focussing and those of P by a multiplepoint dextran-coated charcoal technique. The study shows that more than 80% of the relapses in the poorly differentiated tumors belong to the low E_2 receptor concentration group. Via a combination of low E_2 receptor concentration and myometrial invasion more than one third of the thickness of the myometrium it is possible to select patients at risk of developing relapse. These patients constituted 60% of the women studied and more than 40% relapsed. Thus the determination of E_2 receptor concentration in endometrial carcinomas might be useful for selecting patients likely to benefit from aggressive adjuvant chemotherapy.

08.09.07

Characterization of progesterone receptor in human endometrial adenocarcinoma *in vitro*: Terakawa, N, Aono, T, Ikegami, H, Shimizu, I, Hayashida, M, Tanizawa, O. Dept. Obstet. and Gyn., Osaka Univ. Med. School, Osaka, Japan

The presence of progesterone receptor (PgR) was documented in a newly established cell line (*Ishikawa*), derived from human endometrial adenocarcinoma. The cytoplasmic binding sites had high affinity for R5020 (Kd: 2.0×10^{-9} M, MBS; 175 fmole/mg protein) and typical specificity such as PgR. Sucrose density gradient analysis in a low salt medium revealed the presence of the binder which sediments at both 8S and 4S regions. That this PgR is regulated by progesterone was evident from nuclear translocation of the receptor upon 10^{-6} M of progesterone administration. On the other hand, estrogen receptor could not be detected in these cells and an addition of estradiol-17β to the culture medium failed to induce PgR. The administration of progestin such as medroxyprogesterone acetate caused a marked reduction of the growth in these cells. While, the rate of growth in PgR-negative cells (HEC-IA) was unaffected even in the presence of 10^{-5} M of progestins. These results demonstrate for the first time the presence of the functional PgR in human endometrial adenocarcinoma, *in vitro*, and this cell line appears to be an ideal model for studying the mechanism of the anti-proliferative effect of progestin therapy.

08.09.08

Clinical correlates of nuclear progesterone receptor (PR) concentrations in endometrial adenocarcinoma: Rakar, S, Rainer, S, Lenasi, H, Hudnik-Plevnik, T. Dept. Gyn. and Obstet., Inst. Biochem., Med. Fac., Ljubljana, Yugoslavia

PR concentrations in 48 cases of endometrial adenocarcinoma varied from 0.03 to 5.55 pmol/mg DNA (mean value 1.24; 95% confidence interval 0.88–1.75). PR concentrations in malignant endometrium were significantly ($p < 0.001$) lower than in the normal endometrium of the same patients (16 cases). PR concentrations in endometrial adenocarcinoma did not correlate with the age of patients, menopausal status, parity, carbohydrate metabolism of the patients, clinical stage or lymph node involvement. PR concentrations were significantly ($p < 0.05$) higher in cases of superficial comparing with deeply invasive lesions. PR were present in higher concentrations in well and moderately differentiated tumors than in poorly differentiated, but the difference is not significant because of large variations of individual values and is influenced by the heterogeneity of the tumor samples. There is a significant ($p < 0.05$) negative correlation ($r = 0.43$) between progesterone concentrations in ovarian blood and PR values in well differentiated tumors. This finding can suggest the existence of partly normal regulatory mechanism in well differentiated tumors, and can offer the basis for rational hormonal therapy of endometrial adenocarcinoma.

08.09.09

Identification of T cell subsets and B cell infiltrating in endometrial cancer tissues: Mizuuchi, H, Kudo, R, Hashimoto, M. Dept. Obst. and Gyn., Sapporo Med. Coll., Sapporo, Japan

To identify the distribution of T cell subsets and B cell in 40 endometrial cancer tissues, this study was performed by the immunoperoxidase technique (Avidin Biotin Peroxidase Complex Method). Monoclonal antibodies including anti-Leu1, Leu2a, Leu3a and L26 antibodies were used to detect Pan T cell, cytotoxic/suppressor T cell, helper/inducer T cell and B cell, respectively. The large number of infiltrating lymphocytes in the cancer tissues were T cells which were positive for Leu1. But these were rare in the benign lesion adjacent to the cancer lesion even in the same uterus. B cell infiltration was scarce both in the cancer lesion and in the benign lesion. In stage I, the number of T cells varied according to the case, but in stage III and IV T cells tended to be few in number. T cell infiltration tended to meager in the case where it occupied more than three fourths of an area of the uterine cavity. Leu3 positive cells were dominant in 17 of 19 cases in well differentiated adenocarcinoma and 12 of 15 cases in superficial myometrial invasion. But Leu3 positive cells were dominant in only two of seven cases in poorly differentiated adenocarcinoma and three of eight cases in deep myometrial invasion. The cases with negative lymph node metastasis tended to have a dense infiltration of T cells. The results suggest the possibility that the infiltrating T cells represent a cell-mediated immunity as the local response against cancer.

08.09.10
Hysterosonography in diagnosis and treatment of carcinoma of the endometrium: Clinical applications: Becker, H, Hoetzinger, H. Dept. Gyn. and Radiol., Städt. KH, Passau
Till now the visualization of the structure of the myometrium uteri, the endometrium and its pathologic alterations remained an unresolved problem. Hysterosonography, however, permits the visualization of the normal myometrium, of myomas and carcinomas. In hysterosonography the scanner on the tip of a steel tube is inserted into the uterine cavity and sectional images are made. In a pre-clinical study about 300 uteri were scanned and operated on. In 41 cases of a carcinoma of the endometrium the depth and location of infiltration was correctly defined in 96%. Hysterosonography therefore allows one for the first time to define exactly the target volume for intracavitary radiotherapy, if the patient could not be operated on. Till now we have treated 40 patients after having done hysterosonography before intracavitary therapy – now with an exact information about the real extension of the carcinoma within the myometrium. A computer program which superimposes the necessary isodose curves on the sonographic pictures is demonstrated.

08.09.11
Ovarian steroid production in patients with endometrial cancer: Pelusi, G, Busacchi, P, Moretti, B, Gentile, G, Accolti, A. I Dept. Obstet. and Gyn., Univ., Bologna, Italy
We found an increase of some steroid concentration, especially estrone and testosterone, in the blood flowing from the ovary in some patients with endometrial cancer. Previous studies demonstrated that occasionally areas of luteinizing stromal-holding fatty cells are present in the ovary of patients with endometrial adenocarcinoma. Therefore we examined by traditional histological methods the ovaries of our patients, in order to evaluate possible histological features consistent with a steroidogenetic activity. No aspects of hyperthecosis or ovarian thecomatosis have been found in any cases but one.

08.10.01
Stage I squamous cell carcinoma of the vulva. A malignancy grading system for indication of prognosis: Simonsen, E, Johnsson, J-E, Tropé, C. Dept. Oncol., Gyn. Sect., Univ. Hosp., Lund, Sweden
77 patients with invasive squamous cell carcinoma of the vulva, stage I were followed 4–20 years after surgical treatment. In 87% of the patients external irradiation was given to the inguinal regions in connection with the vulvar surgery. Five-year crude survival rate for the whole series was 81%. Metastases in the surgical lymph node specimens were found in 20% of the patients in whom lymphadenectomy was performed. The future prognoses were estimated from properties of the tumor cell population: structure, differentiation into cell type, nuclear polymorphism, mitoses and the tumor host relationship: mode of invasion, stage of invasion, vascular invasion, cellular response were graded according to a point score system. Each parameter was given 1–3 points resulting in a total of 8–24 points in increasing grade of malignancy. There were more recurrences in patients with high scorings, no patients with a point score value less than 14 points died of the disease before five years and no patients with a point score value less than 12 points had lymph node metastases with primary treatment or later disclosed recurrences. The mode of invasion was the most important factor.

08.10.02
Cancer of the vulva: A 15-year review: Liapis, A, Konidaris, S, Papadias, K, Zourlas, P A. 2nd Dept. Obstet. and Gyn., Univ. of Athens, Areteion Hosp., Athens, Greece
Thirty-four patients with cancer of the vulva were studied retrospectively for a period of 15 years from 1970 to 1984. All the patients were managed in the 2nd Department of Obstetrics and Gynecology of the University of Athens. The main symptom was localized pruritus in 41% of the patients. The stage of the disease was as follow: Stage I, 9 patients, stage II 9, stage III 11, and stage IV 5 patients. The treatment which was given was radical vulvectomy in 10 patients, simple vulvectomy in 12 patients. Radiotherapy was given in 12 patients. The five years survival rate was for stage I 88.8%, for stage II 77.9%, for stage III 56% and for stage IV zero.

08.10.03

An analysis of vulval operations in Govt. Rajaji Hospital, Madurai during the eight-year period 1977–1984: Subbulakshmi, S, Manuel, M. Dept. Obstet. and Gyn., Govt. Rajaji Hosp., Madurai, India

During this eight-year period 47 vulval operations were done. Fourteen cases of radical vulvectomy, 12 simple vulvectomy (nine for leukoplakia vulvae, one for cancer *in situ* and two for Esthiomion) and 21 cases of excision of lipoma vulvae were done. Incidence of cancer of the vulva in this institution is found to be 0.8%. Among the gynecologic malignancies it constitutes 1.4% and it stands fourth. Among the 14 cases who underwent radical vulvectomy 13 were squamous cell carcinoma, one was melanoma. Three patients underwent extraperitoneal lymphadenectomy also. Two cases had skin grafting, one primary and the other delayed. The rest healed by granulation tissue. Mortality and morbidity rate were nil. General condition on discharge was good for all. All leukoplakia cases had primary biopsy and then simple vulvectomy.

08.10.04

Carcinoma of the vulva: Collaborative study in Spain. 1970–1982: González-Merlo, J, Puig Tintoré, L M et al. Dept. Obstet. and Gin., Hosp. Clín. and Provinc., School Med., Univ., Barcelona, Spain

We report a retrospective study of 1337 cases of carcinoma of the vulva with the information furnished by the collaboration of most of Spain's main hospitals. The main epidemiological and diagnosis data are analysed together with the follow-up of the results of treatment. The distribution of carcinoma of vulva by stage was: 0 3.2%; II 33.2%; III 25% and IV 9.1%. The total 5-year survival rate was 40.9%, excluding lost of sight cases and 21.1% counting as dead of carcinoma of vulva the number of cases lost to follow-up.

08.10.05

The "midline incision" in the operative treatment of vulvar invasive cancers: Barents, J W, Lindert, A C M van. Dept. Gyn., Univ. Womens Hosp., Utrecht, The Netherlands

The radical vulvectomy and lymph node dissection using the skin incisions according to *Parry Jones, Way* a.s.o. revealed an important number of local post op. complications and an extended hospital stay. In 40 to 80 per cent of the reported series the patients have a serious necrosis, secondary infection or even a complete breakdown by cellulitis of the skin flaps after the one block dissection of the inguinal and vulvar regions. So we replaced this kind of incision by the midline procedure. We are now able to report an improvement of our post op. complication rate and as a matter of fact a decreased hospital stay for these aged women in mostly poor condition, without making concessions to the radicality in the dissection of the groin. Since 1980 we have used the midline incision in 50 patients. The wide entrance in the dissection area enables us to safe the saphenous vein in the fossa ovalis, cleaning up the femoral vessels from superficial and deep nodes up to the inguinal ligament. Extended suction drainage and pre- and post-operative use of antibiotics and careful control of hyperglycemia and hypoproteinemia will improve the wound healing without necrosis of the skin flaps covering the groins.

08.10.06

Treatment of vulvar cancer: Volk, M, Schmidt-Matthiesen, H. Zentrum Frauenheilk. u. Geburtsh., Univ., Frankfurt

We report on 157 women with invasive vulvar cancer, who were treated in our clinic between 1960 and 1979. No follow-up was possible in seven cases. Of the remaining 150 patients the mean age was 67 years. 14 (9.3%) were younger than 50 years. In 140 cases we found a squamous cell cancer. According to clinical investigation at admission 79 women (52.6%) were in stage I and II, 71 (47.4%) in stage III and IV. On 63 women a radical vulvectomy with bilateral inguino-femoral lymphonodectomy was performed. 39 (62%) survived 5 years, 29 (46%) without signs of recurrence, 8 (13%) with recurrence. From two women we got information that they survived, but none about the question of recurrence. 24 (38%) died within 5 years, 11 (17%) showed recurrence, eight died from other diseases, one from embolism after surgery and from four women no information about the cause of death could be obtained. Non-radical surgery in combination with radiotherapy was performed on 81 women (54%). 18 (22%) survived 5 years, nine without recurrence (11%), seven showed recurrence and from two patients no information could be obtained. 63 (78%) died within five years. 42 (52%) from or with recurrence, 8 (9.8%) from other diseases and four during treatment. From nine women we got no information about the cause of death. Palliative surgery only was performed on six patients. None survived five years and all died from recurrence.

08.10.07

Vulvar reconstruction: Kaplan, A L. Dept. Obstet. and Gyn., Baylor Coll. Med., Houston, TX, USA

Resurfacing the extensive defects following radical vulvectomy has been one of the major challenges to the gynecologic oncologist. The conventional methods of coverage and reconstruction, which included split thickness skin grafting and local and/or distant skin flaps have not been satisfactory to resolve these deep defects. The gracilis musculocutaneous flap has been used since 1977 at the Baylor College of Medicine affiliated hospitals to cover these large defects and experience with 19 cases will be reported. The results have been excellent from the standpoint of decreasing the immediate wound problems and enhancing long-term rehabilitation. The data conclusively shows that this procedure has a definite role in reconstructive surgery for the gynecologic oncologist.

08.10.08

Invasive squamous cell carcinoma of the vulva: An analysis of 114 cases from the University Women's Hospital Zurich/Switzerland (1960–1982): Schreiner, B P, Kunz, J, Genton, C Y*, Schreiner, W E. Dept. Frauenheilk., Univ. Women's Hosp. and *Inst. Path., Zurich, Switzerland

From 1960 through 1982, 114 cases of invasive squamous cell carcinoma of the vulva were treated at the University Women's Hospital in Zurich, representing 5.6% of all genital malignancies seen at this institution during that period of time. Initially 28 tumors were stage I, 25 stage II, 53 stage III and 10 stage IV. The median age at diagnosis was 70 years (29–91 years). The inguinal lymph nodes were metastatic in 61% of patients, 4% of which had bilateral metastases. Metastatic pelvic lymph nodes were found in 18% of cases. Pruritus vulvae had been present prior to diagnosis in 73% of patients, in some instances for several years. The treatment was surgical in 88.6% of cases, with or without postoperative radiotherapy. The remaining patients received radiotherapy only. A radical vulvectomy with inguinal and occasionally pelvic lymphadenectomy was performed in 37% of patients. The adjusted five-year survival rate (102 patients until 1977) was 92.3%, 78.3% and 45.5% for stages I, II and III, respectively. The best results for tumors stage I–III were obtained by radical vulvectomy, the five-year survival rate being 77% for all stages. The additional pelvic lymphadenectomy failed to improve the therapeutic results. Patients treated with radiotherapy only showed a five-year survival rate of 8.3%. The frequency of local recurrences was obviously dependent on the tumor stage at diagnosis. The death rate was highest during the first three years after treatment.

08.10.09

Radiotherapy of carcinoma of the vulva – treatment results of electron therapy in 446 patients 1956 to 1978: Schreer, I, Frischbier, H-J, Thomsen, K. Univ.-Frauenklin., Hamburg-Eppendorf

446 patients with malignant tumor of the vulva were treated from 1956 to 1978. In 432 patients with invasive squamous cell carcinoma, a five-year survival rate of 43.1% was obtained after exclusive exposure to electron radiation. Severe complications were seen in 10.9% of the treated patients. Due to local recurrence 41 patients were treated with secondary vulvectomy after radiation therapy. 36.6% of these patients survived more than three years, 19.5% more than five years. On comparing the results with those obtained after electrocoagulation or vulvectomy, it was seen that a therapy based on electron radiation only yielded more favorable results, especially in cases with advanced stage carcinomas. In younger women with early tumor stages, surgery should be given preference.

08.11.01

Pelvic promontory fixation of the vaginal stump in cases of prolapse: Grünberger, W, Grünberger V. 1st Dept. Obstet. and Gyn., Univ., Vienna, Austria

The choice of operative technique in cases of prolapse of the vagina after hysterectomy is difficult in women still having intercourse. *Amreich's* original procedure of sacrospinal fixation of the vagina, recently recommended by *Richter*, is difficult and dangerous (Geburtsh. u. Frauenheilk. **28**, 321, 1968). We have modified a simple procedure of pelvic promontory fixation, first described by *G.A. Wagner* (Die gynäkolog. Operationen, G. Thieme, Stuttgart 1954). From 1972–1985 we operated on 18 patients (49 to 72 years old) with partial or total prolapse of the vaginal stump. In 11 cases the preceding hysterectomy was done by an abdominal operation, in seven cases by the vaginal route. The promontory fixation, made by a small laparotomy was always finished in less then 45 minutes. In 12 cases the vaginal stump was long enough, in six women the fixation sutures had to be covered by a peritoneal cuff. Of the 18 patients 14 were controlled 0.5–12 years after operation. In all cases there were found excellent results. In three patients 1–6 years after the promontory fixation a colporrhaphy had to be done but a new prolapse of the vaginal stump was never found. Sexual intercourse was possible in all cases.

08.11.02

Management of genital prolapse in nulliparous and low parity women – an abdominal approach: Das, B N, Sen Gupta, P C, Chatterjee, S K, Das Gupta, P, Chowdhury, B. Dept. Obstet. & Gyn., Ramakrishna Mission Seva Pratishthan, Calcutta, India

Forty nulliparous or low parity women with uterine prolapse were selected for cervicopexy by Purandare's technique at Ramakrishna Mission Seva Pratishthan, Calcutta, between 1975 and 1983. The average age was 22.46; 30 were married and 20 were nulliparous. Cervicopexy was carried out by Purandare's technique using an aponeurotic suspension. In addition to cervicopexy, two each had cervical amputation, colpoperineorrhaphy, tuboplasty and myomectomy, eight had plication of round ligament and one repair of rectal prolapse. Seven women became pregnant after cervicopexy; six had normal delivery at term and one miscarriage. No recurrence was noted in 39 women who attended follow-up clinic between one and eight years.

08.11.03

Perineal approach in the management of rectal prolapse – report of five cases: Sen Gupta, P C, Das, B N, Chatterjee, S K, Das Gupta, P. Dept. Obstet. & Gyn., Ramakrishna Mission Seva Pratishthan, Vivekananda Inst. Med. Sci., Calcutta, India

Five cases of large rectal prolapse, treated by a new perineal approach, are presented. Two each were para four and para one and one was nulliparous. One parous women with second degree uterine descent had vaginal hysterectomy and repair of rectal prolapse at the same sitting. The three with minimal uterine descent had only repair of rectal prolapse. The nulliparous patient was treated with cervicopexy by Purandare's technique for second degree uterine descent. The rectal prolapse was repaired by the perineal route at the same sitting. The postoperative period remained uneventful in all five. A follow-up between two and half and five years has revealed no recurrence. The details of the operation are described.

08.11.04
Abdominal sling operation for the treatment of vault prolapse: El Lamie, K, El Maraghy, M. Dept. Obstet. and Gyn., Ain Shams Med. School, Cairo, Egypt
A new operation for the treatment of vault prolapse is presented. The technique is described. The results and follow-up of fourteen cases up to eight years are discussed. Comparison with other methods showed the simplicity and superiority of that operation. The keystone of the technique is suspension of vaginal apex high up in the pelvis away from the genital hiatus. This is achieved through creation of a surgical sling anchoring the vaginal vault to the anterior long-itudinal ligament of the sacrum.

08.11.05
Place of morcellement in vaginal hysterectomy in modern operative gynecology: Drača, P, Miljković, S. Dept. Obstet. and Gyn., Novi Sad, Yugoslavia
There were 136 V.H. operations performed in our Department in the period 1968–1974. In 162 patients (11.87%), V.H. with morcellement was performed. These patients were 40–49 years old (60.49%). V.H. with morcellement was used in only two patients of the senile age. The pathologic conditions requiring this type of surgery are extremely rare in older women. The size of the uterus is the basic indication for morcellement, but some other factors are of importance, like mobility, muscle relaxation of the pelvic fundus, adhesions, fibroma localization, depth and width of the vagina. The largest uterus in which the morcellement was used was 700 g in weight. In all our patients the enlarged uterus was the reason for morcellement. In our opinion the uterus can be extirpated to that of 12 weeks gestational size. Morcellement does not require more frequent administration of blood transfusion during the operation (12.35%); it was 16.84% while compared with V.H. without morcellement. Postoperative morbidity rate in V.H. followed by morcellement was 24.69%; while compared with the total, it was 30.02%. The most frequent complications were dehiscences of the operative wound and infections. It is obvious that morcellement in V.H. does not cause more frequent postoperative morbidity. The more frequent use of V.H. with morcellement has been justified.

08.11.06
A case report: A technique of vaginal hysterectomy for a leiomyoma of fetal head size occupying the whole of the vagina: Kirloskar, S M. Solapur Clin., Solapur, India
Spinal anesthesia was used. The anterior lip of the cervix was exposed by depressing the tumor backwards. By applying retraction the anterior pouch could be opened without injury to the bladder. *Mackenrodt's* ligaments were ligated and cut on either side by an approach through anterolateral pouch. With the descent of uterus, exposure of the posterior lip was facilitated and opening of the posterior pouch. The rest of the steps were same for any other vaginal hysterectomy. The results were rewarding and the patient had an uneventful postoperative recovery. A fetal head size leiomyoma impacted in the vagina can be tackled vaginally without morcellation offering the patient all the benefits of vaginal hysterectomy as against abdominal.

08.11.07
New techniques for gynecological abdominal and vaginal procedures: Dbaly, J, Cimber, H, Leserf, G, Ryser, W. Klin. Beau-Site, Bern, Switzerland
It is possible to shorten the operating time and lower the traumatisation of tissue with the automatic retractor holder "Iron Intern – OCTOPUS". This plays an important role especially in older, obese and high-risk patients. The survey of the entire operating field is guaranteed with its use during the entire time. The change of position of the retractors held by the assistant does not take place with the OCTOPUS, nor the changing pressure and traumatisation of tissue. It is possible to attach a fiberoptic light to the OCTOPUS retractors which enables a steady light in the depth of the operation field. The usually two necessary assistants in vaginal operations can play an active operational role when they do not have to hold retractors. In over 1000 abdominal and vaginal procedures it was proven with the above mentioned advantages of the octopus that the postoperative hospital stay was shortened, less pain medication was necessary and the infection rate was lower. The technical adjustment and assembly of OCTOPUS can be easily learned by the surgeon and his operating team.

08.11.08
Surgical treatment of the prolapsed uterus: Roan, C, Hsu, C. Dept. Obstet. & Gyn., Taipei Municip. Women & Child. Hosp., Taipei, Taiwan
The prolapsed uterus has always been associated with some degree of cystocele and/or rectocele and enterocele. The best treatment of uterine prolapse and its allied condition is still controversial. The most

important factors of the principal of surgical treatment of uterine prolapse in evaluating treatment for an individual are the age and the general physical condition of the patient, the desirability of preserving menstration; the desirability of maintaining childbearing function. In our country, the prolapsed uteri occurred in the multiparous women and old age patient particular in the rural area. In consideration of these factor we proposed a favorite combined procedure which included vaginal hysterectomy, anterior colporrhaphy and plastic of fascicle vaginalis and posterior colporrhaphy. This procedure will be shown in the video betamax system.

08.11.09
Nadkarni's "All in one" operation for prolapse: Shah, K M. Municip. Med. Coll., Univ. Ahmedabad, Gujarat, India
Analysis of 150 cases with reference to its impact on the reproductive function is given. Its aim is to restore the organs to their normal anatomical position. This helps the stretched structures to involute without affecting the reproductive function. Main steps are: plication of the round ligaments including its elongation on Ant. lat. surface of uterus and utero-sacral lig. if necessary; repair of cystocele, pelvic floor and perineum by a different technique (Dr. *Nadkarni's*). All done by vaginal route, portio vaginalis is kept intact. – Results: 100% pregnancy rate with 4% abortion and 2% recurrance rate, 85% of cases had a 2nd or 3rd degree prolapse. Results are compared with various operative techniques.

08.12.01
Fetal outcome in 838 hypertensive pregnancies: Montan, S, Sjöberg, N-O, Solum, T. Dept. Obstet. and Gyn., Univ. Hosp., Lund, Sweden
During six years a strict management program for treatment of hypertension in pregnancy including the β-blocker atenolol as the first drug of choice has been used. Incidence of various forms of hypertension and fetal outcome have been evaluated. Eight hundred and thirty-eight out of 18,006 deliveries (4.7%) were admitted because of hypertension in pregnancy. Moderate and severe pre-eclampsia was seen in 361 and 21 women, respectively. Only one case of eclampsia was observed. Gestational hypertension and pre-existing hypertension were seen in 392 and 64 women, respectively. Antihypertensive treatment with atenolol was indicated in 419 women. In 145 complimentary anti-hypertensive treatment (hydralazine) was given. Labor was induced in 37.9%. Preterm delivery was seen in 13.0%. Cesarean section was performed in 18.4%. The most common indication was ominous antenatal CTG pattern. The total number of SGA infants was 82 (9.6%). A majority of these were term infants. One hundred and eighty-six newborns were referred to the neonatal intensive care unit. The incidence of respiratory disorders was 8.4%. The total peri- and late neonatal mortality in hypertensive women (1.06%) did not differ from the general obstetric population (0.93%). – Conclusion: The results contradict a negative influence of antihypertensive treatment with atenolol during pregnancy.

08.12.02
A stepwise system of hypertension management in pregnancy: Walker, J J, Bjornsson, S, Bonduelle, M, Cameron, A D, Calder, A A. Univ. Dept. Obstet. and Gyn., Glasgow Roy. Maternity Hosp., Glasgow, Scotland
Traditional treatment of pregnancy hypertension consists of admission to hospital of any patient thought to be at risk. This generally means anyone with a blood pressure over 90 mm Hg. Between 10–15% of patients fall into this category. In Glasgow Royal Maternity Hospital we have designed an outpatient assessment area run by a full time midwifery sister. All patients at risk are referred to this unit and are assessed for six hours. Blood pressures are taken every two hours and bloods are taken for urate and platelet count. A cardiotocograph is carried out to assess immediate fetal well-being. Results are assessed at the end of the day and the need for admission decided. We have shown that only 10% of these "at risk" patients require admission and another 20% require further out-patient follow-up. Of the 10% of patients who are admitted about half of them are at an early gestation and benefit from antihypertensive therapy, usually labetalol. By doing this we have reduced our prematurity rate and our perinatal mortality rate. There has been no increase in growth retardation or hypertensive crisis following the introduction of day assessment. This form of management has improved our standard of care for this significantly high risk group and means that we admit only 3% of our pregnancy population because of hypertension and use anti-hypertensives in about 1.5%.

08.12.03
Influence of calcium on blood pressure during pregnancy: Comino-Delgado, R. Depto. Obstet. and Gyn., Fac. Med., Univ., Valladolid, Spain
A daily supplement of two g of Calcium was administered to 36 normal pregnant women for two weeks, assessing blood pressure before and after treatment and we compared the results with those obtained from a control group of 45 comparable pregnant women who were submitted to the same procedure, except for the calcium supplement. The group under calcium treatment showed lower blood pressure values at the end of the two weeks, even though calcemia was not significantly different in both groups. This result suggests that calcium supplementation during pregnancy has a lowering influence on blood pressure levels.

08.12.04

Management of severe pregnancy-induced hypertension with long-term intravenous magnesium sulfate: Mac-Kenna, J, Lentz, S, Dombroski, R, Brame, R, Jones, D. Dept. Obstet. and Gyn., East Carolina Univ. School Med., Greenville, NC, USA

To permit fetal lung maturation delivery can be delayed even in women with severe pregnancy-induced hypertension with appropriate patient selection under carefully controlled conditions. The key to this approach to management appears to be constant supervision of high levels of magnesium sulfate in an intensive care setting. Assuming fetal lung immaturity, absence of clinical evidence of intrauterine growth retardation, and evidence of a stable or improving maternal condition, intravenous magnesium sulfate was continued until fetal lung maturation was identified by lung phospholipid profile. Patients in this study were treated for three to 31 days antepartum and one to ten days postpartum. Sixty patients were treated in this manner. Forty-three of these patients achieved a mature fetal lung profile and were delivered. Deteriorating maternal and fetal conditions resulted in 15 deliveries. The remaining two patients were delivered due to spontaneous labor and one IUFD. A total of 62 infants were delivered with only one NND. Maternal follow-up at three months revealed that all cardiovascular and renal aspects had returned to pre-pregnancy levels.

08.12.05

Management by gestosis: Riedel, H, Grützner, E, Klatt, D. Dept. Gyn. and Obstet. Kreiskrankenh. Großburgwedel, Burgwedel

In 1982 and 1983 57 patients with gestosis delivered in our department, that is 5.9% of the births in our hospital within that time. The patients were controlled by various clinical parameters, the uric acid concentration in serum and the placental hormones HPL and estriol. In cases of blood pressure of 160/100 mm Hg or more, of proteinuria, increase of uric acid concentration in serum or decrease of the placental hormones, growth retardation of the fetus, signs of pre-eclampsia or eclampsia the patients were admitted to hospital. Delivery was managed preterm in 25 cases (43.9%). The most important criterion for preterm delivery was an pathological CTG. Delivery was managed by Cesarean section in 73.7% of the cases, by forceps in 3.5% of the cases and spontaneously in 22.8% of the cases. In most of the cases the Cesarean section was done in the presence of the pediatric team. 21 neonates were transferred to a nearby Childrens Hospital in Hannover (i.e. 36.2%) because they have been small-for-date babies or premature births. All 58 children survived and are well as far as is known. Neither did we lose any of the mothers.

08.12.06

Ambulant prostacyclin therapy for pregnancy-induced hypertension and intrauterine growth retardation: Lang, G D R, Walker, J J, Greer, I A, Belch, J J F, Calder, A A. Univ., Dept. Obstet. and Gyn., Glasgow Royal Maternity Hosp., Glasgow, Scotland

Prostacyclin has been shown to be deficient in pregnancy induced hypertension (PIH) and intrauterine growth retardation (IUGR). Intravenous prostacyclin (PGI$_2$) has been used but studies have been hindered by the need for an intravenous line and the potential side-effects of treatment. We describe a system developed to allow long-term infusion of a mobile patient to study the potential benefits of PGI$_2$ infusion. One patient with severe PIH at 28 weeks was started on PGI$_2$ infusion at 1 ng/kg/min. This was increased to achieve blood pressure control over several days but when the dose reached 7.5 ng/kg/min; side-effects of nausea, diarrhoea and dizziness occurred. The dose was held at that level and labetalol added to help blood pressure control. Patient 2 had severe IUGR at 28 weeks and was started on a dose of 1 ng/kg/min, increasing to 3 ng/kg/min. No side-effects were noted. Growth of the fetus appeared to increase and liquor pool increased. Both patients were initially infused through peripheral lines using a "Pye" battery syringe pump. Both patients were delivered at 30 weeks gestation. The baby from the hypertensive patient was 1.2 kg but unfortunately died of respiratory infection at the age of 9 days. The baby of patient 2 weighed 740 g but has progressed well and is now 9 months old with no apparent defects. Although this system is not of proven benefit, it allows a feasible study of PGI$_2$ infusion to be carried out in these high risk patients where there is little else to offer.

08.13.01

Progestogens action on the breast: Sitruk-Ware, R, Kutenn, F, Mauvais-Jarvis, P. Hôp. Necker, Paris, France

The human breast is a target organ for estradiol (E2) and progesterone (P). From studies performed in animals, it seems likely that E2 and P have synergistic and antagonistic actions on the mammary gland. In the endometrium the antagonistic effect of P on E2 is related to at least three mechanisms: a) it simulates 17β-dehydrogenase (E2βDH) activity, which allows the conversion of E2 to E1, a less active metabolite; b) it inhibits the replenishment of the estradiol cytosolic receptor; c) it inhibits epithelial cell growth and multiplication. Progestins have been shown to act at the breast level just as in the endometrium. In human breast fibroadenomas lynestrenol (LYN), a potent norsteroid derivative, was able to induce the transloca-tion of the progesterone receptor (PR) from the cytosol into the nucleus. This progestin was also able to induce the increase of E2βDH considered to be the marker of PR action. Percutaneous P applied topically on the breast was also demonstrated to stimulate this enzyme activity. Also, it has been reported that R5020 a potent progestogen derived from P decreased DNA synthesis and cell multiplication in human carcinoma

194

breast cells in culture. More recently, the same fact has been demonstrated on normal human epithelial mammary cells in culture. Indeed, the addition of R5020 to E2 clearly slows down cell proliferation as measured by either DNA assay or ^{3}H-thymidine incorporation into DNA. However, in patients treated for benign breast diseases, it has been shown on breast biopsies that LYN does not increase the mitotic activity of mammary cells from a morphological viewpoint. Therefore, progestins able to antagonize the estrogenic effect could have a protective effect against the promoting action of estrogens on susceptible cells. The hypothesis has to be demonstrated in large epidemiologic studies.

08.13.02
Mechanism of action of progestogens: King, R J B. Horm. Biochem. Dept., Imp. Ca Res. Fund, London, UK
The historical development of progestogens from their initial characterization in the 1930s to the synthetic analogues currently available will be described. The modes of action of these compounds will be discussed in relation to their effects on breast and endometrium and by comparing the responses produced by different progestogens. – Endometrium: Different effects occur in epithelium and stroma. Certain enzymes (estradiol dehydrogenase and isocitric dehydrogenase are induced by progestogens in epithelium but not stroma and this parallels histological changes. DNA synthesis and changes in estradiol and progesterone receptor are similar in epithelium and stroma. – Breast: Data are sparse but evidence exists to suggest that human breast epithelium responds to progestogens differently from endometrial epithelium.

08.13.03
Contraception with subcutaneous implants containing 3-ketodesogestrel: Odlind, V, Olsson, S E, Johansson, E D B. Dept. Obstet. and Gyn., Univ., Uppsala, Sweden
Subcutaneous implants for contraception have proven to be highly acceptable due to few side-effects, high efficacy and long duration of efficacy. A single silastic capsule containing a new potent progestogen, 3-ketodesogestrel, which is the biologically active metabolite of desogestrel, was inserted subcutaneously in seven healthy, fertile women and left in place for up to 300 days. The calculated release of 3-ketodesogestrel was around 40 μg per day. Plasma samples were taken frequently and analysed for estradiol, progesterone and 3-ketodesogestrel. Bleeding records were kept by the volunteers. All women had ovulatory pretreatment cycles. During treatment no ovulations were found as judged by constantly baseline progesterone values. Estradiol fluctuations were seen in all volunteers. Two women left the study due to frequent bleeding episodes. The bleeding patterns were characterized by irregular, scanty bleedings in all the volunteers. No other side-effects were reported. The plasma concentrations of 3-ketodesogestrel were slightly higher just after insertion, then they remained on an even level of 0.4–0.8 nmol/l during the study period. This study suggests that it would be possible to develop an implant method with a duration of 1–2 years with 3-ketodesogestrel, with few side-effects other than the bleeding disturbances always seen with continuous low dose progestogen treatment.

08.13.04
Oral contraception for women over 35: Gillmer, M. John Radcliffe Hosp., Oxford, UK
Epidemiological observations of combined oral contraceptive steroids in women over the age of 35 have suggested a significant increase in the risk of death from arterial vascular disease. These data, which have led most doctors to advise against the use of these preparations in women over 35 years of age, were, however, obtained during the 1970s in women who were taking pills with a high progestogen content. In addition, although the risk of death from arterial causes is age related, the risk appears to be concentrated in smokers, and relative risk in non-smokers does not equal that of 35- to 44-year-old smokers at all after 45 years of age. The association between low plasma HDL and high plasma LDL cholestrol concentrations and arterial disease incidence has stimulated much research on the impact of sex steroids on lipo-protein metabolism, in an attempt to assess which formulations are less likely to have an adverse effect. These studies suggest that while the preparations with a high progestogen content, widely used during the 1970s, did have a potentially adverse effect on lipid metabolism, this is not true for currently used pills of low estrogen and progestogen content. These data suggest that the current restrictive advise on the use of combined oral contraceptive pills by women over the age of 35 years, who do not smoke, should be revised.

08.28.01
Prognostic factors among infertility patients with tubal problems: Almeda, L A, Quillamor, R M. Dept. Obstet. and Gyn., Univ. of the East Ramon Magsaysay Memo. Med. Ctr, Quezon City, Philippines
The presence of endometriosis and pelvic peritoneal adhesions are the major tubal problems in infertility. Laparoscopy done in 91 patients out of 684 infertility patients showed endometriosis present in 63% (57/91) and adhesions in 24% (22/91). Pregnancy occurred in 42% (15/36) of patients with mild endometriosis treated with antigonadotrophin alone. Among patients with Stage I adhesive disease pregnancy occurred in 57% (4/7) while none got pregnant in Stage II (0/9). Fifty per cent (4/8) and 4.2% (1/14) of patients with Stage A and Stage B adhesive disease respectively got pregnant after tuboplasty. Among infertility patients with tubal problems the success of having a pregnancy is affected by the staging of adhesions. With the aid of the laparoscope proper staging of adhesions and endometriosis can be made.

The ability to visualize the ovaries, the presence of minimal thin filmy adhesions, the presence of minimal endometriosis and spillage of dye all give optimistic prognosis in tubal disease.

08.28.02

Spray pneumo hysterosalpingography in 500 cases of sterility: Shah, R K, Patel, Y. K. M. School of P. G. Med. & Res., Ahmedabad, Gujarat, India

Spray pneumo hysterosalpingography (S.P.H.S.G.) is a double contrast hysterolsalpingography originally devised by Prof. *Nadkarni* in 1968. The double contrast is created by method of use of contrast medium and gas. The effect of spray pneumography is brought about by gas pressure adsorption and dispersion phenomena. It is a non-invasive method. Study of S.P.H.S.G. was done as a routine in 500 cases of sterility where male factor was found normal. The observations were as follows: Normal uterus and tubes were found in 32% cases. Genital Kochs was found in 17.2% cases. Cornual blockage was seen in 5% cases. Unfolding the fallacies of tubal involvement in H.S.G. by 80% in blocked tubes and by 50% in hydrosalpinx. S.P.H.S.G. is therefore a useful adjuvant to the investigative equipment in cases of sterility.

08.28.03

Hysteroscopy in the treatment of infertile women: Pisarski, T, Sajdak, S. Inst. Gyn. and Obstet. Karol Marcinkowski, Acad. Med., Poznań, Poland

This study aimed at diagnostic tests and hysteroscopic treatment of women with pregnancy failures. The material consisted of 71 patients treated at the Reproduction Clinic, in the years 1983–1984. All the patients had undergone hysterosalpingography and their vaginal biocenosis had been evaluated. The hysteroscopies were performed under general (85%) and local (15%) anesthesia. The cervical canal was dilated up to Hegar no. 8. A Storz hysteroscope was used. In 45 women intrauterine adhesions were diagnosed and 26 patients were found with a total or partial septum dividing the uterine cavity. The adhesions and septa were removed under visual control using oblique optics method. Each time after the operation an intrauterine device (IUD) was inserted into the uterus. In 22 hysterosalpingography control tests in 19 women the uterus was normal. In five patients adhesions recurred and had to be removed again. In 16 patients the treatment resulted in normal pregnancy; seven of these women have already given birth to healthy, full-term babies.

08.28.04

Hysteroscopy for the transcervical resection of the septum uteri: Lindemann, H-J. Deutsches Rotes Kreuz Krankenh., Hamburg

The successful results of the hysteroscopic technic for the removal of a septum uteri provide the justification for a report on the important stages of the procedure. First of all it has to be established if there is a uterus duplex or a septum uteri, in order to prevent an operation for the wrong indications. Before beginning the operation on the corpus uteri different parts of the endometrium are infiltrated with 5 units of POR 8R, a vasopressin derivative, dissolved in 20 ml saline. After about 10 minutes a complete ischemia is obtained. The advantage of this drug is that its action is obtained. The advantage of this drug is that its action is strictly local. We use the 7 mm operating hysteroscope with a straight working channel for inserting rigid scissors, forceps, hooks and high-frequency coagulation probes. As the surgeon is not disturbed by blood and mucus the operation field is clearly recognisable. The operation is concluded by a cleaning curettage with a blunt curette after which a Lippes loop is inserted for eight weeks as a prophylaxis against mechanical adhesions. After our experiences in 45 patients no hysterotomy by the abdominal route has been necessary any more. The results are optimal: no sutures in the wall of the uterus, a normal cavity size and a one-day procedure.

08.28.05

FEMTEST – a new uterotubal insufflator validated against HSG: Alvarado, D A, Kably, A A, Hernández, A R, Bolduc, L R, Gallegos, A J. Obstet. & Gyn. Hosp., C.M.N., I.M.S.S., México City, México, DF

Forty-eight volunteers entered the study. Reasons for attending the clinic were: primary infertility (16), secondary infertility (22) and others (10). All subjects were programmed for routine HSG. Tubal insufflation was performed immediately prior to HSG with the FEMTEST*. The FEMTEST plastic device has a disposable cannula; inside the device housing, an air cylinder containing a maximum of 42.5 ml of CO_2 at 225 mm Hg. Without cervical dilatation, the cannula is inserted into the uterus. With manual activation of a plunger, a small balloon (1–2 cm) inflates inside the uterus; then, the device is gently pulled back, so as to seal the internal cervical os. A valve is depressed releasing CO_2 into the uterine cavity. The entry of gas into the uterus, Fallopian tubes and abdominal cavity was easily read in the instrument. The gas insufflation was safe and no major complications were seen. In one case, a minor and transient vagal reflex was observed. Agreement between procedures (42) cases was 87.5%-BTO in 13 and T.P. in 29; other six cases FEMTEST diagnosed T.P. and HSG T.O. in five. Laparoscopic examination on three of those cases was performed. FEMTEST results were confirmed on two cases. The FEMTEST could be an out-patient clinic procedure causing little patient discomfort, less expensive, faster (2–3 min) and as reliable as the HSG procedure and routinely used by non specialized medical personnel. – *FEMTEST is BioNexus TM for a new hand-carried uterotubal gas insufflator.

08.28.06

Spray pneumo hysterosalpingography: Patel, N M, Patel, Y, Nadkarni, R M. K. M. School of P. G. Med. & Res. Ahmedabad, Gujarat, India

A spray pneumography is a double contrast hysterosalpingography, a method which was independently adopted by *R. M. Nadkarni* in the year 1968. The spray pneumography consists of a method of replacing radio-opaque dye in the uterine cavity by air or gas, thus creating a double contrast in the hollow structures i.e. uterine cavity, tubes, the peritoneal pockets. Small cysts or tumors sprayed over by the gas or air carrying a dye are visualized quite effectively. It is a non-invasive method. The advantages of the spray pneumography are as follows: 1. Endometrial pathology is better visualized as also the endocervical. 2. Tubal status is explored in more details. 3. It helps in visualizing small or big tumors. 4. It is economical and quite safe.

08.28.07

Peritoneal fluid collection in ambulant infertile patients by culdocentesis with the CUPIDO-system: Wiegerinck, M A H M, Moret, E, Laat, W N G M de. Dept. Gyn., St. Joseph Hosp., Eindhoven, The Netherlands

The demonstration of spermatozoa in periovulatory peritoneal fluid provides a diagnostic test of *in vivo* migration of sperm cells to the site of fertilization. Collection of peritoneal fluid by Douglas puncture in infertility patients is not generally accepted because of inconsistent success, pain and the risk of intra-abdominal lesions. The conventional culdocentesis technic was analysed under laparoscopic view. To eliminate the disadvantages (stretching of peritoneum, blocking of the needletop) we developed a new Douglas puncture system (CUPIDO-system). The posterior vaginal wall and adjacent cul-de-sac peritoneum are fixed in a small vacuum cup connected to a guiding tube with finger grip. With a catheter-needle unit a controllable perpendicular puncture through the fixed tissues in a central canal of the cup is made. The needle is withdrawn from the catheter, the catheter tip is positioned in the pouch of Douglas and the peritoneal fluid aspirated in a syringe. 200 Douglas punctures in ambulant infertility patients were performed in the periovulatory period. In nine cases (4.5%) no fluid could be obtained, in 10% only drops, in 78.5% over 1.0 was gained, with a mean of 5.0 cc. 95.5% was suitable to test sperm migration and 84.5% for hormonal analysis. The method was well tolerated. The only complication was a vasovagal reaction in six patients. Culdocentesis with the CUPIDO-system may be a safe, simple and effective procedure in the infertility investigation programme.

08.28.08

Place of laparoscopy in pelvic tuberculosis in infertile women: Deshmukh, K K, Lopez, J A, Naidu, A K, Gaurkhede, M D, Kasbawala, M V. Dept. Obstet. and Gyn., Grant Med. Coll., Bombay, India

In India, where pulmonary tuberculosis is common incidence of genital tuberculosis is also high in females. Genital tuberculosis is generally asymptomatic. Signs and symptoms of tubal disease may occur many years after the initial infection. Thus, genital tuberculosis may be diagnosed for the first time, when they attend infertility clinic. Among women undergoing curettage for infertility, genital tuberculosis has been reported in 4 to 6% of cases after histopathological examination of the endometrium (*Padubidri*, 1980). Laparoscopic examinations diagnose more cases of genital tuberculosis in infertile women. Study was carried out in 500 infertile women, attending 'Infertility Clinic'. Histopathological examination of the endometrium clinched the diagnosis in only 2% of cases, while in 9% of cases genital tuberculosis was diagnosed on laparoscopy. Presence of frank tubercles, caseation, rigid tubes and 'Blue Uterus' with terminal hydrosalpinx were the diagnostic features of genital tuberculosis. Out of 45 cases of genital tuberculosis 10 cases (22.2%) showed evidence of pulmonary tuberculosis. Laparoscopy is an important procedure for the early detection of genital tuberculosis, when only the tubes are involved. Exploratory laparotomy which was a common procedure in the past for doubtful cases of pelvic tuberculosis can thus be avoided.

08.32.01

3β-androstanediol levels in the serum of hirsute women: A valuable endocrine feature in hirsutism?: Bitzer, J, Birkhäuser, M H, Huber, P R. Dept. Obstet. and Gyn., Univ. of Basle, Kantonsspit., Basel, Switzerland

In 38 hirsute women (mean age 25.7 yrs.) venous blood was drawn between 7 and 8 a.m. in the early follicular phase for RIA determination of β-androstanediol (3β-diol), α-androstanediol (3α-diol), total plasma testosterone (T), dehydroepiandrosterone (DHEA), dehydroepiandrosteronesulfate (DHEAS), androstenedione (A), sex-hormone-binding globulin (SHBG) and free testosterone (free T). 26 patients had regular menses, 12 were oligomenorrheic, 16 patients were obese. A clinical hirsutism score was assigned to each patient ranging from 4 to 22. The serum androgen most frequently elevated was 3β-diol (79%), followed by 3α-diol (62%), A (61%); T values were abnormal in 34%, free T in 55%. In 95% of all pat. the combination of 3β-diol, 3α-diol, T, A and SHBG showed at least one abnormal value. The combination of 3β-diol, 3α-diol and A showed elevated levels in 89%, whereas free T + DHEAS was abnormal in only 63%. 3β-diol correlated well with 3α-diol, A, DHEA and DHEAS. 11 out of 12 hirsute women with oligomenorrhea and 15 out of 16 hirsute women obesity showed elevated values of 3β-diol. There was no significant correlation between the severity of the clinical score and the androgen elevation. In 20 patients the effect of combined estrogen-progestin treatment on 3β-diol and 3α-diol levels was studied and a significant decrease of both androgens observed. From these date it can be concluded that 3β-diol is a sensitive endocrine indicator in the assessment of hirsutism probably independently of its origin.

08.32.02

Treatment of infertile hyperandrogenemic women: Westhof, G, Braendle, W, Sprotte, C, Zimmermann, R, Bettendorf, G. Abt. Klin. u. Exp. Endokr., Univ., Hamburg

It is well known that the pregnancy rate of infertile hyperandrogenemic patients treated with clomid (Cl.) is low (*E. Radwanska* and *C. Sloan*, Int. J. Fertil. **24**, 176, 1979). *Steinberger* showed that glucocorticoids are very potent in treating female infertility. So 32 Cl. non-responders were treated with 0.5 mg/d dexamethasone (group I) and 47 with 7.5 mg/d prednisone (group II). The pregnancy rates were 3.1% and 12.8%, respectively. When glucocorticoid therapy alone failed, Cl. was added. Out of 20 patients receiving dexamethasone and Cl. three conceived, and out of 18 patients treated with prednisone and Cl. one got pregnant. In 28 women who did not conceive on the above mentioned treatment hMG/hCG stimulation resulted in a pregnancy rate of 29%. The mean pretreatment plasma testosterone (T) level for group I was 0.76$\pm$0.43 ng/ml and 0.66$\pm$0.38 ng/ml for group II. During glucocorticoid therapy the values were 0.53$\pm$0.25 ng/ml (group I) and 0.32$\pm$0.16 ng/ml (group II). Glucocorticoid administration did not change FSH and LH levels significantly. In spontaneous and corticoid cycles T and LH levels were correlated positively and T and FSH negatively. Higher pregnancy rates during prednisone therapy were achieved in hirsute women (22%) and highest in amenorrheic patients (40%). This means that hyperandrogenemia without hirsutism in Cl. non-responders with spontaneous cycles should not be treated with glucocorticoids but hMG/hCG.

08.32.03

Gonadotropin secretion in patients with irregular menstrual cycle and hirsutism: Pjevic, M, Kovač, T, Aleksić, S. Dept. Obstet. and Gyn., Novi Sad, Yugoslavia

The authors investigated basal serum LH/FSH levels and their levels in the course of LRF test in 31 patients with ovary polycystic disease (PCC), 33 patients with idiopathic hirsutism (IH) and in ten healthy control subjects with normal menstrual cycle (CG). The PCO patients are distributed in two groups by random choice: 17 patients with enlarged ovaries (PCC-I) and 14 with normal size gonads (PCO-II). The mean concentrations of FSH are significantly lower in the patients with PCO and IH than in CG. The consecutive dosage of LH and FSH in two-day intervals, confirmed the lack of the cyclic model of gonadotropin secretion in most patients, accompanied by constantly increased LH concentrations and constantly decreased FSH concentrations while compared with CG. The cumulative increase of LH during LRF test in the patients with PCO and IH was significantly higher than in CG. Basal levels of LH and FSH and the net increase of FSH during LRF stimulation, were significantly higher in the patients with PCO than in IH group. The spectra of disturbances of the gonad axis, significantly coincide in the patients with PCO and IH, while the degree of dysfunction has been significantly higher in the group with PCO than in IH group.

08.32.04

Hysteroscopy; An aid in infertility investigation: Herendael, B-J van*, Pas, H van der**. *Jan Palfijn Gen. Hosp., OCMW, Antwerp; **St. Elisabeth Gen. Hosp., OCMW, Turnhout, Belgium

Hysteroscopy is used to detect and sometimes cure in the same session mechanical problems of implantation. Fibroids with large implantation can be recognised and removed by electro-cautery. Differential diagnosis with myomata are made. Polyps are easily recognised and removed. Differential diagnosis with hyperplastic tissue strands is made. Polyps at the tubal ostia are visualised and removed. Problems at the mechanical or hormonal level are detected. Carbon dioxide hysteroscopy is necessary. Endometriosis interna and endometritis ossificans are diagnosed very easily. The latter can be treated in the same session Malformations of the uterine cavity: The extent of the malformation is better appreciated using the hysteroscope. Flap valve mechanism: The visualisation *in vivo* of the persuffation saves some patients unnecessary microsurgery especially when a Charrière 3 ureteral catheter is inserted in the ostium tubae. Microhysteroscopy: At magnification of X 60 the endometrial vessels are observed and the endometrium can be appreciated. The use of hysteroscopy and microhysteroscopy is a must in the investigation of infertility as a compliment to laparoscopy.

08.32.05

The role of spironolactone therapy in hirsutism: Köksal, A Pabuçcu, R, Akyürek, C. Obstet. and Gyn., Dept., Gülhane Military Med. Fac., Ankara, Turkey

We know that hirsutism usually results from a subtle excess of androgens. There isn't any idea in common on the therapy of hirsutism. Patients have a dramatic improvement of hirsutism with spironolactone therapy. This action comes through because of the competitive inhibition with the dihydrotestosterone receptor. Recent experiments suggest that spironolactone blocks the biosynthesis of testosterone at the 17-hydroxylase step, a microsomal enzymatic reaction dependent upon cytochrome P-450. Ninety patients (mean age 25.1$\pm$7.5) with hirsutism who had attended the Obstetrics and Gynecology Department of Gülhane Military Medical Academy and Faculty were included in this study. 100 mg spironolactone was given orally twice a day in a cyclic manner from the fourth to the 22nd days of each menstrual cycle for six months after the pre-treatment hormonal values and clinical features had been evaluated. 24 patients with hirsutism who were not given any medication, were followed up as the control group. In both of the study groups, the clinical features and hormonal values were re-evaluated at the end of the sixth month. At the end of the treatment we saw that there was no further progression of coarsening and darkening hair, a slow rate of growth of existing hair and a decrease in diameter of the hair shaft. And there was a decrease in hair density ($p < 0.001$). We conclude that spironolactone therapy is beneficial in hirsutism in addition to the advantages of very few side-effects, being a nonhormonal medicine, and having potent anti-androgenic properties.

08.32.06

Cyproterone acetate in severe hirsutism: Results of an ongoing multicentered study by the Canadian Committee for Fertility Research: Belisle, S. Dept. Obstet. and Gyn. Univ., Sherbrooke, Que., Canada

The objective of this current study is to compare the efficacy and safety of ethinyl estradiol (50 µg) combined with a low dose (2 mg: Diane) or a high dose (100 mg: androcur) cyproterone acetate (CPA) in patients with severe hirsutism of non-tumoral origin. 160 women aged 18–35 years were recruited from seven Canadian centers. All presented with severe hirsutism (grade ≥ 18, Ferriman & Galwey Index) with or without menstrual dysfunction and required systemic therapy for their condition. They had been off any prescribed medication for at least 60 days prior to study and presented no contraindications to steroid therapy. After baseline samplings for plasma androgens, gonadotropins, prolactin, cortisol and routine chemistry, all patients received for twelve consecutive months, Diane from day 5–25 of their cycles supplemented through double-blind randomization with either androcur or a placebo from day 5–15. They were then re-evaluated clinically at 1, 3, 6, 9 and 12 months of the study while endocrine testing was repeated at one and 6–9 months of the investigation. A subgroup of patients was also studied more extensively prior to and six month after beginning of therapy for plasma lipid profile, insulin and glucose tolerance tests, and blood coagulogram including thromboelastogram and anti-thrombin III. Throughout the study period, no patient was allowed ancillary therapy for the hirsutism except shaving when appropriate. The results will be presented in terms of longitudinal and cumulative clinical improvements correlated with the observed endocrine and metabolic changes. (Supported by Pentagone).

08.32.07

Treatment of hirsutism with spironolactone, cimetidine and cyperoterone acetate: Buckshee, K. Obstet. & Gyn. Dept., All India Inst. Med. Sci., Ansari Nagar, New Delhi, India

Spironolactone, cimetidine, and cyperoterone acetate were given to hirsute women to evaluate the effect of these drugs on total body hair growth and to compare their efficacy. A total of 75 hirsute women with 25 in each group were chosen for the study. Consistent improvement in total body hair growth, quality of hair and acne was observed in all the three groups. However, the best response was observed with cyperoterone acetate, next was spironolactone and with cimetidine it was least. The face was the most responsive site, chest and back proved resistant to drug therapy. The details of drug regimes, their effectiveness and side-effects will be discussed.

08.32.08

Results of a double-blind study with two anti-androgen containing preparations: Aydinlik, S, Lachnit, U. Schering AG, D Endokr. I, Berlin

A double-blind multicenter study of nine month's duration has been conducted with two combination preparations – Diane and "Diane 35" containing the anti-androgen, 2 mg cyproterone acetate per tablet as progestogen; they differ from one another only as regards the estrogen content; Diane 35 contains 0.035 mg ethinylestradiol per tablet, instead of 0.050 mg, i.e. 30% less than that of Diane. The aim of the study was to find out whether "Diane 35" is as effective as Diane in the therapy of signs of androgenization, like acne, seborrhea in women, and, whether side-effects due to the estrogen component would decline under "Diane 35". Preliminary analysis of the study comprises 2027 cycles; 264 women participated in the study. According to the results there is no significant difference between the two preparations regarding therapeutic effectiveness; e.g. at the end of 9-months therapy, healing and improvement in 87.7% of facial acne have been observed under "Diane 35". The corresponding rate for Diane was 79.1%. Cycle pattern under both preparations was normal. The incidence of intermenstrual bleeding was comparable with that of other progestogen estrogen combinations. The subjective tolerance proved to be good. Side-effects, due to estrogen component like breast tenderness, chloasma, edema, and especially gastric complaints such as nausea and vomiting were less common with "Diane 35". Another interesting fact observed during the study was, that the improvement in acne and seborrhea became evident much earlier (within 4–6 weeks) with "Diane 35" than with Diane, a very agreeable fact for which we have still no explanation. No pregnancy occurred during this study.

08.32.09

Cyproterone acetate versus levonorgestrel combined with ethinyl estradiol in the treatment of acne: Carlborg, L. Dept. Gyn., County Hosp., Halmstad, Sweden

In spite of an abundant literature on anti-androgen treatment of acne with cyproterone acetate (CA), there are no objectively measured results which could prove statistically the possible superiority of CA to regular contraceptive pills. In this study acne lesions over both cheeks were counted by a dermatologist. Three different test combinations were given double-blind at random to volunteers by the gynecologist; 1) CA 2 mg + ethinyl estradiol (EE) 50 μg (Diane®), 2) CA 2 mg + EE 35 μg (Diane mite), 3) levonorgestrel 150 μg + 30 μg EE (Neovletta®) to be used in 21 day cycles. Dermatological evaluation was made during cycle 6 including a subjective statement. As the pre-treatment number of lesions varied considerably, data were expressed as percentage changes. Each group contained 20 subjects. For Diane an average acne reduction of 85% was present, for Neovletta only 15% (p < 0.05). Group data for Diane were within small limits, whereas data for Neovletta had a high spread from a reduction of 70% to worsening Diane mite gave an average reduction of 73%. The subjective evaluation of the treatment was similar for the gyneco-logist, dermatologist and patient. "Poor" corresponded to an improvement below 30%, "moderate" to an interval of 41–50% reduction and "good" to an improvement over 90%. The study has clearly demon-strated the superiority of Diane and "Diane 35" to Neovletta. It is known that Neovletta may cure acne in some patients, but too many get worse, and we do not know how to select them from the beginning.

08.32.10
Hirsutism therapy by a single 300 mg i.m. administration of cyproterone acetate vs. 1000 mg oral treatment: Huber, J, Schmidt, J*, Spona J. 1st Dept. Obstet. and Gyn., *2nd Dept. Derm., Univ., Vienna, Austria
Ten hirsute patients were each treated at random with a single 300 mg cyproterone acetate i.m. injection and with a daily oral dose of 100 mg given for ten days, respectively. Both groups were given orally 2 mg cyproterone acetate and 0.05 mg ethinylestradiol in addition to the above therapy through 21 days. Treatment was started after a control cycle and continued for another six cycles Testosterone (T), dehy-droepiandrosterone sulfate (DHEA-S) and prolactin (PRL) were estimated by radioimmunoassay on day 10 of each cycle. In addition, patients were examined clinically and improvement of hirsutism was evaluated by determination of hair diameter. Statistical evaluation of hormone serum levels revealed a significant decrease of testosterone in the i.m. treated group of patients from 0.61 ± 0.31 to 0.29 ± 0.10 ng/ml serum after six months. DHEA-S declined from 3.8 ± 1.38 to 2.5 ± 1.2 μg% (p < 0.025) in this group. On the other hand, PRL increased from 8.5 ± 5.47 to 18.54 ± 9.7 ng/ml serum (p < 0.0125). Hormone serum levels did not change significantly in the orally treated subjects. Improvement of hirsutism was noted in both groups. Hair diameter reduction to 63% and 88% was recorded in the i.m. and orally treated groups, respectively. Furthermore, no changes in antithrombin III was noted in both treatment groups. Present data combine to suggest a greater efficacy of the i.m. route.

08.32.11
Effect of a combination of ethinylestradiol-desogestrel (Marvelon®) on clinical and hormonal features of hirsutism: Ruutiainen, K, Erkkola, R. Dept. Obstet. and Gyn., Turku Univ. Hosp., Turku, Finland
Oral contraceptives have been used in the treatment of hirsutism because of their ability to suppress the ovarian androgen production and to decrease the plasma free testosterone index by elevating the SHBG level. A group of 22 women with mild to moderate hirsutism was treated for 6 to 12 months with a combination of ethinylestradiol (EE_2)-desogestrel (Marvelon®). The hair growth was graded according to *Ferriman* and *Gallwey* (J. clin. Endocr. Metab. **24**, 1440, 1961). The Wilcoxon matched-pairs signed-rank test was used in statistical evaluation. A decrease of hair growth was demonstrated in total and hormonal scores of hirsutism (p < 0.01) as well as in the face area (p < 0.02). Respectively, a marked elevation of SHBG level and a reduction of T/SHBG ratio (p < 0.01) was noted. There was an increase in total testosterone and LH concentrations (p < 0.02). No significant changes were seen in androstenedione, dehydroepiandrosterone sulfate, estradiol, 17-hydroxyprogesterone, FSH and prolactin values. The treat-ment response was not related to the etiology of hirsutism (ovarian vs adrenal vs idiopathic). These data suggest that EE_2-desogestrel combination is useful in the treatment of mild to moderate hirsutism.

08.41.01
Obstetric performance of Bangladeshi immigrant women in UK: Nysenbaum, A M, Grudzinskas, J G. Dept. Obstet. and Gyn., London Hosp. Med. Coll., London, El, UK
Immigrant women from Bangladesh comprise 40% of the women delivered in this department. Several aspects of their obstetric performance were studied retrospectively using a ten-year data base which was computer stored. Advanced maternal age, high parity, short stature and medical disorders were evident commonly. Perinatal diagnostic techniques were applied more frequently than in the indigenous popula-tion. Obstetric outcome differed with respect to perinatal mortality, an excess of stillbirths occuring in women with high parity. Birthweight charts revealed lower birthweight for gestational age in the immigrant women. Perinatal deaths were not increased in the smaller infants at any given gestational age. These data suggest that birthweight charts derived from Caucasian babies are inappropriate for this immigrant population.

08.41.02
Child health in Bangladesh. Role of N. G. Os.: Begum, S F. Dept. Obstet. and Gyn., Dhaka Med. Coll., Bangladesh
Introduction: Children being a specially vulnerable group of the population susceptible to high risk of

mortality and morbidity and dependent on adults for their health care, deserve special consideration in provision of health care for them. In the last 50 years, there has been a sharp improvement in the health conditions of the people more so in the developed and less so on the developing countries. – Neonatal mortality: Even during infancy (up to 1 year of age), newborns are subject to maximum health risk up to 28 days after birth (neonatal age). Table 2 shows the rate of neonatal mortality per 1000 livebirths found in different studies conducted in rural Bangladesh. The neonatal mortality rate in 1976–77 was found in Matlab and Teknaf upazilas at 73.4 and 89.0 per 1000 livebirth, respectively. The NIPORT studies reported a neonatal mortality of 70.1 and 85.2 for the years 1979 and 1980, respectively. The more recent BAMA-NEH study found the rate at 80.5 per 1000 livebirths. The above rates ranged from 70 to 89, meaning that 7 to 9 per cent of all newborn babies die within four weeks of birth.

08.41.03
Factors affecting the progress of pregnancy in Greek population: Yousef Ayyash H F, Nicky, A, Kakkos, L, Comninos, A, Sofatzis, J. "Marika Eliadis" Maternity Hosp., Athens, Greece
A study was conducted among mothers who in 1982 gave birth to 925 infants in the "Marika Eliadis" Maternity Hospital. The mothers were submitted to a questionnaire investigating various suspected factors, and from the answers the following statistics and conclusions were drawn: 22.8% of the women smoke during their pregnancy, half of them (52.2%) more than 10 cigaretts daily. The percentage of smokers among the mothers of term appropriate-for-dates newborns (gestational age 37 weeks and birthweight 2500 g) was 20.4%; among the mothers of preterm infants (g.a. 37 weeks), 30.2% (P < 0.05); and among the mothers of small-for-date infants (g.a. 37 weeks, birthweight 2500 g), 32,8% (P < 0.05). The socio-economic status continues to be the most adverse factor influencing the progress of pregnancy. Thus we see that only 24.5% of the mothers of term appropriate-for-dates infants have low socioeconomic status as compared to 46.7% of the mothers of preterm infants (P < 0.01) and 44.3% of the mothers of small-for-dates infants (P < 0.01). Other factors found to affect gestation adversely were the age of the mother (high-risk ages 19 and 35 years of age) and heliotherapy. We did not observe any statistically significant differences in nutritional factors (judging from the increase of weight of the mother), consumption of alcohol, previous abortions, and exposure to T.V. radiation.

08.41.04
Reliability of Dutch perinatal mortality statistics: Doornbos, J P R, Nordbeck, H J, Treffers, P E. Univ. Amsterdam, The Netherlands
Despite its shortcomings, the perinatal mortality rate (PMR) is considered indicative for the quality of perinatal care, and at present remains a basis for international comparison. It was suggested that PMRs might not contain what they purport, however, as so far almost no reports on the reliability of a country's statistics have been published. In the Netherlands the Central Bureau of Statistics (CBS) is supposed to include all late fetal deaths (≥ 28 weeks) and all liveborn infants dying before the end of their 7th day of life (according to WHO definitions) in PM statistics. In the present study all 13 Amsterdam hospitals were visited and labor ward records of the years 1981 and 1982 were personally searched for cases of PM. The 360 cases found were individually linked to the cases registered at the CBS. The CBS figures for PM in Amsterdam appeared to be 14.0% lower than the hospital derived figures. This under-recording is due to under-reporting by physicians and not due to errors in statistical book-keeping at the CBS office. Evidence was found that under-reporting is related to birth weight c.q.viability of the infant as well as the socio-economic c.q. immigrant status of the parents. These findings support the hypothesis that the obligation exist in the Netherlands to bury an infant once it is notified affects the quality of PM statistics negatively. Recommendations are made accordingly.

08.41.05
Birthweight and gestation of Nairobi infants: Sanghvi, H C G, Mati, J K G. Dept. Obstet. and Gyn., Univ., Nairobi, Kenya
5293 singleton infants born in Nairobi, Kenya were studied during a seven-week period. The incidence of low birth weight (under 2500 g) was 7.7%. The incidence of LBW was 14.4% in teenage mothers and 12.0% in primigravidae. Hypertensive disease in pregnancy and anemia contributed to higher incidence of low birthweight. Prematurity (gestation under 37 weeks) was found in 14.8% of mothers. Rates of 21.9% were found in teenage mothers. 17.2% in primigravidae, 18% in uneducated mothers and 17.1% in mothers with no income. The weights for gestation percentiles show that the weight at gestation below 32 weeks is similar to Caucasian standards. However, the weights are persistently lower at later gestations. It was concluded that low birth weight and prematurity are more common in teenage mothers and primigravidae and that the western standards for weight gestation are different from those for the Nairobi infant.

08.41.06
Perinatal mortality in Nairobi, Kenya: Mati J K, Sanghvi, H, Aggarwal, V, Lucas, S, Corkhill, R. Dept. Obstet. and Gyn., Univ., Nairobi, Kenya
701 stillbirths and first 24 hour neonatal deaths occurred in City of Nairobi during a seven-month period. The early perinatal mortality rate in Nairobi was 33.4 per 1000. Teenage mother contributed to 30% of these perinatal deaths and primigravidae 35.8%. 18% of the deaths occurred in mothers who had no

antenatal care. Antenatal complications associated with perinatal death were hypertensive disease (in 20.7%), premature rupture of membranes (12.3%), anaemia (15.8%), threatened abortion (9.2%), antepartum haemorrhage (8.5%), febrile illness (7.2%). Labor lasting for over 12 hours was associated with higher mortality. 18.3% of babies who died were delivered by breech. Post mortem was done in 63% of cases. Intrapartum anoxia and cerebral birth trauma contributed to 38.7% of deaths, followed by hyaline membrane disease and pulmonary hemorrhage in 18.7%. Antepartum anoxia was found in 17.1% and congenital malformation in 7.5%. More than 50% of cases had avoidable factors. Inappropriate antenatal care, later referral of high-risk pregnancies and poor intrapartum care were identified as factors leading to perinatal mortality.

08.41.07

Perinatal mortality at the Riyadh Armed Forces Hospital – six-year study: Mesleh, R A. Armed Forces Hosp., Riyadh, Saudi Arabia

Perinatal deaths in single births that occurred among 16,403 Riyadh Armed Forces Hospital patients delivered during a six-year period between 1979 and 1984 were investigated by case record analysis. Causes of death were divided into nine categories (an extended version of the Aberdeen specification being used – *Baird, D, Walker, J, Thomson, A M.* J. Obstet. Gyn. Brit. Empire **61**, 433–448, 1954. Out of 250 perinatal deaths, 79 (31.6%) were due to fetal abnormality which in 19 cases was malformation of the central nervous system. Of the 171 normally formed infants, 127 weighed 1500 g or more, 70 of these died before onset of labor, 29 died intrapartum and 28 were born alive but died during the first week of life. The largest single cause of death was congenital abnormality followed by low birth weight in normally formed babies whose mothers had no complication of pregnancy. The perinatal mortality rate has dropped from 22.1 per thousand in 1979 to 10.8 per thousand in 1984. The lowest perinatal mortality rate was for parities 2 and 3 (11 per thousand) and age groups of 20 to 24 years (12 per thousand). No death was attributed to rhesus incompatibility. Maternal diabetes was not a major cause of perinatal loss. These results were valuable in illustrating that the perinatal mortality rate has fallen to nearly half its former level. The present death rate is low and comparable to that reported by developed countries. This low level has been achieved in great part by attempting to apply the highest quality antenatal and intrapartum care.

08.41.08

A comparison between 1978 and 1984 reproductive profile in the Cipto Mangunkusumo Hospital Jakarta as derived from maternity care monitoring system: Saifuddin, A B, Rachimhadhi, T, Sumapraja, S, Samil, R S. Dept. Obstet. and Gyn., Univ. of Indonesia, Jakarta, Indonesia

The reproductive profile in the Cipto Mangunkusumo Hospital Jakarta during 1978 (analysis of 4470 cases) was discussed in the Ninth WCGO, Tokyo, 1979. This paper will compare the same data with those of 1984 using MCM system. Analysis has been derived from 3668 cases with special emphasis on (1) age and parity; (2) stillbirths; (3) perinatal and neonatal deaths; (4) abortion before these deliveries; (5) anemia and parity; (6) infant births; (7) antenatal visits and stillbirths; (8) the desire to have additional children; (9) post-partum contraception; and (10) post partum sterilization. The results showed evidence of significant improvements in particular in several main factors such as (1) mean parity by mother's age 35–39 years (5.8 to 4.4); (2) births to teenagers below 18 years (3.1 to 1.0%); (3) births to teenagers below 20 years (12.3 to 6.2%); (4) stillbirths (63.9 to 52.5/1000 infants); (5) neonatal deaths before discharge (26.6 to 21.0/1000 livebirths); and (6) perinatal deaths (90.6 to 73.0/1000 infants). However, these figures still surpass those of the developed countries in general.

08.41.09

Perinatal mortality: Description of bi-regional results: Mariona, F G, Galba Araujo, J, Taylor, J. Hutzel Hosp./Wayne State Univ., Detroit, MI; Maternidade Escola Assis Chateaubriand, Fortaleza, Brazil; Dept. Publ. Hlth, Lansing, MI, USA

The purpose of the review is to compare the frequency of low birth weight babies born in two university maternity hospitals that service areas with different populations and resources, and to compare neonatal mortality based on birth weight. Descriptive OB statistics of one year were reviewed. Prenatal care is administered to urban/suburban/rural patients under two different systems. MEAC uses lay midwives for assessment, risk evaluation and low-risk prenatal and delivery care. HH/WSU provides care through physicians in training under the supervision of full-time faculty (board eligible or certified obstetricians/gynecologists or subspecialists in maternal-fetal medicine). MEAC relies heavily on public education and community pressures to entice pregnant women to attend prenatal clinics. Differences noted in the preliminary evaluation my be accounted for by the use of different technological profiles.

Table see page 203 for statistic

08.41.10

The effect of intracranial hemorrhage in the developmental outcome of preterm infants at one year: Morales, W J, Koerten, J, Lennard D, Greenbaun, L D. Dept. Obstet. and Gyn., Orlando Reg. Med. Ctr, Orlando FL

A study was conducted from 1981 to 1984 involving 369 infants under 33 weeks weighing 500 to 1500 g. Infants were monitored electronically during labor. Echoencephalogram was performed during the first 72

	MEAC	HH/WSU
Livebirths	9021	5748
Preterm birthweight (gms):		
< 1000	0.4 %	1.2 %
1001–1500	0.5 %	0.8 %
1501–2000	1.5 %	1.1 %
2001–2500	8.5 %	7.3 %
Stillborns	3.15%	1.33%
Neonatal mortality (0–7 days):		
< 2500 gms	15.74%	1.69%
> 2500 gms	0.7 %	0.07%
Neonatal mortality (8–28 days):		
< 2500 gms	0.9 %	0.02%
> 2500 gms	0.01%	0.03%

Early assessment during pregnancy decreases complications.　　**To Abstract 08.41.09**

hours of life and repeated if intracranial hemorrhage (ICH) was detected. The overall incidence of ICH and mortality was 42% and 22% respectively, both increased for gestations under 1000 g 60% and 48% as compared to 28% and 8% for those over 1000 g. Neuromotor and developmental studies were performed on 158 survivors, 39 under 1000 g through the Bailey test by a multidisciplinary team in addition to ophthalmological and auditory examination. Functional handicaps were identified in 30% of infants and in 42% of the survivors under 1000 g. 82% of infants with no bleed or grade I ICH had normal development as compared to 11% with grade III or IV. Abnormal hearing and ophthalmological findings were identified in 7% and 22% respectively. An obstetrical approach is proposed to decrease ICH and improve outcome of survivors.

08.42.01
Delivery net: Janko, A B. Dept. Gyn. and Obstet., Stanford, Univ., Monterey, CA
A new concept for delivery of the fetal head is presented, employing rotation and traction without the drawback of compression. The proposed delivery net provides inherent qualities of flexion, reduced surface tension, and accommodation to both the fetal head and the maternal birth canal. On reaching the critical pressure, the man-made material is manufactured to break, therefore preventing injury. The stainless steel obstetrical forcep when applied to the moldable fetal head results in an unavoidable compression. Faulty or incorrect application will produce maternal injuries as well. Current obstetrical programs deemphasize use of forceps. Thus, when needed, practitioners are no longer well versed or proficient, therefore both fetal and maternal injuries more likely. Description and presentation of the delivery net with review of the obstetrical forceps development, use, and documented fetal-maternal drawbacks. A theoretical presentation.

08.42.02
Hot tub bath during labor: Lenstrup, C, Schantz, A, Berget, A, Feder, E, Rosenø, H, Hertel, J. Gyn.-Obstet. & Pediat. Depts., Gentofte Hosp., Univ., Copenhagen, Denmark
It has from some countries been claimed that hot tub bath (HTB) during labor through inhibition of pain and fear could improve the effectivity of the uterine contractions leading to labor of shorter duration and less pain (*Tjarkovsky & Odent*). This positive experience is supposed to improve the relation between the mother and the child and improve the condition of the newborn. In a prospective study 64 women after a strictly normal pregnancy ending with spontaneous onset of labor at term bathed in a hot tub from a half to two hours during the first stage of labor. The control group consisted of 62 women fulfilling the same criteria of normality during pregnancy and labor who did not want HTB during labor. Apart from the HTB the two groups followed the usual obstetric procedures of the department. The cervical dilatation in the bath group was 2.7 cm/h compaired to 1.3 cm/h in the control group. Evaluated by a pain score the bath group experienced a pain relief which was not seen in the control group. The use of morphia and the need for stimulation of labor contractions were two times higher in the control group, but this difference was not statistically significant. No difference was observed in frequency of: analgesia during second stage of labor, operative delivery, vaginal or perineal lesions or in bleeding during labor. The total duration of labor was equal in the two groups and no difference in the neonatal condition was recorded. The bacterial contamination of the bath was insignificant and there were no febrile episodes post partum.

08.42.03
The optimum birth position – vertical versus horizontal by the example of the Trobriand people/Papua New Guinea. Results of an ethnomedical field study: Pöschl, U. Frauen- u. Poliklin. re. d. Isar, TU, Munich
Based upon four cases of traditional birth giving among the Trobrianders/Papua New Guinea including

a twin delivery the vertical posture in labor is analysed and discussed. Emphasis will be placed on the advantages of the change of vertical positions according to the different stages in labor. The effect of gravity, pelvic mobility, kyphosis of the lumbar spine, the efficiency of the abdominal muscular pressure, the eased lung ventilation and the long persistence of the intact amniotic sac are important factors which added together have a facilitating, perpetuating and protective impact on the process of delivery. In contrast to the traditional societies where vertical postures dominate in labor the recumbent position is used in most industrialised countries. The latter's insufficient body support for the parturient's bearing down maneuvers, the aortic and caval compression (supine hypotensive syndrome), the hindered turing of the fetus in the birth canal by the fixed pelvis, the postural sacral back pain aggravated by the fetus' weight require a greater need for analgesis and anesthetics, surgical intervention, additional risks at birth and a more painful event for the parturient. Therefore vertical postures are to be preferred especially since technological interventions such as CTG can be applied under these conditions.

08.42.04
"Natural birth" and "time-shift-problems" between mother and child, demonstrated after heterologous insemi-nations: Mutke, H G. Munich
Time indicator for term of birth is presumably the child by inducing oxytocin secretion when it reaches its optimal maturity for delivery. In many cases we observe time-shifts between these three biological systems: mother, child and placenta (and often also the ripeness of cervix), because either the child does not give "the signal on time", when it reaches the optimal maturity, or if the mother does not react adequatly. We have more than one thousand children, spontaneously born after heterologous inseminations, where the day of fertilization of the egg is exactly known. Up to now we have only screened 52 cases with significant time-shifts between mother and child (figures I/II). Mature children weighing between 3300 to 3800 g were delivered spontaneously after a real time of pregnancy of 245–250 days, without any illness of mother. Up to now we are ignorant about prolonged time of pregnancies, or unnecessary overweight of children. It is a common experience to wait 14 days over the calculated day of delivery, and this day has many errors. In cases of such time-shifts, the maturity of a child has to be the time indicator for the obstetrician to deliver early enough and to avoid any complications. Those complications due to unnecessary prolonged delivery time and from an overweight child are mostyl brain damage and difficult deliveries for the mother. Correct timing is a condition for "natural birth".

08.42.05
Intramural uterine administration of PGF_{2a} in postpartum bleeding: Mantalenakis, S, Stamatopoulos, P, Tsalikis, T. 1st Dept. Obstet. and Gyn., Aristotelian Univ., Thessaloniki, Greece
Ninety-two cases of postpartum and postabortion hemorrhage were faced with intramural uterine injection of prostaglandin F_{2a}. In all cases studied the hemorrhage was due to the uterine atony, placenta of the lower segment of the uterus and postabortion evacuation. In 21 cases bleeding was noticed during or after a Cesarean section and prostaglandin F_{2a} (5 mg diluted in 10 cc of normal saline) was injected in 4–6 spots intramurally. In 58 cases of postpartum bleeding the above dose of PGF_{2a} was injected transcervically deeply into the myometrium in 2–4 spots. Thirteen cases of postabortion evacuation and bleeding were treated in the same manner as in the postpartum bleeding group. In all cases the usual uterotonic agents ergonovine and oxytocin were administered before the PGF_{2a} adminstration without satisfactory contrac-tile effect. The above method was not effective in two cases of Cesarean section and in six cases of postpartum bleeding. All other cases responded effectively to the treatment. Side-effects of intramural uterine administration noticed in some cases were mild. The local prostaglandin F_{2a} administration was more effective than the usual uterotonic drugs as it was concluded from this study. We suggest the use of intramural application of prostaglandin F_{2a} in order to manage postpartum bleeding and avoid major surgery in these cases.

08.42.06
Maternal acid-base status during labor and maternal position: Llamas, C, Gallo, M, Reche, A, Arbues, J, Abehsera, M. Dept. Obstet. and Gyn., Hosp. Materno Infant., "Carlos Haya", Badajoz and Málaga, Spain
The maternal acid-base status may be an important factor for the fetal acid-base status during labor. Maternal gasometry was determined in 65 healthy women, 31 during pregnancy, 17 during labor and 17 during early puerperium. Two positions were studied, supine and standing. The acid-base status was determined after 20 minutes in each position, in capillary blood from the finger. There was no differences between both positions during pregnancy and early puerperium, but we found significant differences during labor for the pH (vertical 7.40 ± 0.02, supine 7.37 ± 0.03, $p < 0.01$) and pO_2 (vertical 79.77 ± 11.15, supine 66.67 ± 7.66, $p < 0.001$). That is why we think that the maternal vertical position during labor may be of benefit for the acid-base status of the fetus.

08.42.07
The effect on the separation time of emptying placental blood: Rezai Zadeh, M M, Samiei, H. Dept. Obstet. and Gyn., Emam Khomaini Postgrad. Teach. Hosp., Univ., Teheran
During a period of one year two hundred parturients who were in normal spontaneous labor were selected

randomly for the study. In half of the cases after delivery of the fetus the cord was clamped with two clamps and divided as usual. In the second group, the cord was clamped at only fetal end and maternal end left unclamped and blood allowed to flow freely from the placenta. In the second group, separation time of the placenta was significantly less than the first group. There were no cases who needed manual removal of placenta in the second group in comparison with three cases in the first group. – Result: This study showed that clamping of the maternal end of the cord is not necessary and indeed unclamping of the cord results in rapid separation of the placenta and less manual separation cases.

08.42.08
Therapy of the postpartum hemorrhage (PPH) with the synthetic prostaglandin E_2-derivative Nalador® – report of 111 cases: Gödicke, H-D. Schering AG, Berlin
Atonic PPH constitues a potentially fatal state which calls for rapidly effective therapy. Within the scope of emergency measures tonicising of the uterine muscles is essential. For obvious reasons it seemed justified to employ prostaglandins in addition to the classic oxytocic substances and to begin with the natural PGF_{2a}. The development of synthetic prostaglandins made it possible to treat atony of the uterus with sulprostone, a uteroselective substance which has relatively few side effects and constitutes the active substance of the synthetic PGE_2-derivative Nalador (Schering AG). Emergency situations which require this type of therapy to control the bleeding rule out the possibility of a controlled comparative study. Findings recorded by experienced clinicians in retrospective casuistics were collected and critically examined to determine the efficiency, tolerance and existence of any side-effects. It was confirmed that the administration of Nalador induced powerful tonicity of the uterus, which stopped the bleeding and made it possible to control the situation in conjunction with other emergency measures. A single injection of 500 µg Nalador has proved effective in many cases; it may be necessary to repeat the injection after approximately 60 minutes if the first dose has not had sufficient effect or in order to stabilise the effect obtained. In the case of an intravenous infusion average dose of 4–17 µg/min are effective. The dose can be adjusted to suit the clinical situation, i. e. first increased for a short time and later decreased to maintain the effect. The available data do not indicate any serious side-effects. Nalador can therefore be regarded as a major advance in the management of PPH.

08.79.01
Premenstrual tension (PMT) – diagnostical aspects and classification of patients: Hammarbäck, S, Bäckström, T. Dept. Gyn. and Obstet., Univ., Umeå, Sweden
Women complaining of PMT are a heterogenous group. On history it is difficult to distinguish PMT from an ordinary psychiatric disorder. This study based on prospective daily symptom ratings, is an attempt to find a simple and objective method, to diagnose and classify PMT patients. All women complaining of PMT at the Dept. of Gynec. during eight months (n=47) participated. Age 23–45 years. A somatic and psychiatric case history was taken and the Eysenck Personality Inventory (EPI) was given. 17 symptoms were rated daily for 2 menstrual cycles using visual analog scales earlier tested. Ovulation was detected with weekly serum estradiol and progesterone. Ratings of the 10 pre-ovulatory days were compared to the 10 pre-menstrual days using Mann-Whitney-U-test. 15/47 patients had a significant (P<0.05) symptom cyclicity and more than 80% of the pre-ovulatory days completly free of negative symptoms, (group I). 22/47 patients had in addition symptoms during the pre-ovulatory days (group II). 8/47 patients did not have any significant symptom change, (group III). Two patients were omitted because of poor ratings. Neuroticism, in the EPI, were sign. higher in group II and III compared to I (P<0.05 and 0.025 resp.), but no difference between II and III. Lie and extrovert scores did not differ between groups. Half of the patients in group II and III had earlier psychiatric history while only one in group I (X^2 test P<0.01). With this method it seems possible to separate women with "pure PMT" from those with mostly psychological problems. Such a classificaton is essential before treatment trials can be done as the psychological problems might obscure the results.

08.79.02
Long-term clinical response using danazol in the premenstrual syndrome (PMS): Payne, E S, Watts, J F, Logan Edwards, R, Butt, W R. Dept. Clin. Endocr., Birmingham and Midland Hosp. Women, Birmingham, UK
It has been shown (*J. F. Watts, R. Logan Edwards* and *W. R. Butt.* Brit. J. Obstet. Gyn. In press, 1985) in a double-blind placebo controlled trial involving 40 patients diagnosed as having the premenstrual syndrome (PMS) that danazol (Danol, Winthrop Laboratories) given daily for three months in doses of 100, 200 or 400 mg is effective in controlling the symptoms of irritability, aggression, anxiety, tearfulness, increased appetite and breast tenderness, between 56 and 78% being symptom-free by the third month. In the light of these findings a clinical trial has been undertaken to assess the value of long-term treatment with Danol in patients with PMS who failed to respond to other therapy. Danol was used in dosages of 200 and 400 mg daily for periods of up to 12 months. Maximum benefit was not seen before the third month of therapy and the remission of symptoms continued throughout treatment. During this time no patient withdrew because of any side-effects. After a maximum of 12 months therapy Danol was discontinued. Menses returned promptly but patients remained symptom-free for periods of up to 12 months without further treatment. Recommencement of treatment with Danol of those patients who had previously had a good response produced rapid alleviation of symptoms.

08.79.03

A placebo–controlled double-blind cross–over study of Danazol 400 mg per day for the premenstrual syndrome: Gilmore, D H, Hawthorn, R, McKay Hart, D. Stobhill Gen. Hosp., Glasgow, UK

Few placebo controlled trials have been conducted to assess treatment of the premenstrual syndrome. This study was carried out in 39 women attending a hospital PMS clinic. Patients were monitored for eight complete cycles, the first two being controls to confirm the diagnosis and provide baseline measurements. To assess mood a menstrual distress questionnaire was completed daily. Depression and anxiety in the premenstruum were scored retrospectively. Patients were given Danazol 400 mg per day or matching placebo each for 3 cycles in a double-blind cross-over manner. When compared with placebo Danazol was shown to produce a significant improvement in tension, depression, anxiety, lowered performance, negative affect, concentration, water retention, breast discomfort, swelling, irritability, pain and behavioral change. Danazol is clearly effective in controlling most symptoms of PMS even in women with severe symptoms. The 400 mg dosage was associated with some potentially undesirable side-effects, notably suppression of menstruation. It is suggested, therefore, that lower dosages may be more appropriate for the first line management of milder disease. Further investigation with lower doses are in progress.

08.79.04

Piroxicam in primary dysmenorrhea: Saltveit, T. Dept. Obstet. and Gyn., Haugesund Hosp., Haugesund, Norway

In many cases of primary dysmenorrhea increased synthesis of prostaglandins takes place in the endometrium, and increased excretion of prostaglandins in menstrual blood has been demonstrated (*Pickles, U. R.* Brit. J. Obstet. Gyn. **72**, 185, 1965). Prostaglandin synthetase inhibitors have proved to be effective in the treatment of dysmenorrhea (*Jacobsen, J.* Acta Obstet. gyn. scand. **87**, 73, 1981). Piroxicam is an effective inhibitor of the enzyme cyclo-oxygenase, and thus of prostaglandin synthesis (*Carty, T. J.* Prostaglandins **19**, 671, 1980). Ninety-two patients with primary dysmenorrhea were included in a double-blind randomized cross-over trial to study the efficacy of piroxicam on menstrual pain and associated symptoms with placebo as control. Ninety patients completed the four-month study period. Piroxicam exerted a highly significant relief of menstrual pain and lowering of the need for the supplementary analgesic paracetamol. Piroxicam also had a significant effect on associated symptoms. The drug was well tolerated, with only a few side effects of a mild nature reported and with no difference between the piroxicam and placebo groups in this respect.

08.79.05

The effect of mefenamic acid on coagulation, fibrinolysis and prostaglandins in patients with established menorrhagia: Dockeray, C J, Sheppard, B L, Sharma, S C, Daly, Leisha, Bonnar, J. Trinity Coll. Dept. Obstet. and Gyn., St. James's Hosp., Dublin, Ireland

The coagulation and fibrinolytic enzyme systems and prostaglandins were studied simultaneously in menstrual and peripheral blood in three groups of women: (1) 20 subjects (mean age 36 years) with normal menstrual loss (< 80 ml), (2) 20 patients (mean age 39 years) with excessive menstrual bleeding (> 80 ml) studied in a control cycle and (3) during treatment with mefenamic acid. Menstrual blood was collected directly from the uterine cavity between 24 and 48 hours of menstruation. Significant differences were found between menstrual and peripheral blood in fibrinolytic activity ($p < 0.001$), fibrinogen and plasminogen ($p < 0.001$), antithrombin III ($p < 0.001$), antiplasmin ($p < 0.001$) and the prostanoids PGE_2, $PGF_{2\alpha}$, 6-keto-$PGF_{1\alpha}$, and TxB_2 ($p < 0.001$) in all three groups. No significant differences in the fibrinolytic enzyme system or prostaglandins were detected in peripheral blood between groups 1 and 2, but higher fibrinolytic activity ($p < 0.001$), was found in the menstrual blood of group 3. Treatment with oral mefenamic acid 500 mg/8-hourly (group 3) had no significant effect on the fibrinolytic enzyme system and prostanoids in menstrual blood. These changes in the coagulation, fibrinolytic enzyme system and prostaglandins were accompanied by a 20 per cent reduction in menstrual blood loss during treatment with mefenamic acid.

08.79.06

The use of research data in the treatment of premenstrual syndrome patients: Mozley, P D, Mozley, M D. Dept Obstet. and Gyn., Univ. of Alabama, Coll. Commun. Hlth Sci., Univ., Alabama

The authors established a four visit protocol for all patients referred for evaluation of the premenstrual syndrome. The first visit was a 60 minute interview by the first author who is a board certified gynecologist and psychiatrist. The second visit was to a registered art psychotherapist who administered MMPI and collected drawings of the patient and significant others in her life. The third visit was a complete physical done by the same gynecologist and the collection of plasma gonadal hormone and aldosterone levels during the luteal phase. The fourth visit reviewed a 3-month feelings record, the lab data and the psychological data. One hundred patients were evaluated by this method and the data analyzed. Abnormal findings in any of these aspects were identified and used to set up a treatment protocol for each patient. Most demonstrable abnormalities were intrapsychic conflicts visible only by careful analysis of the art work. The data from the art work are utilized in the treatment program which has been effective in treating these patients. It is necessary to approach each area of abnormality uncovered by each and all of these approaches in the ongoing treatment of premenstrual syndrome.

08.79.07
Nimesulide in dysmenorrhea: Pulkkinen, M O. Dept. Obstet. and Gyn., Univ., Turku, Finland
Thirty patients with primary dysmenorrhea were treated with nimesulide (4-nitro-2-phenoxymethane-sulphonanilide, 100 mg b.i.d.) p.o. for primary dysmenorrhea. In 32 out of 39 treated cycles nimesulide was judged to be very effective or good, but in only 9 of 37 cycles treated with placebo were similar results observed (p < 0.01). In six patients intrauterine pressure (IUP) was monitored with the microballoon-tipped catheter technique for 3 h. The patients received placebo at 0 h and nimesulide 100 mg p.o. at 1 h. During this maximal pain period, nimesulide decreased uterine activity significantly and this was consistent with the relief of pain observed. In six patients, IUP was recorded during two consecutive cycles, one treated with placebo and the other with nimesulide 100 mg b.i.d. on the first day of the cycle (submaximal pain). Nimesulide decreased the duration of the pressure cycle from 150 to 79 seconds (p < 0.01). From ten patients, menstrual blood was collected in a cervical cup over a period of 3 h, both during placebo- and nimesulide-treated cycles. Concentrations of prostaglandin-F will be reported later.

08.79.08
Treatment of the premenstrual syndrome by subcutaneous hormone implants of estradiol – a double-blind, placebo-controlled study: Magos, A L, Brincat, M, O'Dowd, T, Studd, J W W. Dept. Obstet. and Gyn. Dulwich Hosp., London, UK
There are considerable inconclusive data concerning the etiology and management of the premenstrual syndrome (PMS) (*Magos & Studd*. Prog. Obstet. Gyn. **4**, 334, 1984). Certain observations led us to believe that it is the fluctuation of hormones and other metabolites with the ovarian cycle that is of primary importance in the pathogenesis of cyclic conditions such as menstrual migraine and the PMS (*Magos & Studd*. Contemp. Ob/Gyn. **24**, 85, 1984). Subcutaneous hormone implants of estradiol in doses sufficient to suppress ovarian activity should therefore be an effective therapy for premenstrual distress. This hypothesis was tested under controlled conditions in 48 women complaining of the PMS. Treatment consisted of either 100 mg estradiol implants in combination with cyclical norethisterone to induce withdrawal periods and prevent endometrial hyperplasia or identical placebo, with a follow-up period of up to 12 months. Symptomatology was monitored using daily symptom lists (Moos' Menstrual Distress Questionnaire), linear analogue scales and the General Health Questionnaire. Results showed that 100 mg estradiol implants were significantly superior to placebo (p < 0.05 to p < 0.01) for all the major adverse symptom complexes studied despited a placebo response of 97%. The therapeutic effect of placebo was maximal initially, but remained significant throughout the study period. We conclude that (1) suppression of the ovarian cycle with estrogen is an effective treatment for the PMS, and (2) psychological and social factors are also relevant in the pathogenesis of this condition.

09.10.01
Luteinizing hormone-releasing hormone (LH-RH) pharmacokinetics and the corresponding luteinizing hormone (LH) release in men: Fauser, B, Rolland, R, Dony, J, Doesburg, W, Thomas, C. Dept. Obstet. and Gyn., Univ., Nijmegen, The Netherlands
Serum levels of LH-RH and LH were measured following 5 and 20 μg LH-RH injections, given either i.v. or s.c. to 20 healthy men (each group n = 5). Blood samples were collected at frequent intervals for 60 min. The patterns of LH-RH serum levels were similar following both 5 and 20 μg LH-RH injections, with higher levels in the 20 μg group. The area under the LH-RH response curves was not statistically different (P ≧ 0.09) comparing i.v. with s.c. administration. Much sharper LH-RH pulses were found with higher levels between 1–5 min (P < 0.001), but lower levels between 30–60 min (P < 0.05) in the case of i.v. as compared to s.c. administration. In the i.v. group peak levels were reached at shorter time intervals (2 vs 15 min) with a much higher magnitude and a much shorter interval of initial 50% decline. No significant difference was observed in the magnitude (2–2.5 fold) and time occurrence (20–30 min) of maximum LH release as well as the area under the LH response curves comparing i.v. and s.c. administration of both 5 and 20 μg LH-RH. A clear decline in LH levels was not found during the observation time. It is concluded that the i.v. route of administration is preferable in therapeutic regimens using pulsatile exogenous LH-RH, since conditions of intermittent pituitary stimulation are more adequately fulfilled and the risk of dose accumulation is reduced. Futhermore, doses of 5 μg are capable of producing adequate pituitary LH release, whereas increasing the dose up to 620 μg seems to have no additional effects.

09.10.02
Possible role of protein kinase C in the action of LH-RH in the anterior pituitary cells: Hirota, K, Aono, T, Ikegami, H, Tanizawa, O, Catt, K*. Osaka Univ., Med. School, Nara, Japan; *NIH, USA
The actions of LH-RH on LH release in cultured pituitary cells are known to be mediated by calcium and phospholipid dependent manner. TPA (12-o-tetra-decanoyl phorbol-13-acetate) which is known as a potent activator of calium-activated, phospholipid-dependent protein kinase (protein kinase C), also stimulated LH secretion and down-regulated LH-RH receptor (*K. Hirota*, et al. 7th International Congress of Endocrinology 1984). These results suggest the involvement of protein kinase C in hormone actions of LH-RH. To clarify the direct relationship between protein kinase C and LH secretion stimulated by LH-RH, protein kinase C in rat pituitary cells was determined. Protein kinase C was identified and characterized by DEAE-cellulose chromatography and was activated by calcium and phospholipid or TPA

in rat pituitary cells. To study accurate effect of LH-RH on protein kinase C, the anterior pituitary cells were divided into eight fractions by centrifugal elutriation and the gonadotroph-enriched cells were obtained. The maximal change of protein kinase C during LH-RH stimulation was observed in the fraction seven which was mostly composed of gonadotrophs. Stimulation of LH release by LH-RH – correlated well with the decrease of protein kinase C in the cytosol and the increase of protein kinase C in the membrane fraction of the gonadotroph-enriched cells. This change of protein kinase C was an early event in the stimulation of LH secretion by LH-RH. Thus, these results strongly suggest that protein kinase C mediates the hormonal action of LH-RH in LH secretion in gonadotrophs.

09.10.03

Induction of ovulation using pulsatile luteinising hormone-releasing hormone: Soong, Y. Dept. Obstet. and Gyn., Chang Gung Memo. Hosp., Taipei, Taiwan

Induction of ovulation using luteinising hormone-releasing hormone (LH-RH) has been performed in five patients with primary amenorrhea, six patients had secondary amenorrhea. All of them had failed to respond to clomiphene therapy. LH-RH was administered intravenously ($5-20\,\mu g$) in a pulsatile manner using miniaturised automatic infusion systems. Ovulations was successfully induced in most cycles and the rate of ovarian follicular maturation, as monitored by serial pelvic ultrasound scanning, was similar to that observed in spontaneous cycles. The mean diameter of the follicles at presumed time of ovulation was 1.8 cm. Endocrine assessment by serial measurement of gonadotrophins, estradiol and progesterone revealed hormone concentration that was within the normal range. In patients with primary amenorrhea the uterine cross-sectional area before treatment was significantly smaller than in patients with secondary amenorrhea. Anovulation was reflected by lack of uterine growth.

09.10.04

Neuroendocrine regulation of LH-RH and gonadotropin secretion in normal and postmenopausal women: Kumasaka, T, Masaoka, K, Watanabe, H, Mori, T, Ohya, H, Tadokoro, N. Dept. Obstet. and Gyn., Dokkyo Univ. School Med., Mibu, Tochigi, Japan

It is well known that normally cycling women provide a changing pattern of frequency and amplitude pulses of gonadotropin release during the cycle. On the other hand, ovariectomized and postmenopausal women also maintained by an increase in the magnitude of pulsatile pituitary discharge of LH and FSH. To confirm the mechanism, we investigated the difference of gonadotropin and LH-RH pulsatile pattern in plasma between normal and postmenopausal women. Furthermore, we administered LH-RH in form of pulsatile pattern in subjects during the follicular and luteal phase of the cycle. In our studies, there is no different pattern of pulsatile gonadotropin and LH-RH release in the magnitude and frequency. If the frequency of pulsatile LH-RH administration is changed in the luteal phase, withdrawal bleeding was immediately observed during LH-RH infusion. These observations suggest that gonadotropin secretion pattern is not always coincident with LH-RH releasing pulse and is mainly modulated at pituitary level rather than hypothalamus in normal cycling women.

09.10.05

TSH, PRL and E_2 response to double injections of GnRH and TRH in women over 40 years of age at different stages of their menstrual cycle: Malde, J L, Marín, A, Cuadros, J L, Ruiz Requena, E, Salvatierra, V. Dept. Gyn. Univ., Granada, Spain

We studied the response of the hypophysis to double injections of GnRH ($25\,\mu g$) and TRH ($200\,\mu g$) repeated after 60 minutes in women under 35 years of age (n = 15), 40–45 (n = 26) and 46–50 (n = 21). TSH and PRL base levels and those after 20, 30, 60, 80, 90 and 120 minutes were measured by RIA, as were E2 base levels and those after 60 and 120 minutes. The areas formed by the curves of the absolute and incremental values over the base lines were calculated after each dose. There were no significant differences in E2 base values. TSH base values, however, increased between the 11th and 15th day in patients over 45, and PRL values in the first nine days of the cycle. TSH synthesis remained constant throughout the cycle and was not age-related. PRL levels, however, increased from the 16th day, on in patients over 45. In these patients, PRL base levels were also higher. These levels are not related to E2 levels.

09.10.06

Mechanism of action of clomiphene citrate on gonadotropin release in humans: Polak, E, Espinola, B, Romo, A, Guitelman, A, Pozo, E del. Hosp. Alvarez, Buenos Aires, Argentina, and Frauenspit., Basle, Switzerland

Previous studies have shown that clomiphene citrate significantly enhances LH pulsatility in normal subjects (*del Pozo* et al. In: Dopamine and neuroendocrine active substances pp 127–133, 1985). In order to investigate the mechanism of action of clomid (CM) on anovulation, four women with hypothalamic amenorrhea had their LH pulsatile profiles analysed. Blood samples were collected at 15' intervals for 5–6 h in the baseline and in the 9–10 day following standard CM therapy (100 mg/day for five days). LH, FSH and E_2 were measured in all samples. Average LH values and pulse amplitudes were significantly augmented 7.1 ± 2 vs. 19 ± 4 and 3.2 ± 6 vs. $5.7\pm.8$ mIU/ml; p < .0.1/0.5 respectively). Cumulative E_2 (pg/ml) increased from 26 ± 6 to 329 ± 48 reflecting adequate biological activity of LH. FSH was not modified by treatment (5.4 ± 1 basal vs. 6.6 ± 1.4 after CM). The difference in plasma E_2 was significant to the p < .001

level. Pulse frequency was not altered by therapy. Results indicate that CM acts by enhancing LH pulsatile activity which subsequently stimulates sex steroid synthesis by the ovary. The main site of action can be tentatively placed at the level of the hypothalamus. Lack of effect on FSH plasma profiles displaces this gonadotropin to a secondary, probably permissive, role.

09.10.07

Gonadotrophic response to two doses of 25 μg of GnRH in women over 40 years of age in different stages of their menstrual cycle: Cuadros, J L, Marín, A, Malde, J L, Ruiz Requena, E, Salvatierra, V. Dept. Gyn., Univ., Granada, Spain

We studied the response to an injection of 25 μg of GnRH i.v., repeated after 60 minutes, in women under 35 years of age (n = 15), 40–45 (n = 26) and 46–50 (n = 21). FSH and LH base levels were measured by RIA and subsequent levels after 20, 30, 60, 80, 90 and 120 minutes, as were E2 base levels and those after 60 and 120 minutes. We calculate the areas formed by the curves of absolute and incremental values over the base lines after each dose. There were no significant age-related differences in E2 of LH base levels, no matter at which point of the cycle the measurement was made. FSH base levels, however, were significantly higher from the 11th day on, in patients over 45. In these patients there was a more marked FSH response to the 2nd dose of GnRH and a less marked LH response in the 2nd half of the cycle compared with younger women. These responses are not related to E2 levels. We suggest therefore that there is an alteration in central sensitivity.

09.10.08

The forecast value of LH-RH test over the test of clomiphene and the ovulatory conduct of the ovary: Juarez-Aquirre, F, Juárez, R, Marcuello, A C, Oriol, A, Fuente, F de la, Univ. Clin., Navarra, Spain

We have correlated the gonadotropin response of the hypophysis after stimulation with LH-release hormone (LH-RH) and the results with stimulation with clomifen (clomifen test) made in the fifth and ninth day of the cycle. We have analysed the behavior of the ovary during the cycle treated with clomifen effecting a continous echographic and hormonal screening. The monitoring comprises: basal echography (fifth day of the cycle) and successive echography (every 48 hours) until the determination of follicular rupture, luteinization or follicular regression. Estradiol (E$_2$) is determined in each echography and progesterone dosage seven days after temperature raises, if such occurs. The preliminary results indicate that the evaluation of the response to LH in the test of LH-RH is of use and of greater significance forecast the relation of LH/FSH rates. The test has value as index to the ovarian response by stimulation with clomifen.

09.14.01

Activated charcoal prevents enterohepatic recirculation of steroids: Heimer, G M, Englund, D E. Dept. Obstet. and Gyn., Univ., Uppsala, Sweden

Enterohepatic recycling of steroids is a matter of discussion. We have earlier reported on a prolonged effect of orally administered estriol caused by its enterohepatic recycling (1). In this study we wanted to test the hypothesis that administration of activated charcoal could inhibit recirculation of orally given estriol and hence diminish the biological activity of estriol. Plasma concentrations of unconjugated estriol were measured using a specific radioimmunoassay (RIA). Twelve mg estriol given orally to postmenopausal women gives high plasma estriol level still after 24 hours. Plasma estriol fluctuation in relation to meals is seen. When activated charcoal is given three hours after estriol administration the plasma estriol concentration rapidly declines and pretreatment value is obtained after six hours. Our data demonstrate that estriol given orally undergoes enterohepatic recirculation after reabsorption from the intestine since charcoal administration which binds steroids results in a rapidly declining estriol level. Hence enhanced and prolonged estriol elevation is caused by enterohepatic recycling. – (1) *Heimer, G, Englund, D*: Enterohepatic recirculation of estriol studied in cholecystectomized and noncholecystectomized menopausal women. Uppsala J. med. Sci. **89**, 107–115, 1984.

09.14.02

Clinical study of treatment of vaginal atrophy with low-dose estradiol pessaries: Kaalund-Jensen, H, Munck, A M. Dept. Obstet. and Gyn., Svendborg Sygehus, Svendborg, Denmark

Ten postmenopausal women with symptoms of atrophic vaginitis participated. Five patients in group I applied every night for three weeks a pessary containing 25 μg estradiol in a hydrophilic cellulose-derived matrix (NOVO), five patients in group II a pessary containing 10 μg estradiol. At the enrolment and after 1, 2 and 3 weeks of therapy specific symptoms and colposcopy estimation were recorded, and smears taken from the upper lateral vaginal wall for description of Maturation Index and Maturation Value. The subjective symptoms of dryness, pruritus and dyspareunia (8 patients) were relieved or markedly dimished in both groups after therapy, while no considerable effect of therapy on urinary tract symptoms was noted (six patients). Colposcopy revealed the effect of therapy on vaginal mucosa in all patients in group I, but only slight or moderate changes in group II. During treatment the Maturation Index shifted to the right, and the Maturation Values increased toward the status of normally estrogenized epithelium in all patients in both groups. Treatment with low-dose estradiol pessaries result in beneficial effects on vaginal mucosa indicated by increase in the Maturation Value. The clinical assessment and the subjective symptoms are of little importance.

09.14.03

Four different regimens of continuous estrogen-progestogen for climacteric complaints: Sporrong, T, Hellgren, M, Mattsson L Å, Samsioe, G. Dept. Obstet. & Gyn., Univ., Göteborg, Sweden

Continuous therapy with both estrogen and progestogen in the climacteric period is a new regimen. Previous studies showed marked effects on vasomotor symptoms, but intermittent bleeding was a problem. Therefore the clinical efficacy of four different regimens was evaluated. 60 postmenopausal women were randomly allocated to one of four treatment groups. All women were given 2 mg 17β-estradiol (E2) daily along with either norethisteroneacetate (NETA), 1 mg (A) and 0.5 mg (B) or megestrolacetate, 5 mg (C) and 2.5 mg (D). The patients were examined before treatment and after four months of treatment. – Results: All patients experienced a marked reduction of sweats and hot flushes. Nearly half of the women in group A had no bleedings at all. Women in group A recorded bleedings on average 2–3 days per month, the other groups had more frequent bleeding. Group A bled on average 8% of the days during the first three months, and the corresponding figure in the other groups was 15–25%. The amount of bleeding decreased during treatment and heavy bleeding was rare in the last two months. Continuation rate for all groups was 90%. There were no dropouts in group A. Endometrial biopsies before treatment and after four months of treatment showed no hyperplasia. – Conclusion: In the present study continuous hormonal replacement therapy promptly reduced vasomotor symptoms but bleeding disturbances were common. Women given 2 mg E2 and 1 mg NETA had significantly fewer problems in this respect compared to the other groups.

09.14.04

Planning a clinical research center for climacteric studies: Iddenden, D A, Curnyn, P M. Dept. Obstet. and Gyn., Presbyt.-Univ. of Pennsylvania Med. Ctr., Philadelphia, PA, USA

It has been suggested that a clinical research center is an appropriate setting for the evaluation and treatment of menopausal patients (*W. H. Utian*, Menopause in Modern Perspective p. 147, 1980, Appleton, New York; *P. A. Van Keep* et al., The Controversial Climacteric – The Proceedings of the Third International Congress on the Menopause, Ostend, June, 1981). The establishment of such a center requires considerable care in planning and administration if it is to function optimally and to achieve the desired clinical and research goals. This presentation will cover the basic requirements of the planning function, personnel, facilities and financial implications. In addition, methods to attract patients to the center, data collection and sources of funding will be discussed.

09.14.05

Effect of a slow release vaginal estriol preparation on blood estrogen and gonadotrophin levels over two weeks: Weiss, P, Ginsburg, J, Collins, W P, Fink, R S. Cilag AG Switzerland, Royal Free and Kings Coll. Hosp., London, UK

Absorption of estriol (E3) and hormonal changes for two weeks after vaginal administration of two galenic slow release formulations containing 3.5 mg E3 were measured in 22 healthy menopausal women aged 44 to 66 who were not taking estrogen or other therapy for the menopause. Plasma E3 was elevated for 24 to 48 hours after vaginal administration of the slow release E3 preparations, whereas with the standard E3 formulation of equivalent dosage E3 concentration had fallen to base line values by 24 hours. With a second application of the special formulations one week later, i.e. with a "prepared" vaginal mucosa, E3 levels were elevated for up to 84 hours. Blood LH fell after the initial E3 application and then rose rapidly. With the second application LH levels were lowered for up to 60 hours. Insignificant changes were observed correspondingly in plasma estradiol, estrone, prolactin and FSH concentrations. A slow release vaginal E3 preparation weekly could therefore be used for menopausal therapy.

09.14.06

Evaluation of new-styled transuterine instillation as a method for clinical investigation of tubal function: Hayashi, M*, Taguchi, Y*, Ishii, A*, Hamada, H*, Nagae, M**. *Dept. Obstet. and Gyn., **Dept. Clin. Labor., St. Marianna Univ. School Med., Kawasaki, Japan

The diagnosis of tubal disturbances in infertility has been made by Rubin's insufflation, HSG and laparoscopy as well as uterotubal lavage at laparotomy. However the results of these methods are not satisfactory in detecting tubal function. Transuterine instillation of bubbled saline solution and contrast medium with kymographic tracing using a new apparatus was performed in 160 infertile cases, and the results were compared with those of other diagnostic methods. The instrument (Toitsu KH 700) was provided with solid-state pressure sensor instead of a bellows transducer with the advance of medical electronics, and the bubbled liquids were observed by a high resolution real-time scanner (Hitachi EUB 40) instead of by X-ray. Kymographic curves were divided into three categories, normal type (49%), adhesion (37%) and occlusion type (14%), and each of them was divided in turn into five, two and two sub-categories, respectively. These findings accompanied by the observation of HSG and USG were much finer than the results of other examinations up to the present. Analysis could be performed in detail, including the observation of the passage at the intramural, isthmic and ampullary parts of both oviducts with HSG. Peritubal and perifimbrial adhesions were also observed at the transfer of the liquid from uterotubal junction to the pouch of Douglas with USG. High correlation was recognized between these findings and pregnancy rate, and it proved the significance of this diagnostic method.

09.14.07

Histochemical investigation of mucopolysaccharides in testicular tissue from men with fertility problems: Kyroudi, A, Papathanassiou, Z, Paizi-Biza, P, Voulgaris, Z, Terpou, A. Path. Dept., Univ., Athens, Greece

Previous investigations of mucopolysaccharides (MPS) in testicular tissue of men with fertility problems are scarce (*Maseki* et al. Fertil. and Steril. **31**, 456, 1979). For this purpose 100 bilateral testicular biopsies were elected, with criteria the histoligical appearance and the quantitative evaluation of the tissue by the score count method of *Johnsen* (Hormones **1**, 2, 1970). Our material has score count 4 and above, and was classified in four groups. The first group comprises cases graded 9–10, the second 8, the third 6–7 and the fourth 4–5. Grade 4 was selected as the lower value, because under this limit the changes are of no therapeutic interest. The presence of MPS was ascertained by light microscopy. Stains used were PAS reaction, Alcian blue, aldehyde fuchsin-Alcian blue, toluidine blue-testicular hyaluronidase and PAS-diastase. Neutral and acidic MPS were constantly identified. Neutral MPS were traced in the wall of the tubules the germinal epithelium and Sertoli cells. Acidic MPS were traced exclusively in the wall of the tubules. MPS digestible by testicular hyaluronidase were found in all cases. MPS were increased in the low-graded groups, a fact attributed to diminution of the function of the seminiferous tubules. In conclusion, the study of histochemical parameters elucidates these histological changes. The quantitative evaluation on the other hand determines with objective criteria the gravity of the lesion. The increase of MPS chiefly in low-grade cases enhances the significance of the role of the basement membrane in the process of spermatogenesis.

09.12.08

Development of a custom-fitted, valved, cervical cap (contracap): Freese, U E. Univ. of Hlth. Sci.-Chicago Med. School, Chicago; **Goepp, R A.** Univ of Chicago Pritzker School Med., Chicago; **Liao, W C.** Research Triangle Inst., Research Triangle Park, NC, USA

Application of dental techniques resulted in the use of silicone to obtain an impression of a woman's cervix. A plaster mold is cast from the cervical impression. Using a vacuform process, an exact-fitting cervical cap with a built-in valve is then fabricated from a thermoplastic rubber material. Following on-site training of clinical personnel in impression-taking and cap-placement techniques, a multi-center clinical trial of the Contracap was conducted to assess its efficacy, safety and acceptability. The design of this study included concurrent use of a condom during the first month of cap wearing; monitoring for any suspected vaginal infections; ascertainment of causes for dislodgement; colposcopic examinations for a random sample of women prior to cap placement and upon study termination; and materials assessment on a random sample of caps at the end of the study. Preliminary data indicate that impression-taking techniques and individual anatomical variations may be associated with certain cap wearing experiences among the study participants.

09.14.09

"Take me" anticonceptive sponge – a new proper way in family planning: Pickard, E, Knogler, W, Huber, J, Kubista E. 1st Dept. Obstet. and Gyn., Univ., Vienna, Austria

The contraceptive presented in this poster is a sophisticated combination of a diaphragma and a sponge soaked with a spermicide. The use of contraceptive sponge goes back to ancient times and presents one of the oldest methods of contraception. Our sponge consists of two parts, the part directed to the portio is fine and porous, soaked by a spermicide, the other part directed towards the vulva is connected inseparably by an elastomere material, pooling the ejaculated sperms. It is introduced and removed with the aid of an adapter and may be left for up for twenty-four hours. After introduction into the vagina its infolding like a balloon, tightening the vagina in the fornix area. We believe, that this method of contraception is very suitable for a great number of women, especially for women which refuse hormonal contraception, girls who do not have a permanent friend and in general for couples using the periodic abstinence. Our first experience is confined to only 48 couples: in 10 couples we observed seven month, in 16 six, in 9 five and in 3 three month. In some cases a problem was the extraction of the sponge; vaginal inflammatory diseases did not occur, also no pregnancy has been recorded up to now.

09.14.10

Luteal phase after tubal ligation: Cristofaro, D de, Zancanari, C, Pezzoli, C. Dept. Obstet. and Gyn., City Hosp., Desenzano, BS, Italy

A retrospective study of luteal function was performed in 30 patients sterilized according to *Yoon* (Am. J. Obstet. Gyn. **120**, 132, 1975), in 20 patients sterilized with the Pomeroy procedure (*Bishop, E.* N.Y. St. J. Med. **30**, 214, 1930) and in 20 patients sterilized according to *Filshie* (Brit. J. Obstet. Gyn. **88**, 655, 1981). The corpus luteum activity of the study group was compared with the corpus luteum activity of 30 patients waiting for tubal ligation (control group). The interval between tubal ligation and the progestational study varied in all groups from six months to five years. Progestational activity was assessed by the average value of three plasma progesterone obtained in the period from the fifth to the tenth day before onset of menses. Average value of progestational activity were 21.37 ng/ml (S. D. $\pm$ 5.39) in the control group, 22.87 ng/ml (S. D. $\pm$ 5.46) in the Yoon group, 19.80 ng/ml (S. D. $\pm$ 3.83) in the Pomeroy group 19.95 ng/ml (S. D. $\pm$ 3.47) in the Filshie group. There is no statistical difference between the values of control group and patients after

Yoon ring tubal ligation (p > 0.05), between the values of control group and patients after Pomeroy tubal ligation (p > 0.05) and between the values of control group and patients after Filshie clips tubal ligation (p > 0.05). Luteal phase inadequacy should not be expected as a complication of these types of tubal ligation.

09.14.11
Structural and ultrastructural endometrial changes under treatment with an antiandrogenic monophasic contraceptive (SHB209AE, Schering AG Berlin): Fedele, L, Cavalli, G, Zamberletti, D, Carinelli, S, Candiani, G B. Inst. Obstet. and Gyn. "L. Mangiagalli", Univ., Milan, Italy
Endometrial biopsies were obtained in 10 volunteers between 18 and 35 years old, who had used SHB209AE oral contraceptive during the last six months. The biopsies were obtained at variable times during the cycle: three patients were on the 1st week of treatment, four on the 2nd week and three on the 3rd week. Biopsies obtained from ten normomenstruating women in the same period of the cycle were studied as controls. – Histological findings: We have observed three main types of endometrial patterns: 1. Proliferative; very similar to a normal proliferative phase. However, glandular epithelial cells had ovoidal basally placed nuclei and abundant pale to vacuolated cytoplasm. 2. Early secretory; similar to early postovulatory endometrium. Glands were columnar and epithelial cells had elongated nuclei and prominent supranuclear vacuolization. 3. Late secretory; Characterized by diffuse predecidual changes in the stroma. The glands were tubular with small lumina. – Scanning ultrastructural aspects: After one week the endometrial surface appears finely granular with scanty glandular ostia. A great prevalence of nonciliated cells were observed. During the 2nd and 3rd week, the endometrial surface appears still flattened with scanty glandular outlets. Nonciliated cells are still prevailing, some with secretory activity. The endometrial changes produced by the contraceptive seems to be mainly proliferative during the 1st week of treatment, secretory although with immature aspects during the 2nd and 3rd week.

09.14.12
A technique for continuous measurement of inert (argon) and metabolic materno-fetal gas transfer using mass-spectrometry suitable for non-invasive intrapartum placental function testing in man: Johnson, P, Spencer, J A D, Rolfe P. Nuffield Dept. Obstet. and Gyn., John Radcliffe Hosp., Oxford, UK
Only a limited relationship exists between changes in fetal heart rate and acid base balance during labor. Even measurements of total uterine and umbilical arterial blood flows do not relate directly to placental transfer. A more direct measure of placental function suitable for use in man is being investigated by using the maternal inhalation of argon so that maternal and fetal levels can be measured continuously via two inlets of a mass-spectrometer (MM 880 VG gas analysis, WINSFORD UK). Two minutes of argon inhalation gives a sufficient "bolus" of gas into the maternal circulation so that the fetal transfer in and out of argon can be measured every 15 minutes. This is highly reproducible in steady state situations. In chronically catheterised pregnant ewes the effects of graded alterations in uterine and umbilical blood flows, catecholamine, O_2 and CO_2 levels on placental transfer of oxygen and argon (used as an inert tracer) can be differentiated and related to the fetal condition. The use of this technique using skin surface transducers in normal and abnormal human labor will be shown.

09.14.13
Sonographic preovulatory follicle identifcation in fertile AID-cycles: Neuenschwander, E, Ramzin, M, Tschumi, P, Birkhäuser, M H, Näpflin, S. Dept. Obstet. and Gyn., Univ., Basle, Switzerland
To determine accuracy and failure rate of follicle demonstration by ultrasound a prospective study was planned for a duration of twelve months (October 1982 to September 1983). In 150 patients with a total number of 534 BBT-controlled insemination cycles follicular maturation has been documented by transabdominal ultrasound (Superscan 50 Roche, 2.8 MHz). Insemination was done irrespective of sonographic follicle status. 69 of 74 patients with subsequent pregnancies were controlled by ultrasound; five patients are excluded because no ultrasound was done for different reasons. 39 patients became pregnant in spontaneous cycles, 30 patients in clomiphene stimulated cycles. In these 69 patients we found in 91% (63 patients) an adequate preovulatory follicle, in 6% (4 patients) signs of freshly occurred ovulation. In 36% (25 patients) both follicle maturation and ovulation was documented. Only in one case ultrasound showed an inadequate small follicle, in one other case there was no sonographic evidence of a follicle. In the presented study the failure rate of sonographic follicle demonstration was 2.8% in fertile cycles. In conclusion: The sonographic control of follicle maturation is a safe method to plan an insemination; failure of adequate follicle demonstration allows to avoid unnecessary insemination.

09.14.14
The post-coital test: Time to get it right: White, N, Scammell, G, Edmonds, D K, Jeffcoate, S L. Dept. Endocr., Chelsea Hosp. Women, London, UK
The post-coital test (PCT) is frequently used in the assessment of infertile couples. As the characteristics of cervical mucus change during the cycle, and markedly after ovulation, it is important that these tests are well-timed if they are to be interpreted correctly. In this study 33 PCTs were performed on 24 women. They were timed to coincide with ovulation using temperature charts and menstrual histories. The women also collected early morning urine for seven days up to and including the day of the PCT. These were later

assayed for luteinising hormone and the PCTs judged retrospectively to have been well timed or badly timed (either too soon or too late) on the basis of the results. Cervical mucus was scored on a scale from 0–12, a score of 6 or above being considered normal. In 17 PCTs the cervical mucus score was less than 6, and of these 12 were found to have been badly timed. Three of these patients have had repeat PCTs, in two the repeat PCT was well timed with a score of greater than 6 and in one the repeat PCT was also badly timed, again with a score of less than 6. In 16 PCTs the cervical mucus score was 6 or more, and of these 15 were found to have been well-timed. It is clear from this study that poor timing is a frequent cause of a poor PCT.

09.14.15

Histologic reaction to absorbable and nonabsorbable microsutures in reproductive tissue: Sojo, D, Mistal, M, Diez Pardo, J. Labor. Exp. Microsurg., C.S. "La Paz", Madrid, Spain

To contribute some insight into the selection of sutures in microsurgery of the female genital tract, we have studied the histologic reaction to four microsutures in uterine horn of rats. Under microsurgical condition, polypropylene, nylon, Polyglactin 910 and polydioxanone sutures were placed in the wall of both uterine horns of sixteen Wistar rats. After 7, 21, 60 and 90 days the uterine horns were removed for histological study. All sutures were characterised by a very slight tissue reaction. The differences at intervals of time between each suture will be discussed. – Conclusion: All these sutures could be useful in gynecological microsurgery.

09.14.16

Modulation of the vascular response of the uterine serosa by female sexual hormones; An experimental study: Halbe, H W, Gouveia, M A, Schutze Fo, N. Dept. Obstet. and Gyn., Labor. Exp. Path., Labor. Gen Surg. (LIM-62) Fac. Med., Univ., São Paulo, Brazil

Adhesions are one of the major problems in tubal surgery for sterility. Controversy regarding the use of adjuvant therapy to prevent postoperative adhesions led us to investigate the effect of female sexual steroids on the microcirculation of the uterine horn serosa of virgin rats. Experiments were done using conjugated hormones and their influence on vascular permeability was assessed by the colloidal carbon technique. The results obtained show that estrogen has a vessel protecting effect, and inhibits vascular permeability under phlogistic conditions. Progesterone alone is like controls; and has a counterteffect when associated with estrogen, i.e., reduces the inhibition elicited by estrogen.

09.14.17

Fibrinolytic activity – a challenge for the application of fibrin glue in the female genital tract: Spernol, R[1], Szalay, S[1], Riss, P[2], Dinges, H P[2]. 1. Gebh.-Gyn., Abt., LKH, Klagenfurt; 2. II.Univ.-Frauenklin., Wien, Austria

The use of fibrin glue has become a well established technique in reconstructive surgery. Our own experimental work showed that it is useful in tubal surgery. The success of this method depends on the correct mixture of fibrinogen, thrombin and the proteinase inhibitor aprotinin. An imbalance might lead to excessive scarring on the one hand or to dehiscence due to early digestion of the connecting fibrin clot on the other. Practicable concentrations of aprotinin have been worked out for the reconstruction of peripheral nerves, which have a high fibrinolytic activity. In order to find the optimal relation of the glue components for use in tubal surgery we studied the fibrinolytic activity in the Fallopian tubes, uterus and peripheral nerves using a modification of Astrup's method. The activity was found to be even higher in oviducts and uterus than in nerves. A second series: *in vitro* inhibition of the fibrinolytic activity showed the same results in the three tissues studied. Therefore we can assume that the aprotinin concentrations used in nerve surgery might also be suitable for the sutureless reconstruction of the Fallopian tubes.

09.14.18

The tissue reaction of different kinds of suture material in the uterus and the oviduct of the rabbit: Dörr, P U, Hanselaar, A G J M, Herman, C J, Vemer, H M. Depts. Obstet. & Gyn. and Path, St. Radboud Univ., Hosp., Nijmegen, The Netherlands

To verify whether it is preferable to use nonabsorbable suture material instead of hydrolytic absorbable suture material in gynecologic microsurgery, Ethilon, Proleen and Vicryl 8 × 0 and 10 × 0 sutures were placed in the wall of both uterine horns and oviducts of 16 New Zealand White rabbits. The suture material was placed with due regard to microsurgical principles. After 1, 3, 8 and 12 weeks the uterine horns and the oviducts were removed and examined histologically. The histologic evaluation demonstrated, that the tissue reaction from all suture materials was very small and that there were no differences in the tissue reaction between the three tissue materials used. The tissue reaction to the nonabsorbable suture materials (Ethilon and Proleen) persisted after 12 weeks, while the tissue reaction to the absorbable vicryl disappeared with the absorption of the suture. – Conclusion: Regarding the tissue reaction, there is no clear preference for the use of one of the suture materials, because the tissue reaction of the three examined materials was either identical or very small.

09.14.19

A case of hematometra in a rudimentary uterine horn: Maruyama, H, Sato, S, Yamanobe, M, Hatakeyama, Y. Dept. Obstet. and Gyn., Tohoku Kosai Hosp., Sendai, Japan

Introduction: Previous reports indicate the difficulty in finding hematometra in the rudimentary horn pre-operatively. However, we found such a hematometra in a 13-year-old girl, and we then performed the Strassmann's operative procedure. The result was satisfactory. – The patient was brought to our hospital in January, 1984, with the complaint of increasing pain in her lower left abdominal region apart from dysmenorrhea. She had been suffering with this pain since July, 1982. She had visited many gynecologists and pediatricians, but they could not give a correct diagnosis and treatment. After performing a pelvic examination, hysterosalpingogram and ultrasonography, we made a definitive diagnosis of hematometra in the rudimentary horn. In most cases simple total hysterectomy, or simple excision of the rudimentary horn would be indicated. However, we decided to perform the Strassmann's operation for the following reasons: 1) The unicornuate uterus was small. 2) The rudimentary horn consisted of the cavity with functional endometrium and myometrium. 3) She had normal ovaries and her BBT showed ovulatory cycles. 4) The patient was very young and she would like to become pregnant in the future. As a result of the operation, the unicornuate uterus and rudimentary horn now have become on cavity. At present, the patient has normal menstruation with ovulatory cycle, has no complaint and leads a normal life.

09.14.20

Microadenomas and an empty sella: Krzysiek, J. Clin. Gyn. Endocr., Med. Acad., Cracow

Invagination of cerebral fluid cisterns into the sella turcica space if not of congenital origin may probably be caused by both intracranial pressure changes (tumor apoplexy, necrosis of a part of the hypophysis, intracranial hypertension) and an anatomical predisposing factor such as an aperture in the diaphragma sellae. An episode of the invagination may be clearly established in the history or the time of the appearance may remain obscure (*Valenta, L A*, and *Elias, A N*. Am. J. Obstet. Gyn. **143**, 477, 1982). In 58 patients treated because of hypothalamus-pituitary system disorders a computerized tomography of the sella turcica and radioimmunological estimations of a level of FSH, LH and prolactin were performed, and two groups of a partial and a total invagination of arachnoid space were diagnosed. There is a difference in a percentage of microadenomas between these two groups eg: 67% in the partial and 21% in the total invagination ($p < 0.05$). On the base of histories and clinical observations it seems to be likely that the empty sella might be not only a consequence of a tumor apoplexy, but a pre-existing empty sella may play a role as a predisposing factor in the development of microadenomas. In another 20 patients we observed that such intrasellar changes were connected with complications in the course of a subsequent labor and thus revealing of hypothalamic disorders.

09.14.21

Influence of induced hyperprolactinemia on hypothalamic-pituitary-gonadal function in women: Panidis, D, Vlassis, G, Spanos, E, Georgiadis, S, Papaloucas, A. 2nd Dept. Obstet. and Gyn., Aristotelian Univ., Thessaloniki, Greece

We have studied the levels of FSH, LH, prolactin, estradiol and progesterone in six clinically healthy female volunteers, aged 20–23 years, for two cycles (the first cycle under normal conditions and the second under continuous treatment with metoclopramide in a dose of 10 mg every 8 hours). The purpose of this study was, increasing the prolactin levels, to find out the site to which hyperprolactinemia interferes with the hypothalamic-pituitary-ovarian axis. It was found that induced hyperprolactinemia: 1) decreases the level of FSH in the early follicular phase of the cycle, 2) reduces the level of estradiol in the late follicular phase and the midcycle peak of estradiol, which is late by 24 to 48 hours, 3) decreases the midcycle peak of LH, which is late by 24 to 48 hours, and 4) delays the increase of progesterone in the late secretory phase of the cycle and the level of the hormone is reduced, but this is not statistically significant. Our results support the view that hyperprolactinemia suppresses gonadal function due to a direct effect of high hormonal level in the hypothalamic-pituitary area.

09.14.22

Induction of ovulation with pulsatile subcutaneous administration of human menopausal gonadotropin: Kido, S, Nakamura, Y, Hara, S, Nagai, T, Iida, E. Dept. Obstet. and Gyn., School, Med., Keio Univ., Tokyo, Japan

Induction of ovulation with subcutaneous pulsatile (every 90 min) administration of HMG (Pergonal) 75 or 150 IU/day using portable pump (Nipro SP-3I) was performed for three patients (6 cycles), four first grade amenorrhea (Am-I) patients (7 cycles) and four Am-II patients (4 cycles). All patients ovulated except one cycle of Am-I patient and one PCO women conceived. In regard to the duration of administration and total dose of HMG until ovulation, the administration of 150 IU/day (M ± SD = 15.2 ± 5.0 days, 2280 ± 774 IU) is superior to 75 IU/day (43.6 ± 5.9 days, 4395 ± 682 IU), and there was no significant difference between this method and the daily intramuscular injection of HMG. The group treated with HMG in luteal phase revealed longer luteal phase (14.0 ± 2.3 days) than nontreated group (12.6 ± 1.5 days). Ovarian hyperstimulation was observed in one case and subsided spontaneously after admission. There were no other side-effects. In conclusion, this method has many advantages as follows: 1) high ovulation rate, 2) less painful procedure than daily intramuscular injection, 3) possible usual life work by easy insertion and removal by herself, 4) HMG was previously permitted by government for practical treatment, while LH-RH is still not yet allowed.

09.14.23
Induction of ovulation by pulsatile administration of gonadotropin releasing hormone: Berg, F, D, Hinrichsen, M J, Mickan, H, Rjosk, H-K, Zander, J. I. Frauenklin. Univ., München

Ninety-two patients presenting different forms of anovulation – refractory to clomiphen – were treated with gonadotropin releasing hormone (GnRH). 5 μg or 20 μg GnRH were administered intravenously at 90 min intervals by means of a peristaltic pump (Zyklomat, Ferring) until ovulation occurred. The luteal phase was supported by injection of hCG (3×2500 IU). The patients were classified in three groups: (I) 46 women with primary or secondary amenorrhea and normal testosterone values; (II) 26 women presenting anovulatory cycles with normal testosterone values; (III) 20 women with high testosterone levels and anovulatory cycles or amenorrhea. The highest ovulation rates (97%) and pregnancy rates (60%) were found in group I. High ovulation rates (92%) but only few pregnancies resulted in group II. Eight patients of group III (40%) were refractory to therapy. In the rest of the cases, ovulations occurred occasionally, whereby the proliferation phases during the ovulatory cycles were markedly prolonged. Five pregnancies occurred in this group. – Conclusion: The treatment of choice for patients with normoandrogenemic amenorrhea is the pulsatile administration of GnRH; for those patients presenting hyperandrogenemic anovulation, the most suitable treatment at present is the administration of gonadotrophins.

09.14.24
Follicular fluid protein(s) inhibit rat ovary granulosa cell steroidogenesis: Schreiber, J, DiZerega, G. Depts. Obstet./Gyn., Univ., Chicago, IL, and Univ. of Southern California, Los Angeles, CA, USA

Isolated fractions of human and porcine follicular fluid protein(s) can inhibit ovarian response to gonadotropins. To study in detail the action of these follicle regulatory protein(s) (FRP) on ovarian steroidogenesis, we examined the effect of porcine FRP on the production of estrogen (E), progesterone (P), and 20α-dihydroprogesterone (DHP) by cultured rat ovarian granulosa cells (GC). GC from DES-primed hypophysectomized immature female rats were cultured for two days in serum-free McCoy's medium in the presence of various concentrations of FSH (follicle stimulating hormone) and/or FRP. FRP was isolated from porcine follicular fluid by retention on an agarose gel orange A column. At low concentrations of FSH (6.25 ng/ml), 150 μg/ml FRP inhibited E and P production 70–90%, but had little effect on DHP production. There was a stepwise decrease in E production with increasing concentration of FRP (9–300 μg/ml). FRP was heat labile. A saturating dose of FSH (50 ng/ml) prevented the inhibitory effect of FRP. The inhibitory effect of FRP on E production was reversible. When cholesterol substrate in the form of HDL (high density lipoprotein) or LDL (low density lipoprotein) was provided to the cultured GC, FRP inhibited DHP production 50–90%. In control experiments, FRP did not degrade added FSH and eluates off an orange A column not loaded with follicular fluid had no effect on steroidogenesis. These data are consistent with the hypothesis that FRP is an intraovarian factor which can influence folliculogenesis by altering ovarian response to gonadotropins. Grants HD 00401 and HD 17753.

09.14.25
A comparison between prolactin concentrations and pH levels in follicular fluids aspirated by laparoscopy and ultrasound: Lewin, A, Laufer, N, Rabinowitz, R, Barr, I, Margalioth, E J, Navot, D, Schenker, J G. Dept. Obstet. and Gyn., Hadassah Univ. Hosp., Jerusalem, Israel

The current low pregnancy rate in IVF makes it necessary to repeat the procedure several times before pregnancy is achieved and therefore, we observe the expanding role of the ultrasonically guided follicular aspiration under local anesthesia, as being a reliable, safe and cheap procedure. We compared different aspects of follicular aspiration by laparoscopy and ultrasound and found the latter to be, in our hands, a more efficient method in terms of pregnancy rate. All patients included in the present study had mechanical infertility. Super-ovulation was induced with human menopausal gonadotropins, three ampoules a day starting on day 3 of the cycle. Ovarian response was monitored by daily E_2 and ultrasound measurements of the growing follicles. Human chorionic gonadotropin was given when the leading follicle reached ≥ 17 mm in diameter. Patients were then randomly divided into two groups: one group had laparoscopic follicular aspiration under general anesthesia after inflation of the abdominal cavity with CO_2 and the other had ultrasonically guided follicular aspiration. The effect of both methods on follicular fluid prolactin concentration and pH was compared. We found higher prolactin concentration and lower pH levels in the laparoscopy group as compared to ultrasound. The implication of these results on IVF outcome will be discussed.

09.14.26
Possible role of mitochondrial oxidation in ovulation: Koshida, M, Takenaka, A, Okamura, H, Mori, T. Dept. and Obstet., Kyoto Univ. Fac. Gyn., Med., Kyoto, Japan

To investigate the role of mitochondrial oxidation in the ovulatory process, rotenone, a specific inhibitor for respiratory chain, was administered to PMS-hCG treated immature rats. Its effect on ovulation was examined by counting ovulation ova in the tube. Ovarian cytochrome c oxidase (CYO) activities were studied spectrophotometrically as well as histochemically during the ovulatory process. Rotenone inhibited hCG-induced ovulation dose-dependently, with the complete inhibitory effect at the dosage of 0.5 mg/kg. CYO activities in rat ovaries were significantly activated by hCG. This activation was significantly reduced by the administration of rotenone. The ovulation inhibitory effect of rotenone was confirmed by the presence of ova entrapped within the follicle in serial sections of rabbit ovaries. The intense histochemical activities of CYO and 3β-hydroxysteroid dehydrogenase observed in granulosa cells three hours through 12 hours after the hCG injection were significantly suppressed by rotenone concomitantly with hCG, but those in theca cells were not suppressed. These results suggest that activated mitochondrial oxidation in granulosa cells in response to hCG plays an important role in steroid synthesis and ovulation in the ovulating follicle.

09.14.27

Ovaro-uterine implantation. Experimental study of its application in women: Cognat, M. et al. Serv. Gyn.-Androl., Hôp. Saint-Joseph, Lyon, France

The persistance of hormonal function and of ovulation after intrauterine ovarian implantation is not sufficient to allow fertilisation to occur. It has been proved by microscopic studies that a mechanical barrier formed by the endometrium isolates the ovary from the uterine cavity preventing the expulsion of the oocyte and prohibiting its contact with the male gamete. Experiments on 50 female rats submitted to implantation, some pedunculated and some free grafts enable us to support this assertion. Ovario-uterine implants have no place at present in the treatment of tubo-peritoneal sterility. Fertilisation *in vitro* is already perfectly feasible and much more reproducible.

09.14.28

Oxytocin-like immunoreactivity in the ovary of mammals: Weindl, A, Jaenicke, F, Rust, M, Graeff, H. Dept. Neurol., Gyn. and Anesthesiol., TU, Munich

Recently vasopressin and oxytocin, the classical neurohormones of the posterior pituitary gland, have been detected as intrinsic hormones of several steroid hormone producing endocrine glands. The aim of this study was to elucidate the role of the ovary as a site of synthesis of oxytocin and its related neurophysin in various mammalian species. Ovaries of rabbits, rats and sheep were fixed by perfusion; bovine and human ovaries and corpora lutea were fixed by immersion in formaldehyde, glutaraldehyde or Bouin's solution, and embedded in paraffin. Sections of ovaries and, for control, of the rat hypothalamo-pituitary unit were incubated with antisera against oxytocin or neurophysin for the immunoperoxidase technique. Oxytocin-like immunoreactivity was observed in large luteal cells of bovine and rat ovaries. In some luteal cells of the human corpus luteum oxytocin-like immunoreactivity was present. Oxytocin and neurophysin immunoreactivity was abolished after preabsorption of the antisera with oxytocin or neurophysin, respectively. Preincubation with other hypothalamic peptides such as vasopressin, somatostatin or LRH did not abolish oxytocin-like immunoreactivity. These observations suggest that oxytocin is present in the ovaries of various mammalian species including man. (Supported by DFG grant We 608/7.)

09.14.29

Secretion of gonadotropins in superfused rat anterior pituitary cells: Seki, T, Makino, T, Tanimoto, S, Iida, T, Nakamura, J, Iizuka, R. Dept. Obstet. and Gyn., Keio Univ. School Med., Tokyo, Japan

To investigate the secretion of LH, LH-β and FSH *in vitro*, rat anterior pituitary cells were dispersed enzymatically with collagenase, hyaluronidase and viokase, and then cultured on cytodex beads. After three days, the cells attached to cytodex beads were packed in a small column and superfused. Pulsatile stimulation with 10^{-8} M LH-RH induced marked release of LH, LH-β and FSH. The self-priming effect on either LH or FSH release by LH-RH was not significant; in contrast, a desensitization effect was clearly observed in the release of these three peptide hormones when the cells were superfused continuously with 10^{-8} M LH-RH. The superfusion technique was revealed to be useful in analysing the temporal secretion of the gonadotropins from the anterior pituitary cells, and the data suggest that LH-RH induces both LH and FSH release, and that LH-β is released concomitantly with native LH by LH-RH *in vitro*.

09.14.30

Localization of CRH and cholecystokinin (CCK) in the oxytocin (OX) neuron of the hypothalamus: Ajika, K, Arai, K, Okinaga, S. Dept. Obstet. and Gyn., Teikyo Univ. School, Tokyo, Japan

The distribution of OX, CRH and CCK in the paraventricular and supraoptic nucleus was investigated using an indirect immunofluorescence technique. Sprague-Dawley rats were intraventricularly treated with colchicine 24 hours before sacrifice. The brains were fixed by perfusion with 4% paraformaldehyde. Sections were cut in a cryostat and serially incubated in OX antiserum and fluorescence isocyanate (FITC)-conjugated anti-rabbit antibodies. They were examined, photographed in a fluorescence microscope and subjected to an elution-restaining procedure. A distinctive group of OX-positive cells was observed within the paraventricular and supraoptic nucleus. After elution in acid potassium permanganate and restaining with CRH antisera, it was apparent that a significant proportion of OX-positive soma also contained CRH-like immunoreactivity. After elution of anti-OX which was used as the first antibody, the section was restained with CCK antibodies. Considerable number of OX-positive cells also contained CCK-like immunoreactivity. In general, there were rather more OX-positive than CRH- or CCK-positive cells. After elution of anti-CRH which was used as the first antibody, the section was restained with CCK antiserum. Substantial number of the CRH-positive cells also contained CCK immunoreactivity. The present findings indicate that CRH and CCK coexist in the OX-producing neurons of the rat hypothalamus. It may, however, also be possible that some neurons contain only one of these compounds, or other combinations exist.

09.14.31
Induction of ovulation in rabbits by conjugated estrogens "Premarin (x)": Keçecioğlu, Y. Dept. Obstet. and Gyn., Univ. of Istanbul Cerrahpaşa Fac. Med., Istanbul, Turkey
Premarin has selective morphological effects which are different from other steroids (*Keçecioğlu, Y.*: Die morphologische Wirkung der konj. Oestrogene auf das Ovar der alten weißen Ratten und das selektive Lipschutz-Phänomen. Arch. Gyn. **224**, 1977). This experience was applied on eleven adult female rabbits which were 1900–2000 g in weight. Primarily, one of the ovaries was extirpated by laparotomy. Afterwards 10 mg/kg Premarin was injected into the ear veins of the rabbits; 24 hours after this procedure the other ovary was extirpated by second-look laparotomy. Tunica albuginea and stroma were normal in appearance in the ovaries which were extirpated before Premarin injection, but in others which were extirpated after injection, we found black patches on tunica albuginea, one or more splitting follicles in stroma (ovulation!), fresh corpora lutea and in some follicles, ovum which is surrounded by corona radiata was being separated from cumulus oophorus (preparation of ovulation!). In induction mechanism the increase in concentration of intrafollicular estrogen plays a role (direct effect of steroid), rather than indirect LH-surge (LH-Schauer).
– (x) Ayers Lab. Inc., New York N.Y. 10017.

09.14.32
Early sonographic criteria of ovarian hyperstimulation in the FSH- and LH-RH-treatment of PCO-syndrome: Tschumi, P, Birkhäuser, M, Ramzin, M. Dept. Obstet. and Gyn., Univ. of Basle, Kantonsspit., Basle, Switzerland
Thirty-two women suffering from primary sterility due to clinically and biochemically proved polycystic ovary syndrome (chronic anovulation, elevated serum estron and androgen levels, LH : FSH > 2) were treated with either pure follicle stimulating hormone (i.m.) or luteinizing hormone releasing hormone (i. v., pulsatile) in 48 and 16 cycles, respectively. It is well known that patients with PCO-syndrome are at high risk of hyperstimulation. Follicle stimulation was controlled simultaneously by ultrasound and serum-estradiol levels. The following schedule was adopted: after a pretherapeutic control of ovarian size and structure, ovarian reaction was observed between days eight and ten of cycle. Follicle stimulation was then controlled daily until ovulation could be induced. 18% of FSH-cycles and 6% of LH-RH cycles showed hyperstimulation grade II–III (after *Rabau*, 1964). Early prognostic criterion of hyperstimulation was a polyfollicular reaction (more than five) on both ovaries. High estradiol levels gave supplemental confirmation of functional activity of the observed follicles. Severe or moderate hyperstimulation was not observed in case of mono- or oligofollicular reaction. We thus conclude sonographic observation of early ovarian response to stimulation to be the best prognostic sign of possible hyperstimulation.

09.14.33
IVF ET program in Clamart: 100 first births: Frydman, R, Belaisch-Allart, J, Fries, N, Testart, J. Clamart, France
From April 81 to July 84, 100 alive babies were born in our IVF ET program. During this period 142 pregnancies began, 89 women were delivered of 100 babies (among them 11 twins), three ectopic pregnancies occurred, 22 abortions and 27 biochemical pregnancies (defined by hCG ≥ 20 mU/ml and < to 1000 mU/ml). The high percentage of twin pregnancies after IVF is to be noted and is related to the number of embryos replaced. The follow-up of these IVF pregnancies was compared to the one of pregnancies obtained in infertile women or of the patients being delivered in our maternity in 1983–1984. There is no more complication in IVF pregnancies (no more metrorrhagia, no more eclampsia, no more premature delivery); the proportion of breech presentation is higher in IVF pregnancies, the weight of the babies and the sex ratio are identical but the percentage of Cesarean sections is higher in IVF program. Finally, except for the delivery, IVF pregnancies are very similar to normal pregnancies.

09.14.34
Additional infertility factors affecting *in vitro* fertilization: Lindner, C, Lichtenberg, V, Sprotte, C, Braendle, W, Bettendorf, G. Abt. Klin. u. Exp. Endokr., Univ.-Frauenklin., Hamburg-Eppendorf
In a six-month period in 23 patients in 29 cycles ovarian stimulation for IVF was performed. In addition to tubal factors as a primary indication for IVF (19 patients) 10 women had an ovarian insufficiency and in 11 couples a male factor was present. In all 29 laparoscopies (lap) oocytes were found; the mean recovery rate was 3.7. The correlation between follicle volume and oocyte recovery was: < 1 ml 33%, 1–2 ml 26%, 2–3 ml 14%, 3–4 ml 9%, > 4 ml 18%. According to the different stimulation highest oocyte recovery rate was found in hMG/hCG-cycles (80 oocyte in 20 cycles, $\bar{x} = 4.0$), less in clomid/hCG-cycles (19 in 6, $\bar{x} = 3.2$) and in clomid/hMG/hCG-cycles (7 in 3). Highest fertilization rate was found following clomid stimulation (63% of all recovered oocytes, in hMG-cycles 44%). In 22 cycles an embryo transfer was performed (76% ET/Lap), one chemical pregnancy was achieved. Among seven cases in which the oocytes were not fertilized, in three a male factor was existent, in three cycles laparoscopy was performed after spontaneous

LH-surge, and in one cycle ovarian overstimulation after hMG occurred (12 punctured follicles/11 oocytes). Excluding the three cycles with spontaneous LH-surge in all couples with normal spermiogram fertilization of the recovered oocytes could be achieved (13 ET/13 Lap). Out of 23 patients only five exhibited the criteria of exclusively tubal infertility and normal male function. This reflects our group of infertile couples in whom the majority presents multiple causes for the infertility. Further studies have to be done to prove the effect of IVF in patients with multiple infertility factors.

09.14.35
Study on the correlation between self-priming effect of LH-RH and luteal insufficiency by LH-RH two step test: Fukuoka, K, Makino, T, Ohono, T, Suekane, H, Iida, T, Iizuka, R. Dept. Obstet. and Gyn., Keio Univ. School Med., Tokyo, Japan
To clarify not only the releasing function but the self-priming effect of gonadotropins of the anterior pituitary gland, two-step administration of 100 μg of synthetic LH-RH at a 60 minutes interval (LH-RH two step test) was investigated in 19 women with luteal insufficiency, 13 women in puerperium and just after abortion. In luteal phase blood samples were taken every 30 minutes. Δ_1 standing for hormone release = 1st peak level − 0′ level (LH or FSH). Δ_2 standing for self-priming effect = 2nd peak level − 60′ level. $\Delta_1\Delta_2$ ratio = Δ_2/Δ_1. In luteal insufficiency group, Δ_1 was significantly higher and $\Delta_1\Delta_2$ ratio was lower than those in control group. In puerperium group, Δ_1 and Δ_2 responses were not detected. In aborted group, Δ_1 and Δ_2 were similar to those in control group. This study demonstrated that the LH-RH two-step test was capable of evaluating luteal function by measuring gonadotropins release and synthesis.

09.14.36
Stimulation of gonadotropin secretion during acute and chronic dopamine receptor blockade in amenorrheic patients with insulin-dependent diabetes mellitus: Andersen, A N, Djursing, H, Hagen, C, Petersen, K. Dept. Obstet. and Gyn., Rigshosp., Copenhagen, Denmark
The suppression af gonadotropin secretion in amenorrheic patients with diabetes mellitus (DMAM) may in part be due to increased dopaminergic inhibition of gonadotropin releasing hormone (GnRH) secretion. We have studied 12 patients with DMAM and a control group of normally menstruating women with diabetes mellitus (DM). The study involved assessment of pulsatile gonadotropin secretion, and the gonadotropin and prolactin (PRL) responses to the dopamine receptor blocker metoclopramide (MTC) 10 mg i. v. Furthermore gonadotropins, PRL and estradiol were measured during 10 weeks of oral MTC (12.5 mg per day) in 6 patients with DMAM. Patients with DMAM had a significant reduction in pulse frequency ($P < 0.05$), amplitude ($P < 0.05$) and basal ($P < 0.02$) LH levels compared with DM. DMAM had significantly lower basal ($P < 0.02$) and MTC-stimulated ($P < 0.01$) PRL levels than DM and a significant increase in LH and FSH ($P < 0.05$) levels. Chronic oral MTC caused a significant increase in serum FSH ($P < 0.02$) and PRL ($P < 0.001$), but failed to alter serum estradiol or LH levels. The results are consistent with the hypothesis that DMAM patients have an increased dopaminergic inhibition of GnRH, but also suggest that other factors may be operating.

09.14.37
Biochemical study on the effect of bromocriptine in hyperprolactinemic infertility: Yousef, A A, Heshmat, H A, Nour-El-Din, E. Biochem. and Physiol. Dept., Fac. Med. and Vet. Med., Zagazig Univ., Cairo, Egypt.
Serum prolactin levels are the most important criteria for the diagnosis and prognosis in hyperprolactinemic infertility. We report herewith 20 men with oligospermic hyperprolactinemic infertility. Prolactin values of more than 20 ng/ml were considered as abnormal. All patients were treated with 5 mg of bromocriptine daily for a period of 12 weeks. Measurements of serum prolactin, blood glucose and free carnitine in seminal plasma before and during treatment were carried out. The results obtained showed that bromocriptine decreased prolactin levels to normal values as well as return to normal each of serum glucose and free carnitine in seminal plasma. We can concluded, that bromocriptine is an effective drug as antiprolactin agent in subjects with hyperprolactinemic oligospermic infertility.

09.14.38
Treatment of hyperprolactinemias: Results in 187 women: Cristiani, P, De March, A, Frank, G, Jasonni, V, Flamigni, C. Dept. Reprod. Physiol. and Path., Univ. Bologna, and II Dept. Neurosurg., Osp. Bellaria, Bologna, Italy
187 hyperprolactinemic women, 91 with idiopathic disease (ID), 89 with pituitary microadenoma and seven with macroadenoma were studied and treated between 1976–1984. 170 patients underwent medical therapy: 59 ID, 62 micro and two macro assumed bromocriptine (B); 24 ID and eight micro lisuride (L); eight ID and seven micro metergoline (M). Moreover 17 women, 12 micro and five macro, with a relative intolerance to drugs, underwent trans-sphenoidal selective adenomectomy. The three drugs used were effective in lowering the PRL levels and restoring gonadal function. B determined the normalization of PRL levels in 88% of cases (93% of ID and 83% of prolactinomas), L in 96% (95% ID and all micro), M in 73% (75% ID and 71% micro). Surgical treatment lowered the PRL levels to normal values in 47% of cases (60% macro and 41% micro), and a good response to B therapy was recorded in the patients with a pre-operative intolerance. Therefore we think that medical therapy with dopaminergic drugs, especially B and L, should be perferred in patients with microadenoma, while surgical therapy should be reserved for

the patients who present intolerance to medical treatment. In macroadenoma the medical therapy allows the tumor shrinkage and a good cure rate after the adenomectomy.

09.14.39
Menstruation and prolactin secretion in hyperprolactinemic after bromocriptine-induced pregnancies: Rasmussen, C, Bergh, T, Nillius, S J, Wide, L. Uppsala Univ., Dept. Obstet. and Gyn., Akad. Sjukh., Uppsala, Sweden

Today it is well-known that the risk for hyperprolactinemic women to develop serious pituitary tumor complications during pregnancy is very small. However, there are few reports on the long-term effects of the pregnancy on the prolactin hypersecretion. Here we present the result of a long-term follow-up of a large group of hyperprolactinemic women with at least one bromocriptine-induced term pregnancy. – Patients: 58 women with hyperprolactinemia (PRL 24–1470 µg/l, mean 92 µg/l) and long-lasting amenorrhea (median 5 years) were followed-up after a total of 74 term pregnancies. The bromocriptine treatment before pregnancy ranged 1–48 months (median 6). – Results: A decreased prolactin level after pregnancy (> 50% of the pretreatment level) was found in 20 women. Four of them had become normoprolactinemic. Increased prolactin secretion was found in four women who all had had uneventful pregnancies. Return of spontaneous menstruation occurred in 16 of the 58 women. The pretreatment PRL values in this group ranged between 35–116 µg/l (mean 71 µg/l) compared to 8–85 µg/l (mean 39 µg/l, $p < 0.05$) after pregnancy and lactation. Fifteen women had two-term pregnancies. The prolactin level decreased further after the second pregnancy in all 15 women. – Conclusion: Pregnancy did not make the hyperprolactinemic condition worse. After bromocriptine-induced pregnancy the PRL secretion decreased in 34% and regular spontaneous menstruations occurred in 27% of the women with hyperprolactinemic amenorrhea.

09.14.40
Ultrastructure of involutionary mechanisms in endometriotic implants during dydrogesterone (Duphaston) treatment: Cornillie, F J, Brosens, I A, Vásquez, G. Dept. Obstet. and Gyn., Univ., Leuven, Belgium

Thirteen patients were treated for mild or moderate endometriosis with 20 mg dydrogesterone daily for four months. In seven patients, biopsies were obtained from different endometriotic lesions before as well as after therapy, while in six patients biopsies were taken only after treatment. All specimens were processed for light-optic and transmission electron microscopic study. Before therapy, endometriosis could be confirmed by histology in five of seven patients; after treatment, residual endometriotic tissue was found in eleven patients. Before treatment, the morphology of endometriotic tissues is varied and shows focal proliferation and/or secretion in some implants; cystic glandular change was observed in only two patients. After treatment, only few mitoses or small glycogen patches were seen in endometriotic foci of two patients lacking any involution at the subcellular level. However, in endometriotic foci of seven other patients striking involutionary changes are seen such as glandular cystic change, enhanced lysosomal activity, pyknosis and extrusion of nuclei and/or rupture of the apical cell membrane (abortive secretion). In two patients the ultrastructure of endometriotic tissues was compatible with arrested differentiation but lacking obvious involution. Although the cellular response to dydrogesterone is varied – even within the same endometriotic lesion – thus, progestogen causes cellular de-differentiation and/or involution in 70% of the patients studied. Abortive secretion and lysosomal degradation substantiate this involution.

09.14.41
Possible nidation failure associated with endometriosis and infertility: McGuire, J L, Hahn, D W, Carraher, R, Pasquale, S A. Res. Labor., Ortho Pharmaceutical Corp., Raritan, NJ; UMDNJ-Rutgers Med. School, Piscataway, NJ, USA

We have previously reported on the development of a rabbit model for studying endometriosis and its effect on infertility (Soc. Gyn. Invest. **31**, 159, 1984). Several hypotheses have been proposed as the mechanism causing infertility associated with endometriosis, including sperm or embryo phagocytosis, elevated sperm or uterine prostaglandins, luteinized unruptured follicles and spontaneous abortion. We report here on studies examining the effect of endometriosis on pregnancy, from ovulation through day 14 of pregnancy. Endometrial tissue ($3 \times 3 \times 1$ mm) was surgically implanted in rabbits and allowed to grow for 11 weeks without hormonal supplementation. These animals were artificially inseminated with semen from proven bucks, HCG was administered to induce ovulation and animals were sacrificed and the number of corpora lutea (CL), viable fertilized ova or fetuses counted at 1, 4, 8 and 14 days later. Intact, unaltered does and sham-operated animals (without implants) served as controls. The number of CL and fertilized ova were not affected through day 4. However, on day 8 and 14, a significant reduction in the number of normal fetuses was observed. In other studies where peritoneal fluid from animals with endometriosis was transferred to normal rabbits on day I of pregnancy, a significant reduction in the number of normal fetuses was also observed. These studies suggest that nidation failure due to the maternal environment may be a major factor in infertility associated with endometriosis.

09.14.42
The "Kinderwunschpaß": Boschitsch, E. Leodolter, S. Ludwig Boltzmann-Inst. Erforsch. u. Behandl. weibl. Sterilität, Wien, Austria

The "Kinderwunschpaß" is a new documentation form of diagnostic steps for infertility treatment. Each set of information is copied in triplicate. The original for the medical file and one copy each to the patient, referring physician, and data processor. The "Kinderwunschpaß" comprises:

♀ General history
menstrual history
history of pregnancies
socio-economic status
general status
gynecological status
hormone analysis
functional dynamic tests
laparoscopy
hysterosalpingography
pertubation, hysteroscopy
operations
basal body temperature chart
cervical factor, postcoital test
summary of evaluations

♂ general history
socio-economic status
status
hormone analysis
semen analysis
operations
summary of evaluations

The basic purposes are as follows: to give both patients and doctors identical information providing open and reliable communication; to lead to an efficient management by systematic order and availability of results, thus avoiding repetitions of diagnostic procedures and consequent waste of time and material; to enable, by data processing, analysis of a multitude of infertility factors and plan accurate research work through standardized documentation.

09.14.43
Transrectal and transvaginal ultrasonography in gynecology: Kórzycki, J, Marianowski, L, Jakubowski, W. II Clin. Obstet. and Gyn., and Dept. Nucl. Med., Med. Acad., Warsaw, Poland
The clinical application of ultrasound in gynecology has only limited success. The authors present a new method of sonographic examination in gynecology. It means the visualisation of the pelvic woman's organs while using the rotating transducer (USG scanner Brüel and Kjaer 1846 endosonic probe 1850, real-time system) introduced into the rectum and vagina. Transducer is surrounded by the balloon filled with water. USG visualisation is transverse sonogram in which transducer occupies the central part of the area. The organs are shown circularly with the best visualisation of the vaginal or rectal walls. Endosonic technics give the picture of pelvis with similar depth for the examined organs. There were 31 cases of PCO syndrome presented. The full identity of hormonal and postoperative diagnosis was achieved. The evaluation of the level of the advance of cervical cancer was verified by endosonic method in 14 cases. Histopathological verification confirmed the sonographic diagnosis. The nearness of sex organs from the endosonic probe ensures better visualisation of the pelvic organs than by the transabdominal method. The method presented is useful especially while estimating of the parametrium for the verification of the clinical examination of cervical cancer as well as the diagnosis of ovary and diversity of tumors in the area of vagina and rectum.

09.14.44
Diagnosis of ovulation by steroid hormone analysis in peritoneal fluid: Saracoglu, F O, Aksel, S. Univ. of South Alabama, Mobile, AL, USA
Concentrations of estradiol (E2), progesterone (P), testosterone (T) and androstenedione (A) were measured by radioimmunoassays, in serum and peritoneal fluid collected at laparoscopy from 19 ovulatory women during the periovulatory days of the cycle. Serum LH levels were determined to depict ovulation and peritoneal fluid to serum ratios of E2, P, T, and A were calculated.

Cycle Days	Peritoneal		Fluid/Serum	
	E	P	T	A
Late Follicular (N = 8)	1.4	1.5	1	1.9
LH Surge (N = 4)	301	1024	2.4	2.6
Post Surge (N = 2)	93	145	2	5.6
Early Luteal (N = 5)	22	30	2.9	5.7

On the day of LH surge E2 and P ratios rose to 301 and 1024 then fell to 93 and 145, respectively. T and A ratios rose to 2.4 and 2.6 at ovulation and remained at 2 and 5.6 level post LH surge, respectively. There was a significant difference in E2 and P ratios between late follicular phase (1.4 and 1.5) and early luteal phase (22 and 30). These findings suggest that measurement of serum and peritoneal fluid E2 and P concentrations after the LH surge may provide significant information regarding ovulation and may be used as a diagnostic test to document follicle rupture.

09.14.45

Ultrasonographic evaluation of the developing Graafian follicle and signs of ovulation: Dastur, A E, Shah, N M, Dastur, N A. N. M. Med. Ctr., Bombay, India

The technique of evaluation of the developing Graafian follicle by ultrasonography is described. 540 women were serially examined in 720 cycles. The range of the dominant follicular size as determined ultrasonographically was from 20 to 25 mm. Simultaneous record was kept of the B. B. T. charts and cervical mucus. Two consistent signs of imminent ovulation in the Graafian follicle have been identified using ultrasound. These are a line of decreased reflectivity around the follicle. A correlation of 85% was found with the dominant follicular size, the cervical mucus and the B. B. T chart studies. The rate of follicular growth occurring six days prior to the ovulation was studied and estimated to be 2 to 3 mm per day and a rapid exponential growth in follicle diameter was seen during the last 24 hours prior to ovulation. 125 cycles were stimulated for the ovulation. In 13 cycles no follicular growth was seen whilst in 18 the ovaries showed a typical hyperstimulation phenomenon. Ultrasonography also helps to adjust the dose of ovulatory agents in sequential cycles.

09.14.46

Determination of serum Δ^5-3β OH steroids sulfates by combined HPLC and 3β-HSD in column form and its clinical use: Ohsawa, M, Wu, M C, Nakanishi, T*, Okuyama, S*, Narita, O. Dept. Obstet. and Gyn., *Coll. Med. Techn., Univ., Nagoya, Japan

Δ^5-3β OH steroids [Δ^5-androstenediol (5-A-diol), dehydroepiandrosterone (DHEA), pregnenolone, 17-OH pregnenolone] sulfates (S) are secreted almost exclusively from the adrenal gland. DHEA-S is the principle Δ^5-3β OH steroids sulfates, and is the most abundant adrenal steroid in the blood. Serum DHEA-S, therefore, has been acted as valuable tool in assessing adrenal activity. Here, we described the method for determination of Δ^5-3β OH steroids sulfates consisted of HPLC and immobilized 3β-HSD in column form. Sulfate conjugated steroid was hydrolized by sulfatase and then was determined by the method mentioned above. The chromatographic condition was selected to give a complete separation of standard Δ^5-3β OH steroids. Good separation should be achieved on bilepak column using a linear gradient of water-methanol system as mobile phase. The detection limit of Δ^5-3β OH steroids was about 2–10 ng from calibration curve. The recovery rate of added DHEA-S was $87.7 \pm 2.7\%$ (mean $\pm$ S. D.) with 3.1% of interassay CV. Using 1 ml of serum, DHEA-S and 5-A-diol could be measured simultaneously. Good correlation ($r = 0.920$) was obtained between the values of DHEA-S in serum samples determined by the method proposed here and by RIA. The potential clinical use of serum DHEA-S assay in anovulatory women was studied. Concentration of serum DHEA-S in anovulatory women were significantly higher than in control subjects ($P < 0.01$). The data obtained in this study may also point to a possibility that adrenal androgen excess is a cause of anovulation.

09.14.47

The effects of subcutaneous estradiol implants on ovarian and follicular activity: Montgomery, J, Magos, A L, Collins, W P, Studd, J W W. Dept. Obstet. and Gyn., Dulwich and King's Coll. Hosps., London, UK

Anovulatory doses of subcutaneous estradiol implants, repeated every six months, have been shown to be an effective contraceptive agent (*Greenblatt* et al. Am. J. Obstet. Gyn. **127**, 520, 1977), but the timing of this effect following the first implant is uncertain. We investigated the effects on ovarian activity during the first six months of estradiol implants. Fourteen women with regular menstrual cycles (28 ± 2 days) and pre-treatment evidence of ovarian and follicular activity were given either 100 mg (10 cases) or 150 mg (4 cases) estradiol implants together with cyclical norethisterone to induce regular withdrawal periods and prevent endometrial hyperplasia. Ovarian and follicular activity were monitored using daily temperature records, daily early morning urine collections for estrone-3-glucuronide (E1-3-G) and pregnanediol-3α-glucuronide (Pd-3α-G), and twice weekly real-time ultrasound of the ovaries. The criteria for follicular rupture and luteinisation were biphasic E1-3-G excretion, a fourfold increase in Pd-3α-G excretion and follicular growth of > 10 mm on ovarian scanning. Follicular rupture and luteinisation was demonstrated for up to three months after 100 mg and two months after 150 mg estradiol implants. There was no evidence of ovarian activity immediately following a second implant. This mode of contraception is thus not effective during the first three months of therapy and there is no advantage in using a larger dose of estrogen. We recommend that a second dose of estradiol should be administered after three months, and thereafter at six monthly intervals.

09.14.48

Changes of serum concentrations of androgens, estrogens, cortisol, prolactin and gonadotropins in female life: Tomita, Y, Araki, K, Yamashiro, G, Akasofu, K, Nishida, E. Dept. Obstet. &. Gyn., Kanazawa Univ., Kanazawa, Japan

The concentrations of serum dehydroepiandrosterone (DHA), DHA-sulfate (DHA-S), 11-deoxy-17-keto-steroids (11-deoxy-17-KS), cortisol (F), estrone (E_1), estradiol (E_2), testosterone (T), prolactin (PRL), follicle-stimulating hormone (FSH) and luteinizing hormone (LH) were measured by means of RIA in more than 300 female subjects, whose age ranged from 4 to 86. DHA showed a first significant increment at age 8, ahead of all other hormones. The significant increases of 11-deoxy-17-KS, DHA-S and T occurred at age 9, 10 and 10, respectively. After the significant increments, the concentrations of these androgens except T increased progressively and showed the peak at about 20 years of age which was followed by the decreasing trend with advancing age. However, their patterns had a little chronological difference. F did not show any significant variation with age. E_2 increased significantly at age 11 and gradually until the mature period, then decreased at the forties. In the fifties E_2 decreased at one-fourth or fifth of the matured period. E_1 showed gradual decrease in the climacteric period. PRL increased significantly at age 12 but its concentration did not seem to vary very much with age after 9. FSH and LH started to increase after age 9 with their significant increments occurring at age 10 and 9, respectively. In the postmenopausal period FSH and LH showed more than ten times and three or four times of levels of the matured period, respectively. The significance of the changes of these hormones in the pubertal and climacteric periods was discussed.

09.14.49
Experience with TFL-flap in treatment of vulvar cancer: Wilken, H, Schwarz, R, Kasch, R. Women's Hosp., Univ, Rostock

To cover the large defects after radical vulvectomy or resection of recurrent tumors the myocutaneous flap with musculus tensor fasciae latae is a suitable method. The poster presents the applicated operation method, the care after operation and the results. The method was used in 11 patients with radical vulvectomy and in 4 patients with recurrent tumors. Only in 2 cases there were a larger healing by second intention.

09.32.01
Regulation of liver glycogen metabolism in normal developing rat and in type-II IUGR fetal rat: Cheng, K M, Araki, T, Ogawa, T, Yamaguchi, A, Yoshida, Y. Dept. Obstet. and Gyn., Nippon Med. School, Tokyo, Japan

The total amount of liver glycogen increased in parallel with the weight of liver in the normal developing fetal rat, and a rapid increased in glycogen storage between 20 and 21 days of gestation. However, little is known about the glycogen metabolism in Type-II IUGR fetal rat according to the gestation age. In our present work, regulation of liver glycogen metabolism as glycogen synthase total (I + D)-form, I-form, and glycogen phosphorylase total (a + b)-form, a-form were measured. Type-II IUGR rat was induced by ligating the unilateral uterine artery at 17 days of gestation, as orginally suggested by *Wriggleworth*. The opposite uterine horn was left untouched and served as the normal developing rat. The fetuses were delivered by Cesarean section. The results obtained were as follows: i) The glycogen content did not increase in parallel with the weight of liver in Type-II IUGR fetal rat. The glycogen storage increases begin at 19 days of gestation and a slurred increasing between 20 and 21 days gestation. ii) In Type-II IUGR, activity of total glycogen synthase increased 17-fold, and active synthase rose 35-fold, from day 17 to 21, compared to the normal as 20- and 45-fold. A significant difference of active synthase was noted. iii) In Type-II IUGR fetuses, total phosphorylase development pattern as total synthase with a 14-fold increased from day 17 to 21, and the appearance of active phosphorylase showed a lag period compared to total phosphorylase and did not significantly increase until 21 days of gestation.

09.32.02
Purine nucleotide metabolism in perinatal period: Shimura, K, Miyazaki, A, Fujino, Y, Ogita, S, Sugawa, T. Dept. Obstet. and Gyn., Osaka City Univ. Med. School, Osaka, Japan

With high performance liquid chromatographic (HPLC) analysis of human amniotic fluid using an anion exchange resin, a gradual increase in purine nucleotide metabolites (hypoxanthine, xanthine and uric acid) concentration in amniotic fluid was observed correlating with the gestational age. The metabolic changes in purine nucleotide during the perinatal period were investigated in fetal and neonatal rat liver. Inosine 5'-monophosphate dehydrogenase (IMPD) activity as the key enzyme for purine nucleotide biosynthesis and xanthine oxidase (XO) activity as the key enzyme for catabolism were measured by radioisotopic and HPLC method, respectively. IMPD showed high specific activity in early fetal age and decreased gradually through the perinatal period. On the other hand, XO showed markedly low activity in fetal liver and increased toward the end of gestation. These findings indicate that biosynthesis of purine nucleotide dominates in the fetal period and that the catabolic process is induced rather in late gestational age. To clarify the regulatory mechanism, further investigations were performed on the intrauterine growth retarded rats prepared by maternal three days starvation or by intramuscular administration of dexamethasone (0.6 mg/kg/day, for five days). In the dexamethasone group, IMPD in fetal liver showed lower activity while XO revealed higher activity than in the control group. In contrast, no significant changes were observed in the starvation group. These results suggested that corticosteroid may promote the metabolic changes in fetal liver as well as the fetal lung maturity.

09.32.03
Metabolic, cardiovascular and adrenergic response of the fetus to subacute progressive hypoxia – animal experiments: Paulick, R, Kastendieck, E, Weth, B, Wernze, H. Frauenklin. and Med. Klin., Univ., Würzburg

The object of this study was to quantify the fetal metabolic and cardiovascular response to subacute progressive hypoxia and to detect, at which degree of desoxygenation major alterations of the fetal system are induced. In chronically instrumented sheep fetuses (9 experiments) subacute hypoxia was achieved by gradually increasing occlusion of the maternal aorta. The progressive stepwise decrease of oxygen saturation (SO_2) was approximately 10% during a period of 15–30 minutes. When SO_2 was above 20%, lactate concentration increased by 0.01–0.02 mmol/l/min and pH decreased by 0.0003–0.0012/min. A marked increase of lactate production (0.1–0.4 mmol/l/min) and decrease of pH (0.003–0.016/min) occurred when SO_2 fell below 15–20%. With decreasing SO_2 systolic and diastolic blood pressure as well as pulse pressure increased (maximal increase of mean arterial blood pressure: 15 mm Hg). Fetal heart rate showed a tachycardia in most experiments; however, with rapidly declining SO_2 bradycardia prevailed. Fetal plasma concentrations of free norepinephrine, epinephrine and dopamine exhibited a marked increase when SO_2 fell below 20% with exceptionally high values with $SO_2 < 10\%$. For fetal cortisol, a significant inverse relationship was found ($p < 0.03$, whereas aldosterone did not correlate to SO_2. It is concluded that major fetal reactions to subacute hypoxia including a marked stimulation of the sympathoadrenal system, increase of blood pressure and development of metabolic acidosis, take place when fetal SO_2 falls below 15–20%.

09.32.04

L-alanine transfer and prostaglandin effect in the isolated perfused Guinea pig placenta: Goepel, E, Carstensen, M H, Leichtweiß, H-P. Univ.-Frauenklin. Hamburg-Eppendorf

Placental production of prostaglandins (PG) increases with advancing pregnancy in humans and several animals. Biological importance of this hormone in the placenta is still unknown. The study investigates the uptake of PGs and arachidonic acid (AA) from perfusion fluid and the influence of applied PG and AA on placental transport of the amino acid L-alanine (AL). Completely isolated guinea pig placentas ($N = 11$) were perfused artificially on both sides with a modified Ringer solution. After bolus injections of either ^{3}H-PGF$_{2\alpha}$ or ^{3}H-PGE$_2$ or ^{3}H-arachidonic acid together with ^{14}C-L-glucose, the ratio of both isotopes was determined in the venous perfusates. Uptake and transfer of either the PGs or AL were calculated. – Results: 1) PGF$_{2\alpha}$ uptake averaged 15.8% ± 3.4 SEM at the maternal and 13.8% ± 2.9 Sem at the fetal side. 2) PGE$_2$ uptake averaged 28% ± 5.8 SEM at the maternal and 13.5% ± 3.1 at the fetal side. 3) AA uptake averaged 80% ± 3.8 SEM at the maternal and 78% ± 3.1 at the fetal side. 4) Transfer of PG or AA was less than 5% of load in both directions. 5) Uptake of the isotopes was inhibited by not labelled PG and AA, respectively. 6) When PGs or aa were added to the perfusion fluid in a concentration between 0.1 to 5.8 μmol x l^{-1} the placental transport of AL was reduced significantly in a dose dependant manner: the uptake decreases to 62% and the transfer to 80%. – Conclusion: PGs are possibly involved in the transport of amino acids in the hemochorial placenta.

09.32.05

Effects of ovarian steroid hormones on oxytocin receptor and prostaglandin E$_1$ receptor in pregnant rabbit myometrium: Furuya, K, Nagata, I, Sunaga, H, Makimura, N, Kato, K. Dept. Obstet. and Gyn., Nat. Defense Med. Coll., Saitama, Japan

To clarify the mechanism of parturition, we investigated the localization and capacity of oxytocin receptor (OTR) and prostaglandin E$_1$ receptor (PGE$_1$-R) in the rabbit myometrium in late pregnancy, and examined the effects of ovarian steroid hormones on the changes of these receptors. One side of the uterine horn was removed on the 26th day of pregnancy and the rabbits were then treated as follows: (A) ovariectomy + estradiol propionate (0.83 mg/kg i. m.), (B) ovariectomy + progesterone (5.0 mg/kg i. m. for 2 days), (C) estradiol propionate alone, (D) Trilostane (11-hydroxysteroid dehydrogenase inhibitor) 3.0 mg/kg i.v., (E) no treatment. The residual uterine horn was removed on the 28th day of pregnancy. Binding sites of OTR and PGE$_1$-R were found in a subcellular fraction of the myometrium. This fraction was identified as plasma membrane by marker enzyme assays. In group B, OTR concentration was 3154 fmol/mg protein at 48 hours after the treatment. This value was significantly higher than the previous one (584 fmol/mg protein). In the estrogen-dominant groups (A, C and D), OTR concentrations increased by 2.03–3.78 times on treatment, whereas PGE$_1$-R concentrations decreased by 0.52–0.67 times. In group E, however, OTR and PGE$_1$-R concentrations increased by 1.56 and 1.28 times respectively during the 26th and 28th days. These results suggests that OTR and PGE$_1$-R are regulated by ovarian steroid hormones and that estradiol acts to increase the concentration of OTR and to decrease that of PGE$_1$-R in the myometrium.

09.32.06

Changes of adenylate cyclase, guanylate cyclase and GTPase activities associated with the increase of oxytocin and prostaglandin receptors in rabbit myometrium of term pregnancy: Nagata, I, Furuya, K, Sunaga, H, Makimura, N, Kato, K. Dept. Obstet. and Gyn., Nat. Defense Med. Coll., Saitama, Japan

We have already observed that the oxytocin receptor (OT-R) and prostaglandin E$_1$ receptor (PGE$_1$-R) were localized on the plasma membrane of pregnant rabbit myometrium and they increased in number of binding site toward the end of pregnancy. To clarify the signal transmission mechanism of these receptors, adenylate cyclase and guanylate cyclase activities in the membrane fraction were measured by RIA and GTPase activity was assayed by the release of ^{32}Pi from GT^{32}P and the relationship between OT-R, PGE$_1$-R and these enzymes were investigated. Myometrial samples were taken from the same rabbit on the 26th and 28th days of pregnancy. Membrane fraction was obtained by sucrose density gradient centrifugation. Receptors were assayed by filtration-combustion method. The concentrations of OT-R and PGE_1-R increased by 1.2–3.0 and 1.3–2.8 times respectively during the two days. Adenylate cyclase activity was enhanced by PGE_1 more remarkably on the later day. Altough guanylate cyclase activity was not enhanced by OT and PGE_1, it increased in proportion to the amount of OT-R. GTPase activity increased from 51.3 to 118.4 pmol/sec/mg protein by PGE_1 sufficient to saturate the receptors and to 84.3 pmol/sec/mg protein by sufficient OT. These results suggest that although cAMP and cGMP may be the second messengers of myometrial PGE_1-R and OT-R respectively, the signals of these receptors may go down to the messengers in different ways in late pregnancy and that GTPase has a close relationship with the signal transmission.

09.41.01

Studies on tone quality of initial cry of neonate by computer analysis: Hashimoto, T, Furuya, H. Dept. Obstet. & Gyn., Juntendo Univ. School Med., Tokyo, Japan

The phonic nature of the initial cry is considered to be indicative of the vitality of neonate immediately after birth, since repetition of a lively cry is indispensable to establish pulmonary ventilation for extrauterine life. If the amniotic fluid remains in the airway of neonate, this makes the crying more prone to weak or hoarse sound than when it does not. A new system for quantitative analysis of a power spectrum of neonatal cry was developed. – Method: Neonatal cry was recorded on a magnetic tape with a directional dynamic microphone in a quiet room. The analysis of electrical signals was processed by a mini-computer PDP 11/60, after analog filtering (3 Hz–5 Hz) and converting to digital signals at a rate of 10 kHz. The power spectrum was estimated by FFT (fast Fourier transform) method in every 25.5 msec. The changes of the power spectrum were printed out successively with a printerplotter as a bird's-eye view (three dimensional graph). – Results: The pitch of neonatal cry was centered around 500 Hz, the largest power was found at about 1 kHz and smaller power was contained at the frequency more than 2 kHz. Immediately after birth, if the amniotic fluid was still in an airway of neonate, the power was distributed in broad range between 1 and 3 kHz, and the successive changes were irregular. The clinical usefulness of this method will be discussed.

09.41.02

Heel prick blood gases taken from neonate versus its Apgar score as an index of the perinatal status: Terpou, A, Kapetanakis, J, Tsanakas, J, Papathanasiou, Z, Karpouzas, J. Dept. Obstet.-Gyn. and Pediat., Aristotelian Univ., Thesaloniki, Greece

We have studied the fluctuation of the acid-base balance values among blood samples taken from 50 normally delivered neonates and 70 neonates with various problems during delivery. We discuss the advantages of the heel prick method, and its superiority compared with the Apgar score, in estimating the neonates status during the first minutes of life. Because of the facility, simplicity and rapidity of the method we suggest that it could be a useful and valuable supplementary index of the perinatal status of newborn.

09.41.03

Statistical investigations on skin disorders of the newborn: Kimura, Y, Mukubo, M, Shih, S, Ishihara, S. Dept. Gyn. & Obstet., Sanraku Hosp., Tokyo, Japan

In the newborn skin, various kinds of changes different from the adult's can be seen. The skin disorders are apt to change in a short period, so, the clinical significance of these disorders is still unknown. The subjects are 872 cases suffering from some skin disorder out of 1414 babies born during 33 months. – Method: Observation was made macroscopically in newborns twice a week on the skin of the whole body. – Result: The incidence of skin disorders was 61.7%. The total number of skin disorders seen was 1572 (1.8/baby). Twenty-four sorts of skin disorders were observed, and out of them hemangioma was the top disorder seen in 719 cases (50.8%) including 699 cases of salmon patches. They were dominant in female babies born from multipara, and were seen most frequently in the nasal side of the left upper eyelid, followed by the forehead. The second most frequent disorder was toxic erythema seen in 254 cases (18.0%); this was remarkable in the chest and in the babies born from the multipara, but there was no significant difference in the sex of the newborns. Mongolian patches are said to be specific for caucasoids and the "ectopic" Mongolian patches outside of the sacrum were seen in 139 cases (9.8%). The site was the back, the shoulder and the back of the hand in this order. Milium was the third most frequent skin disorder seen in 97 cases (6.9%). This was most frequent in female heavy-weight babies born from multiparae. Purpura was seen in 87 cases (6.2%) and mainly in the forehead and the inguinal region. This was most frequent in male heavy-weight babies born from multiparae.

09.41.04

An under-utilized, yet accurate means of fetal assessment: Cord blood studies: Johnson, J W C, Gordan, A. Dept. Obstet. and Gyn., Univ. of Florida Coll. Med., Gainesville, USA

Although fetal heart rate monitoring, scalp blood sampling and neonatal Apgar scoring are helpful in assessing fetal status, their limitations have been demonstrated repeatedly. In this study, we examined the utility of umbilical cord blood acid-base studies in fetal evaluation, from samples taken at the delivery of 95 term patients. We assessed the relationships of umbilical arterial (UA) and umbilical venous (UV) pH, carbon dioxide tension (PCO_2), and base deficit (B.D.) to Apgar scores and to intrapartum events (fetal heart rate deceleration; umbilical cord entanglement; uteroplacental hypoperfusion). We found that UApH correlated best with one-minute Apgar scores ($r = +.47$; $p < 0.001$) but the association was modest. Cases of uteroplacental hypoperfusion and cord obstruction were both characterized by UA acidosis ($pH = 7.2 \pm 0.07$) but cases of cord obstruction were differentiated by greater arteriovenous (UA-UV) differences ($\Delta pH = 0.12$; $p < 0.025$). The severity of cord obstruction appeared to be quantifiable by the UA-UV PCO_2 difference ($r = 0.93$; $p < 0.001$). UA and UV blood gas acid-base values are useful non-invasive methods of assessing the condition of the fetus, and of reconstructing intrapartum events. These measurements provide a means of auditing the incidence and severity of fetal acidemia, and of evaluating the efficacy of detection and treatment modes.

09.41.05
Changes in the umbilical venous blood flow of human fetus in labor: Murakami, M, Utsu, M, Kanzaki, T, Chiba, Y. Dept. Perinat., Nat. Cardiovasc. Ctr., Osaka, Japan

Previous studies have shown that umbilical venous blood flow is modulated by fetal breathing movements (*Chiba*, Y. Jap. J. med. Ultrasonics 7, 235, 1980). In the present study, we intended to detect the changes in the umbilical venous blood flow of the human fetus in labor and also in chronic hypoxia and with cardiac arrhythmias. The blood flow velocity in the intra-abdominal part of the umbilical vein was recorded continuously using pulsed Doppler ultrasound guided by linear scanning B-mode. At variable deceleration, the maximum blood flow velocity was decreased by 50% or more when compared with that observed between the contractions. Otherwise at late deceleration, there was little or no reduction of the blood flow, and during the reduction of heart rate, the blood flow, which was generally constant, showed a biphasic pattern synchronized with heart rate (hereafter called "pulsation"). This pulsation was also detected in the cases of fetal 2:1 A–V block and bigemina which showed long QRS intervals and in the cases of fetal chronic hypoxia. From these results it is estimated that pulsation would be connected with the ratio of blood flow to heart rate and with hypoxia. The present study has revealed that the umbilical venous blood flow shows characteristic patterns, for example pulsation, with cord compression and when there is utero-placental insufficiency.

09.41.06
Fetal and uterine blood flow during labor: Fendel, H, Pauen, A, Jung, H. Dept. Gyn. and Obstet., RWTH, Aachen

The Doppler technique allows blood flow measurement in uterine arteries and fetal aorta non-invasively. Using the method described by *Campbell* 1983 the blood flow was measure during labor. Doppler wave-forms of uterine arteries show a low pulsatility. Dependent on the degree of the contraction it is changed to a higher pulsatility. The diastolic flow is reduced gradually. At the top of the contraction the systolic shift is slightly decreased and there is nearly no diastolic flow. In a study of 30 cases during labor the mean blood velocity of uterine arteries amounted 60 cm/sec in between the contractions. It decreased to 30 cm/sec during the contractions. Normally the fetal aortic Doppler shifts does not change during the contraction, but during late decelerations the diastolic flow is reduced to zero in the end. Blood flow in uterine arteries is reduced to 50% during the contraction. An imminent intrauterine asphyxia is indicated by a partial or a complete interruption of the diastolic aortic flow.

09.41.07
IgE-screening of atopic diseases in newborns with an enzyme-immuno-assay: Loos, W, Bauer, C P*, Krebs, S, Graeff, H. Frauen- u. Kinderklin.*, TU, München

The determination of IgE in cord blood (cb) may predict the risk for an atopic disease in newborns (nb). In a prospective study 300 nb were registered. IgE in the cb was measured with an EIA (Phadezym) in comparison to a RIA (Phadebas). The test was modified and calibrated for a detection limit of 0.25 kU/l. The results of both methods were statistically comparable ($p < 0.001$). The geometrical mean was 0.246 kU/l and in IgE concentration of 1.5 kU/l was choosen as the cut-off limit as this was the geometrical mean + 2 SD. The IgE values of healthy nb vary in the range up to 1.5 kU/l with a predictability of 95%. 15 nb with IgE values in cb over the cut-off limit were followed up at the age of 12 months and their mothers completed a questionnaire. There was a statistically significant preponderance of nine male to six female children. Nine children manifested obvious atopic diseases (60%), two probable symptoms of the skin (13%). Symptoms of atopic dermatitis (55%) and food allergy (22%) were common. One child suffered from recurrent spastic bronchitis, diarrhea and vomiting, another showed urticaria and itching when exposed to proteins or synthetic materials. Our data suggest that factors like home animals or tobacco smoking of family members probably increased the risk of developing an atopic disease.

09.41.08
Relationship lactate and acid-basic state in fetus: González, Gómez, F, Navarrete, L, Clavero, P, Gilabert, T, Bueno, M. Dept. Obstet. and Gyn., Univ., Granada, Spain

We made 178 lactate and acid-basic blood determinations in 140 labors. Thirty-eight were made in fetus scalp and 140 in umbilical cord. 71 labors were normal and pregnancy and newborn also normal. We have used enzymo-amperometer method after hemolyzed and deproteinized sample of blood to measure lactate and to measure acid-base state. Lactate concentration significantly correlated with pH and base excess but not with pCO_2 and pO_2. After calculating the normal range (3.9 mmol/l) we found 522 which is the cases proportion where it is over 3.9 in different fetal acidosis kind; 82.8% mixed, 76.5% metabolic and 31.7 respiratory. Furthermore 59.4% of fetuses with Apgar under 7 had pH < 7.25 so long as 96.9% of fetuses had lactate over 3.9 mmol/l. The sensitivity and specificity was related to the Apgar score: lactate: 96.9 and 88.1, umbilical artery pH: 59.4 and 70.1.

09.42.01

Ultrasonography and chromosomal abnormalities in early pregnancy failure: Tsuji, K, Sowa, M, Furukawa, K. Dept. Obstet. and Gyn., Wakayama Med. Coll., Wakayama, Japan

Fetal heart movement (FHM) has been assessed by ultrasound scanning to determine the prognosis of abortion. Chromosome abnormalities were present in about half the number of early abortions. We attempted to determine possible relationships between ultrasonic findings and chromosome abnormalities in early pregnancy failure. In such clinical cases with genital bleeding, FHM and maximum diameter of the gestational sac (GS) were determined by ultrasound. Inevitable abortions were diagnosed by the absence of fetal viability. After curettage, placental tissues were cultured for chromosomal studies. In the karyo-typed specimens, 41/71 showed chromosomal abnormalities. There were 31 trisomies, five triploids, three monosomies (45,X), one tetraploid and one mosaic. The GS sizes were compared in the case of normal and abnormal karyotypes. At eight week's gestational age, they were 34.8 ± 8.2 (mean $\pm$ S.D.) mm in normal karyotypes and 19.0 ± 4.8 mm in abnormal karyotypes (P < 0.05). At nine weeks they were 39.4 ± 15.5 mm and 28.1 ± 6.5 mm; at ten weeks, 37.0 ± 6.6 mm and 23.1 ± 5.4 mm (P < 0.05); at eleven weeks, 43.6 ± 11.6 mm and 27.8 ± 6.4 mm. Therefore, GS with an abnormal karyotype (trisomy) is smaller than in case of a normal karyotype.

09.42.02

Cytogenetic studies on Egyptian couples with habitual abortion: Ismail, A A, Abdel Aziz, A A, Kirsch-Volders, M, Abdullaha, A M, Temtamy, S A, Susanne, C. Dept. Obstet. and Gyn., Al Azhar Univ., Cairo, Egypt; Hum. Genet. Labor., Nat. Res. Ctr, Cairo, Egypt; Anthrop. Labor., FU, Brussel, Belgium

Thirty couples of patients with habitual abortion and 15 normal couples as control were investigated. Conventional Giemsa, G-banding techniques were used. Numerical and structural chromosomal abnormalities were detected in nine individuals, giving a frequeny of 30%. No abnormalities were detected in the control group. Chromosomal aberrations included sex chromosome mosaicism (46,XX/45,X0), autosomal mosaicisms; trisomy F20 (2 cases), trisomy G, structural abnormalities (2 cases); one case with deletion of the long arm of chromosome No. 1 and the other one with ring chromosome No. 2. The last abnormality was detected for the first time among habitual aborters. Balanced translocations were detected in three cases. Among couples investigated females were more likely to be the carrier of chromosomal abnormalities than males.

09.42.03

Spontaneous miscarriage subsequent to ultrasound verification of gestational normality and relevance to chorion villus biopsy: Liu, D T Y, Jeavons, B, Pearson, D, Preston, C. Dept. Obstet. and Gyn., City Hosp., Nottingham, UK

Until the spontaneous miscarriage rate for the population subserved is identified, the exact incidence of interference related fetal loss cannot be calculated for chorion villus biopsy. The miscarriage rate subsequent to ultrasound verification of gestational normality is now known to be less than the 10% usually quoted for this complication in the first trimester. Furthermore, maternal age, her medical history and obstetric background all influence the likelihood of this complication. In addition to establishing the miscarriage rate following ultrasound examination for our studied population, the present study attempts to define the miscarriage rate for each gestation in the first trimester and determine the influence of relevant history on this complication. Our findings which suggest useful practical implications will be discussed.

09.42.04

Immunotherapy in habitual abortion: Taylor, C G, Page-Faulk, W, MacIntyre, J A, Hill, J G. Pembury Hosp., Tunbridge Wells, Kent, UK; Southern Illinois Univ., Springfield, IL, USA

Pregnancy is an example of a successful allograft, albeit on a temporary basis. We have attempted to identify immunological defects in couples with three or more spontaneous abortions and have proposed immunotherapy as a means of overcoming some of these problems. Couples were assessed firstly by using the HLA major histocompatibility system as an indication of genetic similarity and secondly by identifying anti-paternal lymphocytotoxins in the maternal blood. Two patterns emerge – primary and secondary aborters. In primary aborters we consider that the increased genetic similarity between couples weakens recognition by the mother of the new fetal material and this leads to failure of activation of blocking factors and suppressor cells which normally prevent rejection of the fetus. We have demonstrated that antigens on the trophoblast are cross-reactive with antigens on the surface of human lymphocytes and therefore have used infusions of lymphocytes from several random donors with the aim of increasing the genetic variation and restoring immunological recognition. Of the 139 couples, 44 women shared two or more HLA antigens with their partners and were therefore suitable for treatment. Twenty-eight women were treated and have delivered 19 babies. Three women are pregnant beyond their previous abortion dates. There have been five failures. Of the patients who have become pregnant 81.5% have had successful deliveries. No adverse transfusion reactions have been observed. In spite of our success rate, we are aware that there is a high expectation of a spontaneously successful pregnancy following three abortions. We aim to collect larger numbers in our ongoing studies in order to confirm our belief that there is a major role for immunotherapy in the management of recurrent abortion.

09.42.05

Habitual abortion: Blocking antibodies and transfusion therapy: Unander, M, Lindholm, A, Olding, L B. Dept. Path. I, Sahlgren Hosp., Univ., Göteborg, Sweden

Pretransplantation blood transfusions increase human renal allograft survival, and are shown to generate both blocking antibodies and suppressor cells. The antiserum against one group of trophoblast antigens blocks reactions in one-way MLC and cross-reacts with antigens on leucocytes (*Faulk, W P.* Proc. nat. Sci. USA **75**, 1947, 1978). Lack of blocking serum antibodies in habitually aborting women has been described earlier and verified by us (Am. J. Reprod. Immun. **4**, 171, 1983). We have tried to change the immunological response of habitually aborting women by giving them transfusions from third party donors. 54 habitual aborters have received three transfusions with intervals of two months, a leucocyte-rich erythrocyte concentrate from one donor each time. They were investigated for blocking serum antibodies before and after the transfusion series. Of 26 women with primary habitual abortion, blocking antibodies were strong in five, weak/absent in 21. Among 18 women with secondary habitual abortion, two had strong blocking antibodies, which were weak/absent in 16. 5/7 women with strong blocking capacity before transfusions have become pregnant, and all aborted again. Of the 37 women with no/weak blocking antibody before transfusions, none has aborted, nine have borne healthy children, and nine are well into their pregnancies. We think that transfusion should not be given to al habitual aborters, since the group of women with strong blocking antibody contains women with autoimmune disease. We conclude that transfusion therapy seems to be beneficial to the women who lack blocking antibody.

09.42.06

Immunogical aspects of habitual abortion: Houwert-de Jong, M H[1], Bruinse, H W[1], Termijtelen, A[2]. [1]Dept. Obstet. and Gyn., Univ., Utrecht; [2]Dept. Immunohaemat., Univ., Leiden, The Netherlands

The observation that fetal and placental weight of allogeneic conceptuses in mice is positively influenced by dissimilarity in major histocompatibility antigens between mother and fetus, supports the suggestion that HLA incompatibility is an important factor in maintaining normal pregnancy (*A. E. Beer* et al. J. exp. Med. **142**, 180, 1975). Similarly, recurrent abortion could be explained by the inability of the compatible fetus to stimulate immunological enhancement, necessary to prevemt reproductive failure. Although indeed an increased incidence of HLA sharing between couples with habitual abortion was found by some investigators, who as a consequence support the use of immunotherapy (*A. E. Beer* et al. Am. J. Obstet./Gyn. **141**, 987, 1981, *C. Taylor, W. P. Faulk*, Lancet **1981, II**, 68), others could not confirm these observations (*M. R. Caudle* et al. Fertil. and Steril. **39**, 793, 1983). Therefore, 16 couples with three or more consecutive spontaneous abortions of unknown etiology and no children were studied. Compared to controls no increased incidence of HL-A-B-C-D antigen sharing was found in the studied couples. During the observation-period 14 patients became pregnant, 8 pregnancies were uneventful, but six patients aborted again. In spite of the high abortion rate, these results indicate that stronger arguments than HLA compatibility are required to support the use of immunotherapy to prevent recurrent abortion.

09.42.07

Ovarian involvement and surgical treatment in acute and severe post partum and post abortion pelviperitonitis: González del Riego, M, Díaz, J H, Gutiérrez, N B, Recavarren, S A, Ferrufino, J C. Univ. Hosp. Cayetano Heredia, Lima, Perú

A retrospective histopathological study of the genital organs of 40 young women operated upon, due to acute and severe pelvic infection secondary to septic abortion or puerperium, was directed to identify the ovarian involvement in these cases. We found ovaries without involvement (22.5%) other ovaries only had superficial involvement (50%) while some (27.5%) had parenchymal involvement (oophoritis abscess). These findings suggested to us routes for the progress of pelvic infection from uterine site to the ovary; one of them is the peripheral inflammatory reaction due to continuity, and the other systemic, through blood vessels of the infundibulo-pelvic ligaments. According to this second option, we believe that this is an important structure to be examined at the time of operation, in order not to resect a gonad in this young patients, whether the ovary is intact of superficially infected, only if the adjacent infundibulo-pelvic ligament appears to be normal. The resection of a gonad or the preservation of the ovary, was so elected in 26 cases, without finding any significant increment in postoperative morbidity rate nor in the postoperative stay in hospital, among 16 patients with one of two ovaries preserved and ten castrated women. Although, in this first group, pituitary hormonal (FSH/LH) and estradiol blood levels did not vary significantly from those found on normal and intact young women. The functional postoperative recovery of these patients was clinically adequate, comparing the ten castrated patients, who developed an abrupt and multisymptomatic climacteric syndrome and due to hormonal changes.

09.42.08

Septic abortions and maternal mortality rates: Babuna, C, Turfanda, A, Ibrahim, L. Dept. Obstet. and Gyn., Istanbul Med. Fac., Istanbul, Turkey

Among 212,314 patients who attended gynecological clinics of Istanbul Medical Faculty during the last ten years, 182 cases (0.08%) of septic abortions have been studied retrospectively. 29 out of 182 cases (15.93%) of septic abortions had developed endotoxin shock, and nine of them died, giving an incidence rate of 31%. Causes of death in these cases were acute renal failure in two, emboli in three, cardiorespiratory failure in three and disseminated intravascular coagulopathy in one case. The maternal mortality rates due to septic abortion was 4.9%. When the distribution of septic abortion cases with respect to the years has been studied, no statistical difference was observed, and all the cases were found to be equally distributed. No decline in the frequency of septic abortions and related mortality rates were found following the liberalization of abortion law in Turkey. This paradoxal result was thought to be due to the psychological condition of the patient who attemps to terminate her unwanted pregnancy. The sense of guilt in these cases usually pushes them into termination of their pregnancy in secrecy as illegal abortion. The liberalization of legal codes, therefore is not sufficient per se to decrease the mortality and morbidity associated with illegal abortion. The education of women on contraceptive methods, the provision of liberal contraceptive clinics, in other words, the prevention of unwanted pregnancies, we believe would be the most effective precaution for illegal abortion, its early complications and long-term sequelae.

10.02.01

Definition of the beginning of human life: Hathout, H. Dept. Obstet. and Gyn., Fac. Med., Univ., Kuwait

A recognized beginning for human life has more than its philosophical value, for its applied implications are obvious in considering abortion policies, experimentation with early *in vitro* embryos etc. Various opinions include the time of fertilization, implantation, attainment of human appearance, quickening, viability, ensoulment and birth (The Council for Science and Society Report, 3/4 St Andrew's Hill, London EC4V 5BY, 1978). We propose that the stage of human life that qualifies to be called its beginning should fulfill all the following five criteria: (1) it should have a reasonably well defined beginning, (2) it should bear the capacity to growth, (3) its growth would take it up to the further human phases of fetus, newborn, infant, child, adult, aged, if it pursues a normal course (4) any preceding phase to it will not *per se* grow to a human being, (5) it should have the genetic endowment that characterizes the human race in general but also characterizes it as a unique individual somehow different from all other individuals since and until eternity. These criteria *in toto* apply only to the fresh fertilized ovum. It is of interest to note that modern laboratory techniques can diagnose fertilization with a few hours by testing maternal serum for an early pregnancy factor (EPF) secreted by the fertilized ovum only a few hours old (*Y. Cheng Smart, I. S. Fraser, R. L. Clancy, T. K. Roberts* and *A. W. Cripps.* Fertil. and Steril. **37,** 201, 1982).

10.02.02

Ultrasonically guided outpatient follicle aspiration as method choice for oocyte recovery for *in vitro* fertilization: Feichtinger, W, Kemeter, P. Inst. Reprod. Endocr. and in vitro Fertil., Vienna, Austria

Ultrasonically guided follicle aspiration is presented as an alternative method to laparoscopy for oocyte harvesting. The method which is carried out under sedative medication and local anesthesia is described in detail and compared to laparoscopic oocyte pick-up. The success rate of this technique reached in 1984 compared to that of laparoscopic oocyte pick-up was the same: the oocyte recovery rate was 93%, the fertilization rate was 58% and the pregnancy rate was 13% (normal ongoing pregnancies per treatment cycle). Ultrasonically guided follicle aspiration is shown to be superior to laparoscopic oocyte recovery as far as ovarian accessibility and complication rate are concerned. With this technique the whole treatment of oocyte recovery, *in vitro* fertilization and embryo replacement may be performed as an outpatient procedure. We may conclude that only cases where additional diagnostic information is required, e. g. idiopathic infertility and cases after previous tubal surgery remain the only indications for laparoscopic oocyte recovery. The vast majority of oocyte harvesting should be performed by ultrasonically guided follicle aspiration.

10.02.03

Pure FSH for ovulation stimulation and in an IVF program: Frydman, R, Belaisch-Allart, J, Testart, J.

The object of ovulation stimulation in an IVF programme is to obtain a high number of mature oocytes, a well developed endometrium and a good luteal phase. Can all these conditions be achieved by the use of pure FSH? In a random study we have compared the results obtained with FSH with the one obtained associating clomifene citrate and hMG that we have used since 1982. Fifty cycles FSH was adminstered according to two protocols (3 ampoules on days 2, 3, 4 of the cycle and then 2 ampoules on 5, 6, 7 – or 2 ampoules in the morning and 2 in the evening from day 2 to day 9). The puncture is performed by laparoscopy or ultrasonically guided puncture. In our first results the number of follicles punctured, of oocytes and embryos obtained were higher with FSH stimulation than with Cld + hMG stimulation, the pregnancy rates by transfer or by puncture were equally higher with FSH, but on the other hand, we noticed a shortening of the luteal phase. Moreover the increase in the number of oocytes obtained helps in the development of freezing techniques.

10.02.04

Gonadotrophin stimulation for oocyte collection and *in vitro* fertilization: Mettler, L, Michelmann, H W, Riedel, H-H, Grillo, M, Semm, K. Dept. Obstet. and Gyn., Univ., Kiel

With the purpose of pelviscopic collection of mature oocytes for *in vitro* fertilization and embryo transfer in a special collective of sterility patients hMG/hCG-stimulation and pure FSH/hCG-stimulation schemes are compared. The endogenous E_2-levels and endogenous LH-levels from day 2 of the cycle on till the time of oocyte collection were compared with the different types of stimulation. It became evident that mature eggs leading to fertilization and consecutive pregnancies after embryo transfer were only collected if basic LH-levels remained below $10\,IU/ml$ and E_2-levels showed a continuous rise still the time of hCG administration. HMG and FSH respectively were given in descending dosages from day 2 of the cycle onwards. The endocrine curves of the evaluated 20 pregnancies demonstrated, that an optimal response was achieved with continuous rising and low LH-levels. No pregnancy occurred when early LH peaks were observed and in cases were hCG was given on the already descending estradiol curve. Thus in contradiction to the increased hMG dosages so far given for oocyte maturation *in vivo*, with *in vitro* fertilization the cohort of follicles seems to be better stimulated with early high dosages of hMG. This may, in the long run, also be the better stimulated schedule for *in vivo* fertilization and consecutive pregnancy.

10.02.05

Hormonal profile of follicular fluid related to the *in vitro* fertilization of human oocytes: Reinthaller, A, Deutinger, J, Müller-Tyl, E, Riss, P, Bieglmayer, C, Fischl, F, Janisch, H. 2nd Dept. Obstet. and Gyn., Univ., Vienna, Austria

The hormonal profile of follicular fluid of 28 fertilized and 24 not fertilized oocytes was analyzed. The follicular fluid and oocytes were obtained by laparoscopy for *in vitro* fertilization. Levels of estradiol, testosterone, progesterone, prolactin, PGF 2alpha, PGE, collagenolytic activity and protein concentration of follicular fluid samples were estimated. We compared the hormonal characteristics of follicular fluid in correlation to the *in vitro* fertilization of the obtained oocytes. No significant difference between fertilized and not fertilized oocytes in regard to the follicular fluid volume could be observed. Levels of estradiol, PGF 2alpha, PGE and protein concentration were approximately equal in both groups. Collagenolytic activity was constantly increased in the group of fertilized oocytes, although no significant difference could be observed $(7.7\pm1:13.1\pm3.6$ arbitr. units). Follicular fluid of fertilized oocytes showed a significant decrease of testosterone $(4.99\pm0.72:7.24\pm0.86\,ng/ml)$ and prolactin $(22.6\pm2:33.3\pm5.1\,ng/ml)$ levels compared to the group of not fertilized oocytes. Progesterone levels were significantly increased in cases of fertilization $(8.54\pm1.04:6.55\pm0.56\,ng/ml)$. Our results show, that follicular fluid progesterone, testosterone and prolactin levels are associated with the oocyte cleavage rate and therefore may represent predictive factors for a successful *in vitro* fertilization of human oocytes.

10.02.06

Thermodynamics of frozen-thawed hamster and human embryos: Hafez, E S E. Reprod. Hlth Ctr, Kiawah Island, SC, and Med. Univ. of South Carolina, Charleston, SC, USA

Various thermodynamic factors affected survival rate of hamster and human embryos; physiological and biophysical characteristics and developmental stage of embryos; time interval and *in vitro* treatment from embryo collection to initiation of cryopreservation; type of computerized freezers and program of cryopreservation; osmotic shock during various steps of cryopreservation; number of embryos in each straw; percentage of serum albumin in Dulbecco phosphate buffer solution; exposure of embryos to excessive light during microscopic examination; crystalloid and colloid osmotic pressures of fluids, prepared media and cryoprotectants, nature and extent of "seeding" and "plunging", possible microbiological contaminants in glassware, freezing, and storage, liquid nitrogen tanks; faults of the freezer, computer, or the operator; and nature and hormonal synchrony of the recipient upon embryo replacement. "Minor", "major", "inconsequential", and "multiple" anomalies were noted in embryos after cryopreservation. A computerized grading system of frozen-thawed embryos, has been based on morphology of blastomeres, vitellus, extruded debris, cellular membranes, perivitelline space and zona pellucida.

10.02.07

The day of embryo transfer (ET) does not affect the achievement of pregnancy after human *in vitro* fertilization (IVF): Tarlatzis, B C, DeCherney, A H, Russell, J B, Boyers, S P, Naftolin, F. Dept. Obstet. and Gyn., Yale Univ., School Med., New Haven, CT, USA

The achievement of pregnancy after IVF/ET depends greatly on successful embryo implantation in a receptive endometrium. After IVF embryos are transferred to the uterus $1-2$ days earlier than after *in vivo* fertilization. In this study we examined the effect of ET day on the pregnancy outcome after IVF/ET. Ovarian stimulation by hMG was initiated in 142 cycles. HCG was given when at least two follicles $>1.5\,cm$ were seen on ultrasonography and serum E2 levels were $>500\,pg/ml$ (day 0). Patients were dropped if E2 was $<500\,pg/ml$ and/or decreased markedly after hCG. Serum E2 on day 0 was $882\pm42\,pg/ml$ and increased to $1109\pm53\,pg/ml$ after hCG injection. A total of 103 laparoscopies were performed, 746 follicles were aspirated (7.2 follicles/woman) and 598 oocytes were retrieved (5.8 ova/woman). The fertilization rate was 61% and the cleavage rate 89.6%. A mean of 3.5 embryos/woman were transferred in 92 patients. From them, 40 were randomly selected to have ET on day $+4$ and 35 on day

+5. Overall 15 women conceived; six (40%) miscarried and one had an ectopic pregnancy. The pregnancy rate per laparoscopy was 14.6% and per transfer 16.3%. Seven women (17.5%) conceived in the day +4 ET group and four (11.4%) in the day +5. Two (29%) miscarried in the former group and three (75%) in the latter. We conclude that ET on day +5 does not seem to offer any advantage over the usual day +4, since it had no impact on the pregnancy outcome after IVF. (B.C.T. is a Lalor Foundation Fellow.)

10.02.08
Gamete intrafallopian transfer (GIFT) as a therapy for infertility: Balmaceda, J, Ellsworth, L, Wong, P, Asch, R. Dept. Obstet. and Gyn., Univ. of Texas Hlth Sci. Ctr, San Antonio, TX, USA
The development of *in vitro* fertilization and embryo transfer as techniques for treatment of infertile couples has improved markedly the ability to obtain mature oocytes and prepare adequate sperm samples. We have successfully utilized the transfer of oocytes and sperm into the fallopian tube, as therapy for infertility. To date, ten couples with infertility (average duration 5.3 years) have undergone GIFT. Women received human menopausal gonadotropin (FSH 150 IU, LH 150 IU daily) from day 3 until at least two 16 mm follicles were visualized by pelvic ultrasound. At that time hCG 10,000 IU IM was administered and laparoscopy for follicular aspiration was performed 36 hours later. Oocytes recovered were assessed for maturity under a microscope. Semen collected two hours before surgery was prepared in Ham's F-10 plus 10% fetal cord serum. Oocytes (1 or 2) and sperm (approximately 100,000) were loaded sequentially, in a catheter and transfered to the ampulla by introducing the catheter through the fimbriated end. Pregnancies were documented using serum β hCG and ultrasound determinations. Of this first series, four patients had serum hCG levels compatible with pregnancies. One is a twin gestation at 34 weeks, a second one is single gestation at 10 weeks. Early pregnancy loss occurred in the other two patients. These results suggest that an alteration in gamete transport mechanisms is involved in some cases of infertility and that GIFT may represent an adequate therapeutic technique.

10.02.09
Induced dichronous delivery of triplets: Brökelmann, J, Diedrich, K, Hansmann, M, Trotnow, S. Univ.-Frauenklin., Bonn and Erlangen
After premature birth of the first triplet, we successfully delayed the delivery of the remaining triplets for 21 days until the 29th week of gestation. The 36-year-old patient from Uganda had spontaneously delivered a girl of 4000 g in 1973. Thereafter she had lost both Fallopian tubes after tubal pregnancies. In July 1984, five embryos, fertilized *in vitro*, were transferred into her uterus. Three embryos implanted as was ultrasonographically diagnosed in the seventh week of gestation. In the 26th week, despite tocolysis, premature labor led to the spontaneous delivery of a 740 g female fetus who died two days later. Immediately after delivery a cerclage was performed under halothane anesthesia. Under intravenous tocolysis and antibiotics, pregnancy progressed and the remaining fetuses showed normal growth ultrasonographically. Premature rupture of membranes of the second triplet occurred in the 28th week. In the 29th week a Cesarean section had to be performed because of uncontrollable contractions and threatened asphyxia of the second triplet. Both infants were female, 1100 g and 1150 g; they have both survived so far without handicaps.

10.02.10
Sperm-quality and success of in vitro fertilization: Diedrich, K, Ven, H v. d., Al-Hasani, S, Krebs, D. Dept. Obstet. and Gyn., Univ., Bonn
Due to the improvement in the conditions of *in vitro* fertilization and embryo culture, appreciable advances recently have been made in this area. For this reason the attempt was made to extent the indication for *in vitro* fertilization and to find new approaches for the treatment of idiopathic, andrological and immunological sterility. In our *in vitro* fertilization program semen analysis was carried out on 490 patients. Of these nearly 70% were able to fertilize at least one preovulatory oocyte *in vitro* and an embryo transfer could be performed. Although, it must be emphasized that of the 57 pregnancies achieved so far after *in vitro* fertilization, 43 were induced by ejaculates from normospermic men. Only in eight cases could a slight reduction in the percentage of motile spermatozoa be discerned. Conventional aspects of semen analysis (sperm count, motility, volume, morphology) and tests of sperm function (sperm swelling-test, zona-free hamster-ova-penetration-test) were performed and compared with the ability of the spermatozoa to fertilize the human oocyte *in vitro*. There was only poor correlation between the fertilization rates of human sperm *in vitro* and any of the standard features of semen analysis. A much better correlation could be observed between the fertilization-rate and the ability of human spermatozoa to swell in hyposmotic medium. The results suggest that this functional test may be useful to assess the fertilizing potential of spermatozoa and to select male patients for *in vitro* fertilization therapy.

10.02.11
The significance of sperm bacteriology for the *in vitro* fertilization of human and mouse oocytes: Langenbucher, H, Riedel, H-H, Mettler, L. Dept. Obstet. and Gyn., Univ., Kiel
Evaluating ejaculates of husbands of patients participating in our *in vitro* fertilization program, we found bacteria concentrations of more than 100,000/ml, i.e. results making treatment mandatory, in about 50% of the samples in 1983 as well as in 1984. 1982/1983 we found no difference in the fertilization rates when inseminating human oocytes with ejaculates free of bacteria or containing bacteria. However, all the

pregnancies obtained so far have only been produced with bacteria-free sperm. In the mouse oocytes system, after incubation of the spermatozoa with various concentrations of Ureaplasma urealyticum or E. coli, we found no difference in the fertilization rates obtained, as opposed to the results of *Frazer* and *Taylor-Robinson* (1977). However, using spermatozoa incubated with Ureaplasma urealyticum as well as E. coli, we saw a marked reduction in culture rates. The deficiencies in embryonic development were significantly correlated with the bacteria concentrations added to the incubation medium. Furthermore, we investigated whether repeated washing of the spermatozoa or the addition of streptomycin to the incubation medium had an effect on the obtained fertilization and embryo culture rates. We found no correlation between bacteriological status of the ejaculates of our patients, sperm cytology, and andrological diagnosis. The bacteria found most frequently were T-mycoplasmas (Ureaplasma urealyticum), Anaerobes and Enterococci.

10.02.12

The problems of cost- and psychosocial stress in an *in vitro* fertilization program: Mao, K, Wood, C. Monash Epworth IVF Unit, Queen Victoria Med. Ctr, Melbourne, Vic., Australia
A survey was made of 121 patients who withdrew from an *in vitro* fertilization and embryo transfer program, and the reasons leading to withdrawal were solicited by a questionnaire. The must common reasons stated by the 91 patients who returned the survey questionnaires were the heavy financial burden and psychosocial stresses that accompanied treatment. Seventy per cent of these patients expressed a desire to re-enter the programme at a later date.

10.02.13

Ultrastructural evidence of microchannels for sperm penetration within the zona pellucida of human oocyte: Cho, D J, Kim, M H, Schmidt, G E, Friedman, C I, Miller, F. Dept. Obstet. and Gyn., Ohio State Univ., Columbus, OH, USA
Human oocytes obtained at the time of laparoscopy, and those obtained for *in vitro* fertilization but failing to undergo cleavage were evaluated by scanning electron microscopy. The morphology of the outer, inner and perpendicularly-cut surface of the human zona pellucida (ZP) was studied before and after hyaluronidase treatment. The outer surface of zona pellucida revealed pores, and it was covered by a thin layer of mucoid material which could be removed with hyaluronidase. Relatively larger pores were demonstrated on the inner surface of the zona pellucida with uniform particulation. The perpendicularly-cut surface of the zone pellucida revealed branching channels connecting the outer and inner pores through zona pellucida. These microchannels were variable in size and course of their directions. Studies of the oocytes having been exposed to spermatozoa in failed IVF demonstrated more than one spermatozoon penetrating through this same pore. The findings confirm the presence of intrazonal microchannels, which may be of importance as a facilitated pathway for sperm penetration in the fertilization process, for transport of nutrients and metabolites of the oocytes.

10.03.01

Primary and reactivated Epstein-Barr virus infection in pregnant women: Costa, S, Terzano, P, Zerbini, M, Gentiloni, G. Musiani, M. II Dept. Obstet. and Gyn., and Inst. Microbiol., Univ., Bologna, Italy
One hundred and two pregnant women were examined on delivery for the presence of primary and reactivated infections due to Epstein-Barr virus (EBV). In the mothers' and cord blood sera, serological signs of primary or reactivated EBV infection were evaluated by the presence of antibodies against EBV-induced viral capsid antigens (VCA), early antigens (EA) and EB nuclear antigens (EBNA), following the criteria stated by *Fleisher* and *Bolognese* (J. infect. Dis. **145**, 537, 1982). A great number of reactivations occurred in patients who were over 30 years (71%), while in patients under 20 years, reactivation occurred only in 11%. The two mothers with primary infection were 19 and 20 years old, respectively. Newborn babies from mothers with serological signs of a reactivated EBV infection did not show clinical signs of birth defects up to one year from the date of birth, while out of the two babies born from mothers with evidence of a primary active EBV infection, one showed a mild congenital defect (epispadias).

10.03.02

Placental transfer of neutralizing antibodies to herpes simplex virus (HSV): Harger, J, Guevarra, L, Armstrong, J. Dept. Obstet. and Gyn., Magee-Womens Hosp., Pittsburgh, PA
Although humoral immunity to HSV does not confer complete protection, it modifies the severity of initial and recurrent HSV infections. Some evidence indicates that higher titers of transplacental anti-HSV antibody in neonates are associated with more favorable outcomes of neonatal HSV infection (*Yeager* et al. Infect. Immun. **29**, 532, 1980). To determine whether maternal anti-HSV titers are predictive of neonatal titers, we measured the activity of neutralizing antibodies against HSV-1 and HSV-2 in 36 pregnant women with culture-proven genital HSV infection and in their neonates at birth. Anti-HSV antibody was assayed by plaque-reduction in VERO cells with HSV-1 and HSV-2. The neutralizing titer was graphically estimated as the dilution of serum that reduced the number of plaques by 50%. Geometric mean titer against HSV-1 was $1:1226$ in maternal serum versus $1:1580$ in cord serum ($p<0.01$), and against HSV-2 was $1:168$ in maternal serum versus $1:229$ in cord serum ($p<0.0005$). Log-log plots show 31/36 (86.1%) fetal

sera had titers $\geq$ corresponding maternal titers against HSV-1 (r = 0.92, p < 0.0005). Against HSV-2, 33/36 (91.7%) fetal sera had titers $\geq$ corresponding maternal titers (r = 0.82, p < 0.0005). In most cases, active transport of anti-HSV antibody results in fetal titers predictably higher than maternal titers.

10.03.03
The problem of rubella during pregnancy in Saudi Arabia: Basalamah, A H, Serebour, F E, Abbas, S, Afonso, R, Al-Amoudi, S. King Abdulaziz Univ. Hosp., Jeddah, Saudi-Arabia

At about 100 deaths per 1000 live births in 1982, Saudi Arabia has one of the highest infant mortality rates in the Middle East. This is in the face of a high per capita income which puts the country as one of the wealthiest in the world. Of the many factors that contribute to infant mortality, viral infections during pregnancy or immediately postpartum has been addressed as a major contributor. Among these is primary maternal rubella infection and the consequent fetal involvement. Using ELISA IgG to determine maternal rubella immunity, 2250 samples from seven centres in various regions were examined. ELISA IgM specific for rubella on elevated cord IgM (total) samples to determine congenital rubella was tested. We found maternal immunity to range from 86.4% in Tabook (north) to 95.4% in Hofuf (east). The mean for the country was 89.5%. Fourteen of 1810 elevated IgM samples showed reactivity to specific IgM to rubella virus. Classical rubella syndrome was noted amongst some of the newborns. We concluded that despite a lack of national vaccination schemes for rubella, most Saudi women have been exposed to the "wild virus" and have immunity by adulthood. The susceptible pregnant mothers are at high risk of contracting rubella. Recommendation for active vaccination should consider the geographical, religious and sociological problems. Only high-risk groups should be immunized against rubella.

10.03.04
Infection rate in mothers and infants after prevention of RDS (respiratory distress syndrome) with betamethasone and ambroxol: Luerti, M, Casolati, E, Rossi, G, Zavattini, G. IV Dept. Obstet. and Gyn., Univ., Milan, Italy

A three-year multicentric randomized study was performed to evaluate the effectiveness of ambroxol versus betamethasone in the prevention of RDS. The incidence of RDS was 31.3% in the betamethasone group and 13.2% in the ambroxol group (p < 0.05). During the study an investigation about the incidence of both neonatal and maternal puerperal infections was performed. The diagnosis of neonatal and maternal infection was based upon the presence of fever 37.5° C, positive cultures, clinical and radiographic evidence of infective pathology. In the betamethasone group 21 babies (21%) developed infections and 3 died. In the ambroxol group 14 babies (10%) developed infections and 1 died. The difference between the two groups was significant (p < 0.025). In the betamethasone group the mean gestational age of infected newborns was significantly lower than that of not infected ones (226.17 $\pm$ 23.6 vs 246.55 $\pm$ 23.7, p < 0.005) while in the ambroxol group this difference was not significant (243.5 $\pm$ 17.5 vs 249.17 $\pm$ 21.3). Moreover the treatment to delivery time in infected babies was significantly lower in the betamethasone group (13.5 $\pm$ 19.5) than in the ambroxol group (20.3 $\pm$ 23.8) (p < 0.005). On the contrary the incidence of maternal puerperal infections was similar in the betamethasone (31 cases, 32.9%) and in the ambroxol (48 cases, 36%) groups (p = N.S.). – In conclusion, it is possible that betamethasone may have a role in promoting neonatal bacterial infections, especially in very low gestational age infants. This could be mediated by a reduced phagocytic, chemotactic and killing capacity of polymorphonuclear leucocytes, as shown by the results of our previous studies.

10.03.05
A sixteen-year follow-up of bacteriuria in pregnancy: Birch, C, Fischer-Rasmussen, W, Vejlsgaard, R. Inst. Med. Microbiol., Univ., Copenhagen, Denmark

In a consecutive study of 2122 pregnant women in 1966/67, 182 (8.6%) were found to have significant bacteriuria (1). This present study is a follow-up of these 182 women. The control group consist of 182 women with sterile urine in the same investigation. We got in touch with 119 women of the bacteriuria group (B) and 104 women of the control group (C). A questionnaire and a urine-agar culture were sent to those women. 88 (73.9%) women from B returned the questionnaire, 85 the urine culture. In C the numbers were 75 (72.1%) and 66. The actual bacteriological investigation demonstrated that 31 (35.2%) of B and 19 (25.3%) of C had significant bacteriuria at present. 63 (71.6%) women of B and 24 (32.0%) women of C reported symptoms of urinary tract infection once or more since 1966/67. Eight (9.1%) women of B reported hematuria once or more since 1966/67. Only one (1.3%) woman of C reported this symptom. Respectively 6 (6.8%) and 5 (6.7%) in the two groups reported hypertension. Nine (10.2%) of the women in B had been treated in hospital for urinary tract diseases. The number in C was three (4.0%). With regard to mortality eight individuals of B and one of C died during the period of observation. However, in no case could the cause of death be associated with any kidney disease or urinary tract infection. It is concluded that screening of bacteriuria in pregnancy may not be recommended in view of the late prognosis. – (1) *Fischer-Rasmussen, W & Vejlsgaard, R.*: Bakteriuri og graviditet, Ugeskr. Læg. **134**, 2000–2007 (1972).

10.03.06

Bacterial colonisation of various sites at birth of babies born in Zaria, Nigeria: Ekwempu, C C, Lawande, R V, Egler, L J. Depts. Obstet. and Gyn., and Microbiol., Ahmadu Bello Univ. Teaching Hosp., Zaria, Nigeria

Because of the high perinatal mortality in Zaria from early neonatal infection some of which began within 24 hours of birth, microbiological studies were carried out on newborns at Ahmadu Bello University Hospital Zaria for bacterial colonisation at various sites: throat (162), skin (161), umbilicus (166), external ear (159), rectum (164), meconium (62), gastric aspirate (116). In all, 17 genera of microbes were isolated from the various sites. The skin showed the highest degree of colonisation (68.94%) while the rectum was the least colonised (5.48%). Predominant organisms colonising the throat, skin, umbilicus and external ear were Gram-negative bacilli, commonest being Escherichia coli and Klebsiella sp. Gram-positive organisms colonised relatively few babies. Candida albicans was predominantly isolated from the throat, external ear, umbilicus and skin. Coliforms were also isolated from gastric aspirates, rectum and meconium. Pathogens such as Salmonella paratyphi and Shigella dysenteriae were recorded in a few instances. The level of microbial colonisation found in the study suggests that the high perinatal mortality from infection observed in Zaria may be due to the fact that babies are born with infections acquired in utero.

10.03.07

Vaginal pH and Papanicolaou smear as screening tools for vaginal flora and pregnancy outcome: Grunebaum, A, Minkoff, H, Feldman, J, Cummings, M, McCormack, W M. Downstate Med. Ctr, Brooklyn, NY, USA

Prematurity is the major cause of perinatal morbidity in the United States. No simple screening tests are currently available to detect carriers of organisms suspected of playing a role in the etiology of preterm labor. We report here on the use of cervical Papanicolaou smears and vaginal pH as screening tests. Vaginal flora cultures, Papanicolaou smears, and vaginal pH measurements were performed at the first antepartum visit in 231 patients. Patients with a vaginal $pH \geq 4.4$ were significantly more likely than patients with a $pH < 4.4$ to be carriers of Trichomonas vaginalis ($p < 0.03$), Bacteroides sp. ($p < 0.01$), and Mycoplasma hominis ($p < 0.001$). Patients with a vaginal $pH \geq 4.4$ were also significantly more likely to have premature rupture of the membranes ($p < 0.01$), and preterm rupture of the membranes ($p < 0.05$). Patients with atypia reported on Papanicolaou smear more frequently carried M. hominis ($p < 0.01$), and had premature rupture of the membranes ($p < 0.01$) than patients without atypia. Patients with inflammation reported on Papanicolaou smear carried Trichomonas vaginalis ($p < 0.01$) and Enterobacteriaceae ($p < 0.01$) significantly more often than patients without inflammation on Papanicolaou smear. Our results indicate that a high vaginal pH and atypia on Papanicolaou smear help identify patients with alterations in vaginal flora and a predisposition to premature rupture of membranes.

10.03.08

The vaginal flora of Irish pregnant women: Vaughan, J, MacDonald, D. Nat. Maternity Hosp., Dublin, Ireland

No satisfactory up to date study of the vaginal flora in pregnancy is currently available. Yet such data are a prerequisite in the investigation and management of genital sepsis. The vaginal flora is modified by local environmental conditions and should, ideally, be established for each population studied. It was considered necessary to make such a survey for Irish pregnant women. To this end a prospective study was undertaken of 1000 pregnant women attending the hospital. The flora was examined on the same patients between the 32nd and 36th week of the gestation, during labor and on the 2nd post-partum day. The survey shows that many pathogenic organisms are regularly present in the vagina, even at the time of delivery. There is a statistically significant increase in the isolation of certain bacteria when the results of pre-term, delivery and post-partum specimens are examined. The survey emphasises the importance of the endogenous pathogen. It highlights the dangers of any invasive procedure, such as amnioscopy, fetal blood samples and unnecessary rectal examination.

10.03.09

A study on the correlation of chlamydia in upper respiratory tract of a newborn infant and in mother's vagina: Maciejewski, Z, Pilawski, Z, Melnyczuk, J, Kopaczyk, M. Inst. Obstet. and Gyn., Pomeranian Med. Acad., Szczecin, Poland

Chlamydia as a pathogenic agent attacks the respiratory system in man, conjunctival mucous membranes, and the genito-urinary organ. The objective of the paper is to study the correlation of Chlamydia in the mother and the newborn infant. The material comprises 47 cases. In the first period of parturition a cytological smear from the posterior vaginal vault was taken in speculum under visual control. In the newborn the cytological smear was aseptically collected from the nose and the throat daily for the first four days of life. The preparations on the microscopical slides were stained by Stamp's method. Chlamydiae were found in cytological preparations from the nose in 42, the throat in 32, and from vagina in 35 cases. A simultaneous presence of Chlamydia in preparations from the nose, throat and vagina was detected in 35 tests, in preparations from the nose and vagina in 31, while from the throat and vagina in 26 cases. It has been revealed that there was always a correlation with regard to the presence of Chlamydia in the upper respiratory tract of the newborn infant in instances whenever Chlamydia was found in vagina of the delivering female.

10.03.10

Usefulness of preventive measures in reducing the incidence of toxoplasma infection in pregnancy: Foulon, W, Naessens, A, Demeuter, F, Lauwers, S, Amy, J J. Dept. Obstet. and Gyn, FU, Brussels, Belgium

To investigate the usefulness of prophylactic measures in the prevention of toxoplasmosis we followed 5026 patients during pregnancy. Group I consisted of 2986 patients investigated during the period 1979–1982. No specific recommendations to prevent toxoplasmosis were given. A second group of 2040 pregnant women (group II) was investigated during the period 1983–1984. All these patients were given the following recommendations: (1) never eat raw or insufficiently cooked meat, (2) avoid touching mouth or eyes after handling raw meat and always wash hands thoroughly, (3) avoid contact with cat feces (or possibly contaminated items e. g. during gardening). Seronegative patients wer serologically screened at 6-week intervals until delivery. In group I a toxoplasma infection in pregnancy was detected in 20 patients (0.67%). In group II an infection was detected in only six patients (0.29%), (p < 0.1). High initial antibody levels indicating a possible infection in the first trimester of pregnancy were found in 17 patients (0.57%) in group I and in 13 patients (0.63%) in group II. Despite this important reduction in the number of seroconverters in the second study group, the difference is not yet statistically significant. However, it is important to note that the decrease in seroconversion rate was equally spread over a period of two years (three patients in 1983 and three in 1984). This finding suggests that simple preventive measures can reduce the incidence of toxoplasmosis in pregnancy.

10.03.11

The prevalence of toxoplasma gondii antibodies in Saudi women and the rate of congenital toxoplasmosis among newborns in Saudi Arabia: Abbas, S M A, Basalamah, A H, Serebour, F E. Dept. Obstet. and Gyn., King Abdulaziz Univ. Hosp., Jeddah, Saudi Arabia

Toxoplasma gondii is a significant pathogen of man and domestic animals. In adults, the infections tend to be mild subclinical and self-limiting. However, the organism is increasingly being recognized as a major contributor to morbidity in the newborn and the immuno compromised host. Recent reports indicate that congenital toxoplasmosis may be responsible for more birth defects than those of rubella, herpes and syphilis in the U.S.A. The classic triad of chorioretinitis, hydrocephalus and intracranial calcification in newborns and the debilitating effect of most acquired infections in later life is becoming an overwhelming burden on medical resourses. Using the indirect latex agglutination test, Toxoplasma antibody prevalence among Saudi women of child-bearing age was determined. A sandwiched IgM ELISA technique, specific to T. gondii has been employed to determine congenital infections amongst elevated IgM cord samples. An average 36.9% of Saudi women posses IgG antibody. This ranges from a low 22.8% in Hofuf to a high 51.2% in Abha. Surprisingly, of the 16.6% (1664 out of 10,033) elevated IgM cord blood, only nine cases were due to T. gondii. Clinical manifestation amongst the infected newborns was not apparent. We conclude that T. gondii infection is widespread in Saudi Arabia but congenital abnormalies in newborns are infrequent. Pregnant women from Abha may be considered as a high-risk group. Seronegative women known to acquire toxoplasmosis during pregnancy should be identified and treated in order to reduce the morbidity in the newborn due to primary maternal infection.

10.03.12

Investigation of intrauterine syphilis by analysis of amniotic fluid (AF): Larsen, B, Glover, D D, Winter, C A, Charles, D. Dept. Obstet. and Gyn., Marshall Univ. School Med., Huntington, WV, USA

Because of the rarity of intrauterine syphilis many aspects of this entity remain obscure. AF, not ordinarily available from such cases, was collected for obstetrical indications from a patient with a positive VDRL at 30 weeks gestation. Non-motile intra-amniotic spirochetes were seen by dark field microscopy 20 hours after Benzathine penicillin G was given. Immunofluorescent staining verified the identity of the spirochete from AF. This has not previously been reported. The AF was VDRL positive and IgM in the AF was elevated. The lecithin : sphyngomyelin ratio was 3.7 : 1 and phosphatidyl glycerol and phosphatidyl inositol were both present. A subsequent amniocentesis showed a decrease in the L : S ratio and phosphatidyl glycerol disappeared. No intra-amniotic spirochetes were observed in the repeat amniocentesis. The fetus at 30 weeks appeared to be growth retarded but by the time of birth at 37 weeks the weight and length of the baby were within normal limits but the head circumference was in the 10th percentile. At birth the cord blood was FTA-ABS positive. This investigation suggests that the fetus is exposed not only by the hematogenous route to the spirochete but also superficially via the AF. Early lung surfactant production and growth retardation appear reversed with penicillin therapy.

10.04.01

A comparative morphologic study between Nepalese and Japanese placentas: Yoshida, K, Soma, H, Matayoshi, K, Yaguchi, S, Malla, D. Dept. Obstet. and Gyn., Tokyo Med. Coll., Tokyo, Japan, and Maternity Hosp., Katmandu, Nepal

In Nepal, the perinatal mortality for infants is extremely high, while the death rate of infants in Japan shows the lowest in the world. The causes of such high perinatal mortality in Nepal may be due to various environmental factors. A pathologic study of 222 placentas collected at the Maternity Hospital in Katmandu was undertaken for comparing perinatal pathology between Nepalese and Japanese pregnant women living at sea level. – Results: 1) The average age of Nepalese pregnant women counts under 20 years old as compared to over 24 years old in Japanese group. 2) Most of the infants and placentas in Nepalese group weighed significantly less than those of Japanese group and their weights correspond to those at 35–37 weeks of gestation in Japanese group. 3) The gross characteristics of Nepalese placentas were represented by extensive lesions such as marked subchorionic fibrin, extrachorial placenta, chorionic cyst, abnormal insertion of cord and chorioangioma. 4) On histologic examination, Nepalese placentas showed prominent inflammation of membranes and cord vessels as well as subchorionic plate. In addition, increased syncytial knots and crowding of the villi suggesting hypoxic state in the intervillous space were also seen. 5) 101 Japanese placentas associated with anemia (Hb < 10 g/dl) during pregnancy were examined as controls and compared with Nepalese placentas. Placenta extrachorialis, maternal site hemorrhage and abnormal insertion of the cord were frequently observed in both groups.

10.04.02

Fetal lung maturity evaluation by maturational changes of the placenta: Sadauskas, V, Baliutavicene, D, Kruminis, V. Dept. Obstet. and Gyn., Kaunas Med. Inst., Kaunas, Lithuania, USSR

It is known that ultrasonic changes occur in the appearance of the placenta with advancing gestation. In our study, maturational changes of the placenta were investigated in 180 patients. We found a great correlation between placental maturity and gestational age ($r = 0.8 \pm 0.03$). Ultrasonic placental changes, amniotic fluid Clements shake test data and percentage of the infants, developed respiratory distress syndrome (RDS) were compared. In cases of grade I placental changes, positive Clements shake test was found in $9.1 \pm 4.4\%$ and the chance for RDS was $65 \pm 11.1\%$; in cases of grade II placental changes, these indices were $60 \pm 13.1\%$ and $6.5 \pm 4.4\%$, respectively. Grade III placentas were indicative for a positive Clements shake test in 100% and none of the infants developed RDS. – In conclusion, ultrasonic placental maturity examination may be helpful in fetal lung maturity determination in pregnancies in which amniocentesis would be technically difficult or hazardous to the mother or fetus.

10.04.03

Studies on the vasculature of the placenta using injection-corrosion method: Kim, W W. Dept. Obstet. and Gyn., Pusan Nat. Univ. School Med., Pusan, Korea

To achieve a morphological study on the placental vasculature, the author made 28 corrosion casts by injecting liquid plastic material (Geon D 11A), dissolved in methyl-ethyl-ketone and mixed with red and blue dyes, into the umbilical arteries and veins. Concentrated hydrochloric acid was used to take the placental tissue away. Placental vessels were divided into primary, secondary and tertiary as well as capillary vessels, and the summary of this study was as follows: The main primary vessels showed two patterns – diffuse (60.7%) and margistra (39.3%). In these subchorionic vessels arteries always run above the veins and the anastomoses between two major arteries were seen in 10.7% of all placentas observed. The ratio of the calibers of vein to artery was about four to three in the primary vessels. Secondary branches showed four different patterns which are diffuse, tree-shaped, straight, and mixed, the distribution of which were 19, 51, 24, and 6 per cent, respectively. Tertiary branches had four different patterns. Those were the shape of spider's leg, tree, and bush clove as well as mixed shape, and were 31, 44, 18, and 7 per cent in their frequency. The branching patterns of the capillary vessels did not have uniformity but they were abundant toward the decidua.

10.04.04

Light and electron microscopy identification of mitotic Hofbauer cells in the human placenta: Castellucci, M[1], Richter, A[2], Steiniger, B[3], Celona, A[4], Schneider, J[2]. [1]Labor. Electr. Micr., [2]Clin. Obstet. and Gyn., [3]Ctr Anat., Hannover Med. School; [4]Clin. Obstet. and Gyn., Univ., Messina, Italy

Twenty human placentae aged 6 to 13 weeks were obtained from normal pregnancies interrupted by legal abortion. Chorionic villi from the central part of the organ were investigated in semi-thin and thin sections. Hofbauer cells in mitotic division were easily identified due to their location inside the stromal channels and to their numerous cytoplasmic vacuoles and flanges. These mitoses were not uncommon, but irregularly distributed throughout the organ. Indeed, in certain areas of the villous stroma they were more numerous. Mitotic division of the Hofbauer cells could be a mechanism to increase their number rapidly where required by the local microenvironment. In addition, the implications of our findings have to be discussed in respect to the current view of the mononuclear phagocyte system which presumes tissue macrophages to differentiate directly from bone marrow derived monocytes.

10.04.05

Early placental maturation and perinatal outcome: Petropoulos, P, Karpathios, S, Koliopoulos, K, Linardos, N. Mitera Maternity Hosp., Athens, Greece

Forty-five pregnant women were found by ultrasonics to have prematurely mature placentas (grade III). The perinatal outcome in these 45 cases was studied and a positive correlation with small-for-dates babies and perinatal asphyxia was noticed. Hypertension was found to be the main clinical cause.

10.04.06

Clinical relevance of morphological investigations on placental villi in pre-eclampsia: Schweikhart, G. Dept. Obstet. and Gyn., Univ., Mainz

Based on a new concept of maturation of the placental villous tree and its various kinds of disorders (synchronous and asynchronous immaturity, asynchronous maturity, hypermaturity and terminal villi deficiency), the problem is studied, as to what effect the placental villous tree could have for mild and severe pre-eclampsia in term and preterm onset of labor. This report describes the investigation of 173 cases as a part of a greater study of 1005 placentas correlated with relevant clinical data on pregnancy, delivery and condition of fetal outcome. In general, pre-eclampsia at term is combined in 30% of the cases (132) with synchronous mature villous patterns, 28% with hypermaturity of the placental villous trees and 19% with terminal villi deficiency. Asynchronous immaturity was seen in only 5% at term. In severe pre-eclampsia at term hypermaturity was found in 57%, whereas terminal villi deficiency decreased to 14%. In prematurely delivered neonates (41 cases) hypermature placental villous patterns correspond with severe pre-eclampsia in 60%. Synchronous immaturity was found in only 15%. About 20–25% of all placentas could not be classified according to this concept of villous maturation. – In conclusion, even a rather simple definition of the histological features, only considering villous development and maldevelopment is obviously sufficient to describe valid correlations between the clinical events of pre-eclampsia and placental structure. Concepts to explain these findings pathophysiologically are suggested.

10.04.07

Morphological and histological pattern of human placenta and umbilical cord in cases of intrauterine growth retardation: Mishra, J, Paul, N A. Patna Med. Coll. Hosp., Bihar, India

Morphological and histological changes in the placenta and umbilical cord were studied in 150 cases of intrauterine growth retardation and 50 control cases of normal pregnancies of compatible gestational age. Placental weight was directly related to fetal weight, small babies usually had small placentae. Placental co-efficient was increased in all the cases of IUGR. Abnormal forms such as circum-vallate, circum-marginate and battledore placentae were encountered in addition to abnormal cord insertion. Gross morphological study revealed ill defined cotyledons, retroplacental hematoma, calcification and placental infacts. Single umbilical artery was found in 6% of the cases of toxemic group. Increased proliferation of Langhans cells, increased syncytial knots (Tennychange) thickness of basement membranes, stromal fibrosis, increased thickening of intervillous capillaries and obliterative endarteritis were common histological observations.

10.04.08

Studies on pregnancy hypertension and IUGR – blood vessels in pregnant SHRSP (stroke prone spontaneously hypertensive rats) placenta: Fuchi, I, Noda, K. Dept. Obstet. and Gyn., Kinki Univ., Osaka, Japan

Object: An important topic in perinatal medicine is clarifying and preventing factors which cause IUGR and accompanying SFD infants. In this study, we used pregnant SHRSP since their conditions of pregnancy hypertension are similar to that of humans and examined the placenta histologically to clarify the factors causing IUGR-SFD. – Materials and methods: Pregnant SHRSP, SHRSP-Na (pregnant SHRSP given 1.5% salt loading after the 11th day of pregnancy), as well as WKY (Wistar-Kyoto rats) as control, were used in the study. On the 20th day of pregnancy, the cross sections of blood vessels in the labyrinth zone in the placenta were measured microscopically using an image analysis system, and the three groups compared. – Results: The labyrinth zone was divided into three layers, I, II, and III, starting from the maternal side and each layer was compared (n = 5). The area of the cross sections of the blood vessels in layers I and II were larger in WKY than in SHRSP or SHRSP-Na. That of layer III was largest in WKY ($165.357 \pm 702\,\mu^2$), second largest in SHRSP ($143.375 \pm 504\;\mu^2$) and smallest in SHRSP-Na ($74.875 \pm 402\,\mu^2$). – Conclusion: It is considered that one of the factors causing IUGR in pregnancy hypertension is possibly a narrowing of the blood vessels in the placenta.

10.04.09

The protective role of placenta for the lead pollution: Georgapoulos, P, Bitos, N, Drimilis, G, Mehleris, D. III Dept. Obstet. and Gyn., "Marika Eliadi" Maternity Hosp., Athens, Greece

The role of placenta for the protection of the fetus against the lead (Pb) pollution was studied in 26 mothers during labor, and in their newborns. Blood lead was determined in the venous blood of mothers, in the cord blood of infants and in the amniotic fluid by the method of stripping voltammetry. The mean value for the mothers blood lead was found $24.8 \pm 12.4\,\mu g/dl$. In the amniotic fluid no traces of lead were detected. The mean value of the ratio Pb fetus Pb mother was $58.0 \pm 19.3\%$. The analysis of our data showed statistical significant correlation between concentration in the blood of mothers and infants cords in 42.6% ($p < 0.001$, $R^2 = 0.426$, $r = 653$). The rest of the range is determined by another factor which might be placenta in a dynamic modus. The higher the lead level in the mother, the more "filtration" of lead by the placenta. This correlation between maternal lead level and the ratio fetus/Pb mother % is statistically significant ($p < 0.001$, $R^2 = 0.926$) and explains 92.6% of the fluctuation of a lead concentration in infants in relation to the contamination of mothers. The correlation coefficient of Pb fetus/Pb mother was r = −0.962. From the regression equation it is apparent that an increase of maternal lead contamination for 1 unit (1 μg/dl) corresponds to a decrease of the ratio Pb fetus/Pb mother % of 1.49%.

10.04.10

Magnesium-levels in the amniotic fluid and serum in normal and pathologic pregnancies: Deichert, U, Schlag, M, Baltzer, G, Daume, E. Dept. Obstet. and Gyn., Univ.-Frauenklin., Marburg

Previous studies reveal a relative lack of magnesium (Mg) in serum and amniotic fluid (a. f.) in abnormal pregnancies because of the positive effects caused by additional Mg therapy during pregnancy (*Conradt* et al. Geburtsh. u. Frauenheilk. **355**, 1983). In 224 pregnancies we measured by atom-absorption spectrophotometry the Mg concentrations in the a. f. recovered in the 16th to the 19th week of pregnancy by amniocentesis and the level was 0.54 ± 0.08 mmol/l. Other authors found 0.55 ± 0.07 mmol/l (*Anastasiadis* et al. J. perinat. Med. **9**, 228, 1981) respectively 0.51 ± 0.07 mmol/l (*Rüttgers* et al. FDM **239**, 1981). In 182 of these patients the Mg level was measured in the serum, this being 0.72 ± 0.05 mmol/l. Until now 57 patients during pregnancy were studied retrospectively. In 30 cases (c.) there were no complications and the Mg level was 0.54 mmol/l in a. f. and 0.75 mmol/l in serum. Similar mean values were observed in 12 c. with bleeding in the first trimester, 7 c. with prematurity, 4 c. with EPH-gestosis and 4 c. with preterm labor. Only in the group with preterm amniotic rupture the values of Mg in serum were low with 0.46 and 0.67 mmol/l, respectively. *Rüttgers* et al. (1981) found high Mg levels in the a. f. of premature babies. *Anastasiadis* and *Rimpler* (Magn. Bull. **1**, 86, 1982) found low Mg values in case of EPH-gestosis but during delivery. The data suggest that no correlation between Mg-levels and complications in pregnancy could be shown.

10.04.11

Amniotic fluid cytology in pre-eclampsia: Fahmy, K, Sammour, M*, Abdel-Razik, M, El-Tomi, H*, Nosair, M. Dept. Obstet. and Gyn., Benha Fac. Med. and Cytodiagn. Unit, Dept. Obstet and Gyn., Ain-Shams Fac. Med.*, Cairo, Egypt

This study aims at using amniotic fluid cytology for the assessment of fetal maturity in pre-eclampsia. Three groups of women, 30–40 weeks pregnant, and each made up of 35 were studied. Groups were normotensive, mild and severe pre-eclampsia. 115 amniotic fluid samples were collected from 30 to 40 weeks, and were analysed cytologically for total number of cells per cmm, % anucleated cells, % orange-stained cells, karyopyknotic index (KPI) and cyanophilic index (CI). All women delivered after the 38th week. In all groups, as pregnancy advanced, there was a statistically significant and progressive increase in mean values of all cytological parameters, except CI. Mean number of total cells per cmm, mean % orange-stained cells and KPI was significantly lower in severe pre-eclampsia than mild pre-eclampsia than normotensive cases. There was no significant reduction in mean % anucleated cells and mean CI. In severe pre-eclampsia, there was a direct correlation between mean fetal weight and mean total number of cells, but none between fetal weight and mean % anucleated cells and mean CI. Amniotic fluid cytology is useful in the diagnosis of fetal maturity in pre-eclampsia.

10.04.12

Amniotic fluid creatinine and fetal lung maturity: Primikiris, D, Deligianni, V, Comninos, A. "Marika Eliadi" Maternity Hosp., Athens, Greece

In the present study, amniotic fluid from 69 normal pregnant women between 36 and 41 weeks gestational age was assessed for the following: 1. Creatinine levels using the method of *Hudsan* and *Raport*. 2. L/S ratio, using the method of thin-layer chromatography (TLC), for fetal lung maturity. The above factors were studied in an effort to prove any possible relationship between amniotic fluid creatinine and fetal lung maturity by correlation of the values attained. This was performed, so that the assessment of fetal maturity in general, can be achieved by measuring only one factor i. e. amniotic fluid creatinine. The results from our study showed that: 1. Amniotic fluid creatinine values increased gradually in correlation with fetal weight at birth, without any statistically significant differences between the values attained. 2. Amniotic fluid creatinine values increased gradually, in correlation with gestational age, although statistically significant increase was between 39th and 40th week. 3. The percentage of respiratory mature neonates increases gradually with amniotic fluid creatinine, from amniotic fluid creatinine values 2.30 mg% and above, all corresponding neonates are respiratorily mature.

10.04.13

Relation between spontaneous abortions of the first trimester and histological alterations of the placenta: Makedos, G, Panidis, D, Vlassis, G, Vakiani, A, Georgiadis, S, Papaloucas, A. 2nd Dept. Obstet. and Gyn., Aristotelian Univ., Thessaloniki, Greece

Histological examination of products of conception from 275 spontaneous abortions and eight terminations of pregnancy for medical reasons during the first trimester were studied. Our material consisted of 275 spontaneous abortions (retained products of conception) and five cases in which the embryonic sac was present but empty (blighted ovum). Histological examination of the retained products showed the following changes: 1) fibrosis (30.5%), 2) hydropic degeneration (28.3%), 3) inflammation (19.4%), 4) hyaloid degeneration (1.5%) and 5) necrosis (9.4%). Histological examination of the five cases of blighted ovum showed evidence of alteration in all of them and specifically hydropic degeneration in three and fibrosis in the remaining two cases. From the eight cases, in which pregnancy was terminated for medical reasons, fibrosis of the placenta villi was identified only in two cases. – Our results show that the frequency of the placenta villum alterations during the first trimester (73.1%) is considerably higher than that observed in cases when pregnancy is interrupted for medically imposed reasons (25%) and that the most frequent histological change is fibrosis.

10.04.14

Histological alterations of the placenta in spontaneous abortions of the second trimester: Moysatat, J, Makedos, G, Papaloucas, A, Vakiani, A, Agorastos, T, Panidis, D. 2nd Dept. Obstet. and Gyn., Aristotelian Univ., Thessaloniki, Greece

We have examined products of conception from 95 spontaneous abortions and from four terminations of pregnancy for medical reasons during the second trimester. The presence of fetus evidenced in only 35 out of 95 spontaneous abortions. Histological examination of the placenta showed the following changes: 1) fibrosis (49.4%), 2) inflammation (24.4%), 3) hydropic degeneration (13.7%), 4) hyaloid degeneration (4.1%) and 5) infarcts (2.1%). In five cases where fetal congenital abnormality identified, changes of the placenta observed in four (two fibrosis, ohne hydropic degeneration and one infarct). Out of the four cases where pregnancy terminated for medical reasons, fibrosis of the placental villi was identified in only one. Our results show that the most frequent histological alteration of the placenta during the second trimester is fibrosis and that the frequency of the placenta villum alterations is considerably higher than that observed in cases when pregnancy is interrupted for medical imposed reasons.

10.07.01

Immunocytochemical detection of estrogen receptors (ER) (monoclonal anti-ER, PAP) in breast cancer tissues and correlation to dextran-coated charcoal method (DCC): Jonat, W, Maass, H, Eidtmann, H, Stegner, H-E. Univ.-Frauenklin., Hamburg

The purpose of the study was to evaluate the relationship between ER determination by immunocytochemical assay (ER-ICA) on frozen sections of human breast cancers and conventional steroid binding assay (DCC) on the same cancers as well as the response to endocrine therapy in the advanced stage of the disease. 40 cancer samples which were stored in a cancer sample bank at $-70\,°C$ were reanalysed utilizing the immunocytochemical technique after primary determination of steroid binding receptor status by DCC. Unaware of patient data including the results for estrogen and progesterone receptors the slides were diagnosed. The preliminary results show an excellent correlation between ER-ICA and DCC assay. Both the specificity and the sensitivity are approximately 90%. The positive staining was seen only in the cell nucleus. From the correlation with clinical response to endocrine therapy in 25 patients it would appear that those breast cancers in which none or very few cells stain for receptors have no chance of responding to endocrine therapy. – We conclude: 1. ER-ICA is a most reliable histochemical method for ER detection. It correlates in more than 90% of the cases with ER-determination by DCC. 2. ER-ICA is useful in predicting the outcome of endocrine therapy in metastatic breast cancer. By analysing more samples we expect to support the idea that patients with receptor rich cancers who failed to respond objectively to hormone manipulations will be those whose tumors contain enough receptor poor and presumably non hormone dependent cells to preclude an objective remission.

10.07.02

Subcellular distribution of phorbol-ester receptors and protein kinase C in human mammary tumor cells: Costa, S D, Fabbro, D, Regazzi, R, Roos, W, Eppenberger, U. Labor. Biochem.-Endocr., Dept. Res. and Gyn., Kantonsspit., Basel, Switzerland

Estrogen-dependent growth of human breast cancer cells has been shown to mediated by tumor-derived growth factors such as α-TGF which act via the epidermal growth factor receptor (EGF-R). It has been reported that the activation of the EGF-R is regulated by specific phosphorylation of protein kinase C (PK-C), the putative phorbol-ester receptor. Therefore we compared the subcellular distribution of the phorbol-ester receptor and PK-C activity between estrogen receptor-containing (MCF-7, T-47-D, ZR-75-1) and E_2-R-lacking (MDA-MB-231, HBL-100, BT-20) established human mammary tumor cells. The amount of specific high affinity phorbol ester binding (app $K_d = 10\,nM$) was similar when measured in intact cells. However, the activity of PK-C and the phorbol ester binding was significantly higher in the cytosol of hormone-independent cell lines ($p < 0.001$). Our results suggest that cytosolic PK-C and phorbol ester-binding activities do not correlate with the amount of phorbol ester bound to corresponding intact cells. – This work was supported in part by the Swiss Cancer League, grant no. FOR.249.AK.83(6).

10.07.03

The relevance of steroid hormone binding proteins for prognosis in breast cancer: Etzrodt, A, Jung, H, Tolxdorff, T. Abt. Gyn. u. Geburtsh., RWTH, Aachen

The intracellular actions of steroid hormones are modulated by receptor proteins. For transport these hormones are bound to plasma proteins, specific or unspecific binding ones such as albumin. In breast cancer albumin can be located in the cells, as previous studies have shown. In 431 primary breast cancers estrogen receptor (ER) and progesterone receptor (PR) and the albumin content were measured. The correlation of these proteins to the axillary lymph node involvement (ax.l.i.) and in 250 patients to recurrence-free survival was evaluated, taking into account tumor diameter and age of patients. For the prognostic relevance or ER a marked difference was found between pre- and postmenopausal patients. In premenopausal patients ER positive tumors showed a significantly higher ax.l.i. and a worse recurrence-free survival than ER negative tumors. In postmenopausal patients those with ER positive tumors did significantly better. For PR this age specific difference was not significant. The albumin content of the primary tumor showed a marked correlation to ax.l.i., tumors with high albumin content had a significantly lower ax.l.i. ($\bar{X} = 1.6$) than those with low albumin content ($\bar{X} = 3.6$). Despite this difference in ax.l.i. no difference was found in recurrence-free survival taking all cancers. If however premenopausal patients were evaluated separately, the recurrence rate was lower in albumin rich than in the albumin poor group (7% vs 29%).

10.07.04

Prognostic validity of prolactin receptor determinations in human mammary tumor tissues: Hoffman, G, Schommer, M, Schweikhart, G, Grill H J, Pollow, K. Dept. Obstet and Gyn., and Dept. Exp. Endocr., Johannes Gutenberg-Univ., Mainz

Determination of prolactin receptors (PrlR) found renewed interest as an additional selection criterion for prognosis as well as therapy of breast cancer. PrlR were quantified with ^{125}I-hPrl as radioactive ligand ± 1000-fold hPrl in 98 human mammary tumor specimens using a partially purified $105,000 \times g$ membrane fraction and a 5-point saturation assay with Scatchard plot analysis of the binding data. Tumors with PrlR levels below 4 fmoles/mg protein were evaluated as receptor negative. PrlR levels were compared to cytoplasmic estrogen (ER) and progesterone receptor (PR) concentrations as well as to histomorphological parameters. Furthermore were 39 patients with non metastasizing mammary tumors, whose primary treatment was at least 18 months before, evaluated clinically with respect to their tumor's PrlR levels. 36.7% of all tumors were ER and 54.1% PR negative. The distribution of PrlR positive and negative tumors was similar. Neither a relation of PrlR status to menopause nor a correlation of PrlR concentrations to the patient's age could be demonstrated. PrlR could also not be correlated to ER or PR concentrations. On the other hand the correlation between histomorphological criteria and PrlR levels was obvious: with increasing tumor mass, positive lymph nodes and metastasisation decreased the number of PrlR positive tumors. During an 18 months observation of 39 patients 5/17 PrlR negative patients developed metastases whereas only 1/22 PrlR positive patients showed progression. The presented results indicate a steroid receptor independent role of PrlR as a beneficial factor of prognosis.

10.07.05

Influence of clinical factors on the response rate of receptor positive advanced breast cancer patients to tamoxifen treatment: Matthiessen, H von et al. Dept. Obstet. and Gyn., Univ., Düsseldorf

Estrogen receptor (ER) status is an important prognostic variable for the response to tamoxifen in advanced breast cancer. Additionally, the probability of response is influenced by certain clinical factors in the individual patient. We analyzed the response of advanced breast cancer patients to tamoxifen in a multicentric retrospective study and correlated it to receptor status, disease free interval (DFI) and age. Patients with ER positive or unknown receptor status demonstrated 34% response rate. None of 11 ER negative patients responded. Response rates related to subgroups of patients with different clinical parameters are shown in the table below. We conclude that response of ER + patients to tamoxifen is influenced by the clinical situation of the individual patient.

All Pat.	52/163 32% Remissions						
DFI	< = 3 Years 18/91 20%			> 3 Years 34/57 60%			
Age (Y)	< = 65 6/49 12%		> 65 12/42 29%		< = 65 14/31 45%		> 65 20/26 77%	
Rec. STAT ?/+	? 1/24 4%	pos. 5/25 20%	? 4/20 20%	pos. 8/22 36%	? 10/24 42%	pos. 4/7	? 17/23 74%	pos. 3/3

10.07.06

Development of resistance to endocrine factors in breast cancer cells: Simon, W E, Albrecht, M, Hölzel, F. Dept. Obstet. and Gyn., Univ. Hosp., Hamburg-Eppendorf

Endocrine treatment of advanced breast cancer is only temporarily successful. The occurrence of relapse indicates the *in vivo* development of resistant cell populations. Our study was aimed at the *in vitro* characterization of growth responses of carcinoma cells derived from patients during relapse under endocrine therapy. The carcinoma cells explanted from solid metastases or pleural effusions were grown in long-term stock cultures. The growth response to various endocrine factors in clinically relevant doses was assayed in multiple experimental cultures. The growth of cell lines derived from patients who had relapsed during treatment with the antioestrogen tamoxifen (TAM) or progestins was not influenced or even

239

enhanced by TAM or progesterone (P). This indicates the occurrence of positive *in vivo* selection for cell populations resistant to the endocrine therapy given. In stock cultures which were kept for five months in the presence of TAM or P equivalent to therapeutic serum concentrations, the initially inhibitory effect of TAM or P on the cell growth disappeared after three months. Further treatment of the cultures provoked stimulatory effects of TAM or P. Apparently, the development of resistance to endocrine treatment *in vivo* and *in vitro* consists in the selection of carcinoma cells which grow independent of or partially dependent on the endocrine factors administered. (Supported by the DFG.)

10.07.07

Monoclonal antibodies to cytoskeletal components for characterization of human breast carcinomas: Kaufmann, M, Jarasch, E D, Böcker, W, Nagle, R B. Univ. Hosp., Dept. Obstet. and Gyn., Heidelberg, Inst. Cell and Tumor Biol., German Ca Res. Ctr, Heidelberg, Dept. Path., Gen. Hosp., Altona, Hamburg, Dept. Path., Univ. of Arizona, Tucson, AZ, USA

Antibodies to cytoskeletal components were analysed by immunofluorescence microscopy on different benign, malignant *in situ* and invasive lesions of human breast tissue. The used antibodies are directed against individual cytokeratin polypeptides or against several related cytokeratins. For comparison antibodies to components of the basement membrane (collagen IV, fibronectin, laminin) to vimentin, actin and myosin, and to epithelial membrane antigen (EMA) were also tested. Antibodies to cytokeratins Nos. 8 and 19 invariably reacted with lobular and ductal epithelial cells of normal breast and also with epithelial cells of benign and malignant lesions. By contrast, monoclonal and polyclonal antibodies to EMA showed positive reaction only with a limited number of cells in epithelial hyperplasia as well as invasive carcinomas. The reactive antigens were analyzed by gel electrophoresis of tissue samples followed by immunoblotting. These findings are discussed in relation to possible different states of secretory metabolism in human breast cancer cells. – We thank Dr. *C. Coombes* and Dr. *M. Ormerod* for the supply of EMA.

10.07.08

Polyclonal antibodies in the study of extra-cellular matrix in the breast disease: Zeferino, L C, Montruccoli, G C, Grigioni, G W, Pinotti, J A. Dept. Obstet. and Gyn., State Univ., Campinas, Brazil

The study of the extra-cellular matrix is the basis for understanding the normal and pathologic biological process in the organs. This is very important and innovatory for the female breast and its alterations. Benign proliferative lesions of the breast from 38 women, 10 cases of *in situ* carcinoma and 20 cases of invasive carcinoma of the female breast were studied through immunohistochemical techniques using polyclonal antibodies of the components of the basement mebrane, collagen III and IV, laminin and fibronectin. The results showed that these components have a different distribution for each kind of proliferative lesion. It was possible to know why a determinate pathologic class differentiates itself in different patients. It was clearly demonstrated: (a) the components of the basement membrane change quantitatively and qualitatively, according to each pathology; (b) the absence of a continuous basement membrane in invasive carcinoma; (c) the presence of a continuous basement membrane in the pre-invasive carcinoma.

10.07.09

Determination of proliferative activity in carcinoma and benign changes of the breast by a monoclonal antibody: Lellé, R J, Heidenreich, W, Stauch, G, Gerdes, J, Peter, H H. Dept. Obstet. and Gyn., Med. Hochsch., Hannover

The monoclonal antibody Ki67 developed by *Gehrdes* and *Stein* is able to mark the nuclei of proliferating cells. So far 70 benign and malignant changes of the human breast were examined histologically and cytologically. The results were compared to the grading (GI to GIII) of *Bloom* and *Richardson*. Well differentiated tumors (GI) showed an average of 10% proliferating cells compared to 28% in poorly differentiated specimens (GIII). Only 6% Ki67 positive cells were seen in benign changes like fibroadenoma or mastopathia. These results seem to demonstrate a prognostic significance for breast cancer and should be studied further.

10.07.10

Retinoic acid enhances cell responsiveness to epidermal growth factor in mouse mammary gland in culture: Wakimoto, H, Komura, H, Chen, C, Aono, T, Tanizawa, O. Dept. Obstet. and Gyn., Osaka Univ. Med. School, Osaka, Japan

It is well known that retinoic acid (RA) plays an important role in maintenance and growth of epithelial cells in mammals. However, little is known about the effect of RA on mammary cells. The present study was undertaken to examine the effects of RA on development and functional differentiation of mouse mammary cells in culture in association with epidermal growth factor (EGF). The addition of EGF to the medium up to 100 ng/ml increased thymidine incorporation into DNA of mammary explants in a dose dependent manner, while RA alone at 10 μg/ml had no significant effect on DNA synthesis. However, an addition of RA enhanced the EGF-stimulated DNA synthesis of the mammary explants. EGF inhibited the synthesis of casein and α-lactalbumin of mammary explants in culture in the presence of insulin, cortisol and prolactin. Simultaneous addition of RA caused complete inhibition of α-lactalbumin synthesis, but not of casein synthesis. Measurement of specific binding of ^{125}I-EGF to mouse mammary glands in culture demonstrated that the pretreatment of mammary explants with RA slightly but significantly enhanced the binding of EGF to its cellular receptors. These results suggest that RA modulates the effects of EGF on the growth and differentiation of mouse mammary epithelium. The regulation by RA seems to be mediated at least in part via enhanced binding activity in the mammary cells for EGF. On the basis of these observations, it is likely that RA stimulates the growth of mammary epithelium and inhibits milk protein synthesis during pregnancy by enhancing the biological effects of EGF on mammary cells.

10.08.01

Epidural anesthesia in obstetrics. Results of a German follow-up: Knitza, R, Sans-Scherer, U, Wisser, J. Dept. Obstet. and Gyn., Ludwig-Maximilians-Univ., Munich

385 German departments of obstetrics participated in our study concerning the current trends in regional anesthesia. We were able to include the results of 260,000 deliveries. 17% of vaginal deliveries are combined with regional anesthesia. Continuous lumbar epidural anesthesia is the most important procedure, used on an average of about 11%. On the contrary continuous caudal anesthesia and spinal anesthesia are irrelevant with an occurrence of about 0.03% for the first and 0.3% for the other technique. The indications for continuous epidural anesthesia in high-risk pregnancies differ with respect to the organizational structure of the participating institutions. Similar distributions concerning the indication for continuous epidural anesthesia are found in patients with pre-planned vaginal delivery after previous Cesarean section. Performance and monitoring of this anesthesiological procedure differ greatly with respect to personal and technical possibilities.

10.08.02

Modification of uterine activity as a result of epidural analgesia: González, N L, García, J A, Santísimo, J L, Parache, J. Hosp. G. y Clin. de Tenerife, Fac. Med. de La Laguna, Tenerife, Spain

Uterine activity as recorded during the period of active dilatation was studied in 60 patients distributed in two groups: One received epidural analgesia and a control group without analgesia. The following variables are observed: basal tone, amplitude, intensity, frequency, duration of contractions and area of active contraction, as well as the maximal and minimal rate of pressure change (dP/dt), and the time intervals T_1, T_2, T_3, T_4 (*Seitchik, J, Chatkoff, M L.* J. appl. Physiol. **38**, 443, 1975). – A statistically significant decrease is shown in basal tone ($p < 0.012$), intensity ($p < 0.041$), frequency ($p < 0.021$), maximal and minimal rate of pressure change ($p < 0.001$, $p < 0.031$). – Statistically significant increases were found in time intervals T_2 ($p < 0.016$), T_4 ($p < 0.008$), $T_1 + T_2$ ($p < 0.031$) and $T_3 + T_4$ ($p < 0.009$), as well as the total duration of contraction ($p < 0.006$). – No significant variations were found in amplitude, area of active contraction and time intervals T_1, T_3, and $T_2 + T_3$. Epidural analgesia modifies myometrial contractile state with no alteration of the uterine labor.

10.08.03

Endocrine response of stress during labor under general or epidural anesthesia: Kalogirou, D, Badalouka, A, Toumbanakis, N, Zourlas, P A. 2nd Dept. Obstet. and Gyn., Univ. of Athens, Aretaiion Hosp., Athens, Greece

The purpose of our research is to compare the reaction of two different methods of anesthesia on the stress of labor. Our study was carried out on 60 healthy women who had normal vaginal delivery. We divided them into two groups based on the type of anesthesia which we gave. The first group is composed of 30 women to whom we gave pethidin and entonox for anesthesia. The second group is composed of 30 women who had a normal birth under epidural analgesia. By processing the endocrine response of labor stress, we measured the prolactin and cortisol hormones. We took four samples from each woman: the first before the beginning of labor, the second during cervical dilatation at 6 to 8 cm, the third immediately following labor, and the fourth 2 hours after that. The hormone levels were measured by radioimmunoassays. From the results we observe a very marked rise ($p < 0.001$) of cortisol level in the blood during labor with general anesthesia, while we do not observe a marked rise in epidural analgesia ($p < 0.10$). As far as the levels of prolactin are concerned we observe a very marked ($p < 0.001$) decrease during labor with general anesthesia, while no marked decrease is observed under epidural anesthesia. The Apgar score of the newly born of the second group was larger than that of the first group. We conclude that the use of epidural analgesia during labor alters the endocrine response to stress of labor and betters the Apgar score of the newly born.

10.08.04

The influence of pethidine on fetal behaviour in labor: Vadas, A, Zimmer, E Z, Divon, M Y, Peretz, B A, Paldi, E. Dept. Obstet. and Gyn. "B", Rambam Med. Ctr, Haifa, Israel

The short- and long-term influences of maternal analgesia during labor on the fetus and infant are still not fully understood. The aim of our study was to find out if maternal pethidine administration during the active phase of labor has an influence on fetal behavioral patterns. Using a specific computer program which was developed in our department, the fetal biophysical parameters – body movements, heart rate and short term beat-to-beat variability – were recorded with internal monitor and ultrasound and correlated to uterine activity. Recordings were performed prior to and after maternal pethidine administration. The simultaneous recording of these four parameters enabled analysis of these variables, and then a look into the interrelation among them. Results were provided both graphically and numerically, and will be discussed.

10.08.05

Epidural injection of fentanyl or morphine for pain relief after vaginal delivery: Aidonopoulos, H, Tzafettas, J, Loufopoulos, A, Boucklis, A, Papaloucas, A. B' Univ. Dept. Obstet.-Gyn., Thessaloniki, Greece

There has been a good number of reports on epidural administration of opiates for post-partum analgesia mainly after Cesarean section, with variable results. In the present work in two different groups of patients delivered vaginally, epidural injection of fentanyl in the one and morphine solution in the other was given after the episiotomy repair. The drugs were given through the same epidural catheter that had been used for continuous intrapartal epidural administration of bupivacaine 0.25%. The duration and degree of analgesia achieved and the additional analgesia required for the first 48 hours postpartum were recorded as well as the vital signs and occurrence of side-effects like respiratory depression, pruritus, nausea and vomiting. The fentanyl group had more effective analgesia compared to the morphine group (additional analgesia required 6% and 14%, respectively) but was of shorter duration. Although there seem to be significant differences with regard to the analgesic result of these drugs tried in this study, their administration for post-partum pain relief seems justified when epidural intrapartum anesthesia is used. The side-effects noticed in these two groups of patients pose no untoward contraindication.

10.08.06

Epidural, on-demand morphine infusion for postoperative pain: Chrubasik, J, Hillemans, H G*. Depts. Anesthesiol. and *Gyn., Univ. Hosp., Freiburg

Previously we have demonstrated that epidural, on-demand morphine infusion could provide analgesia in the early postoperative period (*Chrubasik, J.* Lancet, **1984, I**, 107–108). The aim of the investigation was to test the method in a greater number of patients. – Methods: For constant postoperative analgesia, 50 patients received until 8 p. m. on the 2nd postoperative day (PD) a continuous-plus-on-demand infusion of morphine (*Chrubasik, J.* Anaesthesist, Suppl. **32**, 209–210, 1983) into the epidural space following an initial bolus injection of 2 mg morphine. Subjective pain was assessed on a visual pain analogue scale (no pain = 0, worst pain = 10). – Results (mean ± sem): Morphine demand until 8 a. m. on the 1st PD was 4.8 ± 0.2 mg, the following 24 hours 1.9 ± 0.2 mg and from 8 a. m. until 8 p. m. on the 2nd PD 0.6 ± 0.1 mg. Subjective pain while immobile remained under 1 and pain under stress conditions below 2 on the analogue scale throughout the treatment. – Conclusions: Epidural, on-demand, low-dose infusion of morphine leads to excellent postoperative pain relief. Advantages of the method are: Low morphine consumption, individual pain treatment and no development of respiratory depression (*Chrubasik, J.* Lancet **I**, 793, 1984).

10.08.07

Chronic cancer pain: long-term treatment with epidural opiate analgesia: Naji, P, Naumann, C P, Haller, U, Kern, F. Inst. Anesthesiol. and Dept. Obstet. and Gyn., Kantonsspit., St. Gallen, Switzerland

In patients with progressive incurable cancer the marked deterioration of life quality is rather often caused by severe pain conditions much earlier than disability occurs because of progressing cancer. Since 1981, 26 patients with chronic cancer pain were treated with epidural opiate analgesia. After puncture of the lumbar epidural space and subcutaneous tunneling, the epidural catheters passed the skin in the axillary line. 4 mg morphine in 10 ml saline were injected every 24 hrs up to every 8 hrs if necessary. After one or more days in hospital, treatment was continued as an out-patient. Daily needs of morphine and the quality of analgesia were monitored as well as side-effects and possible complications of the long-term catheter placement. – Results: Initially in all patients there was a good to very good analgesia after injections of 4 mg morphine every 24 hrs. However, after 30 to 180 days, daily dosages had to be increased in all patients, mostly during the terminal stages of the disease. In five patients the daily dosage could be dramatically reduced after interval treatment with local anesthetics. The epidural catheters remained in place up to 311 days, causes for removal were obstruction (8), kinking and subcutaneous infections (2). Side-effects of morphine included itching (4) and transitory urinary retention in a few cases. It is concluded that epidural opiate analgesia is a safe and effective method for long-term use which offers patients with severe cancer pain a very remarkable improvement in the quality of life.

10.08.08

Auriculo-electrostimulating analgesia (AESA) in gynecological operations: Mateva, M, Bobcev, T. Dept. Anesthesiol., 1st Workers' Hosp., Sofia, Bulgaria

The anesthesia was performed in 180 patients by means of ESA-SM8, a creation of Schwa-Medico in Frankfurt a. M., W.Germany. The anesthesia was introduced by standard techniques and continued with $N_2O:O_2$ (2:1) and myorelaxants. Additional analgesics (Fentanyl, DHBP etc.) were seldom used, whereas Fentanyl did not exceed 1–1.5 mg in extraordinary cases. Hemodynamics were stable, substantial pulse deviations were not observed e. g. ±10–15 b/m, and for the AP up to ±20 mm Hg (2.6 kPa). The AESA factors were: 1.5 pulsewidth, 10 mA current power and 30 Hz current frequency. AESA was used to apply postoperative analgesia as well, but with different features (7.5–5.0 mA, 20 Hz) with good results for the first 12 hours.

10.08.09

Morphine superior to bupivacaine in epidural treatment of pain after gynecological operations: Herchenhahn, E, Hillemanns, H G, Chrubasik, J*. Depts. Gyn. and *Anesthesiol., Univ. Hosp., Freiburg

Epidural treatment of postoperative pain is especially indicated after operations under epidural anesthesia. The aim of the present study was to compare the analgesic effectiveness and compatibility of epidural bupivacaine and epidural morphine after gynecological operations. – Methods: For constant postoperative analgesia, 26 women received over 50 hours continuous-plus-on-demand infusions (*Chrubasik, J.* Lancet **1984, I,** 107–108) of either 0.125% bupivacaine (max. flow rate 10 ml/h or 0.25% morphine (max. flow rate 0.31 ml/h) into the epidural space following an initial bolus injection of 12.5 mg bupivacaine or 2 mg morphine, respectively. – Results (mean $\pm$ sem): A total of 413 ± 22 mg bupivacaine and 9.7 ± 1.0 mg morphine was required.

hours of treatment	bupivacaine (mg)	morphine (mg)
0–25	225 ± 7	7.4 ± 0.5
	n.s.	$p < 0.001$
25–50	188 ± 19	2.3 ± 0.6

Side-effects of bupivacaine: paresthesia 12, numbness 13, urinary retention 6, shivering 5, drowsiness 4, hypotension 5; of morphine: urinary retention 3. – Conclusions: Constant analgesia was attainable with continuous-plus-on-demand infusion of bupivacaine as well as morphine. Yet, because of the high compatibility and the low incidence of side-effects, morphine is preferable to bupivacaine in epidural treatment of postoperative pain.

10.09.01

A new tumor marker system for gynecologic cancers using monoclonal antibody derived from endometrial carcinoma cell line: Tsuji, Y, Nakagawa, S, Nishiura, H, Isojima, S. Dept. Obstet. and Gyn., Hyogo Med. Coll., Nishinomiya, Japan

A mouse monoclonal antibody (Mab) C12, was raised against the endometrial carcinoma cell line Ishikawa. Subclass of Mab C12 was IgM, k light chain. Reactivity of this antibody was characterized by indirect immunofluorescence and ABC immunoperoxidase assay against several cell lines and normal and neoplasmic tissues. Mab C12 reacted strongly with all of 20 paraffin tissue sections of endometrial carcinomas but showed extremely weak reactivity with one of six normal endometrial tissues. Immunoradiometric assay by the Sandwich method using Mab C12 could detect tumor associated antigens (MW > 500,000) in the sera of cancer patients, and membrane extracts from Ishikawa cell line using Nonidet P 40. Nine of fifteen sera from patients with ovarian cancer, two of four sera of endometrial cancer and one of six sera of cervical cancer patients were proved elevation of C12 antigen level estimated by radiometric assay using Mab C12. The antigen substance recognized by Mab C12 may be carbohydrate determinant similar to CA 125 and CA 19-9, however it is obviously different from that of CA 125 or CA 19-9.

10.09.02

Discriminant analysis of the level of tumor markers in the early diagnosis of ovarian cancer: Miyoshi, T, Nishimura, H, Nishida, T, Yakushiji, M, Kato, T. Dept. Obstet. and Gyn., Kurume Univ., Fukuoka, Japan

Current advance of the serological methods used in the diagnosis of ovarian cancer is impressive. A new tumor associated antigen CA125 has been the subject of increasing interest as the most reliable tumor marker of epithelial malignancy. Serum level of CA125, however, also rises in other benign gynecological disorders, leading false positive results. To develop the diagnostic value of CA125, combination assay with TPA (tissue polypeptide antigen) and IAP (immunosuppressive acidic protein) was performed, and the results were analysed by statistical methods. Materials were obtained from 97 patients with ovarian tumors, including 40 malignant cases. Among the 40 patients with cancer, serum CA125 level was positive (higher than 35 U/ml) in 80.0%, while seventeen of 57 patients with benign disease (29.8%) also showed positive level of the marker as false positive results. The concomitant measurements of TPA and IAP led to comparatively low false-positive rates, 17.5% and 22.8%, respectively. After making a multivariate analysis of these results, the positive rate increased up to 85.6% in malignant cases, and the false positive rate decreased remarkably to 5.3%. On the basis of these results, this statistical method is thought to be promising. Although the optimal diagnostic method for ovarian cancer is not yet known, this discriminant analysis of CA125 combined with TPA and IAP is supposed to be an acceptable serological method for the detection of ovarian epithelial malignancies in clinical practice.

10.09.03

Phosphohexoseisomerase measurements in sera from patients with gynecological tumors: Auner, H, Lahousen, M, Pürstner, P. Univ. Clin. Obstet. and Gyn., Graz, Austria

The clinical significance of Phosphohexoseisomerase levels (PHI) in patients with malignant gynecological tumors was studied at diagnosis and subsequent to tumor reduction by operation, chemotherapy, radio-therapy and combinations of all three forms of therapy. Forty cases with different tumors were investi-gated: 30 patients with carcinoma of the ovary, five cases with carcinoma of the cervix and five with carcinoma of the vulva. In 70% of all cases significantly elevated PHI was found at diagnosis. The measurements of PHI activity in the ascites fluid were tow to five times higher than in the serum. Tumor reduction correlates well with a decrease of serum PHI. Patients who were clinically without signs of tumor had normal levels (75 U/l). In cases with recurrence and metastasizing tumors increased and abnormal high PHI activities could be measured. Our study documents the clinical value of PHI-measurement as a tumor marker in tumor diagnosis and observation of tumor-bearing patients.

10.09.04
Significance of pre-therapeutic neopterin levels in patients with genital cancer: Bichler, A, Hetzel, H, Reibn-egger, G, Wachter, H. Dept. Obstet. and Gyn., Univ., Innsbruck, Austria

The purpose of this paper is to show the pretherapeutic neopterin values in patients with genital cancer and to prove if they have any significance in predicting the further course of disease. For statistical evaluation the Cox "proportional hazards" model was used. Elevated neopterin levels were found in: cervical cancer (n = 161) in 53%, endometrial cancer (n = 50) in 68%, ovarian cancer (n = 32) in 81%. A correlation with the tumor stage and the neopterin levels was seen. When the 161 women with cervical cancer were divided in two groups according to their pretherapeutic neopterin levels (≤ 400 vs > 400) highly significant different survival functions *(Kaplan-Meier)* were observed. By combining the pretherapeutic neopterin values with the hemoglobin content and the leucocyte count four different groups of patients at risk were formed. A sharper separation of survival functions of these patients with cervical cancer could be achieved regardless of the tumor stage. Therefore patients with low tumor stages but being found in a high risk group according to neopterin levels, hemoglobin content and leucocyte count have to be controlled at shorter intervals than usual in the follow-up because of the higher risk of developing a tumor recurrence.

10.09.05
Urinary cyclic GMP (cGMP) and neopterin (N) evaluation in patients with ovarian carcinoma; A preliminary report on monitoring the response to chemotherapy: Greggi, S*, Villani, L*, Moneta, E*, Flamini, G**, Sambo, A**, Cittadini, A**. *Dept. Obstet. and Gyn., **Inst. Gen. Path., Univ. Cattolica S. Cuore, Rome, Italy

Previous experimental observations have shown that cAMP and cGMP influence cell division and differen-tation *(Friedman, D L.* Physiol. Rev. **56,** 652, 1975). Investigations of the level of urine cGMP in neoplastic patients have provided encouraging results; cGMP elevated urine levels have been detected in over 90% of patients with ovarian cancer *(Turner, G A.* Brit. J. Obstet. Gyn. **89,** 760, 1982). Neopterin (N) is another interesting marker of cell activation and proliferation, and significant correlations have been found between urine N levels and ovarian cancer status *(Bichler, A.* In: Bioch. clin. aspects of pteridines, Ed. *H. Wachter,* de Gruyter, 1982). In our study we report preliminary results about urine cGMP and N values measured in 18 pts. with ovarian carcinoma before and after operation and during chemotherapy. The same two markers were examined in 12 pts. with benign ovarian tumors pre- and post-operation. Urine samples were stored at $-20°$ C until examination. cGMP was tested with an Amersham RIA kit, while N was analysed by HPLC. Results were expressed as μmol cGMP/g creatinine and as μmol N/mol creatinine, respectively. Increased levels for both cGMP and N were observed in ovarian cancer pts., and a reliable agreement was shown between clinical status during chemotherapy and urine values for the two markers. Data from cancer pts. are compared to those obtained from pts with benign ovarian tumors.

10.09.06
Studies on CA 125, CA 19-9, TPA and IAP as tumor markers in patients with ovarian cancer: Negishi, Y, Azuma, T, Sano, Y, Honda, S, Hirata, T, Furuno, K, Okabe, K, Shimizu, K, Ikehata, N, Nakamura, F, Sato, H, Akiya, K. Dept. Obstet. and Gyn., Tokyo Med. Coll., Tokyo, Japan

CA 125, CA 19-9, TPA and IAP were useful for diagnosis of ovarian cancer. The subjects (n = 86) were treated by CAP and FAMT. It was proved that CA 125 was localized on the surface of cancer cells of serous and mucinous cystadenocarcinomas, clear cell carcinomas, endometrioid carcinomas and unclassified tumors, and CA 19-9 localized in mucinous cystadenocarcinomas, utilizing the Avidin-Biotin immunoper-oxidase technique determining reactivity of OC 125 and anti-CA 19-9 antibody. When the cut off value of CA 125 was set by 35 U/ml in the control group, the patients suffering from serous cystadenocarcinoma showed positive in 72.9%, resulting by 1766.5 U/ml as an average value. CA 125 values of ascitic fluids were higher than those of serum in the 3rd and 4th stage. Correlation in CA 125 values was highly significant between the ascitic fluids and serum. As for CA 19-9 having set by 37 U/ml as the cut off value, patients suffering from mucinous cystadenocarcinoma who revealed positive by 50%, were 144.8 U/ml in value on average. Besides, values of TPA and IAP were elevated in those who suffered from ovarian cancers. These markers also decreased in those patients who had a favorable course during treatment. It is considered that measuring values of CA 125, CA 19-9, TPA and IAP are valuable not only to diagnose ovarian cancers but also to evaluate their prognosis.

10.09.07

CA125: A tumor antigen expressed in normal human fetal tissues: Quirk, J G, Norris, J S, Hardin, W, O'Brien, T J. Depts. Obstet. and Gyn. Biochem., Physiol., & Med., Univ. of Arkansas Med. School, Little Rock, AR, USA

CA125, the serious cystadenocarcinoma antigen, has been identified in adult and fetal serosal epithelium. We have established that CA125 is a component of amniotic fluid (AF) throughout gestation and that its likely site of synthesis is fetal chorionic membranes. CA125 is found in much greater concentrations in AF throughout gestation than in serum obtained from patients with cystadenocarcinomas (5 K – 12 K U/ml & 100 – 1000 U/ml, respectively); only background levels are detected in maternal serum. Cord blood and fetal urine contain little CA125 (17 and 25 U/ml, respectively). We have begun to purify and characterize CA125 from AF and chorion. The native antigen (identified by IRMA assay, Centocor Inc., USA) has a mol. wt. > 700 K daltons but is heterogeneous in size and anionic composition based on its elution profile from an FPLC mono Q anion exchange system. CA125 was found to be composed of 2 subunits of mol. wt. 237 K and 186 K daltons detectable by OC125 antibody. The nature of the negative charge heterogeneity was found to be sensitive to neuraminidase and is likely due to the presence of sialic acid in the carbohydrate portion of this glycoprotein. Second antibody studies have demonstrated further subunits of 50–60 K and approximately 20 K daltons.

10.09.08

Diagnostic usefulness of simultaneous measurement of CA125, TPA, IAP, CEA, and ferritin in sera of patients with gynecological malignant neoplasm: Yabushita, H, Masuda, T, Hattori, A, Ishihara, M. Dept. Obstet. and Gyn., Aichi Med. Univ., Aichi, Japan

The values of CA125, TPA, IAP, CEA, and ferritin in sera were measured simultaneously in 68 healthy nonpregnant females and 133 patients with various gynecological diseases, and examined by stepwise discriminant analysis. The usefulness and the limits for diagnosis of various gynecological diseases were investigated for each tumor marker. Also, the diagnostic usefulness of stepwise discriminant analysis employing the values of five tumor markers in sera was studied for the gynecological malignancies compared with that of measuring serum CA125 alone. Because the mean values of CA125 in sera were increased specifically in the ovarian cancer patient group compared with those of other tumor markers in sera, the measurement of serum CA125 was considered to be more useful for diagnosis of ovarian cancer than that of the other tumor markers. The mean values of CA125 in sera, however, were also increased more significantly in the groups of patients with endometriosis and normal pregnancies than in the group of healthy nonpregnant females (p < 0.005). In the stepwise discriminant analysis employing the values of CA125 and four other tumor markers in sera, the diagnostic usefulness of each tumor marker was demonstrated in the early diagnosis, the differential diagnosis, and the determination of complete remission after several therapies for ovarian cancers.

10.09.09

Hormonal influence on the serum level of CA 125: Totani, R, Goto, S, Miwa, T, Suzuki, Y. Dept. Obstet. and Gyn., Nat. Nagoya Hosp., Nagoya, Japan

CA-125 is a cancer related substance, which is recognized in the serous adenocarcinoma of the ovary, by means of murine monoclonal antibody technics. Detection and quantification of this substance in serum is clinically applied as a tumor marker. But recently, it became clear, that this substance shows relatively high concentration in some normal subjects. To analyse the cause of the deviations of serum CA-125, we examined CA-125, estradiol, and progesterone in the following cases: normal menstruating girls, clomiphene-treated patients, HMG-HCG-treated patients, and patients treated with pill or Danazol because of endometriosis or myoma uteri. The analysis of our data indicates, that CA-125 is easily affected by the hormonal circumstances. There is a deviation during the menstrual cycle, in which CA-125 increases during menstruation. This phenomenon is more augmented in cases of HMG-HCG treated hyperovulation syndrome subjects, sometimes exceeding the values of advanced ovarian cancer patients. In conclusion, this study suggests that CA-125 is useful not only as a tumor marker, but also as a more general index of ovarian function.

10.09.10

Significance of immunosuppressive acidic protein (IAP) in patients with ovarian cancer: Shimizu, Y, Miura, S, Kurachi, K, Sawada, M*, Okudaira, Y*. Saiseikai Nakatsu Hosp., Res. Inst. Microb. Dis., Osaka Univ.*, Osaka, Japan

Previously we reported the significance of IAP in patients with gynecologic cancer (Cancer **54**, 652–656, 1984). The purpose of this study is to clarify the characteristics of IAP as a tumor marker compared with conventional tumor-producing markers (CEA, AFP, etc.) and newly established one (CA125). Sera were obtained from 96 patients with ovarian cancer. Controls were 150 healthy females, 92 benign ovarian tumors, 98 uterine myomas, and 84 cervical cancers. Assay of IAP was performed with SRID. The normal limit of IAP of 500 μg/ml was obtained from the mean value plus 2 SD of IAP in healthy controls. The mean value of IAP in patients with ovarian cancer (946 ± 385 μg/ml) was statistically higher than those of both benign ovarian tumors (374 ± 93 μg/ml) and controls (318 ± 86 μg/ml). Positivity of IAP (91.2%) was much higher than that of CEA (27.6%), AFP (17.9%), and CA125 (73.9%). Occurrence of elevated serum IAP values was not affected by tumor histology (different from CEA and CA125), which was very convenient for screening of ovarian cancer. IAP values increased with advanced clinical stage, but no definitive positive correlation with clinical stage was found. As to the relation with clinical course, IAP correlates with the results of therapy and performance state of patients. Most important thing is that IAP values increase earlier than other markers when the condition is exacerbated and this increase occurs before recurrence (or metastasis) is diagnosed clinically. In conclusion, IAP may be a useful marker for both diagnostic purposes and follow-up (early detection of recurrence) of ovarian cancer.

10.09.11

The serum levels of lactic dehydrogenase in ovarian tumors: Özekici, Ü, Babuna, C, Turfanda, A. Dept. Obstet. and Gyn., Istanbul Med. Fac., Istanbul, Turkey

Serum LDH levels were investigated in 196 patients with ovarian tumors who have applied to the gynecological clinics of Istanbul Medical Faculty during the last two years. No differences were present between the LDH levels in cases with benign ovarian tumors and those obtained from normal control patients. The high levels of serum LDH were detected however in patients with malignant ovarian tumors. There were significant decreases in the enzyme levels of operated patients when malignant tumors were successfully removed. Serum lactic dehydrogenase determinations, we believe, might be used as a tumor marker in the follow-up of patients with malignant ovarian tumors.

10.09.12

Estrogen receptor, total tRNA in tissue and serum-hormonal and marker profile in ovarian tumor: Jakowicki, J A, Baranowski, W, Kotarski, J. 2nd Clin. Op. Gyn., Acad. Med., Lublin, Poland

Metabolism of ovarian malignant tumor depends on numerous factors including hormones. Protein synthesis in this tissue can be estimated by tRNA. In nine women aged 42–72 in cancer tissue and in one, aged 22 in dysgerminoma estrogen receptor (ER) by *Gorksi* and *Cannon* method and tRNA by *Deacok* and *Dingman* polyacrylamide gel electrophoresis after phenol-isopropanol extraction by *Sein* et al. was estimated. Serum FSH, LH, E2, E1 as well as CEA, subunits of HCG were performed by RIA. ER in a borderline amount (1–3 fmol/mg prot.) was found only in four patients. ER was not dependent on age, serum LH, E2, E1 and CEA level. Above fifty of age, FSH up to 100 mU/ml correspond with ER(−) in comparison with normal FSH and ER(+ −). Serum alpha-HCG 2-28 ng/ml was noted in patients with ER(−) only. In older women with adenocarcinoma tRNA above 5 OD/0.1 ml indicated greater protein synthesis in contrast to cystadenocarcinoma in younger patients in spite of similar tRNA-5S fraction (20–29%) and more than 1.0 4S : 5S ratio. In the case of dysgerminoma ER 1.6 fmol/mg p, elevated serum LH and beta-HCG, normal FSH, E2, alpha-HCG and CEA was found. Advanced total tRNA 9.6 OD/0.1 ml, tRNA-5S 39% and decreased 4S : 5S ratio (0.64) indicated elevated protein synthesis by tumor tissue.

10.09.13

Monitoring pelvic diseases with CA125: Salvetti, B, Garzarelli, S, De Pascalis, L, Corsini, R, Russo, A. Div. Obstet.-Gyn., Osped. Civ. di Sanpierdarena, Genova, Italy

CA125 is antigenic determinant associated with human epithelial ovarian carcinomas. This study was undertaken to determine whether measurement of CA125 would provide a more precise correlation with tumor than with any other pelvic pathology. Among 200 patients with surgically demonstrable pelvic pathology serum CA125 levels were elevated in case: Of pelvic inflammatory diseases, in ovarian carcinoma, and endometriosis (> 250 U/ml). Consequently we can conclude that CA125 is not specific as a cancer marker, but it can be useful in the study of pelvic pathology.

10.09.14

Amylase production in common epithelial tumors of the ovary: Abe, Y, Ozaki, M, Ueda, G. Dept. Gyn., Ctr Adult Dis., Osaka, Japan

Although it has been reported that some serous carcinomas of the ovary produced amylase which caused hyperamylasemia, no cases of endometrioid carcinoma with hyperamylasemia are known. Recently, we encountered a few cases of serous and endometrioid ovarian carcinomas producing amylase. In these cases, serum amylase levels well reflected the clinical courses. So we studied cellular localization of amylase in various types of epithelial tumors of the ovary by immunoperoxidase method using antibody against human salivary amylase which cross-reacts to human salivary amylase. We found that amylase was present in eight of 34 serous carcinomas and eight of 27 endometrioid carcinomas, while it was not present in any of 34 mucinous tumors, benign to malignant, or any of five malignant clear cell tumors. These findings suggest that amylase, if present, is also a useful tumor marker for endometrioid carcinomas.

10.10.01

DES-associated clear cell adenocarcinoma: Herbst, A L, Senekjian, E K, Rotmensch, J, Anderson, D, Hubby, M M. Dept. Obstet. and Gyn., Univ., Chicago, IL, USA

A registry was established in 1971 to study clear cell adenocarcinoma (CCA) of the vagina and cervix which had previously been found to be associated with intrauterine exposure to diethylstilbestrol (DES). The registry has sought to study all patients with CCA born after 1940, whether or not there is a history of maternal DES. Currently the registry has data on 510 cases of which 63% have evidence of DES exposure. A remarkable peak in the age incidence curve has continued to be present at 19 years. The youngest DES patient was seven years of age at diagnosis, and the oldest 34 years. Newly diagnosed cases of DES-associated CCA continue to be reported. Birthplaces have included the U.S.A., Canada, Mexico, Belgium, Netherlands, France, Great Britain, Czechoslovakia, Ivory Coast and Australia. Factors relating to tumor development and behavior have been analysed. Daughters whose mothers began DES in early pregnancy have a greater risk of developing CCA (and non-malignant vaginal adenosis) than those whose exposure occurred later in gestation. An additional surprising finding was that females with early intrauterine exposure to DES tend to develop carcinomas at a younger age than those whose mothers began DES later. Moreover, patients 19 years or older have a five-year survival superior to younger patients. This in part is related to the prevalence of the tubulocystic form of CCA that appears to be less virulent than the other histologic types. Thus, the time of initial exposure to DES in pregnancy appears to modify both the age at which CCA develops as well as tumor behavior.

10.10.02

Results of adjuvant progestogen therapy in 269 endometrial carcinoma 1971 to 1974: Fournier, D v, Junker-mann, H, Kubli, F. Univ.-Frauenklin., Heidelberg

Since 1971 we have done a prospective study with adjuvant progestogen therapy in endometrial carcinoma. We started with medrogeston or medroxyprogesterone-acetate, 100 mg p. d. Later the dose was increased to 250 MPA p. d. Beginning with 2–3 years of treatment, MPA is given now for five years. Results in 134 patients with adjuvant progestogen and 135 controls show a clear tendency towards a favorable response in the progestogen group. The difference is significant in cases with three or more years of treatment. The rational background is that progestogens can antagonize the gross promoting activities of endogenous estrogens mediated by the progesteron receptor. Severe side-effects were not seen. Four patients stopped therapy because of nausea. Light and medium-light side-effects, which did not interrupt therapy, were: Increase of weight (+3.2 kg) and edema (66%). Thrombosis was not a significant problem in contrast to reports from progestogen therapy in breast cancer (4 cases in both therapy – and control-group). The best results showed the subgroup of carcinomas with high differentiation or with high progesteron receptors. In the whole group (269 patients, stage I or II, all operated, postoperative irradiation) the 5-year-survival was 76% in the therapy-group in contrast to 68% in the control group.

10.10.03

Intra-epithelial neoplasia in the vulvar region: Bock, J E, Andreasson, B. Dept. Obstet. and Gyn. Y, Rigshosp., Univ., Copenhagen, Denmark

From 1978 to 1982, 49 patients with intra-epithelial neoplasia in the vulvar region were included in a prospective investigation. The main purpose was to evaluate the effect of treatment by local excision with a free margin of 2 mm and to estimate the importance of colposcopy. In 28% of the patients, the disease recurred after primary treatment, and in one patient microinvasion was shown. No patients died of cancer. A risk factor of recurrence was involvement of resection margins. Multicentric location of the vulvar disease was found more frequently among patients treated for intra-epithelial neoplasia of the cervix. In 66% of the patients the colposcopic findings were consistent with intra-epithelial neoplasia. Local excision represents an improvement in the treatment of intra-epithelial neoplasia of the vulva, but frequent follow-up is necessary.

10.10.04

Carcinoma *in situ* of the vulva: Kürzl, R, Friedl, G, Baltzer, J, Lohe, K J. 1. Frauenklin., Univ., Munich

From 1971–1982 33 patients with VCIS (vulvar carcinoma *in situ*) were treated at the 1. Frauenklinik der Universität München. The median time of follow-up was 5.9 years. The average age was 56.9 years and the age distribution shows 8 patients under the age of 50 years (though older age groups dominate). Histologically 26 cases were found without early stromal invasion versus seven with early invasion. The labia minora were involved most often and multicentric growth was found in five cases. The primary treatment was not uniform: Most often simple vulvectomy or local excision was performed. Radiotherapy was given in five cases: Four times after vulvectomy, once after local excision. 12 cases were microscopically found to have been incompletely removed. Eight of these cases resulted in recurrences within a time span of 4 to 47 months after primary treatment. The recurrences offer still further details: Three cases again showed VCIS, two had turned into VCIS with early stromal invasion, three had changed into frankly invasive vulvar carcinoma. At the end of the follow-up period, 29 women still lived and four had died. Cause of death was not related to VCIS in three women, but the fourth patient died because of progress to invasive vulvar carcinoma. In summary, this small study allows the following conclusions: 1. Obviously most important for a successful treatment of VCIS is the complete removal of the *in situ* lesion. 2. Microscopic finding of VCIS not completely removed means a high risk of recurrence, combined with possible transition into invasive carcinoma of the vulva. 3. A thorough as well as a close follow-up of patients with VCIS is therefore strongly recommended.

10.10.05

Microcarcinoma (microinvasive carcinoma) of the vulva: Pickel, H. Dept. Obstet. and Gyn., Univ., Graz, Austria

Among 240 patients with carcinomatous diseases of the vulva 12 cases (5%) of true microcarcinomas (MCV) were primarily diagnosed between 1968 and 1984. Three patients were treated with wide local excision of the tumor after the initial diagnostic biopsy. Eight patients underwent a simple vulvectomy. Four patients were treated by a radical vulvectomy and additional lymphadenectomy. Twelve patients remained free from relapse and metastases during the follow-up time between five and ten years. Three patients developed secondary cancerous lesions of the vulva. Based on our morphological and clinical observations the following definition of a true MCV can be suggested: The MCV is a circumscribed small carcinoma with an estimated tumor volume up to $500 \, mm^3$. Generally it is highly differentiated and does not develop regional lymph node metastases. Relapses after the first removing procedures are most likely new primary tumors arising from neoplastic predetermined epithelial fields. Considering these aspects, a conservative treatment of the MCV including total excision of the tumor or simple vulvectomy without regional lymphadenectomy can be justified.

10.10.06

Use of the CO_2-laser in treatment of vulvar condyloma, V.I.N. and V.A.I.N. – a 5-year experience: Meandzija, M. Dept. Obstet. and Gyn., Univ., Bern, Switzerland

Two hundred and sixty-seven patients with vulvar condyloma acuminatum, VIN (vulvar intra-epithelial neoplasia) and VAIN (vaginal intra-epithelial neoplasia) have been treated using the technique of volume destruction or the surface abrasion with CO_2-laser. The average follow-up was 18 months. The high-power CO_2-laser is used as an energy source. This provides a thermal energy whose dissipation in the living tissue is regulated after nonlinear patterns. By reducing the time of laser beam action on tissue and cooling it with pure nitrogen, it is possible to achieve a minimal thermal injury, a faster healing of the wound and a less painful sensation. This is particularly evident when the microprocessor controlled laser beam micromanipulator is used. Among our patients in 23.93% of cases of condyloma acuminatum, 25.0% of cases of VIN and 15.38% of cases of VAIN multiple treatment sessions have had to be performed before the complete eradication of the disease was achieved. The microscope integrated "high-power" laser systems are a promising method for the treatment of vulvar condyloma acuminatum, vulvar intra-epithelial neoplasia and vaginal intra-epithelial neoplasia. It is well tolerated by the patient and reduces the postoperative complications as well as the need for hospital admission.

10.10.07

Experiences of RF hyperthermia by intracavitary applicator (clinical trial) on the treatment of vaginal cancer: Nakamura, R, Nambu, Y, Sou, S. Dept. Obstet. and Gyn., Kyoto Nat. Hosp., Kyoto, Japan

The hyperthermia had never been used practically in gynecology. We had a patient with vaginal cancer suitable for hyperthermia; the progress was shown as follows: Case: 68-year-old female, had radiation on cancer of right vaginal wall 3 years ago (1979) and was diminished completely. The recurrent tumor was found in the same area and patient was admitted for hyperthermia combined radiation on 1982 Oct. 12. – Methods: Intracavitary hyperthermia was performed by 6 MHz RF capacitive heating with Thermotron RF Model 8, which was presented by Yamamoto Vinitor Co. Ltd. The intracavitary RF applicator (clinical trial) consisted of copper wire as electrode in 30 ml capacitive violin type metreurynter filled with cool saline solution. Sizes of external electrode of right hip was selected 20 cm in diameter. Temperature-controlled water ($5-10°C$) was perfused into the electrode. Tissue temperature measured with a thin Teflon-coated thermocouples placed in the tumor through a 21 gauge angiocatheter. Other sensors were placed in the rectum and on the surface of intracavitary applicator in order to protect against local overheating. Temperature measurement was continuously performed during RF irradiation and the distribution of temperature within the tumor were also measured. Hyperthermia was performed once a week, five times in all. – Results: Intratumor temperature above $40.2°C$ was maintained with maximal power 75 Watt for $30 \sim 40$ minutes in each treatment. Maximal temperature of applicator was $40.3°C$, and of rectum was $36.8°C$. Complete response was accomplished after 8 months. – Conclusion: Our case of hyperthermic treatment with intracavitary applicator indicate that RF capacitive heating could be applied effectively and safely to vaginal tumors.

10.10.08

Diagnostic and therapeutic approaches in dysplasias of vulva and uterine cervix: Degen, K W, Bender, H G, Schnuerch, H G. Dept. Obstet. and Gyn., Univ., Düsseldorf

1. Biopsies and cytological smears of ten patients were compared in bovenoid papulosis and morbus Bowen. Two of these showed dysplasias of the cervix at the same time. In cooperation with the Cancer Research Center, Heidelberg (Dr. *Gissmann*) we looked for the papilloma virus DNA content in vulva and cervix of the ten patients. We found almost always an identical virus DAN-pattern. We treated vulva and cervix with CO_2-laser. The advantages of this procedure will be discussed. – 2. Another advantage of the CO_2-laser in treating cervical dysplasias is the negligible impact on child bearing functions. In circumsribed lesions local resection under colposcopic control can be considered as an alternative with the same advantages.

10.11.01

Estradiol and serum lipids – a dose and duration study: Crona, N, Enk, L, Lindberg, U-B, Samsioe, G, Silfverstolpe, G. Dept. Obstet. and Gyn., Sahlgrenska Hosp., Gothenburg, Sweden

Both alkylated and non-alkylated estrogens increase HDL-cholesterol and tend to decrease LDL, effects considered advantageous as regards cardiovascular risk. Alkylated estrogens also increase serum triglycerides (TG), adverse effects in this respect, while non-alkylated like estradiol valerate (E2V) do not, at least not in doses up to 2 mg. 19 oophorectomized women participated in a cross-over study and were given 2 and 4 mg E2V daily, for 6 weeks each. Ten of them continued taking 2 mg and nine taking 4 mg for another 12 weeks. Before treatment and after each treatment period, cholesterol (CH), phospholipids (PL) and TG were determined in serum and in the ultracentrifugally separated VLDL, LDL and HDL fractions. Apolipoprotein A1 (apo-A1) in serum was analysed by electroimmunoassay. Neither dose influenced serum- or VLDL-TG. CH and PL were lower in LDL and higher in HDL after both 2 and 4 mg compared to pretreatment values. No differences were seen between the effects of the two doses. The E2V-induced changes persisted throughout the study. Apo-A1, the main protein constituent of HDL, increased after 2 mg E2V and even further after 4 mg. Thus E2V (2 and 4 mg) has a constant and in terms of cardiovascular risk favorable influence on lipoprotein metabolism.

10.11.02

Lipoprotein lipids and apolipoprotein A1 – effects of ORG OD 14: Silfverstolpe, G, Crona, N, Samsioe, G. Dept. Obstet. and Gyn., Sahlgren's Hosp., Univ., Göteborg, Sweden

Org OD 14 is a steroid which demonstrates weak estrogenic and very weak androgenic/anabolic properties in animal bioassays. It is reported to be suitable for the continuous treatment of estrogen-deficiency symptoms. We have accordingly studied the effects of OD 14 on lipoprotein metabolism. A group of 22 hysterosalpingo-oophorectomized women was given OD 14 2.5 mg/day, estradiol valerate 2 mg/day and a placebo for 6 week periods with a cross-over design in each case. Cholesterol (CH), phospholipids (PL) and triglycerides (TG) were assayed in very-low-density, low-density and high-density lipoproteins (VLDL, LDL and HDL). Apolipoprotein A1 (Apo-A1) was determined by electroimmunoassay. OD 14 substantially decreased all the lipid components of HDL, i.e. CH, PL and TG. Furthermore, OD 14 markedly decreased Apo-A1. These effects indicate that, from a metabolic point of view, OD 14 exerts a rather strong androgenic influence. A decrease in HDL-lipids and Apo-A1, the major protein component of HDL, is associated with a higher incidence of cardiovascular disease. Women with climacteric estrogen-deficiency symptoms belong to an age group in which the risk of developing cardiovascular disease is much higher than in younger women. The use of Org OD 14 for long-term treatment could therefore hardly be justified.

10.11.03

Effects of high dose treatment with estriol in postmenopausal women on serum lipoproteins: Frankman, O*, Rossner, S**, Valldor, G*. Dept. Obstet. and Gyn., South Hosp., Stockholm*; and King Gustaf V Res. Inst., Karolinska Inst., Stockholm**, Sweden

Estriol 12 mg/day was administered orally to postmenopausal women, 1 × 12 mg to ten patients and 3 × 4 mg to ten. Endometrial biopsy was taken before and during treatment for three months and serum proteins and lipoproteins were determined.

Results ($\bar{x}$ mmol/l ± SD):

	Total		VLDL		LDL		HDL	
	Chol	TG	Chol	TG	Chol	TG	Chol	TG
A. 1 × 12 mg, N = 10								
Before	7.92 +1.59	1.34 +0.69	0.42 +0.29	0.62 +0.40	4.83 +1.48	0.48 +0.26	2.01 +0.28	0.19 +0.07
After 3 months	6.93 +1.55	1.41 +0.61	0.46 +0.27	0.77 +0.37	4.62 +1.24	0.45 +0.22	1.87 +0.29	0.20 +0.07
B. 3 × 4 mg, N = 9								
Before	7.54 +1.15	1.21 +0.48	0.47 +0.26	0.68 +0.41	5.09 +1.16	0.37 +0.10	1.81 +0.32	0.15 +0.03
After 3 months	6.75 +1.35	1.33 +0.32	0.44 +0.20	0.70 +0.39	4.61 +1.04	0.41 +0.11	1.79 +0.32	0.17 +0.04

In principle, estrogens increase VLDL and HDL and reduce LDL levels. Although estriol induced mitoses and affected estrogen dependent serum proteins (Maturitas **116**, 6, 1984) little effect was seen on lipoproteins. The estriol half-life is short, however, no lipoprotein differences were observed between the two dose regimens.

10.11.04

Conjugated estrogens, estradiol valerate, estriol and tibolone (ORG OD14) in the control of the climacteric syndrome: Volpe, A, Zirilli, E*, Baralti, R, Campanini, D, Boralti, V*, Grasso, A, Previdi, A M, Borsari, S, Genazzani, A R. Dept. Obstet. and Gyn., Univ. Modena, *Gen. Lab. Clin. Path., Univ. Modena, Italy
113 menopause patients were studied distributed in randomized groups undergoing the following treatments for six cycles each: 1) Conjugated estrogens (CEE) (0.625 mg/die for 21 days) plus norethisterone (NET) (5 mg/die from 12th to 21st day); 2) CEE plus ciproterone acetate (CPA) (12.5 mg/die from 1st to 10th day); 3) estradiol valerate (EV) (2 mg/die for 21 days) plus NET; 4) EV plus CPA; 5) estriol (E) (2–4 mg/die); 6) Tibolone (ORG OD14) (2.5 mg every day); 7) Placebo. Hot flushes were significantly improved during the whole six months, by all other forms of treatment. E, at the dose used, however, was less satisfactory than CEE, EV and OD14. At the end of the six months, histological examination revealed no alteration of endometrial morphology in any of the patients. On the contrary, indeed, addition of a progestin brought about a regression of endometrial hyperplasia in eight of the patients treated. Neither after two nor after six months did the treatment with E or OD14 significantly alter plasma levels of tryglycerides, total cholesterol, HDL or LDL. CEE plus CPA and EV plus CPA increased HDL levels significantly after six months. On the other hand, NET plus CEE and EV decreased total cholesterol and HDL while increased LDL levels. Our data show that CEE, EV, OD14 are all capable of controlling hot flushes. We found that, by adding a progestin it is possible to protect the endometrium. In this regard CPA was found to be as effective and more safe than NET. ORG OD14 is an efficacious alternative to conventional estrogen therapy.

10.11.05

Continuous estrogen/progesteron therapy in postmenopausal women. Effect on vasomotor symptoms, uterine bleeding and plasma lipids: Davey, D A, Berger, G M, Hardie, F E, Yon, D. Univ. of Cape Town, Dept. Obstet. and Gyn., Observatory, S. Africa
This study is aimed at achieving continuous replacement of estrogen and progestogen in physiological doses with relief of symptoms and beneficial effects on cholesterol and bone metabolism but without endometrial abnormality, uterine bleeding or other side-effects. In the 1st phase of a double-blind trial micronised estradiol 2 mg daily (ME) for 28 days followed by ME combined with either 1 or 0.5 mg norethisterone acetate for 28 days (NETA) was administered to 40 menopausal women with hot flushes. The incidence of symptoms, uterine bleeding and side-effects; the levels of plasma estradiol, estrone, FSH, LH; plasma lipoproteins and plasma calcium, phosphorus and alkaline phosphatase were measured. The majority, but not all women, with hot flushes were relieved by ME or ME and NETA but a significant proportion of women experienced side-effects including breast tenderness, abdominal cramps and uterine bleeding though these decreased with continued treatment. No endometrial abnormalities were found. Plasma estradiol and estrone levels were initially low and were restored to normal and high pre-menopausal levels respectively. FSH and LH were initially increased and were reduced on ME but only reached normal levels on combined ME and NETA. ME alone caused a fall in total and LDL cholesterol and a rise in HDL cholesterol and triglycerides and these changes were reversed to pre-treatment levels with ME and NETA. Continuous combined estrogen/progestogen therapy offers the best hope of physiological hormone replacement in postmenopausal women without the risk of uterine carcinoma and side-effects such as bleeding but the ideal estrogen/progestogen combination has yet to be evolved.

10.11.06

Short-term dose response clinical and biological effects of estradiol and estriol (in combination) in postmenopausal women: Erlich, Y, Friedman, M, Peretz, B A. Dept. Obstet. and Gyn. "B", Rambam Med. Ctr, Haifa, Israel
The estrogenic treatment of postmenopausal women with conjugated and semisynthetic estrogens is widely used in comparison to the use of the natural hormones. This study was undertaken to determine the short-term effect (21 days) of a combination of natural estrogens (17β-estradiol and estriol) on the clinical parameters and on the number of biological markers. Two groups of postmenopausal women (12 and 10) suffering from severe menopausal symptoms were studied before and after 21 days on a combination of estradiol and estriol. One group was given 2 mg estradiol + 1 mg estriol, and the second group was given half of it (1 mg + 0.5 mg, respectively). All women reported improvement of subjective signs (hot flushes, insomnia, vaginal dryness, etc.). Serum estradiol increased significantly in both groups. FSH showed a significant decrease in both groups but more in the high dose group. LH decreased significantly only in the high dose group. Both dosages did not suppress these hormones to premenopausal level. The urinary calcium to creatinine ratio (an index of bone resorption) decreased significantly in both groups but more in the high dose group. Vaginal cytology showed an estrogenic effect in both groups. Prolactin increased significantly in both groups. Albumin and globulin did not change. These results express mainly the biological action of the more active hormone – estradiol as estriol was shown to have minimal effect in such a low dose. The biological effects found in this study will be compared to the effects of other hormones used as a replacement therapy in postmenopausal women as found by other authors.

250

10.11.07

Hormone replacement and non-steroid therapy: New approach to the menopausal symptoms: David, A, Weisglass, L. Fertility Ctr and Endocr. Lab., Zamenhoff Centr. Clin., Tel Aviv, Israel

The benefit of estrogen replacement therapy in the treatment of the vasomotor and lower genital tract symptoms is overshadowed by their risk of inducing endometrial and breast carcinoma. The present study reports a new scheme of treatment in 40 patients suffering of the menopausal symptoms. They were treated by ingesting estradiol 2 mg + estriol 1 mg, 21 days, for three consecutive cycles, followed by a 4th cycle of the same estrogen enriched with 1 mg norethisterone acetate resulting in a shedding of the endometrium. Regular endometrial biopsy and hysteroscopy showed that hyperplasia starts to be critical only at the end of the 3rd estrogen cycle. Radioimmunoassays of steroids and FSH, LH could not predict the severity of the hyperstimulation. We concluded for this part of the study that the above schedule prevents the risk of hyperplasia without the monthly side-effects of blood loss, mastalgia and premenstrual tension of a monthly combined therapy. Forty-five other women were treated by a potent elective antagonist of dopamine: the veralipride. Complete relief of their severe complaints were noted in 60 to 75% of the patients. Hyperprolactinemia was transitional. It was concluded that postmenopausal women enduring the vasomotor symptoms only could benefit from this non-steroid treatment especially when there is any contraindication to exogenous estrogen therapy.

10.11.08

LH pulsatility in postmenopausal women under bromocriptine therapy: Kösebay, D, Atasü, T, Çetinkaya, A, Hekim, N. Dept. Obstet. and Gyn., Cerrahpaşa Fac. Med., Univ., Istanbul, Turkey

The aim of our study was to investigate the pulsatility of LH release in postmenopausal women and to determine if treatment with a dopamine agonist, bromocriptine, induces the inhibition of pulsatile LH secretion. Five women aged 45–58, all in postmenopausal state at least for two years, were included in the study. Blood samples from cannulated vein were collected every 15 minutes between 9.00 a. m. and 2.00 p. m. and the LH pulsatility was assessed. PRL levels were also determined. All subjects received bromocriptine 5 mg/day for 17 days. Before treatment, we observed an increase in LH secretion as compared to the premenopausal period. After treatment, LH levels were decreased in two cases and increased in three cases. However, the difference was not statistically significant. There was no significant difference in the number of LH pulses before and after bromocriptine. However, in all cases we observed a decrease in the amplitudes of LH pulses after bromocriptine ($p < 0.05$), i. e. LH secretion became more stable around the average levels. FSH levels were increased as compared to pretreatment levels and there was a significant decrease in PRL values. Postmenopausal women have quite low levels of estrogen so the modulating action of estrogen is negligible on the pituitary. It can be concluded that a dopamine agonist, bromocriptine, has no effect on the modulation of LH pulsatility in postmenopausal women.

10.11.09

Conjugated estrogens and clonidine: A new regimen for the treatment of postmenopausal women: Schindler, A E, Heners, D, Pater, T, Wendel, U, Donath, E M. Dept. Obstet. and Gyn., Univ., Tübingen

The aim of the study was to investigate whether a reduced dose of estrogen combined with clonidine would alleviate climacteric symptoms as effectively as higher doses of conjugated estrogens. A controlled, randomized double-blind study was carried out in 83 patients complaining of postmenopausal symptoms. Treatment with a combination of 0.6 mg conjugated estrogens and 100 μg clonidine daily was compared with a daily dose of 1.25 mg conjugated estrogens alone. The effect of these two regimens on the Kupperman index was evaluated after 2, 4, 8 and 12 weeks of therapy and a statistical evaluation of the results in 65 patients was performed. The number and intensity of hot flushes and sweats, as well as the severity of migraine headaches, improved on both regimens. There were no significant differences in either case. The combined treatment was judged by the patients to be significantly more effective ($p < 0.01$) than estrogen treatment alone. Side-effects were significantly fewer ($p < 0.01$) during combination therapy than with estrogen only. This study demonstrates that lower doses of estrogens can be equally effective in the treatment of climacteric symptoms when combined with low-dose clonidine. Indeed, therapeutic efficacy was even improved and side-effects reduced. Reduced doses of estrogens in combination with clonidine therefore decrease the risk of estrogen-dependent tumor development that is associated with long-term therapy.

10.11.10

Effect of the transient hyperprolactinemia due to the use of Lir 1660 on peripheral androgen aromatization in postmenopause: Fuschini, G, Jasonni, V M, Naldi, S, Cristiani, P, Flamigni, C. Dept. Reprod. Med., Univ., Bologna, Italy

Recently the use of Lir 1660 (Agradil – Vita) has been proposed for the treatment of vasomotor symptoms in postmenopause. However, this drug causes a transient hyperprolactinemia. In this study we attempted to verify the effect of the hyperprolactinemia on the peripheral androgen aromatization. For this purpose the plasma levels of androstenedione (A) and estrone (E_1) were determined before and after 20 days of Lir 1660 administration in 20 postmenopausal women. Obviously the plasma levels of hPRL were also evaluated. In all subjects the hPRL levels raised to 70 ± 15 μg/ml at the end of the treatment. The peripheral E_1 did not show any significant variation, while in six subjects the A plasma levels increased. From these data it appears that the transient hyperprolactinemia due to the use of Lir 1660 does not interfere with the endogenous extraglandular estrogen production.

10.11.11

Treatment of climacteric disorders by low doses of clonidine: Zwiens, G, Sturm, G, Eulenburg, R. Frauenklin., Med. Hochsch., Hannover, Frauenklin., Marburg

Women suffering from intensive climacteric disorders often need a non-hormonal treatment. In the course of an open study we examined 30 patients showing climacteric symptoms and tested the effect of clonidine (Dixarit®) on their complaints. The results obtained were compared with those from ten patients who had received a placebo. Before the treatment and every week during the treatment we wrote down the number of flushes and sweating attacks. Moreover, blood pressure, pulse and bodyweight were measured. The hormones FSH, LH, prolactin and estradiol were measured as well, and a Schellong test was done. There was a significant reduction of climacteric symptoms in 27 out of 30 cases. The patients that were in the perimenopause showed a slower reduction of the symptoms than the other ones who had had their menopause three or more years before. As a result of the Schellong test we found a small orthostatic reaction, but only at the beginning of the treatment. When compared with the values measured without any treatment the hormone profiles showed no significant change. There was no significant reduction of the climacteric symptoms in the group of patients that were given a placebo.

10.12.01

A decidual/endometrial protein (PP14) in early pregnancy: Chapman, M G, Bolton, A E, Yovich, J, Grudzinskas, G. Dept. Obstet. and Gyn., Guy's Hosp., London, UK

The isolation of a 47,000 MW glycoprotein (PP14) which is predominantly of decidual and endometrial origin, has provided a unique tool for investigating the early events of pregnancy. Using a recently developed radioimmunoassay we have observed its production in the menstrual cycle and early gestation. Serum levels are elevated in the luteal plasma (mean $= 45 \, \mu g/l$) as compared with the follicular phase (mean $= 25 \, \mu g/l$). By the 10th day post-ovulation or egg retrieval (in IVF cycles), the levels begin to rise dramatically to peak at levels of $1000 \, \mu g/l$ by 8 weeks of gestation. Serum levels then fall. While the pattern is similar to that of human chorionic gonadotrophin, no correlation between HCG and PP14 exists. Nor does there appear to be a direct correlation with progesterone levels. Further studies of this protein to elucidate its physiological role are in progress.

10.12.02

Pregnancy-associated plasma proteins in hepatic diseases during pregnancy: Břešťák, M, Fuchs, V. Dept. Obstet. and Gyn., Paediat. Fac., Charles Univ., Praha, Czechoslovakia

Biochemical markers (urinary estriol levels, maternal serum hPL and alpha-1-fetoprotein measurements) are said to be inefficient in the monitoring of pregnancies complicated by hepatic diseases, esp. cholestasis of pregnancy. Maternal serum levels of pregnancy-associated proteins were studied in pregnancies complicated by cholestasis of pregnancy, acute hepatitis and chronic progres. hepatitis. The proteohormones hCG, hPL and plasma concentrations of PSbeta-1-G – SP1, alpha-2-PAG – SP3, and six "acute phase" proteins have been measured. All patients after acute hepatitis with an uneventful progress of pregnancy had normal plasma values of the proteins studied. In cholestasis of pregnancy there was a sharp increase in the mean hPL curve when the fetal development was normal, and a relative decrease in IUGR. Plasma concentrations of SP1 were normal in mild forms of hepatosis, mostly elevated in severe forms, but were very low in fetal GR. The plasma levels of SP3 were normal in mild disease, but low in severe ones. The most sensitive response was recognized in "acute phase" proteins in different forms of hepatosis and chronic hepatitis.

10.12.03

Cellular immune spectrum and monocyte function during pregnancy: Rha, J G, Lee, J M, Song, S K, Kim, S J. Dept. Obstet. and Gyn., Cath. Med. Coll., Seoul, Korea

To evaluate cellular immune spectrum during pregnancy, function of monocyte and T cell subset were studied in 36 pregnant women; 11 in 1st trimester, 11 in 2nd trimester and 14 in 3rd trimester of pregnancy. Monocyte and lymphocyte separated from peripheral blood were frozen and kept by using programmed cryosystem with liquid nitrogen and were then thawed for assay at once. Pan T cell and T cell subset were observed by using monoclonal antibody (anti Leu-1, anti Leu-2a and anti Leu-3a) and function of monocyte was also estimated by means of ^{51}Cr release assay system with human 0 type (Rh +) red blood cells as their sole target. Pan T cells (T_p) and helper T cells (T_h) were significantly decreased in the pregnant group (75.0 ± 4.2, 44.5 ± 3.5). Monocyte function was also decreased in pregnant group (13.2 ± 3.5) when compared with normal control group (29.2 ± 3.9). But there was a tendency of the recovery of monocyte function at 3rd trimester of pregnancy. Suppressor T cells (T_s) showed no difference between two groups. T_h/T_s ratio revealed significant decrease in the pregnant group ($p < 0.01$). It is concluded from the above results that pregnancy causes helper T cell deficiency followed by a decreased monocyte function.

252

10.12.04

Monoclonal antibody studies of fetal lymphocytes for prenatal diagnosis of genetic immune deficiency diseases: Holzgreve, W, Beller, F K. Frauenklin., Westf. Wilhelms-Univ., Münster

Monoclonal antibodies provide a tool for the differentiation of lymphocytes bearing distinct cell membrane surface antigens. Using monoclonal antibodies and indirect immunofluorescence we developed an easy and reliable micromethod for the quantitative analysis of fetal lymphocyte markers (*Holzgreve, Golbus* et al. J. Reprod. Immunol., in press). In the present study monoclonal antibodies (Ortho) specific for identification of all peripheral T-lymphocytes (OKT 3), the subclass of suppressor/cytotoxic T-lymphocytes (OKT 8) and for B-lymphocytes (OKI a) were employed. 100 μl blood samples were obtained and the lymphocytes were harvested from a medium/Ficoll-Hypaque interface. 33 μl of a 1 : 32 dilution of monoclonal antibodies was added to the cell suspension, the final cell pellet contained about 1200 cells. The percentages of cells defined by the three different T- and B-cell surface markers are given in the table.

	(n = 19)	(n = 17)
	Newborn	Fetuses
Monoclonal antibody		
OKT 3	75.4±3.2	53.1±9.7
OKT 8	23.7±4.1	20.5±3.7
OKI a	16.3±1.9	18.6±4.9

These results indicate that genetic immunodeficiency states can be identified with monoclonal antibodies and a slide immunofluorescence technique, even in small fetal samples.

10.12.05

A soluble immunosuppressive factor secreted by cultured trophoblast cells: Tanaka, F, Koyama, M, Negoro, T, Saji, F, Nakamuro, K, Tanizawa, O. Dept. Obstet. and Gyn., Osaka Univ. Med. School, Osaka, Japan

The immunologic mechanisms that protect the fetus from rejection are the subject of numerous investigations. The placental tissue especially trophoblasts play a role of an immunological barrier as well as an anatomical one between mother and fetus. In this study immunoregulatory role of trophoblast cells on cell mediated immunity was investigated. Eight-ten weeks human chorion was minced with scissors, treated with collagenase, followed by differential centrifugation, and trophoblast enriched cell suspension was obtained. The trophoblast cells were cultured for periods of 48 hrs and the incubation medium was tested for their immunosuppressive activity. The cultured supernatant of trophoblast cells when added to *in vitro* lymphocyte reaction suppressed their reactivity to lectins (phytohemagglutinin and pokeweed mitogen). The degree of suppression was over 70% at 20% of final concentration and dose dependant. The immunosuppressive effect of the supernatant was not due to the cytotoxicity to lymphocytes. The supernatant also suppressed the mixed lymphocyte reactions and killer cell generation. The results indicate that trophoblast releases a soluble suppressive factor which is a potent inhibitor of cell-mediated immunity and plays an important role in the fetomaternal relationship.

10.12.06

B cell surface receptor differences in rhesus immunized and non-immunized pregnant women: Gupta, I, Ganguly, N K, Gupta, A N, Jolly, J G. Dept. Obstet. and Gyn., Postgrad. Inst. Med. Educ. and Res., Chandigarh, India

Since only about 16 per cent of Rh negative pregnant women produce Rh antibodies when exposed to Rh antigen repeatedly, an attempt was made to find out if there are immunological differences in Rh negative immunised and non-immunised pregnant women. Therefore total B lymphocytes and B cell surface receptors were studied in twenty Rh negative immunised and twenty non-immunised pregnant women matched for age and number of pregnancies. Ten non-pregnant healthy females also matched for age and number of pregnancies were also included to serve as controls. Total B lymphocytes were counted by EAC rosette technique of *Jondal* et al. (J. exp. Med. **136**, 207–215, 1972). B-cell surface receptors were studied by immunofluorescence technique of *Aiuti* et al. (Clin. exp. Immun. **15**, 43–52, 1973). No differences were observed in the total B cell counts and IgG and IgA bearing B cell populations in the three groups. However, IgM receptor bearing B cell sub-population was significantly lower in non-immunised as compared to immunised and controls both during pregnancy as well as post-delivery thereby showing a probable defect in B cell differentiation. Thus it can be hypothesised that there is possibly a defect in B cell differentiation in the non-immunised subjects which is probably responsible for their not being responsive to Rh antigen.

10.12.07

The immunobiological mechanisms of acceptation of the human allogenic egg: Skrzypulec, Z A. Dept. Obstet. and Gyn., Mikołów/Katowice, Poland

Previous investigations allowed us to discover fundamental mechanisms of allotransplantation of the human allogenic egg (*Skrzypulec, Z A.* Zbl. Gyn. **104**, 1503, 1982; **106**, 46, 1984). An original cell culture method was introduced to obtain all the placenta's cells *in vitro*. They were studied as well on cytomorphologic and also on antigenic characteristics by using light-, electron- and immunofluorescence microscope. It was discovered that the so-called syncytium of the chorionic villi is found as a normal epithelial layer, being built of two kinds of nucleiform cells, large ca. $1.5\,\mu$. They do not possess transplantations antigens of the egg (ETA). Also the cells of the amniotic sac, without the endothelium, are also found as one without antigen. The so-called syncytial nuclei and knotes were discovered as large colonies of superantigen cells, possessing AgAbIgG immune complexes. During physiological desquamation of trophoblastic material into the pregnant woman's circulation those AgAbIgG complexes reach her immune systems, causing immune response regulations as: 1. suppression of high synthesis of not complement (C) binding anti-ETA, 2. high synthesis of C-binding anti-AgAb, which block by reaching of equilibrium constant K of complex-Ag the enzymatic activity of the C. Therefore due to the law of mass action the immune cytolysis of egg's allogenic cells is impossible allowing their allotransplantation. It is going first of all under the immunologic, as yet unknown, paramount action of the placenta.

10.12.08

Irregular antibodies, clinical significance: Fadel, H E**, Squires, J E**, Larrison, P J**. Depts. Obstet. and Gyn.* and Path.**, Med. Coll. of Georgia, Augusta, GA, USA

In some practices, only Rh negative patients are screened for antibodies while in others like ours, all prenatal patients are screened. During the years 1979–1983, 8738 patients were screened and 495 (5.8%) had a positive antibody screen. Of the 62 patients with IgG antibodies, 38 had anti-D antibody either singly or in combination with other antibodies, and the remaining 24 patients had clinically significant antibodies other than anti-D, an incidence of 0.27%. If only Rh negative patients were screened, 20 of these patients would have been missed. Out of the 24 patients, six had anti-E, three had anti-C, three had anti-c, one had anti-e, and 13 had anti-Kell antibodies. Anti-Fy^a, anti-JK^a, anti-JK^b, and anti-Co^b antibodies were identified in the remaining four patients, respectively. There was a history of prior blood transfusions in four of these 24 patients. Sickle Cell Disease was the indication for repeated blood transfusions in two of these four patients. These 24 patients were followed by serial antibody titers, seven had undergone amniocenteses 1–3 times for evaluation of fetal involvement. A patient with significant (1/512) anti-Kell titer had serial plasmaphoreses, and three intrauterine transfusions and her neonate survived. Nine of the neonates had positive direct Coombs' tests, six had hemolytic disease of the newborn, three of these were probably due to AB0 incompatibility.

10.12.09

The measurement of alpha-fetoprotein in the serum of the blood of pregnant women with Rh disease, as a non-invasive method of estimating the impediment of the fetus: Majchrzak, J, Dębski, R, Łukaszewicz, E, Marianowski, L. Obstet. and Gyn. Clin., 2nd Dept., Med. Acad., Warszawa, Poland

The method of RIA has been applied to measure the concentration of alpha-fetoprotein in the serum of blood samples collected from pregnant women in the system of Rh (226 designations) as well as from pregnant women with anti Rh antibodies who have given birth to infants with Rh negative factor (150 designations) in the period between 28 and 40 weeks gestation. Most of the patients have undergone the amniocentesis and examination of the optical density of the amniotic fluid. On the basis of the research results the Liley's prognostic chart has been applied. In the case of pregnancies which resulted in intra-uterine death of the fetus caused by severe anemia (7 cases) three or four time increase of AFP density has been observed in comparison with other Rh disease pregnancies. The AFP density noted in the case of patients classified by *Liley* to the 1 and 2 group of impedence who have given birth to infants with Rh negative factor (65 designations) is significantly lower than the density of AFP in the serum of the pregnant women classified in the same groups who have given birth to infants with hemolytic disease. The authors believe that the estimation of AFP density in the serum of the pregnant women's blood is of prognostic value in the prenatal estimation of the impedence of the fetus.

10.12.10

Concentrations of triglycerides (TG), cholesterol (TC) and total protein (TP) in the amniotic fluid in pregnant women with Rh immunization: Marianowski, L, Szostak, W B, Nowicka, G, Cyganek, A, Kłosiewicz-Latoszek, L. Dept. Obstet. and Gyn., II Fac. Med., and Nat. Inst. Food and Nutr., Warszawa, Poland

Concentrations of triglycerides, total cholesterol, total protein were determined in 88 samples of amniotic fluid obtained by amniocentesis. The amniotic fluid was sampled between the 28th and the 36th weeks of pregnancy. The group studied consisted of 72 samples obtained from patients with the diagnosis of Rh immunization. The optic density of the amniotic fluid was determined by spectrophotometry and the risk zone was determined on the basis of these results according to *Liley's* scale. The studied group was subdivided into four subgroups depending on the risk zone. The control group included 16 samples of fluid obtained between the 28th and the 36th weeks of pregnancy from women without evidence of Rh immunization. – Results: A statistically significant difference in the level of TP in the I subgroup – 97.8 mg/dl ($p < 0.001$) and in the II^a subgroup – 199.3 mg/dl ($p < 0.02$) as compared with the control group – 251.2 mg/dl. Statistically significant differences ($p < 0.01$) in TC concentration were found in all four subgroups [I = 4.33 mg/dl, II^a = 5.94 mg/dl, II^b = 4.49 mg/dl, III = 4.79 mg/dl (as compared with the control group) 2.52 mg/dl]. No statistically significant differences were found in TG concentrations in all groups.

10.12.11

Active immunisation of the human fetus to tetanus by immunization of the mother: Tofoski, J, Jurukovski, J, Rukavina, D, Dinulović, D. Dept. Obstet. and Gyn., Univ., Skopje, Yugoslavia

Previous studies have shown that antibodies, cells and antigens can cross the placenta. Experimental studies in animals showed that immunization of pregnant female in appropriate time and dosage of an antigen led to transplacental immunization of her fetuses. Recent studies proved that transplacental immunization in humans also occurs. The pregnant women, unscreened volunteers from the outpatient clinic were immunized twice during pregnancy at either 26 and 30th weeks or at 32 and 36 weeks with toxoid of tetanus (2.5, 5, 10 Lf). The sensitization of the offspring was tested by identification of IgM specific antitetanus antibodies by techniques of *Repetti* (J. immun. Methods **37**, 153–163) in the cord blood at birth and before the first DTP vaccine. The mixed lymphocyte reaction was performed also. The newborns of immunized mothers were sensitized to tetanus, but not those of unimmunized. The study showed that transplacental immunization in humans occurs, and that it enhances the immune response of the offspring to subsequent immunization. Concerning the timing and damage applied there were no significant differences. This method could be very useful in prevention of tetanus neonatorum, especially in developing countries. It can open a new era in the fight against infective diseases very early in life.

10.12.12

Immunoglobulin estimation in bilharzial pregnant women: Yousef, H H, El-Said, A M, El-Assar, S T. Zagazig Fac. Med., Zagazig Univ., Zagazig, Egypt

The immunoglobulins G, A and M have been measured in sera of 39 bilharzial pregnant patients grouped in three groups: 11 in first trimester, 14 in second trimester and 14 in third trimester, in comparison with 30 pregnant non-bilharzial females by the *Mancini's* method of immunodiffusion. IgG decreased in the first trimester and increased in second trimester in bilharzial pregnant women. As regard IgA there was significant increase in second trimester and highly significant increase in third trimester and non-significant increase in first trimester. As regard IgM there was a highly significant decrease in the first trimester and a non-significant decrease in second trimester and third trimester in pregnant bilharzial patients as compared to the pregnant non-bilharzial. The mechanisms causing the variation observed are not clear but dilutional effects, race, and transport across the placenta and the infection with bilharziasis whether it is active or inactive, acute or chronic, and the presence of splenomegaly and ascites or their absence, and whether splenectomy was done for the patient or not, should be considered in looking for an explanation.

10.12.13

Early pregnancy factor in human embryo culture medium: Kuo, T, Sueoka, K, Morisada, M, Kawakami, S, Kobayashi, T. Dept. Obstet. and Gyn., School Med., Keio Univ., Tokyo, Japan

Early pregnancy factor (EPF) is one of the pregnancy associated proteins firstly reported by *H. Morton* in Australia in 1974. EPF is confirmed to be detected from maternal blood six hours after fertilization in mouse and 48 hours after fertilization in the human. Antihuman lymphocyte antibody suppresses E-rosette formation between human lymphocyte and sheep RBC, and EPF acts to amplify the action of the antibody to suppress E-rosette formation. We tried to detect EPF in human embryo culture medium, and identified an EPF activity in the pronuclear stage at the 15th hour after fertilization. We also found higher EPF activity as cleavage of fertilized ovum took place. It was observed that when embryo transfer was performed, an EPF activity appeared in maternal blood on the third day and that in cases being pregnant subsequent activity tended to persist at high levels. EPF seems to be highly helpful in clinical applications such as an early detection of pregnancy, differential diagnosis for failure of fertilization or implantation and prognosis of the embryo.

10.12.14

Identification and purification of β-nerve growth factor (NGF) from human placenta: Koshimizu, T, Takahashi, T, Taga, M, Uemura, T, Minaguchi, H. Dept. Obstet. and Gyn., Yokohama City Univ. School Med., Yokohama, Japan

NGF is a protein that supports growth and maintenance of peripheral sympathetic neurons and development of sensory neurons during the period of development. The presence of NGF in human placenta has been recently reported. In order to study the biological significance of NGF in human placenta, its extraction, purification, and characterization were performed. Placenta was homogenized with cold water, centrifuged and dialyzed. The dialyzed supernatant was passed through a CM-cellulose column equilibrated in 0.02 M phosphate buffer, pH 6.8. The eluate was dialyzed and pH was rapidly reduced to 4.0 to dissociate 7S NGF. The acidified solution was purified by ion-exchange chromatography. Biological activity of NGF was determined by the plasma clot method using dorsal root ganglia of 8–10-day-old chicken embryos in culture plates. Fractions having a NGF activity could be extracted in pH 9.0, 0.4 M NaCl in gradient chromatography of CM 32 cellulose column. Biological activity of extracts had one biological unit in 75–750 ng protein/ml by various lots of purification, which was equivalent to 10 ng/ml of purified mouse β-NGF. 7.5 mg of β-NGF was obtained from 200 g of term placenta. The human β-NGF was further purified by HPLC. The human placental β-NGF did not have any cross-reactivity with antiserum against mouse NGF in radioimmunoassay. In conclusion, we identified the presence of β-NGF in human placenta which was immunologically different from mouse NGF. The presence of β-NGF in placenta suggests its possible involvement in the growth and differentiation of nervous system in human fetal development.

10.13.01
Role of IUD in family planning program in Indonesia: Sumbung, P P. Cawang, Jakarta Timur, Indonesia

Family planning in Indonesia has been given one of the main priorities, and it forms an integral part of the national development program. The execution of the national family planning program pursues various approaches namely integrated approach, community approach, region specific planning approach, decentralized management, active coordination, etc. based on these approaches, efforts are made to attain the program's goals which are formulated as the demographic goals, that is the reduction of fertility rate to 50% in 1990 as compared to the rate in 1971, and the normative goals, namely the establishment of the small, happy and prosperous family norm. To achieve these ultimate goals, one of the main program efforts is contraceptive services which principally follow the "cafetaria system". This system enables the eligible couples to choose any method of contraception which is most suitable for them. At present around 15.5 mln. or 62% of all eligible couples are using contraceptive methods. At the outset of the program in 1969–70, the IUD was the principle method. It was used by 54.7% of the new acceptors. However, as the pill became economically feasible for mass distribution, and as the program expanded into rural areas, in the following five years large number of acceptors chose the pill. The latest data (February 1985) show that among 15,511,153 current users 27.8% are IUD acceptors. The IUD's currently used in the national program are the Lippes loop, the TCu and the multiload. These contraceptives are manufactured in Indonesia. Current program policy is to encourage acceptors to adopt the IUD because of its higher continuation rate and as a means of reducing the costs and logistical problems of pill distribution.

10.13.05
Experiences with the ML Cu 375: Van der Pas, H F M. Rijksuniv., Gent, Belgium

Tatum stated that the antifertility effect of the IUD was more outstanding as the copper surface exposed in the cavum uteri was greater. A matched study is undertaken to control this statement. The object of the study is ML Cu 375 and is compared with ML Cu 250. The contraceptive effect of the ML Cu 375 is significantly greater than with the standard model. This study confirms Tatum's original hypothesis. Two other devices were also compared with each other: the TCu 200 and TCu 220. The observations followed the same trend as with the ML Cu 375. The question is obvious whether the difference of surface area is the major factor in this case. For the copper is not only spread over the surface but it has a volume too. The results of these studies lead to some hypothesis which might explain the greater contraceptive effect of the ML Cu 375. Thus, it could be the mass of copper instead of the surface that has this an influence for the greater contraceptive effect of the ML Cu 375.

10.13.07
Five years of experience with the Multiload Cu 375: A personal series: Beerthuizen, R J C M. Dept. Gyn., Streekziekenhuis Koningin Beatrix, Winterswijk, The Netherlands

From September 1979 until February 1985 the Multiload Cu 375 IUD was inserted in about 600 women with a total of approximately 14,000 woman-months of use. All the insertions, as well as the follow-up visits, were carried out by one investigator. Data were recorded and evaluated for up to 60 months, according to the life table method of *Tietze*. A group of women, who received a second IUD after the first had been expelled, were actively sought out, as well as the group of women, who became pregnant accidentally. The evaluation of this IUD-model confirms its low pregnancy rate and high acceptability. The validity of this study is enhanced by the fact that all cases were treated in one clinic by one investigator.

10.28.01
FSH-therapy in ovarian insufficiency: Braendle, W, Sprotte, C, Bettendorf, G. Abt. Klin. u. Exp. Endokr., Univ.-Frauenklin., Hamburg

In patients displaying an anovulatory cycle or luteal phase defect a lowered FSH/LH ratio during early follicular phase is frequently found. FSH deficiency (*Dizerega, G, Hodgen, G D.* Fertil. and Steril. **35**, 489, 1981) and an elevated LH secretion (*Braendle, W.* et al. Acta Endocr. Suppl. **240**, 79, 1981) have been described in association with insufficient follicular maturation. Patients displaying an FSH/LH ratio < 0.5 were selected for FSH treatment using different treatment schemes. If FSH deficiency during early follicular phase is the cause of the disorder, FSH substitution therapy during this period of the cycle should restore the pathophysiologic situation. 14 patients in 23 cycles received 2–4 amp. of FSH for 4 to 9 days during early follicular phase. In 14 cycles an ovulation occurred, in 10 cycles the luteal phase displayed normal progestin levels and a length of more than 10 days. No pregnancy was achieved. FSH treatment in an individually adjusted treatment scheme according to the ovarian reaction resulted in 22 out of 25 cycles in an ovulation, in 19 cases the luteal phase was normal, six pregnancies were achieved. These data elucidate that not an FSH deficiency during early follicular phase but more probably an elevated LH secretion is responsible for the altered FSH/LH ratio and leads to the disturbance of follicular maturation.

10.28.02

Induction of ovulation by pulsatile administration of LH-RH nasal spray: Hirohashi, T, Sato, Y, Takeuchi, S. Dept. Obstet. and Gyn., School Med., Niigata Univ., Niigata, Japan

This presentation deals with induction of ovulation by pulsatile administration of LH-RH nasal spray, which patients can easily apply effectively by themselves. Ten patients with hypogonadotropic or eugonadotropic hypogonadism, in whom clomiphen or HMG therapy had been proved to be ineffective, were used for this study. Based on the preliminary study, the amount of LH-RH was administered intranasally, 200 μg three times every two hours a day for four to five days, in combination of clomiphen and HMG (Group 1), HMG (Group 2), clomiphen (Group 3) and no combination of these drugs (Group 4). Ovulation was induced in seven cycles out of eight cycles in 6 patients of Group 1, in four cycles of four cycles in 2 patients of Group 2, in no cycles of two cycles in two patients (Group 3), and in two cycles of two cycles in 1 patient (Group 4), indicating excellent efficacy of pulsatile administration of LH-RH nasal spray in inducing ovulation. Combination of HMG with LH-RH nasal spray has been suggested to be more effective.

10.28.03

Five cases of hyperstimulation by pulsatile GnRH: Vervest, H A M, Coelingh Bennink, H J T. Dept. Obstet. & Gyn., and Reprod. Med., State Univ. Hosp. AZU, Utrecht, The Netherlands

Five cases of ovarian hyperstimulation were seen during a consecutive 100 inductions of ovulation by pulsatile intravenous administered GnRH. A dosage of 10 μg was given every 90 minutes by means of a portable autoinfusion pump and treatment was continued during the luteal phase. During all cycles regular estimations of LH, FSH, 17β-estradiol and progesterone were performed. Follicular development was monitored by tridimensional ultrasound measurements. All patients kept a BBT. Multiple follicular development was observed in one patient with a dopamine resistent hyperprolactinemia, one with polycystic ovarian disease and three patients with hypothalamic oligomenorrhea (all with a positive progesterone withdrawal bleeding and inconsistent results with clomiphene). 17β-estradiol serum-levels rose well above the normal limits during the follicular and luteal phase. No pregnancy occurred. We conclude that hyperstimulation remains a risk in anovulatory women when applying pulsatile GnRH for induction of ovulation, especially if signs are present expressing a certain amount of spontaneous endogenous GnRH secretion. The release of LH and FSH by the pituitary is apparently not only related to the pulse interval, but also to the pulse dosage.

10.28.04

Pulsatile administration of GnRH for induction of ovulation: Tanaka, S, Hata, H, Hashimoto, M. Dept. Obstet. and Gyn., Sapporo, Med. Coll., Sapporo, Japan

The method of pulsatile administration of gonadotropin-releasing hormone (GnRH) has been proven to be a useful means for induction of ovulation in various menstrual disorders. Pulsatile secretion of LH and FSH was examined to determine if the frequency of LH pulse, and by inference pulsatile GnRH secretion, varied during the normal menstrual cycle. Pulsatile release of LH was found to occur with a frequency of approximately 120–150 minutes in the follicular phase and a reduced frequency with a higher amplitude during the luteal phase. The pulsatile FSH pattern was not observed in both phases and had no correlation with LH secretion. GnRH was injected at 120 minute intervals in doses ranging from 2.5 to 10 g/pulse, from 07:00 to 23:00 daily. The injection was administered intravenously with a self-administered infuser. Five patients had oligomenorrhea, five patients anovulatory menstrual cycle, five patients secondary amenorrhea, and three patients polycystic ovary syndrome. Twelve out of 18 menstrual disorders ovulated with the pulsatile GnRH treatment. Our data suggest that pulsatile administration of low doses of GnRH is effective for induction of ovulation in various types of menstrual disorders except in the case of polycystic ovary syndrome.

10.28.05

The influence of exogenous progestin on LH pulsatility: Sprotte, C, Braendle, W, Bettendorf, G. Abt. Klin. u. Exp. Endokr., Univ.-Frauenklin., Hamburg

The aim of the present study was to determine LH fluctuation during and after progestin supplementation in anovulatory cycles and cycles with luteal phase defect. The question is if exogenous progestin being present for a period of time similar to the normal luteal phase can influence the LH pulsatile pattern of the subsequent cycle. In four patients presenting an anovulatory cycle or luteal phase defect LH fluctuation first was measured during the early follicular phase of a spontaneous cycle after a preceding insufficient spontaneous cycle. Then the patients were treated with medroxyprogesterone acetate (10 mg/day) for ten days during the second phase of the cycle. The subsequent cycle in three of four patients showed a typical biphasic BBT, normal follicular growth as followed by sonography and normal progesterone values during the luteal phase. The frequency of LH fluctuation was lowered during exogenous progestin administration and the low frequency of LH pulses remaines present for four to six days after progestin medication. It may be concluded that progestin therapy with regard to follicular growth, ovulation, and luteal phase is not only a supplementation therapy during the defect luteal phase but is of influence for the subsequent cycle.

10.28.06

Ovarian stimulation regimens in clomid-induced cycles – a comparative analysis of morphologic ovulation by ultrasound (I): Suh, B H, Lee, J H. Dept. Obstet. and Gyn., Kyung Hee Univ., Seoul, Korea

During 1984, 81 follicle monitorings in clomid-induced cycles were performed by real-time linear scanner. Four ovarian stimulation regimens were used according to cycle day of starting treatment: Group 1. clomiphene 50 mg daily, from day 2 to 6 (22 cycles), Group 2. clomiphene 50 mg daily, from day 3 to 7 (18 cycles), Group 3. clomiphene 50 mg daily, from day 4 to 8 (20 cycles), Group 4. clomiphene 50 mg daily, from day 5 to 9 (21 cycles). We have evaluated aspects of optimal ultrasonic follicular growth following method of timing of controlled ovarian stimulation. Each group had similiar mean and there was no significant difference in leading follicle at the reference day. We expect that possible explanations for implications of these findings will be discussed, with particular reference to follicular endocrine milieu.

Regimens

Days to ovulation	Group 1	Group 2	Group 3	Group 4
−4	12.9±1.7	13.2±2.1	13.4±3.2	13.7±0.5
−3	14.0±2.3	15.6±2.4	14.4±2.8	15.8±0.7
−2	16.3±2.2	17.1±2.0	17.4±1.6	17.6±0.8
−1	18.3±1.8	18.9±1.9	18.3±2.3	19.7±1.4
0	21.4±3.4	19.9±3.9	20.9±2.9	21.1±3.8
(reference day)		Follicle diameter (mm)		

10.28.07

Induction of follicular maturation by "pure FSH" in women with polycystic ovary syndrome (PCO-S): Birkhäuser, M H, Huber, P. Dept. Obstet. and Gyn., Univ. of Basel, Kantonsspit., Basel, Switzerland

In 22 infertile women aged 24 to 34 years suffering from PCO-S characterized by long-standing clomiphen-resistent anovulation, elevated serum estrone and androgen levels and a serum LH:FSH-ratio >2 in the early follicular phase, follicular maturation was induced by i. m. administration of "pure FSH" (Metrodin® SERONO, 150–300 IU/day) and controlled by sonography and serum estradiol determination. Ovulation was induced by i. m. injection of 10,000 IU HCG. Pregnancy occurred in 12 out of 48 treatment cycles. Five women aborted during the first trimenon. The multiple pregnancy rate was 12%. Mild ovarian hyperstimulation syndrome was observed in 12.5% and moderate ovarian hyperstimulation syndrome in 10.4% of the cycles where ovulation was induced. In contrast to earlier reports, the administration of "pure FSH" did not result in a blockade of the luteinizing hormone surge as shown by the occurrence of "premature ovulation" leading to follicular atresia in six patients. In conclusion, "pure FSH" is an efficient new tool in the treatment of clomiphen-resistent infertility in PCO-S. The present study suggests that the pregnancy rate, the incidence of multiple pregnancies and the risk of ovarian hyperstimulation syndrome is comparable to the results obtained in PCO-S by ovulation induction with HMG. It might be speculated that the pregnancy rate following stimulation by "pure FSH" could be ameliorated by the prevention of the encountered premature LH-surge.

10.28.08

Induction of ovulation by hMG/hCG during chronic administration of a GnRH analogue (Buserelin): Geisthövel, F, Bliefert, R, Geyer, H, Breckwoldt, M, Sandow, J*. Dept. Obstet. and Gyn., Univ., Freiburg, *Hoechst AG, Dept. Pharmacol., Frankfurt

In the present study seven patients suffering from luteal phase defect were treated with the GnRH analogue (GnRH-A) Buserelin in order to achieve hypogonadism. GnRH was chronically administered by an external infusion pump (400 μg/day). After decrease of estradiol-17β (E_2) plasma levels the patients were subsequently treated with 150–300 IE hMG/day to stimulate ovarian function. When follicular maturation was completed GnRH-A treatment was discontinued. hCG was injected to induce ovulation (7500–10,000 IE) and support corpus luteum function (2500–12,500 IE). Suppression of ovarian function by GnRH treatment was examined by E_2 plasma levels. Ovarian response to the exogeneously administered gonadotropins was monitored by ultrasonography, plasma levels of E_2 and progesterone (P). Chronic administration of the GnRH-A by an external infusion pump resulted in a rapid and complete depression of ovarian E_2 release (<30 pg/ml) within 6–14 days. Exogeneous gonadotropin replacement was followed by follicular maturation (dominant follicles >20 mm in diameter) ovulation, corpus luteum formation and normal luteal function (P: 16–50 ng/ml) in all cases.

10.28.09

Induction of ovulation with a combined regimen of clomiphene, Pergonal and HCG, using ultrasound: Notay, B, Basu, H K. West Hill Hosp., Dartford, Kent, UK

Induction of ovulation was attempted in 43 infertile women with anovular menstruation in whom prior treatment with clomiphene for, at least, four cycles failed to result in satisfactory ovulation. The treatment regimen consisted of Serophene 100 mg daily for 5 days commencing on the second day. Pergonal 1 amp. was given intramuscularly daily starting on the second day and continued until an ovarian follicle reached 18 mm in diameter, or until 12 injections of Pergonal was given. At this point HCG injection was given. Of the 43 women so treated, 34 (79 per cent) achieved serum progesterone levels of > 30 nmol/l in two or more cycles. The mean progesterone level during the combined treatment was significantly higher $(64.5 \pm 17.2 \text{ nmol/l})$ than that during therapy with clomiphene $(22.2 \pm 7.1 \text{ nmol/l})$ the difference being statistically significant $(p < 0.05)$. There was no clinical occurrence of hyperstimulation. Pregnancy test was positive in 15 of the 35 women and ultrasound evidence of pregnancy was present in all but one of these. Pregnancy ended in miscarriage in three of the remaining 11, four started as twin pregnancies but continued as single pregnancies. The combined regime offers successful ovulation and pregnancy in women in whom treatment with clomiphene alone fails to produce ovulation. Ultrasound assessment was adequate control.

10.28.10
Regulation of fertility by alteration of cervical mucus composition: Gould, K G. Yerkes Primate Ctr, Emory Univ., Atlanta, and **Ansari, A H.** Georgia Baptist Med. Ctr, Atlanta, GA, USA

The physical properties of cervical mucus have been shown to change in a predictable manner with the stage of the menstrual cycle, pregnancy and following sex steroid treatment. Such changes as detected by both conventional (light microscopy and clinical evaluation) and novel (electron microscopy, energy dispersive x-ray analysis and NMR spectroscopy) techniques include alteration in *spinnbarkeit* (threadability), penetrability to sperm, electrolyte concentration and water content. We have demonstrated that it is possible to avoid the use of hormones to induce such changes in cervical mucus by *in vitro* and/or *in vivo* exposure of CM to exogenous electrolytes. In general, polyvalent anions ($NaHPO_4$ or $NaHCO_3$) change the physico-chemical characters of CM toward those associated with the time of ovulation and conversely, polyvalent cations (Fe or Cu salt) promote changes similar to those seen in non-fertile period of luteal phase, pregnancy, or during exposure to contraceptive steroids. We, therefore, conclude that non-hormonal modification of the cervical mucus may provide potential fertility regulation in women.

10.28.11
Ultrasonographic measurement of the ovary: Müller, E, Geier, G R, Franke, H M. City Hosp., Ludwigshafen and Dept. Gyn. and Obstet., Univ., Ulm

In 149 patients, ultrasonographic square measurements of 263 clinically normal ovaries were carried out with a so-called sector scanner the day before abdominal hysterectomy and salpingo-oophorectomy. The largest square area was photographed. Immediately after operation, the unfixed ovaries were photographed on a pane of glass. Both square areas were measured and compared. The correlation factor of the 263 areas was 0.9. The average deviation of ultrasonographic and postoperative areas was 18.9%. In a further part of the study, 44 ovaries from 25 women were investigated by ultrasonography every four days during a one-month cycle. The areas of the ovaries were found to alter by 10% in a 78-year-old woman, and by 300% in a 17-year-old woman. The study convincingly demonstrates that ultrasonography can be used to measure clinically normal ovaries and their cyclical variations. If the supposition is correct that malignant transformation starts with an enlargement of the ovaries, ultrasonography could be a practicable method of screening for the early detection of ovarian cancer.

10.32.01
Existence of calcium channels in the spiral arteries of pregnant Guinea pigs: Kleinstein, J, Renoldi, H J. Dept. Obstet. and Gyn., Univ., Giessen

Uterine blood flow in species with a hemochorial placenta is limited by the vascular resistance of the arteries outside the placenta (*Moll* and *Künzel*, Pflügers Arch. **338**, 125, 1973). Calcium channels regulate the vascular resistance by controlling the rate of calcium influx into smooth muscle cells. Spiral arteries of pregnant guinea pigs were isolated by microsurgical technique. Calcium channels were demonstrated by means of the radioligand binding technique in a particular smooth muscle membrane preparation. Low capacity (B max $= 77.3 \pm 12.3$ fmole/mg protein) and low affinity ($K_D = 1.6 \pm 0.1$ nM) binding sites for the labelled calcium antagonist (^{3}H)-nimodipine could be identified in the membrane fraction. The saturability of the binding sites was achieved in the presence of 2 nM (^{3}H)-nimodipine. Scatchard plot analysis revealed a homogenous group of receptors. A protein concentration of $0.25 - 1.5$ mg/ml in the membrane fraction and an incubation period of 45 min at 30 °C represented the optimal conditions for the (^{3}H)-nimodipine binding. Under these conditions the unspecific binding in the presence of 1 μM nitrendipine represented $40 - 50\%$ of the total (^{3}H)-nimodipine binding. The relatively high percentage of unspecific binding could not be reduced by means of further purification of the membrane fraction in a sucrose gradient centrifugation. The importance of calcium channels for the regulation of uterine blood flow can be determined by means of these binding studies.

10.32.02
Establishment of extrauterine preparation of fetus using extracorporeal membrane oxygenator: Kuwabara, Y, Okai, T, Mizuno, M. Dept. Obstet. and Gyn., Fac. Med., Univ., Tokyo, Japan

Despite the major advances of research methods, it is still difficult to investigate a fetus in utero. In order to reach a fetus more directly, the new incubation system in which a fetus can maintain its life as an extrauterine fetus was developed. Eight goat fetuses (80–145 days of gestation) were incubated in this system with an extracorporeal membrane oxygenator (ECMO). Arteriovenous bypass was achieved using the umbilical cord vessels to keep fetal circulation system. Following systemic heparinization, the catheters were connected with the ECMO circuit which consisted of arterial drainage to a roller pump and a membrane oxygenator. Then, the fetus was moved into an incubator filled up with a balanced electrolyte solution. The perfused blood was recirculated and ventilated with a mixture gas of O_2 and N_2 to get a pO_2 of 30–35 mm Hg and a pCO_2 of 30–35 mm Hg in umbilical venous blood. Flow rate of perfusate was adjusted to between 30 and 100 ml/min according to the fetal size and conditions. Blood samples were obtained intermittently during perfusion for hematological, biochemical and blood gas analysis. FHR, ECG and blood pressure were continuously monitored when fetal death or irreversible conditions were documented. Perfusion were performed in six cases without a reservoir in a circuit and two cases with a reservoir. Duration of perfusion ranged up to eight hours in the former group and 40 hours in the latter. Various fetal movements and reflexes could be observed directly. Many problems need to be solved to keep a fetus in extrauterine circumstances. However, this system will become a useful method for investigating fetal pathophysiology.

10.32.03

Effect of cooling and heating on the regional distribution of blood flow in fetal lambs: Kawamura, T*, Araki, T*, Power, G G**. Dept. Obstet. and Gyn., Nippon Med. School,* Tokyo, Japan; Loma Linda Univ.,** California, USA

The goal of this study was to learn the effect of cooling and heating the amniotic fluid on blood flow to various fetal tissues and organs. In six unanesthetized, chronically prepared lambs cold or warm water was passed through tubing encircling the fetus in utero and blood flow was measured using the radionuclide method with 15 μ microspheres. Following cooling for 30 min, amniotic fluid temperature fell 5.87°C to 33.66 ± 0.14 (SEM)°C, fetal arterial temperature fell 2.13 °C to 37.5 ± 0.33 °C, and maternal arterial temperature fell 0.48 °C to 38.66 ± 0.14 °C. Blood flow through the fetal skin fell significantly ($p < 0.05$) to 12.5 ml/min per 100 g tissue, a 54% fall. Blood flow to the brown fat increased 2.8-fold ($p < 0.05$) when expressed as a percentage of cardiac output. After warming for 20 min, fetal temperature rose to 40.19 ± 0.16 °C and skin blood flow increased 11% when referenced to initial control (n.s.) and 143% when referenced to the cooling phase ($p < 0.01$). During both cooling and heating, blood flow to the adrenals rose significantly ($p < 0.01$) whereas flow to the carcase, brain, kidneys and placenta was not altered detectably. Overall, the blood flow responses are consistent with a thermoregulatory role for the skin and brown fat in the near-term fetal lamb.

10.32.04

^{1}H-NMR of the uterine muscle in pregnant rats: Muraoka, E, Sugawara, N, Fukushima, T, Tsuchihashi, N. Dept. Obstet. & Gyn., Fukushima Med. Coll., Fukushima, Japan

Object: Nuclear magnetic resonance (NMR) is a useful method for a follow-up of changes in the uterine muscle such as physical property and metabolism and NMR-CT have no problem of ionizing radiation exposure. Its use for investigations and management in the perinatal period is therefore expected. – Methods: The subjects were mature nonpregnant Wistar rats, in the 7th, 12th, 14th, 16th, 18th and 20th days of pregnancy and rats in the 1st and 2nd postlabor days. Relaxation time of protons T_1 and T_2 were measured by using a Bruker pulse NMR minispec pc 20 (observation frequency, 20 MHz) and JEOL FX 90Q·FT-NMR (observation frequency, 90 MHz). – Results: 1. At an observation frequency of 20 MHz, the nonpregnant uterine muscle showed T_1 and T_2 of 548 ms and 60 ms, respectively, and the pregnant uterine muscle showed 755 ms and 108 ms respectively. 2. At 90 MHz, the nonpregnant uterine muscle showed T_1 and T_2 of 1.06 s and 45 ms, respectively, and the pregnant uterine muscle showed 1.24 s and 70 ms. 3. No significant difference was found in T_1 and T_2 in stage of pregnancy at both of the observation frequencies. 4. The T_1 value in the postlabor period was the same as that in the nonpregnant period, whereas T_2 values lying at both frequency between those of no pregnancy and pregnancy. – Conclusions: 1. Uterine muscle showed marked changes in physical property due to pregnancy, which were reflected in the relaxation times, T_1 and T_2, in ^{1}H-NMR. 2. The changes by pregnancy in T_2 were greater than in T_1. 3. The changes in T_1 and T_2 were more marked at an observation frequency of 20 MHz than at 90 MHz.

10.32.05

Effect of hypertonic saline on lipoperoxidation in pregnant rat: Yoshioka, T, Motoyama, H, Yamasaki, H. Div. Obstet. & Gyn., Ctr Adult Dis., Kurashiki, Okayama, Japan

Lipoperoxides act harmfully on cell membranes. In severe cases of EPH-gestosis, a significant increase was observed compared with normal pregnant women in the tenth month of gestation. Exessive dietary intake of sodium may be an important factor in the development of EPH-gestosis, and cause the high concentration of blood lipoperoxides during pregnancy. Changes of lipoperoxides in the blood and tissues were investigated in the spontaneous hypertensive rat (SHR). Rats were mated. After checking the spermatozoa in the vagina, the animals were given the hypertonic saline solution (1.0, 1.5, 2.0%) *ad libitum* throughout the pregnancy. In the case of 1.0% solution, there were no significant changes as compared with the control (free of sodium). In the case of 1.5% solution, the fetal body weights were significantly lighter than that of control group. The level of lipoperoxides in maternal and fetal blood were very high as compared with that of control group. In the maternal liver and lung tissues, lipoperoxides and catalase activity were higher, but SOD, glutathione peroxidase activities and vitamin E concentration showed no significant difference as compared with that of control group. In the fetal liver and lung tissues, those anti-oxidant enzyme activities were almost the same activities as that of control.

10.32.06

The effect of different treatments on the post-partum infection of the uterus and retention of the placenta in Egyptian dairy cows and buffaloes: Nasr, M T, Abdel Raheim, A, Eidaroos, A, Hazzaa, A. Dept. Gyn. and Obstet., Benha and Zagazig Fac. Vet. Med., Univ., Benha, Egypt
The bacteriological investigation of the genital discharge of cows and buffaloes suffering from endometritis and cervicitis and/or retention of the placenta, was done on 32 foreign breed cows (Friesian and Brown Swiss) and 28 native breed buffaloes. These animals were aged 3–7 years and gave 1–4 births. The examined animals were divided into four groups and treated with different intrauterine medications. The number of services/conception, the conception rate and pregnancy rate after treatments were recorded. From this study, the bacteriological examination revealed 15 different types of bacteria. Staph. aureus, Str. pyogenes and E. coli were the most prevalent organism isolated from the discharges of the cows and buffaloes with or without retained placenta or uterine prolapse. The fertility rate of either cows or buffaloes suffering from endometritis was regained and the conception rate was increased after the intrauterine treatment with furazolidone S in watery or oily suspension.

10.41.01

In utero cardioversion of fetal atrial flutter: Page, C, Extermann, P, Beguin, F. Dept. Obstet. and Gyn., Univ., Geneva, Switzerland
Antepartum fetal arrhythmias can now be accurately identified with the use of two dimensional echocardiography in tandem with M-mode echocardiography. This also provides a method for detecting associated fetal congestive heart failure and cardiac structure anomalies (C. S. *Kleinman*, Amer J. Cardiol. **51**, 1983). Case report: A 21-year-old white woman GlPO was referred at 29 weeks gestation for antenatal FHR monitoring. She had had insulin-dependent diabetes since she was 12 years old (class. D). Background retinopathy diagnosed at the nineth week of pregnancy had progressed to proliferative retinopathy and was treated with laser photocoagulation. She denied any allergies and received no treatment other than insulin. When she was admitted, FHR was in excess of 200 bpm. A week earlier FHR showed a normal pattern. Fetal realtime and M-mode echocardiography noted a rapid motion of the fetal atrial wall compatible with atrial flutter. Measurements of BP and femur were consistent with a gestational age of 29 weeks. There was no evidence of fetal cardiac anatomic anomalies. Medical cardioversion was performed on the day of admission using digoxin. Twelve hours later FHR converted gradually to a normal pattern. The treatment was controlled by serial serum digoxin level and was continued until delivery.

10.41.02

Nuclear magnetic resonance (NMR), a new non-invasive method to study biochemical changes during fetal hypoxia: Schmidt, S, Langner, K, Dudenhausen, J W, Saling, E. Inst. Perinat. Med., FU, Berlin
We have evaluated *in vivo* NMR spectroscopy as a method for studying biochemical changes after intrauterine hypoxia. In order to measure the pH and the lactid acid concentration in the fetal brain of 9 guinea pigs with a gestational age of 56–62 days as an animal model we used a Bruker-tomograph BNT JS 2430. By means of phosphorus 31 *in vivo* spectroscopy analysis it was possible to calculate the pH in the fetal brain. These pH values correlated with the pH values of simultaneously drawn blood samples. Due to the signal-noise ratio of the *in vivo* technique available today only triglycerides could be identified in our C 13 spectra. Thus, the basis for calculating the lactid acid concentration in the fetal brain as a reference to the enzymatical measured values was insufficient. In the future with further improvement of NMR technology such information in addition to P 31-spectroscopy may become achievable. Our first promising results indicate that NMR has a high potential as a new non-invasive tool to study biochemical changes in the fetus during intrauterine complications.

10.41.03

The management of severe rhesus isoimmunization using fetoscopic blood sampling techniques: MacKenzie, I Z, Castle, B, Bowell, P, Entwistle, C, Ferguson, J. Nuffield Dept. and Gyn., John Radcliffe Hosp., Headington, Oxford, UK
With the introduction of fetoscopy and fetal blood sampling into clinical practice, pregnancies severely complicated by Rhesus isoimmunisation may now be more precisely managed. As well as determining the fetal Rhesus group when the father is known to be Rh D heterozygous, and direct intravascular transfusion into the umbilical circulation, the severity of the hemolytic process has been assessed and further management determined by repeated analysis of fetal hematology and biochemistry. Hematocrit, total protein, albumin and bilirubin concentrations and amniotic fluid Δ.O.D. measurements have been determined for pregnancies complicated by Rhesus isoimmunisation and compared with values for samples obtained from control pregnancies not complicated by Rhesus isoimmunisation. No differences were found in total protein and albumin concentrations between Rhesus complicated and control pregnancies. However,

bilirubin concentrations were always greater than $40\,\mu$mol/litre in Rhesus pregnancies compared with values rarely above this concentration in control pregnancies. In pregnancies severely compromised by Rhesus isoimmunisation there was a poor correlation between amniotic fluid Δ.O.D. values, fetal hematocrit and fetal bilirubin concentrations. The results obtained would suggest that the assessment by repeated fetal blood sampling between 18 and 36 weeks gestation could be superior to repeated amniocentesis or ultrasound examination and might reduce the use of in-utero fetal transfusions.

10.41.04
Fetal blood sampling using a needle guided by ultrasound: Daffos, F, Forestier, F, Capella-Pavlovsky, M.
Dept. Prenat. Diagn. and Fetol., Notre-Dame de Bon Secours Hosp., Paris, France
606 fetal blood samplings were carried out on 562 pregnancies from the 17th to 38th weeks of gestation for various prenatal diagnoses using a 20 gauge needle guided by ultrasound. This procedure was performed on out-patients, under local anesthesia, without medication prior to or after the procedure. Pure fetal blood was obtained at the first attempt in 588 cases. A second attempt was necessary in 18 cases. Maternal blood contamination was never present. Amniotic fluid dilution was noted in 15 cases. Only three fetuses, at the beginning of our experience, could not be punctured. The duration of the procedure was less than 10 minutes in 90% of cases. 58 pregnancies were terminated after considering the results of the diagnosis. 504 pregnancies were continued. The complications found in these pregnancies were 5% of premature delivery, 8% of growth retardation, 1.1% of death in utero and 0.8% of spontaneous abortion. In the future this new procedure could advantageously replace fetoscopy and open an important field of new investigations.

10.41.05
Flow pulsatility of umbilical artery. A non-invasive method for detecting placental pathology: Bruinse, H W, Reuwer, P J H M, Sijmons, E. Dept. Obstet. and Gyn., Univ. Hosp., Utrecht, The Netherlands
Pulsatility of blood flow in the umbilical arteries can be easily measured by continuous or pulsed Doppler techniques. Placental pathology, infarction etc., is in many cases the underlying cause of fetal growth retardation. A decrease in the placental vascular bed will undoubtedly lead to an increased placental vascular resistance. A factor reflecting resistance of a vascular bed is the Pulsatility Index (PI) of its supplying artery as described by *Gosling*. This factor was chosen and normal values were established in the course of normal pregnancy in 50 women. A significant decrease up to the last weeks in pregnancy was found, probably due mostly to a decrease in placental resistance. In almost all cases of already clinically established growth retardation a significant increased PI was found. After this pilot study a prospective study was started to investigate whether this simple method could detect placental pathology before fetal growth retardation is evident with current diagnostics. In an unselected pregnant population the PI as well as biometric variables were measured at 28 and 34 weeks. Results of the first 200 cases indicate that the PI can predict accurately fetal growth retardation due to placental pathology and, more important, at an earlier stage of pregnancy than current diagnostic methods.

10.41.06
Effects of suloctidil in blood flow through umbilical vein in pregnancies with retarded intrauterine growth: Camargo, A, Uranga Imaz, F, Lanari, E. Hosp. M.I.R. Sarda, Buenos Aires, Argentina
The purpose of present trial was that of determining the normal values of flow through umbilical veins both in normal pregnancies with delayed intrauterine growth, measuring as well other factors such as flow of blood though fetal aorta and establishing the corresponding normal curves. The trial was carried out on twenty-five pregnant women, both primiparous and multiparous, whose ages varied between 20 and 35 years, with reliable date of last menstruation and with no added pathology. Variables studied were both flow of blood in umbilical vein and fetal aorta, biparietal diameter, abdominal diameters and abdominal area, for which purpose an echograph was used with type B image of high resolution (Ul. Octoson). Value obtained in present trial on flow of blood through umbilical vein was 113 ml (ml/kg/min). Flow of blood through fetal aorta determined an average of 121 during week number 39. Trial was also performed on twenty-five pregnancies with diminished fetal growth, confirmed through weight an physical exam at birth, obtaining an average value of 105 ml/kg/min (p < 0.01) during week number 40, while averages through fetal aorta during same week reached 126. Therapeutic effects of suloctidil drug of vascular antispasmodic action and of antithrombotic activity, were evaluated on 20 pregnancies with diminished fetal growth, observing an increase in the values of flow of blood through umbilical vein, with an average value of 142 ml/kg/min (p < 0.01) during week number 40. Beneficial effects in the treatment of delayed intrauterine growth are believed to be obtained with suloctidil.

10.41.07
Intrapartum measurement of fetal cardiac electromechanical intervals in high-risk pregnancy: Gintautas, V.
Med. Inst., Kaunas, Lithuania, USSR
Experimental investigations on isolated fetal heart showed myocardial contractility alterations to be one of the earliest signs of hypoxia (*Kilda* et al., 1982). This encouraged us to use measurements of cardiac electromechanical intervals (EMI) for evaluation of fetal well being. Simultaneous recording of fetal scalp ECG and filtered Doppler ultrasound was used for this purpose. In addition, fetal heart rate (FHR),

variability and uterine activity were recorded. 76 women with uncomplicated pregnancies and with no signs of fetal compromise according to the data of FHR monitoring and scalp blood pH, pCO_2, pO_2 sampling served as controls. The mean values of EMI were 72.6 ± 3.6 ms for pre-ejection period (PEP), 31.3 ± 2.9 ms for electromechanical delay time, 41.4 ± 3.3 ms for isovolumic contraction time and 157.3 ± 7.2 ms for ventricular ejection time (VET). Among 64 women with suspected fetal compromise a constant shortening of PEP and VET (less significant) was found in 18 cases. 13 babies with mild hypoxia were born in this group. Prolongated PEP was found for four fetuses. Three of them were born in severe hypoxia. Transient prolongation of PEP simultaneous to variable decelerations of FHR was found in cases of umbilical cord compression. Thus, EMI measurement provide an additional technic for assessing fetal well being.

10.41.08
Fetal heart rate anomalies – incidence and clinical significance: Schlensker, K-H, Breuker, K H, Wolff, F, Glinczewski, B, Bolte, A. Univ.-Frauenklin., Köln

In 19,031 pregnancies between 1969–1982 we recorded persistant fetal heart rate anomalies from the 20th week of gestation till birth in 51 cases (2.6‰). The diagnoses were made by auscultation, fetal ECG, real-time-, time-motion- and Doppler sonography. Cases of sinus tachycardia and bradycardia were excluded. The following diagnoses were made: in nine cases we saw supraventricular tachycardia (0.5‰) and with the same incidence bradyarrhythmia. Two fetuses had a complete AV-bloc (0.1‰) and 31 extrasystoles (1.6‰). That means, extrasystoles were the diagnoses with the highest incidence. In these cases we found no correlation between these anomalies and a heart defect, but in contrast to other authors we found a higher rate of subpartual fetal distress-situations. Two of the nine fetuses with bradyarrhythmia had an incomplete AV-bloc. Only three newborns showed no more heart rate anomalies after birth, two had a heart defect. One of the two fetuses with a complete AV-bloc was suffering from serious organic heart defect and died some days later. In the most of the cases of supraventricular tachycardia (> 200 bpm) the newborns had a normal heart rate up to delivery except three babies, who needed a long-term drug treatment. One of these babies died of multiple malformations. When there were sonographic signs of fetal heart insufficiency, we preferred near at term delivery immediately. In some cases with immature fetuses a successful treatment was done with digitalis and verapamil to the mother.

10.41.09
An approach to intra-uterine fetal resuscitation with theophylline: Ushioda, E, Tsuji, Y, Kosakai, H, Takayama, T, Yoh, S, Oku, M, Kyuma, M, Moriyama, S I, Ichijo, M. Dept. Obstet. and Gyn., Nara Med. Univ., Nara, Japan

The effect of theophylline (Th.), an inhibitor of tissue phosphodiesterase, on the fetal cardiovascular system has been studied. Basic experiments in rat showed that Th. elicits the increase of uteroplacental blood flow, the activation of placental permeability and inhibition of uterine myometrial contractility. However, Th. did not elicit any contraction of the ductus arteriosus. Standing on these results, 250 mg of Th. was administered intravenously to 20 pregnant women who had distressed fetus, to evaluate the possibility of intra-uterine fetal resuscitation. Fetal distress was diagnosed by cardio-tocogram (CTG). After Th. administration, the incidence of fetal heart rate deceleration on CTG showed marked decrease ($3.2 \pm 1.0/60$ min to $0.4 \pm 0.4/60$ min) the depth of fetal heart rate deceleration became shallower than before (36.0 ± 10.1 bpm to 5.3 ± 3.3 bpm), and the duration of deceleration decreased (102.5 ± 28.0 sec to 7.7 ± 7.0 sec), respectively. As control, Th. was administered to 20 normal pregnant women. After Th. administration, the incidence and the mean amplitude of fetal heart rate acceleration showed marked increase ($3.7 \pm 0.9/60$ min to $9.6 \pm 1.5/60$ min and 18.2 ± 3.4 bpm to 26.6 ± 3.0 bpm), respectively. Base line fetal heart rate increased from 138 ± 5 bpm to 154 ± 7 bpm. These results indicate that Th. leads the reinforcement of fetal myocardial contractility and lets the fetus recover from distress. We conclude that Th. administration to fetal distress cases is a very effective way of intra-uterine fetal resuscitation.

10.41.10
Intrauterine fetal resuscitation by the maternal administration of β-agonists in cases of acute fetal distress: Komatani, M, Hidaka, A, Sugawa, T. Dept. Obstet. and Gyn., Osaka City Univ., Med. School, Osaka, Japan

Investigation was made into the efficacy of β-agonists for intrauterine fetal resuscitation in late pregnant dogs, rabbits and women by referring to the effects of β-agonists on the uterine contraction, uteroplacental blood flow and fetal heart rate. In the uneventful uteri, β-agonists induced no significant increase in the placental blood flow, but decrease in the placental vascular resistance. Uterine contraction induced a remarkable decrease by less than 60% of the control level in the placental blood flow. This decrease of the placental blood flow leads to the deteriorating effects of the placental gases exchange. Under such a condition β-agonists were administered intravenously, resulting in the simultaneous improvement in the placental blood flow. Clinically it is possible to observe the improvement in type II dips of the fetal bradycardia. Simultaneously, β-agonists are seen to induce transplacental fetal tachycardiac effects, which bring about less than 10 beats/min. This made us confirm that the efficacy of β-agonists on fetal distress lies chiefly in the improvement in uteroplacental blood flow.

10.41.11

In utero digoxin therapy of the fetus: De Lia, J E, Nappi, J M, Branch, D W. Dept. Obstet. and Gyn., Univ. of Utah Schools Med. and Pharmacy, Salt Lake City, UT, USA

Transplacental therapy of fetal cardiac arrhythmias and congestive heart failure by maternal administration of digoxin has become commonplace. A review of these reports, however, reveals no uniform approach to therapy, variable responses, and multiple methodological problems. Pharmacokinetic data to direct appropriate dosing are lacking. In addition, monitoring of therapy is confounded by the recent identification of a digoxin-like immunoreactive substance in maternal plasma, placental extracts, and fetal plasma of normal pregnancies without digoxin therapy. These reports render most digoxin pharmacokinetic data in pregnancy to date, suspect. We propose an empiric dosing schedule based on existing data from animals and human nonpregnant subjects. Central to this recommendation is a nomogram which adjusts loading and maintenance doses relative to body weight and creatinine clearance to achieve $10\,\mu g/kg$ total-body digoxin stores (*R. W. Jelliffe*, Am. J. Med. **57**, 63, 1974). Although immediate transplacental transfer of digoxin occurs, equilibrium between mother and fetus can be expected only after 8 to 10 days (*J. C. Furon*, Biol. Neonat. **23**, 116, 1973). Response and beweekly determinations of creatinine clearance directs maintenance dose adjustments until delivery is affected.

10.41.12

Management of prolonged fetal bradycardia in labor: Arulkumaran, S, Ingemarsson, I, Ratnam, S S. Univ. Dept. Obstet. and Gyn., Kandang Kerbau Hosp., Singapore

Thirty-three patients with prolonged fetal bradycardia (fetal heart rate-FHR-baseline below 100 beats/min for minimum of three min or 80 for at least two min) in labor were studied. All the cases were treated by a bolus injection of terbutaline $250\,\mu g$ intravenously and scalp pH obtained within 30 min. If the bradycardia lasted 10 min or more, fetal acidosis was common, particularly if the rate was below 80/min and has a flat baseline for four min or more of that time. In 30 cases FHR improved after injection. Twenty-three patients had vaginal delivery with newborns in good condition. Ten had Cesarean section, three for no improvement in FHR, two for cord prolapse and four for ominous FHR later on. These results suggest tocolysis in selected cases can be of benefit for the fetus with prolonged bradycardia. In cases with ominous FHR pattern preceding the bradycardia and abruptio placentae immediate operative intervention without delay is probably better. Administration of terbutaline should be regarded as a temporary measure till it is apparent that the FHR has recovered to the previous baseline. Preparation for emergency delivery should be done while a recovery is awaited.

10.41.13

Down's syndrome and fetal monitoring: Gallo, M, Moreno, F, Parra, V, Torres, A, Abehsera, M. Dept. Obstet. & Gyn., Hosp. Materno Infant. "Carlos Haya", Málaga, Spain

In this paper we studied the fetal heart rate in fetus with Down's syndrome. Nineteen Down fetuses were monitored during labor and seven also during the pregnancy. We found the following result: a) Labor: slight bradycardia in 8 fetuses (41.1%), variable type 0 in four fetuses (21%), type I in 9 fetuses (47.4%), type II in 5 fetuses (26.3%) and type III none fetuses. FHR accelerations in only four fetuses (21%), Dips type II in two fetuses (10.5%), Dips variable in 8 fetuses (42.1%) and rhythm sinusoidal in one fetus. – b) Pregnancy: Six NST were made, 3 fetuses with reactive pattern (50%) and 3 fetuses nonreactive (50%). 3 OCT were made, with one positive test and two negative tests. The "hypothetic pattern" of FHR Down's syndrome would be: slight bradycardia, decreased variability generally type 0–1, no FHR accelerations and variable dips.

10.42.01

Teaching obstetrics and gynecology: Hillemanns, H G, Keller, K. Univ.-Frauenklin., Freiburg

The student planning to be a General Practitioner later on is trained solely to the extent of fulfilling the necessary prerequisites required by the State Examination; in otherwords he receives lectures on theory in addition to one weeks practical clinical experience. Beyond that any further training desired in gynecology and obstetrics is left up to one's individual initiative. He who is planning a future career as Specialist in Gynecology and Obstetrics is trained for a minimum of five years following the M. D. degree, during which time he is working as an assistant in a speciality clinic and is able to account for experience in surgery as well as that of a minimum of normal and pathological births. Following this five-year training time he takes part in a "speciality discussion" whereby the opportunity is offered to demonstrate one's theoretical knowledge. Participation in additional training programs or events such as lectures, congresses, seminars, or work groups is basically a voluntary matter. There is no examination of the resident on a continual basis. Practical training is particularly problematical in our field; instructional films which we ourselves have developed and placed on video have proved to be very beneficial. At the present time consideration is being given toward raising the standards of the speciality examinations as well as providing better opportunities for testing the resident's knowledge on a regular basis.

10.42.02

Teaching in obstetrics and gynecology for the general practitioner and the specialist: Klimek, R. Copernicus Univ. School Med., Cracow, Poland

The fundamental triad of ovulation-anovulation, cancer and pregnancy forms the core of clinical diagnosis in each woman. This concerns the general practitioner as well as the specialist. With increasing frequency the woman may avail herself of opportunities for self-diagnosis of ovulation and pregnancy enabling her to choose a course of action consistent with her desires. Additionally, a great amount of a physician's work entails also prophylaxis and treatment of cancer. This foundation of diagnosis and treatment in obstetrics and gynecology ranges now from the level of cellular to atomic pathology. This means first of all, that advantage must be taken of: 1. advances in medical thermodynamic assessment of all diseases as near and far from equilibrium states, 2. nuclear magnetic resonance, 3. monoclonal antibodies. Finally, recognition of cancer as a biological dissipative structure must change the approach of medical and social research efforts in oncology, especially concerning the relation of complicated pregnancy as a predisposing factor to cancer of the uterine cervix.

10.42.03

The teaching of gynecology and obstetrics in Italy: Pecorari, D. Clin. Obstet. & Gyn., Univ., Trieste, Italy

The teaching of gynecology and obstetrics in Italy is conditioned: 1. by the fact that Italy has a large excess of doctors; 2. by the fact that there is no regulation of the admission of students to the Faculty of Medicine and also that the regulation of admissions to the specialised training departments is not yet sufficiently selective; 3. by the fact that the possibilities of practical teaching for students or for trainees in the specialised departments are extremely limited; 4. by the fact that alongside the specialised departments of gynecology and obstetrics there are also schools of specialisation appearing, with modified and restricted programs (e. g. specialisation in "Pathology of human reproduction"). The implementation of a balanced plan of reform is urgent: fortunately one has the impression that the period of permissive demagogy is in process of disappearing.

10.42.04

Teaching in Obstetrics & Gynecology for general practitioners and specialists: Ratnam, S S. Dept. Obstet. & Gyn., Nat. Univ., Singapore

The trainee in Obstetrics & Gynecology is expected to go through three years of post-registration training – one year of elective posting in a discipline related to Obstetrics & Gynecology and two years of resident training in Obstetrics & Gynecology. He keeps a log book which is reviewed at three-month intervals to ensure that he has adequate clinical exposure. He is expected to write up a number of cases that he has managed and two long commentaries, one in Obstetrics and another in Gynecology. The commentaries are on clinical data that he has accumulated and analysed and only if his case write-ups and commentaries are acceptable by the assessors would he be allowed to appear for the postgraduate degree. The candidates are examined at the end of their residency program. They appear for a paper in Obstetrics comprising four essay questions and a paper in Gynecology also comprising four questions. The candidates are then examined on an obstetric & gynecological case and are subjected to a viva of 40 minutes. A candidate must pass any two of the three sections, must compulsorily pass the clinical and oral in Obstetrics & Gynecology and obtain a minimum of 50% to pass the examination.The academic staff and specialists in the Department are expected to attend four formal postgraduate teaching sessions. In addition, the Department, in conjunction with the Obstetrical & Gynecological Society of Singapore and the Chapter of Obstetricians & Gynecologists of the Academy of Medicine in Singapore, conducts evening lectures, weekend seminars and workshops. There is no formal examination for re-certification nor is there a specialist register in Singapore yet.

10.42.05

Teaching obstetrics and gynecology: Schlaeder, G. Dept. Obstet. and Gyn., Hop. Hautepierre, Univ., Strasbourg; Tournaire, M. Dept. Obstet. and Gyn., Hôp. St Vincent de Paul, Univ., Paris, France

The teaching of medicine in France is now undergoing thorough reform. 1. Future general practitioners in Strasbourg attend 66 hours of lectures in Gynecology-Obstetrics. Their practical hospital training lasts at least one month and may be spread over 2 to 4 months. The reform provides for an improvement in the general practitioner's training. 2. For the training of the future specialists, two parallel systems exist. In the old system, the specialist's training follows two different patterns: the "certificat d'étude spécialisé" testifies "competence" in medical gynecology and obstetrics. The residency of 4–5 years in university hospitals often followed by one or more years of "clinicat" trains "specialists" at a higher level, including practice in gynecological surgery. In the new system, an extended residency will be the only pattern of training for the future specialist. 3. Post-university training is optional. Various local, national or international meetings contribute to it.

10.42.06

Teaching obstetrics and gynecology in Uppsala, Sweden: Victor, A, Lindberg, B. Dept. Obstet. and Gyn., Akad. Sjukh., Uppsala, Sweden

Doctors training for the speciality spend three years in the clinic. Teaching is not formalized. By passing through the different units of the clinic the doctors acquire basal skills and experience in general obstetrics and gynecology including surgery. They serve in specialized units for obstetric risk patients, endocrinology, infertility, oncologic surgery and family planning. They participate in weekly clinical seminars rotating between the different units of the clinic, postdoctoral scientific, administrative and clinical seminars with invited speakers and are invited to research seminars arranged six times a year. They also participate in special rounds with other specialists in perinatology, pathology, radiology, ultrasound and family planning. On request six months of their duties may be arranged in the department of gynecologic oncology. During their training years they also follow six obligatory one week courses arranged on a nation-wide basis. Participation in research project is encouraged. Doctors training to become general practitioners spend four months in the clinic. During this time their duties are arranged so as to get an emphasis on training in general gynecology, mother health care and family planning.

10.42.07

Teaching in obstetrics and gynecology for the general practitioner and the specialist: Lambotte, R. Dept. Obstet. and Gyn., Univ., Liege, Belgium

The MD degree studies extend over a seven-year period in Belgium. Students receive a theoretical course (30 hours) in biology and pathology of gestation and delivery. This teaching includes the current antenatal monitoring and the screening of obstetrical high-risk patients. During the clinical courses (3 × 45 hours), the theoretical course is illustrated by means of clinical cases. The training in gynecology is restricted to the study of major pathologies (15 hours). Finally, during the last two years, each MD student has to spend one to three months of clinical practice under medical supervision in an Ob. Gyn. Department. The training of the specialist is conducted according to the rules of the Department of Health and Welfare. These studies last for five-years during which the candidate actively participates in the clinical duties of an Ob. Gyn. Ward. He must first receives the approval of an "Committee" to undergo this Postgraduate Specialty Program. During the last three years, the candidate must spend six months in a General Surgery Ward. His final qualification of Ob. Gyn. practice is granted by the Secretary of Health and Welfare upon favorable recommendation by the Committee.

10.42.08

Postgraduate training in obstetrics and gynecology for the overseas qualified trainee: Basu, H K. West Hill Hosp., Dartford, Kent, UK

Overseas qualified trainees in the United Kingdom, do not often receive appropriate postgraduate training. A new approach to training has been adopted in a District General Hospital in the U.K. The following check list is used to plan an individuals training: 1. Trainees adaptation to the way of life and practice in the U.K. 2. Clinical obstetrics and gynecology, specifically to suit the requirements of the trainee's country of origin. 3. Special interest areas (where appropriate). 4. Teaching, research and examination methods. 5. Record keeping and documentation – video and photography. 6. Hospital administration. 7. Communication with professionals, media and the patients. A sense of commitment (to teach) on part of the trainers, extensive use of video recording and other aids have made it possible to sustain a comprehensive training programme in a District General Hospital, in spite of various logistical problems. My initial experience confirms the undisputed value to the trainees of such a scheme, which requires for its success a consultant in every district, with time, motivation and facilities to undertake teaching.

10.42.09

Maternal and child health care and education by "rule of ten": Dawn, C S. Med. Coll., Calcutta, India

Dawn's "Rule of Ten" MCH Care and education is innovated as an adequate comprehensive community educative and service providing program. Ten rules are: 1) 10 times antenatal check-ups from 10 weeks of pregnancy with education on food, contraception. To have pregnancy termination by 10 weeks if unplanned. 2) 10 kg maternal weight gain to achieve, during pregnancy by food counselling. 3) 10 hours rest and sleep (two hours afternoon and 8 hours nightly). 4) 10 gm% Hb to achieve before labor by taking daily oral iron folic acid during pregnancy. 5) By 10 months two doses tetanus toxoid immunisation for both nonimmunized wife and husband and third dose postpartum. 6) 10–12 hours labor program in primigravida, 5–6 hours in second gravida with up to 10% Cesarean section rate. 7) Apgar score baby to be delivered. 8) By 10 weeks postpartum, to hand over a contraceptive for 4 years birthspacing and to have voluntary surgical contraception after birth of second child. 9) 10 months breast feeding to be promoted with weaning food to infant on fourth month. 10) By 10 months, infant immunization (inj. BCG, Oral polio, inj. DTP) to be completed. The workup of Dawn's "Rule of Ten" program in 1000 primigravidae showed eight perinatal deaths/1000 births 3.1 kg average neonatal birth weight, only 10% high risk pregnancy.

10.42.10

Teaching pattern in a premier institution in Tamil Nadu, South India: Beebi, N, Pandiyan, A R, Pandiyan, N. Inst. Obstet. and Gyn., Madras, India

Obstetrics and gynecology is a basic speciality which requires intensive training on its fundamental aspects at all levels of medical education. However, unfortunately today, scant attention is paid to the teaching of the subject in the medical colleges in our state. At the undergraduate level, emphasis is laid on medicine and surgery with gross neglect of obstetrics and gynecology. It is introduced only in the final year for three months. At the postgraduate level, undue emphasis is laid on the rarer syndromes at the cost of the common, day to day problems in obstetrics. Re-orientation of teaching in obstetrics is longoverdue in our country, with its limited economic resources and evergrowing population, and particularly in Tamil Nadu, a state with 548 Primary Health centers as sufficient infrastructure to implement the Alma Ata declaration, "Health for all by 2000 A. D.". The paper deals with the current pattern of teaching obstetrics and gynecology for certain reforms, pertaining to its importance, selection of candidates, duration of the course, ideal teaching pattern and the teacher's role. The emphasis is laid on community based teaching with the proper perspective.

10.42.11

Training residents in ambulatory gynecologic surgery at an urban teaching hospital in the USA: Darney, P D. Univ. of California, San Francisco, CA, USA

In the USA economic necessity and patient preference have dictated that more and more operations be performed outside of operating rooms under local anesthesia. Since training programs are hospital based, residents usually have little opportunity to learn these new techniques, although they are certain to require them as practitioners. At a large urban hospital a gynecologic ambulatory surgical unit was organized to accomplish procedures such as tubal occlusion and uterine evacuation and to train residents. Equipment was acquired and a nursing and counselling staff solely dedicated to ambulatory surgery was organized. Residents in the third postgraduate year were selected for training because previous surgical experience was thought necessary to learn local anesthesia techniques. Very specific protocols for analgesic and anesthetic agents and for surgical technique were devised for each of the operations to be performed. Residents were required to follow these protocols and to operate only with attending physicians – not other residents. After introduction of this program, operating room time for more complicated procedures was increased, complication rates, such as tubal occlusion failure and post uterine evacuation infection declined, and residents made increasingly greater use of the ambulatory surgery service for a wider variety of conditions.

10.42.12

Foundations for successful residency program in obstetrics and gynecology in India: Rajaram, P, Omachigui, A. JIPMER, Pondicherry, India

The concept that the medical graduates spend some time in supervised clinical practice with patient responsibility is age old and forms the basis for residency program, the world over. In India the concept is in its infancy. The clinical problems are undergoing constant changes. With the advances in medical sciences and socio-economic changes that are taking place constantly the attitude of the residents and clinicians is also changing. Residency program in our department covers in final year of degree course, during the compulsory rotating internship, non-postgraduate and postgraduate residency level and senior residency level. The present problems are that the resident tends to take things easy in relation to patient care, the problems of the residency are never solved. There is a lack of uniformity in various hospitals and the undergraduate training is more theoretically oriented. Encouraged by the effect of Modified Essay Questions on student learning we have introduced it at the level of selection of postgraduates (*Rajaram* and *Asha*, 1982). This has definitely changed the attitude of interns and non-postgraduate residents to seek for more patient care and contact while they aspire for admission to postgraduate courses. We will present our experiences.

10.79.01

Scoy (Soonawalla copper Y) intrauterine contraceptive device: Dhurandhar, J K, Soonawalla, R P. Nawrosejee Wadia Maternity Hosp., Bombay, India

Study of "Scoy" insertions in 2000 cases over a period of two years. The side-effects, complications, acceptability and failure rates are studied. All the patients were followed up for at least a period of four months. The results were compared with other intrauterine contraceptive devices like Cu T and Lippes loop, comparing percentage of bleeding, pain, expulsion and failure rate. The results show that "Scoy" is a better device than the other intrauterine contraceptive devices. "Scoy" is also easy to insert and hence no incidence of perforation. The acceptability by the patients is excellent. Results show that side-effects and complications are minimal. The efficacy is for two years.

10.79.02

Similarities and dissimilarities between nulliparous and parous women from a multicentre experience with Nova-T: Quartararo, P. Pat. Ost., Univ., Palermo; **Arisi, E.** Clin. Ost. Gin., Univ., Modena; **Volpe, L.** Centro Salute Donna, Milano; **Brambilla, C.** Div. Ost. Gin., Osp. Buzzi, Milano; **Capitanio, G L.** Clin. Ost. Gin., Univ., Genova, Italy

In the present study we evaluated a considerable number of nulliparous women who wore Nova-T in the framework of an Italian multicentre trial. The subjects admitted to the study were 692, mean age 23.9 (±4.8) years. Total women-months of use were 13,677, with a mean duration of 19.8 (±13.7) months. There were six pregnancies (0.9%), bringing about a Pearl Index of 0.53. No ectopic pregnancies were recorded. Expulsion occurred in seven cases (1.0%). Removals were 18 (2.6%) for pain or bleeding, two (0.3%) for PID, and two (0.3%) for other medical reasons. Wish to become pregnant accounted for further 25 removals (3.6%). Main side-effects consisted of spotting (12.4%), pain (4.0%), hypermenorrhea (3.6%) and dysmenorrhea (3.3%). Pre-existing dysmenorrhea, however, disappeared in 6.1% of the women. Ten women had a syncopal attack at the insertion and one exhibited an allergy to copper. On the other hand, in a group of 2891 parous women there were 48 pregnancies (1.7%). The Pearl Index was 1.0 and therefore much more favourable in nulliparous women. Side-effects were slightly more common in nulliparous women. In conclusion it seems that IUDs should not be denied to willing nulliparous women, provided that they do not have multiple partners and are adequately followed up.

10.79.03
A multicentre experience with Nova-T: Arisi, E. Clin. Ostet.-Gin., Univ., Modena; **Caroti, S.** Div. Ostet.-Gin., Osp., Dolo; **Mongelli, L.** Div. Ostet.-Gin., Osp., Vimercate; **Rustichelli, A.** Div. Ostet.-Gin., Osp., Pavullo, Italy

Nova-T is an IUD only recently introduced in Italy, yet already largely used because of its advantageous technical features. The present paper describes a multicentre trial carried out in eight centres belonging to Universities, Hospitals or out-patient Clinics. Insertions of Nova-T were 3583, all performed according to the same protocol; women-months of use were 70,987, with a mean duration of 19.8 (±12.9) months. Analysis of the data was made by the life-table method. Recorded events were: 54 intrauterine pregnancies (1.5%), two ectopic pregnancies (0.1%), 33 expulsions (0.9%), 78 removals, of which 72 for bleeding and/or pain (2.0%) and six for pelvic inflammatory disease (0.2%). Pregnancy rate was higher in the first 12-month period, a similar pattern being observed in expulsion rate. No significant differences occurred between nulliparous and parous women. Pregnancy was more likely when IUD insertion had been difficult. Side-effects were few, not exceeding 20%. The results of the trial suggest that Nova-T is a highly effective, easy to use, and rather safe IUD.

10.79.04
Clinical experience with new copper IUD, Nova-T: Wagatsuma, T. Dept. Obstet. and Gyn., Nat. Med. Ctr, Tokyo, Japan

The paper presents data on a clinical experience with the new copper IUD, Nova-T in Japan. The IUD was inserted in 500 women between April 1981 and December, 1984, at the out-patient clinic of National Medical Center in Tokyo. The net cumulative termination rates at the end of 24 months using the life-table technique are: pregnancy 4.0, expulsion 2.3, removal due to bleeding and pain 1.9, other medical reason 0.4, planning pregnancy 7.8, and other personal reason 0.9, per 100 women. The study revealed that the IUD had excellent antifertility effect with low expulsion rate.

10.79.05
The Canadian experience with the Nova-T IUD: Fugere, P. Dept. Obstet. and Gyn., Hosp. Saint-Luc, Univ., Montreal, Que., Canada

When the Nova-T intra-uterine device (IUD) was introduced in Canada in 1981, we were interested to compare our experience with the results obtained in three Scandinavian countries, Finland, Denmark and Sweden, as reported by *Luukkainen* et al. This study had showed a lower pregnancy rate of the Nova-T IUD compared to a Gyne-T 200. The Nova-T IUD was inserted in 201 consecutive patients consulting in a family planning clinic of a teaching hospital from November 1981 to November 1982. They will be followed for a period of five years. The age of distribution in our study is closer to the group from Finland, while the parity distribution is closer to the group from Sweden. The summary of life-table analysis for the first 12 months shows a pregnancy rate of 1.1 which is not statistically different from the rates of 0.7, 0.68 and 0.67 reported in those countries. Our removal rate of 12.4 for bleeding and/or pain is similar to the rate of 14.5 reported in Sweden compared to 17.7 in Denmark and 3.3 in Finland. The rate of termination for infection is 2.7, very similar to Denmark 2.6 and Sweden 2.5, while Finland is only 0.66. While there was a significant variation in the age and parity distribution in the different countries, all the reports show a constant low pregnancy rate. This study confirms the results reported by *Luukkainen* et al. in the Scandinavian countries.

10.79.06
Seven-year experience of ML Cu 250 IUD use in contraception: Tsalikis, T, Stamatopoulos, P, Kalachanis, J, Mantalenakis, S. 1st Dept. Obstet. and Gyn., Aristotelian Univ., Thessaloniki, Greece

One thousand and thirty-eight patients were fitted with ML-Cu 250 IUDs – over a six-year period. The women enrolled in three groups. In group A were included 224 women in which the IUD was inserted postpartum. In group B were included 352 patients who had the IUD insertion immediately after abortion and in group C of 462 women where insertions were performed at the end of menstruation. All women were followed up every six months for a period of 24 months. The results of the three groups proved a good contraceptive effect in all women. The mean unexpected pregnancy rate was 2.1% (group A = 2.6%, group

B = 2.0% and group C = 1.7%). The mean expulsion rate was 1.8% (group A = 2.2%, group B = 2.0% and group C = 1.3%). The bleeding-pain symptom was apparent in 5.5 per cent. The mean planning pregnancy rate was 3.8%. Removals for medical and personal reasons were 3.6% and 1.9%, respectively. The continuation rate was considered very satisfactory (mean value 78.5%, group A = 76%, group B = 77.6% and group C = 82%). In the present study neither cases of perforations nor cases of ectopic pregnancy have been observed so far.

10.79.07
Multiload Cu IUD at Cesarean delivery: Parikh, M N. Nowrosjee Wadia Maternity Hosp., Bombay, India

Pregnancy occurring in the early post-Cesarean period is not desirable, while its termination carries a high risk of complications. This calls for effective contraception in such patients. An IUD is reliable contraceptive. It would be ideal to insert an IUD six weeks after Cesarean delivery, but very often in developing countries patients do not report for post-partum check-up and are next seen only when they come with unplanned pregnancy. We have developed a technique of temporarily fixing a Multiload Cu IUD at the fundus of the uterus with a catgut stitch during the Cesarean delivery itself. This procedure is intended to minimise the high expulsion rate of IUD which accompanies insertion in the immediate post-partum period. By the time the catgut is absorbed the uterus is well on its way to involution and this results in low expulsion rate. In sixty cases a Multiload Cu 250 was employed and in forty cases Multiload Cu 375. The expulsion rate was 5 per cent. PID was noted in two cases – in one in the second week and in one after 18 months. This technique is not recommended if there is infection. A two-year follow-up of 50 cases showed four per cent medical removal rate and two per cent pregnancy rate. Thus our technique is an effective and satisfactory method of preventing pregnancy after Cesarean delivery.

10.79.08
Five years of experience with the ML Cu 375 intrauterine contraceptive device: Os, W A A van, Nooyer, C C A de, Kleinhout, J, Clements, J. Dept. Obstet. and Gyn., Elisabeth Gasthuis, Haarlem, The Netherlands

This five-year straight evaluation of the ML Cu 375 inserted at interval confirms the efficacy, safety and retainability of this high-load ML IUD model. The analysis concerns 2422 insertions and covers 84,411 women-months of experience. Gross cumulative event rates at five years are: pregnancy 2.9; expulsion 5.4; removal for bleeding/pain and other medical reasons 20.8 and 6.1, respectively. Performance of the ML Cu 375 is influenced by age and parity of the recipient.

10.79.09
Comparison of the TCu 380 Ag and the Multiload Cu 375 in Mehalla Kubra, Egypt: Etman, S, Marper, J M. Sect. Obstet. and Gyn., F.P. Res. Ctr, Misr Company's Hosp., Mehalla Kubra, Egypt

The TCu 380 Ag and the Multiload Cu 375 IUDs were compared in 296 interval women in Mehalla Kubra, Egypt. The IUDs showed similar low rates for undesirable events. There were no accidental pregnancies and continuation rates were better than 93 per cent at one year after insertion. There were no hospitalization subsequent to insertion. There was a significant difference in age distribution between the two IUD groups. Significant differences between the two groups were found in the less than 25 year old age group for the total number of women with one or more pelvic complaints. Age-adjusted, one year gross cumulative life-table rates for pregnancy, expulsion, removals and continuation were not significantly different. Follow-up rates for the two groups were similarly high at one year after insertion.

10.79.10
An IUD with 0% expulsions, less pregnancy, high continuity during three years: Double T Cu 500: Chertkoff, A*, Zimerman, C E, Legal, R R, Mazor, B**, Chertkoff, L E. *Nat. Univ., Cordoba, Argentina; **Haifa, Israel

Our team has been researching 12 years, about how to lower secondary symptoms: abnormal bleeding, expulsion leucorrhea, pain. 5000 insertions with Double T Cu 500: 0% expulsions, also in nullipara it is expelled only if any portion of IUD remains in cervic channel. Double T Cu 500 was designed by uterine microdissection investigations. Thin structures, flexible and well tolerated material lowered abnormal bleeding: treated with phlebotropic and/or riboflavinoid drugs 1200–1500 mg daily: five days. During insertion we used ampicillin 1500 mg daily, three to five days, and control between 6–12 months. After insertion did not show any pelvic inflammatory disease. Leucorrhea we treated previous culture/antibiogram-Lab test indicated proper treatment. Pain during "Adaptation period", three first months – more pain in nullipara. Tolerated by 96.4% with antispasmodic drugs. 97.6% of patients did not want or could not bear children, remain with Double T Cu 500, after three years insertion. High effectivity during four years, after must change. This method accept improvement. 1984–85 a Latin American team begin new investigations with this IUD. We are continuing our research.

11.28.01

Pharmacokinetics and pharmacodynamics of transdermal dosage forms of 17β-estradiol: Comparison with conventional oral estrogen used for hormones replacement: Powers, M S, Schenkel, L, Darley, P E, Good, W R, Balestra, J C, Place, V A. ALZA Corp., USA; Ciba-Geigy Corp., Basel, Switzerland

The pharmacokinetics and pharmacodynamics of three forms of estrogen replacement therapy were compared in postmenopausal women: transdermal systems delivering 17β-estradiol, 0.025, 0.05, and 0.1 mg/day, and oral dosage forms delivering 2 mg/day micronized 17β-estradiol or 1.25 mg/day conjugated equine estrogens. Study design was open-label, multiple crossover. Transdermal estradiol provided serum estradiol concentrations typical of the early follicular phase of the premenopausal woman. Serum levels were similar to those obtained 24 hours after dosing with either oral preparation. Continuous wearing of transdermal systems over three weeks did not result in any accumulation of estradiol. The treated estradiol/estrone ratio with transdermal delivery approximated 1. Both oral dosage forms increased serum estrone to 4 to 6 times serum estradiol levels and to 7 to 20 times the baseline estrone values. The three transdermal delivery rates produced average levels of urinary estradiol conjugated within the range for the follicular phase of premenopausal women. Suppression of gonadotropins by transdermal estradiol and the oral preparations was similar.

11.28.02

Transdermal estradiol substitution in menopausal women, clinical efficacy in a multicenter, open label, dose-finding study: Schenkel, L. Pharmaceutical Div., Ciba-Geigy Ltd., Basel, Switzerland

Efficacy in the control of menopausal symptoms and tolerability of transdermal estradiol substitution (Estraderm TTS) has been studied in 95 menopausal women in a three month open label dose-finding study by a group of practitioners. In the first month the patients were treated with the lowest dose of estradiol (25 µg/day). In the subsequent two months the dose was adapted according to efficacy and tolerability. Treatment was cyclic or continuous, sequential gestagen treatment was recommended. The patients completed a diary twice weekly. Of the 95 patients who entered the study, nine did not fulfil entry criteria, one was not cooperative and seven did not complete the study. In the third treatment month the major number of the patients (46) was treated with Estraderm 50 µg/day, about one third (23) required Estraderm 25 µg/day and the remaining eight 100 µg/day. Skin tolerability was generally good except for transient erythema (19% of application sites). Two patients discontinued treatment due to skin irritation. Systemic toleration of Estraderm TTS was very good.

11.28.03

Biological effects of estradiol (E₂) administered by a transdermal therapeutic system (TTS): Judd, H L, Chetkowski, R, Meldrum, D, Steingold, K, Lu, J, Eggena, P, Randle, D. Depts. Obstet.-Gyn. and Med., Los Angeles, CA, USA

It is recognized that orally administered estrogens can affect hepatic functions leading to undesirable side-effects including hypertension, cholecystitis, and intravascular clotting. We have attempted to avoid these effects by administering E_2 by TTS to 23 postmenopausal women at doses of 25, 50, 100, and 200 µg/day. These systems provide controlled delivery and steady blood levels of hormone. Effects on markers of estrogen action were compared with oral conjugated estrogens (OE) at doses of .625 and 1.25 mg. All doses were given for 28 days. The 50 µg TTS dose had effects similar to .625 mg OE on gonadotropin levels, vaginal cytology, and urinary calcium and hydroxyproline creatinine ratios. None of the TTS doses influenced hepatic markers. Renin substrate, SHBG and CBG were elevated by OE. The ratios of high density to low density lipoprotein cholesterol were also significantly increased with both OE doses. TTS and OE did not alter clotting factors. – Conclusions: 1) Unlike OE, TTS can elicit replacement responses on non-hepatic sites of estrogen action without exerting measurable effects on liver functions. 2) The use of TTS may avoid hypertension and cholecystitis associated with estrogen replacement, while OE may have favorable effects on circulating lipoproteins. 3) Transcutaneous or oral estrogen replacement with appropriate dosages has no measurable effect on intravascular coagulation.

11.28.04

Comparative clinical evaluation of estrogens administered by the transdermal and oral routes: Landgren, B M, Johannisson, E, Diczfalusy, E. Reprod. Endocr. Res. Unit and Dept. Obstet. and Gyn., Karolinska Inst. and Hosp., Stockholm, Sweden

The effects of three estrogen preparations on vasomotor symptoms, endometrial appearance and vaginal cytology were studied in 12 peri- and postmenopausal women. The kidney, liver and thyroid functions were also assessed. The following estrogen preparations were used: estradiol valerate (E_2V, 2 mg/day orally), combined equine estrogen (Premarin, 1.25 mg/day orally) and a transdermal system (TTS-E_2) delivering estradiol at a rate of 50 µg/24 h. Each estrogen was administered for three weeks, followed by one week of medroxyprogesterone acetate (MPA, 5 mg/day orally) and one week of placebo administration. The same sequence was then followed for another five-week period. The effect on vasomotor symptoms was recorded once weekly before, during and after the three 10-weekly treatment periods using *Kuperman's* index. Vaginal smear was taken once daily during the second estrogen treatment with each estrogen formulation for estimation of the karyopyknotic index. Endometrial biopsies for morphometric analyses were taken before treatment and on the 21st day of the second treatment period with each estrogen formulation.

Regular withdrawal bleedings were induced by the treatment in all postmenopausal women; in contrast, the perimenopausal subjects exhibited irregular bleedings. All three estrogen formulations induced significant effect on the karyopyknotic index and a significant endometrial proliferation. A significant effect of all climacteric symptoms was observed with the three estrogen formulations.

11.28.05

A double-blind comparative study of Estraderm™ and Premarin® in the amelioration of postmenopausal symptoms: Place, V A, Powers, M, Darley, P E, Schenkel, L, Good, W R. ALZA Corp., USA; Ciba-Geigy Corp., Basel, Switzerland

Patients whose postmenopausal symptoms were being satisfactorily controlled with conjugated equine estrogens (Premarin®, Ayerst), 0.625 mg/day (n = 57) or 1.25 mg/day (n = 57) of 1.25 mg/day (n = 67), participated in a study comparing the efficacy of these oral regimens with 17β-estradiol, 0.1 mg/day, administered through intact skin (Estraderm™, Ciba-Geigy). The study was a double-blind, randomized, parallel-group trial during which two-thirds of patients receiving each Premarin dosage were changed to Estraderm while the remainder continued with Premarin. A total of 124 patients were included in the analysis of efficacy. The analysis revealed no significant differences between Estraderm and Premarin in control of hot flushes or other postmenopausal symptoms and no statistically significant differences between treatment groups with respect to estrogen-related side-effects. Minor topical reactions to the transdermal systems were reported during only about 20% of study weeks. Thus, Estraderm, 0.1 mg/day, appears to be equally effective for controlling postmenopausal symptoms as Premarin, 0.625 or 1.25 mg/day, and is well tolerated.

11.28.06

The efficacy, acceptability, metabolic effects and endometrial responses to transdermal estradiol in the management of postmenopausal women: Whitehead, M I, Endacott, J A, Padwick, M L. King's Coll. Hosp., London, UK

Oral administration of estrogen to postmenopausal women effectively relieves menopausal symptoms but may cause systemic side-effects which include adverse changes in hepatic metabolism. The transdermal route of administration may minimise these adverse effects. We have studied the efficacy, acceptability, metabolic effects and endometrial responses of transdermal patches delivering 50 μg of estradiol daily in post- and peri-menopausal women over a period of nine months. Transdermal estradiol significantly improved vaginal cytology and climacteric symptoms including hot flushes, sleep disturbance, irritability, poor concentration and optimism. No endometrial hyperplasia was observed. The patches were well tolerated and no systemic side-effects were reported. Local reactions were minimal when present and only occurred infrequently. No clinically significant adverse biochemical changes were observed and plasma renin substrate and renin activity were unchanged during therapy. Transdermal estradiol offers an attractive alternative to oral estrogen therapy in the management of postmenopausal women.

11.28.07

Transdermal resorption of 17β-estradiol: Lauritzen, C. Dept. Obstet. and Gyn., Univ., Ulm

A new transdermal therapeutic system (TTS) was investigated, using plasters containing 2 mg (5 cm^2), 4 mg (10 cm^2) and 8 mg (20 cm^2) of 17β-estradiol (E$_2$). Twelve volunteers with climacteric complaints following oophorectomy or spontaneous menopause received the TTS twice a week on a hairless area of skin at the side of the abdominal wall. Plasma determinations of 17β-estradiol and estrone were performed to measure the speed and the amount of transdermal resorption and to compare these therapeutic concentrations with those of a normal cycle. The resorption of E$_2$ was rapid. There was a significant increase within 2 hours. With a 2 mg plaster the plasma values were between 20–40 pg/ml E$_2$, with 4 mg between 40–60 pg and with 8 mg between 75 and 120 pg/ml E$_2$. Also E$_2$ and E$_3$ conjugates in 24 hours urine were measured. The calculation revealed a mean daily release of 0.025, 0.05 and 0.1 mg E$_2$ respectively per day for up to four days. The plasma concentrations declined between 60 and 90 hours after application. Accordingly an application twice a week seems appropriate. Proliferation of the vaginal epithelium was also monitored and demonstrated the biological activity of the E$_2$ from the TTS. Also climacteric complaints were influenced favorably. The TTS-system was well tolerated. There were no significant subjective and objective side-effects. No skin irritations were seen. Accordingly the TTS for E$_2$ medication seems to yield plasma values similar to those in the normal endogenous cycle and to be effective and suitable for the treatment of estrogen deficiency syndromes.

11.32.01

Monitoring ovarian carcinoma with a monoclonal antibody (CA 125): Torre, G C*, Centonze, A**, Centonze, M**, Farinini, D**, Rosso, G***. Dept. Gyn. and Obstet., Hosp. S. Corona, *Pietra Ligure; **S. Martino, Genova; ***Saluzzo, Italy

A monoclonal antibody (OC 125), investigated by *Bast, R C.* (J. clin. Invest. **68**, 1331, 1981), has been found to react with a circulating antigen (CA 125) derived from ovarian carcinoma cells. With a solid phase RIA we compared serum levels of CA 125 in normal control subjects and in women with benign or malignant uterine and ovarian pathology. Normal values in control subjects ranged from 5.7 to 94 U/ml (37 ± 9.2 mean). In benign uterine and ovarian diseases CA 125 levels were found in a normal range (24 myomas,

17 ovarian cysts); elevated levels were observed in endometriosis (25/25 cases, ranging 50 to 105 U/ml) and in two cases of pyosalpinx (490 and 610 U/ml, respectively). Patients with cervical or endometrial carcinoma showed CA 125 levels within normal range. 28 cases of ovarian carcinoma were examined before surgical treatment. The pre-operative serum CA 125 levels ranged from 110 to 855 U/ml and no correlation was observed with stage, lesion size, ovarian function and patient's age. Two months after the surgical treatment a decrease in serum CA 125 to normal levels was found in all patients. Subsequently, fast increasing levels were found to be strictly bound with a progression of the disease. CA 125 may be a useful marker in monitoring ovarian cancer patients during chemotherapy, allowing early detection of recurrences.

11.32.02

Vaginosonography: An approach to a screening method for early ovarian cancer: Popp, L W, Lemster, S, Müller-Holve, W, Martin, K. Dept. Obstet. and Gyn., Allg. Krankenh. Barmbek, Hamburg

Using two different types of experimental ultrasound probes for vaginal application we have examined more than 300 patients so far. With increasing experience we found it very easy to visualize the ovaries on the screen. The transducer's tip in the vaginal fornix can easily be placed as close as 1 cm or even less to the ovary. Consequently, high ultrasound frequencies with correspondingly high resolution can be applied to the ovary. We used a 5.5 and a 7.0 MHz probe (*Brüel & Kjaer*, Copenhagen). The comparison between morphological sections of extirpated ovaries and their pre-operative sono-morphological sections revealed a striking comparability down to the dimension of about 2 mm. We have studied in this manner normal ovaries of different ages, benign ovarian tumors and also advanced carcinomas. We have not yet had a case of early ovarian cancer. However, as the normal size and sono-morphological pattern of the ovary are defined, early signs of malignancy in the dimension of less than 1 cm must be detectable. Vaginosonography is a very simple and effective diagnostic tool to come for widespread use. Ovarian small-parts scanning by means of vaginosonography is a step in the right direction for early detection of ovarian cancer.

11.32.03

The prognostic significance of morphological parameters for ovarian cancer: Schulz, B O, Werner, A, Baker, E*, Krebs, D, Sellin, D*. Depts. Obstet. and Gyn., Univ., Bonn; and *Inst. Path., Med. Univ., Lübeck

Tissue slides of 225 epithelial ovarian cancers were examined by two pathologic teams to determine the following details: histologic pattern, degree of polymorphy, mitotic index, density of chromatin, presence of nuclei and macronuclei, lymphocytic infiltration, psammoma bodies and necrosis; CEA, TPA, CEA-12/5; and lectin binding sites. For statistical evaluations the data were presented together with stage, age, therapy and survival times and analysed using hazard models (*Cox*, 1972; *Carter*, 1983). – Results: Different parameters were differently correlated with survival times for different stages. The data therefore were analysed in two groups: 1 = stage I and II, 2 = stage III and IV. For the advanced cases age had no effect on survival. Reduced survival prognosis was significantly influenced by polymorphy, histological pattern mitotic index, and density of chromatin and associated with necrosis. Psammoma bodies proved to be a good prognostic factor. For the early stages age was a significant negative prognostic factor. Reduced survival prognosis was significantly correlated with hist. pattern, chromatin density, and degree of polymorphy. Lymphocytic infiltration proved to be a good prognostic factor. The immunohistologically investigated parameters did not influence prognosis significantly. A scoring system is proposed: Grade (1–4) = Polymorphy (1–3) + Necrosis (0/1).

11.32.04

Real-time sonography: A possible early screening test for ovarian neoplasms?: Carstensen, M H, Hüneke, B, Sprotte, C. Univ.-Frauenklin., Hamburg-Eppendorf, Hamburg

The poor prognosis of ovarian neoplasms is attributable to the fact that about 70% already have widespread intraperitoneal metastases at the time of diagnosis. More than 90% of all carcinomas have cystic spaces. These should be detectable by sonography. Using real-time ultrasound (sector scanner) we studied 30 postmenopausal women (41 to 69 y), in whom clinical examination was unremarkable and 14 women (19 to 75 y) with a palpable gynecologic tumor on the day before laparotomy. The three largest diameters of ovaries in orthogonal planes were measured. The ovarian volumes were calculated by: $4/3\,\pi \times (d_1/2 \times d_2/2 \times d_3/2)$. Both ovaries could be displayed in 82% of the postmenopausal women by real-time sonography. Morphology appeared normal in all cases: echogenicity was uniform. The ovarian volumes ranged from 1.9 ml to 37.7 ml with means of 13.9 ± 2.1 ml (SEM) (confirmed at laparotomy) and 14.3 ± 2.1 ml (sonography). The correlation coefficient r between sonar and direct measurement at operation was 0.90. In patients with a palpable tumor r was 0.99. In 13 of 14 cases sonar predictions of the nature of the tumor were correct. In contrast to *Loch* et al. (Ultraschall **5**, 287, 1984) we believe, that real-time sonography is a possible screening test and that this technique warrants further evaluation as a method for early detection of ovarian cancer.

11.32.05

Clinical, prognostic and therapeutic aspects of steroid receptors in endometrial cancer: Kleine, W, König, P, Geyer, H, Pfleiderer, A. Univ.-Frauenklin., Freiburg

In more than 200 endometrial carcinomas estrogen (ER) and progesterone receptors (PR) were determined by the dextran-coated charcoal (DDC) method. A little less than 80 per cent of the adenocarcinomas was receptor positive (> 20 fmol/mg protein). 60 per cent had both receptors. In regard to clinical data stage, histological differentiation and myometrial invasion inversely correlated with receptor status: in early stage, well differentiated carcinomas with minimal infiltration most cases were receptor positive. There was no correlation with age, menarche, menopause and pregnancies. Out of the typical risk factors only obesity could be shown correlating with receptor positive cases. During an observation time up to five years there was no difference of survival time of receptor positive and negative cases in the early stages, but in stage III, IV and recurrences patients with receptor negative tumors died earlier. Regarding the success of receptor dependant hormonal treatment there is only scanty information. However, the knowledge of receptor status opens new therapeutic approaches with anti-estrogens like tamoxifen or gestagens like MPA as an adjuvant or palliative agent in endometrial cancer.

11.32.06

The role of CA 125 as tumor marker in ovarian carcinoma: Krebs, H B, Goplerud, D R, Kilpatrick, J S, Myers, M, Hunt, A. Dept. Obstet. and Gyn., and Biostatist., Med. Coll. of Virginia, Richmond, VA, USA

Thirty-three healthy women (group I), 20 patients with a history of ovarian carcinoma but no manifest disease at the time of the study (group II), and 45 patients with surgically demonstrable ovarian cancer (group III) were studied to establish guidelines for the use of the ovarian cancer antigen CA 125 in monitoring the course of ovarian carcinoma. Although significant differences of the mean CA 125 values determined by three different laboratories were found, 99% of all CA 125 titers of patients in group I and II were ≤ 25 U/ml. By contrast, 96% of patients with manifest ovarian cancer had CA 125 levels > 25 U/ml. CA 125 values rising from the normal range to > 25 U/ml predicted recurrent disease in all of 14 patients provided benign causes (5 cases) for titer elevations such as bowel obstruction could be ruled out. Nine of the 14 patients with recurrent cancer had elevated antigen levels 2 to 5 months before the diagnosis could be made clinically. In patients with CA 125 values > 25 U/ml, titer changes of $\geq 50\%$ compared to reference values predicted tumor response or progression in 41 of 43 patients (95%) with antigen positive tumors. CA 125 correlated poorly with the tumor mass. Antigen levels in normal range did not exclude a positive second look operation in six of 13 patients (46%). It is concluded that the CA 125 is useful for the detection of persistent and recurrent disease, and for the evaluation of treatment response.

11.32.07

Tumoral volume, local extension and prognosis in cervical carcinoma: The significance of the barrier between cervix and parametrium: Dargent, D, Beau, G, Adelaine, P. Hôp. Edouard-Herriot, Lyon, France

In our experience the chances of survival at five years are for cervical carcinoma of 93.5% for stage pI and stage pIIa (n=269) and 54.2% for stage pIIb (n=139). The difference is highly significative. But the question is: isn't this difference due to a difference in tumoral volume? From 80.04.01 to 84.06.30 113 specimens of radical hysterectomy were examined as indicated by *Baltzer*. Local extension and tumoral volume were assessed. It appears that in each volume group prognosis is better for stage pI and pIIa than for stage pIIb. The barrier between cervix and parametrium, as demonstrated in the past by *Kindermann* and *Ober*, is anatomical boundary of a true prognosis signification.

11.32.08

Microcolposcopy in the evaluation of subclinical infections and intra-epithelial neoplasia in relation with HPV: Pace, S, Beau, G, Dargent, D. 2e Clin. Obstet. e Gin., Univ. Studi "La Sapienza", Rome, Italy

Exfoliative cytology and colposcopy are not sufficient for determining if an epithelial abnormality of the cervix is in relation with HPV or not. Microcolposcopy achieved with the microhysteroscope of *J. Hamou* allows a good evaluation. The pathological alterations of connective tissue (papillary growth) are better evidenced with microhysteroscope than with colposcope. The details of epithelial cells are, with the microhysteroscope, studied as good, or nearly as in exfoliative cytology. The correlation between microcolposcopic evaluation and histological diagnosis (serial sections on operative specimens) are, in our recent experience (84.09.01 to 85.02.28) good: 6 false positive for 21 cases and 7 false negative for 21 cases.

11.41.01

Video presentation of anterior target colporrhaphy for female urinary stress incontinence: Browne, A D H. Dept. Obstet. and Gyn., Royal Coll. Surgeons, Ireland

The video demonstrates the technique of anterior target colporrhaphy for use in cases of stress incontinence. Innovative features are as follows: Cystoscopic distension of the bladder to 600 ml of water; insertion of Bonano catheter; performance of the operation with the bladder filled; identification of the target point on the inferior surface of the urethra, at which support controls stress incontinence; exposure of the urethra through anterior vaginal wall incision; insertion of a Nuralon "shoelace" suture at target point; demonstrating the effectiveness of the suture by tightening its ends prior to tying it; tying the stitch and re-testing for efficacy; routine closure of the anterior vaginal wall incision; after-care involving retention of the Bonano catheter until spontaneous emptying can be achieved. The simplicity of the operation, and the advantage of checking that it works are the main advantages claimed for its use. Postoperative results are comparable to those obtained by other methods.

11.41.02
Diagnostic hysteroscopy for endometrial carcinoma: Sugimoto, O, Fukuda, Y, Ikeda, Y. Dept. Obstet. and Gyn., Osaka Med. Coll., Osaka, Japan

In Japan, endometrial carcinoma accounts for about 5% of all uterine malignant neoplasms, but recently it seems the incidence is gradually increasing. In our clinic, hysteroscopy was performed in about 7000 cases in the last ten years and 95 cases were diagnosed as endometrial carcinoma. The hysteroscope used in this study is the panoramic type manufactured by the Machida Company in Japan. The uterine cavity is distended and irrigated by saline or 32% dextran solution. Hysteroscopic diagnosis of endometrial carcinoma was classified into circumscribed and diffuse forms. The circumscribed form was finely classified into papillary, polypoid, nodular and ulcerated types. The papillary type had the highest incidence. This type showed apparently nodular protuberances, but with careful observation many tentacle-like projections were observed. The polypoid type usually consisted of several polyps with a gray-white, uneven surface with atypical venous dilatations in some areas. In the nodular type the protrusion is large with a rough surface and marked subepithelial varicosities. The ulcerated type looked more ragged, fragile and dull on hysteroscopy because of the coating pus and debris. The diffuse form was an invasive ulcerated type. In this series of hysteroscopy, the medium did not flow into the peritoneal cavity and no other side-effects occurred.

11.41.03
Intraoperative prophylaxis of the vaginal descent and prolapse after total hysterectomy: Bobčev, T. Dept. Gyn., 1st Workers' Hosp., Sofia, Bulgaria

Some abdominal and vaginal prophylaxis of the descent and prolapse of the vaginal stump after total hysterectomy is suggested. Intrafascial surgical techniques are recommended to avoid intraoperative complications, such as injuries of the bladder, ureters, incarcerated intestins in the pouch of Douglas etc., whereas extrafascial techniques should be used in carcinoma of the uterus and adnexa. The difficulties in treating postoperative complications such as descent and prolapse of the vaginal stump have proved a good opportunity to suggest a new method. A loop is made by stitching the stumps of the round ligaments. By means of four chromic-catgut No 2 the loop is hidden between the two leaves of the endopelvic fascial cuff. The loop is sewn on the vaginal stump by applying extrafascial operative techniques. The good adhesion between the tissues ensures a reliable fixation of the vaginal stump and prevents from urinary and cohabitational disturbances. The immediate and later results obtained of more than 700 patients appear most encouraging. In cases of vaginal hysterectomy, the vagina is fixed on the stumps of the adnexa, round and sacro-uterine ligaments and on closed peritoneum. Thus the vagina is closed without any paravaginal space which ensures better hemostasis and a good adhesion between vagina, peritoneum and ligament stumps, as well as protection from descent and prolapse. More then 200 patients have been treated with excellent results.

11.41.04
Schauta-Amreich radical vaginal hysterectomy: Reiffenstuhl, G. Frauenklin., Landeskrankenanst., Salzburg, Austria

Demonstration of the technique (30 minutes)

11.42.01
Mastectomy and immediately started breast reconstruction: Vaczi, L. Frauenklin. Prof. Stähler, Siegen

The loss of a breast after mastectomy means not only a confrontation with the cancer, but at the same time it is also a confrontation with the female identity of the patients. In this case, I believe that proper therapy involves not only the mastectomy but also the reconstruction. A one-stage operation – mastectomy and reconstruction – at the same time has several disadvantages: 1. limited radicality because of the expected reconstruction, 2. poor esthetic results, which hardly accepted by the patient. The technique, I am going to report, is based on a modified mastectomy, combined with an immediately started reconstruction with tissue-expander. This technique has the following advantages: 1. The radicality of the mastectomy is independent of the reconstruction. 2. The final results is esthetically accepted by the patient. 3. No difficulties if radiation or chemotherapy are necessary. The 12-minutes colour-movie shows the surgical technique for the mastectomy, how to place the tissue-expander, the exchange of the expander for the prosthesis three months after and an easy new technique of the reconstruction of the nipple. According to my results this easy technique provides the possibility of helping people in this serious life-conflict.

11.42.02
Pelviscopic surgery of tubal pregnancy: Semm, K. Dept. Obstet. and Gyn., Univ., Kiel, and Michaelis-Midwifery School, Kiel

With ectopic pregnancies 80% can be treated by surgical pelviscopy (e. g. endoscopic intra-abdominal surgery). Recently developed techniques such as endosuture with extracorporeal and/or intracorporeal knotting combined with the use of the OP-Pneu-Electronic and the Aquapurator for pelvic washing, guarantee a constant CO_2-Pneumoperitoneum under clear visual conditions. This combination allows the treatment of tubal pregnancy by surgical endoscopy with a similar technique like during laparotomy. The film shows after extended adhesiolysis in the middle abdomen and sucking of blood out of the lower pelvis the new technique of hemostasis called endocoagulation for hemostasis of the extended tube tissue before longitudinal, e. g. antimeso incision. After pulling out the ectopic pregnancy tissue with the newly developed instruments, the tube is washed and cleaned by using the Aquapurator. When hemostasis is achieved, and the lower pelvis cleaned, the wound of the Fallopian tube has to be closed with an endosuture (Ethicon). The physical stress for the patient by all these interventions is nearly the same as during a sterilization. After a short hospital stay of 5 days, after the surgical intervention, the patient can begin with everyday life again immediately. Repeat pelviscopies 6 to 8 months later reveal in about 80% patent Fallopian tubes and no adhesions in the entire abdomen. The typical procedures – here shown in 10 minutes – really need 30–60 minutes like a laparotomy.

11.42.03

Pelviscopic adnexectomy: Semm, K. Dept. Obstet. and Gyn., Univ., Kiel, and Michaelis-Midwifery School, Kiel

For the last six years the newly developed apparatus, instruments and operation methods allow us to remove ovaries or adnexa under pelviscopic conditions. The use of the "OP-Pneu-Electronic" (according to *Semm*) also guarantees a constant pneumoperitoneum, especially in cases of great gas loss, which occurs when sucking blood or fluid out of the lower pelvis or when instruments have to be changed. The film shows the typical way of performing an adnexectomy with the 3-knot-technique in a case of surgical ablative and hormonal treatment in a case of metastatic breast cancer. When ovary and Fallopian tube are ligated three times with e. g. the ROEDER-loop (ETHI-Binder) the adnexa are cut and removed through a trocar sheath of 11 mm in diameter by using the recently developed morcellator. To prevent later adhesions the adnexal stump has to be coagulated with the Endocoagulator according to *Semm* at 100° C (214° F). Bigger ovarian cysts (chocolate-cysts or dermoids) can be removed by using the same method. In this film the technique is shown in ten minutes. The adnexectomy on both sides by pelviscopy needs really about 30 to 45 minutes. The physical stress for the patient is not as great as during a tubal sterilization.

11.42.04

Pathology of the isthmo-interstitial segment of the oviduct: Tran, D K. Hosp. Annexe Républ., Univ., Nice, France

Between 1978 and 1983, we have found 178 patients who presented a pathology of the proximal segment of the Fallopian tube. Pathology of the isthmo-interstitial segment is defined by hysterosalpingography which is compared with laparoscopy and histology of 154 oviducts. Multifocal lesions have a very bad prognosis. When bifocal lesions and pure proximal lesions are not treated, we find more than 50% of ectopic pregnancy. When pure proximal lesions are treated by Danazol, we have the best percentage of pregnancy. When Danazol is not efficient, we use microsurgical isthmo-ostial reimplantation.

11.42.05

Sperm injection by micromanipulation – a new possibility in the treatment of male infertility: Metka, M, Haromy, T, Huber, J, Schurz, B, Kozak, W. 1st Dept. Gyn. and Obstet., Univ., Vienna, Austria

Three couples were selected for this preliminary sperm injection study, with their consent, since in all three cases the zona free hamster egg penetration test was negative and in one couple previous attempts at *in vitro* fertilization were unsuccessful. Of 22 eggs recovered from three patients, nine from each patient, three were injected with sperm, while the others were inseminated by the standard IVF-protocol. Before manipulating human eggs extensive experiments were performed with animal eggs, so decreasing the rate of damage to under 10%. Additionally we optimized the method by using an individual adapted equipment. Manipulation was performed by penetration of the zona pellucida with a $5-7\,\mu$ diameter injection pipette into the perivitelline space – so damage to the egg cytoplasm was avoided. This special technique for sperm injection was not used until now in this indication. From nine eggs – used in this experiment – one egg developed a pronucleus and one egg developed to a four-cell stage. We were not able to achieve a pregnancy.

11.42.06

Creation of a neo-vagina with Müllerian remnants: Şekeroğlu, S, Erez, S, Erez, R. Mimar Sinan Univ., Istanbul, Istanbul Univ. Cerrahpaşa Med. Fac., Istanbul, Turkey

This is the description of a new method for formation of a neo-vagina: A vaginal tunnel is created by dissecting the space around the urinary bladder and rectum and subsequently is covered by peritoneal folds overlying the parametria and the Müllerian remnants. This procedure has satisfactory results comparable to more complicated methods and can be performed by gynecologists with no experience in intestinal surgery. The presence of Müllerian remnants in the walls of this newly created vaginal cavity impedes its subsequent closure.

12.02.01
Interobserver variability: A source of error in obstetric ultrasound: Sokol, R J, Zador, I E, Chik, L. Dept. Obstet. and Gyn., Wayne State Univ./Hutzel Hosp., Detroit, MI, USA

On a busy ultrasound service, scanning is performed by more than one sonographer, with later interpretation by a physician. This system leads to concerns about the quality of reported results on which clinical and research conclusions are based. To determine whether the sonographer had a biasing effect on the results reported, we examined a computerized database of 1094 singleton examinations. Each sonographer had had over four years experience, had used the same model scanner and had been assigned patients for examination randomly. BPD and abdominal diameter (AD) were selected from six recorded measurements; the left kidney was selected from 13 fetal structures examined for on our service. The success rate for obtaining a BPD measurement was found to vary significantly among sonographers ($\chi^2 = 71.5$, $p < .001$). One of the three sonographers failed to obtain a BPD four times more often than expected. In addition, the frequencies with which each sonographer was able to visualize the fetal left kidney varied significantly (by χ^2, $p < .001$). In a three-way discriminant analysis, the sonographers were found to differ in their measurement of AD ($F = 11.4$, $p < .005$); the identity of the sonographer accounted for 6.5% of the variance in the measurement obtained. Thus, the sonographer can have a significant effect on reported results, representing one of several sources of error. This study suggests that the computer can be used effectively as a quality assurance tool. The methodologic implication is that when "field data" are used in clinical research, indicator variables for the identity of the sonographer should be evaluated to avoid missing "cohort effect".

12.02.02
The correlation of ultrasonic fetal biparietal diameter and placental grading with biochemical fetal lung maturity: Park, Y W, Park, T K. Dept. Obstet. and Gyn., Yonsei Univ. Coll. Med., Seoul, Korea

One week before delivery 228 cases were examined utilizing ultrasonography for BPD measurement and placental grade to investigate correlation with RDS development. Three days before delivery 52 cases were examined via amniocentesis to establish the values of the L/S ratio, spectrophotometry at OD 650, and shake test to estimate the fetal lung maturity. If the BPD value ≥ 9.0 cm, 86% had an L/S ratio ≥ 2.0. If the placental grade was III, 65% had L/S ratio ≥ 2.0. If the placental grade was III and the BPD ≥ 9.0, then 100% had an L/S ratio ≥ 2.0 indicating full lung maturity. The limitations of amniocentesis in terms of its invasivenes, time factor, and impracticality in emergencies are well known. We suggest further investigation into extended use of ultrasonography to replace current usage of amniocentesis in estimation of fetal lung maturity.

12.02.03
Ultrasound prediction of shoulder dystocia: Oakes, G K, Williams, J, Kirz, D S, Worthen, N J. Dept. Obstet. and Gyn., Cedars-Sinai Med. Ctr, Los Angeles, CA, and Harbor-UCLA Med. Ctr, Torrance, CA, USA

Shoulder dystocia (SD) is a complication of fetal macrosomia. Accurate methods for prediction of SD have not been reported. This study prospectively assesses our ability to predict SD using ultrasound (UTZ) criteria. 59 patients with singleton gestations at 37–40 weeks were selected for study based upon one of three clinical factors: (1) DM, White class A–C, (2) Fundal height > 42 cm, (3) Clinical estimated fetal weight (EFW) > 4 kg. Biparietal diameter (BPD), head circumference (HC), abd. diameter (AD), abd. circumference (AC), and femur length (FL) were measured on each fetus. Neither the Pt nor her physician were aware of the UTZ results. There were 50 complete Pt records available for analysis. 13 Pts (26%) were delivered by Cesarean section (CS) for cephalopelvic disproportion (CPD) and five (10%) had CS for other indications. Of the 32 Pts who delivered vaginally, nine (28%) had SD. The mean birthweight (BW) in the SD group was 4763 g compared to 3970 g in the non-SD group ($p < 0.01$). The difference between AD & BPD (AD-BPD) was significantly greater in the SD group (2.1 ± 0.6 cm) than in the non-SD group (1.4 ± 0.8 cm) ($p < 0.05$). All cases with SD had AD-BPD of ≥ 1.5 cm and none of the cases with AD-BPD < 1.5 cm had SD. Thus, AD-BPD ≥ 1.5 cm has pos. predictive value = 53%, neg. predictive value = 100%, sensitivity = 100%, and specificity = 70% for SD with vaginal delivery. Non of the other UTZ measurements including BPD, HC, AC, HC:AC ratio, or UTZ EFW had comparable predictive accuracy. These results suggest that fetal UTZ measurement should be performed when there is a clinical risk for macrosomia. If AD-BPD ≥ 1.5 cm primary CS should be considered.

12.02.04
Possibility of early detection of placental insufficiency: Bayer, H, Prenzlau, P. Clin. Gyn. and Obstet. (Charité), Humboldt Univ., Berlin

Placental insufficiency hitherto is mostly not to detect before a retardation of the fetus already occurred. It is reported about a sound-stress-test. Reply to sound irritation takes place in about 90% of the fetuses after 20th week of gestation. These movements are checked up parallel by ultrasound-B-scan and cardiotocography. Fetal reaction is classified by duration, mode and number of the movements. All parameters were lower in those cases in which happened a fetal retardation in further progress of pregnancy. These examinations put as a foundation following consideration. In cerebral activity and muscle action the consumption of oxygen is higher and placenta with trend to insufficiency is not able to supply oxygen adequate as well like a placenta with normal function.

12.02.05
Use of ultrasonography in the diagnosis and management of first trimester bleeding: Purandare, C B, Purandare, N C, Daftary, S N. Bombay, India

The field of ultrasonography has undergone dramatic changes since its introduction. Nowhere are the remarkable advances more evident than in the application of diagnostic ultrasound to the obstetric and gynecologic patient. The role of ultrasound in first trimester bleeding is one such application. We wish to present an analysis of 140 cases admitted at two private nursing homes in Bombay, over a period of 24 months, who were diagnosed clinically as having bleeding in the first trimester. All these cases had an ultrasound examination to confirm the diagnosis. Clinically, these cases were suspected of having threatened abortion, missed abortion, incomplete abortion, vesicular mole and actopic pregnancy. Ultrasonography not only helped us in differentiating the various causes of bleeding due to obstetric etiological factors, but also high-lighted a number of cases where the bleeding was gynecological in origin. From the analysis we conclude that ultrasonography is an irreplaceable diagnostic tool in first trimester bleeding because it is the only non-invasive, imaging technique that gives a specific picture of events in this critical period, thus preventing incorrect diagnosis and management.

12.02.06
Sonographic visualization of the subchorial hematoma: Marziale, G, De Angelis, R, Anelli, L, Grimaldi, G. IV Clin. Ostet. e Gin., Univ. Studi "La Sapienza", Roma, Italy

In this study 17 pregnancies affected by subchorial hematoma, of gestational age from the 8th to the 18th week inclusive have been investigated. The size of the hematomas was from 25×20 mm of width and 20 mm of thickness approximately, up to nearly $60 \times 60 \times 15$ mm. Ten patients presented a blood loss at the first ultrasound examination. In 14 cases the fetal heart was normally recorded, while in three cases internal abortion was diagnosed. The follow-up was possible in nine cases, and in all these a subsequent good outcome resulted. On the periodical ultrasound inspections, the changes of the sonographic features up to the complete recovery, have been observed. While making the diagnosis of subchorial hematoma, it must be born in mind that in the first trimester the amniotic membrane, which divides the embryonic celoma from the amniotic fluid, can be visualized. Furthermore, the differential diagnosis has to be made with the lack of apposition between the capsular and the parietal deciduas, and with the anembryonic gestational sac in twin pregnancy. – Ref.: *Jeanty, P* et al. J. ultrasound Med **1**, 243, 1982; *Kaufman, A J* et al. Proceed 29th Annual Meeting AIUM, Kansas City, USA, 1984; *Mandruzzato, G P* et al. Proceed 5e Congrès EUROSON, Strasbourg, France, 1984; *Mantoni, M* et al. Proceed 4th European Congress Ultrasonics in Medicine, Dubrovnik, 1981; *Shunji, G* et al. Proceed 5e Congrès EUROSON, Strasbourg, France, 1984.

12.02.07
A large, soft echo-free space with daily vaginal bleeding results in a good outcome of pregnancy: Goto, S, Kato, T. Nagoya Nat. Hosp., Nagoya, Japan

It has been reported from our laboratory that vaginal bleeding before 21 weeks of the menstrual age is closely associated with sonographic observations such as echo-free and/or hypoechogenic areas around GS, and irregularity in GS-configuration, and also that the existence of both the vaginal bleeding which lasts more than five weeks and the echo-free space above 3 cm^2 in size which persists for five weeks or longer results in a poor outcome of pregnancy. Now we report on the influence of the size and type of echo-free space and the mode of vaginal bleeding on the outcome of pregnancy in 264 cases. The size of echo-free space and hypoechogenic area was represented as the maximum sectional area in an ultrasonographic film. Viable babies were born in 253 cases, but the rest showed a poor outcome of pregnancy, which included one embryonic (8 weeks) and four fetal (13, 16, 21 and 22) deaths, one stillbirth (24), one abortion (7), and four cases of D&C due to heart failure (15), acrania (14 and 15) and anxiety about prolonged bleeding (15). Intervals between the end of pregnancy, which proved to be poor in outcome, and the time when either vaginal bleeding or echo-free space or both persisting over five weeks disappeared ranged from 0 to 14 weeks. Irrespective of the vaginal bleeding, the existence – exceptional as it was – of an elastically soft echo-free space, which appeared to protrude into the amniotic cavity, always resulted in a good outcome of pregnancy. This type of echo-free space varied in size as well as in the duration of daily vaginal bleeding.

12.03.01
The lysozyme activity in pregnancy: Jevremović, M, Tucović, Ž, Kartaljević, G, Petronijević, A, Momčilov, P. Clin. Gyn. and Obstet., Fac. Med., Univ., Beograd, Yugoslavia

Lysozyme is a bacteriolytic enzyme acting on gram-positive and some gram-negative bacteria. It is being produced in neutrophilic leucocytes and monocytes as well as in placental and amniotic cells and in other cellular structures. Lysozyme activity during pregnancy was measured by using the turbidimetric test using the method of *D. J. Prockop* and *W. D. Davidson* (Testomar-Lysozyme Behringwerke). Our results have shown that the lysozyme values in the maternal blood serum, cervical secretion, maternal milk, umbilical cord, amniotic fluid and in retroplacental blood have characteristic levels. Lysozyme concentrations in the cord blood, amniotic fluid and in retroplacental blood were significantly higher ($p < 0.01$) in relation to the mothers peripheral blood. We have isolated very high levels of lysozyme in the cervical secretion and this appears to be important for the cervical and vaginal ecology in gestation. Our investigations have shown the presence of this antibacterial enzyme in the fetal and maternal compartments and particularly in the cervical and vaginal environment, and confirm the possibility of lysozyme usage in the therapy of infections during pregnancy.

12.03.02

The management of abortion induced septic shock with anti-lipopolysaccharide (anti-LPS) immunotherapy: Lachman, E, Pitsoe, S B, Philpott, R H, Gaffin, S. Dept. Obstet. and Gyn., Meir Hosp., Kfar Saba, Israel; Dept. and Physiol., Univ. of Natal, R.S.A.

Anti-lipopolysaccharide (anti-LPS) antibodies have been shown to lower mortality and morbidity in septic shock in a variety of animal and human studies. We here tested the use of human anti-LPS as a freeze dried plasma preparation in addition to conventional therapy on the morbidity and mortality of patients suffering from septic shock as a result of abortion. Both control and anti-LPS patients had similar morbidities on entry to the study. However, the anti-LPS treated group subsequently had significantly reduced mortality (7.1% vs. 42.85%) and morbidity index (1.64 vs. 4.33). All the patients in the control group required steroids and dopamine to maintain their blood pressure. Only two patients in the anti-LPS group required these agents. Thus anti-LPS appears promising as a useful adjunct to conventional therapy in the management of septic shock.

12.03.03

Materno-feto-amniotic transfer of cephalosporins: Hayasaki, M, Itoh, K, Itoh, T, Matsunami, K, Noda, K. Dept. Obstet. and Gyn., Univ., Gifu, Japan

The assessment of bactericidal efficacy of antibiotics in amniotic infection, materno-feto-amniotic transfer of some cephalosporins, which were cefotiam (CTM), cefmenoxime (CMX) and cephoperazone (CPZ), was evaluated. The drugs of one g were administered intravenously to pregnant women of more than 37 weeks gestation. Maternal serum, umbilical cord serum and amniotic fluid samples were collected simultaneously at the time of Cesarean section. In order to simulate the time-concentration curves of the drugs and calculate pharmacokinetic factors, a three-compartment model was employed, consisting of maternal serum, umbilical cord serum and amniotic fluid. In maternal serum, half-lives of CTM, CMX and CPZ concentration were 0.99, 1.07 and 5.41 hours, and AUC of CTM, CMX and CPZ were 69, 68 and 257 hr $\cdot$ μg/ml. In umbilical cord serum, the peak levels of CTM, CMX and CPZ were 18.7 μg/ml at 0.62 hours, 10.9 μg/ml at 0.80 hours and 16.5 μg/ml at 1.28 hours, and AUC of CTM, CMX and CPZ were 50, 41 and 157 hr $\cdot$ μg/ml. In amniotic fluid, the peak levels of CTM, CMX and CPZ were 18.4 μg/ml at 3.08 hours, 6.78 μg/ml at 3.88 hours and 4.84 μg/ml at 10.04 hours, and AUC of CTM, CMX and CPZ were 179, 91 and 89 hr $\cdot$ μg/ml. The drugs disappeared rapidly from the maternal and umbilical cord serum, but slowly from the amniotic fluid. It was found that CPZ has a longer half-life and higher level in maternal serum than CTM and CMX, but amniotic transfer rate of CPZ is lower than CTM and CMX. It is suggested that amniotic transfer of antibiotics is correlated with fetal urinary excretion.

12.03.04

Pharmacokinetics of antibiotics in the postpartum patient: Charles, D, Larsen, B. Dept. Obstet. and Gyn., Marshall Univ. School Med., Huntington, WV, USA

Despite similar gram negative spectra of activity among piperacillin, cefotaxime, moxalactam and cefoperazone, differences in their pharmacokinetic behavior may affect a physicians choice among these compounds. Four groups of 12 postpartum women volunteered for pharmacokinetic study of these drugs. Intravenous dosage of 1 g of each drug was given on the 2nd or 3rd postpartum day and at six months postpartum. Serum drug concentration was measured at 0.5, 1, 2, 4, and 8 hours after treatment. Bioassay was done in duplicate and employed ATCC strains. Concentration was computed from regression lines of the standards prepared in human serum. The serum levels were analysed by the two compartment open pharmacokinetic model with 95% confidence limits better than 12%. Each patient served as her own control. Results for piperacillin (μg/ml) are as follows:

	0.5 hr	1 hr	2 hr	4 hr	8 hr
2 days postpartum	14.9	4.8	2.2	—	—
3 days postpartum	15.6	5.2	2.4	0.2	—
36 months	24.1	10.4	4.4	2.1	—

Similar results were obtained for the cephalosporins which indicates that the serum levels attained early in the puerperium may be inadequate for the treatment of infections, so that indolent and protracted sepsis may ensue unless the antibiotic dosage is increased by 50 per cent.

12.03.05

Double-blind comparative study of metronidazole I. V. versus placebo in the prophylaxis of sepsis following Cesarean section: Lappas, C A, Leonardopoulos, J. Leto Maternity Hosp., Athens, Greece

No double-blind controlled trials have been carried out so far to test the effect of the prophylactic metronidazole in Cesarean section. Our trial included 100 Cesarean sections according to the protocol. Patients with patent infection, pyrexia $> 38°C$, hematologic disorders, or allergic patients were excluded. The investigator used for each patient four bottles, each of the them containing 500 mg of metronidazole or placebo. The patient received one bottle two hours before the operation, one during the operation and two bottles eight hours after the last one. The follow-up period was four weeks. The prophylaxis was considered a failure even if the infection was proven to be of aerobic origin. Pre-operatively note was made of the indication for Cesarean section, of the time the patient's membranes were ruptured (spontaneous or artificial), of the clarity of the liquor amnii, as well as of any circumstance which might predispose the patient to infection. All the Cesarean sections were performed in the same operation rooms, by the same medical and paramedical staff, the same technique and the same suture materials. Operative difficulty and duration were recorded. Post-operatively wounds, uterine and vaginal discharge and body temperature were inspected. Vaginal and uterine discharge were, if indicated, sent for culture of aerobes and anaerobes. The use of other medicaments and the patient's hospital stay were also recorded. In the placebo group the post-Cesarean infection and febrile morbidity rates were 14%. In the metronidazole group the rates fell to 6%.

12.03.06

The incidence of chlamydial infection in normal and at risk pregnancy: Hetzenauer, A, Trenkwalder, B, Reider, W, Kofler, H. Dept. Obstet. & Gyn., Dept. Derm., Univ., Innsbruck, Austria

There is evidence that genital infections during pregnancy play an important role with respect to perinatal morbidity and mortality, especially regarding premature rupture of membranes and prematurity (*Schachter:* Israel J. med. Sci. **19**, 936–939, 1983). We looked for chlamydial infections in 100 pregnant women. Fifty patients with a pregnancy at risk (PROM, premature labor, dystrophy) and 50 normal pregnant women. Diagnosis was made by determing chlamydial colonisation of the cervix uteri by means of direct immunofluorescence (monoclonal antibody). Preliminary data suggest an infection rate in risk pregnancies of 34%, whereas in normal pregnancy we found an overall infection rate of close to 13%. The difference is statistically significant ($p < 0.025$). At the same time we did a chlamydial culture and stored plasma at $-70°C$ for microimmunofluorescence (data not yet available). As a consequence of the preliminary findings it seems to us to be justified to look for chlamydial infection in all pregnancies at risk, especially premature labor and cerclage patients. If we had diagnosed chlamydial infections, patients were treated with erythromycin 2×1 tbl./d according to the literature.

12.04.01

Patient and doctor attitudes to treatment for vaginal candidosis: Eliot, B W, Tooley, P J H. Northampton Gen. Hosp. and Loddon Hall Hlth Ctr, Twyford, UK

Many studies on the treatment of vaginal candidosis have incorporated a section on patient acceptability. It is generally agreed that in order to produce a high degree of treatment compliance therapies must be in a form acceptable to the patient. This study determined the preference of both pregnant and nonpregnant patients on type and length of treatment. Questionnaires were issued to patients attending ante-natal clinics and general practitioners' surgeries. Patients were asked on their attitude to treatments previously received and preference on treatments currently available. In addition, patient and doctor attitude to therapy was compared. The results show that the patients choice of treatment and that of their doctors did not agree either in length of course of treatment or in type. Patients showed a strong preference towards short courses and oral therapy where as the doctors tended to prefer longer courses and topical therapies. The paper discusses the reasons for this difference focusing on treatment acceptability and doctor and patient expectations.

12.04.02

Oral ketoconazole for treatment of acute vaginal candidosis: Results of open multicentre trial: Dame, W R, Burkart, W. Univ.-Frauenklin., Münster

The purpose of this study was: 1. to study the efficacy of a single daily intake of 400 mg ketoconazole for five days in treating acute vaginal candidosis, 2. to study recurrence rates after the above-mentioned schedule. Patients were divided into two groups: Group 1: with evaluation of therapy at one week after start of treatment (efficacy) and Group 2: with evaluation at one week and one month after start of treatment (efficacy and recurrence). In both groups efficacy of treatment was assessed by scoring of clinical features e. g. leucorrhea, pruritus, vulvitis and by microscopic evaluation of wet smear on presence or absence of Candida albicans. In all patients evaluation of treatment was done one week after start of treatment. In patients of group two evaluation was also performed at one month after start of treatment. Both investigator and patient evaluated therapy at end of assessment period. Interim evaluation resulted in cure rates (both clinical and mycological) of more than 90% at week 1 and in cure rates (clinical and mycological) between 85 and 90% at 28 days (group 2). The results confirm that 400 mg taken in one single intake for five days is an efficacious regimen of treatment.

12.04.03

Systemic treatment with ketoconazole in vulvo-vaginal candidosis: Baraggino, E, Battin, M G, Benussi, G, Pecorari, D. Ist. Clin. Ostet. e Gin., Univ. Studi, Trieste, Italy
The study concerns the ketoconazole treatment (200 mg b.i.d., p.o. for 5 days) on 60 women with vulvo-vaginal candidosis: the diagnosis was confirmed by cultures in Nickerson's medium. Symptoms, i.e. leucorrhea and vaginal pruritus were cured in 61.6% and in 68.3% one week after the end of treatment and in 71.6% and in 81.6% after one month. The mycological examination one week and one month after the end of treatment were negative in 50 patients (83.3%); those findings turned to positive in four patients only at the second check. The drug was well tolerated in 54 patients; three patients complained about nausea; two patients had headache. In one patient the treatment was discontinued because of a skin rash with pruritus.

12.04.04

Ultrastructural features of ketoconazole treated cultures of candida albicans: De Virgiliis, G, Sideri, M. I[a] Clin. Ist. Ostet e Gin. "L. Mangiagalli", Univ., Milano, Italy
Forty women, affected by vaginal candidosis were randomly divided into two groups: the 65 and 80% of the ketoconazole treated, and the 15 and 25% of the placebo treated women were cured after one and four weeks, respectively. In both these groups, the percentages of the positive Nickerson cultures and wet mounts were smaller than those of symptomatic women. Ultrastructural investigation was performed on three positive cultures exposed to $50\ \mu g \cdot ml^{-1}$ for 12 hrs and processed for freeze fracture procedures as usual. a) Placebo treated cultures. In cross sections, a granular dense area was present at the periphery of the cell body. In some instances, the fracture exposed the cell wall of the protoplast. Prominent features were crystal and membrane infoldings, and the presence of crystal-like structures. b) Ketoconazole treated cultures. The most evident alterations concerned the arrangement of the membrane structure, where the typical crystal seemed disrupted, and the crystal-like structures were never seen. Different degree of antifungal activity in relation to different clinical conditions can be discussed. This freeze fracture study adds further evidence to the earlier Raab's report (1), in showing evident alterations after ketoconazole exposure (2). – (1) *Raab, W P E:* The treatment of mycosis with imidazole derivatives. Berlin: Springer-Verlag, 1978: 17 and 44–45. (2) *De Virgiliis, G* et al.: Efficacy of ketoconazole treatment in vaginal candidosis. The cervix e l.f.g.t 1984; **2:** 159–164.

12.04.05

Clinical evaluation and comparison of ketoconazole and clotrimazole in candida albicans vaginitis: Lefebvre, Y, Lapointe, R, Bayardelle, P. Hôp. Notre-Dame, Montreal, Canada
Several foreign studies have shown ketoconazole (KC), the first orally active broad spectrum antimycotic, to be a relatively safe and effective treatment for C. albicans vaginitis (CAV): the present randomized parallel-group study compares its safety and efficacy to that of clotrimazole (CL) in this indication. Women with clinical signs of CAV, without concurrent Gardnerella, Neisseria or Trichomonas infection (as confirmed microscopically and microbiologically) were recruited, and treated with either KC (400 mg PO OD) or CL (200 mg intravaginally OD), for 5 and 3 days, respectively. Repeat evaluations were carried out at 10 and 30 days post-therapy. Those patients still showing clinical signs of infection were offered a second, longer course (10 days for KC; 6 days for CL) of the same medication. Follow-up evaluations were again done at 10 and 30 days post-therapy. Patients used a diary booklet to record their symptoms on a daily basis during both the treatment and follow-up phases. Interim results, evaluating the first 80 patients (total enrollment of 200 anticipated) indicate that comparably good clinical and mycological cure rates, of the order of 85% at the 10-day follow-up, result from treatment with either drug; relapse rates have been of the order of 15%. The incidence of side-effects has been low with both regimens, and in keeping with the known profiles of the drugs: mild gastrointestinal problems have predominated with KC, as compared to symptoms of local mucocutaneous irritation with CL.

12.04.06

Partner treatment and recurrent vaginal candidosis: Derom, R, Thiery, M, Van Kets, H, Parewijck, W. Dept. Obstet., Univ. Hosp., Ghent, Belgium
Due to the increasing number of cases of recurrent vaginal candidosis, and based on the available literature since 1975, the question concerning the necessity of treating sexual partners is being re-examined. Until 1980, little attention was paid to partner treatment probably because of poor compliance with and acceptance of, topical therapy. The intestinal reservoir was regarded as the main source of reinfection and, from the results of one of the rare studies, *Brundin* (1976) concluded that systematic partner treatment did not improve the results. This is of consequence for the social implications of recurrent Candida vaginitis. With the current availability of oral therapies, the problem of partner treatment is again being discussed. Furthermore, in various treatment schedules, advice is given to treat concomitantly at least those partners presenting signs of balanitis. Attention is also being given to the characterization of various Candida species isolated during epidemiologic investigations. The results of studies by *Bisschop* and *Buch*, indicating that partner treatment has no effect on the degree of reinfection, are questionable due to the small sample size of patients involved. Therefore, an investigation is being conducted at the University Hospital of Ghent

involving larger numbers of patients, re-examined three months after treatment, in an attempt to draw more definitive conclusions regarding the benefit of partner treatment.

12.04.07

Management of recurrent vulvovaginal candidiasis (VVC) with ketoconazole (K) prophylaxis: Sobel, J D. Div. Infect. Dis., Med. Coll. of Pennsylvania, Philadelphia, PA, USA

In an open study, 112 women with recurrent VVC presenting with acute vaginitis were treated with K 400 mg daily for 14 days. Following therapy, all 112 women (100%) became asymptomatic and culture negative. Thereafter, subjects were randomized into four groups and evaluated monthly for one year. Group 1 women received daily placebo and had a clinical VVC recurrence rate of 70.5% within six months, and 76.4% at one year. Mean time to clinical relapse was 1.8 months. Intermittent cyclical K prophylaxis 400 mg daily for 5 days with onset of menses was given for three months (Group 2) and six months (Group 3). Evaluation at six months revealed VVC recurrence rate of 51.8% (Group 2) and 33.3% (Group 3); however, following cessation of prophylaxis, symptomatic recurrence was not uncommon in either group and at 12 months, recurrence had occurred in 62.6% (Group 2) and 61.1% (Group 3). Mean time to relapse was 4.5 and 7.2 months respectively. Group 4 subjects received continuous K prophylaxis 100 mg daily for 6 months with significantly lower recurrence rate of 5.9% at 6 months ($p < 0.0001$) and 47% at 12 months ($p < 0.05$). All groups receiving K prophylaxis had significantly reduced clinical attack rates. Apart from one patient who developed mild icteric hepatitis, no serious side-effects were observed, although mild nausea developed in 15%. These results reveal that in spite of initial intensive antimycotic therapy, women with recurrent VVC require and benefit from long-term prophylactic K therapy which is curative in some, but in the majority appears to be protective only as long as the prophylaxis is administered.

12.06.01

Phase II study of a combination of radiotherapy (RT) and chemotherapy (CT) in the primary treatment of advanced uterine cervix carcinoma (CxCa): Wolff, J P, George, M, Haie, C, Pejovic, M H, Horiot, J C, Fenton, F, Le Floch, O, Héron, J F. Inst. G. Roussy, Villejuif; Inst. LeClerc, Dijon; Inst. Curie, Paris, France

A phase II study was initiated in order to determine the efficacy and the tolerance of a combination of split-course RT and CT in patients (pts) with advanced CxCa. RT was given in pelvis in two courses of 25 Gy. External RT could be combined with a brachytherapy boost (BTB). CT consisted of cis-platin (P) 50 mg/m^2 alone for 3 cycles, then with cyclophosphamide 600/m^2. CT started one week before the first course of RT, was repeated between the two courses, after completion of RT and thereafter every four weeks for six cycles. Between July 1981 and April 1982, 36 pts were included by five French oncology centers. Twenty-seven pts were stage III (15 with positive iliac nodes and seven with positive para-aortic nodes at lymphangiogram), seven were stage IVa and 2 were stage IVb. CT was interrupted in 22 pts for the following reasons: refusal (1), leucopenia (2), intercurrent disease (3), protocol deviation (6) and disease progression (10). Thirty-two pts received the two RT courses: median dose 25.5 Gy for the first and 23.9 Gy for the second course. RT was given in 1 course in four pts (median dose = 43.0 Gy). Thirty pts received a BTB and eight pts para-aortic irradiation. Two-year survival rates for stage III and IV were 42.5% and 44.4% (95% CI = 19.8% and 32.5%). Two-year cumulative recurrence and metastasis rates were 15.9% and 32.0% (95% CI = 14.3% and 16.7%). No modification of treatment was due to clinical intolerance. CT was delayed in 15 cases for transient leucopenia and one case for nephrotoxicity. Two-year complication rate was 9.27% for proctitis and 8.6% for small bowel injury. Acute and late toxicities were tolerable, but chosen CT did not improve the survival in patients with very advanced CxCa.

12.06.02

Analysis of complications in five-year survival cases of invasive cervical cancer: Kurano, A, Jimi, S, Watanabe, Y, Imachi, M, Mashiba, H. Nat. Kyushu Ca Ctr, Fukuoka, Japan

During the period of 1972–1979, 564 patients with invasive cervical cancer were treated in our hospital and 373 patients survived over five years. The overall five-year survival rate was 66.1%. 159 cases of these survivors were investigated urological and enterological complications, biochemical findings in blood and immunological responsiveness five years after. These cases were classified in three groups: group A of 68 cases treated with radical operation alone, group B of 45 cases treated with operation and irradiation, group C of 46 cases treated with irradiation alone. Hydronephrosis or unilateral silent kidney was revealed in 10.3% of (A), 11.7% of (B) and 12.2% of (C) by drip infusion pyelography. Urinary bladder complications were found in 40.4% of (C). Rectal disorders were found in 13.3% of (B) and 45.7% of (C) by romanoscopy. The barium enema showed colo-rectal disorders in nine cases of (C). D-xylose tolerance test and Schilling test as the functional examination of intestines were performed. The urinary excretion of D-xylose was 1.78 ± 0.65 g (A), 1.36 ± 0.63 g (B) and 1.21 ± 0.72 g (C), respectively. The urinary excretion rate of ^{57}Co-Vitamin B$_{12}$ in Schilling test was $13.9 \pm 5.6\%$ (A), $11.9 \pm 7.3\%$ (B) and $9.6 \pm 5.8\%$ (C), respectively. Immunological responsiveness was well maintained in some cases. From these results, it was suggested that radiotherapy caused various disorders to the patients, even if they survived over five years.

12.06.03

Sexual dysfunction following treatment for cervical cancer stage Ib and IIa: Poulsen, H K, Kristensen, G B, Hansen, M K. Dept. Obstet. and Gyn., Odense Univ. Hosp., Odense, Denmark

In a prospective study of 67 patients treated for early cervical cancer 53 were sexually active before treatment and did not receive postoperative external radiation. Among these 53 patients a total of 34 were treated with radical hysterectomy only, and 19 patients with intracavitary radium × 2 approximating a dose of 42 Gy in point A prior to radical hysterectomy. It was found that major sexual dysfunction (loss of libido, loss of orgasmic ability, severe persistent dyspareunia or coitus stopped) occurred in 4/34 (12%) patients treated with surgery only, and 8/19 (42%) patients following combined therapy. The corresponding figures for minor sexual dysfunction (reduced libido, reduced orgasmic ability, reduced coital frequency or increased sporadic dyspareunia) were 6/34 (18%), and 3/19 (16%), respectively. As the benefit of combining intracavitary radium × 2 with surgical treatment of early cervical cancer in terms of five-year survival has been undetectable, our results suggest that radical hysterectomy should be the treatment of choice in early cervical cancer. Objective information and increased awareness of the sexual function of these patients might improve the quality of life as well as the quality of sexual function.

12.06.04

5-year results of high-dose rate afterloading with iridium in comparison to radium therapy in cervix cancer: Vahrson, H, Rauthe, G. Univ.-Frauenklin., Giessen

Since 1977 an afterloading unit (*Buchler*) with single source Ir-192 is used for contact therapy with different fractionations and doses to optimize the local control of the cancer and the complications. The preliminary 5-year results are presented in the following table:

stage	primary survivals treated	irrad. %	postop. survivals treated	irrad. %	sum survivals treated	irrad. %
I	$\frac{7}{10}$	70	$\frac{13}{13}$	100	$\frac{20}{23}$	87
II	$\frac{11}{15}$	73	$\frac{7}{9}$		$\frac{18}{24}$	75
III	$\frac{8}{13}$	62	$\frac{0}{2}$		$\frac{8}{15}$	53
IV	0	—	0	—	0	—
I–IV	$\frac{26}{38}$	68	$\frac{20}{24}$	83	$\frac{46}{62}$	74

The 5-year results of radium therapy from 1968–1972 were:
Stage I $\frac{236}{285}$ 83%, II $\frac{72}{147}$ 49%, III $\frac{25}{85}$ 29%, IV $\frac{1}{12}$ 8%, I–IV $\frac{334}{529}$ 63%.

The preliminary high-dose rate afterloading results indicate better cure rates in stages II and III for the future with a comparable number of serious complications (4.2% for primary irradiation). (For congress-presentation an additional 5-year period is in evaluation.)

12.06.05

The outcome in patients with recurrent cervical cancer related to pelvic node metastasis: Ng, H T. Dept. Obstet. & Gyn., Vet. Gen. Hosp., Taipei, Taiwan

Of 804 patients who underwent radical hysterectomy and pelvic lymphadenectomy for invasive cervical cancer from 1973 through 1982, 129 had recurrences. 73 of 129 patients whose pelvic nodes were negative for cancer during the initial operation attained an overall cumulative two-year survival of 32.7%; the five-year survival was 19.5%. Whereas 56 patients with positive pelvic nodes achieved a two-year survival of 5.7% and no five-year survivors. In the former group, 54 of 73 treated with either radiation, chemotherapy, exenteration or in combination, the two-year and five-year survival rates were 40% and 22.7%, respectively. There was, however, a marked decrease in survival to 14.8 in 19 of 73 patients who were not treated. In the later group, 27 of 56 patients treated, obtained a two-year survival of 12.6% compared with zero percent of 22 in 56 patients who were not treated. There was no five-year survival in the later group regardless of whatever method of treatment was employed.

12.06.06

Combination chemotherapy with peplomycin, cisplatin and mitomycin C (PPM) for recurrent and metastatic lesions from cervical squamous cell carcinomas: Katsube, Y, Yorishima, M, Fujiwara, A. Dept. Obstet. and Gyn., Hiroshima Univ. School Med., Hiroshima, Japan

From Nov. 1982 to Dec. 1984, combination chemotherapy of PPM was administrated to eight cases of recurrent and metastatic lesions from cervical cancer. The regimen of PPM therapy was composed of peplomycin at 3.3 mg/m^2 (i.v. infusion) on days 1 to 6, cisplatin at 20 mg/m^2 (i.v. infusion) and mitomycin C at 6.6 mg/m^2 (i.v.) on day 6. This regimen was repeated every two weeks. All the cases with ages ranging 38 to 70 years (median: 51.5 years) had previously received radiotherapy with/without surgery for prior therapy. Clinical stage at time of initial therapy was ranged from Stage Ib to IIIb. Histological type of primary lesions were all squamous cell carcinoma (LNK type-7 cases and LK type-1 case). The lesions studied were four cases of lung metastasis and one case each of liver metastasis, bone metastasis, supra-clavicular lymph node metastasis and recurrent intrapelvic carcinoma. Two courses of PPM therapy was administrated to two cases, three courses in three cases, and five courses in three cases. All the cases were evaluated for toxicity and response. Three cases achieved complete response (CR) following induction, two cases partial response (PR), two no changes (NC) and one case progressive disease (PD). The initial response rate (CR + PR) was 62.5%. The measurable tumor size was less than 3 cm in three cases of CR. The median survival time of five cases of (CR + PR) was 11.8 months and three cases of (NC + PD) was 5.0 months. Hematologic toxicity included leucopenia ($< 10^3$/ml) and/or thrombocytopenia ($< 5 \times 10^4$/ml) in 37.5% of the case.

12.06.07
Effect of local injection of OK432 (immunomodulating agent) on cellular immunocompetence in cervical cancer patients: Yamada, Y, Wakita, K, Mori, H, Shiraki, S, Noda, K. Dept. Obstet. and Gyn., Univ., Gifu, Japan

OK432 has been demonstrated to have antitumor activity in cancer patients, but the mechanism of action is not clarified. Thus, we have analysed morphologically and functionally the changes in cellular immuno-competence at the lesion and the regional lymph-nodes after local injection of OK432 into patients with cervical cancer. OK432 was injected at a dose of 1KE to the area surrounding cervical cancer of 16 patients 14 days and three days prior to the operation. Frozen sections were prepare from cancer tissues and the regional lymph-nodes removed during the operation, and infiltration of macrophages, NK cells and lymphocyte subsets was examined by indirect fluorescent antibody techniques such as biotin-avidin method and ABC method using various monoclonal antibodies. At the same time, lymphocytes of the regional lymph-nodes were cultured in the presence of lectin-free IL-2, and their responsiveness to IL-2 was evaluated from the ^{3}H-TdR uptake. The results were as follows: In many cases receiving local injection of OK432, there was a correlation between the increase in the number of IaI-positive T4 and Leu-7 at the lesion as well as at the regional lymph-nodes and the intensity of IL-2 responsiveness of lymphocytes. These findings suggest that local-injection of OK432 enhance local differentiation of effector cells possessing killer activity.

12.06.08
Immunotherapy using a streptococcal preparation, OK432, for the treatment of cervical cancer (I): Teshima, K, Takeuchi, K, Sawaragi, I, Takashima, H, Tominaga, S, Noda, K. Cervical Cancer Immunotherapy Study Group, Kinki Univ. School Med., Osaka, Japan

The effectiveness of immunotherapy with a streptococcal preparation, OK432, was studied in 387 cervical cancer patients registered from June 1980 to December 1982. There were 206 cases who were surgically treated and 181 cases who were not. Either control treatment regimen (radiotherapy alone, n = 163) or OK432 treatment regimen (radiotherapy as well as intradermal administration of OK432, n = 224) was randomly assigned to patients to maintain the homogeneity in respect to patient's cancer stage by FIGO classification and presence/absence of combined surgical treatment. The three year recurrence-free rate was 72.1% in patients receiving the OK432 treatment (OK432 group) and 57.8% in patients receiving the control treatment (control group), and the recurrence-free interval was significantly longer in the OK432 group than in the control group (p < 0.01). Delayed skin reactions to phytohemagglutinin (PHA) and Su-antigen extracted from Streptococcus pyogenes Su-strain (Su-PS) and peripheral lymphocyte counts were reduced within two months after starting the therapy in both OK432 and control groups. The observed immunological changes were apparently reversed by three months after the start of the therapy in the OK432 group, but took almost a year in the control group, with a significant intergroup difference at six and twelve months of the therapy (p < 0.01). From the results of the present study, OK432 can be considered as one of the most effective and useful immunotherapeutic agents for cervical cancer.

12.06.09
Immunotherapy using a streptococcal preparation, OK432, for the treatment of cervical cancer (II): Hase-gawa, K, Inoue, K, Sekiba, K, Ozawa, M, Chihara, T, Ichijo, M, Tominaga, S, Noda, K. Cervical Cancer Immunotherapy Study Group, Kinki Univ. School Med., Osaka, Japan

It was previously demonstrated that OK432, an antitumor immunotherapeutic agent was remarkably effective for the treatment of cervical cancer. Therapeutic outcome following OK432 treatment seemingly differed among patient groups with different cancer stage and the results were, herein, further analysed in this respect. In the stage II cervical cancer, the three year recurrence-free rate was significantly higher in the OK432 group (77.0%, n = 89) than in the control group (54.2%, n = 64) with p-value less than 0.01. The finding was further supported by longer recurrence-free interval as well as higher peripheral lym-phocyte counts and more intensive PHA skin reaction that were observed in the OK432 group as compared with those the control group (p < 0.01). However, in none of patient groups of stage I, stage III nor stage IV cervical cancer, was any significant difference between the two groups found in these factors. The results may indicate that OK432 shows maximal effectiveness for the stage II cervical cancer but not for the cancer in stage I, III and IV, possibly reflecting the differences across the patient groups of different cancer stage in patient's pathological condition and/or therapeutic regimen which was apparently related to the severity of the disease. Further investigations are necessary in order to elucidate the mechanism(s) for these observations in search of the optimal therapeutic regimen with OK432 that is adjustable to the severity of the cancer.

12.06.10

Neoadjuvant (pre-operative) chemotherapy in the treatment of patients with stage Ib and II squamous cell carcinoma of the uterine cervix. A preliminary report: Kim, D S, Moon, H, Hwang, Y Y, Cho, S H, Kim, K T. Dept. Obstet. and Gyn., School Med., Hanyang Univ., Seoul, Korea

To evaluate the advantages of pre-operative adjuvant chemotherapy such as early treatment of microme-tastasis and reduction of stage of disease in the patients with squamous cell carcinoma of uterine cervix, ten patients (four of stage Ib with high-risk factors, one of stage IIa and five of stage IIb) were treated with neoadjuvant chemotherapy of a single agent of cis-platinum or multiple agents of vinblastin, bleomycin and cis-platinum (VBP). Range of follow-up period is 4–35 months. Complete remission was encountered in four cases (two of Ib and two of IIb), of whom three cases demonstrated chronic cervicitis without any evidence of cervical cancer in postoperative histopathology, and one case refused surgical confirmation but had been doing well without any evidence of malignancy for 35 months. Two cases of stage IIb demon-strated stage reduction to stage Ib making radical surgery possible. One case of stage IIa and one of stage IIb were found to be stable in response. In patients who showed complete remission Papanicolaou smear turned to be negative after 2–3 courses of chemotherapy. Drug induced toxicities were tolerable. This preliminary study strongly suggests that neoadjuvant chemotherapy in patients of stage Ib with high risk factors and stage II is effective in reducing stage of the disease or in curing the disease and may lead a better long-term survival by early treatment of micrometastasis.

12.07.01

Conservation surgery and irradiation of $T_1N_0M_0$ breast cancer: Schreer, I, Frischbier, H-J, Stegner, H-E, Thomsen, K. Univ.-Frauenklin. Hamburg-Eppendorf, Hamburg

From 1972 up to 1981 134 patients with small breast cancer were treated by wide excision followed by irradiation of the breast and regional lymph nodes. Since 1982 the treatment was changed: 139 patients had a segmental resection and complete axillary lymph node dissection in combination with radiation of the breast only. Results of these two groups are compared as regards local and regional tumor control.

12.07.02

Surgical conservative treatment of breast cancer. Indications, early results and complications: Monti, C R, Keppke, E M, Teixeira, L C, Brenelli, H B, Pinotti, J A. Dept. Obstet. and Gyn., State Univ., Campinas, Brazil

The conservative approach to breast cancer is until now a conflicting issue. To classify its role in tumors stage I ($T_{1a}N_{0-1a}$) and stage II ($T_{1a}N_0$, large breast) 70 pts were treated by quadrantectomy/axillectomy/radiotherapy (QUART) between April 1981 and December 1984. QU included the fascia of the muscle and A was realized apart QU with the exception of the tumors located in the upper external quadrant. In attempting to obtain the best possible esthetic results, the plastic surgeon closes the surgical wound. RT began 21 days after QUA using 50 Gy on the breast and boost of 10 Gy in the scar. Twenty-eight pts with axillary involvement and 13 pts without this involvement received adjuvant treatment with chemotherapy (CMF) and antiestrogen (tamoxifen). Thirty pts who presented negative axilla had no therapy. Mean age was 50.6 years (26–72), 39 (55.70%) were pre-menopause, 38 (54.2%) had tumors measuring between 1 and 2 cm, 5 (7.2%) smaller than 1 cm and 27 (38.6%) between 2 to 5 cm. 28 pts (40%) presented axillary metastasis and one pts (1.4%) subclinical inflammatory carcinoma. Moderate radiation dermatitis was present in 18 pts (25.7%). The esthetic results were good in 52 pts (74.2%) with a reasonable appearance in eight pts (11.4%) because of the lateral position of the nipple. Two pts (2.8%) presented local recurrence with a disease-free interval of 12.5 months; both were negative axillary lymph nodes and had no adjuvant treatment.

12.07.03

Conservative treatment for breast cancer. Follow-up protocol: Ferrer Gispert, M, Torralba, I, Ron, A, López-Rodó, L, Fernandez-Cid, A. Inst. Dexeus, Barcelona, Spain

The progressive advances in the diagnosis of breast cancer due to the increase amongst the female population of self-exploration and the periodical check-ups, as well as the complementary technics for the study of the breast, have led us to the early diagnosis of the disease in a high percentage of cases. Ever since Bacclese proposed the conservative treatment for breast cancer diagnosed in the early stages many authors have followed this philosophy which has resulted in results comparable to those obtained with drastic breast surgery. We started this practice in the Dexeus Institute, in 1982, and 103 patients have been treated so far. We were confronted by this problem while trying the early control of the operated area, because, besides the edema due to surgery, external and interstitial radiotherapy, the mammographic alterations of surgical origin impeded the evaluation of this symptom as an early relapse. Because of this we decided to practice regularly the echotomography with cytologic puncture within the operated area six months after the operation. In the 40 patients studied, only in one of them was a relapse suspected, the pathological examination of which was negative. To sum up we consider that this technique is a good immediate way of controlling the evolution of this problem.

12.07.04

Early results and complications in organ-conserving treatment of carcinoma: Bauer, M, Fournier, D von, Kubli, F, Winkel, K zum, Kuttig, H. Univ. Clin. Gyn. and Radiol., Heidelberg

From 1975 till January 1985 280 patients of the University Clinic for Gynecology and Radiology in Heidelberg suffering from clinical stage T1, N0 and M0 were treated in an operative and radiological combination with breast conserving therapy. The early results of 235 patients were analysed up to July 1984. 180 women underwent a quadrant resection while in the case of 31 specially selected patients a tumorectomy was practised (well delimited tumor, no lymphangiosis carcinomatosa). The removal of the axillary lymph nodes was always practised. In the case of 19 women the operative procedure was not typical. The radiotherapy of the remaining breast was done with cobalt-60 gamma-rays. The dose was related to the tumor aggression (histological stage of the lymphatic nodule, lymphangiosis carcinomatosa, hormone receptor stage) and the operative procedure (quadrant resection or tumorectomy). In all cases a dose of 60 Gy was not exceeded. In case of histologic tumor of the lymph nodes (25%) the patients underwent chemotherapy in addition. Up to now four patients died as a result of metastases but without local recurrence. Six patients are still living with metastases without regional recurrence. In the case of four patients a recurrence was found in the axilla and in six patients a recurrence in the remaining breast occurred in the area of the radiological treatment. The locoregional recurrence appeared quite late and their frequency correlated with the classification of the tumor's aggressivity. The organ conserving treatment of breast cancer will be achieved under strict conditions but cannot yet be recommended as a standard treatment.

12.07.05

Place and significance of the lymphadenectomy in mammary oncology: Uyttenbroeck, F. Dept. Gyn., Univ., Antwerp, Belgium

The small or early breast cancer is very controversial. The surgical treatment must give full information on axillary node status. Is this possible with a conservative operation? "Precise information on axillary node status can be obtained only from an axillary clearance and this would seem essential to the proper management of the early disease" (*Hayward*, 1984). The modified Patey's technique used by the author is simple, reducing the risks of bleeding to a minimum and permitting an extensive lymphadenectomy up to the axillary apex and to the pectoralis major. The very important lymph nodes invasion and the effect on the five year survival are described in a personal series of 196 small or early cancers up to 20 mm from a group of 502 patients with 524 cancers.

12.07.06

Radioisotope marking of lymph nodes for axillary dissection: Kubista, E, Skodler, W, Stempel, G, Czerwenka, K, Gitsch, E. Ist Dept. Obstet. and Gyn., Univ., Vienna, Austria

Staging of axillary lymph nodes is the most important factor in the classification, prognosis and postoperative treatment of breast cancer. At the Ist Dept. of Obstetrics and Gynecology, University of Vienna, a new method of marking the axillary lymph nodes by radioisotopes was developed. The axillary lymphatic tissue is marked by a subcutaneous injection of 500 mCi ^{99m}Tc between the second and third finger the day before operation. The operation itself is performed on a gamma camera. 170 patients which have been operated on by this method are compared to a randomized control group of 180 unmarked patients. The method is safe and has no negative side-effects. Because of the intraoperative monitoring in 60% of the patients a complete resection of axilllary lymphatic tissue, controlled and documented by the gamma camera was achieved. The average number of removed lymph nodes was 25% higher in the marked group. That means a better staging, easier prognosis and a better selection for adjuvant therapy. Patients with incomplete removal of axillary lymph nodes had twice as many local recurrences and general metastasis (19.4%) as patients with complete axillary dissection (9.4%).

12.07.07

The significance of complete axillary dissection in early stages of breast cancer: Keramopoulos, A, Giorgiotis, D, Leonardos, V, Akrivos, T, Aravantinos, D. 1st. Dept. Obstet. and Gyn., Univ., Athens, Greece

As *Fisher* described a positive node is a marker of a tumor-host relation which predicts a metastasis rather than the source of a metastasis. On the other hand the number of positive nodes is the only parameter directly related with the prognosis. Of 294 cases St I–II of breast cancer (132 and 162, respectively), 201 underwent a modified radical mastectomy (52 St I and 149 St II) and 93 a segmental mastectomy with complete axillary dissection (71 St I and 22 St II). In both operations a complete dissection of the axilla was performed (mean number of nodes 32.5). In 6.6% (8 cases of St I) and 1.6% (3 cases of St II) positive nodes were found in other levels while the first level was negative. In 12 cases (4% both stages) nodes < 0.5 cm in diameter were found. So in 3.7% of the cases (11 cases) a postsurgical treatment was needed and in all the above cases the prognosis has changed. In early stages of breast cancer a small difference in the number of positive nodes may affect the prognosis and the need for adjuvant treatment. Then the knowledge of nodal status by the examination of a large number of nodes (complete axillary dissection) is much better than by the examination of a smaller number of nodes (sampling of the axilla).

12.07.08

Surgical and histomorphological different procedures as cause of different results in evaluating the nodal status in breast carcinoma: Geppert, M, Pawlowski, Z. Dept. Obstet. and Gyn., Univ., Tübingen

The prognostic and therapeutic relevance of the nodal status of women with breast carcinoma is accepted, since this diagnostic parameter is the most objective possible. The influence of different surgical and histomorphological methods on this important clue to postoperative therapy is investigated in this study. Specimens from 158 patients (group 1) treated in our university hospital were compared with specimens from 170 women (group 2) operated in other local hospitals in regard of number of lymph nodes, extent and rate of metastasis as well as in regard of possible atrophic changes. In group 1 an average of 21.0 lymph nodes per cases was evaluated vs. 11.5 in group 2. All lymph nodes (≥ 5 mm) available in group 1 were examined in layers of 3 mm thickness step by step by the main investigator; the histological slides of all cases in group 2 were reviewed. There was no difference in rate of metastasis in both groups (52.0% vs. 53.8%), however, in women with proven metastasis the number of positive nodes per patient was higher in group 1 (3 pos. nodes: 33% vs. 9%) as well as the rate of tumorous penetration of the capsule (38% vs. 24%). The rate of metastasis was significantly lower in lymph nodes with a size < 5 mm and with signs of fatty atrophy. These smaller lymph nodes were over-represented in group 2 and in women with no evidence of lymph node metastasis, independent of the size of primary tumor. It seems possible that these morphological characteristics could cause a reduced lymphatic flow to the axillary nodes and, in result, metastasis to other locations.

12.07.09

The prognosis of metastatic breast cancer in respect of the first metastatic site: Breitbach, G P, Brachetti, A K J. Dept. Gyn. and Obstet., Univ., Homburg/Saar

Little informations is available about the prognosis of metastatic breast cancer. Therefore we looked retrospectively at 113 patients with recurrent disease in respect of the first metastatic site. In December 31, 1984, we found a) 40 patients with local/regional disease (17.5% dead, survival time $\bar{x} = 20.4$ months, survival range of patients alive $2 - 132+$ months), b) 22 patients with visceral disease (27.3% dead, $\bar{x} = 8.0$ months, survival range $3 - 126+$ months), c) 20 patients with bony disease (30% dead, $\bar{x} = 21.2$ months, survival range $1 - 108+$ months) and d) 31 patients with multi-focal disease (41.9% dead, $\bar{x} = 15.0$ months, survival range $4 - 127+$ months). In this evaluation, the poor prognosis of visceral and bony metastatic disease is almost equivalent. Worst prognosis corresponds to multi-focal disease, best to local/regional recurrence. Possible therapeutic consequences will be discussed particularly regarding patiens who have been treated with adjuvant cytostatic therapy.

12.08.01

The β-HCG-regression after the treatment of active and regressed extrauterine pregnancies: Kontoravdis, A, Kassanos, D, Chryssicopulos, A, Souchleri-Phokas, I, Kilbasanis, H. 2nd Dept. Obstet. and Gyn., Univ. of Athens, Aretaiion Hosp., Athens, Greece

The regression of β-HCG levels was studied in the plasma of 15 cases of tubal pregnancies (6 regressed and 9 active). The measurements of the β-HCG values were made before the operation and after 12, 24, 48, 72 96, 120 and 192 hours. The mean β-HCG values in the groups of the regressed and active cases, before treatment, were 479.4 ± 266.4 mIU/ml and 6334.0 ± 932.1 mIU/ml and after 192 hours were 4.8 ± 0.4 mIU/ml and 115.8 ± 37.9 mIU/ml, respectively. The β-HCG mean values in both groups showed the same exponential function (regressed). The percentage fall of the hormone in both groups, in the period of time between 0 and 192 hours was 98% with the same exponential correlation. The mean values of the hormone in both groups showed a statistically significant difference ($p < 0.0001$).

12.08.02

Neopregnosticon 75 D. Human chorionic gonadotropin (hCG) test for the early diagnosis of ectopic pregnancy: Praest, J, Thorlacius-Ussing, O. Dept. Obstet. and Gyn., Randers Hosp., Aalborg, Denmark

The diagnosis of early ectopic pregnancy without rupture may be difficult and in recent years there has been an increasing interest in non-invasive diagnostic methods. Neopregnosticon 75 D (Organon Teknika) is a selective and highly sensitive hemagglutination test for detection of small amounts of hCG in urine (discriminatory value 75 u/l). The diagnostic reliability of Neopregnosticon 75 D was evaluated in a study comprising 137 patients with a history of unexplained lower abdominal pain and/or abnormal bleeding. All patients had a negative conventional pregnancy test (Pregnostisec, Organon Teknika, discriminatory value 2500 u/l). The diagnostic specificity and sensitivity gave values of 0.97 and 0.88, respectively and a predictive value of positive results of 0.91. We find it a valuable test in the early diagnosis of ectopic pregnancy.

12.08.03

Five-minute, high sensitivity visual Tandem ICON hCG test for diagnosis of ectopic pregnancy: Sasaki, S, Araki, T, Hussa, R O*, Hatano, H, Takahashi, H, Kuraishi, K. Dept. Obstet. and Gyn., Nippon Med. School, Tokyo, Japan; Med. Coll. of Wisconsin*, Milwaukee, WI, USA

Because of the demand for urgency in diagnosis of ectopic pregnancy, it would be ideal to have a rapid test that reliably detects low levels of human chorionic gonadotropin (hCG). The Tandem ICON hCG test

(Hybritech, Inc., San Diego, CA) is a two-site immunometric assay in which antibody is immobilized in the center of a filter membrane in a disposable, self-contained filtration apparatus. Specimens containing more than 50 mIU/ml hCG result in the development of a blue spot on the filter membrane when 5 drops (0.25 ml) of urine are analysed, but we were able to increase the sensitivity of the test to 5 mIU/ml by analysing 2 ml of urine. The present investigation was undertaken to evaluate the diagnostic effectiveness of the visual ICON filter membrane hCG test in patients presenting with the symptoms of ectopic pregnancy. Urine specimens were analysed for hCG in the 5-minute ICON test and in the Hi-Gonavis hCG test (Mochida, Inc., Tokyo), which requires two hours to perform. Serum specimens from the same patients were analysed by radioimmunoassay (RIA) for hCG. Test results were correlated with the clinical outcome of each patient. In our series, the ICON test performed on 2 ml of urine was reliable as a serum RIA for hCG, and more reliable than the Hi-Gonavis test, in predicting the presence of ectopic pregnancy. We conclude that the speed, simplicity, and sensitivity of the visual Tandem ICON hCG test make it ideal for use in diagnosis of ectopic pregnancy.

12.08.04
Significance of serum hCG determinations for conservative management of ectopic pregnancy: Post, K-G, Jaluvka, V, Hammerstein, J. Dept. Obstet. and Gyn., Klinikum Steglitz, FU, Berlin

During the last 8 years (1977–1984) 328 patients were operated on in our department because of ectopic pregnancy. In 220 cases hCG was determined by radioimmunoassay up to eight times prior to the operation, using the β-hCG RIA Kit, Serono. In order to investigate whether hCG determinations can be of help on the way to a less invasive management of either suspected or by laparoscopy diagnosed ectopic pregnancy the hCG values found were correlated to the clinical symptoms esp. to the intensity of pain, to the existence of a hemoperitoneum as well as to the condition of the Fallopian tube (ruptured or not). – As results 1) in patients with ectopic pregnancy there is a positive correlation between the intensity of pain and the hCG level found pre-operatively, 2) cases with hemoperitoneum showed higher hCG levels than those without, and 3) in patients with tubal abortion lower hCG levels were found than in those with ruptured Fallopian tube. – Conclusion: If a patient with suspected ectopic pregnancy is in stable clinical condition which does not require immediate intervention a single value as well as the course of the hCG level can be taken as an indicator of the degree of urgency for further diagnostic or therapeutic steps. Thus, unnecessarily urgent operations can be avoided and rather well prepared possibly even microsurgical interventions can be performed. Under certain circumstances e. g. absolute low values with falling tendency even further diagnostic steps may become unnecessary. Examples are shown to further clarify this subject.

12.08.05
Conservative surgery for tubal pregnancy: Neeser, E, Hirsch, H A, Menton, M. Dept. Obstet. and Gyn., Univ., Tübingen

Salpingectomy has been the traditional treatment for ruptured and unruptured ectopic pregnancies. This radical procedure is being more and more replaced by conservative surgical management in all patients of reproductive age, who desire further pregnancies. At the University Women's Hospital of Tübingen from 1969 to 1983, 333 tubal gestations have been operated upon. In 108 cases the Fallopian tube could be preserved by conservative surgery. In 1983 the percentage of those patients, in whom conservative surgery was desired and possible, rose to 82%. Since 1975, when laparoscopy was used routinely in any suspected ectopic pregnancy, more and more early tubal gestations were found and the percentage of ruptured tubes decreased from 60% to 20%. Seventy-nine patients were treated by salpingotomy as first described by *Caffier* in 1941. In 18 women segmental excision was done and in three patients segmental resection and immediate anastomosis was possible. Eight ampullary pregnancies were expressed from the ampulla or were found to be already tubal abortions. There was one serious complication related to the conservative management: in one patient delayed hemorrhage occurred caused by persisting tubal gestation after manual expression of an ampullary pregnancy. Beta-hCG levels therefore always should be controlled after salpingotomy and tubal abortion to exclude incomplete removal of the pregnancy products.

12.08.06
Conservative management of tubal pregnancy: Ansari, A H. Dept. Obstet. and Gyn.; **Hood, R.** Dept. Obstet. and Gyn., Georgia Baptist Med. Ctr, Atlanta, GA, USA

Recent reports have provided encouraging results with conservative management of most ectopic pregnancies. During the past twelve years we have conservatively managed seventeen cases of tubal pregnancy and have obtained equally satisfactory results. In four of these cases conservative surgery was performed for an ectopic in the only remaining tube (previous unilateral salpingectomy for ectopic pregnancy). We are not in agreement with the two step procedure of segmental excision, followed by a definitive surgery at a later date and firmly believe end-to-end anastomosis can be achieved safely and simply at the time of the initial operation with excellent anatomic and physiologic results. In fact due to significant enlargement of the tubal lumen, approximation is readily achieved by even the less experienced tubal surgeon using a magnifying loup.

12.08.07

Fertility after conservative surgery of tubal ectopic pregnancy: Feiks, A, Dadak, C, Deutinger, J, Reinthaller, A, Janisch, H. II. Univ.-Frauenklin., Vienna, Austria

In the last few years an obvious trend toward conservative technique in tubal surgery is observed. Likewise, at our institution, emphasis has also been placed on preservation of function. Fifty-nine patients had a conservative operation for tubal pregnancies between 1979 to 1982. Seven women were lost to follow-up. 28 patients showed further desire for child-bearing. 20 of them have had a subsequent intrauterine conception (71.4%), 11 women have had term pregnancies (39.3%). 3 patients were pregnant at time of investigation. The abortion rate was 17.8%. Recurrent ectopic pregnancies were found in five cases (9.5%). However, the operated Fallopian tube was involved only in three cases (5.7%). In 26 cases the patency of the tubal lumen was examined by means of hysterosalpingography. 50% of those women had remained childless. The results of HSG showed a patent passage in the operated tube in 11 cases. Our results show a high rate of subsequent pregnancies and a rather low incidence of repeat ectopic pregnancies in cases of conservative surgery and support our option to save the involved tube whenever fertility is desired.

12.08.08

Ovarian transposition and its scope: Mehta, V M, Patel, Y, Nadkarni, R M. K. M. School of P. G. Med. & Res., Ahmedabad, Gujarat, India

The above operative method was adopted by the senior contributor *R. M. Nadkarni* in 1967, for salvaging the problem of the postectopic sterility and repeat ectopics. In ectopic pregnancy prophylactic oophorectomy sometimes results in sterility, if the ovary is atretic or subnormal. In such patients mobilizing the normal ovary with its blood supply in the suspensory ligament well preserved and anastomosing it with the ovary on the opposite side gave gratifying results. Thus a good ovary was made available to a normal tube. Operative procedure was without any complications and could salvage the problem of sterility by one and a half times and reduce the incidence of repeat ectopics by six times. This method also has been found useful in few cases of sterility which posed similar problems to those mentioned above.

12.08.09

Factors affecting conception after tubal pregnancy: Randall, S. St. Mary's Hosp., Manchester, UK

Other studies have shown conception rates to be low after ectopic pregnancy; this study investigated the etiological factors involved. One hundred and eight cases of tubal pregnancy seen between 1979 and 1982 were compared with 100 normal, first trimester intrauterine gestations. The tubal pregnancies were divided into four groups: those at risk of pregnancy, including A, patients who had conceived; B, those trying to conceive and those not at risk of pregnancy, including C, women using contraception and D, those who because of previous tubal pregnancy or damage were considered unlikely to conceive naturally. The following factors were found to be significant in the etiology of tubal pregnancy and subsequent fertility: previous ectopic pregnancy, tubal surgery, pelvic inflammation and infertility. Pathological evidence of tubal disease was significant but could not be compared with the control group and is not included here. The percentages in each group were A 25.2, B 28.9, C 23.4, D 22.5. Scoring 1 for each significant factor, mean scores for each group were A 0.8, B 1.2, C 0.7, D 1.6, control 0.5. Overall conception rate was 25.2%, 46.5% of women at risk of pregnancy (group A, B). Incidence of repeat tubal pregnancy was 5.0% overall, 8.6% of those at risk, 18.2% of all conceptions (group A). Incidence of live offspring was 17.4% overall, 32.7% of those at risk, 70.4% of conceptions. In group A, if only women who had live offspring were considered, mean etiological factor score was 0.6. Patients with an etiological factor score < 1 have a significantly greater chance of conceiving than those whose score is > 1.

12.08.10

Ectopic pregnancy (Schematic diagnosis): Rio de la Loza, F J. Ctro Gin.-Obstet. Mexico, UAEM, Mexico, DF

Due to the risk that is in maternal morbidity and mortality the delay in a patient with an ectopic pregnancy, this study was carried out utilizing the basis of the schematic diagnostic criteria developed by *Wertheimer* and modified by us, with the basical purpose in getting an increase in the number of early diagnosis ectopic pregnancy. Thirty patients were included in this study with a diagnostic possibility of E. P., they were seen at the emergency room of C.G.O. Hospital in Mexico City. Previous studies have shown in the first stage the diagnostic scheme, the incidence of diagnosis was 36.7% for E. P., and 63.3% of correct diagnosis in other problems. In our study, at the final stage we found a 90.0% correct diagnosis in ectopic pregnancy with 9.1% of other diseases with similar clinical picture. Nevertheless they require similar surgical treatment and follow-up. We conclude that with this diagnostic scheme is possible to achieve diagnostic accuracy of 72.7% in unruptured E. P. at an early stage. Other authors have reported 15% of accuracy in the same period. The mortality was 0% which along with the diagnostic certainty confirms the usefulness of this scheme for the diagnosis and treatment of this problems.

12.09.01

Stage I carcinoma of the endometrium: Criteria for a correct treatment: Atlante, G, Pozzi, M, Diotallevi, F, Iacovelli, A. Dept. Gyn., "Regina Elena" Nat. Tumor Inst., Rome, Italy

In the Department of Gynecology of the "Regina Elena" National Tumor Institute of Rome 410 cases of

Stage I adenocarcinoma of the endometrium were treated between February 1, 1965 and December 31, 1984. The survey presents peculiar characteristics of uniformity for were followed in all such cases some clinical and histological criteria, in order to improve FIGO classification, to evaluate the opportunity of eventual associated or complementary therapies whether radio- or chemotherapeutical or hormonal. Indeed an accurate evaluation of the grading, of the myometrial infiltration and of the location of the lesion becomes always more and more important as far as possible lymph node invasion is concerned, this being the most important factor for the risk of recurrence, thus conditioning survival. The very good results obtained employing these clinical observations have given a high survival rate in this group of patients (86.7%) notwithstanding the high age level of the patients (74.7% between the ages of 51 and 70) and frequently encountered associated pathologies. Data regarding relationships between survival and the above mentioned risk factors are also very interesting, given the high number of patients treated. The authors conclude that Stage I carcinoma of the endometrium is a neoplasm which must be treated after an accurate staging which must carefully consider clinical and anatomo-pathological data which characterize the neoplastic lesion, one by one, and which can greatly vary the prognosis.

12.09.02

Intraoperative ultrasonic examination for cervical spread and myometrial penetration in endometrial cancer: Dozono, H, Tanemura, K, Yamada, T, Ohmi, K, Kasamatsu, T. Dept. Gyn., Nat. Ca Ctr Hosp., Tokyo, Japan

Intraoperative ultrasonic examination (IUE) was performed on patients with endometrial cancer to evaluate both cervical spread and myometrial penetration. The ultrasonic apparatus employed was a linear arrayed real time electronic scanning system with specially designed probe. 300–500 cc of warm saline was run into the pelvic cavity and the probe was always kept about 3–5 cm from the uterus. IUE was verified with the pathological findings. (1) The space between anterior and posterior wall of normal uterus showed single line surrounding dark echo zones of the endometrium. (2) The single line, continuing to cervical canal, was without the dark zone. (3) The irregularity or disappearance of the single line eventually showed the location of cancer. (4) Both longitudinal and transverse scans showed that the normal myometrium was filled with moderate-intensity echoes. (5) The different echo levels showed myometrial penetration of the carcinoma which had lower echo level than the normal endometrium. IUE is clinically valuable in assessing the staging and myometrial penetration of endometrial cancer.

12.09.03

Clinicopathological study of 8 cases of endometrial carcinoma with microscopic adenomyosis: Hayata, T, Terao, T, Kawashima, Y. Hamamatsu Univ. School Med., Hamamatsu, Japan

The cause of endometriosis has hitherto been obscure, when one compares it with the possible role of the estrogen on endometrial cancers as a promotive factor. Recently we studied clinicopathologically eight cases which revealed adenomyosis microscopically through the postoperative specimensof 30 endometrial cancers and intended to explore the relationship between these two diseases clinically. – Results: Stage: 2 cases of Ia and 6 of Ib, Menstrual history: Four each of regular and irregular menstruations, three dysmenorrheas and five postmenopausal. Duration from last delivery (pregnancy) to operation: 23–35 (17–33) years, Past history: Three had hypertension and one had diabetes mellitus, Family history: two revealed diabetes mellitus in her father and older brother, respectively, Obesity index (weight × 100/(height − 100) × 0.9): 100–147 (mean 127), Histology: seven are pure tubular adenocarcinomas except for one papillotubular adenocarcinoma. Endometrial backgrounds are proliferative endometrium in five and secretory in two cases. Referring to another 12 cases of endometrial cancers of first stage without adenomyosis, these data showed the possibility of common stimuli to both adenomyosis and endometrial cancer, and moreover gave a good model for studying the histogenesis and uterine myometrial invasiveness of the endometrial cancer.

12.09.04

Prognostic factors in adenocarcinoma of endometrium: Labastida, R, Dexeus, S, Julvé, X. Inst. Dexeus, Depto. Obstet. y Gin., Barcelona, Spain

Other values such as age, myometrial invasion, gland involvement, peritoneal wash, etc. have been gradually added to the classic prognostic values accepted by the FIGO in 1974 (viz: stage, size of uterus, tumor grade) whose influence in neoplastic diseases is undeniable. In order to obtain a homogenisation of diagnosis and treatment a diagnostic guideline has been established using a pre-operative scale of reckoning which enables the treatment to be assessed and determined in each case, and this in its turn is re-assessed in accordance with postoperative prognosis factor which determine the definite complementary treatment. The aforementioned pre-operative guideline includes 11 prognostic factors: age, time elapsed since the first symptom, size of uterus, size of tumor, cervical involvement, isthmian involvement, cornual involvement, tumor grade, histological type, cytological pattern, and hormone receptors, which enable patients to be selected according to their risk, and a decision to be made on the surgical technique and the need for and type of irradiation and adjunctive hormone therapy. After the operation the following postoperative prognosis factors are determined from the pathological findings and the study of the surgical specimen: glandular involvement, peritoneal wash, vascular size involvement, tube imprint, myometrial invasion, tumor grade, cervical stroma involvement, histological type and hormone receptors. Thus, this postoperative classification enables the treatment to be completed in an individualised way, providing systematic cover for those patients with a risk of distant metastasis, or local cover for patients with a risk of recurrence.

12.09.05

Endometrial carcinoma in the gynecological clinic of the São Paulo University Medical School-Brazil: Souen, J S, Bastos, A C, Fonseca, A M, Salvatore, C A. São Paulo, Brazil

The endometrial cancer ist the fourth most frequently found in the Gynecological Clinic of the University of São Paulo-Brazil. The average is 56 years and the majority of the women belong to the sixth decade, and 68% are post-menopausal. The main symptom is post-menopausal bleeding. There was a high percentage of single, virgin, nulliparity and low number of gestation. Quite a larger percentage of obesity, hypertension, and high level blood glucose was found among cancer patients. In 67.4% the tumor was in stage I. We performed exclusively surgery when the neoplasm is at stage I, grade I, uterus lower than 10 cm of height, and superficial myometrium invasion. In other stages circumstances we advised, besides surgery, prior or post-radiotherapy. High doses progestin are indicated in stages III, IV or recurrent tumors. The 5 or more years survival was 55.06%, but in stage I we obtained 87.6% of good results.

12.09.06

Radical surgery in endometrial carcinoma: López García, N, López de la Osa Gonzales, E, Recio Sanchez, S, López de la Osa Garcés, L. Inst. Nac. Oncol., Madrid, Spain

We show here the importance of the pelvic regional lymphadenectomy in the treatment of endometrial adenocarcinoma after fulfilment of the basic anatomical analysis that leads to these possibilities. We analyse the different cases treated with pelvic local and regional lymphadenectomy in the Gynecology Service of the National Oncology Institute and we emphasise the percentages of ganglionic invasion found related with several clinical and histopathological findings.

12.09.07

Thirteen years successful progestagen therapy in histologically confirmed metastatic endometrial carcinoma should be continued indefinitely: Van der Velden, W H M. St. Joseph Ziekenhuis, Eindhoven, Holland

In 1977 the question was raised how long successful progestagen (PG) therapy of metastatic endometrial carcinoma should be continued in the absence of symptoms of recurrence (2nd Int. Symp. Endometrial Cancer, London, 1977) in a patient who, at that time, had already been treated continuously with lynestrenol (Orgametril® Organon) 30 mg daily. In discussion nobody was able to advise a limited period of prescription ("never change a winning horse"). Four years later, 1981, the question was raised again and more definite answers came from *Howard W. Jones* III and *F. Engel* (Management Endometrial Carcinoma, Vrije Univ., Amsterdam, 1981) as both made unequivocal observations that even long-term PG-therapy resulted in remissions only, but not in a definite cure. In the patient observed 1969 (52 yrs) personally a postmenopausal not estrogen-induced endometrial adenoacanthocarcinoma was treated by intracavitary irradiation, followed by total oophorohysterectomy, but as will be described, three years later (1962) she developed a histologically confirmed very large local metastatic lesion in the right iliac fossa for which she was again operated upon. Since then till now she keeps using 30 mg lynestrenol daily. Intercurrently she was successfully treated surgically for obstructions at both carotids, but otherwise she is fine and no deterioration of liver or kidney function could be observed during now more than 13 years of still continuing long-lasting high dosage lynestrenol therapy, not yet seen in literature. It is concluded that, even after 13 years, this successful lynestrenol treatment can and has to be continued.

12.09.08

Endometrial carcinomas: Cianci, S, Russo, I. IIa Ostet. and Gyn., Clin. Univ. di Catania, Osp. S. Bambino, Catania, Italy

After several years spent on studying endometrial carcinoma and after accurately examining literature, we came to the conclusion that such a word includes three kinds of cancer at least, with different natural stories. 1) The most common is the endometrial adenocarcinoma arising more often from the fundus or from the tubal corners. It can spread as far as over the isthmus and here it stops as in front of an impassable border. Such cancer is observed in more than 96% of cases after the menopause and almost always in obese women. 2) Supra-isthmus carcinoma spreading more over the cervix and less over the corpus; it behaves like the cervix cancer. It is observed in patients of any age. 3) Adenocarcinoma in young women – under 40 – generally associated with Stein-Leventhal syndrome, as well as with long periods of anovulatory cycles or with protracted administration of estrogens. It proliferates on the surface, fills up the uterine cavity, does not penetrate the myometrium, does not produce metastasis and it recovers in 100% of cases. This behavior, strange for a cancer, makes us to suspect its biologic malignancy. Actually it responds well to a short therapy with progesterone. Nevertheless many literature data refer to destructive operations with severe consequences for the young women undergoing them. It seems then to be significantly useful to give a correct precise definition of these corpus cancers through a clinical and therapeutical staging better responding to the biologic reality in order to better modulate the treatment according to the true clinical entity.

12.09.09

Hysterosonography in diagnosis and treatment of carcinoma of the endometrium: clinical applications: Becker, H, Hoetzinger, H. Dept. Gyn. and Radiol., Städt. KH, Passau

Till now the visualization of the structure of the myometrium uteri, the endometrium and its pathologic alterations remained an unresolved problem. Hysterosonography, however, permits the visualization of the normal myometrium, of myomas and carcinomas. In hysterosonography the scanner on the tip of a steel tube is inserted into the uterine cavity and sectional images are made. In a preclinical study about 300 uteri were scanned and operated on. In 41 cases of a carcinoma of the endometrium the depth and location of infiltration was correctly defined in 96%. Hysterosonography therefore allows one for the first time to define exactly the target volume for interactivity radiotherapy, if the patient could not be operated on. Till now we have treated 40 patients after having done hysterosonography before intracavitary therapy – now with an exact information about the real extension of the carcinoma within the myometrium. A computer program which superimposes the necessary isodose curves on the sonographic pictures is demonstrated.

12.10.01

Interaction of human ovarian cancer cells with blood platelets: Rogan, A M, Zilla, P, Fasol, R, Heim, K, Dapunt, O. Dept. Obstet. and Gyn., Univ., Innsbruck, Austria

Attachment of malignant cells to the endothelium of blood vessels far away from the site of origin is a main step in the genesis of metastasis. Blood platelets are supposed to play an important role in that process. However, the exact mechanism of platelet-tumor cell interaction is still unknown. We therefore investigated platelet adherence in two established human ovarian cancer cell lines (2780/1847) by means of scanning electron microscopy, transmission electron microscopy and aggregometer tracing. A second wave aggregation was observed with 30×10^4 1847 tumor cells and 10^6 platelets and 65×10^4 2780 and 10^6 platelets, respectively. By means of scanning electron microscopy we were able to demonstrate that only a small number of tumor cells was densely covered with blood platelets. In addition we did not observe any obvious difference in platelet adherence between cell line 2780 and the Adriamycin-resistant subline 2780 AD. Our observations suggest that only particular cells within one and the same tumor cell line are capable of platelet activation probably due to different thrombogenetic properties.

12.10.02

The origin of an epithelial tumor of the ovary in rat: Katabuchi, H, Nishida, T, Sugiyama, T, Yakushiji, M, Kato, T. Dept. Obstet. and Gyn., Kurume Univ., Fukuoka, Japan

A rat ovarian cancer induced by a local application of 7,12-dimethylbenz(a)anthracene (DMBA) is an interesting model for experimental therapeutic study, because of its biologic and histological similarity to the human cancer showing: 1) the primary tumor development in the ovary, 2) intraperitoneal dissemination occasionally with bloody ascites, 3) histology of adenocarcinoma and finally 4) presence of intratumoral steroid receptors. Despite these characteristics of the induced tumor, the origin has not yet been confirmed (*Murphy, E D.* UICC Technical Report Series. **50,** 66, 1980). To identify the origin, the rats were weekly examined from the 15th to 30th week after the DMBA application. From the expectant role of estrogen playing on the surface epithelial proliferation (*Gondos, B.* Am. J. Path. **81,** 303, 1975), some of the rats were set into hyperestrogenic condition and the resulting tumors were examined by immunohystochemical technique. At the time of 17th week the surface epithelial proliferations were noted to show remarkable multistratification with cellular pleomorphism. 20 weeks after the DMBA-treatment, the proliferated surface cells began to infiltrate in the stroma to form irregular gland structures. In estrogen treated rats, the cytoplasms of both the surfcace cell and the infiltrated cell showed similar immunohistochemical reaction suggesting presence of estradiol. On the base of these results, the induced cancer in rat was believed to have a similar histogenetic process to human common epithelial tumor of the ovary.

12.10.03

Monoclonal antibodies to human cervical carcinoma: Yeh, M[ab], Chen, S[ab], Maa, J[b], Han, S[ab], Jiang, S[ab], Hsu, K[c], Shih, M[d], Hsu, C[e]. Dept. Microbiol. & Immun., Nat. Defense Med. Ctr[a], Ca Res. Labor., Tri-Serv. Gen. Hosp.[b], Dept. Obstet. and Gyn., Far-Eastern Memo. Hosp.[c], Dept. Obstet. and Gyn., Tri-Serv. Gen. Hosp.[d], Dept. Obstet. and Gyn., Taipei Med. Coll.[e], Taipei, Taiwan

The existence of antigens associated with human cervical carcinoma has been reported by numerous investigators. However, most of these studies were conducted with conventional hyperimmune polyclonal sera which contained antibodies against a variety of antigens, including normal antigens. In this report, we describe studies on the production of mouse monoclonal antibodies to human cervical carcinoma using hybridoma technique. Because of limit of space, methodology is not to be included here. Two monoclonal antibodies, designated 6A1 and 7T1.1, were selected. Expression of 6A1 antigen *in vivo* was extensively studied by immunofluorescence assay on cryostat sections of 52 samples of normal and 62 samples of tumor tissues. Expression of 7T1.1 *in vivo* was also tested on cryostat sections of 39 samples of normal and 55 samples of tumor tissues. The monoclonal antibodies described here appear to possess sufficient specificity for cervical carcinoma and to be of potential diagnostic and therapeutic use. Studies are in progress to determine the biochemical nature of the antigens recognized by these monoclonal antibodies, and to develop tumor imaging techniques for diagnosis of human cervical carcinoma.

12.10.04
Sex steroid hormone dependency of ovarian dysgerminoma: Ochiai, K, Isonishi, S, Yasuda, M, Therashima, Y, Hachiya, S. Dept. Obstet. and Gyn., Jikei Univ., School Med., Tokyo, Japan

Recent studies have shown that specific estrogen (E) and progesterone (P) receptor (R) exist in some ovarian tumors, suggesting its growth might be affected by E and P. In order to investigate this dependency, we have established an ovarian dysgerminoma line in nude mice (NU) by repeating subcutaneous transplantation. – Materials and methods: Ovariectomized (OVX) NU were prepared and tumor tissue was transplanted subcutaneously. One week later, NU was divided into three groups and subcutaneous injection of 1 μg of estradiol or 1 mg of progesterone in oil or oil alone was given every other day for two weeks and tumor size was recorded during the treatment. NU was then killed and tumor tissue was transplanted to new generation of OVX-NU. Rest of tissue was processed for cytosol preparation and histological study. ER and PR in cytosol were assayed by DCC method. During the course of experiment, some NU died so that cumulative survival rate (CSR) was calculated. – Result: Doubling time of tumor was about seven days. Growth curve was almost identical among three groups until third generation (F3). From F4, however, P suppressed tumor growth significantly, although E had no effect. This is directly correlated to CSR of 10 generations: Control group 18/25 (72%), E-group 17/24 (71%) and P-group 23/25 (92%). ER and PR of original tumor in NU were 5 fmol/mg protein. ER and PR were increased by transplantation and E increased PR significantly. – Conclusion: Since P suppressed the growth of this dysgerminoma and improved CSR, P is considered to be useful as one of therapeutic agents for ER-PR positive ovarian tumors.

12.10.05
A review of 477 granulosa and theca cell tumors of the ovary: Cronje, H S, Woodruff, J D. Dept. Gyn. and Obstet., Johns Hopkins Hosp., Baltimore, MD, USA

A review of 477 patients with granulosa and theca cell tumors from the files of the Emil Novak Ovarian Tumor Registry (OTR) and the Surgical Pathological Laboratory of the Johns Hopkins Hospital was done. The revised diagnoses were as follow: Granulosa cell tumor (GCT) – 100 patients, theca cell tumor (TCT) – 116 patients, granulosa-theca cell tumor (GTCT) – 105 patients, "nonspecific" gonadal stromal tumor (GST) – 63 patients, and 86 patients with "other" diagnoses. In seven patients no slides for review were available. The "other" diagnoses mainly consisted of poorly differentiated adenocarcinoma, with a few cases of mixed mesodermal tumor, sarcomas, Brenner tumor, luteoma of pregnancy, etc. Of the 477 patients, 16 were children, all with benign tumors, and 17 patients were pregnant at the time of diagnosis. Although more than 12 histological patterns of GCT have been described, the following were the most prevalent: diffuse, follicular (micro and macro), cylindroid and a tubular pattern (tubules lined by granulosa cells) in 6% of the patients. A wide variety of treatment regimens were found. The mortality for patients with GCT, TCT, and GTCT combined was only 7% in contrast to 28% in a previous review from the OTR (*Novak, E R* et al. Obstet. Gyn. **38**, 701, 1971). TCT and GTCT were practically benign, but the mortality rate for GCT was 20% and for GST 10%. The most important prognostic factor was the surgical stage of disease. With disease more advanced than FIGO stage Ia(i), the survival was less than 50%.

12.10.06
Origin of immature teratomas of the ovary: Nomura, K, Ohama, K, Okamoto, E, Ihara, T, Fujiwara, A. Dept. Obstet. and Gyn., Hiroshima Univ. School Med., Hiroshima, Japan

Recent genetic studies have shown that mature cystic teratomas of the ovary develop from a germ cell in different ways and have a 46,XX normal karyotype regardless of the mechanism of their origin. However, the mechanism of origin of ovarian immature teratomas has not been studied because of their relative rarity. To determine the mechanism of their origin, six cases of these tumors were karyotyped and analysed for chromosome Q- and R-heteromorphisms, HLA-A and -B specificities and enzyme polymorphisms of phosphoglucomutase-1 and esterase D. Three cases were chromosomally abnormal having a 48,XX,+14,+21, a 47,XX,+20 and a 47,XXX karyotype, respectively. The tumors with a 48,XX,+14,+21 and a 47,XX,+20 karyotype were heterozygous for chromosome heteromorphisms which were identical to those of their host. They, therefore, originated from a premeiotic cell or failure of meiosis I. Both had a poor prognosis. The 47,XXX tumor and three cases with 46,XX normal karyotypes were homozygous for chromosome heteromorphisms found to be heterozygous in their host and either homozygous or heterozygous for HLA and enzyme markers and therefore originated from a failure of meiosis II or duplication of a mature haploid ovum. All four had an uneventful postoperative course. These observations show that immature teratomas are similar to mature cystic teratomas in having at least three separate mechanisms of origin, but they are unlike mature cystic teratomas in having a high proportion of chromosome abnormalities and a high rate of malignant transformations.

12.10.07
Germ cell tumors of the ovary: Fertility after chemosurgical conservative treatment in advanced or recurrent dysgerminoma (D) and endodermal sinus tumor (EST): Bianchi, U A*, Favalli, G*, Pecorelli, S*, Landoni, F**, Mangioni, C**. *Dept. Obstet. and Gyn., Univ. Brescia; **San Gerardo Hosp., Univ. of Milan, Monza, Italy

From 1975 to 1984, 39 patients (90% in the last five years) suffering from recurrent or advanced germ cell

tumors of the ovary (23 D and 22 EST) were treated at our Institutions by different postoperative methods not radiation. When appropriate, in order to preserve fertility with expected satisfactory survival, conservative surgery was followed by chemotherapy in 11 and 12 patients affected by bilateral, metastatic or recurrent D and EST, respectively. In the D group (1 stage IB, 2 IC with microscopic involvement of opposite ovary, one IIB, 5 III, one recurrence; age 9–22, median 14) different well tolerated chemotherapeutic regimens (AC-VAC-PVB**) showed good cure rates: only one patient underwent subsequent radiosurgical treatment; all the patients have no evidence of disease (NED) with a median crude survival of 14 months (range 6–108). Two patients (one a recurrence after conservative surgery for stage IA and the other a stage IB for a microscopic involvement of the opposite ovary) delivered three healthy babies after normal pregnancies occurred five, eight and two years after chemotherapy. In the EST group (2 IC, two IIB, 1 IIC, 4 III, two IV, one recurrence; median age 19, range 12–27) two patients were treated – post conservative surgery – with VAB** and 10 – after 1980 – with PVB**; fertility could be maintained in 10/12: the patients treated by VAB had a recurrence and died after subsequent radiosurgical treatment, otherwise all patients treated by PVB are NED (median survival 22 months, range 3–56) and one delivered a healthy baby one year after chemotherapy for a relapse 18 months after conservative surgery. In conclusion: fertility was preserved in 86% patients after conservative chemosurgical treatment in advanced D and EST; four pregnancies were obtained in all patients (three) who intended to become pregnant.
**AC = ADB + CTX; VAC = VCR + ActD + CTX; PVB = cisDDP + VBL + BLM
***VAB = VCR + ActD + BLM.

12.10.08

Role of second look operation in the management of ovarian germ cell malignancies: Nishida, T, Sugiyama, T, Oda, T, Yakushiji, M, Kato, T. Dept. Obstet. and Gyn., Kurume Univ., Fukuoka, Japan

Although the true clinical value remains unknown, the second look operation (SLO) is widely regarded as an acceptable procedure in the management of ovarian epithelial malignancies. To evaluate the practical value of SLO to patients with malignant germ cell tumors of the ovary, eleven cases managed in our hospital were reviewed. Nine of these patients with elevated serum alpha fetoprotein (AFP) underwent further laparotomy after combination chemotherapy with VAC (vincristine, actinomycin D, cyclophosphamide) or PVB (cis-diamminedichloroplatinum, vinblastine, bleomycin). In four cases, the operation was utilized to debulk the growing residual tumors, and the other five received SLO to decide whether or not therapy should be discontinued. The result of the debulking surgery was equally disappointing. Despite the maximal tumor resection, the invisible residual tumor rapidly developed after the operation. In one of five patients with negative second look, the level of serum AFP rose again postoperatively to result extraperitoneal recurrence. In our cases except for two endodermal sinus tumors mixed with immature teratoma, the level of AFP reflected faithfully the disease activity. Without SLO, one patient is still alive six years from the primary operation. From our experience, the role of SLO in the management of ovarian germ cell malignancy is thought to be questionable. When considering the highly malignant feature of this infrequent tumor, the decision of SLO should demand the more distinct indication.

12.10.09

XY-gonadal dysgenesis, clinical, endocrinological and morphological results: Ruttman, E, Braendle, W, Held, K R, Stegner, H E. Abt. Klin. u. Exp. Endokr., Univ.-Frauenklin., Hamburg-Eppendorf

Eight female patients with XY-gonadal dysgenesis were studied. In six cases a chromosomal status of 46,XY in two cases a mosaicism 45,X/46,XY was found. Only primary amenorrhea led to diagnostic examination in four patients, two patients in addition showed an intersexual external genitalia, one patient presented with gigantism, one patient was operated because of an ovarian tumor. The endocrine parameters showed low estradiol in all cases, in two cases testosterone was elevated. Until the age of 15 all patients had low gonadotropins, beyond the age of 16 they had hypergonadotrophic values. Six patients had a laparotomy at the age of 5 1/2–22 y, only two patients (46,XY) showed neither uterus nor tubes, all other patients had a hypoplastic internal genitalia. Histological examination revealed in two cases streak gonads, in four cases malignant tumors uni- or bilateral (1 gonadoblastoma, three mixed tumors from type of gonadoblastoma-dysgerminoma on both sides). All tumors were encapsulated, max. diameter of gonadoblastoma 2 cm, compared to 3 1/2 cm of dysgerminomas. Female patients with gonadal dysgenesis and XY-chromosome should have a bilateral gonadectomy as early as possible to prevent malignant degeneration and to remove the pathologic source of androgen biosynthesis.

12.11.01

Local treatment of vulval lesions by laser vaporisation: Goodman, M L, Jordan, J A, Emens, J M. Birmingham & Midland Hosp. Women, UK

Fifty patients with superficial vulval lesions were treated by local destruction of the lesion using the CO_2 laser. This study discusses the types of lesion treated, the management of the lasered area, evaluation of response and patient acceptability. The conditions treated included pruritus vulvae, vulval dystrophy, vulval intra-epithelial neoplasia and vulval warts: the laser vaporisation was performed either when more conservative measures had failed or as an alternative to more radical surgery such as simple vulvectomy. The CO_2 laser allowed local destruction to both large and small areas with minimal scarring or disfiguration, factors obviously very acceptable to the patient. The postoperative management of the lasered areas (including 14 cases of skinning vulvectomy) is discussed, and the response to treatment and/or symptoms, measured firstly by the absence of disease following treatment, and secondly by patient acceptability.

12.11.02
A report on intra-abdominal and vaginal surgery using the carbon dioxide laser, August 1983 – December 1984: Rajan, R. Temple Univ. Hlth Sci. Ctr, Philadelphia, PA, USA

One hundred cases of laparotomy using CO_2 laser were evaluated. Transverse abdominal incision and high power density was used in all cases. The skin, fat, rectus sheath and peritoneum were opened by laser beam. Bleeding was remarkably minimal and the operating time was not prolonged. Patients experienced less pain and good healing. Myomectomy – Twenty-five cases of submucous and intramural myoma, multiple and single, sizes varying from 16 cm to 8 cm, were done. Myomectomy was done successfully in all of these cases with minimal bleeding. Ten patients are pregnant currently. Ovarian cystectomy – Ten dermoid and five other ovarian cystectomies were done with laser. Good hemostasis and minimal tissue trauma was obtained. Vaginal hysterectomy – anterior/posterior repair – Fifty cases of vaginal hysterectomy were done using CO_2 laser. Good hemostasis was obtained. Twenty cases of anterior and 20 cases of posterior colporrhaphy were carried out using the CO_2 laser. The blood loss was minimal and the pre-vesical and pre-rectal spaces could easily be dissected out without undue blood loss. The operating time was not unusually prolonged and patients experienced minimal pain postoperatively. Tubal surgery – Fifty cases of hydrosalpinx, 50 cases of peritubal adhesions and 20 cases of tubal anastomosis were carried out in the last year using CO_2 laser. The dissection was easy and operating time was minimized and the postoperative results were satisfactory. – Conclusion: CO_2 laser can be beneficial not only in tubal surgery but also in other intra-abdominal and vaginal surgery.

12.11.03
Application of laser microsurgery for the removal of uterine fibroid tumors: Bellina, J H, Voros, J I, Fick, A C. Laser Res. Found., New Orleans, LA, USA

The application of microsurgical laser techniques for removal of uterine fibroids has proven to be indispensable by our group. Whereas the only treatment previously available for multiple uterine fibroid tumors has been hysterectomy, laser surgical procedures now offer women the choice of myomectomies and uterine reconstruction. Due to the location and multiplicity of fibroids, laser myomectomy has not always been possible and a hysterectomy had to be performed. We have found this to occur in approximately 15% of all fibroid cases we have treated. From 1980 through 1984, a total of 76 myomectomies have been successfully performed by our group. For those women attempting pregnancy after surgery, the gross pregnancy rate has been 64% (follow-up time of six months or more). The mean time to conception has been 11.3 months. This paper reviews surgical techniques, complications, and the feasibility of laser myomectomies in the presence of other pathological factors.

11.12.04
CO_2 laser laparoscopy: a new method for eliminating intraperitoneal smoke: Schmidt, E H, Vancaillie, T. Frauenklin. Diakonissenanstalt, Bremen

Recent technologic progress brought the CO_2 laser into the field of operative laparoscopy. Apart from financial reasons, two major technical difficulties hinder its expansion: vaporization and heat. Both led to a rapid blur of the endoscope. The major problem is the instant elimination of the intraperitoneal smoke. Until now, interrupted suction systems, fitted to the shutter of the laser beam are used. Only small amounts of gas can be aspirated, otherwise the intra-abdominal pressure would fall. Moreover its interrupted character induces a certain instability of the intra-abdominal pressure, leading to more frequent readjustment of the focal distance and therefore waste of time. In cooperation with the company Wolf we developed a closed continous suction-insufflation system, which filters the intraperitoneal gas. The pump is built on the principle of a rotation valve. The intra-abdominal pressure can then be independently monitored by any commercially available insufflator. Beside the stability of the intraperitoneal pressure, the major advantage is the creation of a gas circulation of up to 2 liter/minute at the level of the beam spot, carrying the smoke away instantly. This system therefore provides optimal conditions for a clear view when operating with CO_2 laser by laparoscopy.

12.11.05
CO_2 laser myomectomy: Ovadia, J. Dept. Obstet. and Gyn., Beilinson Med. Ctr, Tel Aviv Univ., Sackler School Med., Tel Aviv, Israel

During a three-year period (1982–1984) 22 patients (age 20–35) underwent myomectomy by means of CO_2 laser. The causes for operation were fibroid uterus with or without a history of infertility. The results were compared to a group of 20 patients treated in our department before 1982 who underwent myomectomy by the cold knife technique. The comparisons of the postoperative morbidity, follow-up and pregnancy rate were discussed.

12.12.01

A randomised trial of the antihypertensive agent, labetalol, against bed rest in pregnancy hypertension: Cameron, A D, Walker, J J, Bonduelle, M, Calder, A A. Univ. Dept. Obstet. and Gyn., Glasgow Royal Maternity Hosp., Glasgow, Scotland

Eighty-five patients with a persistent diastolic blood pressure > 90 mm Hg were randomised into a group receiving hospital bed rest and a group receiving labetalol to lower blood pressure. All patients were hospital in-patients. The effects of the therapy on blood pressure, renal function, hematological and biochemical parameters were assessed along with placental function tests and investigations of fetal well-being. The neonate was assessed for any signs of adverse effects of drug therapy. The blood pressure was obviously lower in the labetalol group. Bed rest had no effect on blood pressure. Renal function improved slightly with drug therapy and the incidence of development of proteinuria was lower. Platelet count remained normal in the labetalol group but fell in the bed rest alone group. There were no adverse or beneficial effects seen in the babies in either group. The morbidity was higher in the bed rest group with 60% developing signs of worsening disease such as proteinuria or diastolic blood pressure > 110 mm Hg compared with only 10% in the labetalol group. However, it is felt that while some apparent benefit was seen in the labetalol group, this is restricted to those patients with diastolic blood pressures greater than 100 mm Hg and this would be the recommended blood pressure level to commence therapy. Treatment did not appear to be harmful to the mother or baby.

12.12.02

The treatment of severe pregnancy induced hypertension with the antihypertensive agent, labetalol: Bonduelle, M, Walker, J J, Bjornsson, S, Cameron, A D, Calder, A A. Univ. Dept. Obstet. and Gyn., Glasgow Royal Maternity Hosp., Glasgow, Scotland

Fifty primigravidae with severe pregnancy hypertension, defined by persistent diastolic blood pressures > 100 mm Hg and proteinuria > 0.3 g/24 hours were treated with labetalol to lower blood pressure. The average gestation at inclusion in the study was 31 weeks and the starting dose of therapy was 200 mg 3 times a day orally increasing to a maximum of 1600 mg/day. Of the 50 patients, four could not be controlled and were delivered within the first 24 hours of starting therapy. The average length of treatment in the rest of the patients was 18 days with the average gestation at delivery being 33 weeks. The treatment appeared to slow the progress of the disease and the platelet count rose in all patients. There were no adverse effects seen on the fetus that could be related to labetalol therapy and all fetuses responded to stress in the normal way. There were two perinatal deaths, one IUD from an abruption at 30 weeks gestation and one 26 week neonatal death and there were two pregnancy related deaths at 3 months of age after long-term ventilation problems. The main reason for delivery was the reaching of the target gestation and blood pressure control was good although the dose had to be increased in most patients. The study shows that labetalol can be safely used to help prolong pregnancy and allow a planned delivery of the high risk fetus.

12.12.03

Effect of labetalol on human myometrium: Ibrahim, M E, Lunell, N O, Moberger, B, Thulesius, O. Dept. Obstet. and Gyn., Fac. Med., Kuwait Univ., Kuwait

Labetalol (L) a combined alpha and beta blocker has been used successfully in the treatment of hypertension during pregnancy. The present study was designed to test the relaxant effect of L on the human myometrium since it has been reported that L prolonged duration of pregnancy and labor in rats. This effect could be explained on the basis of a partial beta-2 agonist activity or alpha blockade. Myometrial specimens were obtained at Cesarean section from uncomplicated pregnancies at term. Anesthesia was pethidine, suxamethonium, tubarine, $NO_2 + O_2$. Immediately following delivery and prior to taking the specimen 0.4 mg of methergin was given i. m. The specimens were cut into 2×6 mm sections and suspended in an organ bath for recording of isometric tension. After spontaneous rhythmic activity appeared L was administered in different concentrations and blocking experiments with the alpha blocker phentolamine and the specific beta-2 blocker ICI 118551 were performed. Labetalol dose-dependently reduced amplitude but not frequency of contractions at a threshold concentration 10^{-6} M. The addition of 10^{-6} ICI 118551 did not significantly reduce the relaxant effect of L. Phentolamine alone or in combination with L did not significantly affect uterine motility. The relaxant effect of L in human uterine preparations could be demonstrated at high concentrations, far above those used during oral or i. v. treatment. Therefore the risk of protracted labor and postpartum hemorrhage should be minimal.

12.12.04

Treatment of chronic arterial hypertension with pindolol: Soto-Yances, A, Hernandez, V, Niebles, R, Barrios-Amaya, J. School Med., Univ., Cartagena, Colombia

We studied 30 cases of chronically hypertensive pregnant women treated with only one daily dose of 10 to 30 mg of pindolol. After an average of ten days of treatment, normotension, or the highest effect of the drug, was obtained. Collateral effects were seen in only three patients, and it was necessary to add a vasodilator and/or a diuretic in 12 cases. At the beginning of treatment the mean systolic pressure was 164 mm Hg and the mean diastolic pressure was 98 mm Hg. At the end of treatment the mean systolic pressure was 142 mm Hg and the mean diastolic pressure was 86 mm Hg. There were four intrauterine deaths, and they all occurred before 37 weeks of pregnancy; there were 19 Cesarean sections and 11 vaginal deliveries. The mean weight of newborns was 2900 g and there were no congenital malformations, nor fetal bradychardia at the moment of delivery. Pindolol appears to be a safe and effective agent in the treatment of chronic arterial hypertension during pregnancy, both for the mother and for the fetus. All patients received doses of human placental lactogen, non-stress and/or stress test, and fetal pulmonary maturity test.

12.12.05
Management of pregnancy-induced hypertension with pindolol: comparative study with methyldopa: Ellenbogen, A, Jaschevatzky, O, Davidson, A, Anderman, S, Grunstein, S. Dept. Obstet. and Gyn., Hillel Yaffe Memo. Hosp., Hadera, Israel

Thirty-two consecutive women with pregnancy-induced hypertension of early onset were allocated to treatment with pindolol or methyldopa. The different parameters considered showed similarity between the groups. There was no difference between the groups as regards the average time of delivery and weight of the newborn. A significant drop in systolic and diastolic blood pressure was observed in the group of patients treated with pindolol as compared with the methyldopa group. In th pindolol group an improvement in renal function was observed, which was not found in the methyldopa group. There were no side-effects from the drugs in the mother or in the newborn.

12.12.06
Atenolol treatment of pregnancy-associated hypertension. Measurement of uterine and fetal circulation: Solum, T, Montan, S, Lingman, G, Marsal, K. Dept. Obstet. and Gyn., Lund/Malmö, Univ., Lund, Sweden

Patients and method: Fourteen women with moderate hypertension associated with pregnancy were examined. The women were observed for three days without medication. During this period the women were examined with an ultrasound Doppler technique. Wave form analysis at the uterine A. arcuata, the fetal descending aorta and the umbilical vessels were performed. Volume blood flow was calculated in the aorta. After three days the patients received atenolol. One and four days after onset of treatment the examination was repeated. During this period the patients were kept in hospital. – Results: Before atenolol treatment no variation compared to normal reference values was found. Both examinations during atenolol treatment showed significant elevation of pulsatility index in A. arcuata and the fetal aorta indicating a rise in peripheral resistance. No changes were found either in the umbilical artery or in the umbilical vein. Volume blood flow in the fetal aorta did not show any significant reduction. – Discussion: The increase in pulsatility index seen during atenolol treatment in A. arcuata of the uterus indicates elevated resistance in the maternal placental circulation. Indications of elevated peripheral resistance were also found in the fetus. Probably because of absence of adrenergic receptors no changes were found in the umbilical vessels. No changes in the volume blood flow in the fetal aorta were observed. It may indicate that the changes are too small to be measured by the method used.

12.12.07
Solcoseryl in intensive treatment of intrauterine growth retardation (IUGR): Kalamaras, E, Džikov, Z, Jovkovski, V. Univ. Clin. Obstet. and Gyn., Skopje, Yugoslavia

The experience of solcoseryl (deproteinised antibody-free dialysate of calf blood) has been presented. The investigation was done in 40 patients in third trimester of pregnancy after the thirtieth gestational week in severe forms of EPH gestosis associated with IUGR. Follow-up of IUGR was performed by sonofetometria and 24 h urinary estriol in pregnancy and Apgar score and neonatal birth weight, after delivery. Solcoseryl in doses of 25 ml by daily infusion (500 ml 5% dextrose) was administered. According to the clinical finding, gestational age and the effect of therapy, the treatment was 10–30 days. In 81.5% the birth weights of babies were 10 percentiles. In 75% Apgar score in 1st minute 7, in 87% of cases in fifth minute 7. After ten days of treatment in 87.5% of cases the urinary estriol came to normal limits. Solcoseryl activates the aerobic metabolism, increases the tolerance to hypoxia and improves the energetic reserves of the cells. It activates the cellular respiratory chain giving improvements in the utilisation of oxygen in the tissue. Solcoseryl, probably, increases the uteroplacental perfusion by influencing the synthesis of prostaglandins, as well.

12.12.08
Efficacy of sublingual nifedipine in the treatment of severe pre-eclampsia: Mendoza, A I, Montaño, A. Gyn. and Obstet. Dept., Gen. Hosp., México, DF

We analyze the results of administering nifedipine sublingual to 30 patients with diagnosis of severe pre- and postpartum pre-eclampsia without any other pathology, with an age range 15 to 34 years. Those with a BP of 160/110 mm Hg or higher were given 20 mg nifedipine sublingually, and we found in all cases a 20% decrease from basal readings with a $p > 0.001$. Its action began at five minutes, with maximum effect at 60 and lasting for 240 minutes. As a secondary effect we found an increase in heart rate of 15.3% at five minutes until 33.4% at 60, decreasing to a 20% at 240 minutes. There was an increase in diuresis in all patients. There was no alteration in FH pattern, the Apgar scores were higher than six at delivery in 90% of neonates, with a normal pediatric evolution. We concluded that nifedipine is effective in severe pre-eclampsia.

12.28.01

Pschodynamic findings in patients with elevated prolactin: Jürgensen, O, Barde, B. Dept. Gyn. and Endocr., Univ., Frankfurt

Twenty-seven females and 11 males with markedly elevated prolactin were submitted to a free psychoanalytical interview and to an object-relation test (ORT); 16/27 females and all the males had pituitary adenomas. – Results: 1) 34/38 patients showed severe psychopathology with a prevalence of depressive or psychotic disorders. 2) Imaginations attached to the disease by the individual were throughout fatal and in contrast to its medially benign nature. 3) Object relations appeared to be unhappy and distorted in the majority of patients. 4) The beginning of the disease appeared to be chronic corresponding to a continuous rather than single acute traumatisation by life-events like separation and loss. 5) Life-long deformation of intrapsychic structures might affect dopamin-metabolism resulting in hyperprolactinemia in females and males alike thus representing an endocrine non sex-linked equivalent of depressive disease. The preponderance of depressive and schizoid personality-structures in 27 females with hyperprolactinemia was statistically highly significant compared to 48 females with merely functional hypothalamic amenorrhea.

12.28.02

Evaluation of the functional capacity of the pituitary in sixteen patients with hyperprolactinemic amenorrhea: Sarris, S, Comninos, A. "M. Eliadi" Maternity Hosp., Athens, Greece

The functional capacity of the pituitary was measured by the response of FSH and LH to synthetic gonadotropin releasing hormone (GnRH) in dose of $100 \mu g$ given intramuscularly before and during treatment with bromocriptine. The study included thirty patients who were divided into three groups. Group A included 16 patients aged from 20 to 35 years (mean 27.6) who had amenorrhea with hyperprolactinemia (250 ng/ml). Group B included 8 patients aged from 16 to 28 years (mean 21) who suffered from post normoprolactinemic amenorrhea. Group C included 6 regularly menstruating women aged from 24 to 31 years (mean 28). The difference (Δ) between basal level at 0' and maximum response at 20' or 60' was used for comparisons. In group A the ΔFSH (3.9 ± 1.8 ng/ml) was significantly increased ($p < 0.01$) when compared to ΔFSH in group C (1.77 ± 1 ng/ml) while the FSH in group B (4.5 ± 2.2 ng/ml) was similar. The ΔLH was the same in all groups. On the 16 patients with hyperprolactinemia on treatment with bromocriptine nine had their prolactin levels reduced to normal (from 250 to 13.9 ng/ml) and started menstruating. The cyclic nine patients of the group A and the six normally menstruating women of the group C were given, while on treatment with bromocriptine, a second injection of $100 \mu g$ GnRH on 1st or 2nd day of their cycles. The ΔFSH (4.6 ± 1.8 ng/ml) and ΔLH (5.5 ± 2.7 ng/ml) before treatment were significantly increased ($p < 0.001$) when compare to ΔFSH (1.9 ± 1.3) and ΔLH (2.6 ± 1) during treatment. From the above findings it can be concluded that the gonadotropic function of the pituitary is unaffected.

12.28.03

Dehydroepiandrosterone sulfate (DHEA-S) levels in women after induced hyperprolactinemia: Vlassis, G, Panidis, D, Makedos, G, Zournatzi, B, Moysatat, J, Papaloucas, A. 2nd Dept. Obstet. and Gyn., Aristotelian Univ., Thessaloniki, Greece

It is known that hyperprolactinemia increases the level of DHEA-S, an androgen secreted by the adrenal cortex. The purpose of this study was to estimate if an artificially induced hyperprolactinemia for short time due to metoclopramide can affect the serum level of the above androgen. Five normal women, aged 25–38 years, who were in the early follicular phase of the cycle, were studied. Blood was taken every three hours for 24 hours, before and during the fourth day of metoclopramide administration in a dose of 10 mg every 8 hours. We found that: 1) there is a circadian periodicity of serum prolactin concentration with maximal values between 2 and 8 a. m., 2) metoclopramide increases prolactin levels on the whole with peak values one to three hours after the dose of the drug, 3) hyperprolactinemia due to metoclopramide increases the mean 24 hour value of DHEA-S. Our results show that metoclopramide – in a dose of 10 mg every 8 hours for four days – causes hyperprolactinemia for 24 hours and affects the circadian periodicity of the hormone. Furthermore, induced hyperprolactinemia for a short period of time increases significantly the mean 24 hour value of DHEA-S.

12.28.04

The correlation of prolactin (PRL)-secreting capacity to episodic pulse of PRL in normoprolactinemic women with ovulatory disturbances: Kato, K, Hoshino, K, Taddokoro, N, Kumasaka, T. Dept. Obstet. and Gyn., Dokkyo Univ., Mibu, Tochigi, Japan

The variaton on episodic pulse of PRL was examined to make clear the cause that bromocriptine (B) is effective to the normoprolactinemic women with ovulatory disturbances (group-1) resting levels of PRL in group-1 were lower than 30 ng/ml, PRL levels were measured every 20 minutes from 9 to 16 o'clock in all cases. The episodic pulse of PRL was provided by the level difference of PRL more than 4.4 ng/ml that was two times of CV (%) 2.2 in intraassay of RIA. Pulse frequency and amplitude of PRL in four women with normal cycle (group-2) were in follicular phase; 2.0 ± 0.8, 10.8 ± 0.8 ng/ml and luteal phase; 1.3 ± 0.3, 12.8 ± 0.99 ng/ml. On the other hand, pulse amplitude and frequency of PRL in three women with hyperprolactinemia (group-3) were 32.9 ± 3.1 ng/ml, 6.3 ± 0.82 during seven hours. Pulse amplitude of PRL in group-1 was 27.2 ± 4.7 ng/ml and frequency was 2.4 ± 0.2. That is to say, pulse amplitude of group-1 increased more than it of group-2, while pulse frequency was not differentiated as compared with that of group-2. Next, group-1 showed hyper-response of PRL to TRH higher than group-2. These results suggested that 1) Pulse amplitude is over 14 ng/ml during seven hours in group-1. These cases will be referred to as latent hyperprolactinemia. 2) Group-1 shows an increase in PRL secreting-capacity that is able to diagnose with hyper-response (Δ%) of PRL to TRH which is over 6.6 times resting level of PRL. And it means the effect to LH·RH of estrogen which increased after administration of B in group-1. B is effective to latent hyperprolactinemia.

12.28.05

Hyperprolactinemia and endometrial changes: Atasü, T, Kösebay, D, Arvas, M, Ertüngealp, E, Hekim, N. Dept. Obstet. and Gyn., Cerrahpaşa Fac. Med., Univ., Istanbul, Turkey

Recently, hyperprolactinemia has been established in some cases as a cause of amenorrhea, anovulatory cycles and luteal phase deficiency leading to infertility. We have carried out an investigation on 85 infertile patients with hyperprolactinemia. Ovalution was evaluated through B.B.T. curves and endometrial biopsies. Prolactin levels were measured by RIA using WHO 75/504 standards and QC was done by WHO referrence program. Out of 85 patients, 11 patients were found to have normal secretory endometrium and normal ovulation (13%), five had hypoplasic endometrium (6%), 23 had anovulatory cycles with endometrium under estrogen influence (27%), 46 had luteal phase defects (54%). Following bromocriptine treatment, the respective rates of pregnancies were achieved: 18% in women with normal secretory endometrium and normal ovulation, 40% in women with hypoplasic endometrium, 30% in women with anovulatory cycles with endometrium under estrogen dominance and 39% in women with luteal phase defect. Concerning the hyperprolactinemic patients with normal secretory endometrium and normal ovulation, we can conclude that in spite of the presence of hyperprolactinemia, there may be cases with no pathological finding other than sterility. The role of prolactin in these patients with a pregnancy rate of 18% following bromocriptine treatment is still unknown and more studies have to be done in this respect.

12.28.06

Metabolic hyperprolactinemia: Hekim, N, Ertüngealp, E, Korugan, Ü, Atasü, T. Maternity Hosp., R. and D. Lab., Obstet. and Gyn. Dept., Cerrahpaşa Fac. Med., Dr. Pakize I. Tarzi, Istanbul, Turkey

Prolactin is very sensitive to metabolic alterations in human body. In our previous works we investigated the response of PRL to the changes in some factors such as glucose, insulin, glucagon, pyruvate, lactate, FFA, glycerol, and physical conditions. In this work our purposes is to show how feeding could change our diagnosis for hyperprolactinemia. The subject matter chosen for this study consisted of 108 women, some of them infertile (n = 48) and some with menstrual irregularities (n = 60). We determined serum PRL and glucose level in all cases before and one hour after the standardized breakfast. 80% of these 108 patients showed a decrease in PRL level after feeding. In 53% of all cases, this decrease was more than 30%. Furthermore, 18 out of 48 infertile women had hyperprolactinemia in fasting state (37.5%), and one hour after feeding only five of these 48 patients still had hyperprolactinemia. As to the other group with menstrual disorders (n = 60), 30% of the patients had hyperprolactinemia (n = 48), but one hour after feeding this figure was found to be 10% therefore, 12 out of 60 patients had transient hyperprolactinemia and only six patients had postprandial hyperprolactinemia. Additionally, there was no significant correlation between fasting hypoglycemia and fasting hyperprolactinemia. However, a mechanism explaining PRL depletion, induced by feeding is unknown. Whether fasting PRL or postprandial PRL is an important criterion for the diagnosis of hyperprolactinemia in infertility and menstrual disorders requires further discussions.

12.28.07

Prolactin and biochemistry of nipple discharges in galactorrhea, and comparison with mother milk: Ertüngealp, E, Atasü, T, Çolgar U, Hekim, N. Dept. Obstet. and Gyn., Cerrahpaşa Fac. Med., Dr. Pakize I. Tarzi Maternity Hosp., Res. and Develop. Labor., Istanbul, Turkey

During the years 1983–1984, 333 patients applied to our Institute with galactorrhea, but only 39% of these patients had hyperprolactinemia. We tried to learn the contents of the nipple discharges in normoprolactinemic and hyperprolactinemic patients with galactorrhea, and compare it with mother's milk. We collected nipple discharges from ten hyperprolactinemic and ten normoprolactinemic women in addtition to colostrum from ten mothers. We determined the followings in all of the collected discharges and colostrum: total protein, albumin, IgG, IgA, IgM, C3, lactoferrin, transferrin, α-lactalbumin, casein, lactose, galactose, sodium, potassium, prolactin, and protein electrophoresis. Our conclusions very briefly: Nipple discharges in galactorrhea were not identical with mother's milk. 1. Nipple discharges contain very large amounts of serum originated albumin (10–80 g/l) relative to the mother's milk (3–6 g/l). This investigation led us to conclude that permeability changes might play an important role in the pathogenesis of galactorrhea. 2. Beta or gamma caseins and lactose levels were in the same amounts both in hyperprolactinemic and in normoprolactinemic groups and in mother's milk. 3. In lactating women, PRL levels in colostrum were very low, and in some instances undetectable, but in normoprolactinemic group (60–435 mIU/ml) nipple discharges contain very large amounts of PRL levels (2000–5000 mIU/ml). In the other features, there were no significant differences between normoprolactinemic or hyperprolactinemic nipple discharges and mother's milk.

12.28.08

Vaginal administration of bromocriptine to treat inappropriate hyperprolactinemia: Spinola, P G, Coutinho, E M, Barbosa, I C, Viana, S. Ctre Rech. Endocr. Moléc., C.H.U.L., Ste-Foy, Qué., Canada

Treatment of hyperprolactinemia by bromocriptine has to be carefully tailored to the individual patient due to the relatively poor tolerance of this drug when administered orally. We therefore decided to test the possibility of administering the drug by the vaginal route. Twenty patients with the syndrome of inappropriate hyperprolactinemia all of whom had prolactin (PRL) levels above 100 ng/ml were chosen for this study. All patients were started with twice daily treatment of 2.5 mg of bromocriptine, which was maintained for three to six months. During the course of these experiments the treatment regimen was increased to 3 or 4 times per day for patients who did not respond to the twice daily routine. After the first month of treatment all patients showed a significant decrease of PRL levels in which 50% of the patients exhibited normal levels. The rest of the patients exhibited a 30% decrease in their PRL levels which were still significantly greater than the normal levels. After three months 60% of these patients exhibited normal PRL levels, while 20% of the patients presented pituitary adenomas and their PRL levels remained above normal even after six months of treatment. The remaining 20% of the patients withdrew from the treatment. Few patients reported transient dizziness, nausea or vomiting commonly associated with oral administration. So we suggest vaginal administration of bromocriptine as a therapeutic option to treat hyperprolactinemia mainly in patients with gastric intolerance to bromocriptine, patients who need high doses of bromocriptine and also patients who need prolonged treatment with bromocriptine. – Acknowledgements: Bromocriptine (Parlodel) and PRL kits (RIA) were kindly supplied by Sandoz S. A. Divisão Farmacêutica, São Paulo, Brazil.

12.28.09

Pergolide and bromocriptine for the treatment of patients with hyperprolactinemia: Kletzky, O A, Borenstein, R, Mileikowsky, G. Dept. Obstet. and Gyn., Univ. of Southern California, Los Angeles, CA, USA

A prospecitve study of 22 women with hyperprolactinemia of various etiologies was performed using bromocriptine (Br) in nine and pergolide (Pr) in 13 patients. Those on Pr were studied for the initial 48 hours of treatment. 50 μg followed by 100 μg of Pr on the second day showed significant decrements (p < 0.01) in systolic and diastolic blood pressure (BP) in either standing or lying position. However, 25 μg followed by 50 μg did not lower BP in other 4 patients. Either 25 or 50 μg of Pr induced a maximal and significant (p < 0.005) inhibition of PRL release at 8 hours and remained suppressed for at least 24 hours. There was also a 30% and 20% temporary suppression of both LH and FSH respectively. Patients receiving either Br or Pr were then treated for 12 months. Both dopamine agonists demonstrated a similar degree of PRL inhibition throughout this time. In contrast, patients treated with Pr had higher levels (p < 0.05) of LH and FSH. Resumption of spontaneous menses and cessation of galactorrhea occurred at about 9 and 8 weeks respectively in both groups. Five patients on Br and 11 on Pr suffered minor side-effects and two discontinued treatment. It can be concluded that either dopamine agonist can be safely given to patients with hyperprolactinemia with or without a pituitary adenoma.

12.28.10

Bromoergocriptine in the management of anovulation due to hyperprolactinemia: Daftary, S N, Desai, S V, Nanavati, M S. Daftary's Total Care Clin., Bombay, India

Over a seven-year period 543 infertile patients were investigated. Of these 126 patients revealed anovulatory cycles and 28 of these showed presence of hyperprolactinemia. Galactorrhea was observed in 14 patients and oligoamenorrhea in 12 patients. Clinical evidence of luteal phase defect was present in three cases. These patients were administered bromoergocriptine in doses varying from 5.0 mg to 7.5 mg daily, and the cycle monitored by *B B T Charts,* cervical mucus studies, and occasionally by sonographic monitoring of the follicle. Ovulation was successfully induced in 22 patients; nine patients conceived. Three discontinued therapy after three cycles only. The menstrual pattern improved in 14 patients. The side-effects observed were nausea in 21 cases, vomiting in 12 cases, headache, vertigo and parched mouth in three cases each, and dry mouth in one patient. Of the nine patients who conceived, two aborted, five delivered full term normal babies and two are currently pregnant.

12.32.01

Human uterine luminal environment: Maas, D H A, Mesrogli, M, Panagiotopoulos, A, Metzger, H. Frauenklin. und Inst. Physiol., Med. Hochsch., Hannover

The culture system used for IVF/ET in the human is derived from tissue culture studies, but as there is little knowledge on the luminal secretions of the human uterus, it is questionable whether the culture conditions for human oocytes reflect the physiological environment. We have therefore started a program to evaluate some basic biochemical properties of the human uterine fluid. The first results are (see page 300).
While the pCO_2 and the lactate concentration is similar to the IVF culture system commonly used, we saw a lower pH, bicarbonate and pyruvate value and a higher protein concentration in the uterine secretion than in HAM's F10 medium. For culture of human oocytes we recommended to use 5% CO_2 in air instead of 5% O_2, 5% CO_2, 90% N_2.

pH	6.5–	7.0	
pCO_2	10	– 50	Torr
pO_2	80	–100	Torr
bicarbonate	0.5–	5	mmol/l
pyruvate		0.09	mmol/l
lactate		1.9	mmol/l
protein	11	– 17	g/l

12.32.02
Regulation of PGF2α, PGE and 6-keto-PGF1α-production in human endometrium monolayer cell culture: Neulen, J, Zahradnik, H P, Breckwoldt, M. Univ.-Frauenklin., Dept. Clin. Endocr., Freiburg

Sexual steroid hormones have been considered to be involved in the regulation of uterine prostaglandin synthesis. The present study describes the effects of progesterone (prog.), estradiol-17β (E2-17β), and clomiphene (clom.) on the accumulation of PGF2α, PGE2 and 6-keto-PGF1α in the medium of monolayer endometrial cell cultures. Subcultured cells of human endometrium obtained by curettage in the proliferative phase were incubated with prog. E2-17β, and E2-17β together with clom. for 24 hours. PGF2α, PGE2 and 6-keto-PGF1α were quantitated in the medium by specific RIAS. Addition of 100 pM E2-17β resulted in an increase of PGE2α (control: 3350 ± 228 pg/ml, 100 pM E2-17β: 6065 ± 780 pg/ml; p < 0.01). PGF2α liberation was reduced by the addition of 1 nM and 10 nM clom. to levels of 1085 ± 263 pg/ml and 1113 ± 188 pg/ml respectively. PGE2 and 6-keto-PGF1α concentration remained unaffected. At a concentration of 100 nM prog. enhanced the levels of PGF2α in the medium (control: 2125 ± 388 pg/ml; 100 nM prog.: 6060 ± 584 pg/ml; p < 0.001). PGE2 levels were also increased (control: 607 ± 153 pg/ml; 100 nM prog.: 1480 ± 209 pg/ml, p < 0.01). The levels of 6-keto-PGF1α remained unchanged. These results indicate that estradiol as well as progesterone stimulate the PGF2α synthesis. PGE2 may be only affected by progesterone.

12.32.03
Ultrasonographic evidence of endometrium in correlation to the follicular development and the hormonal parameters in patients stimulated with clomiphene citrate: Merz, E, Schaller, C, Hoffmann, G, Pollow, K. Univ.-Frauenklin., Mainz

Ultrasonographic monitoring of the follicle allows a good control of the follicular growth and is in combination with the hormonal parameters a useful adjunct in the determination of ovulation. In the present study it should be found out whether the alteration of the sonographic pattern of the endometrium can be an additional parameter for a precise prediction of ovulation. Follicular development and endometrial changes were studied in 50 women with hypothalamic pituitary dysfunction and were correlated with the serum estradiol and progesterone levels. All patients received 100 mg clomiphene citrate per day from day 5 to 9 of the menstrual cycle. Beginning on day 10 of the menstrual cycle pelvic ultrasonography was performed daily on each woman until three days after ovulation. For all studies a real-time-sector-scanner (Kretz-Combison 202) with a 3.5 MHz transducer was used. The interpretation of the endometrial changes was performed with a staging from type I to VI. – Results: The sonographic comparison of follicular growth and endometrial changes showed a good correlation in case of ovulation. One day before ovulation in 63% of the cases endometrium type V and in 26% endometrium type VI was found, the mean diameter of the major follicle was 2.4 cm. In no case was an endometrium type VI, i. e. an endometrial ring sign observed before ovulation, whereas this was seen in most cases after ovulation. The comparison of the different endometrium stages and the hormonal parameters shows an occurrence of type V parallel to the increase of LH. In contrast to the cycles with an ultrasonographic evidence of ovulation in cycles without ovulation no further endometrial development than stage III was found and the major follicle was always smaller than 16 mm.

12.32.04
Dating of the endometrium by microhysteroscopy: Stevens, M*, Flakiewicz, A**, Kula, K***, Herendael, B J van*, Hänsch, C****. *Jan Palfijn Gen. Hosp., OCMW, Antwerp, Belgium; **Lodz Med. School; ***Lodz, Poland; ****Dept. Path., Jan Palfijn, Anwerp, Belgium

In 50 consecutive cases of infertility hysteroscopies the hysteroscope (according to *Hamou*) was used. Hysteroscopy was performed in the second half of the investigated cycle. The hysteroscope was placed in contact with the fundal endometrium. Magnification is standard × 60. The endometrial vessels were visualised and photographed. Endometrial biopsy was taken at the point of contact. After biopsy the hysteroscopy was repeated so as to confirm the exact location of the biopsy. The vessel distribution was compared with the pathology slides. A dating of the endometrium by microhysteroscopy was made. Distribution pattern of the superficial vessels, capillaries, are characteristic whereas the deeper vessels of the stroma have wider and variable diameter and a less characteristic pattern throughout the cycle. The whole of the macroscopic appearance plus the microhysteroscopy enables a dating. The surface is smooth or slightly rough and its colour is yellowish. The visible pores disappear, due to the curling of the glands and edema of the stroma. The superficial vessels form a typical geometrical pattern imitating a net.

300

12.32.05

The perfusion of the human uterus. A model for physiologic and biochemical *in vitro* studies: Bulletti, C, Jasonni, V M, Vignudelli, A, Naldi, S, Flamigni, C. Dept. Reprod. Med., Univ., Bologna, Italy

Thirty human uteri were perfused for 55 h with KRB-G buffer in which estrogens and progestogens were dissolved. Purpose of the study was to demonstrate the feasibility of carrying out physiologic and biochemical *in vitro* studies on the uterine tissues. The perfusions were performed using a perfusion machine that moves the medium into each artery and drawing the perfusate from the veins. The oxygen consumption, as well as the lactate, lactic dehydrogenase and creatine kinase productions showed stability of uterine preparation until the 48th hour of perfusion. Examination of endometrium by light and electron microscopy proved a good preservation of endometrial structures until 36 h. Finally, we studied the uterine uptake of ^{3}H-E$_1$S relative to ^{14}C-E$_1$ injecting a mixture of these compounds in the uterine arteries as a bolus. The results indicated an overall preferential uptake of ^{14}C-E$_1$ and a higher ^{3}H/^{14}C ratio in the endometrium. The low ^{3}H/^{14}C ratios found in the myometrium correspond to the reduced H-E$_1$-S uptake from the perfusion medium.

12.32.06

A successful uterine perfusion for 36 hours: structural and ultrastructural evaluation: La Marca, L, Martinelli, G*, Govoni, E**, Bulletti, C, Flamigni, C. Dept. Reprod. Med., *Dept. Path., **Dept. Electr. Micr., Univ., Bologna, Italy

Thirty human uteri were perfused for 55 hours with KRB-G buffer where estrogens and progestogens where soluted. Endometrium specimens were examined by light and electron microscopy. No significant endometrial structural changes were observed by light microscopy until 36 hours of perfusion. Regressive changes (bacterial colonisation, starting necrosis) were detected after 36 hours. The first submicroscopic reversible changes (dilatation and vesiculation of rough endoplasmic reticulum cisternae, mitochondrial swelling) are found after 24 hours of perfusion. Degranulation of rough endoplasmic reticulum profiles with disaggregation of free lying polyribosomes and mitochondrial matrix, frank cavitation with peripherally placed, disorientated and disintegrated cristae were seen after 36 hours. No submicroscopic changes in smooth muscle cells of the myometrium are seen after 36 hours. When the perfusions were carried out under sterile conditions (two experiments) no ultrastructural degenerations were observed at 36 hours.

12.32.07

Endometria hyperplasia in young infertile women: López, H. Fertil. Clin., Dept. Gyn. "San Juan de Dios", Hosp. General, Guatemala, CA, USA

From January 1981 to January 1985, 72 patients were diagnosed by anatomopathologic studies. Thirty-five of these have completed a follow-up of at least six months after their initial medical treatment. Pertaining the later we have the following data: All patients are less than 36 years old. There are three patients with a diagnosis of cystic hyperplasia and 32 with an adenomatous hyperplasia. It is important to note that 16 patients presented themselves with amenorrhea, 13 had a normal cycle and only six had dysfunctional bleeding. Factors such as age and the will of fertility pointed to a medical treatment. 23 patients were given 100 mg of citrate of clomifen in the usual form plus 200 mg of oleus progesterone in the 20th day of their cycle. Ten patients were given 17-hydroxyprogesterone capronate 500 mg i.m. every eight days for eight doses. Two patients received treatment with medroxyprogesterone acetate P.O. from the 20th day of their cycle for 10 days. Of the 23 patients treated with citrate of clomifen plus progesterone, nine became pregnant, 11 presented a secretory endometrium and three presented a proliferative endometrium by control biopsy. Of the 10 patients treated with 17-hydroxyprogesterone capronate, six presented a secretory endometrium, three a proliferative endometrium and one a cystic hyperplasia. The two patients treated with medroxyprogesterone acetate were also therapeutic failures, summing up a total of three patients in whom it was considered that the medical treatment had failed.

12.32.08

The fibronectin pattern of endometrium in normal and gestational uterus: Alessandrescu, D, Ciobotaru, C, Rusănescu, T. Obstet. and Gyn. Hosp., Bucharest, Romania

Indirect immunofluorescence with rabbit monospecific antibodies of human antifibronectin va. anti-rabbit antibodies conjugated with isothiocynate display an increase of fluorescence of the endometrial structures in the gestation and normal uterus. The fibronectin showed a variable distribution and intensity during decidual morphogenesis. Fibronectin has mainly an intracellular localization in the decidua, but cellular and extracellular localization in the endometrial and myometrial junction. The fibronectin appeared as a glue molecule mediating cell-cell and cell-matrix interaction involvement in the morphogenic changes of normal and gestational endometrium.

12.32.09

A new therapeutic approach for tubal infertility; a large volume hydrotubation under laparoscopy: Seki, M, Yamada, K, Utsugi, T, Tsuchiya, K, Igarashi, M. Dept. Obstet. and Gyn., Gunma Univ. School Med., Maebashi, Japan

The hydrotubation and microsurgery are useful methods for the treatment of tubal infertility, but their effects on conception are limited. Recently, we developed a new therapeutic approach for tubal infertility. A large volume of saline solution, 200 to 2400 ml (999 ± 118 ml mean ± SE), was infused through a balloon catheter inserted in the uterine cavity through the cervix. The infusion was performed with infusion pump or manually under laparoscopic observation. The infusion pressure, recorded with the pressure transducer (0–400 mm Hg) or the pressure gauge (400–1470 mm Hg), was usually from 800 to 900 mm Hg, but sometimes over 1470 mm Hg in severe tubal damage. The saline which ran out into the pelvic cavity was aspirated through the second puncture under laparoscopic control. From October 1983 to December 1984, 27 tubal infertilities, whose duration of infertility ranged from 19 to 144 months (58.8 ± 7.6 months mean ± SE), were treated with this large volume hydrotubation (LVH), and 11 cases (40.7%) succeeded in conception within 3 months after LVH. Among 11 pregnant cases, 3 had LVH alone, 4 had LVH with endocoagulation of pelvic endometriosis and 4 had LVH with laparoscopic adhesiolysis of adnexa. The pressure and the amount of saline which was used were higher and larger than those of former reports. Our new LVH was very effective for patients who had no definite indication for microsurgery.

12.41.01
Fetal monitoring. The application of a modified Fischer score: Vastik, J F de. Univ. Maternal Hosp., Univ., Cordoba, Argentina
Fetal monitoring is a reliable tool in perinatology for fetal assessment. In an attempt to avoid personal bias in the interpretation of fetal monitoring, a scoring system has been introduced, in which several factors can be quantified in the assessment of fetal well-being. From the H.R.A. Department we selected 235 fetal monitoring traces at random, 85 considered as control group and final statistical analysis was applied. It was found that the modified Fischer score is indicative of fetal status, and the lowest scores were observed among hypertensive patients. No predictive correlation when Fischer and Apgar scores were compared. We believe that the Fischer score is useful for medical and paramedical training in fetal monitoring.

12.41.02
Prognostic value of a new scoring system for cardiotocographic patterns: Varanavičiene, N, Sadauskas, V, Puodžius, S, Kilda, A. Med. Inst., Kaunas, Lithuania, USSR
Prognostic value of new scoring system for cardiotocographic patterns was analysed. Fetal heart rate, baseline variability, accelerations and decelerations were evaluated. If normal, each factor was scored 0, if pathologic, depending of its severity, scored 3 or 5 or 10. Cardiotocographic patterns were distributed as follows: normal: score 0, alterations of I° (mild): score 3–6; II° (warning): 8–9; III° (dangerous): 10–20 and IV° (preterminal): above 20. Evaluation of 3516 cardiotocograms and retrospective analyses of fetal outcome was done. In cases the cardiotocographic patterns were considered to be dangerous (III°) – 92.1% of the newborns were compromised in consequence of hypoxic effects upon the fetus: low Apgar scores (16.7%), fetal growth retardation (14.1%), post date delivery (18.3%), fetopathia (7.04%), prolonged hospitalisation (22.5%) and other. Besides, in this group meconium staining of amniotic fluid or hypoxic scalp blood acid-base balance samples were found in 67.1%. Hypoxic conditions were revealed only for 36.9% newborns in cases of normal antepartum cardiotocographic patterns. There was no low (< 7) Apgar score in this group. High prognostic value (92.1%) of scoring system proposed, as well as high sensitivity (76.9%) and specificity (85.7%) makes it of value for clinical use.

12.41.03
Clinical evaluation of fetal heart rate response to sonic stimulation. Comparison with electronic monitoring: Faundes, A, Bacha, S M, Grassiotto, O R, Pinotti, J A. Dept. Obstet. and Gyn., State Univ., Campinas, Brazil
The fetal heart rate (FHR) response to sonic stimulation was evaluated clinically, by counting the FHR during periods of 10 seconds, every 15 seconds, during the three minutes before and the three minutes after sonic stimulation. Sixty pairs of clinical monitoring (CM) and electronic monitoring (EM) of the FHR response, carried out with about one hour interval, were analysed. A very good correlation between the two methods was found. Mean beat FHR was 141.9 ± 11.7 (CM) vs 141.5 ± 11.9 (EM), post-stimulation FHR was 158.3 ± 13.9 (CM) vs 155.1 ± 11.8 (EM), mean increase was 16.1 ± 10.9 (CM) vs 13.6 ± 10.3 (EM). Thus, the clinical monitoring appears to be as valid as the electronic monitoring for the study of FHR response to sonic stimulation, in the evaluation of the fetal condition "in utero".

12.41.04
Influence of the maternal position during pregnancy on fetal heart rate (F.H.R.) and fetal movements (F.M.): Reche, A, Gallo, M, Moreno, F, Abehsera, M, Del Sol, J R. Depto. Obstet. and Gin., Hosp. Materno Infant. "Carlos Haya", Málaga, Spain
The maternal-fetal physiology during pregnancy in relation to the maternal position is a subject that must be studied better. NST was performed on 50 healthy pregnant women, at 38–42 weeks of gestation, in five positions: supine, left lateral, right lateral, sitting and standing. The FHR and FM was recorded on the fetal monitor Sonicaid FM-4 and FM-6. There were no significant differences in the factors: FHR accelerations (omega, lambda, elliptic and periodic pattern), FHR baseline and dips type I. The variability is "better" in left lateral position than supine position, but there was no significant differene between the vertical and horizontal positions. There were significant differences in the factors: total FM (more frequent in left

lateral, less on standing position), single FM (more frequent in right lateral, less on standing position) and multiple FM (more frequent in left lateral, less in standing position). The subjective maternal perception of fetal movements was significantly less in vertical position than in horizontal position.

12.41.05

Advanced quantification of the fetal heart rate variability by spectral analysis: Bręborowicz, G, Moczko, J, Brązert, J, Spaczyński, M, Słomko, Z. Inst. Gyn. and Obstet., Med. Acad., Poznań, Poland

The estimation of variation in the fetal heart rate has become an important method for perinatal intensive care monitoring. It is evident that the fetal heart rate pattern is influenced by many different factors such as the gestational age of the fetus, the use of drugs or different states of fetal activity. In this paper the main aspects of fetal activity will be discussed in relation to antenatal heart rate monitoring. Sixty low-risk fetuses were studied longitudinally at one-week intervals. Fetal body movements visualized by means of real-time ultrasonic imaging, fetal heart rate patterns recorded by means of cardiotocograph were used as state variables. The sequence of intervals was low-pass filtered by analog anti-aliacing filter, a fast Fourier transform program was applied and a power spectrum computed for each record. Different periodical heart rate variations were discovered in the records analysed. A strong low-frequency component (0.03–0.1 Hz) was found in all records. We believe that the spectral analysis of fetal heart rate may be valuable tool in further investigations of the fetal cardiorespiratory system.

12.41.06

Difference in CTG pattern between pre-eclampsia and premature labor diagnosed as fetal distress: Hashimoto, T, Kubo, T, Sagara, Y. Dept. Obstet. and Gyn., Kochi Med. School, Kochi, Japan

Diagnosis of fetal distress during antenatal period was made using cardiotocogram (CTG). The initial change of CTG pattern in case of fetal distress was not clear. In this study, continuous CTG pattern of 14 cases of pre-eclampsia, 28 cases of PROM, and 30 cases of premature labor were retrospectively examined. Sixteen of 72 cases examined were diagnosed as fetal distress. The ratio of fetal distress in the group of pre-eclampsia 9/14 (56%) was higher than that of the group of PROM and premature labor 6/58 (10%) and the initial pattern of fetal distress in the former group was non reactive or smooth baseline whereas the initial pattern of the later group was a mild variable deceleration. In conclusion, the pathophysiology of fetal distress in case of pre-eclampsia and PROM was different.

12.41.07

Direct fetal ECG monitoring in utero: Koresawa, M, Inaba, J, Shibata, J, Kubo, T, Iwasaki, H. Inst. Clin. Med., Univ., Tsukuba, Japan

Fetal electrocardiogram (FECG) has been monitored through the maternal abdominal wall or from the fetal scalp during delivery. However, the quality of FECG is far from satisfactory except the one lead from the fetal scalp after the rupture of membrane. Here we present a direct FECG monitoring method with fine quality and without rupturing the membrane. – Method: A lead was attached to the fetal chest directly through the maternal abdominal wall with a 21-gauged needle, guided by ultrasound in the similar manner to amniocentesis. The electroactivity between the lead and the needle was introduced to the amplifier specially designed to magnify the signal 100 times larger than the conventional ECG monitor. The patients in whom fetal arrhythmia or fetal heart malfunction was suspected ranged from 19 to 34 weeks in gestation. – Results: Nine patients were examined and P waves and QRS complexes were detected clearly in all cases. And three abnormal findings; A–V block type II (Wenckebach phenomenon), complete A–V block and atrial flutter were recorded. No complications due to the procedure have occurred during their pregnancy. – Discussion: When we encounter the cases of fetal arrhythmia or hydrops fetalis, the evaluation of fetal cardiac function is essential for the prenatal or perinatal care. In this field, FECG can give us the fundamental information along with ultrasonic cardiogram. FECG monitoring, presented here, can provide clear diagnostic information with the risk as little as amniocentesis.

12.41.08

Feasibility of two dimensional echocardiographic imaging of the fetal heart in 16–24 weeks of gestation: Haimovich, L, Disegni, E, Levi, A, David, D, Bakst, A, Shapira, H, Bahary, C. Depts. Obstet./Gyn. "B" and Cardiol., Sapir Med. Ctr, Kfar Saba, Israel

Early detection is mandatory for adequate management of fetal malformation. The feasibility of two dimensional ultrasonic imaging of fetal heart (2D echo) in the second trimester of pregnancy (between the weeks 16–24) was assessed. 41 women were studied by 2D echo, and imaging of the fetal heart was obtained in each case. The 4-chamber view was the one most frequently achieved. 90% short axis and long axis views were obtained in 56% of cases. Visualization of the heart was considered diagnostically adequate if at least the four cardiac valves and the four cardiac chambers were imaged. This was obtained in 93% cases. A complete image of the heart including a definition of the relationship of the great vessels and detection of the ductus arteriosus was obtained in 34%. Each heart examined was found to be normal. Physical examination and 2D echo at birth performed in 25 cases confirmed that the heart was normal. In conclusion, a thorough examination of the fetal heart by 2D echo may be carried out as early as at the 16th week of pregnancy. This is of potential value for early detection of cardiac malformations.

12.41.09

Antepartum fetal heart rate monitoring and prognosis of fetal outcome in pregnancies with Rh-iso-immunisation: Yordanov, G, Karagiosova, J, Mateeva, E, Ivanov, S. Inst. Obstet. and Gyn., Sofia, Bulgaria
A correlation was sought between antepartum tocographic data and the spectro-photometric results in cases of immunologically established Rh-iso-immunisation. 91 CTGs have been processed according to the scoring pattern (*Fisher*, 1976). 30 transabdominal amniocenteses have been performed in 21 pregnancies with Rh-iso-immunisation. The results from the spectro-photometric analysis have been assessed according to the chart of *Liley*. With fetuses in Zone 3 and with fetuses with deepening deterioration (shift from Zone 1 to Zone 2 and from Zone 2 to Zone 3) a sinus rhythm has been observed. With fetuses in Zone 1 a Fisher score lower than eight was not observed. With fetuses in Zone 3 Fisher score higher than four was not observed. Cardiotocographic analysis is a valuable auxiliary method of diagnosis of antenatal status of the fetus in cases of Rh-isoimmunisation.

12.42.01

A new cervical catheter for managing premature rupture of the membranes: Ogita, S, Imanaka, M, Matsumoto, M, Hatanaka, K. Osaka City Perinat. Ctr., Osaka, Japan
In the management of premature rupture of the membranes (PROM), there are two principal choices: immediate induction of labor to avoid ascending infection and conservative management to achieve greater fetal maturation. Since the intrauterine environment is more suitable for a fetus than any incubator, it is reasonable to choose conservative managment if such problems as infection and free flow of amniotic fluid can be prevented. With this goal in view, we devised a new catheter with two separated balloons near the cervical tip and a hole between these balloons so that antiseptic solution can flow through to sterilize the cervical canal and the vagina. The catheter, inserted through the cervix after surgical suture of the cervix, prevents almost completely the out flow of amniotic fluid as well as ascending infection. If infection has already developed or is suspected, antibiotics can be infused directly into the amniotic cavity through the catheter. Using this catheter, we treated 20 cases of PROM at less than 32 weeks of gestation until the fetal lung was demonstrated to be mature. No significant respiratory distress syndrome occurred in our cases and no significant correlation was noted between the number of weeks of gestation and the time before the lungs appeared mature. We concluded that PROM can and should be managed according to individual needs until lung maturity is demonstrated.

12.42.02

Intra-amniotic infusion of antibiotics for premature rupture of the membranes: *Imanaka, M, Ogita, S, Matsumoto, M, **Sugawa, T. *Osaka City Perinat. Ctr., **Dept. Obstet. and Gyn., Osaka, Japan
One of the most important problems in the conservative management of premature rupture of the membranes (PROM) is infection occurring during a prolonged latent period, although it has been considered that in some cases amniotic fluid infections may be the cause of PROM rather than the result. Maternal administration of antibiotics and vaginal disinfection have been essential factors in the management of PROM, but the optimal treatment and prevention of ascending infection are not yet established, since administration of antibiotics to the mother results in lower levels in the amniotic fluid. To determine the best method of preventing ascending infection, antibiotics such as CPZ, CTX and LMOX, which have a broad spectrum, are not absorbed by the fetus and are not tissue irritants, were infused directly into the amniotic cavity. A single infusion of 500 mg of each drug resulted in a concentration of $200-1000 \, \mu g/ml$ immediately after infusion, and the concentration remained above $10 \, \mu g/ml$ for 24 hours without significant increase in fetal or maternal blood levels. We estimated the fetal concentration to be below 1% of the amniotic fluid concentration. The results indicate that the amniotic fluid can contain fairly high concentrations of antibiotics which can cleanse every fetal opening and the respiratory and gastrointestinal tracts without entering the fetal blood stream. Thus, we proved that infusion of antibiotics into the amniotic cavity is useful in preventing ascending infection in PROM.

12.42.03

Fibrinolytic activity in amniotic fluid increases at term: Pschera, H, Kjaeldgaard, A, Larsson, B. Dept. Obstet. and Gyn., Karolinska Inst., Huddinge Univ. Hosp., Stockholm, Sweden
According to recent studies on the ultrastructure of amniochorion in late pregnancy the plasminogen content increases with the degree of degenerative changes (*Jenkins, DM* et al. Brit. J. Obstet. Gyn. **90**, 841, 1983). In the present investigation the fibrinolytic activity (FA) was assessed by the fibrin plate technique in 47 amniotic fluid samples obtained at 35 to 39 weeks' gestation. In amniotic fluid FA ($63.1 \pm 2.5 \, mm^2$) was considerably elevated when compared to previously reported serum levels in pregnant women. After centrifugation of the amniotic fluid samples a highly significant reduction of FA in the supernatant was recorded, suggesting that cells of fetal origin are the main source of the high plasminogen activator activity demonstrated in amniotic fluid. A significant rise in amniotic fluid FA was demonstrated beyond the 37th gestational week. Furthermore, significantly higher FA was recorded in amniotic fluid samples from women with spontaneous onset of labor within a week. Thus, plasminogen activators in amniotic fluid may be involved in the yet unknown mechanism of membrane rupture. However, a single FA determination in amniotic fluid obtained by routine amniocentesis was found to be of little value for prediction of the time interval to delivery.

12.42.04

Changes of serum steroid levels in premature infants in the early neonatal period: Kato, H, Kosaki, T, Hashino, M, Yanaihara, T, Nakayama, T. Dept. Obstet. and Gyn., Showa Univ. School Med., Tokyo, Japan

Serum steroid hormone levels in premature infants (n = 21) were measured and compared with those in normal infants (n = 19) at delivery and on the 1st, 3rd and 5th and 30th day after birth. Conjugated dehydroepiandrosterone (DS), 16αOH-DS, pregnenolone (P) and 20αdihydro-P (20P) were measured by newly developed method of gas chromatography-mass spectrometry using deutrated steroid as internal standard and cortisol by RIA. In normal infants, all the steroid showed a highest value at delivery and decreased as days passed except for 16αOH-DS which showed a peak on the first day of life. On the other hand, levels of Δ_5-steroid in premature infants increased significantly on the first day and decreased thereafter. No significant difference was observed in steroid values between normal and premature infants at delivery. The levels of DS, P and 20P in premature infants, however, were significantly higher than those in normal infants till the fifth day of life. On 30th day after birth, no significant difference was observed between two groups in serum steroid levels. Assuming that the Δ_5-steroid levels indicate the activity of fetal zone of adrenal gland, these data indicate that the involution of fetal zone in premature infants was retarded but reached normal levels on the 30th day of life.

12.42.05

Hydroxyproline contents of unruptured and ruptured human fetal membranes at term: Andreucci, D. Labor. Invest. Reumat., Fac Med., São Paulo, Brazil

Membranes from 38 to 41 week pregnancies were selected. 25 had premature rupture with closed cervix and 32 had artificial rupture within the expulsive period. Two samples of amnion were used: one from the free and a second from the placental surface. Bergmann-Laxley method for HOP was used. Dosages were made with lyophilizied matter. The means, standard deviations and maximum and minimum values of HOP are presented for each membrane location, unruptured and ruptured. The comparison of means was performed through an analysis of variance and Scheffé's tests with 5% as the total level of significance. HOP contents show no difference between placental and free amnion in both groups of ruptured or unruptured membranes. HOP contents are higher in the amnion than in the chorion of both groups of membranes. Differences were also found in HOP contents of chorion between both groups. Amnion HOP contents in the unruptured group are higher than in ruptured membranes group.

12.42.06

Effects of premature membrane rupture in some fetal hormonal levels at birth: Muti, A R, Patella, A, *Carta, G, *Ippolito, M. 1st Inst. Obstet. and Gyn., Univ., Roma "La Sapienza", and *School Obstet., Camerino, Italy

Serum levels of TSH, total T4, free T4, T3 cortisol and prolactin in spontaneous delivery were measured in 22 living and vital newborns through blood tests from the umbilical cord. The 22 newborns from spontaneous delivery were born between 38th and 40th week of pregnancy and weight was between 3300–3600 g. The cases studies were divided into two groups: 1) 14 newborns after timely membrane rupture; 2) 8 newborns after premature membrane rupture (RPM was 12–24 hours before labor). TSH and T.T4 levels were significantly higher when premature membrane rupture occurred. No significant difference was noted in other hormones studied. These results are discussed in relationship to the possible role of thyroid hormones favoring fetal pulmonary maturity seeing that RPM reduces the risk of RDS.

12.42.07

Comparison of oral PgE₂ and intravenous oxytocin for stimulation of labor in cases of premature rupture of the membranes: Borisov, I, Starkalev, I. Inst. Obstet. and Gyn., Med. Acad., Sofia, Bulgaria

Double controlled study was carried out to compare the effects of oral PgE₂ and intravenous oxytocin (Syntocinon) on stimulation of labor. All patients had premature rupture of membranes at or near term with more than six hours without labor activity. The results were compared using Friedman graphic analysis. In the groups of nulliparas the augmentation with PgE₂ resulted in shorter stimulation-delivery interval, due to the shortening of the latent phase. Regarding the groups of multiparas oxytocin stimulation was more effective compared with the groups of multiparas, stimulated by oral PgE₂.

12.79.01

Comparison of different treatments of endometriosis in infertile women: Moghissi, K S, Hull, M, Magyar, D, Hayes, M F. Dept. Obstet. and Gyn. Wayne State Univ., Detroit, MI, USA

This study was designed to evaluate the effectiveness of three forms of treatment in the management of stage I and II (AFS classification) endometriosis. A total of 144 patients had complete infertility studies including laparoscopically diagnosed and staged endometriosis. Management consisted of (1) no treatment (controls) in 56, (2) oral medroxyprogesterone acetate (MPA) 30 mg daily for 90 days (N = 36), and (3) Danazol 600 to 800 mg/day for six months (N = 52). All patients were followed up for at least 18 months of exposure to pregnancy during which other infertility problems were also treated. Cumulative pregnancy rates were determined by life table analysis. At 18 months, pregnancies resulted in 36% of group 1 (controls), 34% group 2 (MPA), and 40% of group 3 (Danazol). There were no significant differences between these rates. All together cumulative pregnancy rates were recorded in 39% of stage I and 37% of stage II. Spontaneous abortion rate was 11% in pregnancies achieved with stage I disease and 5.9% for stage II. Abortion rates for various treatment modalities were: MPA 6.3%, Danazol 11%, and no treatment 14.3%. The results of this study do not show a significant difference between MPA, Danazol and expectant therapy of endometriosis associated with infertility.

12.79.02
Low- versus high-dose medroxyprogesterone acetate in the treatment of endometriosis: Willemsen, W N P, Rolland, R, Vemer, H M, Thomas, C M G. Dept. Obstet. and Gyn., Radboud Univ. Hosp., Nijmegen, The Netherlands

The treatment of endometriosis is controversial and the reported cure rates after medical treatment are inconsistent. The purpose of this report is to compare the effect of 20 versus 250 mg medroxyprogesterone acetate (MPA, Farlutal®) daily, on endometriosis and also to test the acceptability of high dose MPA. Twenty women suffering from mild to moderate endometriosis diagnosed by laparoscopy were treated orally for 4 months, at random with 20 mg MPA (11 women) and 250 mg MPA (9 women) daily. At frequent intervals serum MPA levels were measured by specific RIA. Blood pressure, weight and side-effects were recorded and the candidates were asked for complaints with special emphasis on the cycle. – Results: During treatment all patients developed amenorrhea. Mean MPA serum levels during treatment were 6.1 and 81.2 nmol/l in the 20 and 250 mg group respectively. The treatment was well tolerated in both groups. Raised blood pressure, weight gain and spotting did not occur more frequently in the 250 mg group and the treatment was well tolerated in both groups. At the second laparoscopy after four months treatment eight of nine women showed improvement in the 250 mg group: in six of these women endometriosis was no longer present. In the 20 mg group 9 of 11 women showed improvement and in three of them no residual endometriosis was seen. – Conclusion: MPA is effective in the treatment of endometriosis. High dose of MPA even gives a high cure rate after only four months of treatment. Since side-effects are only minor, this type of treatment must be investigated further.

12.79.03
A new approach in the treatment of endometriosis with a gonadotropine-releasing hormone analogue: Andor, J, Szalmay, G, Haller, U. Dept. Obstet. and Gyn.,Kantonsspit., St. Gallen, Switzerland

Results of 20 histological verified cases of endometriosis are reported. As medicament the administration of decapeptyl intramuscular for a total of nine times at three weeks intervals was performed. The effect of this therapy was the following: In the great majority of the cases after the first dose an increase of the FSH- and LH-parameter with consecutive higher estrogen-concentration occurred. In a number of patients an intensification of the symptoms of the primary disease and an increase in frequency and intensity of pains could be observed. Already after the second injection, in most cases a decrease of pain occurred and irregular hemorrhage until the absence of the menstrual cycle. After about the third till fifth injection hot flushes as side-effect were observed, in addition a dry feeling in the vagina. As the application of estrogens is not indicated in endometriosis we treated hot flushes with gestagen-therapy, i.e. MPA as additional medication. This treatment not only leads to a reduction or a disappearing of the hot flushes, but it supports theoretically the effect of decapeptyl in cases of endometriosis. To verify the effect of the trial drug, the hormone status was determined: FSH, LA, prolactin, as well as estrogen and progesterone by RIA. In each of the cases, this hormone profile took place before the beginning of the treatment, after the first, third, sixth and finally after the ninth period of the treatment. In a number of cases, by means of a second look laparoscopy/laparotomy the disappearance of endometriosis sites could be verified histologically.

12.79.04
Effects of LHRH-analog (Buserelin) on the morphological structure of endometriosis: Schweppe, K-W, Cirkel, U*. Univ.-Frauenklin., Münster*, u. Kreiskrankenh. Ammerland, Akad. Lehrkrankenh., Univ., Göttingen

Previous studies have shown that incomplete morphologic response to cyclic hormonal changes may explain the frequent failure of endocrine therapy of endometriosis (*K-W. Schweppe* et al. Am. J. Obstet. Gyn. **148**, 1024, 1984). Histologic data before and after suppressive therapy with danazol have demonstrated, that transient or incomplete suppression may lead only to partial regression of the ectopic endometrium (*K-W. Schweppe, R. M. Wynn.* Europ. J. Obstet. Gyn. reprod. Biol. **17**, 193, 1984). The new LHRH-analog is claimed to eliminate completely the synthesis of ovarian steroids, and to cure endometriosis. Patients with pelvic endometriosis (N = 20) diagnosed by laparoscopic biopsy prior to treatment received LHRH-analogue 900 mcg – 1800 mcg daily. At the completion of six months of treatment laparoscopy was repeated and from remaining scar tissue or endometriotic implants a repeat biopsy was taken. There was a marked improvement in all cases regarding the stage of endometriosis from 2.1 ± 0.7 to 1.1 ± 0.8 using the AFS-classification. But only five patients were healed. The remaining 15 women had peritoneal scars and/or persistent endometriosis. The histology demonstrated characteristic atrophic changes of glandular epithelium and cytogenic stroma, resembling postmenopausal endometrium in nine cases. In six cases however, the implants appeared arrested in an early proliferative stage. Only a few glands showed regressive changes. These findings can be explained by an incomplete suppression of steroidogenesis by the doses of LHRH-analogue in some women, or by the low differentiation and endocrine independent growth of endometriosis in these cases.

12.79.05

Side-effects of medical treatment of endometriosis. A comparison of danazol and LHRH-analogue (Buserelin): Cirkel, U, Schweppe, K-W*. Univ.-Frauenklin., Münster u. Kreiskrankenh. Ammerland, Akad. Lehrkrankenh., Univ., Göttingen*

Danazol is the mostly used drug for treatment of endometriosis in the last decade (*Dmowski, W. P.*, Fertil, and Steril. **31**, 462, 1979). Despite its beneficial effects on symptoms and objective findings there is a 35% recurrence rate and a large number of side-effects reported (*Schweppe*, Endometriose. Schattauer, 1984). Especially metabolic changes of liver function (*Heikkinen* et al. ESCO VII, 135, 1984) and of plasma lipids (*Schweppe* and *Assmann*. Horm. metab. Res. **16**, 593, 1984) have been shown recently. First reports of LHRH-analogue (Buserelin) suggest, that the new substance is effective in the treatment of endometriosis, but there are no data about the side-effects. A total of 82 patients with endometriosis confirmed by laparoscopic biopsy were followed before, during, and after medical therapy. The danazol group ($N = 62$) received 600 mg daily for 6 months, and the LHRH-analogue group 900–1800 mcg daily for 6 months. Examinations and blood samples were done before, every 8 weeks during, and 4 weeks after treatment. There was a transient rise in liver enzymes during danazol intake (SGPT: $p < 0.05$), and normalization after cessation of therapy; but no changes during treatment with LHRH-analogue. A significant HDL decrease ($p < 0.01$) and a rise of LDL caused by danazol was seen during treatment. No significant changes in lipoprotein levels were seen during LHRH-analogue medication. The most frequent subjective complaints during danazol were weight gain (50%), acne, hirsutism, and other androgenic side-effects (up to 20%). Hypoestrogenic effects were mild and rare in the danazol group, but sometimes severe (hot flushes) in the LHRH-analogue group.

12.79.06

Lipids and lipoproteins in the hormonal treatment of endometriosis: Teichmann, A T*, Wieland, H**, Cremer, P***, Kuhn, W*, Seidel, D***. *Dept. Gyn., Univ., Göttingen; **Dept. Intern. Med., Univ., Freiburg; ***Dept. Intern. Med., Univ., Göttingen

Since recent studies of the Lipid Research Clinics Program have proven LDL(β)-concentration to be not only indicator of male's coronary risk but pathogenic agent in the development of myocardial infarction, lipids and lipoproteins have gained a new topicality. It is known, that female sex hormones do influence the serum lipid- and lipoprotein profiles through different metabolic pathways. In a comparative study patients with laparoscopic proven endometriosis were treated for six months with either 600 mg/die danazol ($n = 25$) or 20 mg/die lynestrenol ($n = 25$). In both groups total cholesterol-, triglyceride- and pre-β-lipoprotein cholesterol concentrations remained unchanged. A significant reduction in α-lp.-chol. levels was observed in both groups but was much more marked in the danazol-treated group. β-lp.-chol. concentrations rose slightly under lynestrenol and more significantly with danazol treatment. With the exception of three cases of danazol-patients the hormone-induced changes returned to pretreatment values after cessation of therapy. Taking into account the results of the Göttingen-Coronary-Angiography-Study the elevation of β-lp.-chol. concentrations must be regarded as the most important predictor for the risk of coronary heart disease in women aged less than 50 years. It is concluded that the use of lynestrenol and danazol in the dosages cited above must be based on proven endometriosis, exclusion of coronary-risk factors, and measurement of lipoprotein concentrations before, during and after treatment.

12.79.07

Effects of danazol on lipoprotein metabolism: Sudo, N, Furuya, M, Ueda, M, Miyajima, A, Takahashi, S. Dept. Obstet. and Gyn., and Intern. Med., Nagaoka Red Cross Hosp., Nagaoka, Japan

Lipoprotein profiles were examined in the patients on danazol to see the pharmacological effects on lipoprotein metabolism. The subjects consisted of 20 women taking danazol 400 mg per day for their endometriosis. Fasting blood was drawn pre-administration, during administration (18.9 ± 4.2 weeks) and post-administration (9.9 ± 2.2 weeks). Total cholesterol and HDL-cholesterol (HDL-C) significantly ($p < 0.01$) decreased in 18.9% and 40.4% on average, respectively. LDL-cholesterol was unchanged. Triglycerides markedly (37.1% on average) decreased ($p < 0.01$). LCAT activity significantly ($p < 0.01$) decreased in 46.0% on average, however, cholesterol-ester ratio in HDL increased. Apoprotein A-I, significantly ($p < 0.01$) decreased in 23.9% on average. Decreases of apoprotein A-II and apoprotein B were small amount. β/α cholesterol ratio was considered as athelogenic index (AI). AI significantly ($p < 0.01$) increased from 2.1 to 3.2. These lipoprotein values returned to pre-administration level in 2–3 months after discontinuation of danazol. In summary, danazol reduces both lipid and apoprotein concentrations. The main action of this medicine on lipoprotein metabolism is thought to reduce the synthesis of HDL and VLDL in the liver. Significant decrease of HDL-C and increase of AI suggests that the care must be taken when this medicine is used for a long period.

12.79.08

Estradiol and testosterone implants after hysterectomy for severe endometriosis: Studd, J W W, O'Dowd, T M. Dulwich Hosp. Menopause Clin., London, UK

Details are presented of fifty patients who had a hysterectomy with or without oophorectomy for endometriosis. Conservative surgery (hysterectomy with preservation of some ovarian tissue) was associated with a need for subsequent reoperation in fifteen of twenty-one patients, whereas only one of the twenty-one patients who had complete surgery (hysterectomy plus bilateral oophorectomy) required a further laparotomy. Active endometriosis was not found at this operation. All of the patients were receiving subcutaneous implants of estradiol and testosterone at the time of the study, although twenty-six were given oral replacement therapy initially. Hormone replacement therapy relieved virtually all climacteric symptoms and did not cause reactivation of disease. At the time or reimplantation for returned menopausal symptoms the mean FSH was 7.5 iu/l, the estradiol 2160 pmol/l and the mean testosterone elevated at 4.42 pmol/l. These data demonstrate that when a hysterectomy is indicated for relief of the symptoms of endometriosis it is suggested that bilateral salpingo-oophorectomy should also be performed. This should be followed by implant therapy using estradiol and testosterone. This complete surgical removal of disease plus hormone therapy is a safe effective method for treating endometriosis and avoids the failure of medical and conservative surgical treatments.

12.79.09
Normalization of nocturnal prolactin (PRL) levels during treatment of endometriosis with danazol: Radwanska, E, Dmowski, W P, Henig, I, Rana, N. Dept. Obstet. and Gyn., Rush Med. Coll., Chicago, IL, USA

Exaggerated response of PRL to TRH in women with endometriosis has been recently reported (*Muse* et al. Fertil. and Steril. **38**, 419, 1982). Our own studies (*Radwanska* et al. Fertil. and Steril. in press) indicate nocturnal hypersecretion of PRL in infertile women with endometriosis. It has also been observed that the day-time PRL levels may decrease during danazol administration (*Bohnet* et al. Fertil. and Steril. **36**, 725, 1981). This study was performed to ascertain whether nocturnal hypersecretion of PRL may normalize during treatment with danazol. Thirty-two consecutive infertile women (Group I) with endometriosis and regular cycles were studied before treatment and 15 patients (Group II) during treatment with danazol. Blood samples were drawn during hospital admission throughout the night preceding operation at 8:00 p.m., midnight, 4:00 a.m. and 8:00 a.m. for PRL measurements by RIA. Mean PRL values at 8:00 p.m. were not different for Groups I and II (17.7 and 18.3 ng/ml); at other times they were lower in Group II ($p < 0.05$ at midnight) and not different from the values in normal women. We conclude that the administration of danazol normalizes nocturnal pattern of PRL secretion. This alteration in PRL dynamics may contribute to the therapeutic effects of danazol and endometriosis.

13.14.01
Antibiotic prophylaxis of infections after gynecologic surgery: A prospective randomized trial with cefotetan (cft) vs. piperacillin (pip.): Scalambrino, S, Regallo, M, Consonni, R, Landoni, F, Mangioni, C. Dept. Obstet. and Gyn., S. Gerardo Hosp., Monza, Italy

From January 1985 a prospective, controlled, randomized trial to verify the efficacy and tolerability of cft compared with pip. in preventing postoperative infections after gynecologic surgery is continuing. Patients submitted to vaginal hyst., abdominal simple or radical hyst. and second look clean surgery received a single dose (2 g i. v.) of cft or pip 30 min before operation. Patients submitted to ovarian or uterine conservative surgery, post Rx therapy surgery and operations with opening of bowel or urinary tract receive cft (2 g i. v. before operation and after 8 h) or pip (2 g i. v. before operation after 5 h and after 12 h). We consider a prophylactic failure the occurrence of severe infections morbidity (S.I.M. = fever > 38° C lasting for 48 h at least except the operative day) or by clinical evidence of infection at the operative site. Samples in sites of infection are collected, whenever available for a complete microbiological evaluation. Serum and tissue concentration of cft will be evaluated. About 600 patients (450 and 150 respectively in the two groups) will enter the study. 59 patients entered the study in January: 42 received a single dose prophylaxis (19 with cft and 23 with pip) and a 17 multi-dose one (8 with cft and 9 with pip). One out of 23 and one out of 9 patients in pip group developed infections, compared with 0/19 and 1/8 in the cft group.

13.14.02
A prospective randomized trial of prophylactic ceftezole (cfz) vs. cefoxitin (cfx) in gynecologic surgery: Regallo, M, Scalambrino, S, Mangioni, C, Ortisi, G, Giltri, G. Dept. Obstet. and Gyn., S. Gerardo Hosp., Monza, Italy

From January to December 1984 a controlled, prospective, randomized trial was carried on in order to evaluate the comparative efficacy of cfz and cfx in preventing infections after gynecologic surgery. 211 patients entered the study; 156 women received a cfz or cfx 2 g i. v. single dose 30 min before operation; 38 were submitted to abd. radical hysterectomy, 89 to vaginal hyst., 19 to radical vulvectomy, 12 to simple hyst. and retropubic colposuspension. 55 women submitted to ovarian or uterine conservative operation received cfz or cfx 2 g i. v. 30 min before operation, 5 and 2 h later. The occurrence of severe infectious morbidity (S.I.M. = fever > 38° C lasting for 48 h at least, the operative day excepted) or clinical evidence of infection at the operative site was considered as a prophylactic failure. Altogether a cfz ultra short and short term prophylaxis was performed in 74 and 30 women, respectively; on the other hand 82 and 25 women, respectively, received a cfx ultra-short and short term prophylaxis. 18 patients out of 211 (8.5%) had prophylactic failures without a significant difference between cfz group (7.7%) and cfx group (9.3%). Cfz and cfx single dose and cfz and cfx three-doses failed in 9.5% (7/74), 10.9% (9/82), 3.3% (1/30) and 4% (1/25) respectively. Whenever available samples in sites of infection were collected for a complete, microbiological evaluation. Serum and tissues concentrations of cfz have been evaluated.

13.14.03

Heparin infusion to pregnant women using a portable infusion pump "Zyklomat": Hahn, L. Dept. Obstet. and Gyn., East Hosp., Göteborg, Sweden

Women with a past history of thromboembolism have a risk of recurrence during pregnancy that is about 12%. Oral anticoagulants cross the placenta and should not be used during pregnancy. Heparin has side-effects, mainly a demineralization, which is considered to be dependent on the total dose given. It is usually given s. c. twice daily, which may lead to unnecessary high peak heparin levels. The aims of the study were: 1) to obtain constant heparin levels for long periods of time and 2) to reduce the total dose. A portable pump Zyklomat (Ferring) was used to administer heparin to pregnant women in need of anticoagulation. Fifteen women were treated with the pump for periods from two days up to 22 weeks. – Results: No recurrencies of thrombosis occurred. The treatment was monitored by measuring the actual heparin concentration. A level $0.05-0.20$ IU/ml was considered optimal. This was achieved with rather constant levels. The patient compliance was excellent. The total dose could be reduced with preserved anticoagulation compared with the dose with s. c. injections. – Conclusions: Preliminary results with a portable infusion pump are promising, judged by its ability to maintain adequate levels of heparin for long periods. The patient compliance was excellent. It is foreseeable, that the side-effects of heparin might be reduced compared with s. c. injections, as the total heparin dose can often be reduced. The role of high peak levels of heparin sometimes seen after s. c. injections for the development of osteoporosis is unknown but cannot be disregarded.

13.14.04

Blood coagulation and fibrinolysis during continuous estrogen-progestogen therapy in postmenopausal women: Hellgren, M, Mattson, L-Å, Samsioe, G, Sporrong, T, Stigendahl, L. Dept. Obstet. and Gyn., and Blood Coagul. Lab., Med II, East and Sahlgrens' Hosp., Gothenburg, Sweden

The incidence of thromboembolic complications (TE) increases during estrogen therapy. This study was performed to investigate the hemostasis during continuous estrogen-progestogen treatment. 60 postmenopausal women were randomly allocated to four groups and were given 2 mg 17β-estradiol combined with either norethisteronacetate 1 mg (group I) and 0.5 mg (group II) or megestrolacetate 5 mg (group III) and 2.5 mg (group IV) for climacteric symptoms. Blood samples were collected twice before and after one and four months of treatment. Fibrinogen was analysed photometrically and fibrinopeptide A (FPA) by RIA. Antithrombin III (AT), plasminogen and α_2-antiplasmin were measured with the chromogenic substrates S-2238 and S-2251. – Results: Fibrinogen levels were normal. No increase in FPA levels was observed, but the basal levels were elevated for unknown reason. AT activity was reduced after one month in group I $(-6,6\%, p<0.01)$ and group III $(-7.1\%, p<0.02)$ and after 4 months in group III $(-7.3\%, p<0.05)$. AT levels $<80\%$ of normal were found in 4 women. AT activity decreased $>20\%$ of normal in 11 women. Plasminogen activity increased after one month in group I $(+15.7\%, p<0.001)$. The α_2-antiplasmin levels were normal. One woman with deep venous thrombosis did not differ from the other women regarding the performed laboratory tests. – Conclusion: This study did not show any activation of the blood coagulation, but a decrease in AT activity may suggest an increased risk for TE in individual women. Further studies are needed to explain the increase in plasminogen activity. We recommend control of At before and during postmenopausal estrogen treatment.

13.14.05

Effects of oral contraceptives on fibrinolytic system: Ogino, M, Okano, H, Okinaga, S, Arai, K. Dept. Obstet. and Gyn., Teikyo Univ. School Med., Itabashi, Tokyo, Japan

Recently oral contraceptives (pills) have rapidly come into general use owing to their reliable effects. The relationship between the use of oral contraceptives and occurrence of thrombosis is still controversial. As a result of epidemiological studies and research on blood coagulation, it was shown that the users of oral contraceptives were 5 to 10 times more liable to thrombosis than non-users. An attempt was made to clarify, through animal experiments, the mechanism by which thrombosis was caused by the pill. – Materials and methods: Urinary plasmin-activity was measured by lysine Sepharose affinity chromatography-radiocaseinolytic method. Norethisterone, mestranol, and the both were administered every day to the New Zealand white rabbits. The animals were divided into three groups; 1/20 of the normal dose, the normal dose, and 50 times the normal dose were administered, respectively. – Results: Urinary plasmin-activity did not change in rabbits treated with $1/20 \times$ and $1 \times$ maximal tolerated dose (MTD) of norethisterone or mestranol, but it increased significantly by $50 \times$ MTD of either preparation. On the other hand, when both norethisterone and mestranol were administered simultaneously, plasmin activity did not change with $1/20 \times$ MTD, but significantly increased with $1 \times$ and $50 \times$ MTD. From these results, it was concluded that there was a synergistic action of the two compounds. This fact suggests that the oral contraceptive pills, composed of estrogen and gestagen, have a potential effect to promote hypercoagulability.

13.14.06

Inhibitor effect of placental extracts on ADP-induced platelet aggregation: Matsumoto, T, Katou, K, Ikeda, Y, Sugiyama, Y. Dept. Obstet. and Gyn., Mie Univ., School Med., Tsu, Japan

It has been reported that platelet aggregation rate is decreased in placental extract. In the present study, a specific inhibition of ADP-induced platelet aggregation by human placental leucine aminopeptidase (P-LAP) was detected as reported below. Placental extracts were treated with Triton X-100, zinc sulfate, DEAE-cellulose chromatography, Hydroxyapatite chromatography and then Sephacryl S-300 gel filtration. The eluted fractions was subjected to affinity chromatography with bestatin AH-Sepharose to obtain more purified substance. This sample strongly inhibited platelet aggregation induced by ADP, but did not influence collagen-induced aggregation, and also indicated high P-LAP activity. The alkalified sample after heating (pH 10, 60°C, 1 h) resulted in a loss of inhibitory effect on ADP-induced platelet aggregation. After preincubation with this sample and ADP, the effect of the mixture on platelet aggregation disappeared. Paper chromatographic analysis revealed the hydrolysis of ATP and ADP to AMP by this substance. In conclusion, the potent inhibitory effect of placental extracts on ADP-induced platelet aggregation appears to be due to the ADPase-like action. Attention has been focussed on this action as one of the controlling factors of hemostasis in the fetoplacental circulation.

13.14.07
Coagulation and fibrinolysis in pregnancy studied by the whole blood clotting time and the dilute whole blood clot lysis time: Omsjø, I H, Øian, P, Maltau, J M, Østerud, B. Dept. Obstet. and Gyn., and Inst. Med. Biol., Univ., Tromsø, Norway

In 20 non-pregnant, 29 normal pregnant and eight pre-eclamptic women coagulation was studied by the whole blood clotting time (WBCT) and fibrinolytic activity was assayed by the whole blood clot lysis time (CLT). The results (mean $\pm$ SD) in the non-pregnant and normal pregnant women were as follows:

	non-pregnant	3. trimester	1. day pp	5. day pp
WBCT (min)	19.24 ± 4.35	21.17 ± 3.30	17.08 ± 4.27	19.48 ± 4.39
CLT (h)	3.22 ± 1.09	11.48 ± 6.42	5.32 ± 2.22	4.45 ± 2.13

The first day post partum (pp) WBCT was significantly shortened ($p < 0.05$), but returned to normal on the fifth day pp. The CLT was significantly prolonged ($p < 0.001$) in the normal pregnant compared to the non-pregnant women. The first day pp CLT was significantly shortened ($p < 0.05$) and the fifth day a further return towards normal nonpregnant values was observed. In eight pre-eclamptic patients (data not shown) the WBCT was significantly shortened ($p < 0.001$) compared to normal pregnant women and CLT was considerably prolonged in all patients. In conclusion: A significant shortening of WBCT of the first day pp indicates an increased procoagulant activity of circulating blood after delivery. The significant prolongation of CLT in normal pregnant-compared to non-pregnant women may reflect a marked reduction of the fibrinolytic activity in pregnancy. In the pre-eclamptic patients our preliminary results demonstrate an increased procoagulant and decreased fibrinolytic activity.

13.14.08
The use of bladder retraining in idiopathic detrusor instability: Vignali, M, Riva, D, Casolati, E. 4° Dept. Obstet. and Gyn., Univ., Milan, Italy

Anti-cholinergic drugs are the therapy of choice for bladder instability; they have a recovery rate of 60–70%, but have the disadvantage of several side-effects. Following the method of *Frewen* (1978–1982) bladder retraining has been used for 18 patients who complained of urgency, frequency, involuntary urine loss and proved to be affected by idiopathic detrusor instability. The treatment consisted of filling every day for 12 weeks a voiding sheet in which the patient noticed voiding desires, amounts of urine voided and expecially whether she had been able to delay micturition without urine loss: the purpose was for the patient to lengthen the intervals between micturitions trying volitionally to inhibit bladder contractions. Urodynamic examination was performed before the training and after 12 weeks, while the sheets were checked by physicians also at 2 and 6 weeks. Every patients had also been questionned by a psychologist before and after therapy in order to reval anxiety, problems in her family, etc. Among the 15 patients who completed the trial, 13 achieved continence giving a success rate of 86.6% and two had good improvement of their symptoms and bladder capacity. Mean F. D. (first desire) changed from 110 to 175 cc. ($p < 0.05$) and mean V.S.D. (very strong desire) from 207.8 to 295.9 cc. ($p < 0.05$). The recovery proved to remain stable even three months after the end of the training. We think that bladder retraining proves to be an effective, less expensive and limitation-free therapy for idiopathic bladder instability.

13.14.09
Clinical and experimental studies of a modified Marchall-Marchetti-Krantz procedure: Fianu, S, Larsson, B, Hedström, C-G, Thorgirson, T. Depts. Obstet. and Gyn., and Morphol., Karolinska Inst. and Primate Res. Ctr, Nat. Bacteriol. Labor., Stockholm, Sweden

The Marchal-Marchetti-Krantz (MMK) procedure is a commonly used method for a surgical repair of urinary stress incontinence in the female. In order to avoid relapses and postoperative complications as osteitis, we used a modified MMK procedure. In the MMK it is essential to establish a retained fixation of the urethro-vesical junction to the retropubic periosteum. In the present experimental and clinical study, comprising four monkeys (Macaca fascicularis) and 30 women, the prolonged fixation was established by use of a combination of absorbable sutures and a two-component sealant (Tisseel, Kemi-Intressen, Stockholm, Sweden). The patients were operated upon because of an urinary stress incontinence, confirmed by urodynamic recordings. No relapses or complications have been recorded during a postoperative observation time, ranging up to two years. Histologically verified fibrosis, induced by the sealant, was observed to a certain extent, in the monkeys, which may explain the promising human results. Thus, the modified MMK procedure was found simple and easy to perform and well tolerated by the patients and so far without relapses and complications.

13.14.10
Influence of ions and drugs on the spontaneous mechanical and electrical activities of urogenital preparations: Michailov, M C, Jaud, W, Elsäßer, E, Massinger, H, Lohe, K J. Inst. Biol., GSF, Neuherberg/München

The normal and pathological functions of the urogenital tract depend essentially on the spontaneous electromechanical activities of different tract areas. We observed different specific patterns of spontaneous mechanical activities in isolated human and guinea-pig preparations of myometrium, Fallopian tubes, detrusor and pyeloureter. (Method: Europ. J. Physiol. **402**, R48, 1984; Beitr. Urol. **3**, 188, 1983, Karger, Basel.) Three types of spontaneous electrical patterns were observed in guinea-pig and human detrusor and ureter cells (intracellular recording): (1) single regular spikes, (2) spikes in burst form superimposed on slow waves, (3) burst with a plateau phase. The electrical activity of myometrium and Fallopian tubes is under investigation. The mechanical and electrical patterns can be selectively transformed by elevation or reduction of ionic concentrations (Na^+, K^+, Ca^{++}, Mg^{++}) in rinsing solutions or by hormones (adrenaline, prostaglandins) and drugs (fenoterol, Isoptin®, procaine, Urol®); the ratio (K^+):(Ca^{++}) plays an important role in this transformation. The intra- and extracellular concentrations of ions are probably of essential importance for the specific normal and pathological activities of different areas of the urogenital tract. The differences in the specific spontaneous mechanical and electrical activities of myometrium, Fallopian tubes, detrusor and pyeloureter might be explained by variations in the intracellular ionic concentrations in the different areas.

13.14.11
A prospective study of feto-maternal CO_2 metabolism by estimation of $EtCO_2$ during Cesarean section: Hazato, S. Tokyo Metrop. Ebara Hosp.; **Yamamoto, N, Momose, K, Nishimura, J.** 1st Dept. Obstet. and Gyn., Toho Univ., Tokyo; **Abe, S, Teh, A, Masaki, Y, Okawa, S.** Okawa Maternity Hosp., Matsudo, Chiba, Japan

Purpose: Prospective study of feto-maternal CO_2 metabolism during Cesarean section using anesthesia and brain activity monitor (ABM: Datex, Finland). – Materials and methods: (1) Elective Cesarean section under spinal anesthesia (30 cases) and general anesthesia (30 cases). (2) Application of pre-loading, left uterus displacement device during both spinal and general anesthesia, standard technique for general anesthesia. (3) 100% O_2 for spinal anesthesia, 50% and 66% of O_2 with 14/min ventilation for general anesthesia. (4) ABM recordings during operation for all cases and blood samples from maternal artery and vein and umbilical artery and vein (UA, UV) taken simultaneously for estimation of gas acid base status immediately after delivery of the infants. – Results: (1) A correlation existed between $EtCO_2$ and $PaCO_2$. (2) The homeostasis of UA and UV CO_2 was each maintained by a certain gradient during spinal and general anesthesia. (3) The concentrations of UA and UV CO_2 were directly proportional to the concentrations of the inhaled O_2 and the UA and UV CO_2 had low tendency suggesting of mild acidosis. From the above results, the recording of $EtCO_2$ during anesthesia for Cesarean section is deemed to be an effective index for the prospective study of feto-maternal CO_2 metabolism.

13.14.12
Colposcopy of the vaginal vestibule: Wespi, H J. Suhr/Aarau, Switzerland

The epithelium of the vaginal vestibule is identical with the vaginal and the squamous epithelium of the uterine cervix. It stains brown with 1% Lugol's iodine solution. Studying this staining (Schiller's test) with the colposcope, inflammatory and postmenopausal atrophic changes can be diagnosed.

13.14.13
Radiotherapy and surgery in the treatment of invasive squamous cell carcinoma of the vulva: Stenson, S, Malmström, H, Stendahl, U, Hesselius, I. Dept. Gyn. and Oncol., Univ. Hosp., Uppsala, Sweden

In the treatment of vulvar carcinoma, aggressive surgery may be contraindicated due to poor medical condition of the patient. The purpose of this retrospective study was to analyse survival in patients treated by vulvectomy and postoperative irradiation. 113 patients treated from 1958 to 1981 were included. Median age 65 years FIGO stage: I/27, II/45, III/33 and IV/8. Histologic grading: G1/49, G2/49, G3/15. Tumor size: T1/30, T2/50, T3/33. External irradiation to the vulvar and inguinal regions was given with ^{60}Co or a linear accelerator using a special technique. Five-year corrected survival rate (5YRS) was: Stage I/96%, II/75%, III/62% and IV/29%, overall 68%. According to Grade: G1/78%, G2/70% and G3/22%. Tumor Size: T1/90%, T2/71% and T3/37%. Recurrent disease occurred in 35 patients, most of them within two years of the diagnosis. The 5YRS decreased from 78% to 26% in patients with node involvement. High grade tumors had node involvement less frequently than low grade tumors. The 5YRS acc. to age: 60–69 years/75%, 70–79 years/38%. Single tumors had a better prognosis compared to multiple localizations, 76% and 57%. There was no postoperative mortality and the complication rate was low. The results of this study show, that with less aggressive surgical approach combined with adjuvant radiotherapy, the survival and cure of disease is high with a low morbidity rate. The knowledge of prognostic factors can help in selecting patients for optimal therapy.

13.14.14

Paget's disease of the vulva: Boonyanit, S, Vardananusara, C. Dept. Obstet. and Gyn., Fac. Med., Siriraj Hosp., Mahidol Univ., Bangkok, Thailand

Malignant vulvar Paget's disease is an uncommon disorder when compared with other gynecologic conditions. Up to the present, there have been approximately not more than 150 cases reported in the literature including those cases where subsequent vulvar recurrence or spread to adjacent areas of perineal or lower abdominal skin has been reported in a significant number of patients. The majority of patients appear to have responded relatively well to treatment, except those found to have an underlying apocrine gland carcinoma, and lymph node involvement. Four patients with Paget's disease of the vulva were encountered during the last 18 years. The patients were three Thai and one Sino-Thai, and the average age for the group was 73 years, symptoms of pruritus, bleeding, chronic ulceration, rash, eczema, were prolonged from six months to nine years. The labia majora were involved in all four cases, in two of the cases the perianal skin was also involved. Paget's cells were found in the epidermis in all the four cases, in the pilosebaceous structures of one and in the sweat ducts of the other two. Stains such as Alcian blue, mucicarmine, PAS, Gomori's aldehyde fuchsin and Lillie's ferrous iron reaction were employed to confirm the diagnosis. Definitive surgical treatments were radical vulvectomy in three instances, simple vulvectomy in one. No recurrence has been noted in the period up to eight years following treatment. No instance of an underlying invasive carcinoma were found. A multifocal autochthonous origin of the disease in the epidermis and its appendage is indicated but the exact prototypic cell is still undiscovered. Diagnosis of the vulva by biopsies is the mode of choice.

13.14.15

The anti-androgen cyproterone acetate in the treatment of breast cancer: Hackenberg, R, Schulz, K D, Schmidt-Rhode, P, Hölzel, F, Sturm, G. Univ., Marburg

The anti-androgen cyproterone acetate (CPA) was used in the treatment of 41 postmenopausal patients with breast cancer showing progressive dissemination after different schedules of cytostatic and/or endocrine therapy. CPA was able to induce partial remission or no change status in 34% of these selected patients. In nine patients different serum hormone levels were determined continuously to investigate the influence of CPA on adrenal and pituitary function. FSH, LH, prolactin, estradiol, estrone, cortisol, androstenedione (A), dehydroepiandrosterone (DHA), dihydrotestosterone (DHT) and testosterone (T) were determined radioimmunologically. FSH and LH showed a marked decrease under CPA therapy. The androgens A, DHA, DHT and T decreased by 30–50%. The other hormones showed no significant alterations during treatment. Permanent cell lines derived from human mammary carcinoma were incubated with CPA *in vitro*. A marked decrease of tumor cell proliferation was found at a dose level of more than 100 ng/ml in culture medium after five days of incubation. These results show that CPA may act directly on human breast cancer cells. On the other hand the drug interferes with the serum levels of different hormones partially known as stimulating factors of hormone dependent tumor growth. The positive clinical experience may result from the addition of both direct tumor cell mediated and indirect endocrine effects.

13.14.16

Parallel analyses of steroid hormone receptors in breast cancer: rates and possible explanations for discordant results: Locher, G W. Abt. Gyn. Path., Univ.-Frauenklin., Bern, Switzerland

Histological data on 455 biopsies of invasive mammary carcinoma were recorded, and two analogous tissue specimens selected by one pathologist were sent to two qualified biochemical laboratories for independent steroid hormone receptor analysis. In accordance with the methods of the Quality Control Study in Switzerland (*D. T. Zava*. In: Recent Results in Cancer Research **19**, 122, 1984), each laboratory estimated the receptor status (RS) according to their usual practice as positive (+), borderline (BL), or negative (−). With respect to the estrogen receptors, 310/455 parallel analyses (68.1%) showed complete concordance for designation of (−), (BL) and (+), complete discordance in 63 (13.8%), while 82 cases were within the ranges of either BL/(+) or BL/(−). Progesterone receptors were assayed in 311 double specimens, with complete concordance in 205 (65.9%), and complete discordance in 66 (21.2%). The 455 parallel interpretations of the RS resulted in complete concordance in 376 cases (82.6%) and complete discordance in 54 cases (11.9%). Possible explanations for discordant results relate to a) tissue selection by the pathologist, b) interlaboratory variability, and c) to a "biologic variability", of which tumor heterogeneity is one component. We conclude that the rate of complete concordance of RS when determined in two different laboratories by the same assay method is satisfactory.

13.14.17

Post-mastectomy lymphedema: Göltner, E, Földi, M, Fischbach, J U, Kraus, A. Städt. Frauenklin., Fulda, and Klin. Lymphol./Phlebol., Feldberg-Altglashütten

In spite of less radical interventions in breast cancer therapy, post-mastectomy lymphedema is by no means rare. The regenerative power of the axillary lymphatics, the ability to develop adequate interaxillary and axillo-inguinal anastomoses and the activity of the mononuclear phagocytic system are responsible for the development and for the prognosis of lymphedema. The usual methods of diagnosis and control of lymphedema are unreliable and time consuming. By a new optoelectronic technique, both the early diagnosis and severity of lymphedema can easily be assessed. Spread amounts to no more than 0.5%. – In 65 women, two weeks after modified radical mastectomy, in 12% of the patients lymphedema with a volume above 150 ml was found. In another 200 women investigated, 3.5 years after operation and irradiation, lymphedema was observed in 42%. In 17% the volume of lymphedema surpassed 400 ml. – Every lymphedema has to be treated but only after thorough etiological diagnosis has been established. In benign forms, complex decongestive physiotherapy consisting of a special massage technique, bandages, remedial exercises etc. has to be performed. In malignant forms, in which the transport capacity of the lymphatic systems has been reduced by carcinoma cells blocking lymphatics, the treatment of lymphedema has to come only after the institution of oncological therapy.

13.14.18

Possible histopathological criteria for the evaluation of prognosis in lymph node-negative breast cancer patients: Hilfrich, J, Stauch, G, Siebert, F. Frauenklin. and Path. Inst., Med. Hochsch., Hannover

840 out of 2700 breast cancer patients, treated between 1976 and 1982 in the department of gynecology and obstetrics of the Medical School Hannover were classified as stage $T_{1-2}N_0M_0$. Of this group we were able to record by the end of 1984 26 patients with distant metastases, as well as 40 patients with local recurrences. In addition, we chose a group of 60 patients who have been free of local recurrences and/or distant metastases for at least three years after surgical treatment as a control group. For the description of possible histopathological criteria in relation to the clinical course of those patients the histological slides of the primary tumors and the removed lymph nodes were re-evaluated retrospectively. The following criteria were considered: histological classification, grade of differentiation, tumor growth (invasive-noninvasive), blood vessel invasion, sinus carcinosis or micrometastases in regional lymph nodes. Our evaluation shows so far, that in the group of patients with distant metastases the majority had ductal carcinomas (NOS) with a lower degree of differentiation and a high incidence of blood vessel invasion. In the group of patients with local recurrences the lobular carcinomas with a medium degree of differentiation as well as increased blood vessel invasion seem to be predominant. In comparison to the results in disease-free patients the value of these criteria for the prediction of prognosis will be discussed.

13.14.19

Simultaneous diagnostic curettage during breast cancer surgery: Bieri, J, Genton, C Y, Schreiner, W E. Univ. Women's Hosp., Zurich, Switzerland

The endometrium and the mamary glands are common sites for primary malignant tumors. The increased risk for both of these malignant diseases to occur in the same patient is well known. Performing a diagnostic curettage in 78 successive patients undergoing operation for breast cancer revealed in two cases (2.5%) an occult adenocarcinoma of the endometrium. In these two patients there were neither a history nor any clinical signs pointing towards the diagnosis of uterine cancer, and both patients were in an early operable stage (stage Ia). The simultaneous diagnostic curettage in patients with breast cancer is therefore recommended.

13.14.20

Proposal to decrease the risk and improve the prognosis of breast cancer: Gambrell, R D. Dept. Endocr., Med. Coll. of Georgia, Augusta, GA, USA

This poster will show the ever increasing risk of breast cancer with age and the effect of many different hormones on mammary tissue. Of 256 patients with breast cancer diagnosed between 1972–1981, 102 have expired for a mortality of 39.8%. The mortality in the hormone users (22.2%) was significantly lower ($p \leq 0.01$) than that of the non-users (45.5%). In 162 patients whose diagnosis of breast cancer was made prior to 1979, the five-year survival rate in hormone users was 76.2% compared to 48.1% in non-users, most likely due to an earlier diagnosis. During the prospective phase of the study from 1975–1981, the lowest incidence of breast carcinoma (67.3 : 100,000) was observed in the estrogen-progestogen users, slightly decreased in the estrogen users (141.0 : 100,000) and was significantly lower ($p \leq 0.01$) than that of the non-users (342.2 : 100,000). Methods to detect early malignant changes in the breast are shown including self-examination, frequent evaluation, thermography, xeromammography, ultrasound, needle biopsy, cytologic study, and surgical biopsy.

13.14.21

Pregnancy rate and post-surgical evaluation following reconstructive pelvic surgery using the carbon dioxide (CO_2) laser – report of the multicenter intra-abdominal laser study group: Diamond, M P, Daniell, J F,

Martin, D C, Feste, J, McLaughlin, D S. Nashville, TN; Memphis, TN; Houston, TX; Dayton, OH; Los Angeles, CA, USA

Surgical procedures for the correction of tuboperitoneal causes of infertility include salpingostomy (S), fimbrioplasty (F), lysis of adhesions (LA), and vaporization of endometriosis (VE). It has been suggested that use of the CO_2 laser would improve the outcome of these procedures because of the lasers' attributes including less tissue handling, improved hemostasis, and decreased operating time. To examine efficacy of the CO_2 laser, the outcome of 161 procedures performed with the CO_2 laser were assessed as early second look laparoscopy (within 1–12 weeks). in 48 S patients, tubal patency at second look was present in 92% of patients (90% of tubes). F patients (n = 24) had a second look tubal patency rate of 96% per patient (90% per tube). Tubal adhesions at second look were present at 82% and 51% of tubes in S and F patients, respectively. In 121 women undergoing LA, adhesions were found in 87% of patients at second look. Among 82 women undergoing VE, 15% had endometriosis at second look. With a minimum of six months folllow-up, 32% of patients undergoing CO_2 laser surgery with subsequent early second look laparoscopy conceived. 57 pregnancies occurred in 52 women (two ectopic, five miscarriages and 50 delivered or ongoing pregnancies). Thus compared to previous reports, neither the postoperative assessment nor the pregnancy rates demonstrate superiority of the CO_2 laser in reconstructive pelvic surgery. We conclude that the CO_2 laser represents another instrument for use in infertility surgery, but that such use is not a panacea for the treatment of tuboperitoneal disease.

13.14.22

Increased capacity of Epstein-Barr virus (EBV) activating principle in husbands' semen of cervical cancer and sterility patients: Ida, K, *Tokuda, H, *Ito, Y, Mori, T. Dept. Gyn. and Obstet., *Dept. Microbiol., Fac. Med., Kyoto Univ., Kyoto, Japan

During the screening of natural and physiological product for their EB virus activating potency *Ito* et al. (1984) found that a considerable number of human semen specimens obtained from infertility clinics possess a marked capacity to induce EB virus early antigen (EA) in nonproducer Raji cell system when assayed in combination with n-butyrate. The EBV EA-inducing activity of the semen samples was comparable to that of the most efficient EBV EA-inducer, the plant diterpene esters such as 12-O-tetradecanoylphorbol-13-acetate (TPA). Since such active agents show overlapping with the tumor promotors in their biological reactions. Our recent results showing marked increase in such activity in husbands' semen of servical cancer patients may provide a new insight for assessing the role of semen in the etiology of human genital malignancies. The supernatant of semen samples were diluted to the final concentration of 10, 2, 0.4 mcg/ml. After incubation with Raji cell at 37° for 48 hours EBV activating potency was measured by counting the percentage of cells in the culture expressing EBV EA as detectable by immunofluorescence. Results of semen samples from husbands of cervical cancer patients showed mean EBV EA % value of (7.46), those of sterility patients (6.66), whereas the normal semen samples indicated (1.77).

13.14.23

Molecularbiological comparison of herpes simplex virus type 2 strains isolated in Japan and Sweden: Kawana, T[1], Mizuno, M[1], Sakaoka, H[2], Grillner, L[3]. [1]Dept. Obstet. and Gyn., Univ., Japan; [3]Dept. Microbiol., Hokkaido Univ., Japan; [3]Dept. Clin. Microbiol., Karolinska Hosp., Sweden

In an attempt to classify subtypes of herpes simplex virus type 2 (HSV-2) and to compare international variabilities among HSV-2 isolates, 52 HSV-2 strains isolated from genital lesions in Japan and 30 strains isolated in Sweden were analysed by cleavage profiles of HSV DNA with several restriction endonuclease. According to DNA cleavage pattern of Japanese isolates with Bam H1, Eco R1 and Hind III, we tentatively defined eight subtypes designated as A, B, C, D, E, F, G, and H. Japanese isolates belonged mainly to A, D, E and H, whereas Swedish isolates to A, D and E. Eight out of 52 Japanese isolates but none of Swedish isolates were typed as H. Clinical significance of this classification has not yet been shown. Eight out of 30 (27%) Swedish isolates showed DNA cleavage pattern which had been rarely found in Japan. These results indicate that there is an international difference among the distribution of HSV-2 subtypes and that there may be native strains in each county.

13.14.24

Chlamydial endometritis: Punnonen, R, Aine, R, Teisala, K, Heinonen, P K, Lehtinen, M, Miettinen, A, Grönroos, P, Paavonen, J. Dept. Obstet. and Gyn., Pathl., and Med. Microbiol., Univ. Centr. Hosp., Tampere, and Dept. Clin. and Biomed. Sci., Univ., Tampere, Finland

Chlamydia trachomatis is the most important cause of acute pelvic inflammatory disease (PID). It is also known as a principal cause of acute salpingitis which develops mostly on the basis of ascending infection. In this study the histopathologic manifestations of PID-associated endometritis were evaluated. Endometrial biopsies were obtained from 45 women with suspected PID of whom 31 (69%) had plasma cell endometritis. C. trachomatis was the most common organism isolated from the endometrium. Twelve (39%) of the patients had C. trachomatis isolated from the endometrium (chlamydia group), and 19 did not (non-chlamydia group). Severe endometritis ($p < 0.05$) and lymphoid follicular structures ($p < 0.001$) were significantly more common in the chlamydia group than in the non-chlamydia group suggesting that C. trachomatis is an aggressive endometrial pathogen frequently leading to severe inflammation.

13.14.25

The effect of lactate-gel in bacterial vaginosis: Andersch, B, Forssman, L, Lincoln, K. Dept. Obstet. and Gyn., Univ. of Göteborg, East Hosp., Göteborg, Sweden

In bacterial vaginosis (BV) the lactobacilli mostly are outnumbered by anaerobes. The main symptom is a foul smelling vaginal discharge. The odor arises when vaginal pH rises to 5 to make foul smelling amines volatile. The main purpose of this study was to compare the effect of a locally applied lactate-gel (buffered to pH 3.5) with that of systematically administered metronidazole on symptoms and clinical and microbiological findings in BV. Bacteriological isolation of anaerobes, Gardnerella and lactobacilli was carried out in a group of 54 women with the diagnosis BV. The patients were randomly allocated to one of two treatment regimes: 1. Oral metronidazole 500 mg twice daily for seven days, 2. 5 ml lactate-gel inserted into the vagina once daily every evening for seven days. Objective improvement was defined as lack of one or more of following criteria: 1. Positive amine test. 2. Clue cells. pH $\geq$ 5. The women in both groups became symptom-free and objectively improved after one week of treatment. Four weeks after treatment 69% were objectively improved in the lactate group and 79% in the metronidazole group. The difference was not statistically significant. Anaerobes were significantly reduced (p > 0.0001) in both groups after one weeks treatment but Gardnerella was not significantly reduced. As BV occurs frequently and is generally looked upon as a mild non-inflammatory condition lactate-gel (pH 3.5) seems to be a suitable treatment for this disease.

13.14.26

New vaginal tampon, called Meditamp: Leserf, G, Gimber, H. Bern, Switzerland

In front of the tampon is a compartment which is either air tight concealed for a definite amount of vaginal cream or gel or it can be filled with a variable amount just before use. The advantage of that tampon compared to the direct vaginal insertion of creams, gels and suppositories are: 1. No leakage after vaginal insertion and therefore more comfort. 2. Prolonged local action of the medication. 3. The medication remains concentrated in the vagina over several hours. The latter is especially advantageous when lactacid gel is used in the so called Lactotamp. In gynecological practice Lactacyd has been used for therapeutic purposes in the form of suppositories and vaginal douches. This specifically designed tampon is made for prophylactic use only. In a special preliminary study done for a pharmaceutical Company, 35 cases with yearly recurrent fungal or Trichomonas infection after swimming had no disease after using the tampon prophylactically. This indirectly supports the theory, that fungal or other vaginal infections (Monilia, Trichomonas and Gardnerella) are most likely not caused by direct contact but occur when the normal acidity in the vagina is altered. This happens especially if a person swims frequently or for a prolonged time, or is taking antibiotics or also in pregnancy and in diabetes.

13.14.27

The establishment of criteria for the evaluation of clinical effect of antimicrobial agents in the treatment of gynecological infections: Matsuda, S[1], Kawana, T[2], Tabei, T[3], Obata, I[4], Sakamoto, S[5]. Depts. Obstet. and Gyn., [1]Koto Hosp., [2]Univ., Tokyo, [3]Self Defense Forces Centr. Hosp., [4]Jikei Univ. School Med., [5]Tokyo Women's Med. Coll., Japan

We established a criterion to evaluate objectively the clinical effects of antibiotics in gynecologic bacterial infection. This consisted of five items, such as effects on alleviation of fever, relief of signs and symptoms, normalization of leucocytosis and elevated CRP, as well as bacteriological improvement. Each item was scored as 0, 1, 2, and efficacy was evaluated by summing each scores. Using this criterion, we evaluated the clinical usefulness of cefmetazole (CMZ) in 104 patients with various gynecologic bacterial infections, such as endometritis, adnexitis, parametritis, pelvic peritonitis and bartholinitis from 1982 to 1984 in Tokyo districts. Seventy-eight patients (75.0%) were evaluated as having a favorable response to CMZ therapy. Fourteen patients (13.5%) were not any better than each doctors' subjective evaluation. Since this criterion is easy to score and more objective evaluation can be obtained, we propose to use this in evaluating the clinical effects of antibiotics. We isolated from the lesions mentioned above aerobic gram-positive cocci, gram-negative bacilli and anaerobes which were susceptible to CMZ.

13.14.28

Problems in simultaneous breast reconstruction using the Radovan tissue expander: Walz, K A, Miller, B, Callies, R. Dept. Gyn., Univ. Hosp., Essen

Temporary tissue expansion (Austad, Radovan) is an additional method of immediate breast reconstruction after mastectomy. Although an implant is always needed it includes features of abdominal advancement and myocutaneous flap techniques. The easy to handle inflatable expander as described by *Radovan* (1976) has gained widespread acceptance also for submuscular placement. Since it became available in Germany we have used it up to now in 32 cases of immediate breast reconstructions after mastectomy for breast cancer. We are ready to confirm good results of the method published so far, however we would like to point out some problem areas and to demonstrate problem cases as well. The surgery as such is quite practicable and of little strain for the patient, however two procedures are always needed. The interval which we try and extend to less than three months is very incomfortable for the patient. The implants are very expensive. Early complications as hematoma, infection or dislocation of the implant are very few. There was one spontaneous deflation of an expander, but no problem with connector or reservoir. A higher breast volume could be achieved reducing the rate of contralateral breast reduction, but there are still no good high profile implants of more than 400 cc available. The reconstructed breast mound often has some ptosis from the beginning, but a somewhat flattened form of abdominal advancement technique. It is not possible to achieve as conical breast projection as with the myocutaneous flap technique of *Vasconez*. Nevertheless the importance of the tissue expansion technique has increased to such an extent, that it is becoming more and more difficult not to use it.

13.14.29

Problem areas in breast conserving treatment for invasive carcinoma: Miller, B, Callies, R, Walz, K A. Dept. Gyn., Univ. Hosp., Essen

This report focuses on technical problems of breast conserving treatment for primary and recurrent breast cancer and is based on retrospective chart review and physical examination of 50 patients treated with either lumpectomy (n = 13) or segmental resection (n = 37) axillary clearance and subsequent radiation between 1977 and 1984. All tumors were smaller than 3 cm, 11 patients had axillary metastasis, no signs of dissemination were found in any patient. The medium time of follow-up is 25 months. After lumpectomy the nearly normal appearance of the breast was preserved in 12 cases whereas segmental resection in 15 patients was followed by severe distortion of the breast and asymmetry. Generous mobilisation of the surrounding tissue, separate incision for the axillary clearance, tension free wound closure and partial transposition of the areola will help to circumvent this problem. There was no difference found in the rate of recurrence between lumpectomy and segmental resection, however follow-up time is still too short to draw definite conclusions. Salvage mastectomies had to be performed in five patients. Previous radiation delayed wound healing considerably. Three patients were adamant about simultaneous breast reconstruction. With a latissimus-dorsi flap and silicon implant an adequate breast mound was achieved. Due to the good vascularisation of the flap, healing was undisturbed. In conclusion lumpectomy achieves a better cosmetic result than classical segmental resection. The latissimus-dorsi flap is suited very much for reconstruction after salvage mastectomy.

13.14.30

Effects of prophylactic chemotherapy after hydatidiform mole and the combined chemotherapy in the early stage of invasive mole and choriocarcinoma: Ibuki, Y, Nako, J, Shinkawa, T, Igarashi, M. Dept. Obstet. and Gyn., Gunma Univ., Maebashi, Japan

The occurrence of choriocarcinoma and invasive mole can be prevented by prophylactic chemotherapy immediately after the evacuation of hydatidiform mole. From 1973 to 1983, 1267 cases of hydatidiform mole were treated in Gunma University Hospital and the affiliated hospitals in Gunma Prefecture, Japan. Of 1267 moles, 287 cases (group P) were treated with i. m. or i. v. injection of 15–20 mg of methotrexate (MTX) for five days or 25 mg MTX six times for three weeks or oral MTX 5 mg for five days or injection of 20 mg Adriamycin for five days, immediately after the evacuation of mole, while 980 cases (group C) of mole were treated by only evacuation without any prophylactic chemotherapy. Follow-up results over two years showed the occurrence of choriocarcinoma was two cases (0.7%) in group P and 14 cases (1.4%) in group C and the occurrence of invasive mole was 22 cases (7.7%) in group P and 70 cases (7.1%) in group C. Fishers' exact test demonstrated no significant change between the group P and C. This results demonstrate that prophylactic chemotherapy using MTX or Adriamycin cannot prevent the occurrence of choriocarcinoma and ivasive mole. Our recent protocol for the early stage of clinical invasive mole or choriocarcinoma is five days combined chemotherapy with MTX 0.3 mg/kg/day, Actinomycin-D 10 μg/kg/day, and cyclophosphamide 5 mg/kg/day. The repetition of this early stage combined chemotherapy succeeded in the eradication of choriocarcinoma in 327 cases of hydatidiform mole in the last three years.

13.14.31

Highly specific and sensitive measurements of desialylated forms of human chorionic gonadotropin and their clinical application: Imamura, S, Yamabe, T. Dept. Obstet. and Gyn., Nagasaki Univ. School Med., Nagasaki, Japan

Desialylated forms of human chorionic gonadotropin (ashCG) have previously been detected in the urine of patients with gestational trophoblastic neoplasia in concentrations markedly in excess of those present in the urine of normal pregnant women. Thus, the detection of ashCG may be useful for diagnosis and management of trophoblastic tumors. In order to investigate the clinical utility of such measurement we have developed five different specific and sensitive assays for ashCG in urine. Four of these are lectin-immunoradiometric assays (LIRMA) which utilize peanut or caster bean lectin to selectively extract ashCG which is then directly quantified with a purified and radiolabelled rabbit antiserum or monoclonal antibody. The other is an improved RIA which uses a specific antiserum against desialylated COOH-terminal peptide of the β-subunit of hCG (as β-CTP) to measure ashCG previously extracted with a monoclonal antibody-Sepharose 4B conjugate. These methods can be utilized in order to obtain sensitive measurements of ashCG, as hCGβ and as β-CTP in the presence of excess quantities of hCG or hLH. They have been examined for their abilities to detect desialylated forms of hCG in clinical specimens and the results obtained for patients with gestational trophoblastic neoplasia and normal pregnant women compared.

13.14.32

Radioimmunodetection of human choriocarcinoma xenografts by monoclonal antibody to placental alkaline phosphatase: Mano, H, Kato, S, Kinoshita, Y, Sugiura, M, Goto, S. Dept. Obstet. and Gyn., Nagoya Univ. School Med., Nagoya, Japan

Placental alkaline phosphatase (PLAP)-specific monoclonal antibody (MAb) 11-D-10, which did not react with other isoenzymes of alkaline phosphatase, was raised by hybridoma technique. MAb 11-D-10 were radiolabelled and administered to athymic mice bearing human choriocarcinoma containing PLAP. MAb 11-D-10 could specifically be localized in tumor tissue as compared to normal tissues. Tissue to blood ratio (T B ratio) of MAb 11-D-10 in tumor tissue increased from 1.38 at 2 days to 2.51 at 5 days after administration. On the other hand, T B ratio of isotype control non-immunized IgM in tumor tissue were 0.72 and 0.87 at 2 days and 5 days after administration, respectively. Considerable radioactivity was seen specifically in the syncytiotrophoblastic cells of the tumor section by autoradiography. Iodine-131 labelled MAb 11-D-10 were administered to athymic mice bearing choriocarcinomas with different tumor sizes and different PLAP contents to examine the differences in the radioimage caused by tumor sizes and variations in PLAP content. Tumor less than 0.3 cm in diameter could be imaged clearly by gamma-scintigraphy without any background subtraction. Also, different radioimages, almost correlating to PLAP content, could be demonstrated.

13.14.33

Tissue polypeptide antigen and cancer antigen 125 are oncoplacental and/or pregnancy-associated antigens?: Inaba, N, Fukazawa, I, Ota, Y, Sekiya, S, Takamizawa, H. Dept. Obstet. and Gyn., Chiba Univ. School Med., Chiba, Japan

Tissue polypeptide antigen (TPA) and cancer antigen 125 (CA125), whose clinical usefulness as tumor markers has been evaluated by many investigators in gynecologic malignancies, were studied with special reference to pregnancy. By using commercial radioimmunoassay kits, the levels of these two antigens were measured in the maternal sera through all stages of gestation, paired sera from umbilical artery and vein, and amniotic fluids. In addition, these antigens were investigated immuno-histochemically in the placentae with use of an avidin-biotin immunoperoxidase technique. The results obtained in this study are as follow: 1) In maternal sera, serum TPA levels remained within its normal upper limit (110 U/L) until 30 weeks in gestation, and thereafter increased gradually reaching 170 U/L (mean value), while serum CA125 levels reached the peak in the first trimester, thereafter decreased gradually, and increased again near term. 2) In umbilical artery and vein, mean values of TPA and CA125 near term were 157/177 U/L and 14/11 U/ml, respectively. 3) In amniotic fluids, mean values of TPA and CA125 were 2462 U/L and 2257 U/ml, respectively around term. 4) TPA was located mainly in the trophoblast, while CA125 was found only in the amniotic epithelium. These results suggest that TPA and CA125 are synthesized in the trophoblast and amniotic epithelium, respectively, and leak into amniotic fluids in large amounts and the maternal blood circulation.

13.14.34

Serum-progesterone (P) and -androstenedione (A) as predictors for recurrence of epithelial ovarian carcinoma: Mählck, C G, Bäckström, T, Kjellgren, O. Depts. Gyn. and Obstet., Physiol. and Gyn. Oncol., Univ., Umeå, Sweden

Background: In earlier investigations an increase in P was demonstrated in patients with "non-endocrine" ovarian carcinoma. Furthermore, that P was proportional to the tumor volume and followed the result of therapy[1]. We have found similar results with A. In the present study we have analysed the hormonal changes just before recurrence of the tumor. – Material and method: The material consisted of 13 postmenopausal women with epithel. ovarian carcinoma. The tumor volume was evaluated at regular intervals and blood samples were drawn at the same time for radioimmunoassay. – Results: The hormone concentrations at 1, 2 and 3 months prior to the date of diagnosis of recurrence were significantly lower than those of the date of recurrence. In 4/13 of the patients the lowest P concentration was observed four months before recurrence, and in 2/13 of the cases three months before recurrence was diagnosed. I. e. in 46% there was a rise in P conc. at least two months prior to the diagnosis of recurrence. In 10 of the 13 cases there was a significant rise (= twice the coefficient of variation of the assay) in the P conc. before the date, when the diagnosis of recurrence was made. A. showed a similar pattern, though less pronounced. – Conclusion: P and A may be useful markers for recurrence of epithelial ovarian carcinoma. – Ref.: [1]*Bäckström* et al. Gyn. Oncol. **16**, 129, 1983.

13.14.35

Biochemical, immunohistochemical and ultrastructural studies of four cases with amylase producing tumor: Matsuta, M, Izutsu, T, Kagabu, T, Nishiya, I. Dept. Obstet. and Gyn., Iwate Med. Univ., Iwate, Japan

Four cases of ovarian cancer accompanied by hyperamylasemia were studied biochemically, immunohisto-chemically and ultrastructurally. The results revealed that hyperamylasemia was due to the same type of increase in amylase as found in the saliva and that the isozyme pattern of the homogenate and the fluid of the tumor resembled that of the serum amylase. The serum amylase level returned to the normal level within seven days after operation and there was a close correlation between the tumor burden and the serum amylase level of the patients. The localization of the amylase in the tumor cells was immunohisto-chemically demonstrated. Also, the ultrastructure of the tumor cell cytoplasm showed zymogen-like granules in two cases. These findings supported the concept of the presence, in the cases of ovarian cancer, of a functioning tumor which produces amylase. It is considered that isozyme analysis is valuable in diagnosis and the serum amylase level has become a useful index as a tumor marker. It was founded, however, that the more poorly the tumor cells were differentiated, the less did this characteristic tend to appear. It was concluded that potential for production of amylase in the common epithelium appears in proportion to the progress of malignant change.

13.14.36
Establishment and characterization of human ovarian cancer cell line (undifferentiated carcinoma, FIGO): Yoshiya, N, Tanaka, K, Adachi, S, Kanazawa, K, Takeuchi, S. Dept. Obstet. and Gyn., Niigata Univ., School. Med., Niigata, Japan

Established, well-characterized human ovarian cancer cell lines are valuable for study on nutritional requirement, histopathogenesis and sensitivity to anticancer agents. Recently, in our laboratory, *in vitro* cell line, designated TYK-nu, was established through heterotransplantation of undifferentiated carcinoma of the ovary in nude mice. Dispersed cells were taken from tumor, which was successfully maintained in nude mice, by mincing and dispase-treatment, and cultured in Eagle's MEM with 10% FCS. Selection of cancerous epitheloid cells was completed by the fourth passage through modified colonial cloning method. TYK-nu has been subcultured serially more than 73 times over 17 months and forms monolayer in mosaic pattern with polyhedral or angular cells including several giant cells which have glycogen granules in their cytoplasm. The population doubling time is about 37 hours. Number of chromosome in the majority of cells was hyperdiploidy with a mode of 56 at the sixth passage. Heterotransplantation of TYK-nu into nude mice developed tumor which was histologically similar to the original tumor. TYK-nu was studied for drug susceptibility against cisplatin, adriamycin, vincristine, 5-fluorouracil, etoposide and human interferon using colony forming assay (*Salmon* et al., 1980) and was found to be more sensitive to both cisplatin and adriamycin, than the others.

13.14.37
Incorporation of adriamycin into transplanted ovarian carcinoma by means of sulfatide-containing liposomes: Yagi, K, Kojima, N, Takano, M, Ueno, N*, Ishihara, M*. Inst. Appl. Biochem., Mitake, Gifu, and *Dept. Obstet. and Gyn., Aichi Med. Univ., Aichi, Japan

The clinical usefulness of adriamycin (ADM), an important antineoplastic agent, has been limited by its cardiac and renal toxicities. We have empolyed liposomes containing sulfatide (cerebroside sulfate ester) to reduce the side-effects and increase ADM uptake in ovarian carcinoma. Liposomes consisting of egg phosphatidylcholine, cholesterol, and sulfatide (7:2:1, molar ratio) were prepared as small unilamellar vesicles. ADM, a positively-charged amphiphilic compound, was bound to the sulfate anion of the sulfatide on the liposomes and also inserted into the liposomal membranes in addition to being incorporated into the aqueous compartment of the vesicles, resulting in a higher degree of ADM encapsulation compared with the sulfatide-free liposomes. As compared with free drug, ADM in liposomes was maintained at much higher blood levels by reduced renal clearance and protected from metabolic degradation after administration into nude mice. The liposomal ADM reached a lower concentration in the heart and kidneys than did the free drug. In nude mice receiving ovarian carcinoma transplants, incorporation of ADM into the tumor was increased by means of the sulfatide-containing liposomes after i. v. or i. p. administration. Thus, the negatively-charged sulfatide-containing liposomes which have these advantages are clinically beneficial for use as a carrier of ADM.

13.14.38
Intramuscular administration of hydroxyprogesterone caproate in patients with endometrial carcinoma, pharmacokinetics and effects on adrenal function: Onsrud, M, Paus, E, Haug, E, Kjørstad, K. Norwegian Radium Hosp. and Hormone Labor., Aker Hosp., Oslo, Norway

A radioimmunoassay for the determination of the serum concentration of hydroxyprogesterone caproate (HPC) was established. After a single intramuscular injection of 1000 mg, the serum level reached its maximum (44–81 nmol/l) after 3–7 days. Patients on long-term adjuvant HPC treatment (consisting of 1000 mg daily for five days followed by 1000 mg every two weeks) presented peak hormone levels two weeks after the start of treatment. After a drop at five weeks, the mean serum level again slowly increased to 130 nmol/l after 25 weeks of treatment. Patients being treated by weekly injections had significantly higher serum levels than those treated every two weeks. Considerable inter-individual differences were observed. The serum levels of HPC obtained in this study compare favorably with those previously reported in patients treated with medroxyprogesterone acetate. The patients on adjuvant HPC treatment showed no significant change in the levels of circulating cortisol, dehydroepiandrosterone sulphate, androstenedione, and estrone during the first 25 weeks of treatment.

13.14.39
Screening for endometrial carcinoma by endouterine aspiration cytology with analysis of tumor markers in the aspirates: Niklasson, O, Skude, G, Johansson, R, Stormby, N. Depts. Obstet. and Gyn., and Clin. Chem.,

County Hosp., Kalmar, and Dept. Obstet. and Gyn., and Cytodiagn., Univ. of Lund, Malmö Gen. Hosp., Malmö, Sweden

A new method for postmenopausal screening of endometrial carcinoma was developed (*Niklasson* et al. Acta obstet. gyn. scand. **60**, 1, 1981). The method involves determination of lactate dehydrogenase (LD) isoenzyme activity in the uterine fluid. 18/18 endometrial carcinomas were discriminated by an abnormal LD activity. In the present study another two tumor markers, β_2-microglobulin (β_2-MG) and carcinoembryonic antigen (CEA) were also investigated. Moreover, the LD technique used was simplified and improved since we found freezing of the aspirates awaiting LD analysis not to be necessary. On the contrary, freezing reduced the LD activity. The mean LD activity in proliferative phase plus more than twice the standard deviation was considered "malignant". The corresponding LD activity in climacteric stage was considered "suspicious". – Results: All malignant cases (6/6) were discriminated as "malignant". Significant amounts of β_2-MG and CEA could support the malignant LD diagnosis in 3/3 cases without additional false positives. Out of 22 patients with a normal proliferative or climacteric endometrium one patient with a climacteric endometrium had a "suspicious" LD activity. She was later found to have an ovarian carcinoma. – Conclusion: The results indicate that screening of endometrial carcinoma should be based on the determination of biochemical tumor markers in the uterine fluid.

13.14.40

Tissue plasminogen activators (t-PA) in hydatidiform molar tissue: Tsakok, F H M, Koh, S, Yuen, R, Chua, S E, Ng, B L, Ratnam, S S. Coagul. Res. Labor., Dept. Obstet. and Gyn., Nat. Univ., Singapore

Plasminogen activator apart from being important in the blood fibrinolytic system also plays an important role in other biological processes and is involved in cell migration, tissue destruction and remodelling. Plasminogen activators (t-PA) are involved in malignant tumors such as in malignant melanoma cells. Hydatidiform molar tissue was shown to have fibrinolytic acitivity (FA) (*Tsakok* et al., 1979) and that subsequent development of choriocarcinoma was significantly more in those with decreased FA (*Tsakok* et al., 1983). The t-PA content of hydatidiform molar tissue may be directly related to FA of tissues and may be of importance in the subsequent malignant sequelae of this trophoblastic disease. There have not been any reports of t-PA on hydatidiform molar tissue before. T-PA was measured in hydatidiform molar tissue from seven patients using a plasmin generation method for determining t-PA activity. Hydatidiform molar tissue has been stored from three to seven years at $-70°$ C. They were found to produce either uterine-like or urokinase-like t-PA activity. Molar tissue from two patients produced uterine-like t-PA and FA was high being 50–116 iu/0.5 g of tissue. None of these two patients developed choriocarcinoma. Molar tissue from the five remaining patients showed urokinase-like t-PA. FA was low being 10.5–17.7 iu/0.5 g tissue. Three of these patients developed choriocarcinoma 1–6 months after evacuation and one patient has since died of the disease. It is not possible from this small number of patients to suggest that t-PA activity can help in the prognostication of malignant sequelae p = 0.5. The results encourage more research in this field.

13.14.41

Treatment of dysmenorrhea by rectal administration of two new NSAIDs: Gianella, C, Schmid, J. Klin. Frauenheilk., Kantonsspit., Luzern, Switzerland

A double-blind cross-over trial was carried out to evaluate the analgesic activity of Nimesulide and Naproxen sodium in women suffering from either primary or secondary dysmenorrhea. The patients, who entered the trial after giving their informed consent, were treated for two subsequent menstrual periods, one period with Nimesulide 200 mg suppositories and one period with Naproxen sodium 550 mg suppositories. The sequence in which the patients received the treatments was determined by a randomized schedule. The recommended administration schedule was one suppository on the eve of the beginning of menstruation and the one suppository every 12 hours, for a period coinciding with the mean duration of the symptoms. Both treatments significantly improved the painful symptoms and were very well tolerated even in women with nausea and gastric discomforts, in whom an oral form was contra-indicated. The positive judgements, however, resulted to be more frequent during the second cycle, regardless of the administered drug.

13.14.42

The impact of cytological screening on the incidence and mortality of cervical cancer: Ebeling, K, Nischan, P. Centr. Inst. Ca Res., Acad. Sci., Berlin

The paper describes some early and late outcomes to assess the effectiveness of a cytological screening programme to control cervical cancer having been in operation since 1973 in Berlin. The regular attendance rate increased continuously to more than 70%. Thus, in 1983 about 90% of women aged 20 to 59 had at least one pap-smear since the programme has been started. The age-standardized incidence rate decreased from 49.7/100,000 women (1970–72) to 33.4/100,000 (1980–82). During the same period, the mortality rate decreased from 18.9/100,000 to 11.9/100,000. Evaluating the screening history of 336 invasive cervical cancer cases, the relative risk to get cervical cancer or to die from the disease for non-screened women in comparison to those having been screened at least once during the last 5 years amounted to 3.0 respectively 11.3.

13.28.01

Psychosomatic etiology of non-specific vaginitis, a preliminary report: Berkhout, F J, Bol, J J. St. Ignatius Ziekenhuis, Breda, The Netherlands

Several micro-organisms are known as a cause of non-specific vaginitis. There is a small group of patients left with a non-specific vaginitis, characterised by a vaginal discharge which is malodorous and pruritic in most cases and causes dyspareunia and sometimes dysuria. No known micro-organisms can be isolated and treatment of these patients is without any result. The results and an analysis of interviews with five patients with a therapy-resistent non-specific vaginitis are presented. Known organisms, including Gardnerella vaginalis and Chlamydia trachomatis were not isolated. All patients had psychologic problems and more specific relational disturbances. In a follow-up interview one year later it was shown, that the vaginitis was cured after resolution of the relational disturbances. Possible mechanisms and a theory leading to vaginitis as a psychosomatic complaint are discussed. It is concluded that malodorous and pruritic vaginal discharge is for some women an unconscious excuse to resist and to escape intercourse. Thus besides the well-known causes there is also a psychosomatic entity of non-specific vaginitis and it should be treated as such. Much of the necessary counselling can be performed by a empathic approach of the physician or gynecologist and may be rewarded with a favorable outcome.

13.28.02

Free standing birthing center U.S.A.: Todd, C W, Ormsby, R B, Jukkola, G D. Family Birthing Ctr, Riverside, CA, USA

In response to our patients' quest for more family oriented birthing experiences three board certified obstetricians established the Family Birthing Center of Riverside as an outpatient birthing alternative in April, 1981. Our purpose was to provide a medically safe, home-like environment offering personalized care to the low risk obstetrical patient. Patients were carefully screened initially, during pregnancy and during labor according to written criteria. Patients falling outside the criteria were transferred to the adjacent hospital. In the first 45 months, 745 patients (87%) delivered in the center out of 856 admissions. Intrapartum transfers delivered at the hospital numbered 111 (13%). Fifty-two transferred patients (6%) required Cesarean section. Five patients were transferred post delivery. Eighteen (2.4%) of the 745 infants were transferred to the hospital for various reasons. There were no infant or maternal mortalities. Our experience of 856 consecutive admissions indicates that a responsibly managed out-of-hospital birthing center can offer a medically safe, psychologically rewarding, family centered birth experience to selected low-risk patients.

13.28.03

The influence of maternal hypnosis on fetal movements in anxious parturients: Fuchs, K, Zimmer, E Z, Divon, M Y, Eyal, A, Peretz, B A. Dept. Obstet. and Gyn. "B", Rambam Med. Ctr, Haifa, Israel

Maternal emotions are believed to have influence on the fetus and pregnancy outcome. A correlation was suggested between maternal psychological stress and a variety of obstetrical complications like hyperemesis gravidarum, abortions, toxemia, prolonged labor and fetal distress during labor. The aim of the present study was to examine if fetal activity is influenced by maternal anxiety. The study consisted of healthy women at 35–37 weeks of gestation. They were all subjectively very anxious about pregnancy outcome, although their pregnancies had a normal, uneventful progress. Real time ultrasonic recordings of fetal body movements were performed three hours after lunch. There were two recording periods, 25 min each, before and after maternal hypnosis. Women were hypnotized using eye fixation and arm levitation methods. The change of fetal movements during maternal hypnosis will be discussed.

13.28.04

Changes of self-perception and child-image by ultrasound-examination in early pregnancy: Langer, M, Ringler, M, Reinold, E. 1st Dept. Obstet. and Gyn., and Inst. Psychother., Univ., Vienna, Austria

Ultrasound is a routine examination well known to evoke strong emotions by its vivid imagery. To assess the effect upon self-perception of the gravida and upon her image of her child, we interviewed 58 women, 36 primipara, 22 multipara, with a mean age of 25.1 years. Prior to and after their first US-exam in the present pregnancy they were asked to fill in several polarity profiles concerning self and child image and emotions during the examination. Gestational age at the time ranged between the 12th and 20th week of pregnancy, in all cases before fetal movements could be felt. High-feedback information was given throughout the examination. Results show the US-exam to be well accepted and generally to evoke positive feelings. It contributes to a clearer image of the child and a better understanding of the physical changes in pregnancy. However, there were some major deviations in opinions, which will be discussed in relation to patient's pregnancy problems and social background. A hypothesis concerning the premature loosening of materno-fetal bonds by US and its positive and negative consequences are presented.

13.28.05

Depression, guilt and isolation during the crisis of infertility: Lalos, A, Lalos, O, Jacobsson, L, Schoultz, B von. Dept. Obstet. and Gyn., and Psychiat., Univ. Hosp., Umeå, Sweden

Psychological reactions compatible with a crisis reaction pattern were studied in 30 infertile women with tubal damage, and their men. During a period of two years repeated individual interviews were performed i.e. before reconstructive tubal surgery, during the first postoperative days, at second look laparoscopy and two years after the operation. Among various psychological reactions reported by the participants three main groups were distinguished: 1) Depression (despair, anxiety, depression during menstruation, irritability/sensitiveness, grief, insomnia). 2) Guilt (feeling of being guilty, general inferiority or inferiority in the marital relationship, lack of self-confidence). 3) Isolation (to avoid meeting people or children, difficulties talking about infertility with other people, adverse reactions towards pregnant women, feelings of no genuine emotional support from relatives and friends, defects in the emotional contact between the partners). The crisis reaction was apparent, long-lasting and inhibiting among the women. Depression, guilt and isolation were common both prior to as well as after the surgical treatment. Among the men psychological reactions were rare at the first interview but feelings or grief increased during the two years of the study. Supportive counselling including crisis therapy should be offered throughout the medical investigation and treatment of infertility.

13.28.06

The relationship doctor-patient in tocogynecology: Acosta, J G, Todaro, S, Agrelo, A. Bonet, J M. Univ. Nac. del Noreste, Corrientes, Argentina

Hypotheses of work are here given. They are supported in a theoretical and a referential frame existing between doctor-patient that is, a shared situation where emotional factors belonging to patients even to doctors, play a main rol. As general rule, this is considered to be true. The tocogynecology shows specific features as follow: ones, faces more with life and health than with illness and death. When the doctor at his earliest beginnings meets a "novice couple" the relation results longer and permanent and exclusively remains between the doctor and the couple. As consequence, the chances of projection and identification are deeply close without the prevention that the physical and psychical damage of any one of two will be attended by the other. This emotional "load" not always noticed and individualized on time as constituent of the relation, may affect the relation doctor-patient itself as well as the emotional stability of each of the components. Suggestions are given.

13.28.07

A study of the relation between personality and state of intelligence with the different profiles of dysfunctional urine bleeding: El Attar, A M, El Gharib, M N, Marie, S K, El-Dod, A, Shaheen, O, Bayoumi, S L. Dept. Obstet. and Gyn., Fac. Med., Univ., Tanta, Egypt

This study included 100 women complaining of dysfunctional uterine bleeding (DUB) and 20 normal cases, the latter were normal from the gynecological points of view. The intelligence quotient (I. Q.) and Minnesota multiphasic personality inventory (MMPI) scales were done for each case. Also endometrial biopsy was taken from each case to determine the endometrial pattern. The I. Q. was significantly lower among cases with (DUB) than that of the controls ($p < 0.05$). The incidence of abnormal MMPI scales was 20% among the control cases and 40% among cases of DUB, the χ^2 was significant. The commonest abnormal MMPI scale among cases of DUB was depression in 26% of the cases, followed by masculinity/feminity in 11%. Psychopathic deviation and hysteria scale, each was present in 7% of the cases, schizophrenia scale in 4% and psychasthenia scale in 3% of cases. Most of the cases with abnormal scale were associated with non-secretory endometrium. So it can be concluded from this work that there is a positive relationship between the hormonal and the personality psychopathology or state of intelligence, yet it is difficult to elucidate which change is primary to the other.

13.32.01

Metabolism of estrone sulfate in endometriotic tissue and in uterine endometrium: Carlström, K[1], Bergqvist, A[2]. Depts. Obstet. and Gyn., Huddinge Univ. Hosp., Huddinge[1], and Malmö Gen. Hosp., Malmö[2], Sweden

The metabolism of [^{3}H]estrone sulfate (E$_1$S) into [^{3}H]estrone (E$_1$) and [^{3}H]estradiol-17β (E$_2$) was studied in samples of endometriotic tissue and uterine endometrium obtained simultaneously from patients in different cycle phases. E$_1$S was efficiently converted into E$_1$ and E$_2$ by both types of tissue, and the rates of formation of the unconjugated estrogens were similar in endometriotic tissue and uterine endometrium obtained from the same patient. Since formation of E$_2$ from E$_1$S in uterine endometrium is hormone dependent, with the highest activity in the secretory phase (*Carlström* et al. Acta obstet. gyn. Scand. **69**, 519, 1983), this may reflect a similar response to hormonal stimuli by the two types of tissue.

13.32.02

The effect of treatment on experimentally produced endometrial peritoneal implants: Golan, A, Dargenio, R, Winston, R M L. Inst. Obstet. and Gyn., Hammersmith Hosp., London, UK

Endometriosis was surgically induced by implanting pieces of endometrium in the uterine mesenteries of 50 rats. Their fertility was then assessed following various treatments. Ten rats with endometriosis were treated by microsurgical excision of implants, ten by high-frequency diathermy, ten rats were treated with danazol and ten with intraperitoneal indomethacin. The implants in the remaining ten rats were left untreated. These results were compared with the fertility of ten rats undergoing sham surgery with implantation of fat in the uterine mesenteries. Reproductive performance was better in control animals with sham surgery than in animals with endometrial implants. Maximum restoration of fertility was achieved with indomethacin. Microsurgery and danazol therapy were both effective in preventing residual endometriosis but these animals tended to be less fertile after treatment. Adhesions were most pronounced after diathermy and occurred least after microsurgery or indomethacin therapy. An interesting result was seen in rats treated with indomethacin. In these animals, persistent endometrial cysts were invariably smaller near the site of intraperitoneal injection, suggesting a local antiprostaglandin effect.

13.32.03
Comparative histological studies on the binding and the effect of steroids in endometriotic tissue and uterine endometrium: Bergqvist, A[1], Jeppsson, S[1], Ljungberg, O[2]. Dept. Obstet. and Gyn.[1], and Path.[2], Malmö Gen. Hosp., Malmö, Sweden

Estrogen and progesterone binding to endometriotic tissue and uterine endometrium obtained simultaneously from the same woman was studied histochemically using E_2-BSA-FITC and P-BSA-TMRITC. Thirty endometriotic samples from 21 women were compared with endometrial specimens from 14 of the women. In 97% of the endometriotic samples binding of E_2-BSA-FITC was indicated by specific fluorescence in the epithelial cell population. The corresponding figure for P-BSA-TMRITC was 93%. In endometrial tissue binding of E_2-BSA-FITC was indicated in 93% and of P-BSA-TMRITC in 92% of the samples. Endometriotic tissue and endometrium collected simultaneously from six women were transplanted subcutaneously into 24 nude mice. In each case, specimens were transplanted to four mice; endometrium to one lateral abdominal wall and endometriotic tissue to the other. Of each four mice one was given polyestradiol phosphate, one medroxyprogesterone acetate, one danazol and one remained untreated for eight weeks, after which the mice were killed. Histologic examination of the grafts revealed changes which varied according to given treatment, but were similar in the two types of tissue. Our findings indicate that the steroid binding pattern in endometriotic tissue is similar to that in endometrium and that histological differences between endometrium and endometriotic tissue seen under natural conditions may, at least partly, be due to variations in environmental factors.

13.32.04
Higher ratios of cytosol progesterone receptor (PR) to estrogen receptor (ER) in endometriosis than endometrium: Lyndrup, J, Thorpe, S, Glenthoej, A, Obel, E, Sele, V. Dept. Gyn., Frederiksborg County Hosp., Hilleroed, Denmark

In 14 patients biopsy specimens were taken from abdominal endometriosis as well as endometrium. The specimens were parted, one part for microscopy, the other for analysis of cytosol estrogen receptor (ER) and progesterone receptor (PR). Only patients from whom sufficient material for both receptor assay and microscopy was obtained, and in whom the endometrial specimen proved microscopic endometriosis, were included. PR were detected in endometriosis in all of 14 patients, ER in only 12 of 14 patients. Significantly higher values of both receptors were found in endometrium than endometriosis ($p < 0.01$), and in both tissues significantly more PR than ER were found ($p < 0.01$). To evaluate whether the lower receptor content in endometriosis could be explained solely as a matter of dilution, the ratio between PR and ER (PR/ER) was estimated in both tissues. Significantly higher PR/ER-ratios were calculated in endometriosis than endometrium ($p < 0.01$), rejecting the assumption of simple dilution. Since endometrial stroma is known to contain only small amounts of PR, a deficiency of nutritive stroma in endometriosis might be an explanation. However, the observation might indicate a changed balance of sensitivity to estrogen and progesterone, which could be interesting, since progestogens are known to counteract the proliferative action of estrogens in the endometrium.

13.32.05
Estrogen and progesterone receptor levels in adenomyosis: Paszko, Z, Konopka, B, Chrapusta, S, Goluda, M, Ujec, M. Endocr. Labor., Inst. Oncol., Warsaw and II Clin Gyn., Med. Acad., Wrocław, Poland

Estrogen and progesterone cytosol receptors (ERc and PRc) and nuclear estrogen receptors (ERn) were investigated in 23 cases of adenomyosis and in corresponding normal endometrium and myometrium. The ERc and PRc were determined by dextran-coated charcoal method and ERn were assayed by specific binding of ^{3}H-estradiol in KCl-extracts from nuclear fraction of tissue homogenate at 30° C. It was stated that ERc levels in adenomyosis do not differ significantly from normal endometrium and are higher than in myometrium. PRc levels were significantly higher in adenomyosis than in normal endometrium and myometrium. ERn levels in adenomyosis were also significantly higher than in normal endometrium and myometrium.

13.32.06
Endometriosis: Relevance of retrograde spill, dysmenorrhea and subfertility: Hitchcock, A, Liu, D T Y. Dept. Obstet. and Gyn., City Hosp., Nottingham, UK

Laparoscopic examination of 80 patients during their menstruation was conducted. Retrograde peritoneal spill of menstrual blood was observed in 74% of patients. Dysmenorrhea was not shown to be related to this occurrence nor was the presence of endometriosis an obvious factor. A history or evidence of pelvic sepsis however is associated with dysmenorrhea in 97% of patients studied. Endometriosis was observed in only 58% of patients with retrograde peritoneal spill. If, however, in addition to retrograde spill a history of evidence of pelvic sepsis was also evident, the incidence of endometriosis (84%) was more common and significantly (p < 0.001) different from those patients with no indication of pelvic problems. This study draws attention to the importance of infection in the etiology of endometriosis and reaffirms *Meyer's* 1919 contention.

13.32.07

Limitations of early diagnosis in pelvic endometriosis: Portuondo, J A, Giménez, B, Arregui, E L, De los Ríos, A, Riego, A. Dept. Obstet. and Gyn., Hosp. of Cruces, Univ. of País Vasco, Cruces-Bilbao, Spain

Selective laparoscopy was performed in 444 patients with chronic pelvic pain-dyspareunia-dysmenorrhea and considered to be high risk of having endometriosis. Routine laparoscopy was performed in 957 patients with more than two years of infertility (moderate risk of endometriosis) and in 178 patients with menstrual disturbances considered to be at low risk of having endometriosis. Out of 250 patients with endoscopically proven endometriosis, 112 had peritoneal washings done and 75 had laparoscopically guided biopsy to confirm or rule out the disease; in 19 patients peritoneal washings were performed before and after the biopsy. Results confirmed that mild degrees of the disease were diagnosed when laparoscopy was performed on a routine basis. Cellular exfoliation of endometriotic implants (33% of washings) were not increased while performing the washings either in the follicular or luteal phase. Laparoscopically guided biopsy confirmed the disease in 63 (83.3%) of patients with endoscopically proven disease, and a higher rate (68%) of positive cellular exfoliation was found when the washings were performed after the endometriotic implants were biopsied. We conclude that early stages of the disease can only be diagnosed while performing routine laparoscopy in patients with moderate to severe clinical risk, but there is a limitation of this procedure since a maximum of 23.6% of positive results was obtained. The low rate of cellular exfoliation in endometriotic implants makes peritoneal cytology not a very useful tool in the early diagnosis of pelvic endometriosis.

13.32.08

Incidence of endometriosis discovered during laparotomy or laparoscopy: Trouvas, D, Michalas, S, Politis, G, Diakomanolis, E. 1st Dept. Obstet. and Gyn., Univ., Athens, Greece

Endometriosis is not an infrequent entity in gynecologic pathology during the reproductive life of a woman. In a five-year period 1980–1984 inclusive 5854 laparotomies were performed in our clinic and endometriosis, confirmed by pathology, was found in 189 cases giving an incidence of 3.2 per cent. Endometrial implants were located in both ovaries in 46 cases, in the right ovary only in 48 cases, and in the left ovary only in 74 cases. Other sites such as tubes, peritoneum, appendix, colon, uterosacral ligament were less frequent. The mean age of the patients was 35.4 years with a S.D. 9.35. In the same period 1282 laparoscopies were performed and endometriosis was found in 126 cases an incidence of 9.82 per cent. The most frequent indications for laparoscopy when endometriosis was found were pelvic pain and primary or secondary infertility. The mean age in this group was 30.103 years with a S.D. 5.137 years. Conservative operative surgery in combination with danazol therapy was applied in all women desiring to preserve their reproductive ability.

13.32.09

Low prevalence of the luteinized unruptured follicle syndrome in infertile women with minor degrees of endometriosis: Thomas, E J, Lenton, E A, Cooke, I D. Univ. Dept. Obstet. and Gyn., Jessop Hosp. Women, Sheffield, UK

The prevalence of the luteinized unruptured follicle (LUF) in minor degrees of endometriosis, its relationship to this condition and its role in infertility have been the subject of debate. In order to evaluate this prevalence prospectively, 19 women whose only explanation of infertility was minor degrees of endometriosis were submitted to a detailed study of the menstrual cycle following diagnostic laparoscopy. A daily ultrasound sector scan combined with estimation of the plasma LH, FSH and estradiol was performed from about Day LH-7 to Day LH + 3. Daily salivary progesterone was obtained from about Day LH-2 to menstruation. Using these data only one cycle could be described as LUF. Eleven cycles were normal in every respect. Two cycles demonstrated a follicular cyst. In four cycles there was absent or inadequate folliculogenesis. In the remaining cycle the follicle ruptured prematurely after a prolonged follicular phase. This prospective study demonstrated a prevalence of LUF of only 5.3% in minor degrees of endometriosis. It is concluded that the combination of sequential analysis of follicular dynamics and confirmatory endocrinological data lead to a more accurate diagnosis of LUF. This low prevalence contradicts the hypothesis that LUF is an important cause of endometriosis or the infertility associated with it. The variety of cycle disturbances seen in this group of patients mirrors that seen in patients with unexplained infertility investigated in the department.

13.41.01

Neonatal mortality rates in preterm infants: Relationship to birthweight and gestational age: Verwey, R A, Verloove-Vanhorick, S P, Brand, R, Bennebroek Gravenhorst, J. Depts. Obstet., Pediat. and Med. Statist., Univ. Hosp., Leiden, The Netherlands

In 1983 a nation-wide prospective cohort study was undertaken to collect data on all liveborn infants of < 32 weeks gestational age (GA) and/or < 1500 g birthweight (BW). This cohort comprises 1335 infants who represent 95% of the total very preterm- and VLBW-population in the Netherlands. Because of lethal congenital malformations or uncertain GA 128 infants were excluded. – Results: Total Neonatal Mortality (NM) was 22%. Based on BW alone, NM was 24% for infants < 1500 g (n = 983), based on GA alone, NM was 28% for infants < 32 weeks (n = 905). The relationship of NM to both BW and GA is shown in the contingency table. Application of log linear analysis to these data demonstrated that GA had a significantly larger influence on NM than BW. – Conclusion: GA- rather than BW-stratification should be used in NM statistics of preterm infants.

Neonatal Mortality Rate (%) according to Gestational Age and Birthweight in Very Low Birthweight Infants (actual numbers in brackets)

BW (grams)	GA (wks) 24–25	26–27	28–29	30–31	≥ 32	Total
≥ 1500			19 (6/ 32)	11 (21/198)		12 (27/ 225)
1250–1499		58 (7/ 12)	24 (23/ 96)	8 (10/118)	3 (5/180)	11 (45/ 406)
1000–1249	(2/ 3)	45 (31/ 69)	27 (25/ 91)	19 (13/ 68)	3 (3/ 91)	23 (74/ 323)
750– 999	86 (31/36)	48 (31/ 65)	38 (15/ 39)	19 (7/ 36)	15 (4/ 26)	44 (88/ 202)
500– 749	93 (13/14)	86 (12/ 14)	50 (5/ 10)	33 (3/ 9)	(0/ 5)	63 (33/ 52)
Total	87 (46/53)	51 (81/160)	28 (74/268)	13 (54/424)	4 (12/302)	22 (267/1207)

13.41.02

Risk factors and etiology of low birth weight in a developing country (Columbia, S.A.): Cifuentes, R, Ortiz, I, Martínez, D. Dept. Obstet. y Gin., Univ. del Valle, Cali, Colombia

A group of 1001 low birth weight (LBW) infants was compared with all newborn in general population in the same period (1983) in Cali, S.A. It was found: 1. LBW incidence in general population is 12.6%. 2. Perinatal mortality is four times higher in LBW infants than in general population infants (259‰ and 60.5‰, respectively). 3. Risk factors for LBW were in order: Twin gestation, maternal age less than 15 years old, maternal smoking more than 15 cigarettes per day, pregravid weight less than 40 kg, prenatal controls less than 4, first prenatal control in last third pregnancy, and illiteracy. 4. Morbid etiology associated with LBW were in order: premature rupture of the membranes (38%), hypertension during pregnancy (31%), preterm labor (23%) and urinary tract infection (17%). It is concluded that only by developing means for early identification and treatment of LBW risk factors will it be possible to decrease significantly the unacceptably high mortality and morbidity of low birth weight infants.

13.41.03

A method to evaluate outcome in very premature infants: Sporken, J M J, Boo, J M de*, Boon, J M**, Hein, P R**. Depts. Obstet. and Gyn., Pediat.** and Statist. Consultation*. Dept. Obstet. and Gyn., St. Radboud Hosp., Univ., Nijmegen, The Netherlands

The prognosis of very premature infants depends on duration of pregnancy (D) and weight at birth (W) and both should be taken into account when early termination of pregnancy is considered. Each perinatal intensive care unit should develop outcome curves based on W and D data of own infants who are preferably also recently born. A problem is that in most centers the populations of the infants discussed here are too small to make subdivisions into small groups of infants with the same W and D to do statistical analysis. In our study of the outcome of infants delivered prior to the 34th week of pregnancy we approached this problem by using a linear logistic model, which describes one year survival probabilities of very premature infants, based on D and estimated W. For the calculations a modified version of a program written by *Lee* was used (*E. T. Lee*, Computer Programs Biomed. **4**, 80, 1974). This method presents outcome curves in a continuous way. These curves are plotted in a graph with W on the X-axis and D on the Y-axis. Apart from the advantage that one can read from such a graph the survival probabilities of a yet unborn infant based on D and estimated W, these graphs can also be used to compare the outcome of infants born in different time periods as we did for infants born in two consecutive three-year periods. The improving prognosis for this category of infants can immediately be seen in a surveyable way.

13.41.04

Perinatal morbidity and mortality in preterm and small for dates infants beyond 2500 g: Dadak, C, Neunteufel, W, Gring, H, Janisch, H. 2nd Dept. Obstet. and Gyn., Univ., Vienna, Austria

Out of 10,826 births documented at the 2nd Department of Obstetrics and Gynecology were 575 preterm infants and 310 small-for-dates infants beyond 2500 g. Growth retardation seems to involve premature birth. The part of small for dates babies amounts 26% in the group of babies born before the 28th week of gestation. After the 37th week of pregnancy we found only 5% growth retarded infants. Maternal diseases like liver, lung, heart or renal insufficiency do not influence the dysmaturity. Statistically significant are increased symptoms of gestosis (p = 0.0001). Highly significant was the maternal age (p = 0.0073), primigravidity and primiparity as well. Also maternal size, the height (women less than 1.50 m) and also the pelvic measurements (dist spinarum and dist cristarum) show a certain influence on growth retardation. During delivery in SFD infants there are many more signs of imminent intrauterine asphyxia which are statistically significant; the less the birthweight, the more frequent the operative delivery (p = 0.0001). The highest rate of operative delivery was found in the weight group of 500–1000 g, 30%. The most frequent obstetrical operation in this collective was Cesarean section with 35%, 30% were elective sections. In case of operative delivery because of serious placental insufficiency, 93% of the infants were saved. Babies with a birthweight of 500–2500 g show, if being small-for-dates, a perinatal mortality of 16.7%, non-small-for-dates babies only 12.2%. Our results clearly point out that SFD-babies between 500–2500 g are obviously a high-risk group and have the better chance of surviving after having reached a birthweight of more than 2500 g.

13.41.05

The effect of presentation at birth and mode of delivery on neurodevelopmental outcome (3–5 years), of very low birthweight infants: Altaras, M, Cohen, I, Krikler, R, Ben-Aderet, N. Dept. Obstet. and Gyn. "A", Meir Gen. Hosp., Sapir Med. Ctr, Kfar-Saba, and Neonat. Intens. Care Unit, Beilinson Med. Ctr, Petah Tikva, Israel

The effect of the mode of delivery on the neonatal survival and on short-term and long-term outcome is still controversial. A retrospective study was performed to evaluate the relationship between mode of delivery, presentation at birth and outcome (3–5 years after birth) in 43 VLBW singleton infants born in our department. Overall morbidity was 26% while major neurodevelopmental abnormalities were detected in 21% of the infants. There was no obvious statistical difference in long-term sequelae between those infants with cephalic or breech presentation delivered by vaginal or operative delivery, either among all infants in the study or among those weighing 1001–1500 g (p = N.S.). There was no statistical difference in long-term neurodevelopmental outcome between infants in vertex or infants in breech presentation who were born vaginally. Neither was there any statistical difference between those infants with a vertex or breech presentation who were delivered by Cesarean section (p = N.S.). There was no correlation between Apgar scores at 1 and 5 minutes after delivery and long-term outcome. Among the 11 handicapped children, 3 (27%) and 1 (9%) had a low Apgar score at 1 and 5 min, respectively, while among 32 normal infants in the study, 11 (34%) and 7 (22%) had a low Apgar score at 1 and 5 min, respectively (p = N.S.). Based on the above data it appears that there is no preference in performing Cesarean section for singleton infants weighing 501–1500 g either in vertex or breech presentation with regard to long-term outcome.

13.41.06

Subsequent pregnancy following labor of a viable very low birthweight infant: Cohen, I, Altaras, M, Jaffe, R, Ben-Aderet, N. Dept. Obstet. and Gyn. "A", Meir Gen. Hosp., Sapir Med. Ctr, Kfar-Saba, Israel

It is well known that infants with low birthweight have high mortality and morbidity risk. An obstetric history of abortions, premature births and perinatal death increases the subsequent rate of loss, prematurity and perinatal death. A study was performed to find out what are the chances for a mother who gave birth to a viable very low birthweight infant to have a mature and viable infant in a subsequent pregnancy. 59 liveborn infants weighing less than 1500 g who subsequently survived had a mean birthweight of 1160 ± 263 g and a mean gestational age of 28.7 ± 22.5 weeks (range 25–32 weeks). Twenty-two (76%) of 29 mothers who subsequently became pregnant gave birth to a live infant, with a mean gestational age of 37 ± 3 weeks (range 32–41 weeks) (p < 0.001) and a mean birthweight of 2753.2 ± 570 g (range 1620–3600 g) (p < 0.001). 7 (24%) out of the 29 subsequent pregnancies terminated in a spontaneous abortion in the first trimester. All the 22 infants subsequently born, weighed more than 1501 g. 7 (31.8%) infants born weighing 1501–2500 g and 15 (68.2%) infants were born weighing more than 2500 g. In the control group of 610 mothers (at random chosen) who delivered a normal infant at term, 210 subsequently became pregnant and 208 (99%) gave birth to a normal infant at term. Mean gestational age was 39.54 ± 1.24 weeks (p < 0.001) and mean birthweight was 3299.3 ± 412 g (p < 0.001). There is a 75% chance that the subsequent infant delivered will be more mature and well developed and by that will have better chances to survive and to thrive, but this chance is less than in the normal average population.

13.42.01

Relationship of maternal and fetal lactate levels and FHR changes with duration of second stage of labor: Lunenfeld, E, Katz, M, Bashan, N, Gross, J. Div. Obstet. and Gyn., Pediat. Res. Lab., Epidemiol. Unit, Soroka Univ. Med. Ctr, Beer-Sheba, Israel

The contribution of biophysical and biochemical monitoring of labor in early detection of fetal distress has been recognized for many years. Proper management of second stage of labor with regard to the relationship between maximum length and risk of fetal morbidity or mortality has yet to be determined. In a prospective study the metabolic impact of length of second stage of labor and end stage deceleration on fetus and the mother are analysed. The variables examined included duration of second stage, preceding and concomitant fetal heart rate changes, umbilical artery vein and maternal vein lactate, PO_2, PCO_2, pH, one and five minute Apgar scores and neonatal morbidity. The total number of cases included in the present study was 153. Length of second stage ranged from one to 120 min (with 5 min recording bias, median being 15.4 min). For analysis purposes second stage of labor was divided into three time groups: < 20 min, 20–30 min, > 30 min. Lactate levels in blood samples at delivery, taken from the umbilical artery and vein and the maternal vein show increase with length of second stage of labor ($p < 0.001$). When second stage lasted for > 30 min, the mean lactate was 3.54 mmol/l and 3.65 mmol/l in umbilical artery and vein, respectively. In cases with end stage deceleration of > 20 min the mean umbilical artery rose up to 3.72 mmol/l and vein 3.97 mmol/l ($p < 0.03$ and $p < 0.005$, respectively). Lactate levels in the fetus with previous pathological heart rate were higher than those in the fetus with normal heart rate even if second stage of labor in the last group continued for longer than 30 min.

13.42.02

A comparison between glucose and xylitol for the parenteral energy supply during delivery: Ackermann, R H, Herzog, R E, Baessler, K H. Physiol. and Chem. Inst., Dept. Gyn. and Obstet., Univ., Mainz

The usual supply of glucose or fructose during delivery is supposed to support the labor from the energy side. Recently the simultaneous increase of glucose, free fatty acids, glycerol, and ketone bodies intrapartum is often explained by a reduced peripheral glucose utilisation. Therefore the effects of the parenteral supply of glucose and xylitol were studied in the maternal metabolism and for the fetal outcome. Xylitol was used as the second substrate because it is metabolised at a high rate when glucose turnover is reduced after surgical interventions. To check on the influence of parenteral supplied glucose and xylitol for mother and child the concentrations of glucose, xylitol, pyruvate, lactate, urea, glycerol, free fatty acids, and ketone bodies were measured like insulin including c-peptide in the maternal blood during delivery and in the fetal blood directly after birth: Under the glucose supply the physiological elevated maternal glucose levels increase more and the mobilisation of lipometabolism is suppressed by insulin. Fetal glucose concentrations also increase and the glucose utilisation is nearly doubled. Other maternal energy carriers like a part of free fatty acids and ketone bodies are at a low concentration so that the fetal energy exchange is reduced to glucose. Therefore the fetal situation becomes liable for lactate production and for metabolic acidosis. With a supply of xylitol these typical glucose changes are not found. Summarizing, xylitol is better than glucose for a parenteral energy substitution during delivery.

13.42.03

An analysis of uterine activity during spontaneous labor using a microprocessor system: Fairlie, F M, Phillips, G, Calder, A A. Glasgow Royal Maternity Hosp., Glasgow, Scotland

Detailed knowledge of factors regulating uterine contractility, progress in labor and fetal well-being is crucial if we are to control parturition and achieve the safe delivery of a healthy baby. We have studied spontaneous labor using a *Galtec* intrauterine pressure catheter to provide a continuous indirect measurement of uterine muscle activity and a microcomputer based system to analyse the work done. Patients were Caucasian and randomly selected. We present results derived from the first 17 (10 nulliparous and 7 multiparous). The mean height was 1.59 m (nulliparous) and 1.61 m (multiparous). There was no difference in mean birthweight between the two groups. Mean uterine activity in first stage was 1450 KPA 15 min^{-1} (nulliparous) and 1153 KPA 15 min^{-1} (multiparous). Work done in second stage proved to be greater being 2650 KPA 15 min^{-1} (nulliparous) and 2416 KPA 15 min^{-1} (multiparous). Average length of labor from insertion of catheter (usually at a dilatation of 5 cm or less) to delivery was 5 1/2 hours (nulliparous) and 3 hours (multiparous). Uterine activity was unaffected by analgesia used (pethidine or epidural) and after an initial rise in pressure, the level changed little throughout first stage. There was usually an increase in second stage even in the absence of pushing although this was less obvious in patients with epidurals. This microcomputer based system provides an accurate analysis of uterine activity in labor. It may clarify some of the factors which influence the cause of parturition resulting in a more physiological approach to augmented and induced labor and earlier recognition of abnormal activity patterns.

13.42.04

A topographical investigation of uterine contractile activity in labor: Takagi, S, Sakata, H, Matsuura, M, Takagi, K. Dept. Obstet. and Gyn., Nihon Univ. School Med., Japan

This investigation was undertaken to obtain topographical information, using surface electrodes, concerning strength and duration of uterine contractile activity during labor. We applied 12 bipolar electrodes on the lower abdomens of women in labor and recorded uterine contractive activity by "Data-recorder". This information was assimilated by Fast-Fourier Transforms (FFT) and cyclicity determined by computer. This information was interpreted into electrical activity of the myometrium, then extrapolated graphically into topograms. Our topographic patterns revealed: 1) multiple, 2) isolated, 3) interrupted, 4) regular patterns. These four distinct topographical patterns can be further classified as follows: Types 1 and 2 are most prevalent in early labor and as labor progresses types 3 and 4 become prevalent, however, remain easily reversible. Evaluation of the strength or amplitude of individual contractions revealed that the stronger the electrical activity throughout all 12 electrodes resulted in slighter variation of amplitude between electrodes, with larger high power areas, thus strong uterine myometrial contractions. The originality of this investigation involves the use of non-invasive abdominal surface electrodes to detect variations in electrical amplitude and thus determine the amplitude of myometrial contractions topographically during labor.

13.42.05

Effects of external calcium and calcium antagonist, diltiazem, on pregnant human myometrium: **Kawarabayashi, T, Kishikawa, T, Sugimori, H, Koyanagi, T*, Nakano, H*.** Dept. Obstet. and Gyn., Saga Med. School, Saga; *Dept. Obstet. and Gyn., Fac. Med., Kyushu Univ., Fukuoka, Japan

Spontaneous electrical activity and contraction of pregnant human isthmic myometrium were recorded by the single sucrose-gap method, and effects of calcium and diltiazem (DIL) on the muscle were studied. The muscle obtained at Cesarean section revealed plateau- or spike-type action potential (AP). When external Ca^{2+} was increased from 2.5 mM (Krebs solution) to 7 mM, the duration of the AP was gradually decreased and finally disappeared in both types. Amplitude of contraction usually depended on the duration of AP, however, at 3.5 mM Ca^{2+}, it was larger than that of the control. On the other hand, lower external Ca^{2+} (1.25 mM) shortened APs, and reduced the contraction. 10^{-7} g/ml DIL suppressed APs and plateau duration was gradually shortened, hence the accompanied contraction became small. However, higher Ca^{2+} could partially overcome this inhibition. 10^{-6} g/ml DIL completely abolished the spontaneous activity. In the myometrium, high K^+ contracture revealed phasic followed by tonic phases. 10^{-5} g/ml DIL suppressed both phases. These results suggest that spontaneous AP and contraction are greatly affected by external Ca^{2+} and the optimal concentration may be very limited in human myometrium. High Ca^{2+} might potentiate potassium conductance and stabilizing action of the membrane, consequently AP duration was shortened and finally eradicated. It is also suggested that DIL may antagonize Ca^{2+} mobilization at the membrane surface and intracellular site, hence suppressing the spontaneous contraction and high K^+ contracture.

13.42.06

Use of a new oral oxytocin derivate in labor: **Parikh, S, Garud, M, Parikh, V, Tejani, T.** Cama and Albless Hosp., and **Srivastava, R K.** Wander Limited, Bombay, India

One hundred and seventy patients have been given a new oxytocic derivative – desamino-oxytocin or buctocin – for various indications over a six-month period at the Cama and Albless Hospitals. The major advantage over intravenous oxytocin is that it relieves the patient of various inconveniences like immobilisation and needle pricks. It allows an obstetric patient to move about in early labor and improves her psychological approach to the delivery. This relieves the burden on the labor ward staff – both doctors and nurses. The sensitivity of uterine response of the drug is gauged by initially giving only a half a tablet and observing the frequency, duration and intensity of uterine conctraction and the fetal response. The dose of the drug for uterine inertia and acceleration of labor is 50 I.U. every half an hour up to a maximum use of eight doses i. e. 400 I.U. In induction of labor a much higher dosage i. e. 1000 I.U. in 24–48 hours is recommended. The results of treatment on over 170 patients are discussed. Induction delivery interval was six hours in cases of uterine inertia and 12–20 hours in patients with induction of labor. In 20% of patients alternative methods of delivery had to be performed. Therefore we had 100% results in uterine inertia and 80% successful outcome in induction of labor. Fetal outcome is good.

13.42.07

Neuropeptides controlling uterine smooth muscle function: **Stjernquist, M, Owman, C, Sjöberg, N-O.** Dept. Obstet. and Gyn. and Histol., Univ., Lund, Sweden

The uterine smooth muscle function is controlled by the adrenergic and cholinergic nervous systems. Recent research has revealed further neurotransmitters in the female reproductive tract, namely different peptides. Hitherto three uterine peptides have aroused most interest: vasoactive intestinal polypeptide (VIP), neuropeptide Y (NPY) and gastrin releasing peptide (GRP). These peptides have been identified in uterine nerves by immunohistochemical technique. The highest density of VIP- and NPY-nerves are observed in the cervix. Most GRP-nerves are seen in the paracervical tissue and also within the paracervical ganglionic cells. The smooth muscle effects of these neuropeptides have been studied *in vitro*. VIP has a relaxing effect both upon spontaneous and neurally induced uterine smooth muscle activity. NPY also inhibits neurally induced muscle contractions but leaves the spontaneous activity unaffected. GRP, however, has a strong contractile effect on the uterine musculature, the biological potency being of the same magnitude as that of oxytocin. In conclusion the three neuropeptides VIP, NPA and GRP are all found in nervous elements of the uterine wall, and all have obvious biological effects on the uterine smooth muscle. Thus, the autonomic nervous control of various reproductive functions seems not only to be mediated by adrenergic and cholinergic nerves but also by peptidergic ones.

14.02.01

The fetal-pelvic index: Indicator of fetal-pelvic disproportion: **Morgan, M A, Thurnau, G R, Fishburne, J L.** Dept. Obstet. and Gyn., Univ. of Oklahoma, Oklahoma City, OK, USA

Current methods of assessing fetal-pelvic disproportion (FPD) are imprecise. In order to avoid maternal or fetal sequelae of prolonged and unsuccessful labor trials, a means of prospective recognition of true FPD should prove helpful. The objective of this study is twofold: First, to develop a standardized method of identifying true FPD; and second, to test this method prospectively in a blinded manner. Forty-nine gravidas, at term gestation, with indications for either an induction or augmentation of labor were entered into the study. Fetal ultrasound measurements and maternal X-ray pelvimetry were performed prior to administering i. v. oxytocin. Using individually measured anterior-posterior and transverse diameters, circumferences of the fetal head (HC), fetal abdomen (AC), pelvic inlet (IC) and pelvic midplane (MC) were computed. Based on four circumference differences between the fetus and pelvis (HC-IC, HC-MC, AC-IC and AC-MC), a fetal-pelvic index score was derived from the sum of the two most positive values. Results of these data showed that a positive index score indicated true FPD; whereas, a negative index score indicated the absence of FPD. Following adequate oxytocin stimulated labor trials, 36 (73.5%) patients delivered vaginally and 13 (26.5%) required Cesarean section. All patients requiring Cesarean section for lack of progress in labor had a positive index score (sensitivity = 100%). Of the patients who delivered vaginally, all but two had a negative index score (specificity = 94%). One of these two patients with a positive index score underwent a difficult midforceps delivery of a 4000 g neonate for severe fetal bradycardia. The other one was delivered of a 4050 g neonate by vacuum extractor, also from the midpelvis, for severe fetal bradycardia. – Conclusions: Based on these preliminary data, fetal-pelvic index scoring is an accurate method of prospectively identifying the presence or absence of true fetal-pelvic disproportion (p < 0.001). Furthermore, with this approach, we feel that prolonged unsuccessful labor trials and difficult operative vaginal deliveries from the midpelvis may be avoided in the majority of cases.

14.02.02
Screening for intrauterine growth retardation using symphysis-fundus measurements: Axelsson, O, Cnattingius, S, Lindmark, G. Dept. Obstet. and Gyn., Uppsala Univ., Uppsala, Sweden

A prospective study was performed to evaluate the usefulness of symphysis-fundus measurements as a screening instrument for detection of intrauterine growth retardation. 528 women were followed throughout pregnancy with repeated measurements of the symphysis-fundus distance. All had their gestational age estimated by an early ultrasonic measurement of the biparietal diameter. Fourteen growth retarded (birthweight below – 2SD of the normal mean) infants were delivered by the women studied. Four different types of symphysis-fundus curves were observed. A normal curve (no measurement more than 2 cm below the mean), a static curve (no increase in the last three measurements), a catch-up curve (at least one measurement 3 cm or more below the mean but the last measurement above – 3 cm) and a low curve (the last measurement 3 cm or more below the mean). When static, catch-up and low symphysis-fundus curves were considered pathological 86% of the growth retarded infants were included. There were, however, nine false positives for every correct diagnosis. Therefore only the catch-up and low symphysis-fundus curves were designated as pathological. Then 79% of the growht retarded infants were included and only four false positives for every correct diagnosis were observed. When only catch-up and low symphysis-fundus curves are considered pathological, the number of false positive cases is reduced and 79% of growth retarded infants can be identified.

14.02.03
Changes in the pattern of history and findings concerning risk pregnancies in the course of six years: Stähler, E, Stähler, H. Frauenklin. Prof. Stähler, Siegen

More than 1800 risk-pregnancies were analysed during 1979–1984 in respect to anamnesis and findings of their risk-characteristics. The following changes were observed: Anamnestic risks of all pregnancies increased from 11.6 to 15.5%. An increase was noticed in particular after sterility therapy and operations on the uterus (sectio, metroplastic), in case of pregnancy after the 40th year of life, after adipositas permagna and abnormal increase of weight as well as addiction to tobacco during pregnancy (3.7–8.4%). The findings of risks increased from 42.0 to 44.6%. The most striking changes were noticed in an increase of premature labors (5.7–8.3%), cervical insufficiency (5.3–7.6%) and postmaturity from 3.8–14.1%. A decrease was noticed on EPH-gestoses, on suspicion of fetal growth-retardation (13.2–7.6%), on bleedings during pregnancy (6.5–4.8%). Risks according to history and findings remained unchanged (20%). The results indicate success in the care of expectant mothers (information, motivation etc.) on the one side, whereas on the mother side they show a change in social behavoir which does not always correspond with a way of life necessary for the requirements of the child.

14.02.04
Quickening – a re-evaluation: O'Dowd, M J. Portiuncula Hosp., Ballinasloe, Co., Galway, Ireland; **O'Dowd, T M.** Kings Coll. Hosp., London, UK

Traditionally quickening is said to occur between the sixteenth and nineteenth weeks of pregnancy. We investigated the onset of quickening in a prospective trial, with a carefully selected sample of 100 primigravidae and 100 multigravidae. There were strict criteria for inclusion to and exclusion from the trial. All patients were admitted to the trial by the 12th week of gestation and dates were confirmed by historical and clinical information and by ultrasound. As a further control all babies were accorded a maturity rating by a pediatrician. We found quickening occurred at 19.04 ± 1.55 weeks (mean $\pm$ standard deviation) in primigravidae and at 17.43 ± 1.72 weeks (mean $\pm$ standard deviation) in multigravidae.

14.02.05
Predicting fetal weight from fundal height and abdominal girth measurements – a practical proposition?: Woo, J S K, Ngan, H, Au, K, Fung, K P, Wong, V C W. Dept. Obstet. and Gyn., Univ., Hong Kong

Multivariate regression analysis was performed on measurements of the symphysis-fundal height (SFH) and abdominal girth (AG) in 208 primigravid patients within 48 hours of delivery. The correlation coefficient (R) between the SFH and AG and the birth weight (BW) were 0.705 and 0.557, respectively. The equation $BW = -0.14 + 0.014 \, (SFH) - 9.36 \times 10^{-3} \, (SFH)^2 + 0.017 \, (AG) - 1.38 \times 10^{-3} \, (AG)^2 + 7.58 \times 10^{-3} \, (SFH \times AG)$ yielded the best R value of 0.7400. Using a simpler equation $BW = -1.52 + 0.092 \, (SHF) + 0.016 \, (AG) \, (R = 0.7259)$, the mean percentage prediction errors were $5.7\% \pm 4.2$ (SD) in the fetuses between 2500 and 3500 g (n = 156), $9.4\% \pm 5.25$ (SD) in those > 3500 g (n = 33) and $19.1\% \pm 8.2$ (SD) in those < 2500 g (n = 19). All the equations heavily under-estimated fetal weight in the larger babies and over-estimated in the smaller babies. Logarithmic transformation and inclusion of quadratic functions did not improve the accuracy of prediction or the distribution of errors. A significant correlation (p < 0.05) was also noted between the SFH and AG measurements and the skin thickness and symphysis-xiphisternal distance measured after delivery in these patients. It was concluded that although weight prediction may be reasonably accurate in the range of fetal weight between 2500 and 3500 g, the error is too great to be clinically useful in the smaller and larger babies. Many variables can affect the accuracy of this method of weight estimation.

14.02.06

Antenatal screening for low birthweight in a South Indian population: Mathai, M, Jairaj, P. Christian Med. Coll. and Hosp., Vellore, India

Fundal height (FH) abdominal girth (AG) and total abdominal length (TAL) were measured during routine examination in our antenatal clinic. The ratio (R) of FH to TAL was calculated. Correlation coefficients were calculated on observations on 250 women who were delivered at term. The correlation coefficient was 0.76 between gestational age (GA) and FH, 0.43 between GA and AG and 0.7 between GA and R. Standard FH, AG and R charts were constructed based on these observations. These charts were used prospectively to predict low birhtweight (LBW) in 150 women, of whom 50 were delivered of LBW babies. As the mean birthweight at term in this population is 2872 ± 436 g, any observation falling below mean − 1 S. D. on the chart was considered predictive of LBW. The sensitivity of FH in predicting LBW was 74% while the specificity was 93%. Although the specificity of R was 91% the sensitivity was only 34%. The sensitivity and specificity of AG were 52% and 77%, respectively. The predictive values of FH were 84% for a positive test and 88% for a negative test. It is concluded that FH measurement is a satisfactory method of screening for LBW in routine antenatal care.

14.02.07

Nonstress testing before 30 weeks gestation: Curet, L B. Dept. Obstet. and Gyn., Univ. of Wisconsin, Madison, WI, USA

Fifteen women with normal singleton pregnancies underwent weekly nonstress testing (NST) between 26 and 30 weeks and again at 36 weeks gestation. The average number of total movements did not change between 26 and 30 weeks but decreased significantly at 36 weeks (20 vs 11). The decrease was due solely to a drop in the number of individual movements while the number of multiple movements remained steady. The percentage of individual movements was higher (69% vs 31%) before 30 weeks but slightly lower (44% vs 56%) at 36 weeks. The number of fetal heart rate (FHR) accelerations associated with both types of movement increased from 26 to 36 weeks but at all ages significantly more multiple movements were accompanied by FHR acceleration (9.7% to 55% for individuals and 68% to 97% for multiples). The magnitude of the accelerations associated with individual movements showed no significant change up to 30 weeks and averaged 13 beats per minute (BPM). At 36 weeks it increased to 19 BPM. The number of accelerations associated with multiple movements remained stable up to 28 weeks (16 BPM) and then increased to 22 BPM at 30 weeks and 28 BPM at 36 weeks. Based on these results it would appear that criteria for normal NST prior to 30 weeks are different from those at 36 weeks. In order to minimize the number of false positive tests we suggest that: 1) Only multiple movements be analyzed and 2) The magnitude of FHR accelerations be at least 10 BPM.

14.02.08

Both babies hydrocephalic in twin pregnancy. Single case presentation: Patil, M, Patil, P M. Shree Clin., Sangli, India

The very rare occurrence of hydrocephalus in both the babies of twins is presented. Limitations in diagnosis are discussed. A gravida-4 was routinely attending our antenatal clinic in 1980. By 28th week of gestation hydramnios was noticed, and at 30th week X-ray confirmed the diagnosis of twins, apparently normal. At delivery the first baby presented by breech and the aftercoming head was delivered with difficulty − it was a hydrocephalus. The second baby also presented by breech. Spina bifida was noticed and possibility of another hydrocephalic baby was suspected. This was confirmed by vaginal and abdominal examination. Two separate placentas were removed. Earlier diagnosis of multiple pregnancy on X-rays does not rule out such fetal abnormalities and hence ultrasonographic study in pregnancy for every woman has become a must. Though theoretically possible, and in spite of its very rare incidence in practice and in the literature it was encountered by us and hence is presented here.

14.02.09

Reliability of radiographic pelvimetry: Wilbrand, H, Lundh, C, Lindmark, G. Dept. Diagn. Radiol., and Dept. Obstet. and Gyn., Uppsala Univ. Hosp., Uppsala, Sweden

There is an increasing tendency to let small pelvic dimensions serve as an indication for Cesarean section without trial of labor. In a consecutive series one in ten primiparae had a pelvic outlet within the borderline values. The reliability of radiographic measurements will then be of crucial importance, which warranted an investigation of the method. – Material and method: Radiographs from 20 pelvimetries were sent for assessment to 48 radiologists all over Sweden. They estimated the sagittal inlet and outlet, the interspinous and the intertuberous distances. Ten radiologists also estimated the radiographs once again 6–12 months later. – Results: We found that every third patient will be have her pelvic outlet sum over- or underestimated by at least 4 mm and 3% by more than 10 mm. The random measurement error is about four times greater than the systematic error. The random error did not change significantly over time, but some doctors revealed a substantial change of their systematic error. – Conclusions: Radiographic pelvimetry should not be judged to be more exact than ±0.5 cm. Only in cases with very small pelvic dimensions could it be used as sole indication for operative delivery. Systematic training of radiologists should take place in order to minimize the systematic error.

14.02.10

Korean crown-rump length and the corresponding gestational sac size – ultrasonic measurement in 1st trimester of pregnancy (I): Lee, J H, Suh, B H. Dept. Obstet. and Gyn., Kyung Hee Univ., Seoul, Korea

During 1983–1984, crown-rump length and gestational sac volume in routinely employed pregnancy check were measured by real time linear scanner. These two measurements are the most commonly used in the assigning first trimester gestational age. The gestational sac is the first structure seen on ultrasound examination in pregnancy. We used the longest axis of the embryo for measuring crown-rump length (cm) and an average of antero posterior, transverse, lateral diameter of the sac for determining volume ($4/3\pi \times$ diameter^3). The data we obtained are as follows:

Duration of amenor-rhea; days from last menstrual day	Gestational sac volume (ml)	Crown-rump length measurement (cm)
35–37	0.3	
38–40	0.4(1.1– 0.2)	
41–43	1.0(1.7– 0.5)	
44–46	1.7(6.0– 0.8)	
47–49	2.1(6.5– 0.8)	1.0
50–52	4.0(12.2– 1.5)	
53–55	5.7(18.5– 1.8)	
56–58	9.9(33.1– 3.7)	1.6
59–61	11.5(29.5– 4.7)	1.9
62–64	14.5(40.0– 8.3)	2.0
65–67	21.4(61.2–19.8)	2.0
68–70	29.5(71.2–16.0)	2.2
71–73	37.0(81.3–17.0)	3.1
74–76	45.6(75.9–20.7)	3.0
77–79	56.7(112.3–28.5)	4.0
80–82	59.5(102.3–38.3)	4.3
83–85	72.1(115.2–36.8)	5.1
86–88	72.4(115.7–46.8)	5.5
89–91	89.5(141.3–67.6)	5.8
92–94	88.7(173.9–74.9)	6.0

* Second standard deviation

14.02.11

Pelvimetry with computed radiography: Homma, T, Kato, A, Koh, S, Masuda, H, Eguchi, K, Maeda, G. Dept. Obstet. and Gyn., Doai Fraternity Memo. Hosp., Tokyo, Japan

In obstetrics the risks of ionizing irradiation has been known for many years. Incidence of radiation exposure has markedly diminished since the introduction of ultrasonography, except for pelvimetry. Newly-developed computed radiography (CR) is based on the conversion of X-ray energy pattern into digital signals utilizing scanning laser luminiscence. This system will be expected to reduce the radiation dose in pelvimetry. Utilizing this system we have obtained useful information, whereas the radiation dose was reduced to 1/4~1/6 as compared with the conventional pelvimetry (Kodak Lanex regular/OH). For lateral field measurement of the absorbed doses to the rectum in the patients with high sensitive thermoluminescent dosimeters showed only 0.01 mG.

14.02.12

Seidenschnur. Rostock

Methodical as well as conceptional examinations for the purpose of optimizing evaluation of the ante- and intrapartal condition and monitoring of neonatal adaptation of healthy and asphyctic as well as potentially endangered newly born infants (prematurity, hypotrophy) have been performed on an unselected material of 5724 births of 1983 and 1984. The fetal condition by the help of cardiotocogram can be more accurately evaluated applying an aetiopathogenetic interpretation than by means of descriptions of FHF-patterns and tocograms. Fetal blood gas analysis can be restricted to 2–3% of the deliveries. – Results: At a premature rate of 6.7% (in 1983)/5.9% (in 1984), a rate of hypotrophy of 3.4%/3.4%, admission cardiotocography of 90.8/91.6%, invasive intrapartal cardiotocography of 95.0%/95%, a fetal pH-measurement of 2.7%/1.8% and determination of the state of acidity of 94.7%/95.9% the following rates were achieved: Rate of selections: 3.1%/3.2%, rate of forceps deliveries: 15.4%/14.1%, VE-rate: 1.1%/1.6%, perinatal mortality: deducting non-viable malformations and infants with less than 1000 g of weight: $9.9\%_0/9.2\%_0$, rate of stillbirths: $2.0\%_0/5.4\%_0$, rate of acidosis (pH_{NA} smaller 7.10): 0.3%/0.3%.

14.03.01

Ovarian follicular development in patients taking the combined oral contraceptive pill: Elstein, M, Killick, S R. Univ., Manchester, UK

Serial ultrasonographic measurements of uterine cross sectional area, endometrial thickness and mean dominant follicle diameter were made in 20 spontaneously ovulating women. Ten measurements were made of each factor throughout a single menstrual cycle together with simultaneous serum sampling so that levels of FSH, LH, estradiol and progesterone could be correlated with the ultrasound findings. All cycles proved to be ovulatory. These observations and serum hormone levels were then repeated throughout the first treatment month on a combined triphasic oral contraceptive regime consisting of 6 days 30 mcg ethinyl estradiol and 50 mcg levonorgestrel, then 5 days 40 mcg ethinyl estradiol and 75 mcg levonorgestrel, then 10 days 30 mcg ethinyl estradiol and 125 mcg levonorgestrel. Despite the gradual fall in serum gonado-trophin and ovarian hormone levels consequent upon contraceptive therapy there appeared to be a certain amount of autonomous follicular development in these women. This may be of relevance to anecdotal reports of occasional oral contraceptive failures with this preparation.

14.03.02

Is ovarian activity inhibited during low dose oral contraceptive use?: Vange, N van der, Coelingh Bennink, H J T, Tennekes, H, Haspels, A A. Dept. Gyn., State Univ. Hosp. AZU, Utrecht, The Netherlands

Dosages of estrogen and progestogen in oral combination type contraceptive agents (OCA) have been gradually decreased without loss of contraceptive efficacy. Aim of this study was to investigate whether hypothalamic-pituitary-ovarian suppression is complete during low dose treatment. Fifty healthy volunteers with normal body weight, a regular menstrual cycle (26–35 days), and normal visualizable ultrasound (US) ovarian follicular growth during control cycle were studied. After the control cycle OCA was started containing 30–40 µg ethinylestradiol combined with a low dose of different types of progestogens. During the first, third and sixth cycle of OCA use US examination of the ovaries and endocrine studies of ovarian activity were performed on days −1, 3, 7, 11, 15 and 19. – Results: In 52–56% of OCA cycles US follicular growth occurred. Pre-ovulatory size follicles ($\geqq 18$ mm) were present in 30–32% of OCA cycles. The incidence of US follicular growth did not decrease during the first six months of OCA use. Follicular cysts ($\geqq 30$ mm) were observed in 12 of 150 OCA cycles. A correlation was found between maximal follicular diameter and maximal estradiol level. In seven of 150 cycles post-ovulatory progesterone levels were found. These results support the impression that we are close to the lowest steroid dosages in OCA.

14.03.03

Hormonal profiles and clinical performance of natural estradiol/progestin OCs: Hirvonen, E, Stenman, U-H, Vartiainen, E, Ylöstalo, P. Depts. I and II Obstet. and Gyn., Univ. Centr. Hosp., Helsinki, Finland

The OCs are regarded as contraindicated in women over 35 because of the increased risk of thrombotic and atherogenic complications. We studied the hormonal profiles and clinical performance in forty ovulating women aged between 35–47 (mean 38) and randomized to receive either estradiol valerate/cyproterone acetate or estradiol valerate/norethisterone biphasic regimens. s-FSH, s-LH, s-PRL, s-estrone and s-estradiol were determined on days 12, 14, 16, and 22 of both the pretreatment cycle and the 1st, 3rd, 6th and 12th treatment cycles. In addition, s-progesterone and s-SHBG were determined on day 22 of the cycle respectively. Among the women (n = 20) having completed six treatment cycles to the end of January 1985 no significant differences in the mean values of s-FSH, s-PRL, s-SHBG and s-estradiol concentrations between pretreatment cycle and any treatment cycles were observed whereas s-LH was suppressed on days 12, 14, and 16 of the treatment cycles (p < 0.05) and s-estrone level was increased threefold (p < 0.01). s-Progesterone level fell below 10 nmol/l (normal ovulatory level 21–60 nmol/l) in all but four subjects having raised s-progesterone levels, three in the first, one in the third, but none in the sixth treatment cycle. Four women discontinued the treatment because of irregular bleedings. In the others cycle control was good and no pregnancies occurred in 256 treatment cycles so far. The results are promising but further work will be needed to establish their value in contraception.

14.03.04

Effect of nomegestrol acetate, a new synthetic progestin, on pituitary gonadotrophins, gonadal steroids and ovulation in normal cyclical women: Bursaux, C D. Théramex, Bagnolet; **Thebault, J J.** Applibio, Choisy-le-Roy; **Roger, M.** Fond. Rech. Hormonol., Fresnes, France

Three healthy female volunteers with regular menstrual cycles, normal pituitary and gonadal secretions received nomegestrol acetate: 5 mg/day, from day 5 to day 25 of one cycle. Plasma FSH, LH and estradiol were measured every day from day one to day 25. Plasma progesterone was measured daily from day 12 to day 25. Slight spotting was noted during the treated cycles with an early rise in basal body temperature. There was no mid cycle FSH or LH peak, mean plasma levels obersved between day 5 and day 10 were: FSH: 4.18 mUI/ml, LH: 4.12 mUI/ml, estradiol: 70.3 pg/ml. Between day 20 and day 25 of the same treated cycle they were: FSH: 4.9 mUI/ml, LH: 3.8 mUI/ml and estradiol: 84.4 pg/ml. All these values being in the range of those observed during a normal cycle. Plasma progesterone was undetectable. These results show that ovulation was inhibited as a consequence of the treamtent in the three volunteers. Similar results were obtained in another experiment with a lower dosage of nomegestrol acetate (2.5 mg/day) but with 1.25 mg/day pituitary gonadotrophin blockade was incomplete and plasma estradiol raised in the second half of the cycle. Further experiments are needed to determine: a) the 100% effective dose of nomegestrol acetate for ovulation inhibition, and b) the dose which has no action on ovulation.

14.03.05

Influence of norgestimate and levonorgestrel on SHGB: Hahn, D W, Foldesy, R G, McGuire, J L, Anderson, F, Murphy, R J. Res. Labor., Ortho Pharma. Corp., Raritan, NJ, USA

Norgestimate and levonorgestrel, 18-ethyl gonenes, are both progestational agents utilized in oral contraceptives. In standard bioassays, levonorgestrel is androgenic whereas norgestimate lacks androgenic activity at use levels (J. reprod. Med. **27**, 490, 1982; Contrac. **16**, 541, 1977). It has been suggested that the androgenicity of levonorgestrel in women is a result of its lowering of serum SHBG levels which results in displaced and elevated serum levels of free testosterone (Fertil. and Steril **38**, 48, 1982; J. clin. Endocr. Metab. **52**, 138, 1981; Contrac. **29**, 261, 1984; Acta endocr. **86**, 430, 1977). Laboratory and clinical studies were conducted to examine the effect of norgestimate in serum SHBG. When rabbits were given norgestimate and levonorgestrel, levonorgestrel induced a decrease in serum SHBG levels. Norgestimate had no effect. In *in vitro* studies, norgestimate did not displace ^{3}H-testosterone from human SHBG whereas levonorgestrel, like unlabelled testosterone, did. These results suggest that in clinical use norgestimate will not create imbalances in the free and bound fractions of endogenous steroids which bind to SHBG.

14.03.06

Metabolic effects of oral contraceptives in long-term users: Reinprayoon, D, Tangkeow, P, Nitichai, Y, Kankeerati, W, Virutamasen, P. Chulalongkorn Univ. and WHO CCR Chulalongkorn, Bangkok, Thailand

A cross-sectional study of fasting serum glucose, oral glucose tolerance tests (OGTT), triglycerides (TG), cholesterol and the liver function tests were assessed in three groups of women treated with combined oral contraceptives (OC): Group I – women on OC for 2–3 years, Group II – women on OC for 3–5 years, and Group III – women on OC for 5 years and 57 healthy non-OC users. The mean fasting serum glucose was unchanged among long-term OC users. The deterioration in glucose tolerance seem to be increased with the increasing duration of OC use. The mean OGTT area under the curve for Group III was significantly greater than those on other two groups and the controls. A statistical significant increase in TG seen with all groups of long-term OC users, though the change seen with the control was not. Metabolic impact on OGTT and TG of the high dose products (EE 50 µg and LNG 250 µg) in long-term OC users was significantly greater than that of the lower-dose preparations. No statistical significant difference could be observed among the three groups of long-term OC users and the controls for cholesterol level, total bilirubin, SGOT, SGPT and alkaline phosphatase.

14.03.07

The effect of a new triphasic low dose oral contraceptive on the glucose tolerance and lipid metabolism: Pedersen, K R, Dreisler, A, Skouby, S O. Dept. Obstet. and Gyn., Herlev Univ. Hosp. and Diabetes Ctr, Dept. Obstet. and Gyn., Rigshosp., Copenhagen, Denmark

An oral glucose tolerance test was performed in ten healthy female volunteers before and after cyclic intake for two and six months of a triphasic hormonal compound containing ethinyl estradiol and gestoden (Δ15-levonorgestrel). Besides the determination of plasma glucose and insulin also fasting levels of total cholesterol, triglycerides, free fatty acids, lipoproteins and cortisol were measured. In all volunteers the SHBG concentrations and the estrogen/androgen profiles were investigated to examine any possible relation to changes in the lipoprotein concentrations. Fasting levels of glucose and insulin as well as the areas under the glucose and insulin curves did not change during the hormonal treatment and no influence on the triglyceride levels or HDL-cholesterol/total cholesterol ratio could be observed. Judged by the SHBG concentrations and the androgen/estrogen profiles the hormonal preparation exhibited total luteal suppression and no unfavorable androgenic activity. The results indicate, that the triphasic combination of gestoden and ethinyl estradiol possess some important qualities which are demanded from oral contraceptives of tomorrow.

14.03.08

Effect of low dose oral contraceptives on glucose tolerance: Comparison of triphasic and monophasic formulations in normal and previous gestational diabetic women: Skouby, S O. Diabetes Ctr, Dept. Obstet. and Gyn. Y, Rigshosp., Copenhagen, Denmark

In two groups women with previous gestational diabetes (GDM) (n = 9 and n = 10) and two groups of non-diabetic women (controls) (n = 8 and n = 10) oral glucose tolerance tests (OGTT) were performed before and during 6 months intake of hormonal compounds containing ethinyl estradiol (EE) and levonorgestrel (LNG) in monophasic and triphasic combinations. Before treatment the previous GDMs had significantly impaired glucose tolerance compared to the controls (AUC: 1372 ± 100 (SEM) mmol $\times$ min $\times$ 1 and 1218 ± 49 (SEM) mmol $\times$ min $\times$ 1^{-1} vs. 1038 ± 41 (SEM) mmol $\times$ min $\times$ 1^{-1} and 944 ± 44 (SEM) mmol $\times$ min $\times$ 1^{-1} (p < 0.05). No differences in glucose, insulin or glucagon levels wer observed between the two groups of previous GDMs and controls. During the study no deterioration of glucose tolerance was observed in any of the groups investigated. The glucagon responses to glucose remained unchanged during the whole treatment period. However after six months treatment both the previous GDMs and the controls taking the monophasic EE/LNG preparation displayed elevated insulin concentrations during OGTT compared to the pretreatment test (AUC: 69 ± 11 (SEM) nmol $\times$ min $\times$ 1^{-1} and 65 ± 6 (SEM) nmol $\times$ min $\times$ 1^{-1} vs. 49 ± 9 (SEM) nmol $\times$ min $\times$ 1^{-1} and 53 ± 5 (SEM) nmol $\times$ min 1^{-1}, (p < 0.05). No changes in insulin response to glucose were recorded in either the control or the women with previous GDM during intake of the triphasic preparation.

14.03.09

Hormonal and histopathological patterns in post-pill ovarian suppression: Askalani, A H, Ibrahim, I I, Badrawi, M H, Yossef, M A. Al Azhar Univ., Cairo, Egypt

Post-pill ovarian suppression (PPOS) is infrequently encountered among pill users (*Shearman, R P.* Lancet **1971, II,** 64). Correlation of the hormonal status with the histopathological endometrial patterns was performed in this study in a trial to determine a causal relationship between these two factors. Twenty-eight females presenting with post-pill amenorrhea, hypomenorrhea, oligomenorrhea or oligohypomenorrhea were subjected to endometrial biopsy and hormonal determinations by radioimmunoassay procedures according to the WHO-RIA matched program 1978 using their antisera and tracers. Hormones studied were serum prolactin (PAL), follicle stimulating hormone (FSH), luteinizing hormone (L.H.), estradiol (E2), progesterone (P) and testosterone (Testost.). The average duration of oral contraceptive use was 44.9 ± 8.0 months. The patients were divided according to the endometrial picture into two main groups PPOS-proliferative and PPO-atrophic. The age of the patients and their parity did not influence the development of PPOS. There was no relationship between the length of usage of contraception and the incidence of PPOS or its duration. Hormonal data conformed with the idea of ovarian dysfunction with a general feature of ovarian suppression more marked in patients with atrophic endometrium.

14.03.10

Scanning electron microscopy studies of the effects of the progestogen only pill on the surface epithelium of the human endocervical canal: Hammad, M K, Sheppard, B L, Bonnar, J. Trinity Coll., Dept. Obstet. and Gyn., St. James's Hosp. and Rotunda Hosp., Dublin, Ireland

Biopsies of endocervix were obtained from three groups of patiens after hysterectomy. Group 1 was a control, group 2 and 3 were patients receiving either $350 \mu g$ norethisterone or $30 \mu g$ levonorgestrel daily for a minimum of eight weeks before hysterectomy. The biopsies were examined by scanning electron microscopy. In the control group, the surface of the endocervix was lined with ciliated and non-ciliated secretory cells, the majority of cells were of secretory type covered by microvilli. The luminal surface of both types of cells was convex, and the cells varied in shape from round to ovoid with diameters from $3 \mu m$ to $5 \mu m$. In patients receiving progestational steroids micropolyps were a common finding. The columnar epithelium lining these micropolyps was formed of ciliated and secretory cells. The surface topography of these secretory cells varied in (a) size from $3 \mu m$ to more than $10 \mu m$ (giant cells), (b) shape from polygonal or angular to pleomorphic in appearance and (c) contour of either flat or collapsed cells with degenerative changes. Their microvilli were reduced in number with drumstick appearance and irregularity in length. Some of these columnar cells were defined by prominent intercellular parts which may represent terminal bars. Similar but less pronounced changes of the secretory cells appeared in focal areas of the endocervix. The effect on ciliogenesis was variable with some areas of deciliation and other areas which were highly ciliated.

14.03.11

Oral contraceptives and bleeding irregularities: Wagner, H-H, Wagner, A. Dept. Obstet. and Gyn., Roskilde County Hosp., Roskilde, Denmark

A different approach to evaluation of spotting and breakthrough bleeding under hormonal contraceptive medication. An oral contraceptive containing $30 \mu g$ ethinyl estradiol and $150 \mu g$ D-norgestrel was tested in 72 women during 760 cycles. Spotting occurred in 34.7% in the first cycle and 12.9% in the 12th cycle. Breakthrough bleeding in 2.6% in the first cycle and 3.2% in the 12. cycle. This is concordant with other investigations. This apparent decrease could be caused by a high drop-out rate in the first cycles. We have tried to evaluate this problem statistically by using Fishers exate 2 $\times$ 2 test which showed no significant decrease (p = 0.05). We question the generally accepted opinion that bleeding irregularities will decrease after continuous use, especially after the third month.

14.03.12

Vitamin B₆ metabolism in hormonal contraceptive users: Amatayakul, K, Supapang, A, Sriruk, N. Res. Inst. Hlth Sci. and Dept. Obstet. and Gyn., Fac. Med., Univ., Chiang Mai, Thailand

Tryptophan oral load test and erythrocytic aspartate aminotransferase activity (EAspt.) were assessed synchronously in 135 healthy non-lactating female volunteers before, during and after 12 months administration of either a combined oral contraceptive (OC containing 150 μg of d-norgestrel + 30 μg of ethinyl estradiol), or long-acting injectables (DMPA and NET-EN). These results were compared with those obtained from other groups of subjects who used a Lippe's IUD for contraception. EAspt. activities remained unaltered in all of the studied groups, while urinary xanthurenic acid (XA) excretion following a 2G oral loading of L-tryptophan underwent significant increases in OC users. These effects were not seen in those who employed other form of contraception. Abnormal XA excretion, though corrected by daily supplementation with 10 mg of vitamin B₆, appears not to be related to true vitamin deficiency.

14.04.01

Arginine vasopressine in amniotic fluid, arterial and venous cord plasma and maternal venous plasma: Johannesen, P, Pedersen, E B, Rasmussen, A G. Dept. Gyn. and Obstet., Aarhus Kommunehosp. and Aarhus Univ., Aarhus, Denmark

High concentrations of arginine vasopressin (AVP) in arterial umbilical cord blood at the time of delivery has been attributed to either a generalized increase in the activity of the fetal endocrine system at the onset of labor or to fetal asphyxia. We measured AVP in amniotic fluid, arterial and venous cord blood and in maternal venous blood from 13 patients at 38–40 weeks of gestation at the time of elective Cesarean section with a non-asphyxic fetus (group I), in amniotic fluid from 19 patients at 15–17 weeks of gestation (group II) and in venous blood from 13 non-pregnant control subjects (group III). Our results showed a high concentration of AVP in the amniotic fluid both at the middle and end of normal pregnancy and at the same level as in arterial cord blood, whereas AVP in the venous cord blood was significantly lower and at the same level as in the maternal venous blood and in the control group. It is concluded that the fetus produces AVP and this is at least not solely caused by fetal asphyxia or related to parturition.

14.04.02

Influence of aminophylline on glucose utilization by human placental tissue in the _in vitro_ perfusion system: Żrubek, H, Bednarek, W, Oleszczuk, J. I Op. Gyn. Clin., Inst. Obstet. and Gyn., Med. Acad., Lublin, Poland

Studies were carried out on 36 term placentas born spontaneously after normal pregnancies. The method of extracorporeal perfusion of the fetal placental circulation was employed. Aminophylline was administered to the arterial side of the perfusion circuit in doses 12.5, 25 and 37.5 mg. Concentration of glucose, lactic acid and pyruvic acid were determined in samples collected from the various effluents at 0, 30, 60, 90 and 120 minutes of the experiment. On the basis of these data the utilization of glucose and the ratio of lactate/pyruvate was calculated. The results of the investigations of perfusion pressure put on record on the kymograph, lactic acid, pyruvic acid, ratio lactate/pyruvate were converted into percentage of value in minute 0 of the experiment. Aminophylline administered only once, independently of the dose, lowers perfusion pressure in the placenta. Analysis of value of utilization of glucose and a quotient lactate/pyruvate showed that aminophylline decreased utilization of glucose by placenta and increases regeneration of its energetic material as a result of intensification of oxygen decomposition of glucose.

14.04.03

Activities of coagulation- and fibrinolysis-factors in the amniotic fluid and their significance: Oberheuser, F, Kleinbauer, D, Wagner, T, Klink, F. Dept. Obstet. and Gyn., Med. Univ., Lübeck

Recent studies suggest estimation of global coagulation tests as an additional test to estimate the degree of fetal lung maturity, as a direct relation between phospholipids and prothrombin activity has been established. Our study was concerned with estimation of the single coagulation- and fibrinolysis-factors in the amniotic fluid, trying to find out, whether this increase in the procoagulatory activity is only related to the increased phospholipids and thromboplastins or whether it is related to the increase of coagulation-factors in the amniotic fluid. This study was carried out on collectively 120 samples of amniotic fluid and maternal sera at different gestational ages. The following factors were estimated by chromogenic method: Prothrombin, factor III, plasminogen, antithrombin III, α_2-antiplasmin, α_2-macroglobulin, α_1-antitrypsin. 1) No correlation between the individual factors in the amniotic fluid and maternal serum could be found. 2) A direct correlation between the increasing prothrombin/tot.prot. quotient from the 28th week on and increasing gestational age was detected. A concomitant estimation of L/S-ratio has been shown to correlate with the increase in prothrombin/tot.prot. quotient during normal pregnancy. No such correlation could be found with other individual coagulation-factors. In cases of intrauterine fetal retardation a negative correlation between L/S-ratio and prothrombin/tot.prot. quotient was found. Thus it seems that the prothrombin/tot.prot. quotient is not only a valuable parameter of fetal lung maturity but also an interesting indicator of fetal dystrophy, taking into consideration that the fetal liver is the site of prothrombin synthesis.

14.04.04

Thromboplastic activity of the amniotic fluid in term and preterm pregnancy: Fernández-Sepúlveda, R, Araneda, H. Hosp. Gmo Grant Benavente, Concepción, Chile

Thromboplastic activity of the amniotic fluid (T.A.A.F.) was measured by the Jaffé method in 74 amniotic fluid (A.F.), coming from equal number of pregnancy, whose gestational age were 34 to 42 weeks. Measurement of the T.A.A.F. were compared to the gestational age by cytology (Brossens) and with the Clements test. T.A.A.F. showed a negative correlation of 0.866. T.A.A.F. less than 71 sec concentrates mature fetus, with 98% of reliance. Values equal to or greater than 71 sec concentrate immature fetuses and 78% of reliance. Negative false were 9% and the positive ones 5%. The sensitivity of the method was 90% and the specificity 95%. The χ^2 test for the T.A.A.F. and the Clements test or the gestational age with a degree of liberty, gave an association of 47.61, with $p = -0.0005$.

14.04.05

Umbilical cord metabolism: Activities of enzymes of energy production in Wharton's jelly: Herrmann, U, Degiampietro, P, Peheim, E, Bachmann, C. Dept. Obstet. an Gyn., and Dept. Clin. Chem., Univ., Berne, Switzerland

In Wharton's jelly (WJ) of the umbilical cord, a connective tissue involved in mechanical support, various enzymes have been found by histochemical methods (*Benedetti* et al. Europ. J. Obstet. Gyn. reprod. Biol. **3/6**, 185, 1973). This finding has evoked the hypothesis that WJ is involved in the transfer of nutrients and in hormone metabolism. For testing if enzymes of energy production (carbohydrate, fatty acids) are active in WJ we determined glycogen phosphorylase (GLP), hexokinase (HK), phosphofructokinase (PFK), lactate dehydrogenase (LDH), hydroxyacyl-CoA-dehydrogenase (HAD) and succinate dehydrogenase (SDH) and compared them to placental activities (PL) at term ($n = 11$). Results: Median values U/g protein mg/g wet weight). $^*p < 0.01$

	GLP	HK*	PFK*	LDH*	HAD*	SDH	protein*
WJ	2.5	9.3	76	1734	7.3	3.8	18.4
PL	3.2	20.4	157	834	21.9	4.2	58.0

Considering the low soluble protein content of the umbilical cord, the specific activities of the enzymes being in the same range as in the placenta indicate that metabolic function beyond local needs cannot be attributed to these enzymes because of a limited total amount.

14.04.06

Nucleic acids, acid soluble nucleotides and proteins in the placenta of normal pregnancies and pregnancies with EPH gestosis: Aleksić, S, Pjević, M, Dordević, M, Gudelj, S, Višnjevac, V. Dept. Obstet. and Gyn., Novi Sad, Yugoslavia

The authors present the results of their investigations of nucleic acids, acid soluble nucleotides and proteins in 30 pregnancies with EPH gestosis and 30 normal pregnancies of the control group. Acid soluble nucleotides were determined by spectrophotometry while ribonucleic acids (RNA) and deoxyribonucleic acids (DNA) nucleotides were determined by spectrophotometry after alkaline and acid hydrolysis. The proteins were estimated by *Fallin's* reaction. The results obtained show that acid soluble nucleotides were increased in the placenta of the pregnant women with EPH gestosis and that this increase was statistically significant. The nucleic acids as well as the proteins were also increased in the placenta of the pregnant women with EPH gestosis in relation to the control group. There was a significant increase of DNA (31.79%) in relation to the control group. We named this increase "the malignancy of the placenta tissue", because DNA increase was a characteristic of the malignant processes. The authors suggest that the disturbance of purine metabolism in EPH gestosis causes the increase of acid soluble nucleotides and nucleic acids.

14.04.07

Cadmium concentrations in the human placenta: Klose, B-J, Schramel, P, Kailer, G. Gyn. Hosp. Erding and Ass. Radiat. and Environm. Res. (GSF), Neuherberg/Munich

Cadmium is one of the most frequently discussed heavy metals in the environment. It will be mostly incorporated in food and some of the chronic effects in the organism are well known. Previous studies have shown that the placenta can be seen as a very good indicator for environmental load during pregnancy. The placenta works as a filter for the non-essential trace elements like cadmium and others. Therefore an accumulation of these "toxic" metals can be observed in the placenta. The concentrations of the different heavy metals reflect the environmental situation during the nine month period. Data, especially for Cd, will be given for different regions in Germany with different environmental influences, over a period of more than ten years.

14.04.08

Study on purification of human placental oxytocin: Sugahara, M, Makino, T, Nakayama, A, Nakazawa, K, Nakamura, J, Iizuka, R. Dept. Obstet. and Gyn., Keio Univ. School Med., Tokyo, Japan

The extract solution from freshly obtained human term placenta by Cesarean section before onset of the labor was gel-filtrated through Sephadex G-25 column ("fine" grade, Pharmacia Ltd., Uppsala, Sweden; column size; 2.5 × 100 cm) with solvent of 0.2 M acetic acid and 0.0005 M $CuSO_4$. The fractions collected were divided by Lowry method into seven groups including the void volume as the first peak. Each of them were lyophilized and examined for both immunoreactivity by our own radioimmunoassay and bioactivity by Magnus apparatus using rat uterus. The first, second and fourth pooled fractions showed both high immunoreactivity and synthetic oxytocin-like bioactivity, whereas others not. The retention constant of the substance in the fourth fraction also well corresponded to that of synthetic oxytocin. These results suggest that both oxytocin-neurophysin complex and/or big hormone including oxytocin structure and presumably free oxytocin may exist in the human term placenta.

14.04.09

Studies on L-glutamate transport mechanism in human placental trophoblast microvilli membrane vesicles: Iioka, H, Moriyama, S I, Ichijo, M. Dept. Obstet. and Gyn., Nara Med. Univ., Nara, Japan

The uptake of L-glutamate in brush border microvilli vesicles prepared from human term placenta was studied using the rapid filtration technique. The uptake of L-glutamate into the vesicles occurred osmotically, and preincubation with L-glutamate increased the uptake of amino acid. These findings indicate that the uptake of L-glutamate by placenta trophoblast brush border membranes represents the transport into membrane vesicles. A Na^+ electrochemical gradient (extravesicular > intravesicular) stimulated the initial rate of L-glutamate uptake about three times. Pre-equilibration of the vesicles with K^+ stimulates L-glutamic acid uptake. Imposition of a K^+ gradient ($[Ki^+] > [K_0]$) further enhances Na^+-dependent L-glutamate uptake. Changes in membrane potential incurred by anion replacement markedly affect Na^+-dependent L-glutamate uptake only in the presence of K^+. The data indicate that Na^+-dependent L-glutamate transport can be additionally energized by a K^+ gradient. Furthermore K^+ renders Na^+-dependent L-glutamate transport sensitive to changes in the transmembrane potential difference. The initial rate of transport exhibited saturation kinetics with respect to L-glutamate concentration; an apparent Km of 0.15 mM and V of 70 p mol/mg protein in 20 seconds were calculated. The uptake of L-glutamate into the vesicles was competitively inhibited by L-glutamate and L-cysteate (acidic amino acid). These results indicate that a Na^+-dependent acidic amino acid specific transport system exists in the placental trophoblast microvilli membrane.

14.04.10

Effects of indomethacin, methylergometrine maleate, isoxuprine-HCl on the human placental 15-hydroxyprostaglandin dehydrogenase activity *in vitro*: **Nagai, K, Mori, N.** Dept. Obstet. and Gyn., Miyazaki Med. Coll., Miyazaki, Japan

The first step in the metabolism of PG (prostaglandin) is oxidation at C15 by NAD-linked PGDH (15-hydroxyprostaglandin dehydrogenase). We examined the effects of three drugs on PGDH activity. The supernatant of human placenta homogenate was used as the source of PGDH. Enzyme activity was measured by the spectrophotometric assay for the chromophore of 15-keto-PGE_2. Indomethacin concentration for 50% inhibition (I_{50}) was 40 μM, at pH 8.4, which was higher than that of PG synthetase (0.75 μM) reported by *Vane*. It seems that PGDH inhibition by indomethacin requests higher concentration than PG synthetase. The inhibition pattern by indomethacin was competitive and non-competitive with regard to PGE_2. Km value for PGE_2 was 5.87 μM, and Ki value for PGE_2 was 14.33 μM. PGDH was found to be inhibited by methylergometrine maleate with I_{50} of 1.18 mM at pH 7.4. Isoxuprine-HCl is one of drugs that relax the uterine muscles, and placental PGDH activity increased 10% to 50% by adding 1.48 mM isoxuprine-HCl at pH 7.4. These drugs showed neither inhibition nor activation of PGDH at pH 7.8. On the basis of the fact that PG stimulates the uterine activity, suppression and stimulation of PGDH activity might possibly be involved in the mechanism of their uterotonic and uterorelaxant actions.

14.04.11

Biochemical markers of the aging of placenta in prolonged pregnancy: Laudanski, T, Armatys, A. Perinat. Dept., Med. Acad., Łódź, Poland

The aim of this study was to verify the hypothesis that the prolongation of pregnancy may be caused by blockade or limitation of biosynthesis of prostaglandins by intensified lipid peroxidation. Consequently it can lead to the non-appearance of myometrial contractility. Additionally the authors tried to confirm the theory that in postmaturity the process of atherosclerosis takes place in placental vessels. The biochemical investigations of 17 placental homogenates in prolonged pregnancy and 13 in pregnancy at term were performed. The level of lipid peroxidation products were estimated by the colorimetric test with thiobarbituric acid and the level of cholesterol as a characteristic marker of atherogenesis. The reagents of Boehringer Mannheim GmbH were used. Statistically significant higher values of lipid peroxidation products were found in pregnancies terminated by the birth of postmature newborns ($13.8 \pm 0.16 : 10.6 \pm 1.8$ nmol MDA/g; MDA = malondialdehyde). Similarly statistically significant higher values of cholesterol in postmature pregnancies were found ($0.80 \pm 0.16 : 0.53 \pm 0.13$ mg/g). No significant differences were noted in other placental structures (amnion, chorion). The results confirm that the process of lipid peroxidation may take place in placenta and the increased level of peroxidation products may indicate the aging of placenta.

14.04.12

Placental function in cases of placenta praevia: El-Said, A M, Yousef, H H, Moustafa, E Y, Soliman, E M, Aly, M M. Zagazig Univ. Hosp., Zagazig, Egypt

In an attempt to see the effect of placenta praevia on placental function, a case control study of 42 cases of placenta praevia and 32 cases of normally implanted placenta were followed up prospectively. The placental function was decreased in cases of placenta praevia where the serum levels of human placental lactogen, free estriol and heat-stable alkaline phosphatase were decreased and the decrease was more with the increase in the grade of placenta praevia. The results of this study may be of value in managing cases of placenta praevia.

14.04.13

Steroid sulfatase activity in human leucocytes: Miyakawa, I, Taniyama, K, Yamaguchi, M, Mori, N. Dept. Obstet. and Gyn., Miyazaki Med. Coll., Miyazaki, Japan

Pregnancies with SS (steroid sulfatase) deficiency were first described by *France & Liggins* (JCEM **29**, 138, 1969) by *in vitro* study of placental tissue. For the rapid diagnosis of SS deficiency, SS activity was assayed in peripheral blood leucocytes from patients with SS deficiency (X-linked ichthyosis) and normal controls. SS activity was measured by desulfation of (H^3)-DHA-S using a modification of the method of *Burstein & Dorfman* (J. biol. Chem. **238**, 1656, 1963). Protein content of the enzyme solution was measured by the Bio-Rad method. Using our method, the coefficients of variation of intra- and inter-assay were 3.5% and 11.4%, respectively. SS activity in leucocytes was significantly ($p < 0.01$) greater in pregnant women in the 3rd trimester (n = 21, 0.139 ± 0.029 pmol/mg protein/8 h, mean $\pm$ SD) than normal females (n = 12, 0.108 ± 0.028) and males (n = 18, 0.088 ± 0.014). Also, SS activity was very much lower in leucocytes from patients with X-linked ichthyosis (n = 7, < 0.005) than normal fetuses (umbilical cord blood, n = 15, 0.116 ± 0.024) and other groups. We found only a small difference in leucocyte SS activity in women who are carriers of recessive X-linked ichthyosis (n = 6, 0.079 ± 0.018) and normal females. These results suggest that our assay of SS activity in leucocytes offers a fast and simple method for the diagnosis of placental SS deficiency and the identification of patients with X-linked ichthyosis.

14.06.01

Hormonal studies of women with normal and EPH-gestosis pregnancies: Mantov, S, Bogdanov, N, Liniova, V A, Mirkov, K, Kurtev, I, Kozhuharova, M. Med. Acad.-Ctr Cardiovasc. Dis. and 3rd City Hosp., Sofia, Bulgaria

Twenty-five women with EPH-gestosis in the second half of pregnancy and 36 women with normal pregnancy were studied for plasma levels of cortisol, aldosterone, progesterone and estradiol. – Method: Radioimmunologically, by means of a complex of reagents of the "Hoechst" Firm, West Germany. Average age of women investigated has been 23.7 ± 3.8 and 24.5 ± 4.7 years of age, while average arterial blood pressure was 15.99/10.43 kPa (120.3/78.4 mm Hg) and $22.42 \pm 1.22/14 \pm 1.61$ kPA (163.6 $\pm$ 9.2/105.3 $\pm$ 12.1 mm Hg), hyper- to normotensive, respectively. Considerably higher medium of plasma cortisol (x = 26.07 ± 6.28 and 22.74 ± 7.54 mg%), plasma aldosterone (x = 27.32 ± 10.09 and 24.2 ± 14.16 pg%), plasma progesterone (x = 37.79 ± 5.6 pg/ml) and plasma estradiol (x = 1883.84 ± 439 and 1451.78 ± 370.88 pg/ml) have been observed. Higher rates of hormones tested dominate in both groups of pregnant women. The mineral corticoidal glucocorticoidal and corticosteroidal overproduction, thus, increased in both groups of pregnant women investigated, does not give us any grounds for discussing their direct participation in the genesis of arterial blood pressure of pregnant women with EPH-gestosis.

14.06.02

Effect of advanced labor on concentration of estrogen in uterine, umbilical and placental blood: Takahashi, K, Endo, H, Ikeno, N, Watanabe, M, Shima, I, Yamamoto, H. Dept. Obstet. and Gyn., Sendai Nat. Hosp., Sendai, Japan

Peripheral venous, uterine venous, retroplacental and umbilical cord venous blood were collected from 20 pregnant women (33–42 weeks) undergoing Cesarean section, who were divided into three groups: 10 non-labor, five advanced labor and five gestosis non-labor women. Serum levels of estrone (E_1), estradiol (E_2), estriol (E_3) and progesterone (P) were determined by RIA and compared among these groups. Serum E_1 levels in peripheral, uterine and umbilical cord blood of the advanced labor women were significantly higher than the levels of the other groups. No significant differences in these levels were observed between the non-labor and gestosis women. However, serum E_1 levels in retroplacental blood of the gestosis women had a tendency to be lower than the level of the non-labor women. Serum E_2 levels in all blood samples from the advanced labor women were significantly higher than the levels in the other groups. There was no significant difference in these levels between the non-labor and gestosis women. Serum E_3 levels in the gestosis women slightly decreased as compared to the levels in the other groups. A ratio of P to E_2 in the advanced labor women was lower than in the other groups. These results suggests that production of estrogen is influenced by labor and gestosis.

14.06.03

Significance of sex steroids, prostaglandins and oxytocin in blood and myometrium in pre- and post implantation period: Satoh, N, Kodaira, H, Suzuki, H, Fukasawa, M, Katoh, H, Den, K, Takagi, S. Dept. Obstet. and Gyn., Nihon Univ., Itabashi, Tokyo, Japan

During the period of implantation, there are marked changes in the endocrine homeostasis in the maternal circulation, endometrium and myometrium. In these compartments, sex steroids (estrogen, E; progesterone, P), prostaglandins (PGF, PGE) and oxytocin (OT) may conceivably interact to establish a successful implantation. The present study was performed to study the changes of these hormonal events. Timed pregnant Wistar strain rats were used and E, P, PGF, PGE and OT in the circulation and receptors (R) of these hormones were determined chronologically. Serum E showed two peaks on day 3 (81 pg/ml) and 6 (121 pg/ml) postconception (pc). P started to rise on day 3 pc (73 ng/ml) and the nuclear PR on day 4 pc (400 fmol/mg DNA) and maintained these levels. PGE levels on day 1 and 3 pc were 2.0 and 1.8 ng/ml and PGE-R started to decrease on day 3 pc. PGF peaked on day 5 pc but PGF-R started to decrease on day 1 pc. OT also had peak on day 2 pc (290 μIU/ml) but OT-R began to fall on day 1 pc. These results suggest the presence of integrated hormonal changes both in the circulation and intracellular receptor levels during the period of implantation.

14.06.04

Quick measurement of unconjugated estriol and estradiol by high performance liquid chromatography (HPLC) and its application for management of abnormal pregnancies: Kondo, Z, Makino, T, Uchida, N, Takahashi, M, Fukuoka, K, Iizuka, R. Dept. Obstet. and Gyn., Keio Univ. School Med., Tokyo, Japan

By utilizing newly developed HPLC apparatus that is capable of measuring serum unconjugated estriol (E3) and estradiol (E2) within 22 minutes, alterations of these two steroids were analysed in 61 normal pregnant women at 20 to 41 weeks of gestation and in various kinds of high risk pregnancies. Serum levels of E3 gradually increased from 2.9 ng/ml at 20 weeks to 12.9 ng/ml at 40 weeks (mean values), concomitantly unconjugated E2 also increased 10.7 ng/ml to 28.2 ng/ml. The correlation of values with HPLC and RIA is E3:Y = 0.875X-0.172, the coefficient of correlation is 0.899, E2:Y = 0.972X + 6.791, the coefficient of correlation is 0.841 (Y = RIA values, X = HPLC values). Thus it is expected that HPLC method is useful for evaluating feto-placental function. In high risk pregnancies including with diabetes mellitus, sever toxemia, anencephalus, IgA nephropathy and previous poor obstetrical history, lower levels of serum unconjugated E3, especially progressive decline of this hormone strongly indicated feto-placental dysfunction following severe fetal distress. These findings suggest that frequent measurements of blood levels of unconjugated estriol and estradiol by this device improve perinatal management in high risk pregnancy.

14.06.05

Serum estriol assays and intrapartum fetal heart rate testing in predicting fetal outcome: Becker, G, Gerhard, I, Runnebaum, B, Kubli, F. Women's Hosp., Univ., Heidelberg

As part of a prospective study, intrapartum fetal heart rate monitoring was performed in 687 women with singleton pregnancies. For the interpretation of the cardiotocogram (CTG) the Meyer-Menk score was used; number and type of accelerations, decelerations and contractions were separately evaluated. During the last trimester of all these pregnancies blood samples were routinely taken for the post-partum determination of free estriol (E_3) in serum. The results of the hormone assays and of the fetal heart rate tracings were compared with the fetal state at birth and to the infants' development up to two years of age. There was a significant correlation between abnormal fetal heart rate tracings and premature delivery, low Apgar scores, acidosis and postnatal complications, especially pulmonary disorders (p = 0.01). Serial or single E_3 determinations during the third trimester exhibited a stronger association with the above mentioned factors than CTG (p = 0.0001). In addition, infants of mothers with low E_3 levels showed significant retardation of physical and intellectual development in the first two years of age, while there was no correlation with the intrapartum CTG. The E_3 levels of the third trimester showed no correlation to the CTG. Only after high E_3 concentrations in the week of birth, there was evidence of significantly fewer decelerations and better intrapartum CTG scores (p = 0.05). Our data suggest a better prognostication of the state of the newborn and of the infant up to two years, if antepartum E_3 assays are performed in addition to intrapartum fetal heart rate tracings.

14.06.06

Physico-chemical characteristics of progestin binding protein in human chorion and term placenta: Asai, M, Fukunaga, T, Sagara, Y. Dept. Obstet. and Gyn., Kochi Med. School, Kochi, Japan

Although progesterone (P) is recognized as an essential steroid for maintaining pregnancy, the mechanism of action of P has not been proved in human trophoblastic tissues. We report here our attempt in elucidating the mechanism of P in human chorion and term placenta. Cytosol from chorion or term placenta was labelled with 3H-R5020. The dissociation constant and the concentration of progestin binding site were determined. For a qualitative study, the progestin binding protein (PBP) analysed by an analytical isoelectric focusing (IEF). Scatchard analysis demonstrated progestin binding of high affinity (Kd = 13.4 $\times$ 10^{-9} M for chorion and 17.7 $\times$ 10^{-9} M for placenta) and low capacity (57.7 fmol/mg protein for chorion and 729 fmol/mg protein for placenta). The PBP from chorion was focused as two peaks at pI 6.0

and 5.3, whereas that from placenta was focused as single peak at pI 5.3. Progesterone receptor (PR) of human endometrium was focused as two peaks at pI 6.3 and 6.0. And the peak at pI 6.0 correlated significantly with the binding affinity of PR to chromatin. Our data show that although PBP exists in human chorion and placenta, it may be different in physico-chemical characteristics from PR in human endometrium. Furthermore, it was suggested that the action of P might be regulated by qualitative change of cytosolic PBP in human trophoblastic tissues through pregnancy.

14.06.07

Hyperandrogenism: Total and free testosterone (T), dihydro-T (DHT) during pregnancy: Moltz, L, Hollmann, K-J, Schwartz, U, Hammerstein, J. Dept. Gyn. Endocr., Sterility, Family Planning, UFK, Steglitz, Berlin
Free and total T (pg/ml; mean $\pm$ SD) and DHT were measured by equilibrium dialysis and RIA, resp., in 30 androgenized patients at monthly intervals from week (wk) 5 of gestation until delivery, since such data are lacking. Compared to 388 non-hirsute gravid controls, free and total T were significantly higher. Total T rose considerably during the first trimester, reaching a peak between wk 9–12, followed by a slight decrease and another increase between wk 37–40. Similar pattern were observed with free T and DHT. Representative examples are:

Gest. age	total T	free T	DHT
non-gravid	670 ± 240	9.8 ± 7.6	–
9–12 wk	1375 ± 836	12.2 ± 12.7	398 ± 238
13–16 wk	1173 ± 510	7.6 ± 7.2	396 ± 246
37–40 wk	1283 ± 643	3.8 ± 3.6	327 ± 148
post-partum	617 ± 356	3.5 ± 2.2	300 ± 162

The values were not influenced by infant sex. Total T was elevated throughout pregnancy; it exceeded the critical value suspicious of tumorous hyperandrogenism (non-gravid patients: 1.5 ng/ml) in 14 cases. Free T surpassed the upper limit of normal (7.2 pg/ml) only during the first 16 wk. Clinical signs of hyper-androgenism improved in 27 patients. It is concluded that the estrogen-induced rise in SHBG during pregnancy causes an increase of total T, but prevents an equivalent rise of its biologically active fraction. Free T may possible be a helpful index to rule out tumorous hyperandrogenism when total T exceeds 1.5 ng/ml after wk 16 of pregnancy.

14.06.08

Hormone markers for spontaneous abortion in women with vaginal bleeding during the first half of gestation: Pantos, C J, Stathis, P, Tzingounis, V A. 1st Dept. Obstet. and Gyn., Univ., Athens, Greece
Serum levels of progesterone (P_4), estradiol (E_2), prolactin (PRL), and human chorionic gonadotropin (hCG) were measured by radioimmunoassay (RIA) in 48 pregnant women with vaginal bleeding episodes between the 6th and 20th weeks of their pregnancy. After statistical analysis of the data obtained we observed that serum P_4 levels less than 10 ng/ml were markers for spontaneous abortion in 88% of the cases studied. A strong correlation was found between serum P_4 and E_2 levels. On the other hand serum PRL levels were not found to be of any value in predicting the outcome of pregnancy. However, serum E_2 levels showed a significant correlation with serum PRL levels on those women who did not abort. Serum hCG levels less than 8000 mU/ml between the 6th and 12th weeks of gestation were markers for spontaneous abortion in 87% of the cases studied. But after the 12th week of gestation serum hCG determinations were without value in predicting the outcome of pregnancy. We believe that the combined determinations of serum P_4, E_2 and hCG in pregnant women with vaginal bleeding during the first trimester of gestation increase the accuracy of the prognosis of these pregnancies.

14.06.09

The relation between growth of fetal adrenal gland and steroid values in maternal serum: Matsumura, I, Hashino, M, Kondo, H, Maruyama, S, Yanaihara, T, Nakayama, T. Dept. Obstet. and Gyn., Showa Univ. School Med., Tokyo, Japan
Fetal adrenal glands were sonographically evaluated and maternal steroids were measured to study the role of fetal adrenal gland on the steroidal environment during pregnancy. Forty normal pregnant women at 28–40 weeks of gestation were selected for the study. Real-time ultrasonography was used and the length (L), circumference (C) and area (A) of fetal adrenal glands were measured. Maternal serum steroids including DHA-S, 16αOH-DHA-S (16DHA-S), estradiol (E_2), estriol (E_3) and 16αOH-pregnenolone (16P) were measured by gas chromatography mass spectrometry. L, C, and A increased as gestational weeks advanced reaching the values of 20.1 ± 2.0 mm (L), 62.0 ± 7.2 mm (C) and 1.8 ± 0.5 cm^2 (A) at term. A significant correlation was observed between the values and weeks of gestation. Although there was no correlation between the levels of DHA-S, 16DHA-S, E_2 and the measurements of fetal adrenal glands, a significant correlation was observed between serum E_3 levels and L as well as A ($r = 0.398, 0.445$). 16P levels also correlated well with A and L ($r = 0.449, 0.443$). These results demonstrated that the fetal adrenal glands develop in size from 28 weeks till term and the size of fetal adrenal glands correlates well with the maternal E_3 and 16P values.

14.06.10

Prostaglandin production from human decidua of normal pregnancy and missed abortion: Ishikawa, M, Kasamo, M, Shimizu, T. Dept. Obstet. and Gyn., Asahikawa Med. Coll., Asahikawa, Japan

We have investigated the production of PGE and PGF by human decidua *in vitro* obtained from induced abortion group and missed abortion group, trying to consider the role of PGs in the early period of human pregnancy including implantation. The PGE production was not significantly different between the induced abortion group and the missed abortion group. The PGF production of induced abortion group was significantly higher (p < 0.01) as compared to that of missed abortion group. In conclusion, it may be stated that the results from the present study suggest that the PGF produced by decidua may play an important role in the early stages of human pregnancy, including implantation.

14.06.11

First trimester nausea and vomiting as related to steroid hormones: Järnfelt-Samsioe, A, Bremme, K, Eneroth, P, Samsioe, G. Depts. Obstet. and Gyn., Sahlgren's Univ. Hosp., Göteborg and Karolinska Univ. Hosp., Stockholm, Sweden

Nausea and vomiting associated with early pregnancy is extremely common. The cause of this condition is still unknown, but endocrine factors have been suggested as playing some part. Previous studies have shown a relationship between emesis gravidarum and intolerance of oral contraceptives as well as gall bladder disease (Gyn. Obstet. Invest. **16**, 221, 1983; Sth. med. J. in press). In this study circulating levels of cortisol, testosterone, dehydroepiandrosterone-sulfate (DHEA-S), progesterone, estradiol as well as total and free estriol were determined in early and late pregnancy in 102 healthy, pregnant women. 62 subjects complained of emesis gravidarum. During pregnancy a significant rise in serum levels of cortisol, testosterone, progesterone and estriol were found in all subjects. A significant fall in serum concentrations of DHEA-S were noted as pregnancy advanced. In early pregnancy significantly lower levels of cortisol and progesterone were observed in women with emesis gravidarum compared to non-affected subjects. Higher levels of estradiol were seen in gestational week 14 in women hit by nausea and vomiting. In late pregnancy significantly higher values of DHEA-S and lower levels of testosterone were found in women who had suffered from nausea and vomiting earlier in the pregnancy. In conclusion our results demonstrate that hormonal factors may have a role in the pathogenesis of the condition, emesis gravidarum.

14.07.01

Treatment of mastalgia. A prospective randomized trial: Eppel, W, Kubista, E, Müller, G, Genger, H, Spona, J. 1st Dept. Obstet. and Gyn., Univ., Vienna, Austria

About 10–15% of women suffer from mastalgia. In a prospective randomized trial 121 patients with mastalgia were treated with gestagens (2 × 5 mg lynestrenol/d), mastodynon®, a phytopharmacon and a placebo medication. Three groups of 55 patients with mastodynon therapy, 28 patients with gestagen therapy and 38 patients with placebo medication can be compared. Therapy was given for three months. RIA-measurements of E_2, P and HPRL were performed before therapy and every month after the onset of therapy. Mammography and thermography before and the end of treatment was done. Successful treatment with pain relief was observed in 74.5% of the mastodynon group, 82.1% of the gestagen group and 36.8% of the placebo group. An interesting observation was the significant rise of HPRL levels in the patients with gestagen medication in comparison to the other groups (p < 0.05, Wilcoxon test). This fact should be considered when long-time gestagen medication is planned. The drop-out rate from therapy was the highest in the gestagen group (31.7%) because of side-effects followed by the mastodynon group (22.5%) and the placebo group (20.8%).

14.07.02

Comparative trial of danazol and tamoxifen in mastophathy: Junkermann, H, Legler, U, Lellig, U, Fournier, D v. Univ.-Frauenklin., Heidelberg

Since 1981 we have compared danazol and tamoxifen for the treatment of symptomatic mastopathy in a prospective open trial with alternating respectively randomized allocation. Patients complaining of long-standing breast pain were entered into this trial. Danazol was given continuously 200 mg/day per os. Tamoxifen was given 10 mg/day per os from day 5 to day 25 of the cycle. Control visits were scheduled after 3 and 6 months of treatment. 104 patients were evaluable, 52 in each treatment arm. Half of the patients in each group experienced complete relief of pain (50% with danazol and 54% with tamoxifen). 38% of patients on danazol and 33% of patients on tamoxifen reported partial relief. Only 6 patients (12%) in the danazol group and 7 patients (13%) in the tamoxifen group reported no improvement of pain. Nodularity was improved in both groups equally well. In a group of 30 consecutive patients (15 of each group) mammography before and at the end of treatment was compared. Four patients of the danazol group and six patients of the tamoxifen group showed massive reduction of dysplastic densities in the mammogram. Five further patients in the danazol group and three patients in the tamoxifen group showed slight improvement. Objective regression of dysplastic masses could be demonstrated on mammograms in 60% of patients. In 12 patients (6 in each group) no change could be detected. In our experience tamoxifen 10 mg/day and danazol 200 mg/day are equally effective and they are the prefered treatment in severe cases of symptomatic mastopathy.

14.07.03

The treatment of the cyclic mastodynia: Ioannidou-Mouzaka, L, Toufexi, H, Skrapari, M, Mandonakis, J. Breast Ctr, Hellenic Soc. Found., Athens, Greece

We would like to report the therapeutic effect of lynestrenol and bromocriptine in the women with cyclic mastodynia but no other pathological findings. Our study concerns 400 women with mastodynia from which 249 women with apparently normal cycles form the group "A" and were treated with lynestrenol 10 mg/d for 10 days and repeated for four months. The group "B" consists of 151 women with abnormal cycles who have been treated with bromocriptine 5 mg/d without interruption for three months. The results were controlled by thermography, personal opinion of the woman and hormone determination. The results obtained were: I) Before treatment: a) In group "A" progesterone was low ($\bar{X} = 6.3 \pm 4.1$ ng/ml, $p < 0.001$) but estradiol and prolactin were between normal ranges. b) In group "B" FSH and PRL were elevated ($\bar{X} = 9.05 \pm 6.5$ ng/ml and $606.6 \pm 366\ \mu$U/ml, respectively) and LH was low ($\bar{X} = 6.8 \pm 5.4$ ng/ml). – II) After treatment: a) The intensity and the extension of vascular hyperthermias in the thermography decreased in both groups. b) In group "B" FSH and PRL decreased ($\bar{X} = 4.96 \pm 1.4$ ng/ml and $283.4 \pm 150\ \mu$U/nl), while on the other hand LH increased ($\bar{X} = 14.1 \pm 3.7$ ng/ml). c) In group "A" good results 77.9%, medium 13.7%, bad 8.4%. d) In group "B" good results 80.8%, medium 11.9%, bad 7.3%. e) Relapse of mastodynia after 6–12 months, 49% in group "A", 28.5% in group "B".

14.07.04

Bromocriptine therapy in benign breast conditions: Souka, A R, El-Gendi, M. Dept. Gyn. and Surg., Alexandria Univ., Alexandria, Egypt

The therapeutic effectiveness of bromocriptine in treating benign breast conditions was evaluated in this study. Thirty cases of cyclical and non-cyclical mastalgia and fifteen cases of fibrocystic breast disease (FBD) were enrolled. Pretreatment investigations included serum prolactin assays, mammography, needle biopsy and cytology for any nipple discharge. Two dose regimens of bromocriptine (the low dose and recommended dose) were tried in mastalgia cases for two cycles; while cases of FBD received three cycles in a dose of 7.5 mg/day. Three parameters were stressed during therapy, namely: pain, nodularity discharge. The mean serum prolactin level in studied cases before therapy was significantly higher than our normal controls. Pain was completely or partially alleviated in more than 90% of the cases. Small breast nodules became painless, softer and smaller in size but they did not disappear. Big cystic nodules needed surgical removal. Breast discharge, in the presence of normal serum prolactin, responded poorly to bromocriptine. The low dose regimen gave moderately good results and excellent tolerance. It is suggested that mastalgia cases could receive the low dose regimen first to be shifted to the recommended dose in case of poor response. Bromocriptine therapy is mainly indicated to alleviate breast pain.

14.07.05

Reproductive improvement in patients with benign breast disease (BBD) treated with bromocriptine: Melis, G B, Paoletti, A M, Petacchi, F D, Mugnetti, C, Fioretti, P. Dept. Obstet. and Gyn., Univ., Pisa, Italy

Previous studies by many authors have demonstrated that BBD is accompanied by reproductive disorders like anovulatory cycle, luteal inadequacy and altered prolactin (PRL) secretion. However, treatment with bromocriptine, a dopaminergic drug with PRL lowering effect, has been proposed in these patients. The aim of this study was then to evaluate the effect of bromocriptine on BBD both from a clinical and endocrinological point of view. Bromocriptine (2.5 mg twice/day) or placebo treatment for three months were performed in 80 patients. Hormonal evaluation (progesterone [P], PRL, LH, FSH during the menstrual cycle) and clinical examination were repeated during and after the withdrawal of the treatments. With a drastic decrease of PRL levels, a significant increase of mean luteal P values was found during bromocriptine treatment in comparison to placebo. The improvement of P secretion was confirmed by the increase of progesterone/estradiol ratio (PEL index) during luteal phase in treated subjects. After therapy P secretion and PEL index appeared significantly higher than the values observed before the treatment, whereas PRL levels were similar to those measured before the onset of the therapy. Clinical evaluation confirmed the efficacy of bromocriptine therapy to correct subjective symptoms as mastodynia and premenstrual tension, and to reduce edema and the size of microcysts and macrocysts. These data indicate that bromocriptine therapy may favourably improve breast symptoms in BBD patients through its action on gonadal function.

14.07.06

Can bromocriptine be useful in the treatment of fibrocystic breast disease?: Parlati, E, Polinari, U, Liberale, I, Giorlandino, C, Salvi, G, Fiorella, G*, Dell'Acqua, S. Univ. Catt. S. Cuore, Rome; *Sandoz, Prodotti Farmaceutici, Milan, Italy

Previous investigations have demonstrated that bromocriptine may be useful in the treatment of cyclical mastalgia and fibrocystic breast disease (FBD). However, owing to the lack of a control group in these studies, a possible placebo effect, particularly in the reduction of the subjective symptoms cannot be excluded. Moreover the improvements of breast lesions found at clinical examination were often not confirmed by mammography. Thus, to verify the efficacy of bromocriptine as treatment for mastalgia and FBD, we devised a double-blind trial. Thirty normal menstruating women, suffering from cyclical mastalgia and FBD, were included in the present study. Bromocriptine (2.5 mg) or placebo tablets were administered three times daily for three months continuously. The evaluation of subjective symptoms, clinical examination of the breast, echo mammography and thermography were performed in the luteal phase of the cycle before, during and at term of the trial. At the same time estradiol, progesterone and prolactin plasma levels were measured in the follicular and luteal phases of the cycle. Our results have shown that mastalgia was significantly reduced in the treated group. Also the breast lesions appeared significantly reduced in size in the group who received bromocriptine in respect to controls. However echo mammography and thermography did not show differences between the two groups. A marked decrease in prolactin levels was observed in the treated group, while estradiol and progesterone levels did not show any significant variation. Therefore we can conclude that the positive effects observed in the treated group are probably mediated by a reduction in prolactin plasma levels.

14.07.07

Effect of bromocriptine in the treatment of cyclic mastalgia: Shin, M W, Ji, S B, Kang, S B. Dept. Obstet. and Gyn., Seoul Nat. Univ., Seoul, Korea

A total of 45 patients suffering from severe cyclic mastalgia participated in a double-blind cross-over trial. The patients received at random either bromocriptine or identical placebo tablets, each for a period of two months. The initial dosage of bromocriptine was 1.25 mg at night, gradually being raised to 2.5 mg b.i.d. in order to minimize side-effects. Mean serum prolactin levels before treatment were within the normal range (13.9 ± 1.3 ng/ml), and were reduced significantly when bromocriptine was discontinued. Symptoms were completely or almost completely relieved in 29 of 36 patients during two cycles of bromocriptine treatment, and did not reappear in seven of 17 patients on placebo treatment who had shown a response to bromocriptine. The prolactin produces a variety of effects on breast tissue and is capable of mammotrophic effect. We assume therefore that lowering the serum prolactin concentrations decreases to the total stimulatory effect on the breasts and thus stops the pain. Side-effects observed were significantly increased during bromocriptine treatment, but were tolerable in view of the relief from the symptoms of severe mastalgia. Bromocriptine appeared a very useful drug for the treatment of cyclic mastalgia.

14.07.08

The treatment of severe mastalgias with anti-estrogen therapy: Figueira, A S S, Carneiro, M H, Tscha, V B. Breast Unit, Fac. Med. Sci., Recife, Brazil

The mastalgias occurring in women suffering from mammary dysplasia, although not particularly serious, do acquire significance when the number of sufferers is borne in mind. Among such women there is a small percentage in whom the breast pain was resistant to the different treatments employed. The authors present an analysis of 100 patients suffering from severe mastalgia who were submitted to anti-estrogen therapy (tamoxifen 20 mg/day) for a period of three months, with a clinical follow-up of 93.1%. About 92.5% of the patients presented an objective improvement in their symptoms. The side-effects of the drug, which are slight and transitory, are also discussed.

14.08.01

Clinical, morphological and biochemical aspects of cervical ripening by intracervically applied sulprostone-gel: Rath, W, Adelmann-Grill, B C*, Schauer, A, Hilgers, R, Harder, D, Kuhn, W. Dept. Obstet. and Gyn., Univ., Göttingen; *Max-Planck-Inst., Biochem., München

Intracervical application of prostaglandins (PG) in viscous gel is an efficient method for cervical ripening. In a randomized, double-blind study 30 patients were given intracervical applications of 25 μg, 50 μg or 100 μg sulprostone gel in order to soften the cervix prior to first trimester termination of pregnancy. The cervical ripening effect of PG-gel was measured objectively by a special electronic-force monitor. The 50 μg-dose proved to be highly efficient independently of any significant uterine activity. Morphological studies of cervical biopsies showed a marked multifocal loosening of the collagen fibre bundles after PG treatment. For biochemical investigations specimens were obtained from the pregnant cervix of sulprostone-treated and untreated patients. Collagenase activity was measured by a specific technique using highly purified ^{125}I-labelled native collagen type I. Noncollagenolytic proteolytic activity was determined with commercially available ^{14}C-methemoglobin as substrate. There was no evidence for a significant increase in collagenase and protease activity after PG application. No typical collagen degradation products were found in the SDS-polyacrylamide electrophoresis. PG-induced ripening of the cervix is unlikely to be associated with a heightened degradation of collagen by collagenases and proteases.

14.08.02

Induction of labor with prostaglandin E$_2$ vaginal pessaries: Vengadasalam, D. Dept. Obstet. and Gyn., Alexandra Hosp., Singapore

The vaginal route for the administration of prostaglandin (PG) for cervical ripening has taken precedence over other routes since it is convenient and could be expected to provide a high concentration of PG close to the cervix for a local effect, without undue uterine stimulation. Vaginal pessaries containing 3 mg of prostaglandin E$_2$ were used to induce labor in 40 patients. Patients with a modified Bishop's score of 0–4 were included in the study. Period of gestation varied from 37 to 43 weeks. Static weight was the most frequent indication for delivery. Labor was closely monitored clinically and by CTG. Thirty patients (75%) were primigravidae and ten patients (25%) were multiparous. Vaginal delivery was achieved in 38 patients

(95%). There were two failed inductions in this series. Cesarean section was performed in both the cases. In five patients (12.5%) labor was augmented with oxytocin. There was no perinatal mortality and the maternal side-effects were nil. Increased uterine activity was not noted in any of the cases studied. The 3 mg prostaglandin E_2 was found to be safe and effective for ripening the pregnant cervix at term. This method of cervical ripening does not produce any adverse effects on the fetus. Nevertheless patients with suspected placental insufficiency should be monitored closely for the first few hours after insertion of the pessary in case of possible fetal compromise.

14.08.03
Cervical ripening by administration of 16-phenoxy-prostaglandin E_2 methylsulphonilamide: Gulisano, A S, Garozzo, G, Garofalo, A, Giardinella, S, La Greca, M, Panella, M. Gyn. and Obstet. Dept., Univ., Catania, Italy

16-phenoxy-prostaglandin E_2 methylsulphonilamide was administered to 31 pregnant women, seven in the first trimester, eight in the second trimester, and 16 in the last. Indications for treatment were: missed abortion, intrauterine fetal death or therapeutic abortion. Cervical modifications were begun immediately after treatment and ripening was completed after an average of eight hours and 30 minutes. Abortion or delivery was accomplished by all patients within 24 hours, with the exception of one case in which treatment failed. Side-effects were almost completely absent.

14.08.04
Continuous extraovular prostaglandin $F_{2\alpha}$ instillation for second trimester pregnancy termination: Atad, J, Sorokin, Y, Rofe, A, Abramovici, H. Dept. Obstet. and Gyn., Carmel Hosp., Haifa, Israel

One hundred late pregnancy terminations were successfully induced with continuous extraovular infusion of prostaglandin $F_{2\alpha}$ ($PGF_{2\alpha}$). The solution was infused to the extraovular space with a new double balloon catheter. The mean instillation abortion time (IAT) was 12.9 hours. Abortion was completed in 48% of the patients within 12 hours, and in 96% within 24 hours. The mean total dose of $PGF_{2\alpha}$ instilled was 12.4 mg per patient. Only four patients aborted within more than 24 hours from the insertion of the catheter and instillation of the $PGF_{2\alpha}$. Side-effects were few. Thirteen patients (13%) had nausea and vomiting, 14 patients (14%) had transient pyrexia (above 38°C). No major complications occurred. It appears that this method has a high success rate, good patient tolerance, and an acceptable safety factor with few minor side-effects.

14.08.05
Induction of an abortion by intra-amniotic instillation of NaCl in combination with PGE-2: Atanasov, A, Sabev, A. Inst. Obstet. and Gyn., Med. Acad., Sofia, Bulgaria

The induction of abortion by intra-amniotical application of prostaglandins or different types of salt solutions is known to be with relatively low effectivity. In the present study we present data about the use of a combined method for the induction of abortion using NaCl solution together with PGE-2 derivative (Nalador-100, Nalador-500). These were applied intra-amniotically. Amniocentesis was done according to a method previously described by us, through the posterior vaginal wall, extraperitoneally. After aspiration of 60–120 ml liquor amnii we performed instillation of 160–180 ml NaCl solution (25%) together with one ampoule Nalador. This method of induction of an abortion we applied to 49 pregnant women during the 16th–24th week of pregnancy. The interval between the instillation and the expulsion of the fetus was estimated to be 20 h 8 min (mean value). In the control group, treated with salt solution only, the expulsion of the fetus was shown to be for 34 h. No side-effects were observed after the use of the combined method for the induction of abortion in the second trimester of pregnancy.

14.08.06
Comparison of prostaglandin E analogue and vacuum aspiration for termination of early pregnancy: Hingorani, V, Kinra, G, Prasad, S, Basu, K. Dept. Obstet. and Gyn., All India Inst. Med. Sci., New Delhi, India

The efficacy of a prostaglandin E analogue "Sulprostone" administered intramuscularly was compared to vacuum aspiration, in termination of early pregnancy. In one group of 40 women, with 45 days amenorrhea and positive pregnancy test, the pregnancy was randomly terminated by vacuum aspiration in 20 women and the other 20 women received two sulprostone injections intramuscularly, one of 500 µg and another of 1000 µg after four hours. In all of them serum HCG levels were done before the start of treatment and two weeks later. These tests were negative after two weeks in all of them. However, as in three women in the injection group, bleeding was persisting after two weeks, they underwent a curettage. In second group of 30 women who had two weeks delay of menstruation, menstrual induction was done randomly by vaccuum aspiration or by three intramuscular injections of sulprostone, 500 µg given at three hourly intervals. In all women serum HCG was done before induction and two weeks later. Of the 15 women in vacuum aspiration group, five were found to be not pregnant and in sulprostone group three were not pregnant. In vacuum aspiration group, in one, the pregnancy had continued and repeat evacuation was done. One other patient in this group developed Asherman's syndrome. In sulprostone group success rate was 100% as determined by onset of bleeding both in pregnant and nonpregnant women, and HCG level fell in all the pregnant women. Even though 10% incidence of vomiting and abdominal cramps were observed in women receiving sulprostone, this method was accepted as a good alternative to surgical procedures for menstrual regulation.

14.08.07

Induction of second trimester abortions with sulprostone: Changes in maternal plasma and amniotic β-endorphin concentrations: Segre, A, Petraglia, F, Facchinetti, F, Santoro, V, Genazzani, A R. Dept. Obstet. and Gyn., Univ., Modena, Italy

The participation of maternal and amniotic β-endorphin (β-EP) in the events leading up to and during parturition has been suggested. The aim of this study was to evaluate the changes of β-EP concentrations in maternal plasma and in the amniotic fluid during the induction of abortion of the second trimester with new synthetic prostaglandin E_2 derivative (Sulprostone, Nalador, Schering, Berlin, W. Germany) (500 mcg i. m.). Ten pregnant women (22–31 years), admitted between the 15th and the 22nd week of pregnancy for therapeutic abortion, participated in the study. The drug was firstly injected at 9 a. m. and blood samples collected every 15 min for the first two hours and hourly later on. The amniotic fluid was collected by amniocentesis before, and one and three hours after the drug injection. The measurement of the hormone was performed by RIA, after extraction and column chromatography. Only slight side-effects were recorded, and the fetal delivery occurred in 6–10 hours from the first dose. Plasma β-EP levels showed a rapid and significant rise, which remained constantly in a range three-four fold higher than basal levels, until the delivery. In the amniotic fluid collected after Sulprostone injection β-EP levels appeared significantly higher than before. These data indicate that: prostaglandins represent a strong stimulus for maternal β-EP circulating levels and are able to activate the mechanisms leading to the fetal secretion of the peptide. This evidence reinforces the concept that β-EP may play a role in the feto-maternal events preceding delivery.

14.08.08

Clinical experiences with Sulprostone: Fioretti, P, Fruzzetti, F, Strigini, F, Melis, G B. Dept. Obstet. and Gyn., Univ., Pisa, Italy

A new PGE_2 derivative, Sulprostone (Schering AG, Berlin, W. Germany), was administered to pregnant women at different gestational ages to induce cervical dilatation only, or complete abortion. When a single dose of 50 mcg of Sulprostone was injected bilaterally into cervical walls (at 3 and 9 o'clock) cervical dilatation was greater than 8 mm in three of ten patients after 3 h, in two of three subjects after 6 h and in 18 of 23 subjects after 12 h from Sulprostone administration. In patients treated with 500 mcg intramuscularly cervix dilated > 8 mm in 62.5% and 83.3% of subjects examined after 3 and 6 h respectively. In the attempt to induce abortion, Sulprostone was administered intramuscularly (500 mcg every 4 h) to four patients with impending abortion, to 15 patients with missed abortion and to four patients with fetal death. Uterine evacuation was achieved in all but one patient after a mean time of 2 h 11 min ± 42 min in patients with impending abortion, after 6 h 54 min ± 1 h 46 min in patients with missed abortion and after 11 h 48 min ± 4 h 22 min in patients with fetal death. In another group of six patients with fetal death 1 mg of the drug was infused intravenously. Uterine evacuation was observed after 6 h ± 1 h 30 min. As for side-effects, eight patients had vomiting and two diarrhea. These data confirm the efficacy and acceptability of Sulprostone in different obstetric conditions.

14.08.09

Missed abortion and intrauterine fetal death the use of 15-methyl prostaglandin $F_{2\alpha}$: Lailla, J, Fortuny, A, Iglesias, X. Hosp. Clin. Univ., Barcelona, Spain

Intramuscular administration of 15-methyl prostaglandin $F_{2\alpha}$ has proved to be effective in emptying the uterus in cases of intrauterine fetal death. The study includes 43 patients in which the diagnosis of fetal death was made by clinical and echographic criteria. Group I included patients of less than 28 completed weeks of pregnancy (15 patients) and group II those beyond the 28th week (28 patients). No differences between group I and II as to the number of doses required to complete evacuation, and no significant differences were found in the induction period between primigravidae and multiparous. Biochemical studies carried out have shown no statistically significant differences. Progesterone and 17β-estradiol in plasma declined immediately after evacuation in both groups. The plasma cortisol values increased after evacuation, to return to normal levels after 24 h. Although stress may be responsible for the rise, it is also possible to speculate that prostaglandin itself may increase synthesis and release of cortisol by the adrenal or the placenta. This effect has been found in experimental studies using $PGF_{2\alpha}$ in the sheep.

14.08.10

Prophylactic antibiotic treatment with doxycycline prior to induced abortion: Strålin, E-B, Darj, E, Nilsson, S. Dept. Obstet. and Gyn., Falun Hosp., Falun, Sweden

A prospective double-blind study was performed in order to evaluate the effect of prophylactic antibiotic treatment prior to induced abortion. Eight hundred women who were admitted for first trimester abortion were included in the study. Women with clinical signs of genital infection pre-operatively or who were treated with antibiotics within three weeks before the operation were not included in the study. Four hundred mg of doxycycline (Vibramycin®) or placebo was given in a single oral dose 10–12 hours before vacuum aspiration. If any complications occurred the women were instructed to return to the clinic as soon as possible. Twenty-six of the women were excluded because of non-compliance. Ninety-one (11.7%) of the women returned to the hospital because of suspected complications after operation and 32 (4.1%) of these were diagnosed as having endometritis and/or PID. Six weeks after their operation 683 women reported that they were feeling well. Of the 32 women with endometritis eight had taken the active drug (doxycycline) and 24 placebo. This difference is statistically significant ($p < 0.01$). – Conclusion: The incidence of post abortum endometritis was significantly reduced when 400 mg of doxycycline was given 10 hours prior to vacuum aspiration.

14.08.11

Advances in cervical dilatation: Burnhill, M S. Dept. Obstet. and Gyn., Rutgers Med. School, New Brunswick, NJ, USA

A variety of changes influencing the practice of Obstet. and Gyn. has refocused interest on the process of safe cervical dilatation. The occurrence of vast numbers of elective induced abortion as well as the numbers of induction of labor (for medical conditions occurring in late pregnancy) have again focused attention on the methods of cervical dilatation. A series of controlled studies comparing a new osmotic dilator made from an exceptionally hydroscopic polymer will be presented. The studies were conducted at two locations and consisted of short-term studies in which the dilators were put in place for two hours and long-term studies in which the dilators were used for an average of fourteen hours. The plastic dilators were compared to conventional laminaria. The studies were analysed with respect to the amount of cervical dilatation, cervical softening, patient response, and overall efficacy of the procedure. The dilators apparently worked both by direct dilatation of the cervix and also by producing softening by an as yet unexplained mechanism. The discussion will review current data known on the mechanism of cervical dilatation as well as what is known about the similarities and differences between the three main types of osmotic dilators now known.

14.09.01

Study on the uterine isthmus: Suzumura, M, Kikuchi, S, Ishiwara, K, Ogata, E, Takahashi, T, Iwasaki, K. 2nd Hosp. of Nippon Med. School, Kanagawa, Japan

The uterine isthmus is a canal covered by endometrium, located between the anatomical international os and the histological internal os. The anatomical internal os is situated at the narrowest part of the uterus, while the histological internal os is a junction between the endometrium and endocervix. On the hysterogram, we have taken as the isthmus the straight or curved line between the uterine cavity and the spindle-shaped cervical canal. The length of the isthmus is 10.0 mm on the average and its width is 4.5 mm. However, the above mentioned length and width are what are measured on the films and the real figures may be somewhat different. It is supposed that the anatomical internal os is dilated to be cup shaped after the 4th month of gestation, but this has not been clinically proven. The authors inserted a microballoon catheter into the uterine cavity to measure the length of the isthmus. The length gradually increases as the gestation advances; that is, from 37 mm at 6 weeks, 41 mm at 7, 43 at 8, 43.6 at 9, 45.5 at 10 and to 46.3 at 11, but it decreases as 37.3 mm at 12 weeks, 30 at 15, and 29 at 22. We also measured the length of the isthmus by ultrasonography. The length is 35.2 mm at 6 weeks of gestation, 46 at 7, 46.2 at 8, 46 at 9, 45.2 at 10, and 46.2 at 11, but it is shortened to 41.5 at 12, 39.5 at 13 weeks. Thus we have proven clinically that the isthmus is 10 mm in length and is clearly shortened after the 12th week of gestation. Uterine isthmus has no dilating mechanism in structure and it remains unknown how it can be rapidly dilated during labor and how it repairs so quickly after labor.

14.09.02

A double cervical cerclage: Treatment of placenta praevia: Semchyshyn, S. Prof. Rutgers Med. School, St. Barnabas Med. Ctr, Livingston, NJ, USA

The application of cervical cerclage is based on the hypothesis that bleeding in cases with placenta praevia is due to cervical effacement and dilatation. At the level of the internal os, a merciline tape is applied as described by *Shirodkar* in his original report, with personal modification. The tape is fixed to the cervix. One end of the tape is left protruding from the vaginal mucosa to facilitate its removal at the conclusion of pregnancy. A proline (encircling) suture is placed about 1.5 cm below the tape in a purselike fashion as described by *McDonald*. In this study, a series of 20 women with placenta praevia diagnosed by ultrasound (15–19 weeks), underwent a double cervical cerclage procedure. No bleeding necessitating transfusion occurred, and all patients delivered live infants at 37–40 weeks gestation. Eight patients needed C/S because of central placenta praevia while the remainder delivered vaginally. It is felt that thus applied, double cervical cerclage reconstructs the anatomic cervix, provides physiological function and prevents preterm delivery. Also, the risk of maternal morbidity due to hemorrhage is reduced. This therapy offers an alternative to a well established current therapy of restrictive and incapacitating bed rest, blood transfusions and preterm delivery. This method has been effective in reducing both maternal and fetal risks emanating from placenta praevia while permitting patients their usual activity at considerable cost reduction.

14.09.03

Early diagnosis of cervical incompetence by ultrasonography: Kuroda, K, Kobayashi, M, Kato, K. Div. Perinat. and Matern. Med., Nat. Defense Med. Coll. Hosp., Saitama, Japan

Cervical incompetence frequently causes second trimester spontaneous abortions. The objective of the present study is the early detection of cervical incompetence by using ultrasonography, thereby preventing abortion or premature delivery. The patients included in this study are almost all those with the past history of second trimester spontaneous abortions. From about eight weeks on pelvic examination and ultrasonography are performed on these patients at two-weeks intervals. We have established four cervical factors related to cervical incompetence. Ultrasound scanning was always performed with the full bladder. These factors are: (1) length of cervical canal, (2) diameter of dilated internal os, (3) diameter of dilated external os, (4) internal angle of the internal os on the longitudinal plane. The last factor is specific to ultrasonography and is considered especially important. Each of these factors was given certain scores (2 points, 1 point or zero according to the severity). It was shown that in scores of 3 points or more abortions may occur with higher incidence and cervical cerclage may be indicated.

14.09.04
Ultrasonography of the uterine cervix as an aid for the retrospective and prospective judgement of the correctness of the indication for prophylactic cerclage operations: Ulbrich, R, Kuhn, W. Dept. Obstet. and Gyn., Univ., Göttingen

Ultrasonography is not only a valuable tool in the detection of cervical incompetence. Furthermore it is possible to identify the site of the surgical sutures in cases of cerclage. After having established normal values of the length of the uterine cervix in 106 normal pregnancies the same method was used in 35 patients with cervical cerclage because of suspected cervical incompetence, of which 32 were done as a prophylactic and 2 as an emergency procedure. Measurements of the distance between the internal os or the lower pole of the gestational sac respectively (upper distance) and the plane of the cerclage sutures was 2.1 cm as a mean value in the prophylactic group, whereas it was below 1 cm in the emergency cases. Further follow-up showed no decrease of the upper distance indicating that most cases of prophylactic cerclage had not been necessary and could have been avoided. The distance between the external os and the plane of the sutures (lower distance) was found to be 1.3 cm as a mean value indicating that in cases of prophylactic cerclage the internal os of the cervix was never reached. The site of the suture was found at the border of the lower to the middle third of the entire cervix. This sonographic method is recommended as a valuable tool in further studies in attempt to decrease the high number of obviously unnecessary cerclage operations when an effacement of the cervix by means of palpation findings is thought as an indication for surgical treatment of suspected cervical incompetence. Our own frequency of cerclage operations is about 4%; a decrease during the last years can be confirmed.

14.09.05
Histopathology of the cervix in cases of cervical insufficiency: Mahran, M, Iskandar, S, Barsoum, D. Dept. Obstet. and Gyn., Ein Shams Univ., Cairo, Egypt

Cervical insufficiency as a cause of late abortion and premature delivery is a well-documented entity in obstetrics. Histopathology of the cervix in 40 human uteri removed by total hysterectomy was studied. 20 cases known to have a history of incompetent cervix and the other 20 cases were control cases with competent cervix. Three blocks at different planes were prepared and stained with H & E Masson's Trichrome, Verhoff, van Gieson and Jordan Silver impregnation methods. The ratio of fibrous tissue and muscle fibers was evaluated in different fields, in both groups. A definite increase was noticed in the percentage composition of the muscle fibers in the incompetent group which were arranged in bundles. There was also an increase in the muscle tissue of the blood vessels, in comparison to the finding seen in the control group, in which the cervix was composed mainly of fibrous tissue and muscle tissue was scattered in minute amount. Elastic tissue inside the wall of the blood vessels was a prominent feature, in the healthy cervix, in comparison to a deficiency of elastic tissue in the incompetent group.

14.09.06
Congenital uterine malformations as indication for cervical suture (cerclage) in habitual abortion and premature delivery: Abramovici, H, Atad, J, Pascal, B, Sorokin, Y. Dept. Obstet. and Gyn., Carmel Hosp., Haifa, Israel

Twenty-one women with diminished fertility as a result of various congenital uterine anomalies were treated by cervical suture (cerclage) in the 11th–12th week of pregnancy without surgical correction of the uterine anomaly. None of these women had either clinical or radiological evidence of cervical incompetence. As a result of the treatment 13 women delivered live full term infants, three of the women aborted and five of the women delivered prematurely but the infants were alive and well. Comparison of these good results to the very poor outcome of previous pregnancies in these women (80 per cent pregnancy wastage) points to a distinct advantage to be gained by cervical suture. As a result of this experience we recommend cervical suture in cases of diminished fertility as a result of congenital uterine anomaly. We recommend that the suture be performed before considering surgical repair of the anomaly and irrespective of lack of evidence of cervical incompetence. Only in cases where cervical suture is unsuccessful would we recommend surgical correction according to the accepted techniques.

14.09.07

Changes in uterine cervix during pregnancy – measurements of elasticity by ultrasound and collagenous fiber by image analyser: Saga, M, Onizawa, S, Sato, I, Honma, T, Hamada, H. Dept. Obstet. and Gyn., St. Marianna Univ. School Med., Kawasaki, Japan

The uterine cervix becomes increasingly soft during pregnancy and at parturition in comparison to the non-pregnant state. However, it is difficult to measure elasticity objectively. The changes in consistency were evaluated by two new methods of measurement: measurement of ultrasonic velocity through the cervix and quantification of collagenous fibers in the cervical stroma. The former method showed gradual decline of sound velocity with the progress of gestation, reflecting the softening of the cervix. In the latter study, involving automatic image analysis of sections stained by Masson's trichrome stain, showed a decrease of collagenous fibers during gestation. The above results suggest that decrease in collagenous fibers may be involved in the process of the ripening of the cervix.

14.09.08

Collagenolysis in human vaginal tissue during delivery: A light and electron microscopic, and immunofluorescent study: Manabe, Y, Yoshida, Y, Kasai, K, Kawanami, D. Dept. Obstet. and Gyn., Shiga Univ. Med. Sci., Shiga, Japan

Biopsy specimens of the vagina obtained from non-pregnant and immediately after delivery were studied by light and electron microscopy, and an immunofluorescent technique. The vaginal wall is composed of epithelium and mainly a collagen fiber layer, below which bundles of smooth muscle are intermingled. In the non-pregnant vagina, collagen fibers were tight and regular. In the post-delivery vagina, edema was pronounced and collagen fibers were irregular and more dispersed. Interstitial hemorrhage and granulocyte infiltration were rare, though vascularity was increased with thrombus. Electron microscopically, compact and thick collagen fibers in non-pregnant vagina dissociated into thin fibrillar components in post-delivery vagina. These are markedly sparce around fibroblasts. Hydroxyproline content in connective tissue was significantly less ($p \leq 0.05$) after delivery than that in non-pregnancy. Prostaglandin E specific immunofluorescence was observed in collagenous stroma in both non-pregnant and post-delivery vagina but the reaction was far stronger in the latter. These findings suggest that widespread collagenolysis occurs during delivery, through which fetal delivery is permitted with minimal vaginal damage. Thus, the stretch-induced release of prostaglandins, more than granulocyte infiltration, may be involved in these processes.

14.10.01

Using 4'-o-tetrahydropyranyladriamycin (THP-ADM) to treat patients with gynecological cancer: A phase II study: Nishimura, H, Umezu, J, Yakushiji, M, Kato, T. Dept. Obstet. and Gyn., Kurume Univ., Fukuoka, Japan

The results of animal experiments have shown that the anthracycline derivate 4'-o-tetrahydropyranyladriamycin (THP-ADM) developed by *Umezawa* in Japan has a carcinostatic action equivalent to that of ADM and that its cardiac toxicity is extremely low. We conducted a joint phase II study in 76 patients with gynecological cancer (41 patients with ovarian cancer, 23 patients with cervical cancer, ten patients with endometrial cancer, two patients with vaginal cancer). The response rate was 25.0 per cent in the patients with ovarian cancer, 13.3 per cent in those with cervical cancer, and 28.6 per cent in those with endometrial cancer. The overall response rate was 23.1 per cent. When the patients were classified according to dose schedules, the highest response rate was obtained in the group given THP-ADM at a dose of 60 mg per body by single i. v. injection at 3-week intervals. Such side-effects as myelosuppression and gastrointestinal disturbances were observed, but alopecia, a marked side-effect of ADM administration, was mild, and no cardiac toxicity was seen in any of the patients.

14.10.02

Peplomycin sensitivity of cultured cells from female genital malignancies: Ueda, M, Maeda, T, Yamada, T, Ueki, M, Sugimoto, O. Dept. Obstet. and Gyn., Osaka Med. Coll., Osaka, Japan

Various kinds of tumor cells from female genital malignancies were cultured and tested for sensitivity to peplomycin (PEP) by the regrowth assay method and morphological observation. Bleomycin (BLM)-hydrolase activities of these cell lines were also compared in cell-free extracts by assaying the conversion of BLM into its deamidated form (HPLC method). SKG-I, SKG-II and SKG-IIIb cells, derived from squamous cell carcinoma of the cervix, and RKN cells, derived from myosarcoma of the ovary, were much more sensitive to PEP than other cell lines. The cell-kill-kinetics of PEP showed that their effect was mainly concentration-dependent, but also time-dependent. Their effect on cell morphology was characterized by the appearance of enlarged cells with swollen nuclei and vacuolized cytoplasm. The specific activities of BLM-hydrolase in SKG-I, SKG-II and SKG-IIIb cells were relatively lower than those in other cell lines. These results suggested that cervical squamous carcinoma cells and ovarian myosarcoma cells were sensitive to PEP, and BLM-hydrolase activity was one of the factors which decided the PEP sensitivity of human gynecological cultured tumor cells.

14.10.03
The long-term follow-up studies on advanced uterine and ovarian cancer patients in treatment with S.S.M. (an extract from human tubercle bacilli, so-called Maruyama vaccine): Fujita, K, Arai, Y, Hirai, T, Maruyama, C. Inst. Vaccine Ther. Tumors and Infect. Dis., Nippon Med. School, Tokyo, Japan

From 1964 to February 1985, 213,000 cases of various advanced malignancies, mostly in terminal stages, were submitted to S.S.M. non-specific cancer immunotherapy, generally after conventional treatment had failed. Among 91,050 cases treated from 1979 to April 1984, there were 3947 cases of the uterus and 2065 cases of the ovaries; 599 cases of the former (15.1%) and 150 cases of the latter (7.2%) survived more than three years, receiving the subcutaneous injections of S.S.M., usually alternating the type A (2.0 μg/ml) with the type B (0.2 μg/ml) every other day for the first three years, then twice a week for the following two years and only the type A once a week thereafter, as long as possible. No adverse side-effect has been reported. The clinical data were followed through the entire course of the therapy. In some of the long-surviving cases, the laboratory data were classified by Status Index advocated by *Kadota, Masaoka, Nishikawa* et al., more simply representing the general conditions of the patients. Some clinical examples are shown, including uterine sarcoma under treatment with S.S.M. more than five years postoperatively.

14.10.04
Enzymatic activity in normal and neoplastic human uterine tissues: Montoneri, C, Iachello, R, Sanfilippo, A, Geremia, E, Vanella, A. Gyn. and Obstet. Dept., Inst. Biochem., Univ., Catania, Italy

Ornithine decarboxylase, the initial enzyme in polyamine biosynthesis, and transglutaminase which is involved in the regulation of ODCase, may play a role in tissue growth. A comparison of these two enzymes in human uterine tissues was carried out by determining the picomoles of $^{14}CO_2$/min/mg proteins for ODCase; and the picomoles of ^{3}H-putrescine/min/mg proteins for TGase.

	ODCase	TGase	ODC/TG
Normal prolif. Endometrium (6)	12.2$\pm$ 3.7	0.42$\pm$0.2	29
Normal secret. Endometrium (8)	1.8$\pm$ 0.5	1.35$\pm$0.7	1.3
Endom. carc. (9)	206 $\pm$81	0.7 $\pm$0.3	294
Cervic. carc. (8)	11.2$\pm$ 2.1	1.4 $\pm$0.2	8
Fibromyoma (11)	2.2$\pm$ 0.8	1.2 $\pm$0.4	1.8

The increased ODC activity corresponds to reduced TG activity, and the ratio ODC/TG seems to relate to rate of tissue growth and malignancy.

14.10.05
***In vitro* chemosensitivity testing of gynecologic tumors with the human tumor colony forming assay (HTCFA): Umbach, G E, Poethen, J, Koldovsky, U, Matthiessen, H v.** Dept. Obstet. and Gyn., Univ. Med. School, Düsseldorf

So far, 54 fresh tumor samples derived from patients with breast (36 patients), ovarian (15), tubal (1), cervical (1), or endometrial (1) malignancies were disaggregated by mechanical and enzymatic (collagenase/ DNase) procedures and passed through a 60 μm mesh. 26 samples resulted in cell suspensions with an insufficient number of dispersed cells and 3 samples in suspensions with inadequate cell viability. The remaining 25 samples were plated in a bilayer soft agar system similar to that of *Salmon* et al. (New Engl. J. Med. **298**, 1321–1327, 1978), and continuously exposed to various cytotoxic drugs. Inadequate growth of colonies (less than 20 colonies larger than 100 μm) occurred in 13 samples and contamination in 6 samples, so that only six samples were evaluable for chemosensitivity studies. Using 50% inhibition of colony formation as the criterion for drug-induced cytotoxicity, only three of the evaluable six tumors were noted to be sensitive to any drug. Because of the low yield of sufficient single cells and the low growth rates found in our laboratory, the HTCFA has only limited value in the prospective assignment of chemothera-peutic treatments for patients with gynecologic malignancies treated at our institution.

14.10.06
The "human tumor necrosis factor", an important possibility of immunological treatment of human cancer: Limburg, H. Women Hosp., Univ. of Saarland Med. School, Homburg/Saar

Previous clinical studies since 1976 have shown that cytostatically pretreated human carcinoma cells may be used in the treatment of patients with mammary, ovarian and other cancers (Excerpta Medica No. 512, p. 516). In more than 30 cases of these tumors mostly in stages T4 (T$_3$) we noticed after this new immunotherapy a subjective and objective amelioration of health and an inhibition of tumor growth, partly with tumorlysis. The mean survival time of all these patients was more than four years. This phenomenon was attained with the treatment of ultrafiltrates of cultured carcinoma cells even from different patients. The results were obtained by repeated intramuscular injections of 10 ml calf serum containing 10^6 partly necrotic cells. There have never been any side-effects whatsoever as to produce interruption of treatment. These findings are now basically completed by the report of the "Human tumor necrosis factor" (TNF): Precursor, structure and homology to lymphotoxin – found by a US scientific group in California (Nature **312**, 1984). This tumor necrosis factor has been associated with *in vivo* and *in vitro* killing of tumor cells.

14.10.07

Nuclear magnetic resonance imaging of the female pelvis: Initial experience with 0.6 T system: Lovecchio, J*, Stein, H**, Fenton, A N*. Dept. Obstet. and Gyn.*, Div. Gyn. Oncol. and Radiol.**, North Shore Univ. Hosp., Cornell Univ. Med. Coll., Manhasset, NY, USA

Nuclear magnetic resonance (NMR) imaging has emerged as a non-invasive method of visualizing visceral organs without exposure to ionizing radiation. A pilot study was undertaken to survey the clinical applicability of *in vivo* NMR imaging in those patients who possessed gynecologic neoplasms. Seventy-five patients with either benign or malignant disease of the uterus, cervix, vulva, and ovary were entered into the study protocol. All candidates underwent abdominal-pelvic CT scans for comparative purposes. Images were produced utilizing a Picker Synerview 1200 fourth generation CT scan and Technicare 0.6 T NMR imaging unit. Single and multi-slice sagittal, coronal and transaxial images were obtained utilizing spin echo technique and various pulse sequences. Analysis of the NMR images demonstrates that both benign and malignant pelvic neoplasms can be identified. Assessment of these data suggest that an accurate characterization of the nature and extent of various pathologic gynecologic conditions is possible. However, additional studies must be conducted to elaborate upon the specificity of these findings.

14.10.08

Magnetic resonance imaging of gynecologic tumors: Weitzel, H, Albig, M, Hamm, B, Wolf, K-J. Dept. Gyn. and Radiol., FU, Berlin

The application of magnetic resonance imaging (MR) to the diagnosis of gynecologic tumors has been studied presurgically in 30 patients with different gynecologic tumors. MR was performed with a 0.35 Tesla superconductive magnet. Images were obtained in axial, sagittal and coronal planes. The findings were compared with computed tomography and ultrasound examinations. MR has the advantages of avoiding completely the use of ionizing radiation, penetrating bone and air without attenuation and imaging in three planes. The pelvis is suited for the investigation because the images are not degraded by respiratory motions. Therefore MR provides a clear picture of the pelvic organs. It permits a clear differentiation between the myometrium and endometrium of the uterine corpus. In malignant tumors it shows the extent of the tumors and the involvement of surrounding organs such as the bladder, bowel and pelvic lymph nodes. However, the resolution does not suffice to exactly identify small structures like normal ovaries (postmenopausal) or small lymph nodes. The ability of the three methods to distinguish cystic, solid and calcified structures and the delineation of surrounding organs are compared. The best images of the ovaries and pelvic lymph nodes were obtained in the coronal plane, of the uterus in the sagittal and of the parametrial structures in the axial plane.

14.10.09

The effect of ritodrine i. v. infusion on: The lipid metabolism, the protein and Ca^{++} levels, and the fetal activity: Athanasiadis, A, Tzafettas, J, Plevrakis, G, Fasekis, D. B' Univ. Dept. Obstet. and Gyn., Thessalonica, Greece

There has been evidence that β-mimetics also affect the lipid metabolism in addition to carbohydrates. This effect, as well as the changes in the protein levels and of certain electrolytes, seem to be a matter of controversy in the studies reported. In this group of patients the levels of glucose, cholesterol, triglycerides, total lipids, α-lipoproteins and of total proteins and Ca^{++} were measured both before and after two hours of ritodrine hydrochloride i. v. infusion. All the patients were pregnant women between 25 and 36 weeks and the principal indication for the administration of ritodrine was to suppress labor and postpone delivery. It was found that lactic acid increased, ($p < 0.01$) and protein concentration decreased ($p < 0.05$) while there was no significant change detected in the other parameters measured. The fetal activity was also monitored and was found to be increased during the ritodrine therapy in comparison to the period after the discontinuation of the drug. The latter was attributed to the hyperglycemia ($p < 0.01$) caused by β-mimetics and perhaps the improvement of the placental perfusion reported.

14.10.10

Magnetic resonance of the breast – what can be expected?: Kaiser, W, Zeitler, E. Radiol. Ctr, Nürnberg Clin., Nürnberg

Magnetic resonance (MR) has been used successfully for about 5 years as a new imaging method avoiding X-rays. By the use of surface-coils the investigation into the surface-areas (e. g.breast, eyes, ears, limbs) can be dramatically improved. Since March 1984 we have been testing the significance of Magnetic-Resonance-Imaging concerning diseases of the breast and employing therein special breast-coils. MR and mammography were compared up until June of this year with an investigation of 85 breasts; most of the results were confirmed by a postoperative histopathological examination. The most important fact about MR is the question of its capability to detect early cancers. By the selective imaging of thin slices in different planes (avoiding tissue overlapping), the high tissue contrast and the possibility of tissue characterisation a high probability of correct results can be achieved. The detection and differentiation of benign and malignant lesions is especially important and superior compared with mammography in dense breasts of young women and in the area near the thoracic wall.

14.10.11

Rectosonography of local recurrencies of gynecologic tumors: Application in diagnosis and treatment: Wischnik, A*, Hoetzinger, H**. *Dept. Gyn., Rot-Kreuz-KH, München; **Dept. Rad., Städt. KH, Passau
Rectosonography is a new diagnostic procedure which allows the visualization of the internal female genitalia, especially of lesions near the transducer. The method seems to be of great value for detection of postoperative local recurrencies of gynecologic tumors (carcinomas of the cervix, the corpus uteri and the ovaries). 30 patients with local postoperative recurrencies were scanned, the results were verified cytologically and by the clinical course. The tumor masses appeared in 100% as areas of low echogenicity. The extension could be correctly defined in correlation to CT in all cases. The therapy of local recurrencies presents great problems because in most cases neither a new operation is possible, nor percutaneous radiotherapy is effective. Rectosonography, however, allows the application of local brachytherapy with ultrasound guided installation of afterloading needles. 13 cases have been treated till now. The procedure is presented.

14.11.01

Apolipoproteins A₁ and B during continuous hormonal replacement therapy (HRT) with four progestationally different regimens: Mattsson, L Å, Samsioe, G, Sporrong, T, Hellgren, M. Depts. Obstet. and Gyn., Univ., Göteborg, Sweden
Recurrence of bleedings is one problem of modern HRT. Continuous treatment with estrogen-progestin combinations, which induce endometrial atrophy, provides an intriguing possibility of avoiding this. However, long-term treatment demands due consideration to possible metabolic effects of which lipid metabolism is a sensitive indicator with proved clinical significance. Apolipoproteins A_1 (ApoA$_1$) and ApoB are the main protein moieties of HDL and LDL and therefore accurately reflect lipoprotein metabolism. Low levels of ApoA$_1$ and/or high concentrations of ApoB in serum are regarded as risk factors for coronary heart disease. 60 postmenopausal women were randomly allocated to one of four oral estradiol (2 mg)-progestin regimens containing either NET (1 mg = prep. A, 0.5 mg = prep. B) or megestrol ac (5 mg = prep. C, 2.5 mg = prep. D). Apolipoproteins A_1 and B were determined by electroimmunoassay before as well as after one and four months of treatment. No significant changes were noted in ApoB. A transient decrease (prep. A) and a transient increase (prep. B) were encountered in ApoA$_1$ (p < 0.05). The ratio ApoA$_1$/ApoB showed a transient increment of 13% (p < 0.02) on prep. B. As no significant changes persisted after four months none the preparations seems to induce lipid metabolic effects of clinical significance.

14.11.02

Combined action of tamoxifen, danazol and medroxyprogesterone on the endometrium and sexual hormone levels in cases of perimenopausal hemorrhage: Salvatierra, V, Cuadros, J L, Beltran, E, Malde, J L, Salvatierra-Cuenca, J. Dept. Obstet. and Gyn., Hosp. Clin. Univ., Granada, Spain
Daily administration of 20 mg of tamoxifen to 37 women with perimenopausal menstrual disorders and/or uterine myoma, stopped the hemorrhage, and frequently caused endometrial atrophy and increased FSH, LH, progesterone, testosterone and, especially, estradiol levels. Tamoxifen was administered for a further month in 27 of these cases, in combination with 400 mg of danazol daily. This resulted in more frequent and intense endometrial atrophy. FSH, LH, P and T levels dropped, while estradiol levels increased slightly, but not significantly. In 23 of these cases, tamoxifen, danazol plus 20 mg of medroxyprogesterone were administered daily for another month. While endometrial atrophy persisted in some cases, most patients showed a pseudodecidual transformation of gestational type. FSH, LH, E2 and T levels dropped. Progesterone levels showed a modest increase. Tamoxifen and danazol did not suppress the action of medroxyprogesterone on the endometrium.

14.11.03

Progestins in the postmenopause: Short-term hormonal and metabolic effects: Schwartz, U, Baumgarten, S, Moltz, L, Arntz, H, Hammerstein, J. Abt. Gyn. Endocr., UFK Steglitz, FU, Berlin
Sequential progestin addition to estrogen replacement therapy (ERT) decreases the risk of endometrial cancer, but may induce potentially adverse metabolic reactions, e. g. lipoprotein patterns associated with atherosclerosis (decreased HDL and increased LDL cholesterol). This study examined the effects of medrogestone (MG) in combination with conjugated estrogens (CE). Eight postmenopausal patients participated, serving as their own controls. Four oral regimens were given consecutively for 20 days each, always followed by a 1-week drug-free interval: CE 0.6 and 1.25 mg daily alone (phases I and III) and with cyclic MG 5 mg daily for the last 10 days (II and IV). Hormonal changes included CE-dose dependent increases of estradiol and estrone and decreases of FSH and LH. MG acted synergistically on both gonadotropins, but inhibited the slight rise of prolactin observed with CE alone. Monitoring of lipid metabolism revealed no significant alterations of total, HDL, LDL and VLDL triglycerides with any regimen. The changes of total, HDL and LDL cholesterol were only minor. MG addition did not cause

a significant fall of HDL cholesterol or a rise of LDL cholesterol. Antithrombin III also remained unaffected throughout phases I–IV compared to pretreatment values. Thus, in combination ERT the use of progesterone derivatives such as MG may offer advantages over 19-nortestosterone derivatives which elicit a significant drop of HDL cholesterol even during short-term administration (*Hirvonen* et al. New Engl. J. Med. **304**, 560, 1981).

14.11.04
Use of danazol in the treatment of post-menopausal uterine bleeding: Jasonni, V M, Bulletti, C, Citti, P, Tabanelli, S, Flamigni, C. Dept. Reprod. Med., Univ., Bologna, Italy

The synthetic steroid danazol may act on human endometrium inducing atrophic changes. In the present study we attempted to verify the efficacy of danazol on the treatment of uterine bleeding in post-menopause which is often associated with an enhanced estrogen stimulation of the endometrium. For this purpose 200 mg/day were administered per os to 12 post-menopausal women with uterine bleeding and with histologically proven endometrial hyperplasia (N.8) or proliferative endometrium (N.4). All subjects underwent endometrial biopsy after 30 days of therapy. In five subjects the plasma levels of estrone sulfate (E1S) and estrone (E1) were determined before and at the end of the treatment. All subjects showed atrophic aspects of the endometrium and the bleeding disappeared after 6–10 days of treatment. The E1S/E1 ratio increased, probably from an impaired peripheral sulfatase activity that was observed by others for DHAS. The direct action of danazol on the endometrium – interaction with androgen and progesterone receptors – and the influence on the peripheral sulfatase activity produce an endocrine environment that inhibits the endometrial growth. These preliminary results indicate that danazol should be considered in the treatment of uterine bleeding especially in presence of an endometrial estrogen stimulation.

14.11.05
The effect of estrogen-progestin treatment in two different doses in premenopausal women: Ylöstalo, P, Vartiainen, E, Stenman, U-H, Widholm, O. II Dept. Obstet. and Gyn., Univ., Helsinki, Finland

The effect of replacement treatment on ovarian function was studied in 35 premenopausal women (aged 40 to 56; mean 47 years). Estradiol valerate 1 mg/d was given to 17 women (group A) on 21 consecutive days, and levonorgestrel 0.125 mg/d during 10 last estradiol treatment days, with a pause of seven days between treatment cycles. Group B (18 women) received same therapy but the dose was doubled. Three treatment cycles and two before and two after treatment were studied. Subjective symptoms were relieved in 62% of women during treatment. Menstrual cycles were regular in 71% and 77% before and after treatment and in 94% during treatment. Normal secretory phase was observed in 39% before and in 35% at the end of the treatment. Serum FSH decreased slightly during treatment particularly in group B. The frequency of serum progesterone > 5 nmol/l was 79% in group A and 74% in group B. During treatment it decreased significantly in group B. The frequency of serum progesterone > 15 nmol/l decreased in both groups during treatment. In ultrasonic studies the average volume of ovaries, in which no follicles were found, was 7.6 cm^3, and in ovaries, in which follicles were found, it was 10.5 cm^3 (p < 0.001). Follicular growth was often defective also in ovulatory cycles.

14.11.06
Comparison of two estrogen/progesterone formulations in the treatment of peri-menopausal women with climacteric symptoms: Kolvik, R, Schiefloe, A, Jerve, F, Dalaker, K, Hoevik, P. Nordland Sentralsykehus, Bodø, Norway

The study was set up to compare two hormone replacement therapies with different estrogen/progesterone dose with regard to symptom control, adverse effects and acceptability. It was a multicenter, single-blind six-months study where 54 patients entered randomly into one of the two treatment groups. The hormones used were estrone and norethisterone given in sequential order and the patients on high-dose treatment were given tablets containing a double dose. Both the tested treatments were effective in alleviating specific symptoms like hot flushes and sweating and also unspecific symptoms like mood changes, irritability and insomnia. The improvement was significant for the most common and severe climacteric symptoms. Also menstrual irregularities and excessive bleeding showed significant improvement. No serious adverse reactions were observed during the study. There was a small tendency to weight-gain. No significant change in blood pressure, although the low-dose group had a slight lowering of blood pressure. Both the high and low-dose treatment exerted significant effects on the climacteric syndrome. High dose treatment was slightly more effective in the regularization of the bleeding pattern.

14.11.07
Measurement of cytosolic and nuclear progesterone receptors in premarin primed human endometrium after single-dose progesterone administration: Gorodeski, I G, Beery, R, Geier, A, Lunenfeld, B, Bahary, C. Dept. Obstet. and Gyn. "B", Meir Hosp., Sackler Med. School, Univ., Tel-Aviv, and Inst. Endocr., Sheba MCR, Israel

Progesterone receptors (RP) were measured in normal endometria of premarin treated perimenopausal women, following single dose progesterone administration, using [^{3}H] R5020 as the ligand. Following progesterone injection (test group, n = 11) nuclear RP (measured in the 0.4 M KCl nuclear extract) were significantly higher than in the control group (n = 6) and comprised $50 \pm 19\%$ and $25 \pm 9\%$ respectively, of the total RP. A wide range of individual values of total RP was found in both the test and control groups, i. e. 6781 ± 4386 and 7527 ± 5583 fmol/mg DNA, respectively. These results indicate a change of distribution of the RP in premarin primed hormonal human endometrium following progesterone injection. This may be either a result of induced translocation *in vivo* of the RP (according to the 2-step model theory) or increased affinity of the RP to the nucleus (according to the nuclear receptor theory).

14.11.08
Effects of medroxyprogesterone acetate (MPA) on HDL cholesterol during estrogen replacement therapy: Ottosson, U B, Schoultz, B v. Dept. Obstet. and Gyn., Univ. Hosp., Umeå, Sweden

The choice of progestogen is important during estrogen replacement therapy. 17-hydroxy progesterone derivatives like MPA are often preferred because they have few androgenic side-effects and are supposed to have a slight or even a beneficial influence on blood lipids. Subfractions of HDL cholesterol and its apolipoproteins were followed in 58 postmenopausal women during three cycles of unopposed estrogen therapy with estradiol valerate 2 mg daily. During the last ten days of the following three cycles the women received sequential addition of either levonorgestrel 250 μg, medroxyprogesterone acetate 10 mg or natural micronized progesterone 200 mg. At the end of the third treatment cycle serum levels of HDL cholesterol and of HDL_2 cholesterol were significantly reduced (p < 0.01) in women receiving medroxyprogesterone acetate. Though less pronounced the pattern of the decline for the different lipoproteins was quite similar to that in women receiving levonorgestrel. Data suggest that doses and relative biological activity of 19-nor steroids and 17-hydroxy progesterone derivatives are more important for their metabolic effects than are qualitative differences and that the two groups of progestogens are probably equally suitable for sequential addition during estrogen replacement. Natural progesterone had no apparent influence on HDL cholesterol or its subfractions.

14.11.09
Continuous combined treatment with conjugated estrogens and either medroxyprogesterone acetate or norethisterone: Siddle, N C, Padwick, M L, Endacott, J A. King's Coll. Hosp., London, UK

Standard regimens for post-menopausal women involve withdrawal bleeding. It is possible to avoid withdrawal bleeding by giving both estrogens and progestins continuously. Previous studies of this approach have been associated with a high incidence of bleeding problems. The most successful study to date achieved control only by using doses of norethisterone up to 2.1 mg daily. We have studied 80 women taking 0.625 mg of conjugated estrogens daily who were randomised to receive either norethisterone 0.35 mg b. d. or medroxyprogesterone acetate 2.5 mg b. d. Psychological and endometrial status and pattern of bleeding were observed while on sequential therapy and then on continuous combined therapy. Eighty per cent completed six months and had either no bleeding (30%) or acceptable bleeding (50%). Acceptable bleeding was defined as either less than 5% of the total time studied, bleeding restricted to the first two months or bleeding occurring due to failed compliance with the regimen. Six per cent of patients withdrew because the estrogen dose used was insufficient or for psychological reasons. At the six months endometrial biopsy of all patients, 82% had endometrium that was too scanty for assessment and 18% atrophic late secretory endometrium. The rationale for b. d. prescription of progestin, the comparison between the two progestins and the psychological effects of this type of regimen will be discussed.

14.11.10
Oral replacement therapy with estradiol-cyclo-octylacetate – a new estradiol analogue: Dahlgren, E, Crona, N, Janson, P O, Samsioe, G. Dept. Obstet. and Gyn., Univ. of Göteborg, Sahlgrenska Sjukhuset, Göteborg, Sweden

Treatment with estrogens, most frequently non-alkylated, to alleviate climacteric estrogen deficiency symptoms is well established. Given orally, the most convenient route of administration, there is a rapid liver metabolism of the drug and the dose has to be rather high to be effective, which leads to untoward side-effects. An estrogen compound that is absorbed by the chylomicrons, thereby avoiding the first liver passage would therefore be of interest. Estradiol-cyclo-octylacetate (E2-CoA) dissolved in arachis oil has in animal test models shown promising results. In this study 0.5 mg E2-CoA dissolved in arachis oil was given orally to 11 oophorectomized women for 21 days. The study was performed in two steps. In the first step the effect of E2-CoA administered after an over-night fast, on plasma estrone, estradiol, FSH, LH, prolactin as well as on serum proteins, fatty acids, oral glucose tolerance test and on the cervical and endometrial morphology were compared to the effect of daily oral intake of 25 μg ethinylestradiol (EE) in an cross-over study. In the second step the effects of E2-CoA non-fasting conditions on plasma estrone, estradiol, FSH and LH were studied. E2-CoA alleviated climacteric estrogen deficiency symptoms in all women. It showed an estrogenic effect on cervical and endometrial morphology and depressed FSH, though to a lesser extent than EE. No side-effects were seen. The unchanged metabolic parameters after 21 days of E2-CoA treatment may support the assumption of a weak estrogenic effect and the relatively slow resorption and the low estradiol-estrone ratio does not support the hypothesis that the drug is resorbed by the chylomicrons.

14.11.11

Triphasic estrogen/progestagen formulation in the treatment of women with climacteric symptoms: Jacobson, J B. Södertälje, Sweden; **Schoultz, B v.** Umeå, Sweden; **Suhonen, S.** Helsinki, Finland; **Kolvik, R.** Bodø, Norway; **Schiefloe, A.** Bodø, Norway

In a six-month double-blind parallel comparison 191 patients were randomly entered into two treatment groups: low-dose replacement treatment, presented as a sequential pack holding five 0.5 mg estrone tablets and seven tablets containing 0.5 mg estrone and 0.5 mg norethisterone followed by nine tablets containing 1 mg estrone and 1 mg norethisterone. The high-dose treatment was presented as a similar pack holding the same number of tablets, each containing the double dose of estrone and 1 mg norethisterone. Ninety-seven patients received high-dose treatment, 94 received low-dose treatment, and in all 168 of the patients could be evaluated. Both tested treatments were effective in alleviating both specific and unspecific climacteric symptoms. The relief of vasomotor symptoms was most evident. The psychic symptoms were also reduced in both patient groups. The improvement was significant for the most common and most severe unspecific climacteric and perimenstrual symptoms, whereas for the less common and less severe symptoms the amelioration mostly fell short of being significant. Excessive bleeding and amenorrhea became less common during the treatment period. More than 95% of the patients had regular cycles. The high-dose treatment had a statistically significant more effective regulation of the bleeding pattern. No unexpected adverse reactions were seen. Both triphasic hormone replacement regimes were shown to be highly effective in reducing the climacteric symptoms.

14.12.01

Thirteen years, 14,000 laparoscopies at a community hospital: Kleppinger, R K. Reading Hosp. and Med. Ctr, Reading, PA, USA

Of 14,000 laparoscopies performed at our institution from 1972 to date, 74% were tubal sterilizations and 26% diagnostic procedures. The complications reflect the chronology of our program; of those requiring laparotomy (0.18%), most occurred in the first 18–24 months of our experience. Evolution from unipolar to bipolar and mechanical tubal occlusion, with emphasis on reduction of complications, is demonstrated. Our continuing concern with laparoscopic sterilization is a failure rate of 3–4/1000 and, particularly, the occurrence of a peritoneal tubo-uterine fistula at the cornu. These accounted for all 15 ectopic pregnancies. Each was located in the blunted, occluded, distal tubal segment. When high-frequency coagulation is the method, coagulation at the cornu should be abandoned. The three contiguous areas of coagulation should be so placed that 2.5 cm of isthmus remains uncoagulated. For the method of mechanical occlusion with the Hulka clip, the criteria of "appropriate" clip application must be mastered. The slightly higher failure rate with the Hulka clip may reflect the difficulty of this procedure and the longer learning period.

14.12.02

Importance of laparoscopy in gynecology: Izzo, V M, Souza, A Z, Salvatore, C A. Gyn. Clin., Univ. of São Paulo Med. School, São Paulo, Brazil

The results of 522 laparoscopies that have been performed at Gynecologic Clinic of São Paulo University Medical School, between 1978–1982, permit the following conclusions: 1) Laparoscopy should be indispensable for investigation of infertility, among other propedeutic methods. 2) Among 224 patients with clinical gynecologic symptoms, we found pelvic abnormalities in 175 (71.7%) cases. Otherwise, 69 (28.3%) cases showed no laparoscopic evidence of pathology. 3) Complaint of chronic pelvic pain occurred in 43 patients. Twenty-five (58.1%) had normal genital system and in 18 (41.9%), the laparoscopy was able to establish a diagnosis related to the symptoms. 4) Among 183 patients with infertility, only 20 (10.9%) had normal laparoscopic findings. The remaining 163 (89.1%) showed several pelvic abnormalities. The most frequent were tubal occlusion, tubal adhesions, peritoneal adhesions previous sterilizations and endometriosis. 5) Ninety-five laparoscopic sterilizations were performed with silicone rings. This procedure is mainly indicated in severe medical diseases such as arterial hypertension, diabetes or cardiopathy. Failures were found in 2.1% cases due inadequate technic of insertion. 6) There was no mortality in this series of 522 gynecologic laparoscopies.

14.12.03

Laparoscopy under local anesthesia: Gordon, A G. Princess Royal Hosp. Hull, UK

Few gynecologists in Britain have experience of laparoscopy under local anesthesia. The advantages of the technique are improved safety, less postoperative discomfort and an earlier return to normal activities. Pre-operative counselling and medication are essential. The importance of gentleness in theatre is stressed. The injection of local anesthetic is described and also the insertion of instruments as the patient voluntarily distends her abdomen to prevent damage to intra-abdominal vessels and viscera. The main contraindications are fear, obesity and the possibility of intra-abdominal adhesions. The technique is advocated for tubal sterilization and also for the assessment of pelvic pain and the suitability for reversal of sterilization. The chief complication is unexpected pain or encountering adhesions. An anesthetist must always be present to allow rapid induction of general anesthesia if problems should arise as they do in about 0.7 per cent of cases.

14.12.04

Dr. Gadhvi's laparoscopic technique: Gadhvi, C K. Sir T. Hosp. and Bhavnagar District, Bhavnagar, Gujarat, India

This is a modified laparoscopic sterilization operation technique which is presented after performing about 1000 operations at Sir T. Hospital, Bhavnagar, Gujarat, India. This method is superior to the conventional method as initial pneumoperitoneum is not done by using a Verrie's needle. After giving pre-operative sedation (pethidine and phenergan by injection), the trochar is introduced directly through a small sub-umbilical incision. Local anesthesia is not used. The laparoscope is introduced directly through a small sub-umbilical incision. Local anesthesia is not used. The laparoscope is introduced through the cannula and a minimum amount of air is introduced under direct vision through the cannula till the operative field becomes clear. The rest of the method remains as usual. This method removes all the fear of all the complications caused by local xylocaine, Verrie's needle and blind induction of pneumoperitoneum. As no operative complications have been recorded, and as follow-up shows no morbidity or mortality this should be the method of choice.

14.12.05

Second-look laparoscopy after treatment of acute salpingitis: Teisala, K, Punnonen, R, Heinonen, P K, Aine, R, Miettinen, A, Lehtinen, M, Grönroos, P, Paavonen, J. Dept. Obstet. and Gyn., Univ. Centr. Hosp., Tampere, Finland

Long-term sequelae of acute salpingitis (AS) are common and often severe, including infertility, chronic pelvic pain and increased risk of ectopic pregnancy. Hysterosalpingography is in common use for examination of the postinflammatory tubal passage. Its value, however, is limited. In the present ongoing study, second-look laparoscopy has been used for evaluation of treatment results of laparoscopically verified AS. We also collected microbiologic specimens from the lower and upper genital tract and obtained endometrial biopsy to confirm the effect of antimicrobial treatment. Second-look laparoscopy was performed for ten symptomless women 15–23 weeks after acute stage of AS. Chromotubation showed unilateral distal tubal occlusion in two patients. Tubal adhesions were detected in three cases. At the acute stage of AS, pelvic adhesions were found in three cases. In all these cases adhesions were milder at second-look laparoscopy. The vascularity of the Fallopian tubes was still increased in all cases, although no sexually transmitted pathogens were isolated and endometrial biopsy showed no signs of inflammation. This finding is important in differential diagnosis of AS, because the postinflammatory erythema can be confused with mild AS.

14.12.06

Complications of laparoscopy after previous abdominal surgery in gynecological practice: Petrikovsky, B, Pillari, V, Khulpateea, N, Cohen, M. Coney Island Hosp., Brooklyn, NY, USA

Previous abdominal surgery had been traditionally considered a contraindication for laparoscopy. This study examines the effect of previous abdominal surgery on closed laparoscopies performed under strict supervision of the same experienced surgeon. One hundred and fifty consecutive patients were studied. In group I, 95 patients had laparoscopy performed without abdominal surgery; 55 patients (group II), underwent laparoscopy after prior abdominal surgery with only minimal deviances in routine laparoscopic technique. In group I, 38.5% of patients had laparoscopy for elective voluntary sterilization, while in group II, 47.5% were performed because of chronic pelvic pain. Pelvic adhesions were found three times more often in the patients in group II. Cesarean section, cholecystectomy, herniorrhaphy and laparoscopy were associated with fewer adhesions than appendectomy, ovarian and tubal surgery and exploratory laparotomy. Febrile morbidity was higher in group II. Unintended major surgery was performed for two reasons: 1. Dense pelvic adhesions which made it impossible to visualize pelvic structures (in 22.5% in group II vs. 3.6% in group I, $p < 0.05$), though pneumoperitoneum was successfully created and laparoscopic and auxiliary instruments introduced in all patients. 2. Intraoperative bleeding that required laparotomy (2.3% in group II vs. 1.8% in group I). In conclusion, laparoscopies by closed technique can be safely performed on patients who have had previous abdominal operations.

14.12.07

Laparoscopic study of vermiform appendix at the time of diagnostic laparoscopy: Gogate, S G. Surlata Hosp., Bombay, India

Diagnostic laparoscopy provides an excellent opportunity to study the ileo-cecal area and appendix. Paucity of such studies in medical literature prompted this study of 255 cases in last year and a half. All the cases were for diagnostic or operative laparoscopy. The indications varied from sterility to suspected ileo-cecal or appendicular pathology. Laparoscopies were performed using double puncture set up. A long Verrie's needle was used to probe the ileo-cecal area. In difficult cases a right lateral tilt to the table in addition to lithotomy position was used. Most of the cases were done under local anesthesia with sedation. The vermiform appendix was observed in its various anatomical positions in more than 90% cases. Appendicular pathology was detected in 24.5% of cases (many of them unsuspected). In contrast in nine cases with suspected appendicitis endoscopy showed normal appendix and ileo-cecal junction. Eight cases underwent appendicectomy after laparoscopic study. This small study shows the value of laparoscopic study of the appendix, particularly in those "doubtful" cases, as it can easily avoid unnecessary laparotomies and appendicectomies.

14.12.08

Evaluating the symptom of pelvic pain by peritoneoscopy: Cangello, V W. Providence Hosp., Oakland, CA, USA

This report describes the author's experience with 600 patients who underwent peritoneoscopic examinations to evaluate the symptom of pelvic pain. Age range was 17 to 63 year; 270 patients were nulliparous, 210 patients had one to four previous surgical procedures. The pain was chronic in 520 patients. Patients with positive findings were: endometriosis 130, pelvic adhesions 122, hemorrhagic and/or ruptured cysts 48, pelvic infections 39, pelvic varicosities nine, tubal pregnancy nine, and appendicitis five. Retrograde menses were seen in numerous patients with no other positive findings. Negative examinations were found in 15% and occurred more often in the chronic pelvic pain patients. In the group with positive findings were 44 patients with endometriosis not suspected prior to the procedure, and 13 cases with subsiding pelvic infection. Twelve patients reported relief of pain following lysis of adhesions performed during the examination and two patients with actively bleeding hemorrhagic corpus luteum were treated by electrocoagulation. Patients with acute pain frequently do not require any major operation, others with pain and/or infertility may need a major operation when unexpected pathology is discovered. The author's conclusions are: Laparoscopy is an excellent procedure for the investigation of pelvic pain. Previous surgery did not prove to be a contraindication. Retrograde menstrual bleeding was found to be common cause of pelvic pain. Endometriosis, pelvic infection and appendicitis may be found when abdominal and pelvic examinations are inconclusive.

14.12.09

Microcolpohysteroscopy: Tolosa, H A de, Pinotti, J A. Dept. Obstet. and Gyn., State Univ., Campinas, Brazil

Although microcolpohysteroscopy is a well-known method, the possibility of performing the examination without anesthesia and on an ambulatory basis opens up a new field for its use in gynecological practice. Microcolpohysteroscopy with Hamou's microhysteroscope which is 0.4 cm diameter, and using CO_2 as distension medium was performed in 470 patients on an ambulatory basis. Main indications were menstrual alterations – 26.8%, sterility – 25.7%; bleeding – 19.7%; check-up on high risk patients for endometrial carcinoma – 13.8%. Main findings are listed on tables II, III and IV. For example, atrophic endometrium was found on 23.6% of the patients with a complaint of bleeding. In these cases, when hormonal treatment was not satisfactory we performed hysterectomy. This saved the patient the trouble of previous D + C. The diagnostic capacity of the method is established when compared to histology. Out of 29 histological examinations, 23 were already diagnosed by microcolpohysteroscopy. According to the tables presented, M.C.H. is a valuable aid to gynecological practice, and its role, yet to be fully determined, will be of relevant importance to the practical gynecologist, its importance being mainly focused on: sterility, bleeding and endometrial pathology.

14.12.10

Hysteroscopic diagnosis of submucous fibroids and the evaluation of vaginal twisting myomectomy: Fukuda, Y, Sugimoto, O. Dept. Obstet. and Gyn., Osaka Med. Coll., Osaka, Japan

Uterine submucous fibroids are one of the most common diseases which causes menometrorrhagia. The diagnosis was carried out by hysteroscopy or ultrasonography, which may occasionally be misread. Hysteroscopy made it possible to diagnose submucous fibroids easily, correctly and promptly. We have found 135 cases of submucous fibroids by hysteroscopy in the last three years. Of the 135 cases, 47 were of the pedunculated type, 83 of the protruded type and 5 of the combined type. Of 52 cases of the pedunculated type and the combined type, 27 cases were successfully treated using vaginal twisting myomectomy. The procedure of which was to catch the pedicle of the fibroid at its root with hysterectomy or hemostatic forceps of various kinds. All these procedures were done in the outpatient clinic under local anesthesia of the paracervical block. The indication for myomectomy is that the pedicle is under 2 cm and the fibroid is under 8 cm in diameter. Bleeding after myomectomy was scanty and stopped within seven days in all cases but one. Re-examination by hysteroscopy after myomectomy was carried out in 21 cases. Five of them were found to have minor retention of the pedicle which was removed by curettage.

14.12.11

"The single-hand hysteroscope", a new instrument for ambulant hysteroscopy: Van der Pas, H F M. Rijksuniv., Gent, Belgium

The hysteroscopic examination has been an important step forward in medical diagnosis. However, the intervention will not be a real acquisition until it can be done in the gynecologist's consulting room, without difficulty and ambulant. The instruments and the experience play a prominent part beside a correct indication. First of all the preparation of the patient is dealt with, including the possibilities of local analgesia. The risk and safety norms of this anesthesia are discussed as well. If the proper instruments are used, dilatation and analgesia can even be omitted.

14.12.12

Evolution of adnexal cystic tumors identified through echography: Marussi, E F, Pinotti, J A. Dept. Obstet. and Gyn., State Univ., Campinas, Brazil

The use of echography being more and more common in the gynecological propedeutic, besides the improvement in the evaluation of texture, topography and volume of several gynecological pathologies, has aroused the question of what to do when diagnosing pelvic cystic lesions with no clinical or echo-structural worrying signs, and if there might be echographic criteria that could guide the next steps of the action to the taken. Trying to answer these questions, 14,525 women between the age of 13 and 84 (mean age 38) were examined and 30,749 pelvic echographies were performed in a period of five years – from March 1979 through March 1984. Using a real-time ultrasound set, with linear probes, and *Donald's* and *Abdulla's* technique, 499 adnexal masses were detected: 438 of cystic texture, 21 cystic-septated tumors, 21 solid-cysts and 19 cysts with bizarre texture. The authors analyse in this paper the 438 tumors of cystic texture, 21 of the cystic septated echo-structure tumors that are larger than 30 mm in diameter, and indicate echographic criteria for a surgical approach to adnexal masses. They also evaluate the evolution of these adnexal masses with an echographic follow-up in cases of conservative procedures, concluding that 60.6% these tumors involuted in the first three months. The echographic evaluation of the pelvis will allow the avoidance of unnecessary operations on cystic masses, but it requires that precise criteria for the interpretation of ultrasound anatomy be established and followed.

14.12.13
A technical review of over 40,000 laparoscopies: Wadia, B J, Joshi, N U. J J Hosp., Univ., Bombay, India
An experience of over 40,000 cases followed up from 3 months to 5 years. Discussions on: (1) mode of anesthesia, (2) pneumoperitoneum, (3) uterine elevation, (4) technicalities of tubal occlusion. Analysis of results includes morbidity. Follow-up of the cases is high. It is even 100% in the first 15 days. One-year follow-up is achieved in over 80% of the cases. A large number of cases are followed up even for 5 years.

14.28.01
Gamete intrafallopian transfer (GIFT) in rhesus monkeys: Wong, P C, Heitman, T, Balmaceda, J P, Ellsworth, L R, Asch, R H. Dept. Obstet. and Gyn., Univ. of Texas Hlth Sci. Ctr, San Antonio, TX, USA
Recently, *Asch* et al. (Lancet, 1984, II, 1034) reported the first pregnancy resulting from translaparoscopic GIFT in humans. To complement our understanding of the new procedure, we have applied the technique of GIFT to a group of ten Rhesus monkeys. Six monkeys (group 1) received human menopausal gonado-tropin (hMG; FSH 37.5 IU and LH 37.5 IU) daily from day 2 of the cycle. When serum estradiol levels were above 250 pg/ml, laparoscopies were performed to assess follicular development. In the presence of pre-ovulatory follicles, human chorionic gonadotropin (hCG; 1000 IU) was administered and laparotomy and follicular aspiration were performed 36 hours later. Semen collected three hours before operation was prepared in TALP/HEPES with bovine serum albumin. After capacitation for two hours, the final concen-tration was adjusted to $100,000/10 \, \mu l$. Two oocytes mixed with $10 \, \mu l$ of sperm preparation were loaded into a catheter and transferred immediately to the ampulla by introducing the catheter through the fimbria on each side. In animals in which more than four oocytes were aspirated, GIFT was carried out in four other synchronized non-stimulated periovulatory monkeys (group 2). Pregnancies were documented by macaque chorionic gonadotropin (mCG) levels and ultrasound. Of the six monkeys in group 1, three conceived. One is presently 90 days post-GIFT. The second pregnancy was a twin gestation and culminated in a spontane-ous abortion at 73 days post-GIFT. The third was an early pregnancy loss at 38 days post-GIFT. Of the four synchronized recipients in group 2, one conceived. She had four positive mCG levels at 18, 21, 24, and 27 days post-GIFT. She resumed menstruation 35 days after GIFT. These results support those obtained in our human GIFT program, and suggest that the Rhesus monkey is an excellent animal model in which to study new techniques to improve the efficiency of GIFT.

14.28.02
Studies on pituitary and hypothalamic dopaminergic mechanism in rats with estrogen-induced pituitary tumor: Takahashi, T, Satoh, S, Osada, H, Satoh, K, Minaguchi, H. Dept. Obstet. and Gyn., Yokohama City Univ. School Med., Yokohama, Japan
The mechanism of hypothalamus-anterior pituitary dopaminergic system during the development of estrogen-induced pituitary tumor was not well clarified. Hypothalamic DA turnover and pituitary DA receptor were studied in rats following estrogen treatment. Estradiol dipropionate (E2, 5 mg/kg, i. m.) was injected every two weeks up to 12 weeks. Bromocriptine (BC) was administered (1 mg/kg, p. o.) daily for seven days before decapitation. Dopaminergic receptors were estimated in partially purified pituitary membrane preparations by using [3H]spierone (SPIP). Dopamine concentrations were measured by HPLC. Dopamine turnover was calculated by using α-methyl-p-tyrosine (300 mg/kg, i. p.). Anterior pituitary weight and plasma prolactin concentration increased as numbers of E2 injection and the increment was reduced by BC. Specific [3H]SPIP bindings were demonstrated in the anterior pituitaries of both nontreated and estrogen-treated rats with pituitary tumors. The binding affinity was not significantly different in all groups (Kd; 0.06–0.09 nM). The numbers of binding sites (Bmax) in the pituitary were lower in estrogen-treated rats than in nontreated controls. Both BC and short-term E2 (estradiole benzoate 25 μg/kg for 5 days, s. c.) treatment significantly decreased the Bmax. Dopamine content of the hypothalamus decreased and dopamine turnover rate increased in rats with pituitary tumors. These results suggest that estrogen injection increases dopamine turnover of the hypothalamus to induce a reduction of pituitary dopaminergic receptors during the development of a pituitary tumor.

14.28.03

Characterization of epidermal growth factor (EGF) receptor in human endometrium and its cyclic changes during the menstrual cycle: Taketani, Y, Mizuno, M. Dept. Obstet. and Gyn., Fac. Med., Univ., Tokyo, Japan

EGF, a potent mitogenic peptide, is known to be present in the fluid of the uterine cavity. Therefore, in an attempt to clarify its physiological roles, we investigated the EGF receptor in human endometrial tissues. The membrane fractions from endometrium possessed the capacity to bind EGF in a specific, saturable and reversible manner. The Scatchard plot was linear, showing a single class of the receptor ($Kd = 3.8 \times 10^{-9}$ M). Trypsin and plant lectins inactivated the receptor. α-methylmannoside reversed the decreased EGF binding by concanavalin A, indicating that the receptor is glycoprotein. The amount of specific EGF binding was very low during menstruation and increased gradually, reaching its peak in the late follicular phase. There was an abrupt drop in the binding after ovulation. However, Kd value was unaltered throughout the menstrual cycle. In a primary cell culture system of human endometrium, the addition of estradiol into culture media resulted in a significant increase in the EGF binding to endometrial cells. These studies demonstrate the presence of EGF receptor in human endometrium and its cyclic variation in the menstrual cycle, thus implying the possible involvement of EGF in the proliferation of endometrial tissues in concert with estradiol.

14.28.04

Effect of clomiphene citrate on implantation in the rabbit: *Birkenfeld, A, Mootz, U, *Schenker, J G, Beier, H M. Dept. Reprod. Biol., Med. Fac., RWTH, Aachen; *Dept. Obstet. and Gyn., Hadassah Univ. Hosp., Jerusalem, Israel

The induction of ovulation with clomiphene citrate (CC) in human patients results in a high ovulation rate but achieves a relatively low pregnancy rate. In order to clarify the possible role of CC in interfering with normal reproductive physiology, we have transferred four-day-old rabbit blastocysts from untreated donors to CC treated pseudopregnant recipients and from CC treated donors to untreated pseudopregnant recipients. Each group was further subdivided into two subgroups, one receiving CC before and the other after ovulation. CC was administrated subcutaneously in three consecutive doses of 10 mg/kg body weight. Ovulation was induced with PMS and HCG. The implantation rate of the control group, evaluated on day 8 of pregnancy, reaches 62.0%. When recipients were treated with CC before ovulation, implantation rate is reduced to 18.8% (p < 0.0005) and to 20.0% (p < 0.007) when CC was administrated after ovulation. The implantation rate of blastocysts transferred from donors, treated before ovulation, is 22.2% (p < 0.02), however, reaches 70.8% when treatment was started after ovulation. All implantations are analysed microscopically and show normal morphological features. Our results demonstrate that CC altering endometrial receptiveness for the implanting conceptus, and possibly by an effect on other reproductive processes prior to implantation leads to a rapid decrease in the establishment of implantations and to the relatively low pregnancy rates observed with CC treatment.

14.28.05

Effects of tyrosine ingestion on circulating concentrations of dopamine metabolites in normal men and women: Ishizuka, B, Hirata, K, Hamada, H, Minegishi, A, Ishizaki, T. Dept. Obstet. and Gyn., St. Marianna Univ., Kawasaki, and Div. Clin. Pharmacol., Clin. Res. Inst., Nat. Med. Ctr, Tokyo, Japan

Since it has been suggested that increased tyrosine (TS) concentrations can accelerate the brain dopamine system, we have investigated the acute effect of oral TS ingestion on plasma levels of DOPAC and HVA in serial double-blind placebo-controlled studies in fasting healthy men and women. In all studies, blood was drawn at 15 min intervals between 1100 and 1430 h and TS (90 mg/kg) or lactose placebo was given at 1200 h. Plasma DOPAC and HVA levels were measured by HPLC and electrochemical detection. – Results: (men, n=4) DOPAC and HVA levels decreased significantly from basal levels (DOPAC 1.94 ± 0.24 ng/ml, HVA 10.2 ± 1.5 ng/ml at 1200 h) during the control studies (DOPAC 1.69 ± 0.09 ng/ml at 1400 h, p < 0.05, HVA 8.8 ± 1.3 ng/ml at 1245 h, p < 0.05), but TS ingestion nullified these changes in levels of both metabolites (women, n=4). Mean basal concentrations of DOPAC were significantly (p < 0.05) elevated during the luteal phase (follicular phase 1.47 ± 0.25 ng/ml, luteal phase 2.45 ± 0.3 ng/ml). There were no measurable changes in DOPAC levels following both TS and placebo ingestion. Mean basal HVA levels were comparable during the follicular and the luteal phase (8.7 ± 1.16 and 8.82 ± 0.9 ng/ml, respectively). HVA levels were lowered significantly (p < 0.01) when subjects consumed placebo; however, no corresponding changes were observed following TS ingestion. – Conclusions: These results suggest that the oral ingestion of tyrosine may exert acute effects on dopamine systems within the brain.

14.28.06

Effect of gonadal hormones on intestinal functions in ovariectomised rats: Dhall, G I, Singh, R, Nagpaul, J P, Majumdar, S, Chakravarti, R N. Dept. Obstet. and Gyn., Postgrad. Inst. Med. Educ. and Res., Chandigarh, India

The effect of sex hormones on intestinal digestive and absorptive functions were studied in ovariectomised rats by administering intraperitoneally low and high doses of 17β-estradiol and progesterone for two weeks. The uptake of glucose was significantly enhanced after ovariectomy and was restored to normal level following treatment with these hormones. Neither the uptake of L-leucine nor calcium was affected either by ovariectomy or treatment with gonadal hormones. The alkaline phosphatase (AP) activity of ileum was significantly elevated with both low and high doses of 17β-estradiol but in jejunum; such increase obtained only with a high dose. Progesterone enhanced significantly the jejunal and ileal AP activities only in combination with 17β-estradiol. The AP activity appears to be under the control of 17β-estradiol. The kinetic studies revealed that increased specific activity of AP is due to increase in enzyme content (Vmax) rather than affinity constant (Km) following treatment with sex hormones. The activity of ileal disacchariases and leucine aminopeptidase were enhanced at high doses of 17β-estradiol alone or in combination with progesterone, whereas in the jejunum only AP activity was increased significantly in such conditions. Therefore, 17β-estradiol plays an important role in regulating the activities of intestinal digestive enzymes and the ileal enzymes are more prone to alter in the presence of gonadal hormones.

14.28.07

The stimulation of 3β-HSD activity by hCG in PMS treated immature rat ovary: Yoshida, Y, Sano, Y, Kambegawa, A, Okinaga, S, Arai, K. Dept. Obstet. and Gyn., Teikyo Univ., School Med., Itabashi, Tokyo, Japan

Progesterone production in mammalian ovaries increases from the preovulatory phase to the luteal phase, and this phenomenon is widely accepted to be due to the LH effect to stimulate cyclic AMP mediated ovarian cholesterol side-chain cleavage enzyme (CSCC) activity and to increase the transport of cholesterol to this enzyme. We demonstrated that hCG stimulated not only CSCC but also 3β-HSD (Δ^5-3β-hydroxysteroid dehydrogenase and Δ^{4-5} isomerase) in ovarian cells from PMS treated immature rat. In this study, *in vivo* effect of hCG on the 3β-HSD activity was studied in the time course experiment. HCG or saline was injected to PMS treated immature female rats. The ovaries were removed at 0, 3, 6, 9 and 21 hours after the administration of hCG. The 800 × g supernatant of each group of the ovarian homogenate was incubated with ^{14}C-pregnenolone (10.8 nmol) in 1 ml of 0.25 M sucrose solution containing 0.2 μmol of NAD at 37° C for 60 min. At the end of the incubation, steroids were extracted and separated by TLC. Then the radioactivity of each metabolite was measured. 3β-HSD activity was expressed as the sum of the amounts of progesterone and its metabolites produced from ^{14}C-pregnenolone per unit weight of protein per hour. The enzyme activity in the hCG group was 1.5 times of that in the control group at 3 hours after injection and approx. twice at 6–9 hours. But at 21 hours, they reached to the same level. The result indicates that hCG increases 3β-HSD activity several hours after its administration, and it is suggested that this activation contributes to the increase of progesterone secretion.

14.28.08

In vitro effect of danazol® on follicle-stimulating hormone and luteinizing hormone secretion in rat anterior pituitary cell cultures: Kowaguchi, Y, Siraishi, S, Tanabe, K*, Nakamura, Y. Dept. Obstet. and Gyn., School Med., Keio Univ., Tokyo; *Tokyo Women's Med. Coll., Tokyo, Japan

The purpose of this study was to determine if danazol has its direct inhibitory action on FSH and LH secretion, employing a rat anterior pituitary cell monolayer culture as reported previously (JCEM 57, 24, 1983). After cells were exposed to 10^{-10} to 10^{-5} M of danazol for 24 hours, conditioned culture media (CCM) were collected and 10^{-9} M of luteinizing-hormone releasing hormone (LRH) was again added to cultures. After five hours with LRH, CCM and cell lysates were stored frozen until analysis. LH contents in LRH-free CCM (basal) significantly decreased with increment of danazol concentrations, while FSH contents markedly increased at concentration higher than 10^{-7} M. The critical points of concentrations during which FSH and LH response to LRH was suppressed by danazol were 10^{-10} to 10^{-6} M, and 10^{-10} to 10^{-5} M, respectively. Danazol suppressed LRH-stimulated total LH level (LH contents in CCM plus in cell lysates), although total basal LH level was not affected by danazol. In contrast, total FSH level with or without LRH increased at high doses of danazol. These data suggest that danazol may exert its direct inhibitory action on pituitary gonadotropine secretion in LH synthesis. This study was supported in part by a Rockefeller Foundation grand RF83002 to K.T.

14.28.09

Morphological and physiological aspects of organ preservation of the female genital tract in rats: Wiedemann, R, Strowitzki, T, Scheidel, P, Hepp, H. Dept. Gyn. and Obstet., Ludwig-Maximilians-Univ., Klinikum Grosshadern, München

In 110 white inbred rats a standard model of preservation of uterus, Fallopian tube and ovary for a period up to 24 h was established. The genital organ tract was preserved *en bloc* under hypothermic conditions after initial *in vivo* perfusion with different media according to the Collins technique for renal preservation. Ringer-Heparin, Euro-Collins and a special solution (TPM II) were tested in standardized conditions. Organ preservation was evaluated by light microscopy (including semi-thin cuts) and TEM. Ionic concentrations of tissue after preservation was analysed by NAA and AAS. Morphological damage of the uterus, Fallopian tube and ovary varied significantly, indicating that the mucosa of the ampulla is the most sensitive structure which allows histological grading of preservation effects. Excessive shifts of the ionic concentrations, especially potassium, were found in all media, thus indicating, that similar ionic shifts in different media do not correlate with the grade of morphological damage. Immediate transplantation of the genital organs after initial perfusion resulted in a 40% transplant survival (n = 20).

14.28.10

Induction of ovulation in the hypogonadotropic hypogonadism with "pure" urinary FSH: Nappi, C, Rosa, M de*, Quagliozzi, L*, Del Giudice, M, Lombardi, G*, Montemagno, U. Dept. Obstet. and Gyn. and Endocr.*, 2nd School Med., Univ., Naples, Italy

Past data suggested that both gonadotropins (FSH and LH) are synergically required to induce ovarian steroidogenic response in hypogonadotropic patients. Recently it has been reported that "pure" urinary FSH alone was able to stimulate follicular maturation and E_2 production in monkeys with reversible hypogonadotropic state induced by a Gn-RH antagonist treatment (*Kenigsberg* et al., 1984). Four patients affected by idiopathic hypogonadotropic hypogonadism were treated with purified urinary FSH (HU-FSH, Serono) monitoring ovarian response by rapid E_2 RIA and ultrasound scanning of follicular development. In all the patients the treatment induced an increase of E_2 secretion and follicular maturation. Ovulation occurred in three patients after exogenous HCG administration, while one patient had a spontaneous LH surge and a subsequent ovulation. These findings demonstrate that exogenous FSH alone may be effective for induction of ovulation also in the idiopathic hypogonadotropic hypogonadism.

14.28.11

Steroid secretion pattern of tertiary bovine atretic follicles in a superfusion system: Zimmermann, R[3], Westhof, G[1], Peukert-Adam, I[2], Braendle, W[1], Grunert, E[2]. [1]Abt. Klin. u. Exp. Endokr., Univ., Hamburg; [2]Klin. Geb. u. Gyn., Hannover; [3]Yale Univ., New Haven, CT, USA

A superfusion system as previously described (*Zimmermann* et al. Horm. Metab. Res., in press) was applied to 13 atretic follicles, which were removed from cows 12 h, 24 h, 48 h, 72 h, 84 h after $PGF_{2\alpha}$ induced luteolysis. After termination of each experiment the follicles were histologically processed and classified according to *Marion* et al. (J. Anim. Soc. **27**, 451, 1968). Aromatase activity of all follicles was very low (E2 < 0.01 ng/ml) whereas the secretion of testosterone (T) and progesterone (P) was in the range of P and T concentrations of periovulatory dominant follicles. Follicles with early or contraction atresia always showed higher T than P levels. In contrast, P was greater than T for cystic, cystic + contraction, and late atresia. Steroid secretion did not correlate with follicular size and time interval after PG injection. It is concluded that atretic follicles in addition to dominant follicles contribute significant amounts to peripheral T and P levels during the periovulatory phase and characteristic steroid secretion patterns were found in defined histological entities.

14.28.12

The influences of weight loss and subsequent regain on rat hypothalamo-pituitary-ovarian (HPO) function: Kotsuji, F, Goto, K, Aso, T, Tominaga, T. Dept. Obstet. and Gyn., Fukui Med. School, Fukui, Japan

Twelve weeks of age female SD rats were restricted to 8 g/day feed intake for two months followed by feeding ad libitum for three weeks. Feed restriction resulted in weight loss (56%) and constant diestrous. Serum LH, FSH and PRL levels reduced throughout the under-fed period, while the decrease of serum and ovarian E_2 levels were initially detected on the 14th day. Persistent increase of hypothalamic GnRH contents was observed during the period. Anterior pituitary showed significant response to GnRH + TRH (0.5 and 1.0 μg/300 g B. W.) during the course, and the relative increases of LH, FSH and PRL were greater than those of pretreatment rats. In the course of re-feeding, the body weight returned to the control level and regular estrous cycles were re-established on the 15th and 21st day, respectively. The changes in pituitary-ovarian axis were; prompt rebound elevations of serum FSH and PRL levels and pituitary FSH content, delayed regains of serum and pituitary LH levels and serum and ovarian E_2 levels, marked increase of serum and ovarian progesterone levels on the 16th day. Elevated hypothalamic GnRH content returned to the control level on the 16th day. The relative increases of LH, FSH and PRL after GnRH + TRH injection in re-fed period were smaller than those in under-fed period. The present study revealed the detailed sequence of events in HPO function accompanying weight loss and regain induced by the change of feeding regimens. It is indicative that weight loss primarily disturbs the releasing mechanism of endogenous hypothalamic factors, and the normalization of this mechanism with weight regain is a prerequisite for restoration of the HPO axis.

14.28.13

Plasma renin activity in normal menstrual cycle: Michalas, S, Stamatiou, G, Aravantinos, D. 1st Dept. Obstet. and Gyn., Univ., Athens, Greece

Plasma renin activity (P.R.A.), luteinizing hormone and progesterone were measured by radio-immunoassay in 25 normal young women during the menstrual cycle. The blood samples were drawn every second day from day 2 to day 26 of the cycle and every day during the periovulatory time. It was found that P.R.A. presents a first peak two days before ovulation, a second higher peak the day of ovulation, corresponding with the LH peak, and after a short decline the next day after ovulation a progressive rise reaching a plateau in the secretory phase. From these data it is concluded that P.R.A. is another parameter for the determination of the day of ovulation. On the other hand when P.R.A. is measured in a woman in the reproductive life, the value must be taken into consideration according to the appropriate phase of the menstrual cycle.

14.28.14

Neuropeptides and female reproduction: Ottesen, B, Bardrum, B, Fahrenkrug, J. Inst. Med. Physiol., Panum Inst; Dept. Gyn. and Obstet. Y, Rigshosp. and Dept. Clin. Chem., Bispebjerg Hosp., Univ., Copenhagen, Denmark

During the last few years, a number of "brain-gut peptides" have been demonstrated in the nervous structures of the female genital tract by immunological methods, raising the question of their physiological significance as neurotransmitter substances. We have examined the effect of vasoactive intestinal polypeptide (VIP), PHI-27 (the peptide with N-terminal histidine and 27 amino acids), substance P (SP), somatostatin, enkephalins and avian pancreatic polypeptide (APP) on non-vascular uterine smooth muscle and blood flow in rabbit and cat. SP caused a dose-dependent increase in mechanical and myoelectrical activity, an action which could be antagonized by VIP. SP, leu-enkephalin, VIP and PHI induced concentration-related increase in blood flow of the uterus where VIP and PHI seem to be the most potent vasodilators with additive effects. Moreover, VIP and PHI caused a dose-dependent relaxation of non-vascular smooth muscle with superimposable dose-response curves. Neither the effect on vascular nor on non-vascular smooth muscle was inhibited by adrenergic or cholinergic blocking agent. APP was able to inhibit the VIP-induced vasodilation in rabbit. These findings suggest that several peptides are involved in the local nervous control of both uterine contraction and hemodynamic event. Thus, besides the cholinergic and adrenergic systems, the autonomous nervous system has a third component, the peptidergic nerves which are of importance in reproductive physiology.

14.28.15

The modulating effect of estrogens on luteinizing hormone release in complete androgen insensitivity syndrome: Göretzlehner, G, Scholz, B, Wodrig, W, Weber, M, Sas, M, Morway, J. Depts. Obstet. and Gyn., Ernst Moritz Arndt Univ., Greifswald, German Democratic Republic, and Med. School, Szeged, Hungary

The complete form of the androgen insensitivity syndrome (AIS) is a useful model for study the effect of estrogens on gonadotropin release before and after gonadectomy. The present study is a report for the modulating effects of estrogens and CMA on LH release after gonadectomy in a different time of age in three patients with a complete AIS and a karyotype 46, XY. None of the subjects had received any medication known to exert an influence upon the hypothalamic-pituitary-gonadal axis. To assess LH release in on estrogen provocation test, 0.5 mg estradiol bencoate per kg body weight was administered intramuscularly between 8 and 9 a. m. and blood samples were collected at 12 hour intervals over the next 96 hours. This test was performed after gonadectomy and three month after 18 month of therapy with Sequenz-Ovosiston (mestranol 100 μg 9 pills, mestranol 80 μg and CMA 2 mg 12 pills). In the first test no LH secretion could be provoked by estrogen stimulation. A positive feedback was induced in two patients three months after the long time therapy with steroids.

14.32.01

Cytogenetic findings in prenatal diagnosis: A collaborative study in Japan: Tamura, S[1], Fujimoto, S[2], Hayashi, K[3], Maeda, K[4], Kenjo, T[5]. [1]Keio Univ., Tokyo; [2]Hokkaido Univ., Sapporo; [3]Kyoto Univ., Kyoto; [4]Kitasato Univ., Kanagawa; [5]Tokai Univ., Kanagawa, Japan

The collected data of 2579 prenatal chromosome determinations performed by five university hospitals in Japan are reported. The main indication groups were: Advanced maternal age (1322 cases), previous child with a chromosome abnormality (610 cases), parental chromosome abnormality (85 cases), and miscellaneous (562 cases). A total of 81 fetuses with a chromosome abnormality was detected. These included trisomy 21 (23 cases), sex chromosome aneuploidy (11 cases), balanced structural rearrangements (26 cases), and other autosomal anomalies (21 cases). Among 915 mothers from 35 to 39 years old, 1.2% had abnormal fetuses, and among 407 mothers 40 or more years, 3.4% had aneuploid fetuses. Among 610 mothers who had had a previous child with a chromosome abnormality, eight (1.3%) were found to be carrying a fetus with a chromosome abnormality. There were three fetuses (9.1%) which had unbalanced translocation among 33 families in which one parent was carrying a Robertsonian translocation, whereas in 46 families with a reciprocal translocation, six fetuses (13.0%) showed an unbalanced karyotype. The number of women undergoing amniocentesis because of advanced age has increased rapidly in recent years.

14.32.02

Ultrasound scanning for transcervical chorion villus biopsy: Richardson, R, Liu, D T Y. Dept. Obstet. and Gyn., City Hosp., Nottingham, UK

It is becoming increasingly clear that ultrasound scanning is essential for successful chorion villus biopsy. Ultrasound examination can define normality and stage of gestation besides identification of the most appropriate site for biopsy. Adverse sequelae such as trauma or excessive bleeding and particularly perforation of the gestation sac can be minimised when scanning is maintained during the biopsy procedure. Studies were conducted to determine which of the currently popular 3.5 and 5 MHz linear array, convex or sector probe is the most suitable facility. Examples of pitfalls associated with the use of ultrasound for this purpose will be indicated.

14.32.03

Chorion villi sampling – a comparison of different sampling methods: Zahn, F W, Müller-Holve, W, Popp, L, Stoeckenius, U, Martin, K. München and Frauenklin., A. K. Hamburg-Barmbek, Lehrkrankenh., Univ., Hamburg

360 cases of chorion villi sampling are reported. Different sampling methods were used such as catheters of different diameters, cytological brushes and chorionoscopic technics. Advantages and disadvantages of the different technics in relation to complication and practicability are reported.

14.32.04

Chorion biopsy in early pregnancy – laboratory experiences with 312 specimens: Purandare, H, Chakravarty, A, Purandare, C B. Med. Genet. Diagn. Ctr, Bombay, India

Chorion biopsy was performed in 312 cases at 7–11 weeks pregnancy. In 52 cases biopsy was performed prior to MTP (control group). Biopsy was performed in 46 cases for genetic reasons. Fetal sexing was performed in 214 cases by using X and Y chromatin assay. In all the cases direct chromosome preparations were done. In the diagnostic group results were compared in 28 cases by amniotic cells culture (16–18 weeks). Fetal sexing by sex chromatin studies was also compared with direct chromosome preparation (karyotype). Overall a good mitotic index was observed by direct preparation in 80% of the specimens. In 51 cases repeat biopsy was performed to get good quality of tissue. Result of sex chromatin and direct preparation was found to be accurate (100%) in all the cases delivered and those who opted for abortion (110). In diagnostic specimens two cases of late maternal age showed an abnormal karyotype (trisomy-21) and were also confirmed by amniotic cell culture (16 weeks). Both the patients opted for an abortion and diagnosis was confirmed. Pregnancy resulted in timely delivery of full term healthy infants. Therefore the method described is valuable means of diagnosing inherited disorders in early pregnancy.

14.32.05

Indian experience of first trimester chorion biopsy: Purandare, C N, Purandare, H M, Chakravarty, A. Med. Genet. Ctr, Bombay, India

Chorion biopsy can be used for antenatal diagnosis of sex and chromosomal abnormalities in the first trimester of pregnancy. The procedure consists of taking an aspiration biopsy of chorionic tissue under ultrasound control from the chorion frondosum. The entire procedure is done as an out-patient procedure by a special apparatus without needing any anesthesia, with hardly any fetal or maternal morbidity. It is an easy and safer method as compared to amniocentesis done at 16 weeks gestation. Preliminary report of 150 cases done in private practice in Bombay showed accuracy of sex diagnosis at 100%. There were no abortions resulting from the procedure within 72 h but one abortion after ten days. Patients who continued pregnancy showed no evidence of abortion with eleven patients already delivering a healthy normal child. This method can also be used for diagnosing chromosomal abnormalities.

14.32.06

Chorion villi sampling: Klink, F, Froster-Iskenius, U*, Grzejszczyk, G, Schwinger, E*, Oberheuser, F. Dept. Obstet. & Gyn., and Dept. Humangenet.*, Med. Univ., Lübeck

Fetal diagnosis has become an important tool in the prevention of genetic diseases. A new method of prenatal diagnosis during the first trimester of pregnancy is reported. First trimester fetal diagnosis reduces the anxiety of the long interval of waiting the sampling in the second trimester and minimizes the technical and physiological consequences of a late termination. The gynecological and cytogenetic aspects of more than 100 experimental cases and 22 diagnostic cases of transcervical trophoblast samplings are studied. Two different preliminary methods of sampling were carried out in the first series, the failure rate was 12.5%, whereas sampling of the second series was completely successful. The cytogenetic study of the aspirated samples proved to be very reliable. The short culture time of the chorion villi showed in general very good results concerning partly the mitosis and the quality of the metaphase plate. A drawback of this method is that, it does not allow the estimation of α-fetoprotein or acetylcholinesterase which are part of the prenatal diagnosis of neural tube defects. This, however, can be postponed to the 16th week of gestation or done by estimation of α-fetoprotein in the maternal serum.

14.32.07

Patient compliance for transcervical chorion villus biopsy as an out-patient procedure: Pearson, D, Jeavons, B, Liu, D T Y. Dept. Obstet. and Gyn., City Hosp., Nottingham, UK

First trimester diagnosis and earlier results will undoubtedly promote chorion villus biopsy as a valid alternative to amniocentesis. Despite the many advantages of villus biopsy, general acceptance and use will not be forthcoming unless the procedure is well tolerated by patient and can be accomplished with the same ease as amniocentesis. The responses of 80 patients undergoing chorion villus biopsy as an out-patient procedure was compared with 30 patients undergoing amniocentesis. Discomfort at each stage of the procedure for both techniques were sampled by use of a linear scale ranging from 1 to 10. Results suggest that on average, chorion villus biopsy is well tolerated and compares favorably with amniocentesis for pre-natal diagnosis.

14.32.08

Prenatal diagnosis: First experiences with transcervical aspiration biopsy of chorion villi: Eelen, C, Buytaert, P, Loquet, P. Dept. Obstet./Gyn., Acad. Hosp., Univ., Antwerp, Belgium

Prenatal diagnosis by chorion villi sampling (CVS) has many advantages: villi are removed at an amenorrhea of 8 to 10 weeks; results of direct chromosomal analysis are known in a few hours. An eventual early interruption of pregnancy has many advantages, medical and psychological. Recent advances in DNA technology make CVS necessary. However, CVS is a delicate technical procedure. On 70 women, who wanted interruption of their pregnancy for social reasons, we took off chorion villi, by means of chorion aspiration and under echographic control by real-time sector scanning, before the vacuum aspiration was performed. Next we removed chorion villi for diagnostic reasons in ten women. With the results obtained we discuss the optimum period for CVS, problems and thus absolute contra-indications for CVS, influence of quantity and quality of villi on successful chromosomal analyses. The period, most successful for CVS is at an amenorrhea of 9 to 10 weeks. Before pursuing CVS with success for diagnostic reasons, experience on patients who decided to interrupt their pregnancy is necessary, just as careful selection of patients, who, by obesity, position or malformation of the uterus, localisation of the placenta can be considered well or not as a candidate for CVS. The percentage of successful chromosomal analyses is maximal if more than 10 mg villi are obtained.

14.32.09

Chorionic villi sampling in the management of severe blood group immunisation in pregnancy: Bennebroek Gravenhorst, J[1], van't Veer, M B[2], Bernini, L F[3], Kanhai, H H H[1]. [1]Dept. Obstet. and Gyn.; [2]Centr. Lab. Neth. Red Cross, Amsterdam; [3]Dept. Hum. Genet., Univ. Hosp., Leiden, The Netherlands

In pregnancies complicated by severe blood group antigen sensitisation, early identification of fetal red cell antigen could be of great importance. Pregnancy termination at an acceptable duration of gestation could be considered and unnecessary invasive diagnostic procedures prevented. Studying material, obtained by chorionic villi sampling (CVS) before pregnancy termination, we found that many chorionic villi contain blood vessels from which fetal red cells could be obtained for blood group antigen determination. Fetal erythrocytes were identified by staining with a specific anti-HbF antibody. D positive erythrocytes could be detected by the minor cell population technique (1:500). In three severely sensitised Rh neg women with a bad obstetrical history and a Rh (D) heterozygous partner CVS was performed. In two of the biopsy samples D positive red cells were identified. After pregnancy termination the diagnosis could be confirmed. In the biopsy material of the third patient 1.5% fetal cells were detected, no D positive cells could be identified. This pregnancy is still proceeding without signs of hemolysis. Recently we developed an immunofluorescence technique by which positive cells can be detected up to 1 in 4000. Besides Rh D also A, B, Kell, C, c, and E antigen have been identified in material obtained by CVS. We believe CVS can be of considerable help in the management of severe blood group immunisation in pregnancy.

14.32.10

Prenatal diagnosis of Hunter syndrome: Granat, M*, Zlotogora, J, Zeigler, M, Bach, G. *Dept. Obstet. and Gyn., and Dept. Hum. Genet., Hadassah Univ. Hosp., Jerusalem, Israel

Hunter syndrome (mucopolysaccharidosis II) is a lysosomal storage disease caused by the deficiency of iduronate sulfate sulfatase (ISS) leading to lysosomal accumulation of mucopolysaccharides principally in connective tissue. The disease is characterized by severe disability and shortened life span. It is inherited as an X-linked recessive disorder and has been found in increased frequency among the Jewish population in Israel. The disease is incurable, but prevention of birth of affected babies is possible by prenatal diagnosis. In the last five years we examined 25 pregnancies at risk for Hunter syndrome. Ten fetuses were identified as affected and their families elected to undergo abortion. Prenatal diagnosis of Hunter syndrome is performed by enzyme determination directly in the amniotic fluid, and sex determination by karyotyping the cultured amniotic fluid cells. The diagnosis has therefore been usually completed only after the 18th week of pregnancy. Chorionic villi sampling (CVS) makes the diagnosis possible at the first trimester of pregnancy. Determinations of enzyme activity and embryo sex are performed directly on the specimen obtained by transcervical aspiration, and can be accomplished within 48 hours. Preliminary data on the determination of ISS activity in samples of chorionic tissue obtained by CVS is presented, serving as a baseline for future prenatal diagnosis of pregnancies at risk in the early stages of pregnancy.

14.41.01

Fetal movements and heart rate associated with fetal malformations: Sadovsky, E, Navot, D, Mor-Yosef, S, Granat, M. Dept. Obstet. and Gyn., Hadassah Univ. Hosp., Jerusalem, Israel

An exceptionally high Cesarean section rate with malformed fetuses together with low salvagability calls for reduction of inappropriate interventions in these pregnancies. Out of 822 cases of high risk pregnancies there were 55 cases with decreased fetal movements (DFM), nine of whom had congenital malformations (16.5%). Among the remaining 767 patients (without DFM), eight had malformation (1.04%). Antenatal fetal heart rate monitoring of 20 fetuses with major congenital malformations revealed loss of long-term variability (LLTV) in 11 (55%) and an isolated, abrupt-onset fetal heart rate deceleration in 13 (65%). In ten (50%), loss of variability coexisted with periodic fetal heart rate decelerations. These fetal heart rate changes were significantly more prevalent in the malformed group than in a control population. Perinatal mortality was 75%, reflecting the lethal nature of the malformations. When DFM, and/or LLTV associated with abrupt fetal heart rate deceleration appear every effort should be made to exclude fetal malformations before termination of pregnancy especially by Cesarean section.

14.41.02

Validity of ultrasound scanning for fetal congenital abnormalities: Sollie, J E, Geijn, H P van, Bruyn, K, Arts, N F T. Dept. Obstet. & Gyn., Acad. Ziekenhuis, Vrije Univ., Amsterdam, The Netherlands

From 1980 onwards, ultrasound scanning for fetal congenital anomalies has been performed in 516 pregnant women, according to a schematic protocol. The women were referred by other hospitals (53.6%) or attended our out-patients clinics (46.5%). Scanning was done at 17 and 24 weeks of gestation in women with an obstetric or family history of fetal congenital abnormalities (37.6%) and as early as possible in complicated pregnancies (44.5%) i. e. early intra-uterine growth retardation, polyhydramnios or premature labor. Major structural defects were found in 80 fetuses, 25 had neural tube defects, 17 urinary tract anomalies, 11 hydrops or associated signs and 8 skeletal dysplasia. Many fetuses had more than one anomaly. Abnormalities were particularly found in the group developing complications during pregnancy (58.2%), and fewer in the group with an obstetric or family history of congenital anomalies (10%). The positive predictive value of this type of scanning was 100%, the negative predictive value 97%. The specificity of the indications applied for performing an ultrasound scanning was 91%, the sensitivity 97%. Systematic ultrasound scanning for congenital anomalies should be an essential part of obstetric practice. In this way unnecessary obstetric procedures can be omitted in pregnancies producing children with anomalies, incompatible with life. On the other hand, planning of time and mode of delivery and immediate neonatal care in a multidisciplined approach may lead to a better prognosis for the infant.

14.41.03

Prenatal ultrasonic diagnosis of short rib polydactyly syndrome (SRPS) type III: A case report and a proposed approach to the diagnosis of SRPS and related conditions: Meizner, I, Bar-Ziv, J, Holcberg, G. Div. Obstet. and Gyn., and Dept. Pediat. Radiol., Soroka Univ. Hosp., Ben-Gurion Univ. of the Negev, Beer-Sheva, Israel

The diagnosis of skeletal dysplasia using only ultrasound is possible. Several cases of these pathologies have already been described in the past. We present a case of short rib polydactyly syndrome type III which to the best of our knowledge, is the first report of a prenatal ultrasonic diagnosis of this condition. SRPS type III is a lethal dysplasia characterized by severe shortening of the ribs and hypoplasia. Polydactyly is present in all cases, the long bones are shortened with widened metaphyses characterized by marginal spurs. Genital anomalies in the external genitalia and cardiovascular anomalies are often present. Other conditions associated with dwarfism and polydactyly include SRPS type I (Saldino-Noonan syndrome), SRPS type II (Mayevski syndrome) Ellis-van Creveld syndrome (chondro-ectodermal dysplasia) and Jeune syndrome (asphyxiating thoracic dystrophy). The differential diagnosis between these conditions will be discussed and prenatal ultrasonic algorithmic guidelines for correct diagnosis will be presented.

14.41.04

Fetal urinary tract anomalies diagnosed by ultrasound scanning: Antoli, A, Cabo, A, Domene, J, Mico, J M, Beamud, A. Dept. Obstet. and Gyn., La Fe Hosp., Valencia, Spain

High-resolution real-time ultrasound was routinely used to examine 20,000 pregnant patients, and fetal urinary tract anomalies were encountered in 18 cases that were serially scanned to term of pregnancy, and further confirmed by a postnatal urologic and anatomical study. In this report, two cases are excluded: a fetus with bilateral polycystic kidney and an anephric fetus, both stillborn. The 18 cases are classified into three groups according to the anomaly: uretero-pelvic stenosis: nine case, polycystic renal dysplasia: four cases, posterior urethral valve: five cases. Ultrasound images are described and all the findings of amniotic fluid, mictional rhythm and renal enlargement are appraised in order to make a differential diagnosis of these anomalies, as well as clarifying the unilateral or bilateral involvement that will be essential in regard to adequate treatment at a later stage.

14.41.05

Fetal macrosomia: Demographic analysis and perinatal performance in a Chinese population: Li, D F H, Wong, V C W. Dept. Obstet. and Gyn., Univ., Hong Kong

A retrospective analysis of the demographic and perinatal data of 332 macrosomic infants (≥ 3.8 kg) born of Chinese mothers in a teaching hospital in Hong Kong was performed. Results were compared with similar data from 334 normal weight infants (> 2.5 to < 3.8 kg) randomly selected in the same year. The incidence of fetal macrosomia was 5.7% of the annual deliveries. Significant maternal risk factors were increased maternal age, high pre-pregnant weight and ponderal index, positive history of previous macrosomic babies and presence of maternal diabetes. The incidence of diabetes mellitus was 13.6%. Clinical suspicion of macrosomia before delivery was positive in only 31.0% of cases. The uterine volume index (UVI) at term was calculated by the formula: UVI = (Fundal Height $\times$ Abdominal Girth^2)/4π. When the UVI was ≥ 34.0 litres, the predictive value for macrosomia was 40% with a false positive rate of only 2.2%. Meconium stained liquor and Cesarean section were more common. First stage of labor was comparable but second stage was significantly prolonged. Among the macrosomic infants, male : female ratio was 2 : 1.

Birth trauma and neonatal jaundice were more common. Fetal macrosomia is less common in Chinese mothers. Maternal diabetes is a significant contributory factor which may justify screening of the maternity population to allow early detection and treatment.

14.41.06
Fetal pulmonary hypoplasia: Report of a case: Murayama, K, Jimbo, T. Tokyo Seamens' Hosp., Tokyo, Japan

We wish to report a case of fetal pulmonary hypoplasia with a large amount of pleural fluid, diagnosed by ultrasound examination at 28 weeks gestation and managed by aspiration of the pleural fluid after premature delivery at 33 weeks. The neonate grew up without any subsequent eventful episode. This case appears to be the first one in the world. T. K., a 29-year-old woman, presented with abdominal fulness at 28 weeks gestation. She was admitted with the diagnosis of hydroamnios and threatened premature delivery. Ultrasound examination at 28 weeks demonstrated hydramnios, a large amount of pleural fluid in the fetal pleural cavity, the fetal lung looked like a small mass probably through compression by pleural fluid, and a normal fetal cardiac activity. Amniocentesis and aspiration of fetal pleural fluid, 200 and 25 ml, respectively, were done. On the cytologic examination, there was no malignant cell. Fetal pleural fluid analyses were as follows: specific gravity, 1.013; positive Rivalta reaction; amounts of protein, 1.4 g/dl. L/S ratio of amniotic fluid aspirated at 32 weeks was 5.67. Premature rupture of the membrane occurred at 33 weeks, and labor began spontaneously. A premature female infant weighing 2060 g was delivered spontaneously. The infant was transfered to NICU and managed by continuous aspiration of the pleural fluid. She was discharged uneventfully weighing 3094 g. A large amount of pleural fluid was thought as the etiology in this case. It appears too hasty to do artificial interruption of pregnancy in such a case. Whether the continuation of pregnancy is proper or improper should be referred to the phospholipid fraction value in amniotic fluid.

14.41.07
Prenatal diagnosis of Ellis-van Creveld syndrome with ultrasound: Gollop, T R, Eigier, A. Serv. Genét. Hum., Ass. Matern., São Paulo, Brazil

Chondroectodermal dysplasia or Ellis-van Creveld syndrome is an autosomal recessive trait characterized by: short limb dwarfism, postaxial polydactyly, dysplastic nails and teeth and upper-lip frenula, in addition to congenital heart disease in half the cases. To the best of our knowledge the first and unique report of prenatal diagnosis of Ellis-van Creveld syndrome was done by *Mahoney* and *Hobbins* (1977) using both fetoscopy and ultrasound. We report the prenatal diagnosis of Ellis-van Creveld syndrome with ultrasound in the 16th menstrual week of a 29-year-old Japanese female. Her husband was also Japanese and they were nonconsanguineous. The couple had had two previous fetal deaths at 32 weeks which showed dwarfism, and a normal girl. Ultrasound findings at 16th week of pregnancy showed long bone shortening with all long bones below two standard deviations of the normal, fetal scalp with double contour probably secondary to heart disease. The aborted fetus showed hexadactyly of hands and feet. The association of dwarfism, hexadactyly, double contour of fetal head and histological findings gave us the prenatal diagnosis of Ellis-van Creveld syndrome.

14.41.08
Antenatal detection of a rare fetal tumor: Ultrasound and histologic findings in a case of embryonal rhabdomyosarcoma (case report): Pfeiffer, K H, Bachmann, F F. Univ. Frauenklin., Tübingen

An echogram of a 27-year-old primipara in the 31st week of gestation showed a solid tumor (diameter, 8 cm) on the right side of the fetal thorax. Concomitant findings were hydramnios and pleural effusion, right worse than left. Intra-uterine death occurred three days after diagnosis. Labor was induced with prostaglandin. At delivery, a large soft-tissue tumor extending as far as the pleura and infiltrating the right shoulder and neck was found on the right side of the thorax. Subsequent histologic evaluation showed the tumor to be an embryonal rhabdomyoscarcoma. This extremely rare embryonal tumor is shown on the antenatal echogram and the postnatal histologic picture. The differential diagnosis from other fetal tumors with similar localization (i. e., hygroma, teratoma, struma congenita) is presented.

14.41.09
Fetal urinary tract study by ultrasound: Perez, E, Cabo, A, Domene, J, Mico, J M, Beamud, A. Dept. Obstet. and Gyn., La Fe Hosp., Valencia, Spain

The standard ultrasound findings in fetal biometry enable one to recognize early urinary tract components. Routine ultrasound fetal evaluation to term, after identifying kidneys at the 19–20th gestational week, allow their development and size to be known. The bladder can be also measured and valued in its filling, emptying and correlation with the state of the upper urinary tract. Renal function is indirectly evaluated through the mictional rhythm. The normality of the whole urinary tract can be stated only if mictional rhythm and amniotic fluid are both normal, taking their functional relation into consideration. Misdiagnosis in fetal ultrasound scanning can be very serious, therefore a through study must be performed. We describe the normal findings based upon our large experience in ultrasound scanning of more than 90,000 pregnant patients, and also considering the reports of other authors. Obviously that experience has been improved by new technology.

14.41.10

Prenatal evaluation of anatomic and functional lesions of the urinary tract: Kozlowski, P, Terinde, R. Dept. Gyn. and Obstet., Univ., Düsseldorf

Lesions of the fetal urinary tract may be grossly divided into two major groups: 1) anatomic lesions such as agenesis, dysgenesis, stenosis and atresia and 2) functional disorders in a macroscopically normal shaped urinary tract. At present we survey 36 cases of urinary tract malformations. Unilateral or bilateral cystic degeneration of the kidneys, megaureter or stenosis of the urethra are – in most cases – easily to detect by sonographic examination, because the amount of amniotic fluid is not altered. In case of anhydramnios, however, it is nearly impossible to differentiate between anatomic and functional lesions. Stimulating the fetal kidneys by administration of frusemide to the mother fails in most cases of anhydramnios. To improve ultrasound imaging we considered an imitation of physiological conditions of the fetus in utero to be useful. We replaced the missing amniotic fluid by instillation of a solution into the amniotic cavity. This artificial amniotic fluid is of a similar electrolyte concentration as physiological amniotic fluid. Comparing several infusions, we evaluated "Normofundin sK" as the least problematic fluid. At present (Jan. 1985) we report eight cases of artificial amniotic fluid instillation for diagnostic purposes. Depending on the gestational age we used between 40 and 80 ml of fluid. There are three main effects which can be achieved by this technique: 1) The fetus is surrounded by fluid and can be examined by ultrasound, thus further malformations may be detected, 2) artificial amniotic fluid is swallowed by the fetus and can be demonstrated within the stomach and intestines, 3) it facilitates the evaluation of the function and anatomic size of the kidneys, either by fluid instillation alone, or – if this fails – by a subsequent frusemide provocation test.

14.41.11

Prenatal diagnosis of defects of the fetal abdominal wall: Rabe, D, Leucht, W, Schmidt, W. Dept. Obstet. and Gyn., Univ., Heidelberg

Omphalocele, umbilical cord hernia and gastroschisis are surgically correctable defects of the abdominal wall. This paper reports the prenatal ultrasonographic diagnosis, coexisting malformations, course of pregnancy and delivery. From 1975 to 1983 266 congenital fetal malformations had been diagnosed in our department. Of these cases 27 showed an anterior abdominal wall defect (10.2%). 26/27 underwent antenatal ultrasound examination. In 23 patients (89%) the congenital abdominal wall defect was identified by ultrasound, in 16 cases prior to the 24th week of gestation. In seven cases the patients had been admitted to our department after 24th week. In three cases the diagnosis was missed by ultrasound. There were 17 cases of omphalocele, of which 13 cases (77%) had been accompanied by associated malformations. The four cases of gastroschisis had no further anomalies. Six cases of extensive malformations of the abdominal wall (neither omphalocele nor gastroschisis) had also been associated with abnormalities of other organ systems. Chromosomal aberrations could be found in six of all 27 fetuses (22%). They were all combined with an omphalocele. – Conclusions: The prenatal diagnosis of an abdominal wall defect by ultrasound is possible in most of the cases. However, it often seems difficult for us to distinguish between omphalocele and gastroschisis. Therefore we suggest amniocentesis and fetal karyotyping in all of the cases.

14.41.12

Consequences of antenatal detection of fetal malformations for obstetrical and neonatal management: Wisser, J, Bald, R, Knitza, R. Dept. Obstet. and Gyn., Klinikum Grosshadern, München

Technical improvement of high-resolution B-mode ultrasound and increasing experience of the examiner allows the antenatal diagnosis of fetal malformation with increasing accuracy. Between Oct. 1983 and Oct. 1984 we examined 38 fetuses with fetal malformations. In 34 cases (89.5%) we put forward the correct diagnosis. These figures are in good agreement with those published by *Hansmann* who found the correct diagnosis in 270 out of 304 fetuses (89%). According to the antenatal diagnosis our obstetrical and neonatal management is divided in four groups: 1. In case of a fetus suffering from a non-viable disease, labor is conducted without fetal monitoring and with minimal risk to the mother (osteogenesis imperfecta typ II). 2. The fetus with a deteriorating intra-uterine condition, which can be treated post-partum is delivered prematurely (ileal atresia). 3. Postnatal emergency therapy is planned for fetuses with a correctable but life-threatening condition (diaphragmatic hernia). 4. Postnatal diagnostic procedures are planned for the fetus with a morphological malformation (cystic adenomatoid malformation of the lung type I). Antenatal diagnosis, obstetrical and neonatal decision-making are illustrated and discussed in typical case reports.

14.41.13

Fetal sex determination by amniotic fluid cells examination (prenatal): J. S. Trezza. Obstet. and Perinat. Clin., Fac. Med., Córdoba, Argentina

In experimental medicine and biology, several prenatal diagnosis can be done by the study of amniotic fluid or chorionic membranes tissues. Certain alterations affecting the chromosoms, the neural tube and the fetus metabolism, have been diagnosed by this method. As shown in the following results, the amniotic fluid can also be used for prenatal sex determination in humans. In this work, fifty pregnant women, requiring amniocentesis for different pathological reasons (hydramnios fetal ... etc.) were subjected to amniotic fluid study. A 5 ml aliquot of amniotic fluid was centrifuged at 800 g for 10 minutes and the containing cells were five times concentrated by resuspension of the cells pellet in only 1 ml of supernatant fluid. From each case, two or more slides were prepared for 2% Giemsa stain. At least 500 cells were microscopically examined at 50 × magnification in the search of Barr corpuscules carrying cells. The fetus was considered female (chromatin positive) when at least 10% of the cells were Barr corpuscules carriers. The following results were obtained: 31 amniotic fluids were chromatin positive, 16 chromatin negative, 1 doubtful and 2 were not studied because of severe contamination. The correlation of these results with the final sex determination after delivery was 98%. The doubtful case was a male baby. According to these findings it seems reasonable to state that the described method is a very simple way of prenatal sex determination to be applied every time sex. Linked pathological conditions make it desirable (hemophilia, Hunter syndrome, etc.).

14.42.01
The value of the intraurethral pressure transmission ratio in the assessment of female stress incontinence: Farghaly, S A, Shah, J, Worth, P. Inst. Urol., Univ., London, UK
With the rise in intra-abdominal pressure, intravesical pressure usually exceeds the maximal urethral closure pressure. If the pelvic floor remains intact and urethral wall unchanged, continence is retained even under stress conditions. In females with stress urinary incontinence this mechanism is impaired. Pressure transmission is jeopardized when the bladder neck slides down either anteriorly or posteriorly and out of the abdominal pressure zone. Forty female patients with stress urinary incontinence were urodynamically assessed with videocystourethrography. A separate urethral pressure study was performed. A size 9 Ch Gaeltec Catheter with 5 microtip transducers was used for the measurement of the intraurethral pressure in both lying and standing positions. A Sirius 1 microprocessor system with an interface was used to record and digitally store the pressure wave form. This enabled greater flexibility and accuracy in both display and analysis. Fifteen normal females acted as control group. The aim of the study was to compare the radiological appearance of the bladder neck and urethra during cough stress with the information provided by urethral profilometry. The use of the Pressure Transmission Ratio providing useful predictive information. This study has demonstrated that the pressure transmission ratio is higher in premenopausal than postmenopausal females.

14.42.02
Ultrasonographic determination of bladder volume and residual urine: Segal, O, Segal, S. Barzilai Med. Ctr, Ashkelon, Israel
The purpose of this study was to evaluate the use of ultrasound to assess bladder volume and residual urine in gynecological and obstetrical patients. Abdominal and vaginal surgery is associated with urinary retention and frequent catheterization. Ultrasound can be of great value in avoiding those catheterizations and infection by assessing residual urine volume. The study was based on 145 ultrasound measurements in 69 women. An initial study included nine patients following vaginal hysterectomy. Their bladder was filled stepwise and scans were done at volumes of 0, 50, 100, 150, 200, 300, 400 ml. 50 ml had been chosen as the minimal volume for clinically significant residual urine. Volumes were calculated as a product of three internal bladder diameters (height, width and depth). A group of 60 patients after vaginal and abdominal surgery or during early pregnancy, had scanning of their bladder before and after micturition. The volume was calculated by a simpler method of measuring longitudinal and transverse dimensions. The formula used was: $4/3 \pi [1/4L_1 + 1/4L_2]^3$ using a correction factor of 0.9. The accuracy of this method was shown to be limited to an average errow up to 30% and more accurate for residual volumes of 50 to 100 ml. False negative readings were found for volumes less than 50 ml. Our experience indicates that ultrasound assessment of residual urine offers a safe alternative to catheterization for most clinical purposes.

14.42.03
Computer programmed investigation of urethral closure function employing a catheter with six microtransducers: Kauppila, A, Penttinen, J. Dept. Obstet. and Gyn., Univ., Oulu, Finland
In simultaneous urethrocystometry a urethral pressure profile is recorded by one urethral microtransducer withdrawn through the urethra at a predetermined speed. This method gives qualitative information of urethral closure function during stress. To avoid harm owing to movement of the catheter and to record pressures in the bladder and the whole urethra quantitatively and at the same time we started to use a special catheter which is comprised of six microtransducers, one in the bladder and 5 in the urethra (0.5 cm apart from each other). The amplified pressure information from each transducer is transmitted to the microcomputer 300–500 times a second. Using a specific programme, the urethral pressures are compared with the simultaneous pressure in the bladder during a test cough or during several consecutive test coughs. Investigation of 16 women with stress urinary incontinence revealed that the maximal negative urethral closure pressure was -3.2 ± 4.1 (mean SD) mm Hg with a bladder pressure of 61 ± 19 mm Hg, and the negative urethral closure pressure lasted for 0.35 ± 0.32 sec during one cough. In 11 continent women the minimal urethral closure pressure during the cough was 23 ± 12 mm Hg with a bladder pressure of 56 ± 24 mm Hg. In stress urinary incontinence the negative urethral closure pressure was not always apparent before the second – fourth cough, which indicates that the urodynamic circumstances of the lower urinary tract change during repeated stress. According to our results the new method is practical for dynamic investigation of normal and disturbed function of the urethra and bladder.

14.42.04

Role of altered urethral resistance in postoperative voiding difficulties: Bhatia, N N, Bergman, A. Dept. Obstet. and Gyn., Harbor/UCLA Med. Ctr., Univ. of California, Los Angeles, CA, USA

Determination of outflow urethral resistance to voiding requires simultaneous measurement of true detrusor pressure and the peak flow rate. Seventy women with stress urinary incontinence underwent simultaneous voiding urethrocystometry using microtip transducers and 8-channel recorder, before and 3–12 months following Burch (48/70) or Pereyra (22/70) retropubic urethropexy. Increase in urethral resistance ($p < 0.005$) was more marked following the Pereyra procedure (0.057 ± 0.05 to 0.099 ± 0.05; 30% experienced voiding difficulties) when compared to Burch procedure (0.047 ± 0.04 to 0.073 ± 0.05; 20% with postop voiding difficulties). Fifty per cent of patients who voided without detrusor contraction prior to operation (35/70), developed a detrusor contraction ($p < 0.05$) and overcame increased urethral resistance with no postoperative voiding difficulties. The remaining 50% failed to develop a detrusor contraction during postop voiding and 90% of them needed prolonged postoperative bladder drainage prior to resumption of spontaneous voiding ($p < 0.005$). In conclusion, inability to develop a detrusor contraction (true detrusor atony) during voiding in face of increased urethral resistance provided a suitable explanation for postoperative voiding difficulties in 20–30% of patients.

14.42.05

Urinary incontinence in elderly women: Kralj, B. Obstet. and Gyn. Dept., Univ., Ljubljana, Yugoslavia

The incidence of urinary incontinence increases with age. In order to assess the incidence of urinary incontinence in elderly women, an enquiry was carried out among 306 women over 65 years of age, living in homes for the aged. The study covered only women capable of independent mobility and self-care and of such psychic condition that permitted them to take part in the inquiry. 57.2% of the participating women were found to be incontinent. Out of 175 incontinent women over 65, 58 (33.1%) were found to have stress incontinence, 63 women (36.0%) had urge incontinence, and 54 women (30.9%) had mixed incontinence. Because of the frequency of urge and mixed incontinence, at least 66.9% of elderly women may be treated conservatively, this is by functional electrical stimulation (FES). FES treatment was performed by means of pelvic floor muscles stimulators. Although 83.4% of incontinent women (146 out of the total number of 175 incontinent women) felt to be inconvenienced by incontinence, only 54.3% of the women wanted to be treated. Elderly women are capable of using stimulators of pelvic floor muscles for treatment by FES in 78.9%. 54 elderly women (over 65 years) were treated by FES. The results of treatment by FES are satisfying: 12 patients (22.2%) were cured, and in 36 patients (66.7%) the condition improved.

14.42.06

Measuring the postoperative urethral closure by simultaneous urethrocystometry: Kujansuu, E, Wirta, P, Ylä-Outinen, A. Dept. Obstet. and Gyn., Univ. Centr. Hosp., Tampere, Finland

To measure objectively the urethral closure after treatment of stress urinary incontinence (SUI) 31 women were investigated after an Ingelman-Sundberg operation. The results were evaluated by the patient's history and urethrocystometry (UCM). Subjective result was called either as successful (continent or markedly improved) or failed. The severity of the residual SUI was clinically quantified as follows: Leakage on coughing, fast movements, walking or standing gave 1, 2, 3, or 4 points respectively. Use of pads, inconvenience at job or hobbies and avoiding social events gave 1 point when occasional and 2 when regular. The sum of the points was called the SUI score (0–10). UCM was done by the perfusion method. Urethral pressure profiles were measured at stress during coughing. Several UPP's were measured with the patient coughing more heavily each time. Urethral closure was measured by the SUI threshold indicating the bladder pressure increase at coughs producing zero urethral closure pressure in the whole urethra. The median of the SUI threshold was 85 cm H_2O after successful operations ($n = 18$) and 57.5 cm H_2O after failed ones ($n = 13$, $p < 0.05$). The SUI threshold had a significant correlation with the SUI score (Kendall's tau $= -0.43$, $p < 0.001$). The results indicate that the SUI threshold can be used as an objective measurement for urethral closure function after SUI surgery.

14.42.07

Colpocystographic study of urinary stress incontinence in women: Chakmakov, D, Lazarevski, M. Clin. Gyn. and Obstet., Univ., Skopje, Yugoslavia

The authors describe their experiences with colpocystographic examination performed as a routine method of investigation at the Clinic in all cases of urinary stress incontinence. The material encompasses 1185 cases examined in the period from 1968–1984. The analysis of colpocystographic aspects using the classification of *Béthoux-Lazarevski* (Am. J. Obstet. Gyn. **22**, 704, 1975) shows that the stress incontinence of the anterior type was found in 195 cases (16.5%), its anterior section in nine (0.8%), posterior type with concomitant bladder prolapse in 126 (10.6%), posterior type with sliding bladder prolapse in 336 (30.9%), mixed type with concomitant prolapse in 141 (11.9%), and mixed type with sliding bladder prolapse 348 (29.4%). After presenting some technical details the authors emphasize that colpocystography is simple, easy, inexpensive and safe procedure. Its use in surgical gynecology assists in evaluating the tactical and technical indications, assessing the effectiveness of the operations and studing recurrences and postoperative complications.

14.42.08

The incompetent bladder neck in continent postmenopausal women: Cardozo, L D, Versi, E, Brincat, M, Studd, J W W. Dulwich Menopause Clin. and Urodynamic Unit, King's Coll. Hosp., London, UK

Female urinary continence is said to be maintained by the internal and external urethral sphincters. At the time of the menopause, genuine stress incontinence (GSI) is the most common cause of incontinence and so we have examined the status of these sphincters in untreated postmenopausal women. Assessment consisted of history taking, examination, urine culture to exclude infection, pad test, uroflowmetry, videocystourethrography and urethral pressure profilometry. Of 93 consecutive patients presenting to the clinic, six refused to have urodynamic studies, 21 had GSI, nine had detrusor instability and two the mixed condition. The remaining 55 were found to be continent on a pad weighing test and on video-cystourethrographic imaging. However, 28 (51%) of these had an incompetent bladder neck on coughing but contrast medium did not pass the midurethral point. Analysis of urethral cough pressures revealed that in these women continence was maintained by the use of the distal urethra. Proximal urethral shortening was compensated for by augmentation of cough transmission pressures to the distal urethra and thus maintenance of the stress functional urethral length. The fact that half of continent postmenopausal women have an incompetent bladder neck devalues the role of the internal sphincter in these women. It is not known whether the compensatory mechanisms are learned subsequent to the postmenopausal malfunction of the internal sphincter or whether the incompetent bladder neck is a normal variant. Studies on perime-nopausal and estrogen treated women are in progress to resolve this question.

14.42.09

Urodynamic studies in gynecological patients: Prevedourakis, C, Nestoridis, N, Daskalou, C. Gyn. Dept., Tzanion Gen. Hosp., Piraeus, Greece

In 161 women (23 to 28 years of age, parous 0 to 12) admitted for several gynecological problems to our Department from 1980 to 1982 routine urodynamic studies of the urethra and bladder were performed in order to find or not coexistent urinary disturbances. The whole material was divided according to the clinical picture in group A (34 cases) with no symptoms of urinary disturbances and group B (127 cases) with concomitant urinary dysfunction. The urodynamic studies performed include: 1. For the urethra, determinations of the involuntary and voluntary sphincter pressures, the differences of the above pressures, the intra-urethral pressure during bearing down efforts and the length of the urethra by using the technique described by *Nestoridis*. 2. For the bladder, determinations of the first sensation of filling, the first urge to void, the strong desire to void and the holding pattern by using the method of filling liquid cystometry. The obtained results revealed: 1. Lower m. values (group B) for vol. sphin. pressures, the press. diff. ($p < 0.001$) and intra-ureth. press ($p < 0.03$). 2. Lower m. values (group B) for first sens. fill ($p < 0.065$) and first urge to void ($p < 0.09$).

14.42.10

Para-urethral mass in a woman. A case report of leiomyoma: Youssef, H. London Hosp., Mile End Acad. Unit, London, UK

True benign para-urethral neoplasms in women are so rare, that there is scant literature regarding their diagnosis and management. They present incidentally in the course of vaginal examination or maybe are the cause of obstructive or irritative urinary symptoms (*Harry* et al. J. Urol. **116**, 451–453, 1976). Differential diagnosis must include urethral diverticulum, ureterocele and para-urethral cysts. *Das, S.* presented a comprehensive classification of para-urethral cysts and case reports with their management (J. Urol. **126**, 41–43, 1981). – Case report: A 45-year-old multiparous woman was referred from well woman clinic as a case of cystocele. She presented with a vaginal mass and symptoms of stress and urge incontinence. Examination revealed a firm para-urethral mass in the anterolateral aspect of the vagina. She was referred to the urologist for cystometric studies and evaluation. The studies were normal. Cystoscopy was performed under general anesthesia and showed normal urethra and bladder with no urethral attachment. Enucleation of the para-urethral mass transvaginally was performed. The mass was quite firm 3 × 3 cm. She had an uneventful postoperative period. Her symptoms had disappeared completely, six weeks post-operatively. Histology report showed a benign leiomyoma. Cystourethroscopy will help define the nature and extent of para-urethral lesions. A pre-operative needle biopsy is recommended in some centers. Urethrography will often provide the picture characteristic of a urethral diverticulum.

14.42.11

Estrogen treatment for genuine stress incontinence; Collagen as a prognostic index: Versi, E, Cardozo, L D, Brincat, M, O'Dowd, T, Studd, J W W. Dulwich Hosp., Menopause Clin. and Urodynamic Unit, King's Coll. Hosp., London, UK

The incidence of female urinary incontinence increases with age and at the time of the menopause; genuine stress incontinence (GSI), is the most common underlying condition. This is due to urethral sphincter weakness and so studies on continence mechanisms necessitate analysis of urethral pressures. Urologically asymptomatic women were recruited from the menopause clinic and underwent urodynamic assessment to ascertain normality. Assessment consisted of urine culture, a pad test, uroflowmetry, videocysto-urethrography, and 55 patients were found to have no abnormality. These then had urethral pressure profilometry allowing several measures of urethral function at rest and during coughing. The patients then had a full thickness 3 mm skin biopsy from the right thigh and this was assayed for collagen content. Multivariate analysis revealed that collagen content of skin is significantly correlated with most parameters of urethral sphincteric function. This implies that patients with a higher skin collagen content have better sphincters. We have previously shown (*Brincat* et al. Brit. med. J. **287**, 1337, 1983) that skin collagen content declines after the menopause in untreated but not in treated patients. Response to oestrogen replacement therapy depends on the initial pretreatment collagen content in that patients with low levels derive the most benefit. We can therefore use these data to predict which postmenopausal patients with GSI are likely to improve with oestrogen treatment.

14.42.12

Anal electrostimulation in female urinary incontinence using Incontan: Eriksen, B C. Dept. Obstet. and Gyn., Univ., Trondheim, Norway

An integrated automatic electrical stimulator has been developed to treat urinary incontinence. The purpose of this study was to evaluate the therapeutic effect in women with stress-, urge- and mixed incontinence who had used the stimulator for at least three months. The evaluation was based on a clinical, urological and urodynamic examination before and after the treatment. Ninety-six women used the stimulator for at least six hours a day for an average of eight months. No serious side-effects were registered. Incontinence charts showed a significant reduction in frequency, urgency, nocturia and number of leakages. Stress provocation test changed from positive to negative in women with stress incontinence who were cured. In the same group a significant increase in functional urethral length was found, but no significant change in maximum urethral closure pressure. However, it changed from negative to positive during cough in women with stress- and mixed incontinence who were cured. A significant increase in bladder volume at first desire to void and at maximum capacity was found in motor urge and combined stress- and motor urge incontinence. About one-third of the bladders with a hyperactive detrusor were stable after the treatment. 60% of the patients became continent and 31% improved significantly. Only 9% recorded no effect of the treatment. Electrostimulation therapy should be the first choice of treatment in women with genuine stress- and combined stress- and urge incontinence. Primary operation should be reserved for women with a marked cystocele or a marked descent of the anterior vaginal wall.

14.79.01

Sexual behaviour of 117 girls in a Japanese reformatory: Matsuzawa, K, Mizutani, T, Kihira, M, Suzuki, M, Tomoda, Y. Dept. Obstet. and Gyn., Nagoya Univ., School Med., Nagoya, Japan

Nowadays sexual behaviour and subsequent pregnancy in adolescence is not only one of the greatest social problems but medical ones, but the approach from the gynecologists has been not enough for new trend. Therefore we had investigated with questionnaire in one of the greatest reformatories near Tokyo what these girls had thought and done before their misdeed. 117 sentenced to more than one year punishment are between 15 and 20 years old. 48 were caught for amphetamine abuse, 35 threat, 27 injury (inc. murder). 74 have both parents and 92 had only junior high school education. Their physical maturation and psychological development toward sex was almost the same as with other Japanese teenagers but their sexual behaviour was much more active. Almost all of them experienced petting and 13.2 was the mean age of first sexual intercourse. The first partners were acquaintances (44), boyfriends (41), gangsters (12) and others (incl. family). 54 found their first partners in the thriving town. 69 prostituted themselves. No more than 17 always took contraceptive measures, they said, but seven failed. 40 girls had never prevented conception. Then 45 got 81 pregnancies (5 had 4 times) but only five babies were born. Our study could not be directly introduced in our society because of its singularity, but more than half of D & C of the unmarried in Japan are now already teenagers. Abundance of curiosity toward sex but lack of adequate knowledge of contraception brings these girls unexpected pregnancy followed by abortion, sterility and other problems.

14.79.02

Ovarian function in adolescent females following chemotherapy for malignant diseases: Distler, W[1], Graf, M[1], Kuhrke, H[2], Juergens, H[2], Goebel, U[2]. [1]Dept. Obstet. and Gyn., [2]Dept. Pediat./Sect. Pediat. Oncol., Univ., Düsseldorf

Chemotherapy for malignant diseases can cause gonadal dysfunction (Ann. intern. Med. **93**, 109, 1980). However, little is known about the reversibility and severity of those effects in girls being treated during puberty. Therefore clinical data and endocrine parameters (FSH, LH, PRL, E_2, progesterone) of 51 adolescent females were investigated. Our clinical data show that girls treated before the menarche failed to start menstruation while on chemotherapy, but all had their menarche shortly after cessation of the treatment. Most of the girls treated after their menarche developed amenorrhea, some had irregular cycles unless they were on a very mild drug regimen. The most remarkable endocrine parameters (high FSH and LH, low E_2) were seen in girls treated for advanced Hodgkin's disease with chemotherapy plus total nodal radiation and in one girl with an extensive Wilms' tumor who had total abdominal radiation in addition to intensive four-drug chemotherapy. All girls who were off chemotherapy and had regular monthly bleedings showed hormonal evidence of anovulation or an inadequate luteal phase. From our data we concluded: (1) Primary ovarian failure is rare and occurs in adolescent females only while on a combined chemo- and radiotherapy, (2) after chemotherapy the incidence of anovulation or an inadequate luteal phase is high, and (3) hormone replacement therapy should be restricted to girls with high gonadotrophins only.

14.79.03

Problems in precocious puberty: Ortner, A, Glatzl, J, Karpellus, E. Univ.-Klin. Frauenheilk., Univ.-Klin. Kinderheilk., Innsbruck, Austria

Twenty-five girls with precocious puberty attended our special out-patient clinic for Pediatric and Adolescent Gynecology. We propose a classification in view of the newly findings in recent literature. As to date we still differentiate between pubertas praecox vera (complete form) and pseudopubertas praecox (incomplete form). The incomplete form of precocious puberty should however be subdivided into a "combined form" with premature thelarche and pubarche as well as in an "isolated form", when the cause of precocity is to be found either in the ovary or in the adrenals, e. g., in tumors of these organs. Physical examination, hormonal studies before and after stimulation, and hormonal cytology of the vaginal epithelium are fundamental diagnostic procedures. The newly introduced procedures of sonography and computerized tomography are of essential value. The chosen therapy for cases of pubertas praecox vera was to give cyproteronacetate. Danazol was given additionally in some selected cases. In some cases no therapy was given, but the patients were re-examined at closely spaced intervals. The results of the follow-up controls are discussed.

14.79.04

Significance of an early diagnosis, treatment and long follow-up among of cases primary amenorrhea: Dramusic, V. Dept. Obstet. and Gyn., Kandang Kerbau Hosp., Singapore

In a group of 134 teenagers referred for primary amenorrhea, after extensive investigations, particularly genetical and endocrinological, it was found that predominant group refers to ovarian dysgenesis: 63 cases (47%), with either numerical or structural aberrations of sex chromosomes. Hypothalamo-pituitary failure of various origin was found in 24 patients, followed by uterine and vaginal dysgenesis or other anomalies in 29 cases. Other causes are far more rarer: testicular feminisation four; resistant ovary syndrome one; CAH three; POS two; hermaphrodite one; true gonadal agenesis two; only five were normal but late maturers. With exception of five infants, all patients were seen first as teenagers. Follow-up of these cases revealed paramount importance of early diagnosis and timely treatment which has multiple beneficial effects: physically visible maturation, increase in growth, improved self-image, acceptance of the idea of their future sexuality. Particularly sensitive topic is problem of permanent infertility in the majority of the cases, what is vitally connected with timely professional orientation of such patients. Also replacement treatment should be balanced to be closest to physiological, which imposes regular laboratory follow-up. Cancer risks should not be neglected, particularly if a Y chromosome is present. Those undergoing corrective operations face significant emotional problems concerning their marital life and infertility. In conclusion: Our experience throughout 15 years points that early diagnosis and treatment, extensive professional and marital life counselling and practically life long follow-up only gives chances to such patients to lead a relatively normal and satisfactory life.

14.79.05

Getting pregnant of adolescents that have come for artificial abortion and for delivery of legitimate child: Demerdžiev, K, Dimitrov, V, Adamova, G. Gyn.-Obstet. Clin., Med. School, Univ. "Kiril and Metodij", Skopje, Yugoslavia

Our research refers to two groups adolescents (A) aged 15–19 years from the region of SR Makedonia, Yugoslavia which belong to Macedonian nationality, chosen by change. One group is represented by A which have come for artificial abortion (AA), and the other group coming for delivery of a legitimate child (P). Group A for AA got pregnant on average ($\bar{X}$) within 10.1 months after start of sex. activity, with remarkably high SD 11.65 of $\bar{X}$ and with medium error (SE) 0.73. With the group coming for P $\bar{X}$ is 5.5, SD 6.65 and SE is 0.42. The difference between $\bar{X}$ of the two groups examined is of maxim. statistic importance ($\bar{X}$ t = 6.40, p < 0.001). In the first month of sex. life the A coming for AA got pregnant in 16.4%, the ones from A coming for P protecting themselves and not wanting pregnancy, got pregnant 8.7% and the ones with no protection but wanting pregnancy got pregnant with first sex. relation in 27.4%. Getting pregnant within first six months of sex. life for the three groups is in percents: 52.4, 53.1 and 88.9. Between A for AA and P not protected and unwanting pregnancy there is nearly no difference in time of getting pregnant although intensity of sex. life is different. The P wanting pregnancy got pregnant in first sex. relation. Group A for AA used regularly contraceptives only 0.8% and 4.4% irregularly, occasionally. The patients of this group asking for advice of a medical authority for prevention of unwanted pregnancy was only 1.6% (4 of them).

14.79.06

Diagnostic approach in adolescent patients with secondary amenorrhea: Bila, S. Clin. Gyn. and Obstet., Med. Fac., Beograd, Yugoslavia

Measurement of gonadotropin and steroid concentrations in blood has proved to be particularly significant for differentiation and classification of patients with secondary amenorrhea. Fluctuations of serum FSH, LH, PRL, E_2 and progesterone levels were analysed and the patients were divided into five groups:

370

1. patients with the elevated prolactin levels, 2. patients with low levels of both gonadotropin hormones, 3. patients with low FSH levels but with relatively high LH levels, 4. patients with high FSH and LH levels, and 5. patients with normal basal FSH and LH values. Estradiol and progesterone variations in blood are shown within each group represented. Classification of patients represents a contribution to more complete understanding of this problem and to the possibility of giving the appropriate therapy. The success in treating secondary amenorrhea in adolescents depends on the duration of disorder and on timely detection of its cause.

14.79.07
Secular trend in menarche over a period of 150 years: Helm, P. Dept. Gyn. and Obstet., FAC, Hilleröd, Denmark

The Scandinavian countries have a long tradition of collecting data on sexual maturation. Recent recalculations on Norwegian data indicate, unexpectedly, that the greater part of the acceleration towards earlier age at menarche occurred during the first half of this century. Moreover, the data suggest that the trend has come to a halt, since menarcheal age remained constant at 13.3 years in Oslo from 1952 to 1970. Scrutiny of the Danish literature revealed 23 sets of data concerning menarche scattered over a period of one and a half centuries. On the basis of a new method of recalculation on recall data an almost linear decrease in age at menarche was demonstrated, from 17.4 years in 1835 to 14.4 years in 1945, that is, on average 0.30 years per decade. From the middle of this century data collected by the status quo method is available. A continued decline in menarcheal age was observed, though at a slightly slower rate, from 13.8 years in 1950 to 13.0 years in 1983, that is, on average, 0.23 years per decade. The latest part of this period was covered by the author's data collected in the same region and by identical methods in 1966 and 1983, respectively. During this period age at menarche decreased from 13.4 to 13.0 years, i. e. with a similar rate of 0.22 years per decade. Obviously, the secular trend in menarche may have ceased before the last investigation in 1983; but conclusions as to the state of the trend will have to await future studies.

14.79.08
Ovarian tumors in children and adolescents: Bregun, N, Vuleta, P, Djurdjević, L, Ićurup, Z, Bujas, M. Dept. Gyn. and Obstet., Fac. Med., Novi Sad, Yugoslavia

During the last 24 years 26,356 abdominal and vaginal operations were performed, including 46 operations for ovarian tumors done in children and adolescents. Of five tumors operated in girls below 14 years of age, two cases were torsion of follicular and dermoid cyst, in one case it was torsion of healthy adnexa, two ovarian tumors were malignant: chorionepithelioma and malignant ovarian dysgerminoma. The following cases occurred in 41 girls aged 14–18: one malignant ovarian tumor and 40 benign ovarian tumors, including 26 dermoid cysts, 14 follicular cysts, 12 torsions of dermoid cyst and in two cases intra-uterine pregnancy was complicated by torsion of an ovarian tumor. These 46 operations done in children and adolescents were as follows: unilateral cystectomies – 6, resection of ovary and suture – 2, unilateral ovariectomy – 3, unilateral ovariectomy and resection of ovary – 2, unilateral adnexectomy – 27, unilateral adnexectomy and enucleation of cystic ovary – 1, unilateral adnexectomy and resection of ovary – 3, subtotal hysterectomy with bilateral adnexectomy – 2. Of these 46 ovarian tumors in children and adolescents, 43 were benign and three were malignant, their proportion being 93.57% to 6.52%.

15.13.01
Introduction: Pathogenesis and treatment of osteoporosis: Dambacher, M A, Rüegsegger, P. Res. Labor. Calcium Metab. and Inst. Biomed. Engineer., Univ., Zurich, Switzerland

Osteoporosis is the most frequent metabolic bone disease. Because osteoporosis is a heterogenous syndrome, therapy cannot be a uniform one and has to be adapted to the different forms of osteoporosis. The most important period of time for the development of osteoporosis seems to be the perimenopausal phase, characterized by an increased rate of calcium efflux from bone into the extracellular fluid, and a PTH decrease. The fact that calcitonin, in spite of the increased serum calcium, is not elevated in postmenopausal women indicates that a reduced calcitonin secretion may be one of the mechanisms by which the immediate postmenopausal rapid bone loss is induced. In this perimenopausal state of osteoporosis development, estrogen with or without progesteron, is usually used until now to block further bone loss. In acute osteoporosis, defined as an acute dramatic bone loss with painful new fractures, calcitonin inhibits further bone loss and has furthermore an analgetic effect. The treatment in the future may be an intermittent schedule based on the "bone multicellular unit"-hypothesis. In a first activation step the basic multicellular units must be stimulated, i. e. by an increase of endogenous PTH through elevated phosphate intake, the bone resorption shall be reduced by estrogens or calcitonin. But the stimulation of bone turnover seems to be a major problem. In short-term studies with osteoporotic patients we were unable to increase PTH levels by high phosphate intake. This in contrast to findings in a healthy control group who have increased PTH levels during the phosphate administration.

15.13.02
The non-invasive assessment of individual bone loss in pre-, peri-, and postmenopausal women: Rüegsegger, P, Müller, A, Dambacher, M A. Inst. Biomed. Engineer. and Res. Labor. Calcium Metab., Univ., Zurich, Switzerland

Since there is still no effective treatment available for PM osteoporosis precise and safe methods are required to establish early diagnosis, and to assess the course of the disease, enabling preventive procedures. To this end we have developed a high precision, low dose bone densitometer. The special purpose computed tomography system allows to quantify bone density at peripheral measuring sites with a precision of 0.3% at a radiation dose of 10 mrem. With this technique the bone mineral loss in 120 women was assessed serially to establish the course of bone density in healthy pre-, peri- and postmenopausal women as well as in PM osteoporosis. Groups of approximately 20 patients were followed for 4 years. In healthy premenopausal women aged 20 to 50 year found that bone density remains stable. In the years immediately following menopause the individual bone loss varies in the range 0 to 10% per year with the majority of females in the range 0 to 2%. Healthy PM women aged 64 to 76 year lose 0.95%, untreated osteoporotics in the same age range 2.7% per year. Bone is lost step-wise with long phases of relative stability and brief phases of rapid loss. – In conclusion: Low dose high precision computed tomography allows a detailed analysis of the individual bone loss. It is especially useful in the assessment of the severity of osteoporosis, the identification of risk patients and the evaluation of the effectiveness of treatment.

15.13.03

The reduction of risk for osteoporosis: Lindsay, R. Reg. Bone Ctr, Helen Hayes Hosp., New York, NY, USA

The identification of causative and associative risk factors for osteoporosis at an early age holds the promise for risk reduction. The earlier risk analysis is performed, the greater the benefit which might be achieved. Presently, since we do not sufficiently understand the processes controlling skeletal growth and maturation, the prevention of bone loss is the prime focus. Although insufficient data suggest the concept of premenopausal bone, it is still important to change these life style and dietary factors at as early an age as possible. Increasing dietary calcium, adequate exercise, and reduction of cigarette, alcohol, and caffeine consumption may be important for other health care reasons as well as for maintenance of calcium balance. After the menopause, estrogen therapy remains the single most important pharmacological approach to prevention. The use of bone mass measurements may allow further clarification of risk potential and efficacy of therapy. Among the elderly, reduction in the risk of falling and/or trauma is probably the single most important factor in fracture prevention.

15.13.04

Bone density assessment in hyperprolactinemic subjects: Pepperell, R J, Seeman, E. Dept. Obstet. and Gyn., Royal Women's Hosp., and Dept. Med., Austin Hosp., Melbourne, Australia

Oestrogen deficiency is a recognised risk factor for accelerated bone loss. Nevertheless, bone mass in hyperprolactinemic patients has been found to be unaffected or only minimally diminished despite amenorrhea of prolonged duration. To clarify these discrepant observations, and to identify factors which may substantially influence bone mass in these patients, bone mineral density (BMD) was measured at the lumbar spine (LS), femoral neck (FN) and midfemoral shaft (FS) using the technique of Dual Photon Absorptiometry in 47 female hyperprolactinemic patients, mean age 35 years (range 18–48 years), mean during of amenorrhea 97 months (range 24–248 months) and 55 healthy controls matched by age and sex.

Region	Hyperprolactinemic Patients			Control Subjects (n = 55)
	All Patients (n = 47)	Nulliparous Patients (n = 17)	Parous Patients (n = 30)	
LS	36.05 ± 0.77	32.36 ± 1.40	37.73 ± 0.84	38.73 ± 0.83
FN	2.41 ± 0.06	2.32 ± 0.10	2.41 ± 0.06	2.50 ± 0.05
FS	3.27 ± 0.06	3.16 ± 0.11	3.27 ± 0.07	3.36 ± 0.07

Compared with controls, statistically significant observations were restricted to measurements at the lumbar spine. For all hyperprolactinemic patients, lumbar spine-BMD was 7% less than controls only ($p < 0.02$). By contrast, lumbar spine-BMD in nulliparous hyperprolactinemic patients was 16% less than controls ($p < 0.002$) and 14% less than lumbar spine-BMD in parous hyperprolactinemic patients ($p < 0.005$). However, lumbar spine-BMD in parous hyperprolactinemic patients did not differ from controls. Moreover, lumbar spine-BMD did not differ between parous and nulliparous controls. In hyperprolactinemic patients parity, but not the duration of amenorrhea, correlated significantly with lumbar spine-BMD. We conclude that nulliparous hyperprolactinemic patients are at risk of bone loss at the axial skeleton and parity appears to confer a substantial protective effect.

15.41.01

SPACER-technique in breast reconstruction: Audretsch, W. Klin. Landeshauptstadt Düsseldorf, Frauen-klin., Düsseldorf

The use of a silicone SPACER (*Audretsch*, 1978), as a preliminary distancing prosthesis in breast reconstruction followed by insertion of a silicone gel prosthesis six month later is demonstrated by typical examples of subcutaneous – (S.C.M.) or modified radical mastectomy (M.R.M.) and flap techniques.

Surgical refinements after seven years of experience in this new surgical technique are explained by typical intraoperative stages. Definite advantages of the two stage methods are: Use of the wide entrance by immediate s. c. or s. musc. insertion of the SPACER after M.R.M. or S.C.M. Wound-healing without tension on the scars in cases of skin reduction and S.C.M. Short insertion time of gel prosthesis after removing the SPACER. XRT and/or Chemo T. possible without complications. Security of local control by palpation and s. c. biopsy from the former tumor area before insertion of the gel prosthesis. Reformation of fat tissue to cover Silicone-implant in case of subcutaneous insertion after flaps. Potential advantages of the SPACER-technique: Possible contribution to reduce capsular fibrosis in combining the SPACER with Silastic II – Silicone-gel prosthesis. Positive psychological influence on the patient by conceivable reconstruction.

15.41.02

Colposcopy clinic set-up in the Academic Medical Center: Struyk, A P H B. Dept. Obstet. and Gyn., Univ., Amsterdam, The Netherlands
This video-tape with a duration of 21 minutes, recorded in colour on U-matic system presents an introduction to colposcopy. It shows the place colposcopy is beginning to take in the Netherlands in relation to cytology and histology. It also shows how colposcopy is performed in our hospital. The theory behind colposcopy and the flow-chart used in the evaluation and treatment of patients with abnormal PAP-smears are illustrated. Both normal and abnormal patterns in colposcopy are demonstrated as well as diagnostic procedures such as directed punch biopsy and endocervical biopsy. Various modern video-techniques were used to obtain an esthetic, entertaining and instructive educational program. Accordingly this video-tape might be of interest to those who are engaged in teaching obstetrics and gynecology.

15.41.03

Laser laparoscopic treatment of diseases of the reproductive organs: Nezhat, C. Fertil. and Endocr. Ctr, Atlanta, GA, USA
In this 25 minute video, varying degrees of pelvic adhesions and also hydrosalpinges are being treated via laparoscope with the help of CO_2 laser.

15.41.04

Pelviscopic surgery with the carbon dioxide laser: Sutton, C J G. St. Luke's Hosp., Guildford, Surrey, UK
Video film on U-MATIC format lasting 20 mins. – The video shows the technique of pelviscopic (laparoscopic) laser surgery using the single portal and double portal approach. The disadvantages and advantages of each approach are discussed and attention drawn to the potential hazards of using a carbon dioxide laser beam down a pelviscope. Sequences are shown of laser adhesolysis in patients with pelvic pain and infertility and the technique of laser vaporisation of endometriotic deposits. Another sequence shows the technique of emptying ovarian cysts and aspirating fluid. The safety of the procedure is discussed and a review of the first hundred consecutive patients treated by this technique in Guildford are shown.

15.42.01

Investigation on the pathogenesis of fetal death in the shark and rabbit by toxic agents affecting the terminal vascular bed: Fischer, H. Univ.-Frauenklin. (Charité), Berlin
Acid products of metabolism – histamine and allyl compounds – cause a fatal collapse of blood circulation of the fetus by blood stasis of the peripheral terminal vascular bed. This may well be demonstrated in the shark's yolk-sac and fetus, as a living model which is 30 mm long and transparent. It has been put into seawater, to which poison has been added, as narcose (MS 222) and the horny skin has then been removed. As a model for numerous noxas, which can also affect human beings, pregnant rabbits received injections of histamine and allyl. The injections cause a severe disturbance of the permeability of the fetal terminal vascular bed, combined with stasis, necrosis of the vascular bed and sclerosis. This can be seen in a sequence of histological pictures and special effect drawings. In an astonishingly short period the injections lead to edema, fibrinoid exudation, and already within a few hours to sclerosis and augmentation of the mesenchyme of the fetal placenta stroma, later to stasis in the maternal blood area of the trophoblastic tubes of the rabbit's placenta. Peripheral disturbances of the circulation after application of histamine and allyl cause cataract of the lens of rabbit's and shark's fetus. This is a new proof of the unspecific etiology of phenocopies of well known patterns of deformity (histamine 3 mg/kg and allyl/formiate 50 mg/kg).

15.42.02

A Cesarean section with Uchida's abdominal retractor: Uchida, H, Uchida, M. Uchida Hosp., Kanazawa, Japan
Recently the rates of Cesarean section are rising and some unexpected operative difficulties may confront the operator. In order to solve the difficulties, the author would like to introduce his techniques and his specially designed retractor, based on over 2000 cases, focusing on the following points by the film which presents the whole duration of one operation. 1) Where the uterine incision should be made to obtain the upper and lower incised edges of the same thickness in the uterine wall for complete suturing. 2) How the fetal head can appear smoothly through the uterine wall by avoiding lacerate scars. 3) How to obtain a wide operative view as closely as possible to the pubes.

15.42.03

Delivery from a dynamic sitting position using the CRADLE (cybernetic recliner for assisted delivery and labor ease): Tanaka, Y. Tanaka Women's Clin., Tokyo, Japan

The first part of this 14.5 min film shows the mechanisms and explains the operation of new automated equipment, the CRADLE, which allows the doctor and the patient to adjust an extremely variable sitting delivery position. The second part of the film outlines the researched benefits of using the CRADLE. Tests on 20 women revealed that this equipment allowed a mean maximum intrauterine pressure during bearing down of 79.13 ± 33.78 mm Hg. 61.15 ± 15.48 mm Hg was recorded for the same women bearing down from the semi-supine position and 55.33 ± 14.18 mm Hg was recorded for the lithotomy position. In 200 CRADLE deliveries between June '83 and Sept. '84 mean duration of the first stage of labor was 286 ± 162 min and of the 2nd stage was 31 ± 20 min. In 100 deliveries using a conventional fixed position apparatus first stage of labor was 338 ± 192 min and 2nd stage was 56 ± 32 min. Blood-loss in CRADLE deliveries was 195 ± 147 ml and in fixed position semi-supine deliveries was 271 ± 198 ml. Mean Apgar scores for CRADLE delivered newborn was 9.7 ± 1.1 and for others was 9.4 ± 1.1. Compared with delivery in the lithotomy or semi-supine positions this equipment allows greater intrauterine pressure during bearing down. Labor is shorter, particularly in the 2nd stage. The flexibility of the CRADLE allows easy return to a relaxed position, preventing congestion in the pelvic region. Using the CRADLE mean blood-loss was significantly lower and mean Apgar scores were slightly higher.

15.42.04

Prenatal diagnosis of congenital malformations: Sidiropoulos, D, Negri, P. Perinat. Div., Dept. Obstet. and Gyn., and Unit. Instructional Media, Med. Fac., Univ., Bern, Switzerland

The rapid evolution of prenatal detection of hereditary diseases and congenital defects implies adequate training of physicians involved in counselling families who are at increased risk of having congenital malformations, in their offspring. The tape slide show conveys basic knowledge of genetic counselling and describes the standardized methods of prenatal diagnosis. The following techniques and their indications are demonstrated in detail: 1. ultrasound to assess gestational age and for diagnosis of some major malformations, 2. amniocentesis to detect chromosomal abnormalities, inborn errors of metabolism and neural tube defects, 3. fetoscopy for fetal visualization (in the example of Apert's syndrome), fetal blood sampling (in the example of thalassemia) and fetal skin biopsy (in the example of congenital ichthyosis). Because of the crucial nature of the decision the involved parties have to make, prenatal diagnosis warrants adequate timing and performance of the techniques described here.

16.03.01

A new superagonist of gonadotrophin-releasing hormone for contraception in women: Gudmundsson, J A, Nillius, S J, Bergquist, C. Dept. Obstet. and Gyn., Univ., Uppsala, Sweden

Ovulation can, paradoxically, be inhibited in women by chronic treatment with stimulatory analogs of the hypothalamic gonadotrophin-releasing hormone (GnRH), a new promising approach to contraception (*Nillius, S J.* In: Update on Contraception, *Newton, J R.* [Ed.] Clin. Obst. Gyn. **11**, 545–566, 1984). Here we present results from a contraceptive study with a new, highly potent stimulatory analog of GnRH, nafarelin acetate. – Materials and methods: Forty-seven regularly menstruating women used the new GnRH superagonist nafarelin acetate (D-[Nal]2^6-GnRH, Syntex) for inhibition of ovulation during six months. The superagonist was administered intranasally in daily doses of $125 \mu g$ to 24 women and $250 \mu g$ to 23 women. Estradiol and progesterone in blood were measured weekly. – Results: No pregnancy occurred during 262 completed months of treatment. One presumptive ovulation occurred. Estradiol levels gradually decreased to early follicular phase values during the treatment. Hot flushes were reported by some of the women. Ninety per cent of the women developed amenorrhea or oligomenorrhea. Ovulation promptly returned after discontinuation of therapy. – Conclusion: Continuous intranasal nafarelin treatment for inhibition of ovulation proved to be an effective method for contraception. Further investigation of this superagonist for peptide contraception, is clearly warranted.

16.03.02

Endometrial morphology in women during treatment with nafarelin acetate – a new GnRH superagonist: Lundkvist, Ö, Gudmundsson, J A, Bergquist, C, Nillius, S J. Dept. Obstet. and Gyn., Univ., Uppsala, Sweden

Intranasal GnRH agonist treatment for inhibition of ovulation is one of the new leads to peptide contraception. However, there has been concern that the induced anovulation and subsequent unopposed endogen estrogen secretion may provoke endometrial hyperplasia. The present study was undertaken, to investigate the effects of a continuous intranasal treatment with a new GnRH superagonist on the morphology of the endometrium. – Materials and methods: Nafarelin acetate (D-[Nal]2^6-GnRH, Syntex) was administered intranasally in daily doses of either 125 or $250 \mu g$ to twenty-five fertile women. Endometrial biopsies were taken after 4–6 months of treatment. Results: Inhibition of ovulation occurred in all the women resulting in early follicular phase serum estrogen levels. Most of the women had either oligo- or amenorrhea during therapy. Light microscopy showed an inactive or weak proliferative endometrial patten. There were no signs of endometrial hyperplasia. Mitoses were seldom seen. Ultrastructurally the endometrial cells of all biopsies displayed signs of low metabolic activity. The epithelial cells contained a poorly developed Golgi apparatus, single ribosomes and only few membranes of endoplasmic reticulum. – Conclusion: Continuous intranasal nafarelin treatment for contraceptive purposes did not induce endometrial hyperplasia. Thus, with the dosages used in the present study there seems to be no need for gestagen supplementation.

16.03.03

Clinical and laboratory experiments on a contraceptive combination containing desogestrel: Gáyan, P B, Gálan, G C, Tisne, L B. Hosp. del Salvador, Santiago, Chile
During the last 15 years, progress in oral contraception has been achieved by reducing the dosages of the compounds rather than improving the quality of the substances in use. A combined oral contraceptive containing a recently developed progestogen desogestrel (150 mg/EE 30 mcg) with the claim that the preparation has effects on lipid metabolism, especially an elevation of the HDL-cholesterol, that could be considered potentially beneficial, was studied in 78 multiparous women. From the 78, 28 used a combined contraceptive combination containing 500 mcg norethindrone and 35 mcg EE before entering the study (group B), the remaining 50 did not use a hormonal contraceptive in the three months before the study (group A). Free T, SHBG, LDL-C and HDL-C were determined at 0, 6 and 12 months. In both groups there was an increase in SHBG, with subsequent reduction of free T levels ($p < 0.05$). In addition there was an increase in HDL-C in both groups ($p < 0.05$), and a reduction in the level of LDL-C in group B at 6 and 12 months. It is concluded that the progestogen desogestrel will offer both short-term (acne, hirsutism) and long-term (low cardiovascular risk) advantages.

16.03.04

Comparative effects of a desogestrel or levonorgestrel oral contraceptive preparation: Lavín, P A, Bravo, C L, Cerón, M D, Sanhueza, L, Henriquez, A. Serv. de Salud Metrop. Sur & Fac. Med., Univ. de Chile, Santiago, Chile
Previous studies have shown deleterious effects of a reduced plasma HDL-cholesterol level on cardiovascular disease (thrombosis, stroke and myocardial infarction). Progestagen component of oral contraceptives (OCs) such as the norethisterone and levonorgestrel have been detected as producers of this lowering of HDL-cholesterol in plasma of OC users plus androgenic effects by alteration of the level of sex hormone binding globulin too. A new progestin, desogestrel, have been shown to affect these plasma levels inversely, so that the long-term deleterious effects of OCs should be expected to slow down. In Chile for some years a 0.150 mg levonorgestrel with 0.030 mg ethinyl estradiol (EE) (Microgynon®) has been freely distributed to some of the 30% OC users by governmentally run family planning clinics with good acceptance by patients. Thinking of the beneficial effects of desogestrel, in two of these clinics a total of 195 – healthy 17 to 40 year old patients were randomly assigned to either Microgynon® or Marvelon® (0.150 mg of desogestrel + 0.030 mg EE), and planned to be followed for the first 12 cycles, checking for adverse symptoms, clinical effects and acceptability. In the starting groups (desogestrel n = 101; levonorgestrel n = 89) there were no differences in age (24.7 ± 0.43; 26.5 ± 0.55); education (8.5 ± 0.24; 8.5 ± 0.30); parity (1.7 ± 0.11; 1.9 ± 0.11); and hematocrit (40.9 ± 0.55; 42.2 ± 0.28). There were no pregnancies in either group and acceptability and continuity of use was similar. Based on these data and the biochemical affects already known we think that biochemical effects already known we think that for the long-term OC user the desogestrel preparation should be the choice.

16.03.05

Injectable contraceptives: A national concern: Jhaveri, C L. Bombay, India
Injectable contraceptives have been in use the world over for the last 20 years as accepted by the World Health Organisation and other concerned authorities. The two common available injections are Depo-Provera Aqueous 150 mg (DMPA) and NET-EN 200 mg in oily solution. Government of 80 countries have granted the use of an aqueous solution while the Government of 30 countries have allowed use of NET-EN, an oily solution. The Federation of Obstetrics and Gynecological Societies of India and Indian Association of Fertility & Sterility have recommended the release of both types of injections to the concerned authorities. Ultimate choice which injection to use is left to the physicians. It is felt that the injection can be administered fairly and freely compared to subcutaneous implants. It is felt that all developing countries should accept this challenge of population explosion by accepting the use of injectable contraceptives in National Program for Family Planning and Welfare.

16.03.06

Clinical and metabolic study of depot-medroxyprogesterone acetate (DMPA) in long-term users: Chutivongse, S, Virutamasen, P, Reinprayoon, D. Dept. Obstet. and Gyn., Fac. Med., Chulalongkorn Univ., Bangkok, Thailand
A longitudinal observation for clinical changes in 223 Thai women, who voluntarily requested DMPA as injectable contraceptive continuously for more than five years, was carried out. Fifty-seven clients were randomly allocated for metabolic evaluation and a cross-sectional study was chosen. No significant changes in blood pressure were noted even after ten years of use, while amenorrhea and irregular bleeding were the most common undesired effects. The incidence of amenorrhea gradually increased in relation to the duration of practice and 94% of them were amenorrheic at the end of ten years. Body weight, in most of the cases, was steadily on the increase in the first five years of use and became quite stable there-after.

There were no significant changes in the routine liver function tests between the DMPA users and the controls. However, it was found that alkaline phosphatase and cortisol levels were significantly higher in DMPA users. Abnormal oral glucose tolerance tests (OGTT) were observed in four women. After stopping DMPA, two women had normal OGTT within six months while the rest returned to normal within twenty-three months. (Partly supported by WHO-Special Program of Research in Human Reproduction.)

16.03.07
Clinical results comparing Norplant® with two covered rods releasing levonorgestrel: Olsson, S-E, Odlind, V, Johansson, E D B. Inst. Obstet. and Gyn., Univ., Uppsala, Sweden
The Norplant® contraceptive system consists of six silastic capsules releasing levonorgestrel. The dose of levonorgestrel is 30 µg/24 hours. The capsules are implanted subdermally. Covered rods are manufactured differently and have a higher release rate than Norplant®. With two covered rods, the same dose will be delivered as with Norplant®. The aim of this study was to investigate if there were any differences between the two contraceptive systems with regard to efficacy and frequency of side-effects. 240 healthy parous women, 18 – 40 years old, volunteered for the study. They were randomized to two groups. 171 women used covered rods and 69 women used Norplant®. – Results after one year: No pregnancies occurred. In the group with Norplant® implants 39% discontinued during the first year. In the group with two covered rods 23% discontinued during the first year. This difference is significant ($p < 0.5$) using χ^2 test. The main reason for discontinuing was menstrual problems (24% for Norplant® and 14% for two covered rods). Other reasons for discontinuation were mood changes, nausea, headache or planning pregnancy. The plasma concentrations of levonorgestrel were with Norplant® 1.1 ± 0.1 nmol/l ($n = 21$) and with two covered rods 1.3 ± 0.2 nmol/l ($n = 20$). This difference was not significant. – Comment: The systems seem to be equally effective. Two covered rods might have fewer side-effects than Norplant®.

16.03.08
Two years experience with a long-acting contraceptive levonorgestrel implant: López, G, Rodríguez, A, Rengifo, J. Ctro Mèd. de Los Andes – Ctro Reg. de Población, Bogotá, Colombia
The clinical trial of a long-acting levonorgestrel implant-Norplant®, as a reversible method of contraceptive in the out-patient clinics of two hospitals in Colombia, has had promising results. It was the first time this method was used in the country. In close to 400 acceptors, in 593 women-years, the pregnancy rate has been nil. Results of users which completed two years are summarized, illustrating characteristics, acceptability, primary and secondary effects. Life table at 12 and 24 months showed high continuation rates, 91.6% and 76.5%, respectively. Local infection and complications were minimal. Causes of termination at 24 months included: amenorrhea and irregular bleeding: 14%; other medical: 6.4%; planning pregnancy: 1.2% and other personal: 1.9%, for a total termination rate of 23.5%. Differences between the two clinics and different factors are analysed, with comments related to insertion, extraction and future of the method.

16.03.09
Norplants' insertion and removal by paramedical personnel: Affandi, B, Santoso, S S I, Hadisaputra, D W, Moeloek, F A, Samil, R S. Dept. Obstet. and Gyn., Univ. of Indonesia/Dr. Cipto Mangunkusumo Hosp., Jakarta, Indonesia
To assess the performance of paramedical personnel in inserting and removing Norplants, a comparative study between doctors and paramedical personnel in inserting and removing Norplants was conducted in Klinik Raden Saleh, Department of Obstetrics and Gynecology, University of Indonesia, Jakarta. From 828 women who had been recruited to use Norplant, 285 were inserted by doctors and 543 inserted by paramedical personnel. There was no significant difference between the two groups regarding the age, parity and education. The average insertion time for the groups were 7.6 minutes for doctors and 7.1 minutes for paramedical personnel ($p > 0.01$). Regarding the average removal time, were 21.2 minutes for doctors and 22.5 minutes for paramedical personnel. It was concluded that paramedical personnels can insert and remove the Norplant as well as doctors do.

16.03.10
New regimen of injectable contraceptives: Prem, C, Chao, P A. Abhai Bhu Bejhr Hosp., Prachin-Buri, Thailand
In previous studies depo-medroxyprogesterone acetate (DMPA) had a higher incidence of spotting and amenorrhea than Norethisterone enanthate (NET-EN) but NET-EN had a higher pregnancy rate. The contraceptive efficacy of NET-EN had been improved by given it on a modified dose schedule. This study, as a new regimen of them, was set to solve all these problems. NET-EN 200 mg every 12 weeks was given to 150 Thai Prachinburi women after the first two DMPA 150 mg of 12 weeks intervals. Another 150 Thai Prachinburi women were injected 150 mg of DMPA every 12 weeks as a control group. No pregnancy occurred in either group. Amenorrhea was significantly more frequent with the control group than with the study group. The study group had a significantly greater number of acceptable cycles than the control group. Only 4.7% of the study group had unacceptable cycles during the first year of study. The continuation rate was 94.7% at the end of the study. The discontinuation rate was 5.3%, 80% had dropped out for irregular spotting, 10% for amenorrhea and 10% for weight gain over 5 kg. This new regimen was proved to be an effective and acceptable method of fertility control.

376

16.04.01

Single dose antibiotic therapy for asymptomatic bacteriurea in pregnancy: Jakobi, P, Neiger, R, Merzbach, D*, Friedman, M, Paldi, E. Depts. Obstet. & Gyn. "B" and Microbiol.*, Rambam Med. Ctr, Haifa, Israel

The prevalence of asymptomatic bacteriurea (ABU) is approximately 5% in pregnant women. About 30% of the untreated bacteriuric pregnant women subsequently develop acute pyelonephritis with all the known associated complications for the mother and the fetus. So, antibiotic treatment for ABU in pregnancy is mandatory. The standard way to treat ABU patients is a short course (one week) of drug therapy or even continuous suppressive treatment until delivery. Several reports on non-pregnant women indicate that single dose antimicrobial therapy may be as effective as a 7-day therapy. 41 pregnant women with confirmed ABU were treated with a single dose antimicrobial regimen (Moxypen 3.0 g or Keflex 2.0 g), according to *in vitro* disc diffusion tests for determining the sensitivity of the urinary pathogen. Urine cultures were taken 1, 2, 4 and 8 weeks after the therapy. Overall, the immediate success rate for the single dose antimicrobial therapy was 82.5%. Relapse occurred in one case (2.5%) and in four (9.5%) reinfection appeared, 60% of these recurrences were successfully treated by another single dose antibiotic treatment. 75% of the failures were cured by a 7-day therapy. In two cases which did not respond to either form of therapy, a pathological IVP was found after delivery. No patients in the study group developed symptomatic UTI, in spite of the expected 30% rate of symptomatic disease. We suggest that single dose antibiotic therapy is a satisfactory form of treatment for ABU of pregnancy and may even identify the group of high risk for developing symptomatic infection.

16.04.02

Antibiotic prophylaxis in surgery for stress urinary incontinence: Bergman, A, Bhatia, N. Harbor/UCLA Med. Ctr, UCLA School Med., Los Angeles, CA, USA

A prospective randomized study was undertaken to determine, (1) the clinical efficacy of antimicrobial prophylaxis for reducing postoperative febrile morbidity and, (2) the benefit-cost analysis when compared to a non-prophylaxis group. Twenty-six women, aged 27–70 years, undergoing retropubic urethropexy for stress urinary incontinence, were randomly assigned to a prophylaxis (14) and a non-prophylaxis group (12). Antibiotic prophylaxis consisted of a total of three intravenous doses of cefazolin sodium (Ancef) of 1 g each given before, during and after completion of surgery. In both groups, the paravesical and retropubic spaces were drained for 2–3 days after the operation. Based upon established criteria for postoperative febrile morbidity (wound infections, abscesses, UTI's), three patients with subfascial abscesses and two with UTI accounted for $\geqq 40\%$ postoperative febrile morbidity in patients without prophylaxis (p < .01). These patients needed a prolonged stay in hospital (2–5 days more than prophylactic group, p < .05) expensive laboratory and bacteriologic workups, additional diagnostic and surgical procedures. – In conclusion, our study, for the first time, demonstrates the clinical efficacy and tremendous cost effectiveness of prophylactic antibiotics and strongly suggests their use in patients undergoing incontinence surgery.

16.04.03

Cefoxitin versus placebo in the prophylaxis of postoperative infection in abdominal hysterectomy: Davi, E, Ausín, J, Escofet, C, Mensa, J, García-Sanmiguel, J. Dept. Obstet. and Gyn., and Infect. Dis., Hosp. Clin., Barcelona, Spain

In a prospective, randomized and double-blind assay, we compare the efficacy of cefoxitin versus placebo in the prevention of postoperative infection in abdominal hysterectomy. One hundred and fifty patients received 2 g i. m. of cefoxitin, 30 min before the operation and 6 and 12 hours after the first dose and other 160 received placebo. Both groups were statistically homogeneous. The postoperative (wound or pelvic) infection rate was 4% in the first group and 8.13% in the second group. Fifteen patients (10%) of cefoxitin group and 30 (18.75%) of placebo group (p = 0.02) had fever with no apparent cause and they needed antibiotic treatment. Twenty patients in the cefoxitin group and 41 of placebo group had urinary infection (p = 0.005). There was no difference in the postoperative stay and tolerance. In post-menopausal patients, the infection rate was 8.6% and before the menopause 24% (p < 0.005). The postoperative stay in complicated patients was 8.43 ± 3.25 days versus 6.89 ± 1.5 days in uncomplicated patients (p = 0.002). – In conclusion cefoxitin versus placebo really lowers the incidence of infections in abdominal hysterectomy. Premenopausal state is a risk factor of infection.

16.04.04

Prophylactic mezlocillin in patients undergoing radical hysterectomy: Micha, J P, Kucera, P R, Sheets, E E, Rettenmaier, M A, DiSaia, P J. Dept. Obstet. and Gyn., Univ. of California, Irvine, Med. Ctr, Orange, CA, USA

Prophylactic antibiotics (PA) and suction drainage significantly decrease febrile morbidity after vaginal hysterectomy. Simple abdominal hysterectomy PA studies have often but not always shown benefit. The role of PA in radical hysterectomy patients has not been extensively studied. A double-blind randomized prospective study of mezlocillin (Miles Pharmaceuticals), a broad spectrum semisynthetic penicillin versus placebo, was conducted. Patients received 4 g of mezlocillin or saline placebo intravenously, one half hour preoperatively, a second dose 4 to 6 hours later, and a final dose 6 hours after that. The difference in infectious morbidity between placebo and mezlocillin groups reached statistical significance after only 30 patients were enrolled, and the study was then terminated for ethical reasons.

	Mezlocillin (n = 15)	Placebo (n = 15)	p Value
Febrile Morbidity	4	11	< 0.005
Fever Index (°F-hr)	94	136	
Wound Infections	0	7	< 0.005
Pelvic Cellulitis	1	3	

No significant differences were noted between the two groups in estimated blood loss, duration of operation, or weight. Short-term perioperative antibiotic prophylaxis is indicated in patients undergoing radical hysterectomy.

16.04.05
Ticarcillin/clavulanic acid treatment of gynecological infections with special reference to the blood and tissue concentrations: Gutschow, K, Weißenbacher, E R, Adam, D, Schneider, A, Wachter, I, Lühr, H G. Frauenklin., Klinikum Grosshadern, LMU, München
Ticarcillin/clavulanic acid combination was taken by 20 women with soft tissue infections such as pelvic inflammatory disease, wound infections after hysterectomy etc. E. coli was the most frequent strain. Eighteen of 20 women were cured. No side-effects were noticed. The highest serum levels of ticarcillin were reached 15 minutes after injection of 3 g i.v. (213.3 mcg/ml). The highest serum levels for clavulanic were obtained 15 minutes after injection of 200 mg i.v. (5.5 mcg/ml). The highest tissue concentrations were measured in the Fallopian tube 15 minutes after a bolus injection for ticarcillin (59.4 mcg/g).

16.04.06
Ofloxacin versus doxycyclin in gynecological infections: Schneider, A, Weißenbacher, E R, Gutschow, K, Wachter, I. Frauenklin., Klinikum Grosshadern, LMU, München
In a randomised study 20 patients received either 2 × 200 mg ofloxacin (daily p. o.) or 2 × 100 mg doxycyclin (daily p.o) for seven days. All patients suffered from soft tissue infections e.g. wound infection, pelvic inflammatory disease etc. E. coli was the most frequent strain isolated. One patient in the ofloxacin group and two in the doxycyclin group were not cured. There was one side-effect in the doxycyclin and none in the ofloxacin group.

16.04.07
Prophylactic topical cefamandole in radical hysterectomy: Miyazawa, K, Hernandez, E, Dillon, M B. Tripler Army Med. Ctr, Honolulu, HI, USA
From July 1, 1978 to June 30, 1984, 45 radical abdominal hysterectomies were performed by the authors at Tripler Army Medical Center. Management was uniform except for the use of prophylactic antibiotics. Three patterns of practice were identified. Group I, no antibiotics were used; Group II intravenous (IV) antibiotics were given in the induction room and for less than 48 hours postoperative; Group III, prophylactic IV antibiotics were given and the surgical site was irrigated with a cefamandole and saline solution. The three groups were found to be similar with regards to age, parity, height-weight index, pre- and post-operative hematocrit, pre-operative white blood count, operative and anesthesia times, estimated blood loss and amount of blood transfused. Groups I and II had a higher surgical site infection rate (87.5% and 63.6%, respectively) than Group III (3.8%). The mean 10-day fever index in degree hours for Group I was 109, 71 for Group II and 30 for Group III (p < 0.000001). Irrigation of the surgical site with a cefamandone and saline solution in addition to i.v. antibiotics seems to have a role in decreasing the infectious morbidity of radical hysterectomy.

16.06.01
Exogenous TRH effects on prolactin secretion of human decidua-chorion, amnion and placental parenchyma by organ culture: Song, S K, Hur, P H, Namkoong, S E, Kim, S J. Dept. Obstet. & Gyn., Cath. Med. Coll., Seoul, Korea
In order to evaluate the main secreting site of hPRL in amniotic fluid during pregnancy and the effects of exogenous TRH on hPRL secretion, the explants of decidua-chorion, amnion and placental parenchyma of placenta expelled from 15 normal term pregnant women were cultured *in vitro*. The control was one without TRH in culture medium and the experimental group was one with added synthetic TRH in different (1, 5 and 10 μg/ml) concentrations and measured hPRL in culture medium by using radioimmunoassay. In control group, the mean daily secretion of hPRL (mean ± SEM) in decidua-chorion, amnion and placental parenchyma were 107.60 ± 6.40, 10.89 ± 1.38 and 3.23 ± 0.58 ng/100 mg, respectively. In experimental group with addition of 1, 5 and 10 μg/ml of TRH, mean daily secretion of hPRL were 155.52 ± 6.8, 171.86 ± 8.23 and 194.82 ± 9.32 ng/100 mg in decidua-chorion, 13.72 ± 1.53, 15.86 ± 1.69 and 18.81 ± 1.91 ng/100 mg in amnion respectively. But the above patterns of secretion of hPRL failed to show

in placental parenchyma. The above results showed that the main secreting site of hPRL in amniotic fluid during pregnancy is decidua-chorion but amnion is also shown to secret a small amount of hPRL and it is also believed that TRH is involved in the control of secretion of hPRL from decidua-chorion and amnion.

16.06.02

Relationship of maternal and fetal TSH, total T4, free T4, T3, cortisol and prolactin levels and type of delivery: Patella, A, Muti, A R, *Carta, G, *Ippolito, M, Arzano, S. 1st Inst. Obstet. and Gyn., Univ. of Roma "La Sapienza", and *School Obstet., Camerino, Italy
TSH, T4T, FT4, T3, cortisol and prolactin were measured during delivery in 23 healthy patients and relative living and vital fetus of 37–42 weeks single fetus pregnancies. Weight of newborns was between 3000–3800 g. Case studies have been divided into two groups: 1) 18 spontaneous vaginal deliveries: Blood tests on maternal plasma were effected at beginning of labor, the length of which was between 2–8 hours. 2) Five elective Cesarians: Blood tests were performed on maternal plasma before the operation. Blood tests on fetal plasma were done on the umbilical cord after birth. No significant differences were noted in the hormones studies in mother and in fetus in relationship to parity and week of pregnancy. Furthermore only a slight increase of FT4 in maternal plasma was noticed in the patients with spontaneous delivery. This confirms the homogeneity of the two groups. However T4T, T4F, T3 and cortisol levels were higher in newborns of vaginal delivery with significant difference. In conclusion, labor stimulates fetal production of thyroid hormones and cortisol which justifies a major frequency of RDS in Cesarian newborns after delivery.

16.06.03

The dating of gestation by measurement of placental lactogen (hPL), chorionic gonadotrophin (hCG) and Schwangerschaftsprotein 1 (SP₁): Klopper, A. Dept. Obstet. and Gyn., Univ., Aberdeen, Scotland
The serum concentration of the placental proteins hPL, hCG and SP_1 increases steeply with advancing gestation. Single assays of each protein were done in early pregnancy to determine whether the concentration was a reliable indicator of the stage of gestation. It was found that gestation could be accurately determined by hCG assay up to 9 weeks and by hPL and SP_1 assay up to 16 weeks. The placental protein concentration compared favorably with ultrasound measurement as a means of forecasting the date of spontaneous onset of labor and was at least as accurate as the last menstrual period for this purpose.

16.06.04

Hypophysial hormones in human placenta and fetal membranes: Takagi, T, Otsuki, Y, Mori, M, Yamaji, K, Tanizawa, O. Dept. Obstet. and Gyn., Osaka Univ. Med. School, Osaka, Japan
Recently, oxytocin (OT) was found in extrahypothalamopituitary regions such as rat spinal cord, human ovary, bovine corpus luteum and human placenta. Moreover, human placenta contains various other hormones such as LH-RH, PRL and CRF besides hCG and hPL. From these findings, we suggested that vasopressin (VP) might be present in human placenta and fetal membranes. Immunoreactive OT and VP was identified and measured by radioimmunoassay (RIA) in extracts from human placenta and fetal membranes. Tissue extraction was performed in 0.1 M acetic acid containing enzyme inhibitors. The homogenate was heated in boiling water for 5 min and then centrifuged at 3000 g for 15 min at 4°C. The supernatant was adjusted to pH 7.0 with NaOH, recentrifuged and frozen at −20°C until assayed. Maternal and cord plasma OT and VP were measured by RIA. Biochemical properties of tissue extracts were the same as those of synthetic OT and VP except that it contained a component of high molecular weight that was separated on a Sephadex G-25 column. The immunoreactivities in these tissues were much higher than circulating level in pregnant women at term or that in cord blood. It is suggested that OT and VP may be produced in the placenta or fetal membranes and may have a local role in maintenance of pregnancy or initiation of labor.

16.06.05

The studies on the inhibiting effects of LH-RH analog in early pregnancy: Yaoi, Y, Ohkura, T, Sono, S, Hayashi, M, Takahashi, K, Takamizawa, M, Kumasaka, T. Dept. Obstet. & Gyn., Dokkyo Univ. School Med., Saitama; **Kubota, T, Oiyama, H, Teh, A, Saito, M.** Dept. Obstet. & Gyn., Tokyo Med. & Dent. Univ., Tokyo, Japan
From our previous experience, we found that the LH-RH analog had the so called "paradoxical effect" and the administration of LH-RH analog disturbed the progress of early pregnancy. In this study we tried to find out the inhibiting effects of the analog in experimental animals both endocrinologically and morphologically. In various stages of gestation in rats, the LH-RH analog (D-Leu[6]-LH-RH-EA) was administered for five days and then blood samples and uterus were collected for endocrinological and morphological studies. Plasma estrogen (E) and progesterone (P) levels and P/E ratio decreased in the analog group. E-receptor (E-R) were low and P-R/E-R ratio was 0.2. In the control group, however, the P-R/E-R ratio was 1.0. The development of the endothelial cells in the gestational myometrium was poor and atrophic in the analog group. These results suggested that a certain hormonal homeostasis was necessary for maintenance of normal pregnancy, and the administration of LH-RH analog disturbed this hormonal environment including the uterine wall, resulting in the interruption of early pregnancy.

16.06.06

Evaluation of dopaminergic neuroendocrine control of anterior pituitary hormones release during labor in human: Nishii, O, Takeuchi, T, Takahashi, M, Okamura, T, Yaginuma, T, Kobayashi, T. Dept. Obstet. and Gyn., Fac. Med., Univ. of Tokyo at Mejirodai, Tokyo, Japan

Eight women with normal term pregnancy were given 10 mg metoclopramide (M) i.v., dopamine antagonist, before and during labor. Serum prolactin (PRL), TSH, GH and cortisol levels were measured at -30, 0, 30 and 60 minutes of M administration by specific radioimmunoassay. Basal serum PRL levels before labor, 287.5 ± 28.6 ng/ml (M $\pm$ SE), significantly declined to 237.0 ± 22.4 and 216.4 ± 22.9 ng/ml ($P < 0.05$ at both) at -30 and 0 minutes of M administration, respectively, during labor. The increments in serum PRL at 30 and 60 minutes after M administration during labor (209.5 ± 33.9 and 120.0 ± 27.1 ng/ml, respectively) were not significantly different from those before labor (202.1 ± 48.7 and 89.9 ± 30.1 ng/ml, respectively), suggesting that the decline in serum PRL levels during labor is not due to the dopaminergic control. Basal serum TSH and GH levels were not significantly changed by labor and M administration both before and during labor. Serum cortisol levels tended to increase during labor, but not significantly. The data suggest that the anterior pituitary hormones releases are not controlled by dopaminergic mechanism during labor.

16.06.07

***In vitro* effect of LHRH on human normal and malignant trophoblasts:** Kim, S J, Park, J S, Kang, B C, Lee, J W, Namkoong, S E. Dept. Obstet. & Gyn., Cath. Med. Coll., Seoul, Korea

To observe certain difference of hormonal production between normal and malignant trophoblasts, we evaluated *in vitro* hormonal responses of trophoblasts to LHRH stimulation. The placental tissue at 10 weeks gestational age, the tissue of choriocarcinoma which obtained from the patients and established choriocarcinoma cell line (BeWo) were cultured and serially diluted LHRH of 1, 5 and 10 μg/ml were added to the media for five days. The concentrations of β-hCG, LH, FSH, estradiol-17β and progesterone in culture medias before and after LHRH stimulation were measured by radioimmunoassay. The results were as follows: 1. In the cultural media of placental explants at ten weeks gestational age, the normal trophoblastic cells significantly responded to LHRH stimulation to produce β-hCG (869.2 ± 29.4 to 1277.6 ± 129.9 mIU/ml), LH (495.5 ± 12.6 to 633.8 ± 38.5 mIU/ml) and progesterone (203.0 ± 8.9 to 318.0 ± 16.7 ng/ml). 2. In the cultural media of the tissue of choriocarcinoma, the malignant trophoblastic cells significantly responded to LHRH stimulation to produce β-hCG (1182.0 ± 46.2 to 1961.0 ± 100.0 mIU/ml) and LH (918.0 ± 22.4 to 1194.0 ± 35.5 mIU/ml). 3. In the cultural media of established choriocarcinoma cell line (BeWo), the production of β-hCG, LH, FSH, estradiol-17β and progesterone were not stimulated by LHRH, although the baseline levels of estradiol-17β (817.0 ± 11.8 pg/ml) and progesterone (43.7 ± 9.2 ng/ml) were much higher than in normal and malignant trophoblastic cells.

16.06.08

Plasma ACTH, β-lipotropin and β-endorphin in the human fetus and their mother during delivery: Furuhashi, N, Suzuki, M, Hiruta, M, Tanaka, M, Takahashi, T. Dept. Obstet. and Gyn., Tohoku Univ. School Med., Sendai, Japan

Plasma ACTH, β-lipotropin (β-LPH) and β-endorphin (β-EP) were measured by high sensitive radioimmunoassay in maternal and umbilical cord plasma samples which were obtained simultaneously in 12 cases. Mean ACTH levels in cord (97.1 ± 7.9 pg/ml, $\pm$ S.E.) and maternal plasma (135.9 ± 35.8 pg/ml) were significantly ($p < 0.05$) higher than that of normal adults ($n = 8$, 48.5 ± 6.9 pg/ml). Mean β-LPH in maternal (690.1 ± 138.6 pg/ml) and cord palsma (1111.4 ± 94.2 pg/ml) were significantly higher than that of normal adults ($n = 8$, 93.0 ± 8.2 pg/ml). Mean β-EP in maternal (125.8 ± 24 pg/ml) and cord plasma (130.6 ± 20.6 pg/ml) were significantly higher than that of normal adults ($n = 8$, 6.0 ± 0.9 pg/ml). There were significant positive correlations between β-LPH and β-EP levels in maternal and cord plasma. Mean β-EP to β-LPH molar ratio of 0.19 ± 0.03 in maternal plasma was significantly ($p < 0.05$) higher than that of cord plasma (0.13 ± 0.01). These data suggest that ACTH, β-LPH and β-EP were elevated during delivery responding to the stress. Beta-LPH and β-EP in cord plasma were fetal and/or placental in origin.

16.07.01

Histologic and histometric aspects of the breast in polycystic ovary syndrome: Fonseca, A M, Souza, A Z, Bagnoli, V R, Celestino, C A, Salvatore, C A. Gyn. Clin., Univ. of São Paulo Med. School, São Paulo, Brazil

The author has performed a microscopic study of breast tissue of 28 women with diagnosis of polycystic ovary syndrome and has observed that: – The breast tissue in the women with polycystic ovary syndrome has presented gross disorders in the qualitative study of the lobular architecture. The intralobular and the interlobular connective tissue were hypertrophic and partially hyalinized. – The volume occupied by the acinar tissue in the women with polycystic ovary syndrome was not found in the ductal, connective, vascular or adipose tissues. – The middle surface of the acinus in the mammary gland did not differ in both of groups. – The middle diameter of the excretory ducts was greater in the patients with polycystic ovary syndrome. – The number of nuclei in the acinar tissue was not different in both of the groups; hence we may conclude that there is no lobular hyperplasia.

16.07.02

Dysplasia and breast cancer: Blanchard, O. Aeronautic, Centr. Buenos Aires, Argentina

In the Department of Gynecology of Aeronautic Central Hospital from 1969 to 1982 230 carcinomas of the breast have been verified. The relation and simultaneous presence of dysplasia and carcinoma of the breast noticed in 41 cases (17.82%) were investigated. Statistics are shown of the patients who consulted us about those with mammary dysplasias and in addition to the mammary carcinomas, as regards age, menarche and menopause. The parity shows that when it increases the carcinomas and dysplasias decrease. The proportion of the volume between the carcinoma and the dysplasia was greater in a 68% for the dysplasias above the dimension of the mammary carcinoma. The prognosis and evolution were more unfavorable for patients in whom the dysplasia predominated over the carcinoma. Only in one patient (2.43%) could we verify the evolution of a mammary adenosis. After three years of follow-up it showed a papillary carcinoma with metastasis in axillary nodes.

16.07.03

Ten-year prospective follow-up study of histologically proven mastopathia: Opri, F, Weitzel, H. Hosp. Gyn. and Obstet., FU, Berlin

The research and better understanding of the pathological and biological characteristics of preneoplastic lesions helps to prevent certain types of carcinoma. From 1968 to 1978, we followed 1725 patients with histologically proven mastopathia: Type I – 833 cases, Type II – 610 cases, Type III – 92 cases. The observations took place in a special breast clinic. The average age of the patients was 45.6 years. In 463 cases, it was necessary to obtain a second surgical specimen because of suspicious tumors on palpation. In this group microscopic evaluation showed an increase of the degree of cellular proliferation and a certain percentage a malignant transformation. It is of practical importance (1) to identify the facultatively preneoplastic transformation, (2) to classify them as high-risk cases and (3) to include them in a special follow-up program.

16.07.04

Tubal sterilization in relation to fibrocystic disease and breast cancer: Vorherr, H, Vorherr, U F, Argubright, K F. Dept. Obstet.-Gyn., Univ. of New Mexico, School Med., Albuquerque, NM, USA

Disturbance of vascular, nervous, local neurohormonal and lymphatic physiology may play an etiologic role in ovarian dysfunction (estrogen predominance, progesterone deficiency) following tubal sterilization. Of 322 premenopausal patients with fibrocystic breast disease, 130 (40.4%) had preceeding tubal ligation and 47 (14.6%) a hysterectomy; 145 (45.0%) patients had no history of sterilization. Mastodynia and fibrocystic breast changes develop within one to two years after sterilization. In general, 25% of premeno-pausal patients undergo sterilization. In our population with fibrocystic disease, 55% of patients have undergone sterilization; i. e., the risk of development of fibrocystic disease after sterilization is more than twice the normal rate. The risk of developing fibrocystic disease is increased sevenfold for women who had undergone tubal sterilization as compared to a nonsterilized age-adjusted control population. Within 1 ½ years, breast cancer has been diagnosed in six patients (age range: 37 to 47 years) in whom fibrocystic disease developed following sterilization; this number is in excess of the expected rate. Thus, patients with both sterilization and fibrocystic breast disease require close follow-up by clinical examination, sonogra-phy, and mammography. Consequently, sterilization techniques (endotherm coagulation) should be chosen with a minimum of interference with tubal-ovarian physiology.

16.07.05

Hormonal status of dysplasia mammaye: Nedeljković, B, Sajdl, V*, Kapor, S*. Med. Ctr, Zrenjanin, Hosp. "Djordje Jovanović"; *INEP – Labor. Biophys. and Anal. Chem., Zemun, Yugoslavia

The relations between 12 urinary steroids were investigated in premenopausal patients with dysplasia mammale. These values were compared with the control group. In the dysplasia mammale patients the (Pd) and (Pt) concentrations were significantly decreased in the luteal phase compared to normal control values. Different indexes of hormones or groups of hormones were tested and it was established that the index $A + HE/E + HA$, as well as the function log Pd versus log (F_2/F_1) most fully reflect the differences between patients with dysplasia mammale and the control group. The results of this study suggest that the steroid ratio (indexes) rather than the extent of steriod excretion was often more sensitive in the characterization of the hormonal status of the illness (dysplasia mammale). A – androsterone; E – etiocholanolone; HA – 11-hydroxyandrosterone; HE – 11-hydroxyetiocholanolone; Pd – pregnanediol; Pt – pregnanetriol; F_1 – sum of androgens; F_2 – sum of Pd, Pt, HA and HE.

16.07.06

A clinical approach to the puerperal and non-puerperal mastitis cases with the bromocriptine treatment.: Durmuş, Z, Gökmen, O, Ulaş, G. Ankara Maternity Hosp., Ankara, Turkey

This study is the evaluation of a clinical trial for benign fibrocystic mastopathies and puerperal mastitis. Seventy patients were included in the study between December 1983 and July 1984 in Ankara Maternity Hospitaly, 45 being puerperal and 25 being non-puerperal. Dopamine agonist, BC (bromocriptine), was used in the treatment. The results yielded 80% success in non-puerperal mastitis and 92% success in puerperal mastitis. These results indicated that bromocriptine can be effectively used in the treatment of puerperal and non-puerperal mastitis without causing an interference in the lactation process.

16.07.07

Bacteriological aspects of mastitis: Souza, A Z, Tomioka, E, Hegg, R, Kesselring, G L, Salvatore, C A. Gyn. Clin., São Paulo Univ. Med. School, São Paulo, Brazil

We have studied 23 patients with a diagnosis of mastitis. All of them were submitted to bacteriologic study to investigate the aerobic and anaerobic agents. Seven cases (30.4%) were associated with lactation, one case (4.3%) was diagnosed during pregnancy and 15 (65.2%) were not related either to pregnancy or lactation. Anaerobic agents were recovered in four (17.4%) patients, aerobic in 15 (65.2%) and aerobic plus anaerobic in one (4.3%) case. The culture was negative in three (13.4%) patients. Anaerobic flora were more frequently related to non-puerperal mastitis although one case of puerperal mastitis showed only anaerobic agents. Staphylococcus aureus was the most common among aerobic agents, and it was obtained from the abscess of 11 (47.8%) patients. Ten different species of anaerobic organism were recovered from the five patients but the same agent was never recovered twice from different patients.

16.08.01

The lack of indication for screening colposcopy in patients with cervical ectropion: Fejgin, M, Goldberger, S B, Markov, S, Cohen-Alloro, J, Ben-Nun, I, Ben-Aderet, N. Dept. Obstet. and Gyn. "A", Meir Gen. Hosp., Sapir Med. Ctr, Kfar-Sava, Israel

To the gynecologist in the community who has no access to a colposcope, the finding of cervical ectropion may be suspicious. Two-hundred such patients were referred to our screening colposcopy clinic for evaluation. In addition to colposcopy and biopsies when indicated all had a Papanicolau smear. The results were compared to 460 patients that were referred for screening colposcopy for various other reasons (routine, chronic cervicitis and contact bleeding) and that served as control. Thirty patients (14.6%) had colposcopic directed biopsies compared to 96 (20.9%) in the control group. Only five dysplasias were found (2.4%), three of them mild (CIN I) and two moderate (CIN II). There were 30 dysplasias in the control group (6.5%). We therefore conclude that women with ectropion only have a low incidence of cervical intra-epithelial neoplasia and screening colposcopy is not indicated when there is abnormal cervical cytology.

16.08.02

An evaluation of the usefulness of columnar cells of endocervical origin (CE) and metaplastic cells (MC) as indicators of effective cytological sampling: Woodman, C B J, Williams, D R, Yates, M, Jordan, J. Dept. Obstet., Univ., Birmingham, UK

Cervical smears which accurately predicted the presence of cervical intra-epithelial neoplasia were compared with those that failed to do so. Adequate smears were more likely to contain CE and MC. This difference was only significant for MC ($p < 0.01$). The Rocket and Ayre spatula were compared. Cervical smears taken with the Rocket spatula were more likely to contain CE ($p < 0.1$) but less likely to contain MC ($p < 0.1$). Smears taken following cone biopsy were less likely to contain CE or MC ($p < .001$); no difference was observed following laser vaporisation. Smears taken in a colposcopy clinic were more likely to contain CE or MC than smears taken in Family Planning Clinics, Gynecology Clinics or by General Practitioners ($p < .001$). Smears taken in an ante-natal clinic were less likely to contain EC or MC when compared with those taken from other sources ($p < .001$). This has important implication for cervical cytology screening programmes.

16.08.03

Lectin binding in smears of the cervix uteri during menstrual cycle: Zippel, H H, Klein, P J, Tillmann, C, Würz, H. Univ.-Frauenklin., Marburg; Path. Inst., Univ., Freiburg; Univ.-Frauenklin., Köln

The aim of the study was to demonstrate the binding of FITC-conjugated peanut-agglutinin (PNA) in smears of the cervix uteri ($n = 60$). The intensity of staining was evaluated by a quantitative method of fluorescence microscopy. During the normal menstrual cycle the PNA binding capacity exhibited different patterns. In the proliferative phase a maximum of binding was detected, whereas in the secretory phase reduced levels were observed. The PNA binding correlated with the cytologically defined hormonal grade and with the serum estradiol values. Furthermore the distribution of PNA binding was comparable to the levels of estrogen (ER) and progesterone (PR) receptors in the endocervical mucosa during the menstrual cycle. From these observations it may be concluded that peanut agglutinin binding in cervical smears is an expression of hormonal stimulation. Analogous findings have been described for mammary gland and endometrium.

16.08.04

Comparison of effect on cervical erosion with cryotherapy and M. S. A. M.: Liu, C T, Liu, T S. Huiiying Gyn. Private Clin., Taipei, Taiwan

Up to the present, here are mainly three types of method being commonly used for the treatment of cervical erosion, these are: electrocauterization, cryotherapy and laser therapy. Only limited symptomatic improvements in such as leucorrhea, abdominal pain, foul odor have been reported, the improved effects commonly only last up to six months. Using of metacresol sulphonic acid with methanal (M. S. A. M.) get very excellent results (normal physiological state of cervix, endocervix, vagina) with five years follow-up. Since M. S. A. M. is a selective action on necrotic and pathologically altered tissue which is coagulated and cast off, and destroys the pathogenic bacterial mixed flora of the vagina without affecting the Döderlein's bacilli, thus reestablishing physiological conditions. Total 582 completely healed cases under five years observation made no complaints of recurrent cervical erosion except taking D&C and/or delivery; abdominal pain, bearing down sensation, foul vaginal discharges seems to be very scarce here. Hence, it can be stated that the success rate is nearly 100%. From the past ten years clinical experience, no cervical stenosis is found out as in post-cryotherapy cases when the endocervix was treated. In brief, normal menstruation and pregnancy can be assured after complete healing. The most important preventive method is to have regular follow-up with correct sanitary habits.

16.08.05
Presence of immune reactive relaxin in uterus and ovaries of non-pregnant humans: Lippert, T H, Burghardt, A, Seeger, H, Reus, W, Voelter, W. Dept. Obstet. and Gyn., Univ., Tübingen

So far, relaxin has been found almost exclusively in pregnancy. Since smaller amounts can now be detected by radioimmunoassay (RIA), the presence of relaxin has been investigated in the uterus and ovaries of non-pregnant women. Tissue samples were obtained from patients undergoing gynecological surgery with removal of uterus and ovaries. The average age of the patients was 45 years. The samples (minimal weight of 0.2 g) were frozen immediately at $-65°C$. The extraction consisted of defreezing and disintegrating the tissue with a scalpel, addition of phosphate buffer, homogenisation, centrifugation and filtration. Relaxin was estimated in the supernatant using a heterologous RIA for pig relaxin and protein content was measured according to *Bansadoun* and *Weinstein* (Anal. Biochem. **85**, 295, 1978). The following relaxin values per g of wet weight tissue or protein were found (mean values $\pm$ SEM): myometrium (n=15): 1.7 ± 0.3 ng/g tissue and 45.6 ± 8.7 ng/g protein; cervix (n=6): 2.4 ± 0.4 ng/g tissue and 63.0 ± 21.6 ng/g protein; fibroid (n=9): 5.5 ± 1.7 ng/g tissue and 150.2 ± 38.5 ng/g protein; ovary (n=6): 3.2 ± 0.7 ng/g tissue and 76.7 ± 14.7 ng/g protein. In summary, it can be said that relaxin was found in measurable concentrations in all the tissues examined, with fibroid tissue having the highest values.

16.08.06
Presence of immunoreactive relaxin in human female urine: Fuchs, U, Lippert, T H, Seeger, H, Voelter, W. Dept. Obstet. and Gyn., Univ., Tübingen

Little is known about the occurrence of relaxin in urine. Since it is now possible to detect very low levels of relaxin by radioimmunoassay (RIA) excretion of relaxin in urine was examined. Morning urine was collected from 31 women with mammary carcinoma and from a control group of ten non-pregnant women of childbearing age. Determination of relaxin content was carried out with a heterologous RIA for pig relaxin. Investigations have shown that there is a cross-reaction between pig and human relaxin. The following results were obtained (mean values $\pm$ SEM): mammary carcinoma: 399 ± 77 pg/ml and control group: 636 ± 159 pg/ml. Thus, immunoreactive relaxin was found in both groups, larger amounts being present in the control group than in the patients with carcinoma. Further, acid-acetone extraction of the urine was performed and after column chromatography an elution profile was obtained. By RIA examination, one peak with relaxin activity was identified. A dilution series was also prepared from urine of patients who showed high relaxin values. The results showed a linear relationship with low standard deviations. Because of the low concentrations of immunoreactive relaxin in urine, it has not yet been possible to obtain sufficient amounts for biological testing. However, according to the present investigations relaxin seems to be present in urine.

16.08.07
Behavior of sliding knots in mono- and multifilament suture material: Trimbos, J B, Rijssel, E J C van. Dept. Gyn., Univ. Med. Ctr, Leiden, The Netherlands

Knots in surgical sutures can be divided into flat knots (square knot; granny knot; surgeon's knot) and sliding knots. It has been shown that the vast majority of knots routinely made in surgical practice are sliding knots (Obstet. Gyn. **64**, 274–280, 1984). In this study six different sliding knots were tested. Knot failure was defined as breaking of the knot or slippage exceeding 2 mm. Two resorbable multifilament suture materials (Vicryl®; Dexon-Plus®) and three monofilament materials (Prolene®; PDS®; Maxon®), all size 3–0, were tested. Every knot was tested ten times after soaking the sutures in human plasma for 15 minutes. Knot failure levels differed widely, and some knots proved to be more than eight times stronger than others. Knots with identical throws around the same suture were the weakest. Throws alternately tied around each of the two thread ends resulted in the most reliable knots although the difference with knots composed of non-identical throws around the same suture was relatively small. These differences were for the greater part statistically significant. Adding two extra throws to three-throw sliding knots increased the knot holding power considerably, especially in the monofilament suture materials. When the knot properties of the materials were compared Dexon-Plus® proved to be superior to Vicryl®, and Maxon® to be superior to PDS®. It is emphasized that sufficient knowledge of the mechanical properties of different knots and suture materials should be regarded as an important aspect of surgical performance.

16.08.08

Spontaneous occurrence of adenocarcinoma of the uterus and suppression of natural killer (NK) cell activity in neonatally androgenized SD rats: Morikawa, S, Naito, M, Takamizawa, H. Obstet. and Gyn., Chiba Univ. School Med., Chiba, Japan

In a previous studies, we showed that a persistence of both hormone imbalances and dysfunctional uteri in neonatally androgen-sterilized rats (ASR) spontaneously induced abnormal uterine proliferation at a late age. In SD female rats sterilized by a single injection of testosterone propionate two days after birth, three atypical hyperplasias, three adenocarcinomas and one adenosquamous-cell carcinoma were detected in 61 ASR 500 days after birth. In contrast, in 162 normal control rats (NR) no abnormal uterine proliferation was detected during a 770 day observation period. We examined the sex-steroid values and NK activity in ASR. The plasma estrone/progesterone and estradiol/progesterone ratios in 300-day-old ASR were twice as great as in NR. Estradiol/progesterone in 550-day-old ASR with adenocarcinoma was 2.5 times and 4.6 times greater than in ASR without adenocarcinoma and NR, respectively. Splenic NK activity (% specific lysis) was determined in a 4-hr 51Cr release assay using YAC-1 cells as targets. NK activity in ASR was significantly depressed when compared with that in NR at both 250 and 500 days of age. Such hormone imbalance produced both depression of NK activity which may facilitate the development of malignant tumors, and endometrial carcinogenesis in ASR.

16.09.01

Action of magnesium sulfate (MgSO$_4$) on platelets and umbilical vessel prostacyclin (PGI$_2$): Briel, R C, Lippert, T H, Zahradnik, H P*. Dept. Obstet and Gyn., Univ., Tübingen/Freiburg*

High dose intravenous MgSO$_4$ is recommended for its anticonvulsive action in pregnancy induced hypertension (PIH). In PIH vascular synthesis of PGI$_2$ and platelet sensitivity to prostacyclin (PSP) are supposed to be decreased. Mg is known to exert an inhibitory effect on coagulation and platelet function, but, so far, little is known about its influence on PGI$_2$ metabolism. Therefore, the influence of MgSO$_4$ on PSP and vascular PGI$_2$-synthesis was investigated. Blood specimens from 12 healthy volunteers and arteries from eight umbilical cords of normal term deliveries were used for the investigations. Mg concentrations of 4, 8 and 16 mVal/l were tested. Evaluation of PSP was carried out after spontaneous and ADP-induced aggregation (according to *Breddin* and *Born*) using a stable PGI$_2$-analogue (Iloprost, Schering AG, Berlin). PGI$_2$ production of the umbilical artery was estimated by a radioimmunoassay for its stable hydrolysis product 6-keto-PGF$_{1a}$. Results: MgSO$_4$ enhances inhibition of platelet aggregation induced by the PGI$_2$-analogue Iloprost. If Iloprost plus MgSO$_4$ are added to platelet rich plasma there is additional inhibition of spontaneous and ADP-induced platelet aggregation caused by MgSO$_4$. MgSO$_4$ induces an increase in release of PGI$_2$, measured as 6-keto-PGF$_{1a}$, from the umbilical artery. There is a concentration dependent and statistically significant increase in the mean levels of 20 to 36%. Further studies are warranted to demonstrate whether MgSO$_4$ is also able to improve the impaired PGI$_2$-production and platelet function found in pre-eclamptic patients.

16.09.02

The influence of local therapeutic irradiation on platelet aggregation and platelet sensitivity to prostacyclin in patients with uterine cancer: Kieback, D G, Briel, R C, Schneider, A I, Schmucker, R G A. Dept. Obstet. and Gyn., Eberhard-Karls-Univ., Tübingen

During radium therapy a high rate of thromboembolism has been observed. Alteration of platelet function and prostacyclin metabolism might be important as a pathophysiological mechanism under these conditions. Spontaneous and ADP-induced platelet aggregation as well as platelet sensitivity to prostacyclin have been determined in 21 patients treated with intravaginal radium applications after hysterectomy for adenocarcinoma of the corpus uteri stage I and in ten patients submitted to combined intravaginal and intrauterine irradiation for squamous cancer of the cervix uteri stage IIa to IIIb. The intravaginal irradiation dose was 960 mgeh in all patients, the additional intrauterine dose for patients with carcinoma of the cervix ranged from 960 to 1200 mgeh. The time of exposure to radiation was 24 hours. All patients were on low-dose heparin prophylaxis. Blood samples were taken before the start of radium therapy and 1 and 24 hours after its termination. In both groups spontaneous and ADP-induced aggregation did not show any systematic changes. In patients treated with intravaginal radium only, platelet sensitivity to prostacyclin was significantly reduced. The effect was most pronounced after 24 hours, by then reaching an average of 20% (p < 0.025, t-Test). Combined intrauterine/intravaginal treatment did not affect platelet reactivity to a significant degree. Lowering of platelet sensitivity to prostacyclin is considered to be a possible radiogenic alteration of platelet function *in vivo*. It may reinforce the thrombogenic effect of decreased prostacyclin formation in irradiated vessels.

16.09.03

Hemostatic system changes with progestogen only pill compared with combined oral contraceptives: Sabra, A, Bonnar, J. Dept. Obstet. and Gyn., Univ., Assiut, Egypt and Univ., Dublin, Ireland

Serial changes in blood coagulation were studied in 74 women using different types of oral contraceptives. Group A: 31 women treated with Norinyl-I (50 mcg mestranol + 0.1 mg norethisterone) for 48 weeks. Group B: 21 women treated with Micronor (350 mcg norethisterone) for 48 weeks. Group C: 15 women treated with Orthonovin (50 mcg mestranan 0.1 mg norethisterone) for, 24 weeks followed by Micronor for

24 weeks. Group D: 7 women treated with Micronor for 24 weeks followed by Orthonovin for 24 weeks. Group A showed a highly significant increase in factor II, VII, X and platelet count and drop in at-III and anti-Xa from the 6th week of treatment onwards compared with group B which remained unchanged. Women started on Orthonovin (Group-C) showed significant increase in Factor VII, VIII, X and VII + X complex from the 6th week of treatment onwards. A significant drop in anti-Xa was also found. No significant change was found in factor V or at-III. However, when they changed to the progestogen only pill Micronor, factor VIII, X and VII + X complex activities droped to levels less than the pretreatment values. The coagulation inhibitors anti-Xa increased with Micronor therapy. Women started on Micronor (Group-D) showed no significant change in factor II, V, VII, VII + X complex and at-III. However, they showed increase in factor III and gradual decrease in anti-Xa activities. Factor II, VII, VIII, X and VII + X complex increased while the coagulation inhibitor at-III and anti-Xa droped significantly after the change-over from Micronor to Orthonovin. These results suggest that the progestogen only pill is having no discernible effect on the coagulation factors compared with that of combined oral contraceptives.

16.09.04

Longitudinal study of the effects of a combined estrogen-progestogen administration on hemostasis: *Bruni, V, *Bucciantini, S, *Rosati, D, **Abbate, R, **Pinto, S. *I Clin. Obstet. e Gin., Univ., Firenze; **I Clin. Med., Univ., Firenze, Italy
This investigation has been planned in order to study the effects of a combined estrogen-progestogen administration (EE 0.035 mg + cyproterone acetate 2 mg) on blood coagulation, platelet functions and fibrinolysis. Thirty subjects have been investigated before and after 1, 3, 6 and 9 cycles of administration. Blood withdrawals have been performed on the 25th and 26th day of menstrual cycle. The activation of blood coagulation has been investigated by fibrinopeptide A assay (RIA), reliable and sensitive index of thrombin action. Activity of coagulation inhibitors has been explored by assay of antithrombin III. Platelet activation has been studied by β-thromboglobulin, platelet specific protein released in plasma, and by measuring the formation of platelet aggregates in circulating blood. Fibrinolytic activity has been evaluated by euglobulin lysis time both before and after venous stasis in order to explore fibrinolytic capacity. The same investigation will be performed during the administration of a monophasic and a triphasic formulation with gestoden.

16.09.05

Partial purification of placental coagulation inhibitor: Murata, M, Shidara, Y, Maki, M. Dept. Obstet. & Gyn., Akita Univ. School Med., Akita, Japan
The coagulofibrinolytic system during pregnancy is thought to be thrombotic, especially in toxemia. Platelet count, ADP induced aggregation were decreased and plasma-TG which shows platelet release reaction was increased in severe toxemia. AT-III was decreased according to severity of toxemia and discrepancy between antigen and heparin cofactor activity was shown in severe cases. These phenomena could be explained by the formation of thrombin *in vivo*, and placental infarction was often seen in these patients. On the other hand, in normal pregnancy, placental thrombosis is rather rare in spite of a slow blood stream in the choriodecidual space and of maternal thrombotic tendency. So anti-thrombotic mechanism would play an important role in the circulation of choriodecidual space. As an anti-thrombotic substance, we already reported "Anti-platelet aggregating substance" at Xth World Congress; now we have identified another protein which inhibited blood coagulation, especially prolonged prothrombin time, from the microsomal fraction of placental homogenate. It was soluble in Triton X-100 or NaI and purified by several steps of chromatography. It had a molecular weight of approximately 45,000 daltons by the method of gel filtration chromatography. This protein may have an important role in preventing thrombosis in the microcirculation.

16.09.06

Acting point of the placental coagulation inhibitor: Shidara, Y, Murata, M, Maki, M. Dept. Obstet. & Gyn., Akita Univ. School Med., Akita, Japan
We isolated a new protein having the inhibiting activity of blood coagulation from placental extract. The inhibiting mechanisms of this placental coagulation inhibitor (PCI) in the clotting systems were studied, and the following results were obtained: (1) Immunological examination revealed that the PCI was not capable of cross-reaction with AT-III, α_1-AT, α_2-MG, and C_1-INA. (2) PCI had neither heparin-like characteristics nor platelet aggregation inhibiting activity. (3) The activities of fibrinolysis and antifibrinolysis were not demonstrated in PCI. (4) Echis carinatus venom time and thrombin time were not affected by PCI. (5) Factors XII, XI, X, IX, VIII, VII and V were not inactivated by incubation with PCI. (6) In the extrinsic pathways, activation of factor X was markedly inhibited, when tissue thromboplastin was preincubated with PCI. It seems to be likely that PCI keeps the placental circulation unthrombotic. The lack of PCI would be suspected in such cases as severe toxemia, IUGR, and unknown placental infarction.

16.09.07

Correlation between fetal blood states and fetal acidosis: Sakuraba, M. JSW Memo. Hosp., **Shimizu, T.** Dept. Obstet. and Gyn., Asahikawa Med. Coll., Asahikawa, Japan; **Saling, E.** Inst. Perinat. Med., Berlin
Perinatal acidosis or hypoxia is one of the major causes of intracranial hemorrhage in the early neonatal

period. In the present study, we have checked a correlation between fetal acidosis and intracranial hemorrhage by the blood coagulability and fibrinolytic activity. We have measured umbilical arterial blood pH, Normotest (N.T.), Fibrin Degeneration Product (FDP), Soluble-fibrin-monomer-complex (SFMC) by ethanol-method-Anti-Thrombin III (AT-III) at Mariendorfer-Lying in West Berlin from October 1982 to February 1983. Total patients were 178 cases and were sampled at random. In this period, we have diagnosed by ultrasonic echography five intracranial hemorrhage infants in the same group. The results are following: 1) In the non-acidotic group whose U.A. pH values showed more than 7.30, N.T. values were $5.47 \pm 11.2\%$ (n = 70), on the contrary, in the acidotic group, whose U.A. pH value showed less than 7.19, N.T. values were $24.2 \pm 7.3\%$ (n = 11). The significant difference was recognized by Student-t-test (p < 0.01). In five ICH infants, two infants were acidotic. 2) There were five infants whose U.A. pH value showed less than 7.19, and four of five (80%) infants showed high FDP value more than 80 units. And all of them were diagnosed as ICH. On the contrary, in the normacidotic group, high SFMC levels were not recorded. 3) In the acidotic group, SFMC were recognized in high concentration (66.7%), and three infants were diagnosed as ICH. 4) There are no significant differences between U.A. pH value and AT III. Thus, fetal acidosis changes the blood coag. and fibri. act., and is probably the major cause of ICH.

16.09.08.

The absorption, excretion and transplacental transport of vitamin K in the perinatal period: Suzuki, S. Dept. Obstet. & Gyn., School Med., Hokkaido Univ., Sapporo, Japan

It is a well-known fact that hemorrhages are observed in wholly breastfed infants beyond the neonatal period. In order to clarify vitamin K (VK)-deficiency, it is necessary to follow-up the absorption and excretion of VK_2. 1. To 128 cases of newborns. i) The activity of VK-dependent factors (II, VII, X) were determined by Hepaplastin test (HPT). ii) Using Latex-test, PIVKA-II was tested. We found values of HPT (Y) and PIVKA-II (X) to be inversely proportional in the relation. $Y = 61.9 - 6.7 X$ (r = -0.3). 2. These 15 cases of hypoprothrombinemia, VK_2 6 mg, VK_2 2 mg were given, and plasma VK_2-concentration was measured by gas chromatography. After 3 hours VK_2 6 mg concentration was 1030 ng/ml; VK_2 2 mg, was 224 ng/ml. This clearly shows a dose-response relation. 3. VK_2 transplacental transport was also proved by using umbilical venous blood after Cesarean section. (Before Cesarean section, VK_2 60 mg was given.) In umbilical venous blood, relatively high doses of VK_2 (50–120 ng/ml) were demonstrated. Additionally, the γ-carboxylglutamic acid-concentration in the urine of newborn, who received VK_2-syrup was higher than those who did not receive it.

16.09.09

Conservative and operative treatment of deep vein thrombosis in pregnancy and the puerperium: Hugo, R von, Stelzer, S, Theiss, W, Dörrler, J, Stiegler, H, Graeff, H. Frauen-, I. Inn. Med., Chir. Klin., TU, München; Chir. Klin. Grosshadern, LMU, München

We report our results in 21 patients who had suffered DVT in pregnancy (n = 13) or postpartum (n = 8); the diagnosis was verified by Doppler ultrasound or phlebography. All patients received anticoagulants for at least six months; in addition, 11 patients were treated by venous thrombectomy in the acute phase. All patients whose DVT occurred in pregnancy were brought to full term and delivered vaginally without complications regardless of the initial form of therapy. Long-term sequelae were looked for at a mean interval of two years after the acute episode. Patients were examined by clinical inspection, Doppler ultrasound, venous occlusion phlethysmography and venous pressure measurements. Phlebography was performed in few patients. Nine of 11 patients treated by thrombectomy were free of any post-thrombotic damage, the remaining two suffered from a moderate post-thrombotic syndrome. In contrast, only three of the ten patients treated with anticoagulants alone were free of any post-thrombotic sequelae, while seven suffered from post-thrombotic changes, which were moderate in two and severe in five.

16.09.10

The field trial of preventing neonatal vitamin K (Vit. K) deficient intracranial hemorrhage in Shizuoka prefecture: Okada, K. Shizuoka Ass. Obstet. & Gyn.; **Kawashima, Y, Terao, T, Sumimoto, K.** Dept. Obstet. and Gyn., Hamamatsu Univ. Med., Shizuoka, Japan

Vit. K deficiency can induce neonatal intracranial hemorrhage (NICH) which usually happened between two weeks and two months after birth. The incidence of NICH in Japan is about 1/4000 babies especially in breast feeding cases (1/1700 babies). To detect the Vit. K deficiency, field trial is performed in Shizuoka prefecture where is near Mt. Fuji in Japan and about 45,000 babies are born in a year. NICH happened in 16, 5, 9 cases in 1979, 1980, 1981, respectively. Since Feb. 1982 to July 1984, 26,944 neonates were checked by Hepaplastin test (HPT, normo test) which was performed at least twice after delivery, in one week and at one month. The lowest HPT level is shown at the third day after birth and then gradually increasing to 48.3% at one week and 77.6% at one month. Vit. K is administered to 5049 cases in neonatal stage in which 3539 cases are for prophylactic and 1510 cases are for therapeutic management because of low HPT. HPT levels are increased after therapy. But in 103 cases (6.8%) of the therapeutic group, HPT levels could not be increased or remained at low levels after Vit. K administration, so follow-up is necessary. The HPT levels of 291 cases are under 40% (1.08%) at one month HPT levels of 46 cases are under 10%, of which 38 cases were not treated by Vit. K before. After this field trial, no NICH has happened. It is clear that prophylactic, or therapeutic Vit. K administration could prevent NICH, but low HPT level may persist after taking Vit. K in some cases. So HPT at one month might be necessary to check up these low HPT cases.

16.10.01

Regression of leiomyomas with long-term treatment with the anti-estrogen, anti-progesterone gestrinone: Coutinho, E M. Fac. Med., Fed. Univ. of Bahia, Salvador, Bahia, Brazil
One hundred and four women with uterine leiomyomata were treated with Gestrinone for periods of one to three years. The drug was administered either by the oral or vaginal route and the dose varied from 2.5 mg three times weekly to 5.0 mg twice weekly. The first group of 39 women received 5 mg twice weekly orally. The second group of 38 women received 2.5 mg three times weekly also orally. The third group of 27 women received 2.5 mg three times weekly vaginally. Seven patients were treated for three years; twenty patients were treated for two years and 77 for one year. 136 woman years of treatment were recorded. Among the 78 women treated by the oral route, uterine volume decreased in 66 (85%). Among the 27 women treated by vaginal route, reduction in uterine volume occurred in only 15 (55%). With few exceptions amenorrhea occurred in all patients during the treatment. Major side-effects were seborrhea, acne and weight gain, which was promptly reversible after stopping treatment. Of 46 patients who wished to conceive but could not because of the myomatous uterus, nine conceived after Gestrinone treatment. Seven of these pregnancies were brought to term successfully. The study shows that treatment by Gestrinone allows postponement of surgical removal of leiomyomata and may in selected cases result in complete regression of the tumors.

16.10.02

Endocrine profile in patients with uterine fibromyomata: Abdalla, M I, Osman, M I, Bayad, M A, El-Shenofi, O, Ibrahim, I I. Reprod. Endocr. Res. Unit., Dept. Obstet. and Gyn., Univ., Cairo, Egypt
Although evidence of associated ovarian dysfunction and anovulation prevail in patients with uterine fibromyomata, the majority of published data were based on clinical and/or pathological grounds. The aim of this study was to demonstrate the pituitary-ovarian relationship in uterine fibromyomata patients as judged by the premenstrual serum level of FSH, LH, prolactin, estradiol-17β, progesterone and testosterone. The subjects comprised 40 healthy, regularly menstruating and fertile females as control and 77 patients with uterine fibromyomata diagnosed on clinical and histopathological basis. Both groups had the same specifications as regards age, freedom from chronic disease or apparent endocrinopathy and non-use of drugs that affect hormone homeostasis. Fifty patients were regularly menstruating and the rest had menorrhagia. Premenstrual venous blood samples were collected at days M-7 to M-4 considering M O as day of menstrual onset. Sera were analysed for the assigned hormones by RIA procedures. Mean $\pm$ SE levels of FSH, LH, PRL, estradiol, progesterone and testosterone in control were: 3.72 ± 0.38, 3.60 ± 0.19 miu/ml, 14.26 ± 1.84 ng/ml, 139.31 ± 7.67 pg/ml, 8.06 ± 0.53 ng/ml and 0.37 ± 0.12 ng/ml, respectively. In patients group: 8.15 ± 1.34, 10.40 ± 1.14 miu/ml, 17.01 ± 1.93 ng/ml, 101.42 ± 11.56 pg/ml, 2.25 ± 0.21 ng/ml and 0.48 ± 0.03 ng/ml, respectively. Significant increase in FSH and LH mean values and significant decrease in estradiol and progesterone mean values were observed in patients as compared to control.

16.10.03

Characterization of aromatase activity in uterine leiomyoma and the inhibitory effects of aminoglutethimide and Δ^1-testololactone on the enzyme activity *in vitro*: Yamamoto, T, Takamori, K, Fujii, M, Honjo, H, Okada, H. Dept. Obstet. and Gyn., Kyoto Prefect. Univ. Med., Kyoto, Japan
Uterine leiomyoma is a benign tumor that appears frequently in fertile women and has a tendency to grow gradually until the termination of ovarian function. Furthermore, the growth of uterine myoma is closely dependent on estrogen. Recently, we have reported that myoma tissue has the ability to aromatize androstenedione to estrogens and the enzyme activity is significantly higher than that in the normal myometrial tissue of the uterus (*T. Yamamoto* et al. Horm. metab. Res. **16**, 678, 1984). Therefore, in this study, we investigated the distribution of aromatase activity in myoma node, and the kinetics and the localization of the subcellular fractions. We also examined the effects of aminoglutethimide and Δ^1-testololactone, inhibitors of breast cancer aromatase, on aromatase activity in uterine myoma tissue *in vitro*. Aromatase activity in leiomyoma was high in the order of surface "middle" center, and was inversely proportional to the tissue estrogen concentrations. The activity was mainly located in the 105,000 g pellets of tumor tissue. The product, estrone, was increased in parallel with the incubation time, reaching a plateau after 1 hour. Aminoglutethimide and Δ^1-testololactone showed a dose inactivated 10 to 50% of myoma enzyme activity. The results suggest that the growth of uterine leiomyoma is dependent upon the aromatase activity and that it is possible to terminate or reduce the growth by the local application of breast cancer aromatase inhibitors. (Supported by Grant-in Aid, No. 59570718, from the Ministry of Education, Science and Culture, Japan.)

16.10.04

Myomectomy: Suzuki, M, Furuhashi, N, Kyono, K. Dept. Obstet. and Gyn., Tohoku Univ. School Med., Sendai, Japan
Myomectomy has a logical and useful place in gynecological practice when we find that removal of the

myoma will enhance the patient's chance of being able to become pregnant and deliver a normal child. Our indications are 1) the couple should be young enough to bear a child, 2) they should have a strong desire to have a child, 3) the husband should be confirmed to have no finding of sterility, 4) the wife should not have any cause for sterility except uterine myoma. Before the decision for myomectomy, semen analysis of the husband is necessary to confirm his fertility. Hysterosalpingography is an important pre-operative examination to understand the status of the uterine cavity and Fallopian tubes. Obstruction of the Fallopian tubes bilaterally obviously provides a contraindication for myomectomy. The most important technique in myomectomy is that the myoma should be removed as one mass and that a healthy muscle layer surrounding the myoma should be kept intact. The cavity created by removal of the myoma is closed using a mattress suture in two layers. The buried sutures of the cavity with Dexon should be as shallow as possible inside muscle layer to preserve the blood vessels of the normal muscle tissues. This procedure should be repeated several times to close the deep layer. Care should be taken to avoid suturing through the endometrium. Each stitch should not be too close. Too many stitches will disrupt the blood supply of the uterus. After myomectomy, we usually examine the passage infusing indigo carmine from the uterine cervix into the tubes.

16.10.05

Ultrasonographic diagnosis of sarcoma in gynecology: Kozuma, S, Okai, T, Mukubo, M, Baba, K, Shi, S, Mizuno, M. Dept. Obstet. & Gyn., Fac. Med., Univ., Tokyo, Japan

Six cases of sarcoma were ultrasonographically examined and operated on in the Dept. of Obstet. & Gynecol., Univ. of Tokyo during 1978–1983. There were five cases originating in the uterine corpus and one case in the Fallopian tube. Pre-operative clinical diagnosis was uterine sarcoma in three cases, ovarian tumor in two cases and peritonitis in one case, respectively. Ultrasonographically sarcoma had irregular hyperechoic parts in central portion of the tumor mass which were surrounded by irregularly shaped echo-free spaces. Polypoid echo existed protrusively into the echo-free spaces. One case pathologically diagnosed as Mullerian adenosarcoma of the uterus had a hyperechoic area which looked like a honeycomb. Ovarian carcinoma and degenerated uterine fibroid should be differentiated from uterine sarcoma. Ovarian carcinoma has usually an echo-free space in the central portion of the tumor mass with papillary mural echo pattern. In addition, there is the uterine echo in the other part of the pelvis. Severely degenerated fibroid is most difficult to differentiate from sarcoma. Degenerated fibroid has echo-free spaces in the central portion of the tumor mass and/or dispersed hyperechoic areas. Sarcoma has both hyperechoic area in the central portion and irregular shaped echo-free spaces in the periphery. The boundary of the irregular shaped echo-free space is clearer in sarcoma than in degenerated fibroid. It is concluded that the rather precise diagnosis of sarcoma can be made pre-operatively, based on the above mentioned characteristic echograms.

16.10.06

Propensity to retroperitoneal lymph node metastasis in patients with stage I sarcoma of the uterus: Chen, S S. SUNY, Stony Brook, NY, USA

The incidence of regional nodal spread and its clinical implication in stage I sarcoma of the uterus is not available. The purpose of this prospective study is to provide such information. Sixteen patients were treated by primary operation of surgical staging, total abdominal hysterectomy, bilateral salpingo-oophorectomy, and selective biopsy of para-aortic and pelvic nodes as well as any abnormal site. Histologic types in this series were mixed mesodermal tumor six, leiomyosarcoma four, carcinosarcoma four, and stromal sarcoma two. Stage Ia was nine and stage Ib seven. The grades were G 1, one; G 2, five; and G 3, ten. The incidence of nodal involvement was 50%. 62.5% had both positive para-aortic and pelvic nodes and only 37.5% had pelvic involvement. This high rate of nodal involvement is associated with G 3 tumor 70%, those uteri larger than 8 cm 71.4%, leiomyosarcoma 75%, and deep myometrial invasion 75%. Among 15 patients who had been followed for more than 18 months, all (8) with positive node succumbed to their disease. This result indicates that incidence of nodal spread in stage I sarcoma of the uterus is a frequent occurrence, associated with many prognostic variables and related to their ultimate survival. Furthermore, it suggests that lymphatic permeation might precede hematologic spread in sarcoma of the uterus. Similar studies are urgently needed.

16.10.07

Treatment of uterine leiomyosarcoma: Malmström, H, Tropé, C, Simonsen, E. Dept. Gyn. and Oncol., Univ. Hosp., Lund, Sweden

The survival rate after treatment of uterine sarcoma is poor. In this retrospective study, survival and recurrence rate were analysed in pts treated with surgery in combination with irradiation and/or chemotherapy. 65 cases treated from 1955–1984, median age 55, FIGO stage: I/38, II/9, III/10, IV/8. Grade: 1/19, 2/5, 3/16, not stated 25. Myometrial invasion < 1/3: 10, > 1/3: 52. TAH was performed in 59 cases. External irradiation to the pelvis in 40 cases, mean dosage 30 Gy. Adriamycin, cisplatinum, 5-FU, methotrexte, cyclophosphamide and melphalan were given as single drug or in combination. Recurrences were diagnosed in 30 pts, local rec. 11 pts, pulmonary and hepatic metastases in 21 and 8 pts, respectively. Crude overall survival rate at 5 years was 52.8%. Five year survival rate according to stage: I/72%, II/22%, III/22%, IV/33% and acc. to myometrial invasion: < 1/3 68%, > 1/3 46% and acc. to pre- or postmenopausal state at diagnosis: 58% and 37%. According to treatment in pts with tumor confined to the uterus (St I–II): surgery and radiotherapy 85%, without radiotherapy 46% (p < .003). There was also a higher survival rate in pts treated adjuvantly with chemotherapy (p < .02). The complication rate of therapy was low. We conclude that uterine leiomyosarcoma in early stages treated adjuvantly with irradiation and/or chemotherapy may show improved survival. Thus, adjuvant therapy should be considered in all patients with poor prognostic factors and high risk of recurrence.

16.11.01

Ultrasonographic study of puerperal uterine involution by volume and cavity analysis: Carta, G, Patella, A*, Indraccolo, S R, Ippolito, M, Muti, A R. School Obstet., Camerino; *1st Dept. Obstet. & Gyn., Univ., Rome, Italy

Sixty-three women who breast fed normally and gave birth to single, full-term fetuses were studied. They were divided into two groups: 35 women treated with methylergometrine maleate (first group) and 28 who did not receive uterotonic therapy (second group). Echographic examinations, 309 in all, were carried out over the postpartum period, from the second to the fourteenth day. Uterine volume was determined using the formula for ellipsoids. The difference between the two groups of women was statistically significant only on the second postpartum day: variance analysis gave $F(1.17) = 13,617$. The uterine cavity was studied using longitudinal scanning and showed different echographic features during the first postpartum week as compared to the second. These differences were independent of the use of the uterotonic drug. Methyl-ergometrine maleate has an influence on the uterine volume/cavity dimension ratio.

16.11.02

Echographic changes in the cervix during the early puerperium: Indraccolo, S R, Carta, G, Patella, A*, Ippolito, M, Muti, A R. School Obstet., Camerino; *1st Dept. Obstet. & Gyn., Univ., Rome, Italy

Changes in the internal orifice of the uterus and in the cavity of the cervix during the first week postpartum (early puerperium) were observed by ultrasonography. 192 examinations were performed with a real-time ultrasonographic scanner on 27 healthy primiparas who gave birth to single living children at term. Uterine involution went on rapidly and regularly in all cases. Ultrasonic investigations were performed far away from breast feedings and from a uterotonic drug administration. The internal orifice of the uterus showed a vary peculiar behaviour: sometimes it was seen to be open and sometimes closed with no relationship with the day of puerperium and the contents of the uterine cavity and even in the course of a single day in the same patient. On the contrary, the canal of the cervix showed a gradual and progressive narrowing during the first seven days after delivery.

16.11.03

Effect of dopaminergic agents and TRH on the endocrine profile in labor and early puerperium: Kubota, T, Kamata, S, Nishi, N, *Yaoi, Y, *Kumasaka, T, Saito, M. Dept. Obstet. and Gyn., Tokyo Med. and Dent. Univ., School Med., Tokyo, and *Dokkyo Univ., School Med., Tochigi, Japan

The purpose of this study is to investigate the effect of the prolactin (PRL) releasing mechanism on the hypothalamo-pituitary axis during labor and early puerperium. – Methods: 1) 10 mg metoclopramide (MCP) was given intravenously to five full-term women in labor and 22 women in early puerperium. 2) 2.5 mg bromocriptine (BC) was given to four women in early puerperium. 3) 10 mg MCP or 500 μg TRH was given i. v. to 12 women in early puerperium who had received 5 mg/day of BC for five days. Plasma hormone levels were measured by RIA for three hours. – Results: The plasma PRL levels increased significantly (p < 0.001) after MCP. The peak values of PRL increase were 609.3 ± 194.1 ng/ml during labor and 447.0 ± 62.3 ng/ml in early puerperium. However, there were no significant differences of PRL response to MCP between these two groups. The plasma PRL decreased significantly (p < 0.001) after BC in puerperium. The PRL release from the pituitary by MCP was suppressed significantly (p < 0.001) by pretreatment of BC, but the PRL release by TRH was not suppressed by BC. No significant changes in plasma estradiol, progesterone and cortisol levels could be observed after MCP. – We concluded that the control mechanism of PRL secretion remained unchanged during labor and early puerperium, and revealed the different mechanism of PRL release between MCP and TRH.

16.11.04

Effects of low-caloric diet in puerperium on prolactin (PRL) and milk secretion: Okamura, T, Takeuchi, T, Nishii, O, Takahashi, M, Yaginuma, T, Kobayashi, T. Dept. Obstet. and Gyn., Fac. Med., Univ. of Tokyo at Mejiroadi, Tokyo, Japan

Ten puerperal women were given 1200 cal diet per day for three days followed by normal 1800 cal per day for three days (LC group). Fifteen puerperal women were given 1800 cal diet per day for six days [control (c) group]. All of the women took breakfast at 7:30 a. m., were drawn blood samples at 9:30 a. m. and then milked from breasts from two minutes by a breast pump starting from the day of delivery (Day 0) to Day 6. Four women of LC group and C group underwent a thyrotropin-releasing hormone (TRH) stimulation test on Day 1 and 3 of puerperium. Serum PRL levels in LC group tend to be much lower than in C group but not significantly. The ratio of serum PRL levels on Day 1, 3 and 4 to that on Day 0 (0.64 ± 0.78, 0.68 ± 0.29 and 0.61 ± 0.29, respectively) was significantly low in comparison with that in C group (1.45 ± 0.78, 1.76 ± 1.24 and 1.79 ± 1.59, respectively) (p < 0.05). Milk volume in LC group was significantly less than in C group on Day 2 (p < 0.01). Analyses of milk specimens components were not significantly different between both groups. Serum PRL release responses to TRH in LC group were much lower than in C group but not significantly. Body weight of infants was not significantly different between LC and C group every day. These results suggest that low-caloric diet may suppress PRL and milk secretion probably not through the effect on the pituitary.

16.11.05
Oxytocin concentrations in milk and its origin: Takeda, S, Kuwabara, Y, Mizuno, M. Dept. Obstet. and Gyn., Fac. Med., Univ., Tokyo, Japan
It is noticed that there are various peptide hormones in milk. However, oxytocin (OT) in milk has not been described in any reports. We have ascertained the existence of OT in milk and determined OT concentrations in human milk. Furthermore, the origin of OT in milk and its absorption into the blood of neonates were investigated using ^{3}H-OT administrated to rat mothers. – Materials and methods: Samples of human milk were obtained from women with normal delivery in early postpartum period and OT concentrations were measured by RIA, following extraction procedures with Florisil. Degradation rate of ^{3}H-OT in milk and molecular size of OT immunoreactive substance in milk were analysed by Sephadex G 25 column chromatography. After administrating H-OT to rat mothers, starved neonates were left with the mothers to suckle freely for 1 hr. Then blood and gastric contents were taken from neonates. OT in neonates plasma was purified by column chromatography, to compare with the elution pattern of ^{3}H-OT. – Results: Mean OT concentrations in human milk at postpartum day 1 to 5 were 4.5±1.1, 4.7±1.1, 4.0±1.3, 3.2±0.4, 3.3±0.6 μU/ml (±SE), respectively. And the OT levels were increased by suckling. ^{3}H-OT in human milk was stable even after incubation at 37°C for 2 hr. Dilution curve of the OT immunoreactive substance in milk was parallel to the curve of OT. The chromatographic fraction of the substance was identical to that of ^{3}H-OT. The counts of radioactivity in neonatal blood and gastric contents were 21.9 and 13.5% of the counts in maternal blood, respectively. It was made clear that OT exists stably in milk and that OT in maternal blood can be transferred into milk and then into neonatal blood.

16.11.06
Natural steroid transfer in breast milk: Fayad, M M, Abdalla, M I, Bayad, M A, Lahzy, N, Ibrahim, I I. Dept. Obstet. and Gyn., Cairo Univ., Cairo, Egypt
The excretion of administered synthetic steroids in breast milk has been previously reported. The milk content of natural steroids has not been clarified yet due to problems of estimation. This study was undertaken to determine breast milk levels of estradiol and progesterone in comparison with serum levels in fully lactating mothers. Hormonal estimation were done by modified RIA techniques based on double extraction with ethanol and diethyl ether. Serum and milk samples were collected from 53 fully lactating and amenorrheic mothers six weeks postpartum. Mean ± SE serum levels of estradiol and progesterone were in the range of early follicular phase of menstrual cycle (40.52 ± 2.62 pg/ml and 1.21 ± 0.30 ng/ml). Breast milk had significantly lower estradiol and higher progesterone mean ± SE values (10.63 ± 0.25 pg/ml and 3.66 ± 0.34 ng/ml, respectively). These data suggest the presence of a mechanism of conjugation and/or binding of progesterone in the milk secreting glands.

16.11.07
Lactation during pregnancy: Badraoui, M H H, Hefnawi, F, Essa, I, Abdalla, M, Bahgat, R. Al-Azhar Univ., Cairo, Egypt
Breast feeding is the main source of babies' nutrition in developing countries. Interruption of breast feeding occurred when pregnancy started during lactation. The purpose of the study is to estimate the amount and chemical composition of milk yield and the hormonal profile during pregnancy in lactating mothers. A comparison was also made between lactating mothers who got pregnant before and after six months postpartum. Milk samples were collected from each breast after suckling the other on two occasions. Blood samples were collected before suckling, a total number of 101 cases were followed. Collection of milk and blood samples were performed every two weeks from cooperative mothers. The amount of milk yield showed a continuous decrease from the 8th week (27.5 ± 15 g) to the 26 weeks (4.5 ± 2.5 g) of pregnancy. It was significantly higher in mothers starting pregnancy during the first six postpartum months. The protein content increased gradually from the 8th week of pregnancy (0.8 ± 19 g/100 ml) until the 28 weeks (1.22 ± 0.27 g/100 ml). There was a significant rise at the 28th weeks only. The amount of carbohydrate fluctuates between 5.77 ± 0.8 g/100 ml and 4.9 ± 1.61 g/100 ml without a significant differences. The milk fat remained almost stable. F. S. H. levels were 8.12 ± 1.9 mIU/ml at eight weeks and did not change significantly until the 28th week of pregnancy. PRL level ranged from 1226.9 ± 295 nmol/l to 1850 ± 749.7 ng/ml at 26 weeks. LH levels were 11.37 ± 1.9 and 11.08 ± 5.87 mIU/ml at 8 and 12 weeks, respectively. Progesterone increased from 1.81 ± 0.93 at eight weeks to 2.65 ± 0.42 mg/ml at 28 weeks. Cortisol increased from 12.93 at eight weeks to 21.81 ± 9.742 μg% at 28 weeks.

16.11.08
Mercury concentrations in human milk, fatty tissue and maternal serum: Goetze, S, Beier, F, Karkut, G, Weitzel, H, Braetter, P*, Weigert, P**. Inst. Gyn. and Obstet., FU, Berlin
Mercury concentrations were measured by atomic absorption spectrometry using a hydride-system in fatty

tissue (taken from the vulva at episiotomy) in human transitional milk, maternal serum 3–5 d after delivery and in mature milk 14 d after delivery in women who had and had not been treated with Merfen®, a disinfectant containing mercury phenyl borate, 0.66 g/l, typically on the vulva before episiotomy. No differences were found between the two groups of women for all types of samples except for a few cases of direct contamination of the fatty tissue in the treated groups (not reported). Levels in transitional milk were 20.8 ± 16.0 ng/g dry weight (mean $\pm$ SD) (n = 125) for the untreated group and 20.0 ± 10.0 (n = 17) for the treated group; for mature milk untreated 11.1 ± 6.0 (n = 98), treated 11.6 ± 10.0 (n = 14); serum 20.0 ± 11.0 (n = 118) untreated, 15.6 ± 10.6 (n = 18) treated; and for fatty tissue in untreated women 29.3 ± 23.7 ng/g (n = 38). All values were closely grouped except for one untreated woman who had high mercury levels in both transitional milk and serum. The lower values in mature milk are attributed to the different properties of cellular and aqueous components. It was concluded that the topical application of mercury phenyl borate is without effect on the mercury levels of the mother in all investigated compartments. – *Bundesgesundheitsamt (ZEBS), Berlin; **Hahn-Meitner-Inst. Kernforschung, Berlin

16.11.09

Transfer of resistance to experimental autoimmune disease EAE by breast feeding: Evron, E, *Ovadia, H, *Abramsky, O. Hadassah Univ. Hosp., Dept. Obstet. and Gyn. and *Labor. Neuroimmun., Jerusalem, Israel

Spontaneous remission of putative autoimmune diseases during pregnancy and postpartum has been demonstrated in a number of mammalian species, including women. The immunological transfer of such resistance to experimental allergic encephalomyelitis (EAE) was evaluated in correlation to pregnancy and postpartum breast feeding. Outbred female rats were sensitized with CNS antigen and adjuvant during the second week of pregnancy. The litters were similarly immunized either 30 or 70 days after birth. 25 of 26 (96%) immunized litters born to normal mothers developed moderate or severe EAE. Only 38% 21/55 of litters born to sensitized mothers developed mild EAE when immunized 30 days after birth. But, when immunized 70 days after birth 10/16 (62%) developed moderate or severe EAE. When litters born to sensitized mother were fed since birth by a normal mother 17/19 (89%) they developed EAE following immunization at day 30 after birth. None (0/19) of the litters born to normal mothers and fed by sensitized-mother developed EAE following immunization. It is concluded that 1) Sensitized-mother transfer immunological resistance during pregnancy and this is present in the newborn and disappears with time. 2) Resistance to EAE may be transferred postpartum by breast feeding.

16.12.01

A controlled trial of treatment of recurrent spontaneous abortion by immunisation with paternal cells: Beard, R W, Mowbray, J F, Gibbings, C, Liddell, H, Reginald, P W, Underwood, J L. Dept. Exp. Path. & Obstet. and Gyn., St Mary's Hosp. Med. School, London, UK

Recurrent abortion is a condition which has failed to respond to many treatments because of the lack of understanding why the condition occurs. Our theory has been that occasionally a high degree of sharing of Class 1 and 2 HLA antigens between couples results in a failure of the formation of blocking antibodies in the mother which have a protective role in normal pregnancy. Some substance has been given to this hypothesis by the apparent success of the immunising of women with a history of recurrent abortion by transfusing small amounts of blood during pregnancy from multiple donors (*Taylor & Faulds*, 1981). We have carried out a paired sequential double-blind trial of immunisation in 105 women, with a history of three or more consecutive abortions with the same partner who did not have detectable antibody against paternal HLA antigens. Analysis of the results of this trial showed a preference for paternal immunisation (p < 0.01) with a successful pregnancy (> 28 weeks of gestation) in 17 out of 22 women in this group as compared with such an outcome in 10 out of 27 women who had been given their own cells. The significance of these results will be discussed.

16.12.02

Lymphocyte subpopulations in cord blood of anencephalic and normal newborns: Analysis with monoclonal antibodies: Escobar, I E, Céspedes, G M de, Kumate, J. Div. Immunoquím., Unid. Invest. Biomèd., Ctro Méd. Nac., IMSS, México, DF

Monoclonal antibodies (OKT3, OKT4, OKT8) were used for the determination of lymphocyte subpopulations in the peripheral blood of 25 normal non-pregnant women, 19 normal pregnant women and their normal newborns and 15 anencephalic newborns and their mothers. Women ranged in age from 20 to 30. Newborns (normal and anencephalic) were products of full-term pregnancy (37–40 weeks) with normal deliveries. There were difference (p < 0.001) statistically significant in the OKT4/OKT8 ratios, between non-pregnant controls (1.1 to 1.9) and the other two groups (0.4 to 1.0). However, there were no significant differences between normal pregnant women and women with anencephalic pregnancies. Although, normal and anencephalic newborns had lower OKT4/OKT8 ratios than the normal women, there were no demonstrable differences between both groups. Pregnant women who give birth to normal or anencephalic infants have reduced numbers of helper T cells. These findings may help to explain why the fetal-allograft is not rejected in utero.

16.12.03

Suppressor cells – a requirement for successful pregnancy?: Daya, S, Clark, D A. McMaster Univ., Hamilton, Ont., Canada

Survival of the mammalian fetus in an immunologically hostile host has been shown to be determined by the properties of the tissue at the maternal-fetal interface. Suppressor cells have been found in the decidua in both murine and human systems. This study was carried out to further characterize these cells and to determine whether they were present in abnormal early pregnancies and in the endometrium at the time of implantation. Decidual lymphocytes were obtained from women who underwent a D & C procedure for missed abortion and also from women who had therapeutic abortions. Lymphocytes were also obtained from the endometrium in women who had normal menstrual cycles. These lymphocytes, both separated by velocity sedimentation and unseparated, and the factors released by them were tested for their ability to suppress the response of peripheral blood lymphocytes to concanavalin A in *in vitro* cultures. Normal pregnancies at 10–11 weeks gestation suppressed (mean $34.0 \pm 6.0\%$) compared with no suppression in missed abortions at this gestation (p = 0.02). Decidual lymphocytes from successful pregnancies released a soluble factor which was highly suppressive. Suppression was associated with a small lymphoid cell with a modal sedimentation velocity of 4.0–4.3 mm/hr. Luteal phase endometrium also suppressed (mean $33.4 \pm 11.4\%$) whereas none occurred in the proliferative phase (p = 0.008). Suppression in endometrium was associated with a large lymphoid cell with a sedimentation velocity of 7–8 mm/hr. The level of suppression increased as the menstrual cycle progressed towards menses. Suppressor cells appear in the endometrium following ovulation and their activity is present in the decidua of successful pregnancies but is absent in missed abortions. Two types of cell have been identified. An early phase large cell appears to be hormone-dependent and a later phase small cell appears to be trophoblast-dependent. This would suggest that suppressor cells may play a role in protecting the fetal allograft, from the time of implantation, against maternal immunity thereby allowing a pregnancy to succeed.

16.12.04

Clinical use of early pregnancy factor analysis: Berger, M, Wolf, M. Dept. Obstet. and Gyn., Univ., Bern, Switzerland

The T-lymphocytes rosette inhibition test (RIT), first described by *Halle Morton* for proof of the early pregnancy factor (EPF) in the serum or – as we found – also in the urine, enables the earliest diagnosis of a pregnancy with a viable embryo. Advantages over the HCG test: a) definite diagnosis 24 hrs. post coitum; b) 24 hrs. after demise of the embryo the RIT is negative. Disadvantage: The analysis takes 6 hrs. The RIT has the following practical applications: 1. With an abortion history the new pregnancy can be protected with Gravibinon (Schering, W. Germany) right after conception. 2. Medication: In the second half of the cycle, medication with a possible teratogenic effect can be avoided. The opposite is also possible when a pregnancy can be excluded so early with the RIT. 3. Vaccinations: Same principle as in two. 4. X-ray exposure: If a pregnancy is not suspected hyperemesis symptoms can be mistaken for intestinal disorders and many X-ray pictures could be taken. X-ray damage to the embryo can be avoided with the RIT. 5. Artificial insemination: 24 h after successful insemination proven by the RIT further inseminations can be avoided. 6. Dead embryo: After demise of the embryo choriongonadotropin is still produced as long as villi are attached to the uterine wall, and the HCG test stays positive. Therefore the false diagnosis of an imminent abortion leads to wrong therapy. The RIT is helpful in that situation.

16.12.05

Complement system in pregnancy and malignant disease: Ohkawa, K*, Ohkawa, R**. *Nippon Med. School; Hosp., Ushiku; **Hosp., Shiroi, Japan

In normal pregnancy the cellular immunity of the mother is generally suppressed, because the fetus must develop in the uterus. From the phylogenetic point of view, when cellular immunity is suppressed, the C3-system of complement must be enhanced. – Methods: The study group consisted of 491 cases of normal pregnancy, 250 cases of threatened abortion, 80 cases of hydatidiform mole, 22 cases of chorionic pregnancy, 35 cases of severe toxemia, 11 cases of abruptio placentae, 25 cases of normal gravida during labor. For delayed hypersensitivity P.P.D., candida, varidase, D.N.C.B., hemocyanin, croton oil were used as antigen. For measurement of factor the CH50, C4, C3 and C3-proactivator were used. For immunostimulation the B.C.G., OK-432 and T.G.D.S. were used. – Results: In cases of normal pregnancy CH50-60, C3-98, C3-proactivator-27, Al-CH50-27.5 increased. In cases of threatened abortion with poor prognosis, of toxemia and of apoplexia uteroplacentaris the activity of alternative pathways was low, and in cases of hydatidiform mole and choriocarcinoma C3-activator decreased. For activation of pathway, T.G.D.S. is very useful.

16.13.01

Calcium intake and bone health: Heaney, R P. Creighton Univ., Omaha, NB, USA

Ca is a threshold nutrient: Below its threshold bone mass is limited by intake; above, intake has no effect. There is controversy concerning where the threshold lies with respect to actual Ca intakes. Most population-based studies show a statistically significant relation between intake and bone mass, but the effect is small. By contrast, most physiological and intervention studies in middle-aged and elderly persons indicate that high Ca intakes reduce age-related bone loss. Loss from some skeletal regions (e.g., distal forearm) seems insensitive to Ca intake, but most diaphyseal regions show dependence on Ca intake. Peak adult bone mass at age 35–40 is probably intake-dependent and may be a principal protection against future fracture. Ca absorption efficiency falls with age, and thus, quite high Ca intakes are often required to produce therapeutically interesting absorbed Ca loads. The decline in absorption efficiency is probably intrinsic, but a part is probably the result of marginal vitamin D deficiency, since serum 25(OH)D levels fall strikingly with age, and Ca retention can regularly be improved by providing additional D or 25(OH)D. Age-related bone loss, leading to premature structural failure, is now seen to be heterogeneous problem. Progressive decreases in mechanical loading of the skeleton, effective Ca intake, and solar exposure play interactive roles. Thus, unless a patient is D-replete, ordinary Ca supplements will not be of much help; and disuse following development of fracture aggravates bone loss, largely irrespective of Ca and D status. While the physician needs to be aware of such relationships, these problems can be best solved at the level of national nutritional policy.

16.13.03

The analgesic activity of calcitonin – results of controlled clinical studies: Welzel, D. Nürnberg
In 20 patients with bone cancer exhibiting a positive analgesic response to calcitonin a double-blind trial was performed aiming at the differentiation of calcitonin from placebo. In the framework of a cross-over trial patients were applied 200 I.U. of calcitonin i.v. and placebo with a drug-free interval of at least 24 hours. The results show that calcitonin suppresses pain as reflected by pain interviews and the individual need of analgesics. On that background a dose-finding study was carried out in another 30 patients with bone cancer. The dosage regimen consisted in 50, 100 and 200 I.U. of calcitonin that were applied by daily infusions during a period of 8 days. Each sub-group comprised 10 patients. During the first 4 days of inter-patients comparisons 200 I.U. calcitonin proved superior to 100 and 50 I.U. as well. Afterwards the differences in activity between the three dosage regimens gradually vanished with all of them initiating comparable pain relief as reflected by pain interviews and the individual need of analgesics. In summary, our results demonstrate that onset of analgesic action is dependent on calcitonin dosage whereas the "steady-state" analgesic potentials of the three dosages appear equi-effective. Overall tolerance was good. Episodes of flush, nausea and vomiting were restricted to the first 2–3 days of therapy and did not necessitate its stoppage.

16.28.01

A new approach in the diagnosis or hyperthecosis ovarii: Darwish, N A H, Thabet, S M A, Shaarawy, M, El Mallah, S Y. Dept. Obstet. and Gyn., Fac. Med., Cairo Univ., Cairo, Egypt
Clinico-endocrinological studies were performed in three cases of hyperthecosis ovarii and 14 cases of genuine polycystic ovarian disease. Measurements of serum LH, FSH, progesterone, testosterone, DEAS and prolactin; as well as urinary total estrogens, total and fractionated 17 oxosteroids and 17 osogenic steroids were carried out. Moreover, two dynamic tests were performed on both groups. The first: Dexamethasone suppression test to identify the source of androgens, the second: LHRH estrogen amplification test for the choice of therapy. The characteristic endocrine profiles for cases of hyperthecosis ovarii are the following: a) disproportionately high LH/FSH ratio, exceeding 2, b) significant elevation of serum testosterone, c) normal level of serum DEAS, d) significantly elevated levels of urinary androsterone and etiocholanolone, e) normal levels of urinary DEAS and 11β-hydroxy-androsterone, f) negative estrogen amplification to LHRH response.

16.28.02

Clinical and endocrinological evaluation of a new combination SH B 209 AE (ethinylestradiol 0.035 mg and cyproterone acetate 2 mg) in women suffering from polycystic ovary syndrome: Falsetti, L*, Dordoni, D*, Gastaldi, C.** Clin. Ostet. e Gin., Univ., Brescia*; I Clin. Ostet. e Gin., Univ., Milano**, Italy
Twenty-eight women suffering from polycystic ovary syndrome (PCOS) whose ages ranged from 16 to 34 (mean $\pm$ SD 23.5 $\pm$ 4.7) were treated with SH B 209 AE for 12 cycles without interruption (318 cycles in all). During the course of this study, two patients interrupted their therapy at the 6th cycle for personal reasons and two others at 9th due to side-effects. The PCOS diagnosis was made according to the clinical and endocrinological aspects. The endocrinological and clinical follow-up was made during the 3rd, 6th and 12th treatment cycle by evaluating the following hormonal (LH; FSH; PRL; progesterone; estrone; estradiol; androstendione; total and free testosterone; DHEA-S) and clinical features (acne, seborrhea, hirsutism and possible side-effects). According to a quantitative score, acne and seborrhea were classified as being mild and severe, while hirsutism was classified as mild, moderate and severe. Furthermore, the sex hormone binding globulin (SHBG) was studied. During the administration of the drug, a highly significant decrease of LH; FSH; estrone; estradiol; total and free testosterone; androstendione; DHEAS-S was noticed both at the 6th and 12th cycle, while no differences were noted for PRL and progesterone. As far as the clinical aspects are concerned, the changes in the hyperandrogenism symptoms seem to be of considerable interest. Acne, seborrhea and hirsutism showed significant improvement during the 6th and 12th cycle of therapy, as follow (before treatment/6th/12th): acne (85% – 42% – 9%) – seborrhea (100% – 64% – 50%) – hirsutism (78% – 65% – 30%). The endocrinological and clinical results allow us to conclude that SH B 209 AE is well-indicated for PCOS therapy.

16.28.03

Polycystic ovaries identified by ultrasound: A common finding in anovulatory women and those with idiopathic hirsutism: Franks, S, Adams, J*, Polson, D W. Dept. Obstet. and Gyn., St Mary's Hosp. Med. School; *Dept. Ultrasound, Middlesex Hosp., London, UK

We have used high-resolution ultrasound imaging (US) of the ovaries to define polycystic ovaries (PCO) in a series of anovulatory women who presented to a gynecological endocrine clinic. A total of 171 consecutive patients were studied: 73 with amenorrhea, 74 with oligomenorrhea and 24 with idiopathic hirsutism (IH). The ovaries were found to have a polycystic pattern in 19 (26%) of women with amenorrhea; only three of these women complained of hirsutism (three others had acne). PCO was found in 64 (86%) of women with oligomenorrhea; 31 (45%) were hirsute. Twenty-one (88%) women with idiopathic hirsutism had PCO. Mean LH levels were elevated in PCO women with amenorrhea (14.5 ± 1.7 [SE] μ/l) and oligomenorrhea (15.6 ± 1.1) compared with normal women (6.7 ± 1.0). Likewise the mean ratio LH:FSH was raised (> 3:1) in PCOS women with amenorrhea or oligomenorrhea. However, 50% of ovulatory women with PCOS had normal levels of LH and a normal LH:FSH ratio; of the women with IH, only one had a raised serum LH and the mean LH and LH:FSH ratio were normal. In summary, PCO as defined by pelvic US is very common, occurring in 58% of anovulatory women, and is not necessarily associated with hirsutism or a raised serum LH. On the basis of US scanning most women with hirsutism and regular menses have polycystic ovaries.

16.28.04

Lipid metabolism in women with a polycystic ovary syndrome. Effects induced by an oral contraceptive: Cullberg, G, Mattsson, L Å, Hamberger, L, Mobacken, H, Samsioe, G. Depts. Obstet.-Gyn. and Derm., Univ., Göteborg, Sweden

Women with a polycystic ovary syndrome (PCO) could be at increased risk for coronary heart disease (CHD). Oral contraceptives (OC) are commonly used in PCO women but such a treatment could deteriorate lipid metabolism. Twenty women with a PCO-syndrome were compared to a control group of 13 regularly menstruating women. They were treated with a low dose OC containing 0.030 mg ethinylestradiol and 0.150 mg desogestrel (Marvelon, Organon). All patients were examined before treatment and after three months of treatment as regards body weight and blood pressure. Lipids in serum and in the lipoprotein fractions VLDL, LDL and HDL were also assessed. – Results: Compared to regularly menstruating women the PCO women had significantly higher body weights and blood pressures as well as elevated levels of triglycerides in serum and VLDL before treatment. During treatment a reduction in body weights was recorded in 14 out of 20 PCO women. In the PCO group moderate increments in serum cholesterol, phospholipids and triglycerides were induced. The changes in serum and lipoprotein lipids in PCO women were of the same type and magnitude as those found in the control group apart from an HDL cholesterol increase in the latter. The difference between the two groups in VLDL triglycerides remained after treatment. – Conclusion: Thus, similar changes were induced in lipid and lipoprotein patterns in PCO and regularly menstruating women by the desogestrel/ethinylestradiol combination. A positive influence on lipids and lipoproteins cannot be added to the list of indications for OC treatment in PCO women.

16.28.05

Serum prolactin and dehydroepiandrosterone sulfate levels in polycystic ovarian disease: Lee, J Y, Yoon, B K, Moon, S Y, Chang, Y S. Dept. Obstet. and Gyn., Coll. Med., Seoul Nat. Univ., Seoul, Korea

Serum LH, FSH, prolactin (PRL), estradiol (E_2), testosterone (T) and dehydroepiandrosterone sulfate (DHAS) levels were measured radioimmunologically in 43 PCO patients and 20 normal, regularly cycling women to evaluate the prevalence rate of hyperprolactinemia and the effect of hyperprolactinemia on adrenocortical function in polycystic ovarian disease. Mean levels of LH, T and DHAS were significantly higher in PCO as expected, whereas no significant differences were observed in either FSH or E_2 levels between PCO and normal control. Hyperprolactinemia was present in 16.3% of PCO (7 among 43 cases). Mean T levels in hyperprolactinemic and euprolactinemic groups were 0.69 ± 0.01 ng/ml and 0.62 ± 0.05 ng/ml respectively, and there was no difference statistically between both groups. Mean DHAS levels in hyperprolactinemic and euprolactinemic groups were 2904 ± 500 ng/ml and 1839 ± 134 ng/ml respectively, and there was a significant difference between the two groups. Since DHAS is virtually an exclusive product of the adrenal cortex, it is suggested that increased DHAS levels in hyperprolactinemic PCO are a consequence of a prolactin effect on the adrenal cortex.

16.28.06

Polycystic ovarian disease and hyperprolactinemia: Garud, M A, Parikh, V, Parikh, S, Tejani, T, Rodrigues, A*. Cama & Albless Hosp.; *Sandoz (India) Ltd., Bombay, India

One hundred patients of suspected anovulation attending our Gynecological Out-Patient Department have been selected for study with a view to find out the incidence of anovulation. Of these 30 patients had clinical and laparoscopic evidence of polycystic ovarian disease (P.C.O). The menstrual pattern of these patients has been studied in detail. We wanted to see the incidence of raised prolactin levels in patients with polycystic ovarian disease. Galactorrhea was present in nine of 30 patients – the incidence of galactorrhea in polycystic ovarian disease is 30%. These patients were primarily treated with Parlodel (bromocriptine) as a first choice of treatment. Laparoscopy was performed on all the patients. The incidence of silent tuberculosis in 100 patients with anovulation was 34%. Galactorrhea and hyperprolactinemia were present in 34% patients. 10/30 patients conceived of whom six were primarily treated with bromocriptine. Details of results will be discussed.

16.28.07

Ovulation and pregnancy after "pure" FSH therapy in sclerocystic ovarian change: Sallam, H, Scammell, G, Massam, G, Katz, M, Curzon, R, Collins, W, Jeffcoate, S, Ginsburg, J. King's Coll., Chelsea, Princess Anne Southampton, Royal Free and Univ. Coll. Hosp., London, UK

Thirty-one women with sclerocystic ovarian change (SCO) who had hyperstimulated or failed to conceive on clomiphene citrate or human menopausal gonadotrophin containing LH and FSH, were treated with an FSH extract from menopausal urine containing less than one 1 iU LH per ampoule. Ovulation occurred in 91 out of 113 courses and 10 women conceived. Mild hyperstimulation, observed on ultrasound scanning, occurred in only 12 cycles and moderate hyperstimulation in three, in two instances in pregnant women. FSH dosage and course duration per cycle were significantly greater in women who conceived than in those who did not but there was no significant difference in cycles associated with hyperstimulation compared with those in which no excessive ovarian activity was observed. LH levels and the LH/FSH ratio fell during FSH administration to within the normal range in most cycles. Plasma estradiol and sex hormone binding globulin increased markedly after FSH; serum prolactin increased slightly. There was no change in plasma testosterone. Pure FSH seems effective and safe therapy for infertile women with SCO, reducing the elevated LH/FSH ratio characteristic of the condition and inducing adequate follicular development in the absence of hyperstimulation in the majority of cycles, with a pregnancy rate of 30% in a group of women with prolonged infertility.

16.28.08

Correlation between the ultrasonic appearance, clinical, laparoscopic findings and hormonal profile of patients with PCOD: Aleem, F, ElTabbakh, G, Lotfi, I, Azab, I, Rahman, H A. Dept. Obstet. and Gyn., New York Med. Coll.-Metrop. Hosp. Ctr, New York, NY, USA; Alexandria Fac. Med., Cairo, Egypt

Few reports have been published about the ultrasonic (US) appearance of polycystic ovaries. Most of the reports, however, did not correlate the US picture to the clinical, laparoscopic and hormonal findings. The following paper reports the US appearance in 20 PCOD patients. Scanning was performed with a 3.5 MH^3 sector scan real-time transducer. The mean ovarian size of the group studied was 9.75 ± 3.38 cm^3. 75% had enlarged ovaries, 25% had normal-sized ovaries. 55% showed multiple small cysts (< 1 cm), 25% showed single cyst (> 1 cm) and 20% showed no discernible cysts. The ovaries were hypoechoeic in 80% and isoechoeic in 20%. Ovarian capsule was thick in 90%, ovarian margin was regular. US findings regarding ovarian size, surface and capsule were all confirmed by laparoscopy. The US ovarian size in the hyperprolactinemic was enlarged in 77.8%, 11% had isoechoeic and 89% had hypoechoeic ovaries. In the normoprolactinemic, 72.7% had hypoechoeic ovaries. Comparison between normal-sized vs. enlarged ovaries showed that obesity, amenorrhea, hirsutism, high prolactin, elevated testosterone, elevated dehydroepiandrosterone sulfate, low estradiol were more in the group with enlarged ovaries (93% vs. 40%, 46.7% vs. 40%, 80% vs. 60%, 46.7% vs. 40%, 86.7% vs. 60%, 20% vs. 0% and 86% vs. 60% respectively). Oligomenorrhea, elevated LH/FSH elevated androstenedione, elevated estrone were more in the group with normal-sized ovaries. These findings support the role of ultrasound in diagnosing PCOD.

16.32.01

Prenatal diagnosis and treatment of intrauterine growth retardation: Kaneoka, T, Taguchi, S, Shirakawa, K. Dept. Obstet. and Gyn., Fukuoka Univ. School Med., Fukuoka, Japan

Intrauterine growth retardation (IUGR) is one of the most important complications in perinatology. In a prospective study of pregnancies with fetal body weight ultrasonically determined to be less than the 10th percentile of population, double-blind fashion trial of maternal allylestrenol therapy was carried out. In our clinic, the gestational age was routinely confirmed in the first trimester by ultrasonic measurements of the crown-rump length. Both the biparietal diameter (BPD) and abdominal circumference (AC) were also routinely measured in the third trimester. When the fetal body weight, estimated from BPD and AC values in accordance with the method of Warsof's equation, was less than the 10th percentile of the intrauterine growth curve at more than two ultrasonic determinations separated by two weeks, the prenatal diagnosis of IUGR was made. Maternal biochemical determinations of plasma and urinary E$_3$, plasma hPL, and serum HSAP were made on these pregnancies. All IUGR cases were instructed to have daytime bed rest and a high-protein diet. In addition, 75 cases in the trial were allocated in randomized double-blind fashion to treatment with oral intake of allylestrenol in a dose of 30 mg/day until the time of delivery. Other 75 cases had no medications. Both ultrasonic and biochemical measurements were repeated bi-weekly on those 150 pregnancies. In the treated group, only 22% were small-for-gestational age at birth, far less than 64% in the non-treated group: the difference was statistically significant. Perinatal mortality was also reduced in the treated group.

16.32.02

How do obstetric risk factors influence the risk of neonatal respiratory diseases?: Wennergren, M, Karlsson, K, Hjalmarson, O, Krantz, M. Dept. Obstet. and Gyn., and Dept. Pediat., Univ., Göteborg, Sweden

The clinical impression has been that after obstetric conditions associated with "antenatal stress" the incidence of neonatal respiratory diseases (Rd) is unexpectedly low. This has been explained by a favorable effect of corticoids and catecholamines upon lung maturation and adaption. An obstetric risk group with either of the following criteria was identified: High score according to a scoring system indicating IUGR (*Wennergren* et al. Brit. J. Obstet. Gyn. **89**, 520, 1982), hypertension, ultrasound indicating IUGR or biochemical evidence of placental dysfunction (n = 142). The incidence of Rd in this group and for all infants with birth weight $< -2SD$ were compared with the incidence for all infants born the same year (n = 4659). The study was made prospectively one year. The infants from the risk population had a significantly higher incidence of Rd than the infants in the total population (27% versus 5% in newborns $\geq$ 37 weeks). This difference could not be explained by a higher Cesarean section rate in the risk group, since the same difference remained after vaginal delivery (24% v 3.7%). The IUGR infants also had a surprisingly high risk of Rd, 25% after vaginal delivery and $\geq$ 37 weeks. Thus, contrary to our preliminary hypothesis obstetric risk factors seem to increase the risk of neonatal respiratory diseases.

16.32.03

Significance of fetoplacental function tests in IUGR pregnancies: Murata, T[1], Kuwabara, Y[2], Mizuno, M[2]. [1]Dept. Obstet. and Gyn., Aiiku Hosp.; [2]Dept. Obstet. and Gyn., Fac. Med., Univ., Tokyo, Japan

In IUGR pregnancies the prenatal assessment of fetal status is of considerable clinical importance. This study was designed to see whether fetal outcome could be predicted by using plasma concentration of fetoplacental products. Peripheral serum levels of unconjugated estriol ($U.E_3$), hPL, 11-deoxycortisol, cystine amino-peptidase (CAP) were determined in 30 pregnant women who subsequently gave birth to infants with birth weight less than the 10th centile and in 102 normal pregnant women as a control group. Blood samples were taken serially from 28 weeks gestation onwards. Each patient delivered between 37 and 41 weeks. In this study the cases with birth weight less than the 5th percentile were diagnosed as severe IUGR. In 30 IUGR patients there were 15 cases of severe IUGR and 11 cases with evidence of fetal distress. In severe IUGR patients mean $U.E_3$ concentration was significantly lower than the control value. It is considered that 11-deoxycortisol is derived from the fetal adrenal and its maternal levels reflect fetal production of corticosteroids. In IUGR patients 11-deoxycortisol levels were significantly elevated between 28 and 30 weeks. In IUGR groups mean hPL levels of the cases with F. D. were significantly lower than those without F. D. between 35 and 36 weeks. In severe IUGR patients the mean values of CAP were significantly lower than those in the mild IUGR patients and the control. It is concluded that maternal serum $U.E_3$ levels can be used for diagnosing the severity of growth retardation and hPL for the antepartum evaluation of fetal conditions in IUGR pregnancies.

16.32.04

The predictive value of estrone (E_1) in DHEAS loading compared to HPL and SP_1 in intrauterine growth retardation (IUGR): Delaloye, J-F, Churchod, A, Rey, F, Weihs, D, Bossart, H. Dept. Gyn. and Obstet., CHUV, Lausanne, Switzerland

We compared the predictive value of E_1 elevation after dehydroepiandrosterone-sulfate (DHEAS) loading (50 mg i. v. bolus injection) with human placental lactogen (HPL) and Schwangerschaftsprotein 1 (SP_1) basal levels in 36 pregnant women, half of them presenting an IUGR. E_1 and HPL measurements are performed by radioimmunoassay (RIA) and SP_1 by enzyme-immunoassay (EIA). 120 and 180 minutes after DHEAS loading, we observe a significatively diminished response of E_1 conversion (ΔE_1 120 and ΔE_1 180). ΔE_1 120 = 42.3 nmol/l $\pm$ 9.9 SEM in normal pregnancies versus 15.1 nmol/l $\pm$ 3.0 SEM in IUGR (p < 0.02). ΔE_1 180 = 37.2 nmol/l $\pm$ 7.2 SEM in normal pregnancies versus 17.9 nmol/l $\pm$ 3.8 SEM in IUGR (p < 0.05). Among IUGR 17/18 have a ΔE_1 120 < 28 nmol/l, 10/18 a low HPL and 9/18 a low SP_1. Among normal pregnancies 8/18 have a ΔE_1 120 < 28 nmol/l, 4/18 a low HPL and 7/18 a low SP_1. 5/18 IUGR present a ΔE_1 120 < 28 nmol/l with normal HPL and SP_1. In conclusion, the dynamic ΔE_1 elevation has a more predictive value in IUGR than any static determination.

16.32.05

Impaired estriol levels in methadone addicted pregnant women: Facchinetti, F, Comitini, G, Petraglia, F, Volpe, A, Genazzani, A R. Dept. Obstet. and Gyn., Univ., Modena, Italy

The plasma levels of human chorionic somatomammotropin (hCS), estriol (E_3), dehydroepiandrosterone-sulfate (DHA-S), cortisol and the circadian changes of the two last adrenal hormones were studied in 25 pregnant methadone addicted women (MA) and 21 pregnant drug-naive controls (C) at different periods of gestation and in 13 non-pregnant women (seven MA and six drug-naive). MA pregnant women showed normal plasma levels of hCS while those of E_3 at term were lower than normal (MA: 4.4 $\pm$ 0.8; C: 8.1 $\pm$ 1.0 ng/ml, p < 0.01). DHA-S plasma levels of MA pregnant women were half the normal values in the three trimester of gestation, while there were no differences in non-pregnant subjects. Circadian variations of cortisol and DHA-S plasma levels were present in both MA and C. The blunted DHA-S, while normal cortisol plasma levels found in MA pregnant women indicate that opiate abuse interferes with adrenal function, mainly of the fetus. Since the scarce availability of adrenal precursors, these data suggest that E_3

measurements should be not considered as a useful index of fetal well-being in the presence of opiate addiction.

16.32.06

Smoking affects the fetal development: Endler, M. 2nd Dept. Gyn. and Obstet., Univ., Vienna, Austria

Most obstetricians advise their pregnant patients to quit smoking during pregnancy. The records of 7541 pregnant women who were delivered between Jan 1, 1976 and June 30, 1982 at the 2nd Dept. of Ob/Gyn, Univ. of Vienna, were reviewed. Among them were 4937 nonsmokers, 1751 smokers, and 853 women who quit smoking as soon as they knew they were pregnant. Weight, length, and maturity of the newborns was significantly different in the three groups while there were no differences in the average gestational age at the time of delivery. The mean birth weight and length were 3243 g/49.2 in nonsmokers, 3179/48.9 in smokers who stopped smoking during pregnancy, and 3055/48.3 in smokers. Simultaneously the rate of low birth weight infants was significantly higher in mothers who quit smoking during pregnancy and still higher in smoking mothers. It appears therefore reasonable to advise women who smoke to quit this habit during pregnancy in order to reduce the risk of delivery of low birth weight infant.

16.32.07

Prevention of low birth weight by flunarizine given to smoking mothers: Janssens, D. Dept. Gyn. and Obstet., St.-Elisabethziekenhuis, Turnhout, Belgium

In a randomized double-blind setting, a preventive pharmacotherapy was tested in pregnant women unwilling to give up smoking, a pilot group with an increased risk of low-birth-weight babies. The selective calcium antagonist flunarizine shows an interesting pharmacological and pharmacodynamic profile which might antagonize chronic fetal hypoxia leading to an increased dysmaturity and prematurity risk in the babies of smoking women. One hundred pregnant women were given orally either a placebo (n = 50) or flunarizine (n = 50) in a single daily dose of 10 mg from the fifth month of pregnancy until confinement. There was no significant difference between the two groups with regard to age, parity, smoking habits, duration of treatment and weight at the start of pregnancy. In the placebo group the mean birth weight was 3011 g, against 3291 g in the flunarizine group. That difference is statistically significant (p = 0.0024, Mann Whitney U-test, 2-tailed). The mean duration of pregnancy is not significantly different: 279 days in the placebo group against 282 days in the flunarizine group (p = 0.2, same test). When in multiparae of both groups the difference in birth weight between the studied pregnancy and the average birth weight after previous pregnancies is calculated, the mean of the flunarizine group (+ 252 g) is again significantly higher than that of the placebo group (− 52 g) (p = 0.03, same test). Further investigations will be required to show a simular eutrophic effect of flunarizine on the fetus in other obstetrical risk situations.

16.32.08

A preliminary study of alcohol detoxification in pregnant women: Jacyszyn, K, Woytoń, J, Rzepka, Z, Zalewski, J. Dept. Toxicol., II Clin. Obstet., Med. Acad., Wrocław, Poland

A preliminary study was conducted for the purpose of evaluating detoxification dynamics of ethyl alcohol in pregnant women and their fetuses. The study was performed in 21 hospitalized women between the 37th and 38th week of pregnancy. The control group consisted of ten non-pregnant women. Alcohol was given intravenously as one 3.3 g dose and was followed by known methods for evaluating blood and kidney clearance. The results of the research indicated that most probably ethyl alcohol distributes freely between the blood of the mother and the fetus as the biological half-life was found to be shorter and the renal clearance smaller in the pregnant women group. This preliminary study indicates that alcohol detoxification in pregnancy is shared by the developing fetus.

16.32.09

Effect of DDT on fetal outcome: Mehra, P, Das, V, Seth, T D. Dept. Obstet. and Gyn., K.G's Med. Coll. and Indust. Toxicol. Res. Ctr, Lucknow, India

DDT continues to be used as a pesticide in our country whereas its use has been given up in developed countries. However, the clinical implication of DDT exposures in humans are still controversial. We have studied the relationship of maternal blood levels of DDT and its metabolites (DDE & DDD) to fetal outcome (abortions, intrauterine growth retardation and still birth). Blood from 27 mothers giving birth to full-term normal babies, six cases of unexplained intrauterine growth retardation, nine cases of unexplained still births and 17 cases of unexplained abortions were collected. The levels of DDT, DDE and DDD were measured by GLC. The levels in women giving birth to normal babies i. e. values in control cases were 0–65.2 ppb (median 6.3 ppb) for DDT, 2.09–47.75 ppb (median 9.09 ppb) for DDE and 0–17.21 ppb (median 3.17 ppb) for DDD. It was found that seven (77.81%) cases of still births and 10 (58.8%) cases of abortions had DDT and DDE values respectively higher than the 95% confidence limits of values of mothers giving birth to a normal baby. Four out of six cases of IUGR had higher DDE levels than controls. Since raised DDE values reflect a long-term exposure to DDT, it appears that chronic exposure to DDT may be associated with unexplained abortions and IUGR in some instances. On the other hand in cases of still births, DDT levels were raised suggesting a more recent exposure to DDT in these patients.

16.32.10

Role of chlorinated hydrocarbon pesticides in intrauterine growth retardation: Chopra, U, P, Chandravati.
Dept. Obstet. and Gyn., King George Med. Coll., Lucknow, India
Organochlorine pesticides (BHC, Aldrine, P P'DDE, P P'DDT, DDTR) were measured in the maternal blood, fetal blood, placental tissue and amniotic fluid of women undergoing full-term normal labor and intrauterine fetal growth retardation and the results were compared. Levels of these organochlorine pesticides were detected using an electron-capture gas chromatographic method. One conclusion of the work is that most of the pesticides act as antagonists to the pregnancy and cause fetal growth retardation in utero. A plausible explanation for the facilitatory role of organochlorine pesticides in causing intrauterine fetal growth retardation is hypothesized.

16.32.11

Limb malformations in a case of hydrops fetalis with ketoconazole use during pregnancy: Lind, J. Sint Franciscus Gasthuis, Rotterdam, The Netherlands
There are no documented cases of human anomalies with the use of ketoconazole during pregnancy. A hydrops fetalis (HF) was diagnosed at 29 weeks of gestation in a Turkish woman how had used ketoconazole, 200 mg daily, during conception till seven weeks of gestation. Echocardiographic examination did not show any abnormalities except for generalized edema of the fetus. Fetoprotein levels in the amniotic fluid and maternal serum were elevated. Other laboratory tests and cultures were negative; chromosomal analysis of the cells of the amniotic fluid showed a normal karyogram, 46,XX. Digoxine therapy was started without any results. At $30^1/_2$ weeks of gestation labor started and a hydropic girl was vaginally delivered showing multiple anomalies of the limbs. High ketoconazole levels are correlated with embryotoxocity and teratogenesis in rats, especially female species. Ketoconazole seems to block the synthesis of androgen and corticosteroids *in vivo* and *in vitro* and the action of this drug may last for several weeks, when used for a longer period. Ketoconazole may in this case have caused the congenital anomalies of the limbs and the disturbance of the fluid homeostasis of the amniotic fluid and the fetus. The need to perform a punctilious echographic examination of all the limbs when screening for congenital anomalies is stressed. Strict contraceptive advice is essential during ketoconazole use.

16.32.12

The teratogenecity of progestagens given during the first trimester of pregnancy: Lancet, M, Katz, Z, Skornik, J, Chemke, J, Mogilner, B M, Klinberg, M. Dept. Obstet. and Gyn., Clin. Genet. Unit, Neonat. Intens. Care Unit, Kaplan Hosp., Rehovot, Israel
In order to examine possible teratogenic effects of exogenous progestational agents given during early pregnancy, a controlled historic prospective study was done, including a total of 2754 babies born to mothers who had bled during the first trimester of pregnancy. The study group comprised 1608 newborns whose mothers had been treated with progestational agents (mostly medroxyprogesterone acetate) beginning in the first trimester, and in the control group there were 1146 babies whose mothers remained untreated. Thorough examinations were done during the first days of life, looking for malformations classified according to the different anatomic systems. In most systems, the rate of malformations was somewhat higher in the control group, but in no case was a statistically significant difference found between the two groups, either way. The overall rate of malformations was 120.0 per thousand in the exposed group and 123.9 per thousand among the controls. Major malformations were 63.4 and 71.5 per thousand, respectively. These findings prove that those clinicians who think it useful to administer progestagens in early pregnancy for any clinical reason, need not fear an increase in the incidence of malformations in the newborn.

16.41.01

Sensitivity and specificity of the diagnosis "fetal distress": Eskes, T, Jongsma, H, Crevels, J, Houx, P. Inst. Obstet. and Gyn., St. Radboud Hosp., Univ., Nijmegen, The Netherlands
Prospectively the diagnosis "fetal distress" leading to operative delivery was evaluated in 1983 on 1584 neonates. Umbilical artery blood gases were used as a criterion: pH < 7.16, base deficit > 11.3 mmol/l being 1 SD below the mean. Complete values were available in 85%. All fetuses were electronically monitored. The frequency of microblood analysis was 4.1% and instrumental deliveries 26.7%. The results are given in the table.

		Neonatal acidemia		
		Yes	No	Total
Fetal	pos.	20	51	71
Distress	neg.	88	1188	1276
Total		108	1239	1347

Sensitivity $\frac{20}{108} \times 100 = 18.5\%$ Specificity $\frac{1188}{1239} \times 100 = 95.9\%$

Pos. predictive value $\frac{20}{71} \times 100 = 28.2\%$

Neg. predictive value $\frac{1188}{1276} \times 100 = 93.1\%$

Prevalence $\frac{108}{1347} \times 100 = 8.0\%$ Likelihood ratio $\frac{18.5}{4.1} = 4.5\%$

It was concluded that specificity (95.9%) was high but sensitivity (18.5%) too low.

16.41.02
Clinical randomised trial: Stimulation of fetal surfactant production by carnitine combined with a reduced betamethasone dose: Vytiska-Binstorfer, E*, Salzer, H*, Langer, M*, Lohninger, A**, Simbruner, G***. *1st. Dept. Obstet., **Dept. Med. Chem., ***Dept. Neonat., Univ., Vienna, Austria

Stimulation of the surfactant production in fetal lung cells by carnitine (gamma-trimethylaminobeta-hydroxybutyrate) combined with a betamethasone standard-dose has been shown both in animal experiments and also in human. In animal experiments a differentiation of the alveolar epithelial cells with a reduced steroid dose and a stimulation of dipalmitoylphosphatidylcholine (DPPC) by carnitine was found. Based on these results and on the lack of any toxicity carnitine combined with betamethasone has been used in our clinic for RDS-prophylaxis with good success for three years. Following doses for the new clinical trial were used: day 1: 2 mg betamethasone i. m., day 1 to day 5: 6 g carnitine i. v. daily. In a prospective randomised study this dose was compared with the standard steroid dose: day 1 and day 2: 8 mg beta-methasone i. m. In all cases (n = 25) amniotic fluid samples were taken before and after therapy on day 1 and 6. Excluded were women after the 35th week of gestation and pregnancies with premature rupture of the membranes. We investigated L/S ratio, DPPC, dynamic surface-tension measurement in amniotic fluid and postpartum the compliance of the respiratory system of the newborns. First results (n = 20) show a clear benefit of carnitine therapy. Group A: Carnitine-combination, group B: Standard-cortis.

Increase of L/S-ratio:	4.1(x)	2.1(x) p < 0,05
Increase of y-min:	9.3(x)	4.3(x) p < 0,05
Increase of DPPC:	4.3(x)	1.7(x) p < 0,05

16.41.03
Carnitine metabolism during pregnancy and the perinatal period: Genger, H, Legenstein, E*, Lohninger, A*, Sevelda, P, Salzer, H. 1st Dept. Obstet. and Gyn., *Dept. Med. Chem., Univ., Vienna, Austria

Carnitine (2-hydroxy-3-trimethylamino butyric acid) and its acylesters are present in all living cells. They are necessary for the transport of fatty acids into mitochondria and for other metabolic functions of the cell. High doses of carnitine for pregnant women with imminent premature delivery have been reported to activate surfactant synthesis and provide a better postnatal prognosis for the newborn. For further investigation blood samples from 95 women between the 8th and 40th week of pregnancy were analysed for free and short-chain acyl carnitine according to *Cederblad*. Carnitine was found to be reduced in blood plasma and in whole blood during all trimesters of pregnancy. Compared to nonpregnant women the decrease in plasma carnitine is about 50%, while whole blood carnitine drops only 30%. These results suggest an important role of erythrocytes in carnitine transport. The distribution of carnitine between blood plasma and erythrocytes in the maternal blood and umbilical cord blood is under investigation. Together these results might indicate an increased need of carnitine during pregnancy which is necessary for the biosynthesis of surfactant and for the growing of the fetus. Therefore carnitine therapy of pregnant women with premature labor or placental insufficiency should be considered. It must be stressed that no known side-effects are caused by carnitine therapy.

Total carnitine	(μmol/l)	1st trim	2nd trim	3rd trim
plasma	mean $\pm$ SED	20.0 ± 3.9	16.4 ± 4.0	13.3 ± 2.9
whole blood		19.8 ± 4.3	17.3 ± 7.3	16.3 ± 5.9

16.41.04
Evaluation of the fetal pulmonary maturity by thin layer chromatography: Argeri, N, Darbón, H, Uranga Imaz, F, Koremblit, E. Univ., La Plata, Argentina

208 samples of amniotic fluid were examined and 94 of these were analysed by semi-quantitative technic, extracting the phospholipids and separating these by thin layer chromatography. They were visible evaluating the phosphatidyl glycerol (FG) presence and the lecithin-sphingomyelin (L-S) relation by comparison to a standard. The other 114 samples were analysed by a quantitative method similar to the former one by comparison to a standard and quantitated in a scanning densitometer. The results suggest that estimation of FG correlated with the LS ratio and has provided a more reliable prediction of the risk of hyaline membrane disease causing respiratory distress. In presence of FG and without LS ratio it was possible, in 96.5% of the newborns, to predict the absence of respiratory distress. The absence of FG was associated

in 89% with respiratory distress. The precision and reproducibility of the method becomes more significant with the incorporation of the LS ratio. In presence of both methods, FG positive and LS ratio with high values none of the newborns had respiratory distress, however, 5.8% had respiratory distress when the LS ratio was immature in presence of FG. The authors conclude that the determination of both the FG and the LS ratio it is very important in the high risk pregnancies to predict the respiratory distress in newborns.

16.41.05

Nuclear magnetic resonance (NMR) – a noninvasive technique for the diagnosis of fetal lung maturity: Langner, K, Schmidt, S, Dudenhausen, J W, Saling, E, Herbst, R. Inst. Perinat. Med., FU, Berlin

We studied the lungs of six guinea pig fetuses with a gestational age of 45 to 65 days with help of nuclear magnetic resonance. Using a Bruker Tomograph BNT IS 24/30 or 24/40 we succeeded in obtaining magnetic resonance-tomographic cross-sections with 2 DFT-technique (2 dimensional Fourier transformation) as well as T 2-relaxation time-technique. Additionally, we were able to measure *in vivo* P 31-spectra of the lungs of fetuses with defined gestational age. Phosphatidylcholine, a main component of surfactant, was identified in the P 31 spectra due to its characteristic chemical shift. Ultramicroscopical analysis of the fetal lungs was performed and the morphological result was compared to the NMR spectra. We found that by means of NMR spectroscopy phosphatidylcholine is already detectable, before it is found in the lamellar body of the pneumocyte type II. These results prove that NMR spectroscopy as well as NMR imaging techniques can provide information about fetal lung maturity. In contrast to the difficulties in studying the lung after birth with help of nuclear magnetic resonance, this technique has high potential as a tool to achieve information about the fetal lung.

16.41.06

Study of serum prolactin in newborns with RDS – a preliminary report: Mukherjee, T K, Lala, R, Rajegowda, B K, Lala, V. Dept. Obstet. and Gyn., Lincoln Hosp. Ctr, New York Med. Coll., Bronx, NY, USA

There is scant information regarding the changes in prolactin (PRL) level in the first few days of life in newborns (NB) with severe RDS. PRL levels were assayed in cord, day 1, 2 and 3 after birth in 19 NBs who subsequently developed severe RDS (GrA); four NBs developing mild RDS (GrB) and eight control NBs with no RDS (GrC).

		PRL levels ng/ml		
Gr.	Cord.	Day 1	Day 2	Day 3
A.	156.5±13.7	128.2±14.4	115.6±11.5	120.9±16.3
B.	226.2±47.6	207.7±17.0	187.7±19.5	153.0±36.7
C.	206.9±26.8	224.5±28.0	173.7±27.4	148.7±25.1

The cord PRL is significantly lower in GrA females compared to GrC (p < 0.02). There is significant fall in day 1 PRL in GrA when compared to GrC (p < 0.001). The decline was also noted on day 2 vs. day 1 in GrA and also in GrC (p < 0.05). The severity of fall in day 1 PRL is apparantly proportional to the severity of RDS: 52% drop in two NB who expired due to severe RDS; 19.6% in NB with severe RDS who survived and 10.5% in GrB with mild RDS. It seems important to observe PRL for first few days after birth to identify high risk category amongst premature newborns susceptible to develop RDS.

16.41.07

Impact of fetal distress on neonatal respiratory disease: Lilja, H, Wennergren, M, Karlsson, K, Hjalmarson, O. Dept. Obstet. and Gyn., and Dept. Pediat., Univ., Göteborg, Sweden

In a recent paper intrauterine stress, expressed in terms of abnormal CTG pattern was unexpectedly correlated with decreased incidence of neonatal respiratory disease (Rd). This was suggested to be due to a favorable effect of catecholamines on the fetal lung. Because of this finding a detailed analysis of continuous CTG recordings during 52 deliveries was carried out. The CTG patterns were analysed blindly by a senior obstetrician according to changes in basal heart frequency, heart rate variability and the presence of decelerations. All 52 infants were > 38 weeks and vaginally delivered. In 28/52 cases the CTG patterns were abnormal, while umbilical vein pH values were < 7.20 in 12/52. Four infants had Rd. One of these had an abnormal CTG pattern and low pH values, whereas the other three had normal CTG patterns, normal pH and lactate values. The incidence rate of Rd was 3.5% in the group with abnormal CTG vs. 11.5% in the normal CTG group. In the previous study the CTG classifications were based on routine examinations. Also all deliveries in that study ended in Cesarean section, which might have influenced the development of Rd. In this study the infants were vaginally delivered and with the exception of one, they all had a normal Apgar score. In spite of this CTG changes occurred in 54% and low umbilical pH in 23%, indicating moderate intrauterine stress. Thus, the present study confirms earlier findings, which suggest that the effect of a certain intrauterine stress might alert the baby and prevent development of Rd.

16.41.08

Shift of pacemaker as a sign of fetus hypoxia: Puodžius, S. Med. Inst., Kaunas, Lithuania, USSR

Experimental investigations have shown pacemaker shift to be one of the earliest signs of hypoxic affect on the fetal myocardium (*Sadauskas* et al., 1981; *Kilda* et al., 1982). Thus, the aim of our studies was to define the frequency and character of pacemaker shift under hypoxic conditions. 25 experiments on isolated human embryo hearts with perfusion via aorta were carried out. ECG and intra-atrial delay (IAD) periodograms were recorded using special devices under normoxic and hypoxic conditions. It was found that starting already with the first minutes of hypoxia frequent and significant changes of IAD (previously stable) are observed, which points out to pacemaker shift. The average frequency of shifting is 3.12 ± 1.98 min^{-1}. Pacemaker shift was registered in all experiments by the seventh min of hypoxia. Every shift is related to the change of R-R duration and atrial ECG complex morphology. The early hypoxic stages (up to 14–15 min) reveal smooth wave-like changes of R-R interval and P wave without shortening of P-Q interval. Later on R-R interval reveals spike-like changes, while P wave changes are accompanied by shortening of P-Q interval. This indicates a more marked shift of the pacemaker. Pacemaker shift manifesting in early hypoxic stages allows to consider it as a valuable clinical sign for the diagnosis of fetal hypoxia.

16.41.09

Fetal lung maturity correlated to ultrasonic detectable epiphyseal centers: Deutinger, J, Bernaschek, G, Reinthaller, A. 2nd Dept. Obstet. and Gyn., Univ., Vienna, Austria

In 62 cases of high-risk pregnancies amniocentesis was performed to analyse amniotic fluid and estimate the lecithin: sphingomyelin ratio. At the same time measurement of the epiphyseal centers in the area of the fetal knees was done. The present study was undertaken to evaluate, if fetal bone maturity is correlating with lung maturity. Amniocentesis with following measurement of epiphyseal centers was done in 62 cases of pregnancy between the 31st and the 39th gestational week. Before 34th week of pregnancy sonographic proof of the distal epiphyseal center of the fetal femur was possible in 6 of 13 cases, after the 34th week the distal epiphyseal center could be detected in all cases. In our investigation the size of the visualized epiphyseal centers increased from the 32nd to the 39th week of pregnancy from 3 mm to 8 mm. In 15 of the 62 cases an epiphyseal center could be detected in the proximal area of the tibia. In those cases gestational age was more than 35 weeks. If it was possible to detect an epiphyseal center in the proximal area of the fetal tibia, in all cases – except two patients with diabetes mellitus – prenatal lung maturity could be demonstrated. Detection and measurement of epiphyseal centers of fetal knees seems to be a valuable method for determinating date of birth. In addition in cases with positive proof of epiphyseal center in the proximal area of the fetal tibia or in the distal area of the femur with a size of more than 6 mm fetal lung maturity could be presumed.

16.42.01

May urinary incontinence with bladder instability be cured by surgery?: Algeri, M, Vigano, R, Quadri, G, Scalambrino, S, Milani, R. Monza, Italy

Thirty-six incontinent women with bladder instability and vaginal prolapse underwent operation from October 1982 to December 1984. Pre-operative and postoperative (3–5 months) work-up included history, clinical examination, cystoscopy and a complete urodynamic investigation; a detrusor pressure rise more than 15 cm H_2O during filling cystometry was assumed as diagnostic of detrusor instability (I.C.S.). Average age was 60.3 years (range 42–75) a mild cystourethrocele was present in 17 cases and a severe cystocele in 19: the last group underwent anterior repair (A.R.), the former underwent retropubic colposuspension (R.C.). Altogether 55.5% of the patients were dry after operation and 52.7% had a normal bladder function; a normal vaginal anatomy was restored in 33 patients. The successful operation rate was analysed according to pre-operative cystometric figures of three different types of instability: Dry patients were 31.2%, 48.8% and 92% when a pre-operative filling instability (U.D.C.), a postural instability or a high pressure bladder (steep) was demonstrated. Into the three groups bladder instability disappeared in 12.5, 83 and 29%, respectively. No statistically significant difference was observed between the two surgical procedures. Incontinence surgery may be, with a high probability, a failure when uninhibited detrusorial contractions are present, and a success in cases of high pressure bladder.

16.42.02

A magnetic urethral closure system for treatment of urinary incontinence: Grüneberger, A D, Hennig, G R*, Geier, G. Dept. Gyn. and Obstet., Univ. Ulm; *Gauting/München

The new urethral closure system consists of a retropubic magnet and another removable intravaginal magnet. The urethra is closed by the mutual attraction of both magnets. The pressure on the tissue can be modulated by the size and strength of the removable magnet. Thus, pressure action time is limited to the actual needs of the patient. The system showed according to previous experimental work in merino sheep that continence can be achieved in female patients without complications.

16.42.03

The control of stress incontinence: Comparison of anterior colporrhaphy and colposuspension: Stanton, S L, Chamberlain, G V P, Holmes, D M. Dept. Obstet. and Gyn., St. George's Hosp. Med. School, London, UK

To resolve the controversy of whether a vaginal or suprapubic operation is more effective in controlling

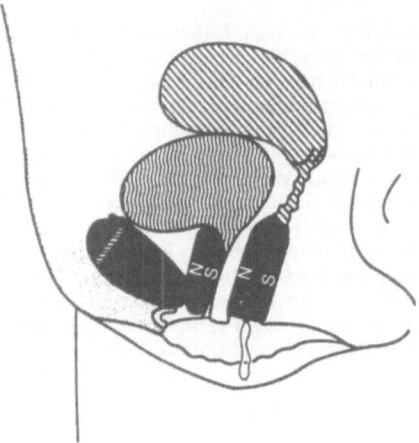

Fig.: Magnetic system with bone screw, implanted magnet, bladder-urethra, and intravaginal magnet.

stress incontinence due to urethral sphincter incompetence, a prospective randomised study was performed to compare an anterior colporrhaphy and a colposuspension. Fifty-two patients, without previous bladder neck surgery, were randomly allocated to either an anterior repair or a colposuspension: each patient was randomly allocated to either GVPC or SLS for the operation. Pre- and postoperative urodynamic studies were performed and follow-up ranged from three months to two years. There was no difference in mean age, weight, parity, operating time or postoperative complications between the two groups. Intra-operative blood loss was significantly higher with the colposuspension operation (p < 0.01). Both the symptomatic and objective (urodynamic) cure of stress incontinence was significantly greater with the colposuspension (p < 0.01). There was no significant difference in the incidence of postoperative voiding difficulties, detrusor instability or anterior vaginal wall prolapse between the two groups. The colposuspension was found to be a more effective operation to control urethral sphincter incompetence in the follow-up so far.

16.42.04
Randomized surgery for incontinence and prolapse: Retropubic colposuspension vs anterior repair: Quadri, G, Scalambrino, S, Boisio, N, Marchesin, R, Milani, R. Monza, Italy
From October 1981 to January 1985, 103 incontinent women with moderate to severe prolapse were submitted to a randomized operation: retropubic colposuspension (R.C.) versus anterior repair (A.R.). 48 patients had a R.C. (34 with moderate prolapse and 14 with severe prolapse) while 55 had an anterior repair A.R. (25 with moderate prolapse and 30 with severe prolapse). Mean age was 54 (range 36–75) and 58 (range 38–76) in R.C. and A.R. group, respectively. A complete clinical and urodynamic evaluation was done before operation, after operation (3–6 months) and whenever a relapse of urinary incontinence occurred. Pre-operatively bladder instability was diagnosed in seven cases of R.C. and 12 cases of A.R. One woman had a 12-month mean follow-up (range 3–33 months). In 13 out of 48 women submitted to R.C. the prolapse relapsed (moderate to severe urethrocystocele in seven cases, vaginal cuff in six cases) while only in three out of 55 women submitted to A.R. prolapse relapsed (moderate cystocele two, vaginal cuff one). Urinary incontinence recurred in quite similar percentage after the two surgical procedures (5 out of 48 R.C. and 6 out of 55 A.R.). Significantly menopausal status appears to be more advanced in patients who had a relapse than in patients successfully cured. The two surgical procedures showed a quite similar effectiveness in curing incontinence, while a prolapse relapse followed R.C. significantly more frequently.

16.42.05
Comparative study between the Marshall-Marchetti-Krantz operation and the endoscopic suspension of the bladder neck for surgical correction of stress urinary incontinence: Palma, P, David, S, Pinotti, J A. Dept. Obstet. and Gyn., State Univ., Campinas, Brazil
The present study covers two groups of patients presenting stress urinary incontinence, who were submitted to surgical correction. Group I: 30 patients were submitted to surgical correction using the Marshall-Marchetti-Krantz technique. Group II: 20 patients submitted to endoscopic suspension of the bladder neck. Analysis of the results obtained, after an average period of two years, has shown that the endoscopic suspension of the bladder neck achieved good results in 93% of the cases; however, the Marshall-Marchetti-Krantz technique achieved only 80% of cure of the disease. The above results indicate that the endoscopic suspension of the bladder neck is superior to Marshall-Marchetti-Krantz technique in the surgical correction of stress urinary incontinence.

16.42.06

Evaluation of our surgical material in urogynecology from 1982 to 1984: Giambanco, V, Alio, L, Accursio, M C, Cappello, F, Monastra, A, Cabibbo, R*. Dept. Obstet. and Gyn., Dept. Serv. Radiol.*, Osp. G. F. Ingrassia, Palermo, Italy

Women complaining of urinary stress incontinence were submitted to surgical treatment from 1982 to 1984. Pre-operative evaluation, devoted to the selection of the most suitable operation, consisted of a patient history, a general clinical and pelvic bimanual examination and cysto-urethrography. Post-operative evaluation consisted of a cysto-urethrographic follow-up after one month, six months and one year. We performed 162 operations; of those, five according to operative technique of *Ingelman-Sundberg, 57* according to *Marshall-Marchetti-Krantz*, 50 according to *Burch*, 40 according to *Kelly-Kennedy* and ten according to *Pereyra*. In the authors' experience the highest objective and subjective success rates were obtained with Burch colposuspension and with Pereyra's operation. The high recurrence rates of stress incontinence induced the authors to abandon the other operative techniques.

16.42.07

About 411 modified Burch's operations in treatment of urinary stress incontinence in female: Lazarevski, M B, Čakmakov, D A. Clin. Gyn. and Obstet., Med. Fac., Skopje, Yugoslavia

A modified technic of Burch's operation is elaborated to achieve the requirements of our conception that stress incontinence is due to deterioration of a not-permanently acting suburethral support, created by the upper leaf of the midpelvic fascia, pubo-urethral ligament, perivaginal fascia and urethro-vaginal septum. In the period from 1968 till 1984, 411 modified Burch's operations were performed in the Service, of which 348 in cases of manifest or masked stress incontinences and 63 as a preventive procedure with potential stress incontinences. A hydromechanical analysis of the effects of the suburethrally created support is presented and the indications and technical details of such a procedure with different colpocystographic aspects of stress incontinence are discussed. The operation should be performed in all cases of stress incontinence, radiologically Types A and Aa, incontinence associated with a slight degree of intravaginal prolapse, recurrent stress incontinence and cases where an associated genital pathology could be more easily handled by an abdominal approach. With a series of 264 mainifest and masked stress incontinences, followed for minimum of 24 months, the recurrency rate showed up to be 3.0%.

16.42.08

The role of elevation versus fixation of the internal urethral meatus in the Burch colposuspension procedure: Valsecchi, A, Dolci, F, Tucci, E. Dept. Obstet. and Gyn., Valduce Hosp., Como, Italy

In order to evaluate the role of proximal urethra elevation and fixation in the Burch colposuspension procedure, we have reviewed the pre- and postoperative cysto-urethrographic findings of 73 female patients with SUI urodynamically assessed. The position of the internal urethral meatus (IUM) at rest and the amplitude of its vertical descent during Valsalva maneuver have been compared before and two months after therapy. Three cases with postoperative detrusor instability are excluded. In 65 out of 70 patients, who became dry after operation (92.9% success rate), the IUM appears located at a significantly higher level after surgical correction ($p < 0.001$) and the IUM descent during Valsalva is significantly reduced ($p < 0.001$). In the five patients not cured by operation, the level of IUM is not significantly higher after operation ($p < 0.05$), whereas the IUM descent during Valsalva is significantly reduced ($p < 0.01$). While the Burch colposuspension procedure is therefore effective in both elevation and fixation of the proximal urethra, the elevation more than fixation seems to be the clue to success.

16.42.09

Clinical and urodynamic evaluation of oxybutynin chloride (Ditropan) in the treatment of incontinent women with bladder instability: Milani, R, Marchesin, R, Boisio, N, Merlo, E, Algeri, M. Monza, Italy

The efficacy and side-effects of oxybutynin chloride were evaluated in a clinical trial involving 40 incontinent patients with detrusor instability. The presence of uninhibited detrusorial contractions (U.D.C.) and/or a detrusor pressure rise more then 15 cm H_2O during filling cystometry was assumed as diagnostic for admission to the trial. 15 mg per os of the drug were administered daily for 30 days; before and after treatment patients were submitted to a complete clinical and urodynamic evaluation. The average age of the patients was 53.5 years and parity 2.6; a mild urethrocystocele was present in 12 patients. Altogether, diurnal and nocturnal frequency were improved by Ditropan in 68 and 55% of patients; urgency and urge incontinence were improved in 62 and 90.5%, respectively; stress incontinence was improved in 65% and enuresis in 89%; on clinical examination 55% of patients were dry or free of symptoms at the end of treatment, 29% and 16% respectively were improved or unchanged. On cystometric findings U.D.C. disappeared in 15 out of 15 patients, while altogether a normal detrusorial activity was demonstrated in 13 out of 25. Only in two patients severe side-effects caused the interruption of therapy. Oxybutynin chloride proves to be successful in controlling urinary symptoms in incontinent women with uninhibited detrusor instability.

16.42.10

Regeneration of transitional epitheleum on the surface of de-epithelialised intestinal loop used for urinary diversion – an experimental study on goats: Sharan, M, Sharan, U K. Sharan's Inst. Surg., Obstet. and Gyn., Rajendra Med. Coll. & Hosp., Ranchi, India

Introduction: Among the tribes dwelling in the hilly regions of the Chhotanagpur Plateau (India), damage to the bladder, urethra and vagina due to prolonged obstructed labor is at times so extensive that it is impossible to close the rent. Ileal or colonic conduit is very happily accepted by such patients in preference to their perpetually wet life which even makes them social outcastes (*Sharan & Sharan*, 1977). An intestinal conduit is also an integral part of any anterior or total exenteration operation in which the bladder is removed. It is also required in a few patients with intractable urinary frequency or urethral incompetence which may follow any gynecological operation when there is destruction of the bladder neck closing mechanism or even in some cases of intractable stress incontinence (*Howkins* et al., 1983). There is, however, one great drawback with the intestinal conduit, i. e. there is always some amount of reabsorption of the urinary solutes by the endothelium of this isolated loop producing extra strain on the kidneys. If this endothelium can somehow be replaced by the transitional epithelium of the urinary tract, this problem will be overcome. – Experimental work: A small segment of the ileum or a portion of the caecum in a goat was isolated with its blood-supply intact and, after scraping away the endothelial layer, it was anastomosed to the bladder. After a lapse of four to six months, the anastomosed loop together with the adjoining bladder wall was excised and the abdominal wound was closed, after closing the bladder. The excised tissue was subjected to histopathological examination. – Observations and conclusions: There had been complete coverage of the de-epithelialised intestinal surface by the transitional cell epithelium of the bladder. In cases where complete de-epithelialisation of the intestinal segment could not be achieved, islands of intestinal mucosa could be seen surrounded by the regenerated urothelium.

16.42.11

Pudendal nerve blockade for urethral catheterization in bucks: Attia, M, Othman, G M. Depts. Anat. & Histol. and Surg., Fac. Vet. Med., Benha Univ., Moshtohoer, Egypt

The origin, course and distribution of the pudendal nerve (N. pudendus) have been studied in bucks. Moreover, the surgical anatomy of the perineum has also been studied in this animal. The findings showed that from the ventral tuberosity of the tuber ischii, the nerve passes for about 3.5 cm cranio-ventrally along the dorso-lateral aspect of the penis at a depth of 3–4 cm from the skin. These findings served for determination of the proper site for blocking such a nerve using 5 ml local analgesic solution (3% procaine HCl with 1:10,000 adrenaline). Double injection for both pudendal nerves was seen to be necessary in each animal. A consequent temporary paralysis of the retractor penis muscle then effacing the sigmoid flexure of the penile urethra was encountered within five minutes of injection of the second side. Under the influence of this sort of analgesia, complete urethral catheterization was facilitated and afforded after excision of the processus urethrae. Moreover, full analgesia of the perineum was effected.

17.04.01

The office automation and network in the antenatal care: Korenaga, M, Sumioki, H, Kadota, T. Med. Inst. Bioregul., Kyushu Univ., Beppu, Japan

The purpose of this study is to develope the computer aided chartless system for antenatal check-up at out-patient clinic (OPC). This system is composed of Omninet network, hard disk (20M bytes) and four intelligent terminals. Intelligent terminals are equipped with Apple II computer for doctors' and patients' use at OPC as well as in ward and doctor's office. We newly developed file control program and I/O control program using assembly language (32K bytes). The former program is designed to accept and edit the many items of clinical records which vary in length and number in each individual patient. The latter is to enter the data more easily, using mark sheet, light pen and keyboard. At the OPC, patient's comprehensive data and graphic presentation can be immediately displayed by the input of patient's number and selection of the initial menu. The physicians in ward can also obtain access to the summary of the above follow-up on her admission. At the end of the consultation at OPC, patients are prepared to print out the pregnogram, fetal growth curve and gestational calender. Above summaries are transfered to the larger data bank through the modem for the statistical analysis. Universal I/O port (RS-232C) makes this terminal possible to attach the other network and media. This software enables the prospective use of chronological data and ongoing data of each patient and is totally different from the traditional programs which are designed for statistic use only.

17.04.02

Delivery in the sitting-position: Our experiences: Vallerino, G, Garzarelli, S, Cirillo, R, Corsini, R, Salvetti, B. Dept. Obstet. and Gyn., Hosp. S.P.D'Arena, Genova, Italy

The authors want to show, by studying the methods used to assist women in labor from the prehistoric age until now, how people started using the supine position in labor and how it is only now that there is a critical change in the use of this method by many doctors. In our department we used the sitting position during labor for low obstetric risk patients (21 women). For the sitting position we used a semi-solid cushion on which the woman could be supported by her husband. All the women so assisted had a regular delivery, felt more comfortable, and, more especially, felt a more active participation in the birth. We are satisfied by our experiences of using this type of assistance. Therefore we would like to extend the use to many more women.

17.04.03

Embryoscopy and chorionic villus samples for first trimester fetal diagnosis: Garzarelli, S F, Corsini, R, Vallerino, G, Cirillo, R, Spinelli, G. Div. Ostet. and Gin., Osp. Civ. Sampierdarena, Genova, Italy

Our study concerns 83 cases of C.V.S. In the first phase 70 cases were investigated. In 30 cases the "Portex" catheter technique was used while for 35 cases the "Wolf" biopsy forceps was employed and in five cases "Wolf" biopsy forcep together with hysteroscopy was utilized. Following this initial experimental phase, the "Portex" catheter was used for diagnostic purposes in 13 cases. Three babies have been born following sampling and seven women are pregnant as of March 1985. As a result of our study we can conclude that the catheter guided by ultrasound is the best, and the least dangerous diagnostic method for C.V.S. Increased knowledge about embryonic anatomy along with advances in technology will certainly create a new approach to C.V.S. Consequently, we have made a videocassette showing the different anatomic structures and membranes of an eight weeks gestation including the procedure necessary in order to have a good chorionic villus sample using "Wolf" biopsy forceps together with hysteroscopy.

17.04.04

Laparoscopic tubal occlusion with Hulka clips – three different techniques: Kleppinger, R K. Reading Hosp. & Med. Ctr, Reading, PA, USA

The first portion of the tape allows the viewer to observe from within the abdomen the penetration of the Veress needle, trocar and sheath, and the clip applicator. The use of the original single-puncture 10 mm Hulka clip applicator with the standard 5 mm telescope, and the new 7 mm Finger-grip type handle clip applicator which can be used either through the 10 mm operating laparoscope or through a second puncture 7 mm trocar sleeve are demonstrated. The proper finger movements required to open, close and lock the clip with each applicator are explained. Intra-abdominal photography demonstrates the application of local anesthesia applied to each Fallopian tube and the ideal technique of clip application to each tube. This is repeated three times to allow the viewer to observe the proper technique of clip application with each of the three techniques. The final portion of the tape demonstrates that whatever method or technique is used for sterilization, a laparoscopy is not genuinely complete without a diagnostic component. Thorough inspection of the genital organs has been accomplished prior to performing the tubal occlusion. The peritoneal cavity is explored with the laparoscope for congenital anomalies, effects of abnormal physiology, subclinical inflammatory processes and unexplained pathologic entities. The proper method of visualization of the appendix, liver, gallbladder, stomach and subdiaphragmatic surfaces is demonstrated. The final portion of the tape reveals that "the laparoscope is the 'picture window' in the abdomen".

17.04.05

Urethral suspension with vaginal flap (Mermut method) in female urinary stress incontinence: Mermut, S. Obstet. and Gyn. Dept., Gülhane Military Med. Fac., Ankara, Turkey

Twenty consecutive female patients with urinary stress incontinence treated by urethral suspension with vaginal flap according to the method of *Mermut*. After following up all patients for a mean of several months (minimum 5 months) 100% were free of symptoms or at least markedly improved. There were not any complications. The patients were 25–70 years old and follow-up has been from 3 to 18 months. Of these, 16 patients had a classic history of urinary stress incontinence alone and four had also vaginal prolapse. The pre-operative work-up included urodynamic procedures. The operative technic may be described briefly as follows: The anterior vaginal wall was dissected partially from the bladder base in rectangular form. This flap is rolled in and sutured with polyvinyl to the pubic rami bilaterally by its two ends.

18.04.01

Creation of artifical vagina: Papanicolaou, N A. Gen. Hosp. Alejandroupolis, Aristotelion Univ., Thessaloniki, Greece

We refer to our technique of vagina creation in 20 cases with congenital lack of vagina and to the postoperative results as compared with the results of other techniques.

18.04.02

Ectopic pregnancy in its different forms including unruptured extra horn pregnancy: Patel, N M. N.H.L. Municip. Med. Coll. & Sheth K.M. School Postgrad. Med. and Res., Ahmedabad, India

This video film on different types of ectopic pregnancy, namely acute type, subacute and chronic types and unruptured extra horn pregnancy is presented as a teaching aid to undergraduate and postgraduate students. This is because it is difficult for the students to see all the varieties at one occasion. In the last part of this film – film on unruptured extra horn pregnancy, it is shown how even an experienced gynecologist can make a mistake in coming to the diagnosis of this rare condition. This film has an educational purpose.

18.04.03

The soft vacuum extractor – the modern alternative to forceps delivery: Pelosi, M A. Univ. of Med. and Dent., New Jersey Med. School, Bayonne, NJ, USA

The development of the silicone obstetrical soft vacuum cup has made possible a simple and safe method for mechanically aided vaginal delivery (when indicated). The benefits of the instrument include minimal risk of maternal and fetal trauma when compared with the complications that may be encountered with the use of forceps and metal vacuum extractors. Its use as a safe and easy alternative to forceps and metal vacuum extractors in assisting and shortening the second stage of labor will be illustrated, and two innovative uses of the instrument-delivery of the fetal head at Cesarean section, and the manipulation and delivery of large solid pelvic masses at operation will be also presented.

18.04.04

Intrauterine puncture of pleural effusions in a 32th-week hydropic fetus – a case report: Wurster, K G, Pfeiffer, K H. Dept. Obstet. and Gyn., Univ., Tübingen

In a 32-year-old II-para, III-gravida we found in the 30th week of pregnancy a generalized fetal hydrops with large pleural effusions and hypoplastic lungs. During amniocentesis in the 32th week we also punctured the two fetal pleural cavities to decompress the lungs. From each side 50 ml of transudate could be aspirated. The pleural effusions returned to a lesser extent within 24 hours. Further punctures were refused by the patient. In the 34th week the fetus died *in utero*. The fetus had a generalized hydrops, pleural effusions on both sides, hypoplastic lungs and a 3 mm ventricular septal defect without any other malformations, but we found no explanation for the hydropic changes in the fetus. The fetal karyotype was also normal, 46,XY. Because the patient refused further active treatment, we were unable to prove the positive influence of intrauterine pleural puncture for fetal survival, as has been mentioned in the literature. The procedure will be demonstrated by video.

19.04.01

Mass laparoscopies tubal ligation: Wadia, B J. J J Hosp., Univ., Bombay, India

Film of a typical ligation camp by the author experience of over 40,000 ligations, done. – Modus operandi: (1) Complete general anesthesia is given (thiopentone). (2) Cold sterilization of all endoscopic equipment (up to 9 sets are used). (3) Vaginal elevation/manipulation for all cases. (4) Cold sterilization of vaginal instruments. (5) Rapid insufflation methods (up to 35 litres per minute). (6) No skin stitching (special skin clamps) with Benzoin Seal. (7) Post-operative recovery. (8) Film shows an operative output of 50–60 cases per hour.

19.04.02

Conservative management of uterine prolapse by lateral sling: Joshi, N, Wadia, B J. J J Hosp., Univ., Bombay, India

A lateral sling done on a study of 400 consecutive cases spread over the last 15 years. The idea of using a nylon tape is followed from Prof. *V. N. Shirodkar* with whom the author had worked. The procedure is simplified by anchoring the sling behind the insertion of the cervico-uterine junction at the level of the insertion of the utero-sacral ligament. (The technicalities are shown in the film.) The second anchor is to the aponeurosis of the external oblique and the periosteum of the anterior superior iliac spines on both the sides. (The technicalities are shown in the film.) The sling runs within the broad ligament and in the pelvic cellular fascia. The uterus becomes anteverted and the sling maintains the uterus at a fixed position in the pelvis preventing it to come out of the abdominal incision and accordingly not allowing it to prolapse out of the vulva. Overall success rate is over 80% in nulliparous and parous prolapse. The cases are followed up for many years and even after delivery. Analysis of results shows that this simple procedure is highly effective and should rank high in management of prolapse when the child bearing function is required.

19.04.03

Treatment of intrauterine adhesions: Papanicolaou, N A. Gen. Hosp. Alejandroupolis, Aristotelion Univ., Thessaloniki, Greece

We refer to our own technique of breaking adhesions (Asherman's syndrome) in 400 cases, using a special catheter, and to the results of this procedure.

Authors Index

For Woman After Woman After

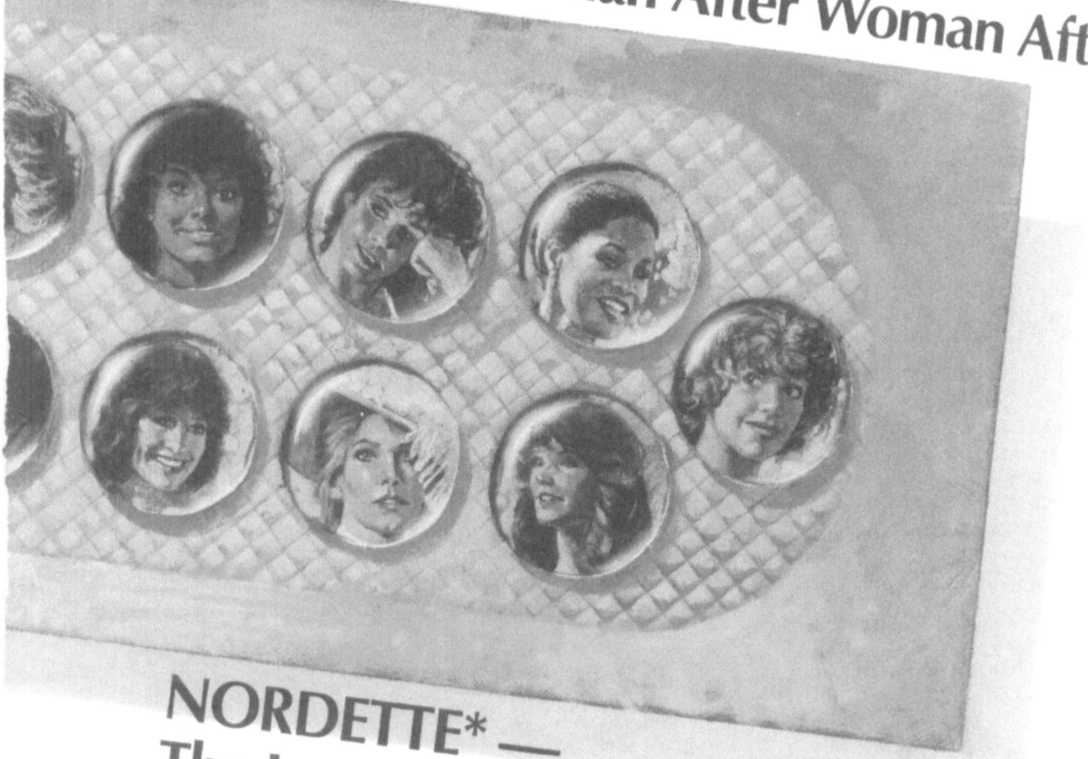

NORDETTE* —
The Lowest Dose Monophasic Oral Contraceptive Formulation

Proven in more than **450,000,000 cycles** of actual use, in more than **100 countries,** and in clinical trials involving more than **10,000 women.**

- ● **The lowest dose monophasic**
- ● **Outstanding clinical performance**
- ● **Confirmed long-term safety**
- ● **Excellent patient comfort and acceptance**

NORDETTE

(150 mcg levonorgestrel and 30 mcg ethinyl estradiol)

The NORDETTE formula
#1 in the world

Wyeth
Wyeth International Limited
Philadelphia, PA 19101 U.S.A.

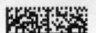